To my mother, for being an exemplary model of successful aging and love. You are an inspiration to me and so many others.

Dale Avers

To my husband, Al, for his unwavering support and encouragement, and to my children and grandchildren, who grow more precious every day.

Rita A. Wong

FOURTH EDITION

Guccione's Geriatric Physical Therapy

DALE AVERS, PT, DPT, PhD, FAPTA
Professor
Department of Physical Therapy Education
College of Health Professions
SUNY Upstate Medical University
Syracuse, New York

RITA A. WONG, PT, EdD, FAPTA
Professor
Associate Provost, Research and Graduate Education
Marymount University
Arlington, Virginia

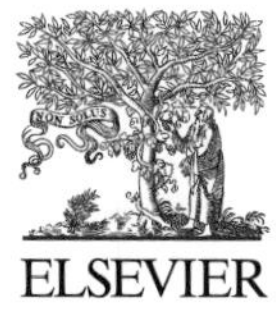

ELSEVIER

Elsevier
3251 Riverport Lane
St. Louis, Missouri 63043

GUCCIONE'S GERIATRIC PHYSICAL THERAPY, FOURTH EDITION ISBN: 978-0-323-60912-8

Previous editions copyrighted 2012, 2000 and 1993.

Library of Congress Control Number: 2019952355

Content Strategist: Lauren Willis
Content Development Specialist: Elizabeth McCormac
Publishing Services Manager: Deepthi Unni
Project Manager: Srividhya Vidhyashankar
Design Direction: Ryan Cook

Printed in United States of America

Last digit is the print number: 9 8 7 6 5 4 3 2 1

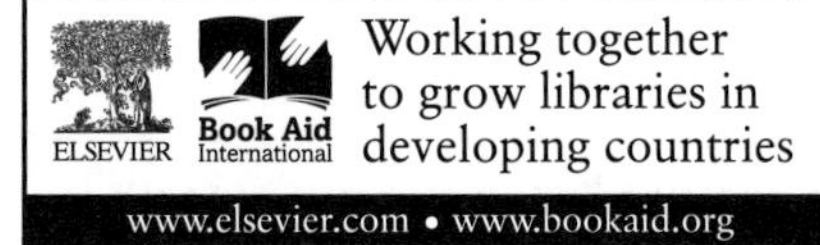

CONTRIBUTORS

Alia A. Alghwiri, PT, PhD
Professor
Department of Physical Therapy
School of Rehabilitation Sciences
The University of Jordan
Amman, Jordan

Brady Anderson, PT, DPT
Physical Therapist
Jackson Memorial Hospital
Miami, Florida

Dale Avers, PT, DPT, PhD, FAPTA
Professor
Department of Physical Therapy Education
College of Health Professions
SUNY Upstate Medical University
Syracuse, New York

Katherine Beissner, PT, PhD
Professor and Dean
College of Health Professions
SUNY Upstate Medical University
Syracuse, New York

Elizabeth J. Bergman, PhD
Associate Professor & Chair
Department of Gerontology
Ithaca College
Ithaca, New York

Marghuretta D. Bland, PT, DPT, MSCI, NCS
Associate Professor
Program in Physical Therapy
Program in Occupational Therapy
Department of Neurology
Washington University School of Medicine
Saint Louis, Missouri

Richard Briggs, PT, MA
Principle Consultant
Hospice Physical Therapy Associates
Chico, California

Lawrence P. Cahalin, PT, PhD, CCS
Professor
Department of Physical Therapy
University of Miami Miller School of Medicine
Coral Gables, Florida

Tzurei Chen, PT, PhD
Assistant Professor
School of Physical Therapy and Athletic Training
College of Health Professions
Pacific University
Hillsboro, Oregon

Cory Christiansen, PT, PhD
Associate Professor
Physical Therapy Program
School of Medicine
University of Colorado – Anschutz Medical Campus
Aurora, Colorado

Kevin K. Chui, PT, DPT, PhD, GCS, OCS, CEEAA, FAAOMPT
Director & Professor
School of Physical Therapy and Athletic Training
College of Health Professions
Pacific University
Hillsboro, Oregon

Charles D. Ciccone, PT, PhD, FAPTA
Professor
Department of Physical Therapy
College of Health Sciences and Human Performance
Ithaca College
Ithaca, New York

Cathy Haines Ciolek, PT, DPT, GCS, CDP, CADDCT, FAPTA
President
Living Well with Dementia®, LLC
Wilmington, Delaware

Moira Gannon Denson, MA, ASID, IIDEC, IIDA, LEED
Associate Professor
Department of Interior Design
School of Design, Arts, and Humanities
Marymount University
Arlington, Virginia

Cathy S. Elrod, PT, PhD
Professor
Department of Physical Therapy
Malek School of Health Professions
Marymount University
Arlington, Virginia

Christine E. Fordyce, PT, DPT, GCS
Executive Director
Kindred at Home
Liverpool, New York

Jenny Forrester, PT, DPT
Core Advanced Physical Therapist
University of Maryland Medical Center
Department of Rehabilitation Services
Baltimore, Maryland

Christian Garcia, PT, DPT
Physical Therapist
West Gables Rehabilitation Hospital
Miami, Florida

Rosanna Gelaz, PT, DPT, GCS
St. Catherine's West Rehabilitation Hospital
Hialeah Gardens, Florida

Jared M. Gollie, PhD, CSCS
Postdoctoral Research Fellow
Polytrauma/TBI Rehabilitation Research Program
Washington DC Veterans Affairs Medical Center
Washington, DC
Adjunct Faculty
Department of Health, Human Function, and Rehabilitation Sciences
School of Medicine and Health Sciences
The George Washington University
Washington, DC

Greg W. Hartley, PT, DPT, GCS, FNAP, CEEAA
Director of Rehabilitation & Assistant Hospital Administrator
Assistant Professor of Clinical Physical Therapy
University of Miami Miller School of Medicine
Department of Physical Therapy
Coral Gables, Florida

Catherine E. Lang, PT, PhD
Professor
Associate Director for Movement Science PhD Program
Program in Physical Therapy
Program in Occupational Therapy
Department of Neurology
Washington University School of Medicine
Saint Louis, Missouri

Paul LaStayo, PT, PhD, CHT
Professor
Department of Physical Therapy and Athletic Training
College of Health
University of Utah
Salt Lake City, Utah

Alan Chong W. Lee, PT, DPT, PhD, GCS, CWS
Professor
Physical Therapy Department
Mount Saint Mary's University Los Angeles
Los Angeles, California

Sin Yi Lee, PT, M Appl Geron
Principle Physiotherapist
Tan Tock Seng Hospital
Singapore

Daniel Liebzeit, RN, PhD
Advanced Fellow in Geriatrics
Geriatric Research, Education and Clinical Center
William S. Middleton Memorial Veterans Hospital
Madison, Wisconsin

Robin L. Marcus, PT, PhD, OCS
Professor
Department of Physical Therapy and Athletic Training
College of Health
University of Utah
Salt Lake City, Utah

Caitlin Miller, PT, DPT
Physical Therapist
Department of Physical Therapy and Athletic Training
Department of Orthopaedics
University of Utah
Salt Lake City, Utah

David M. Morris, PT, PhD, FAPTA
Professor and Chair
Department of Physical Therapy
School of Health Professions
University of Alabama at Birmingham
Birmingham, Alabama

Karen Mueller, PT, PhD
Professor
College of Health and Human Services
Department of Physical Therapy
Northern Arizona University
Flagstaff, Arizona

Cynthia E. Neville, PT, DPT, CWS
National Director of Pelvic Health & Wellness
FYZICAL Therapy & Balance Centers
Bonita Springs, Florida
Adjunct Professor
Department of Rehabilitation Sciences
Marieb College of Health & Human Services
Florida Gulf Coast University
Fort Myers, Florida

Brian W. Pulling, BS
Masters by Research Candidate
Body in Mind Research Group
School of Health Sciences
University of South Australia
Adelaide, South Australia, Australia

Paul Reidy, Msc, PhD
Postdoctoral Fellow
Department of Physical Therapy and Athletic Training
College of Health
University of Utah
Salt Lake City, Utah

Julie D. Ries, PT, PhD
Professor
Department of Physical Therapy
Malek School of Health Professions
Marymount University
Arlington, Virginia

Elizabeth Ruckert, PT, DPT, NCS, GCS
Assistant Professor
Program in Physical Therapy
School of Medicine & Health Sciences
George Washington University
Washington, DC

Carol Sames, PhD
Associate Professor
Department of Physical Therapy
College of Health Professions
Upstate Medical University
Syracuse, New York

Ellen Strunk, PT, MS, GCS, CEEAA, CHC
President and Principal Consultant
Rehab Resources and Consulting, Inc.
Birmingham, Alabama

Anne Thackeray, PT, PhD, MPH
Assistant Professor
Department of Physical Therapy and Athletic Training
University of Utah
Salt Lake City, Utah

Martha Townsend, PA-C, DPT
Lead Advanced Practice Provider
US Acute Care Solutions
Arvada, Colorado

Chris L. Wells, PT, PhD, CCS, ATC
EBP & Research Coordinator
Department of Rehabilitation Science
University of Maryland Medical Center
Baltimore, Maryland
Clinical Associate Professor, Adjunct II
Department of Physical Therapy & Rehabilitation Science
University of Maryland, School of Medicine
Baltimore, Maryland

Susan L. Wenker, PT, PhD, GCS-Emeritus, Advanced CEEAA
Assistant Professor (CHS)
Department of Family Medicine and Community Health
Doctor of Physical Therapy Program
University of Wisconsin–Madison
Madison, Wisconsin

Susan L. Whitney, DPT, PhD, NCS, ATC, FAPTA
Professor
Department of Physical Therapy, School of Health and Rehabilitation Science, and Department of Otolaryngology, School of Medicine
University of Pittsburgh
Pittsburgh, Pennsylvania

Christopher Wilson, PT, DPT, DScPT, GCS
Assistant Professor
Physical Therapy Program, Human Movement Sciences Department
School of Health Sciences
Oakland University
Rochester, Michigan

Rita A. Wong, PT, PhD, FAPTA
Professor
Associate Provost, Research and Graduate Education
Marymount University
Arlington, Virginia

Sheng-Che Yen, PT, PhD
Associate Clinical Professor
Director, Laboratory for Locomotion Research
Associate Director, PhD Program in Human Movement and Rehabilitation Sciences Department of Physical Therapy, Movement and Rehabilitation Sciences
Bouvé College of Health Sciences, Northeastern University
Boston, Massachusetts

PREFACE

Remarkably, much of the science that underpins geriatric physical therapy is less than 30 years old. It was only in 1990 that Fiatarone published the study that described the profound effects of progressive and high-resistance exercise on frail elders, initiating an avalanche of research about the effects of exercise on aging adults as well as spurring investigations to challenge beliefs about the inevitability of the downward health trajectory of older adults. In every area of geriatric science, remarkable strides have been made in the understanding of the systemic, clinical, and psychosocial effects of the aging process. Of particular interest to physical therapy clinicians are the intended and unintended consequences of lifestyle on the aging process. But understanding the science isn't sufficient to provide interventions to an older adult. The physical therapy clinician also uses psychosocial and clinical skills to help the older adult manage individual complexity. The fourth edition of this textbook reflects the breadth of knowledge and interventions necessary to provide best practices in the delivery of physical therapy for older adults. The development of competent, reflective geriatric physical therapy professionals, a continued focus of this text, is fostered through analysis, synthesis, and application of current science and expert opinion within a functional context in this edition. Additionally, the text has increased its international focus with the addition of several international authors, reflecting the globalization of geriatric physical therapy care.

The fourth edition includes several new chapters that reflect the application of science to clinical practice. While the basic organization of the text has not changed, the reader will note changes in each section. For example, in Part I, Foundations, a chapter on Psychosocial Aspects of Aging has been added, reflecting the wholistic nature of patient care.

Part II presents the core practices and interventions used for every older adult, across systems and pathology. New chapters in this section include Functional Performance Measures and Patient Education. Evaluation, diagnosis, and plan of care is the focus of Part III. New chapters include the Frail Older Adult, Older Patient with Neurological Conditions, and Older Patient with Cardiovascular and Pulmonary Conditions. Part IV chapters address special issues and their interventions with new chapters on Caregiving and Postsurgical Orthopedic Conditions. The continuum of care is reflected in Part V and includes a new chapter on the Acute Management of the Older Adult. Finally, Part VI provides a chapter on health policy and advocacy that addresses the role of the physical therapy professional within a societal framework.

This fourth edition reflects a change in the title to *Guccione's Geriatric Physical Therapy*. Andrew Guccione, the first editor and conceptualizer of this text, always had the goal of providing a text about geriatric physical therapy that was of the highest credibility based on current science and expert clinical thought and that would advance the provision of the physical therapy care of older adults. We are indebted to him for his vision and encouragement and hope this text reflects his intent and commitment to excellence.

Dale Avers, PT, DPT, PhD, FAPTA
Rita A. Wong, PT, EdD, FAPTA

ACKNOWLEDGMENTS

This textbook is a creative collaboration of the best scientists and clinicians in geriatric physical therapy. We are indebted to this highly respected and passionate team of individuals and proud to call them colleagues. We welcome our new authors and are grateful for the expertise of former and current authors. We are also indebted to those who have inspired us along the way, whose thoughts and examples have influenced our thinking, especially Davis Gardner (1926–2019) and our patients and students, from whom we continue to learn.

Elsevier's commitment to excellence is demonstrated through the thoughtful and conscientious attention Elizabeth (Betsy) McCormac has paid to the intent and content of this text. Her unending patience and advice are beyond value.

Dale Avers, PT, DPT, PhD, FAPTA
Rita A. Wong, PT, EdD, FAPTA

CONTENTS

CHAPTER

1

Geriatric Physical Therapy in the 21st Century: Overarching Principles and Approaches to Practice

Cathy Elrod

OUTLINE

INTRODUCTION

All physical therapists, not just those working in settings traditionally identified as "geriatric," should possess strong foundational knowledge about geriatrics and be able to apply this knowledge to a variety of older adults. Although the fundamental principles of patient management are similar regardless of patient age, there are unique features and considerations in the management of older adults that can greatly improve outcomes.

The first wave of the baby-boomer generation turned 65 years old in 2011. This group, born post–World War II, is much larger than its preceding generation, in terms of both the number of children born during this era (1946 to 1965) and increased longevity of those in that cohort. The 2008 landmark report of the Institute of Medicine (IOM) *Retooling for an Aging America*[1] provides a compelling argument for wide-ranging shortages of both formal and informal health care providers for older adults across all levels of the health care workforce (professional, technical, unskilled direct care worker, and family caregiver). These shortages include shortages of physical therapists and physical therapist assistants. The report provides numerous recommendations for enhancing the number of health care practitioners and the depth of preparation of these practitioners. The goal of this textbook is to provide a strong foundation to support physical therapists who work with older adults.

The U.S. Census Bureau reports that in 2016, 15% of the population was age 65 years or older; by 2030, one in five Americans is projected to be an older adult.[2] Undoubtedly, with very few exceptions, the majority of the caseload of the average physical therapist will soon consist of older adults. Despite this, physical therapists still tend to think about "geriatrics" in terms of care provided to frail individuals in a nursing home, hospital, or home care setting. Although these are important practice settings for geriatric physical therapy, physical therapists must recognize and be ready to provide effective services for the high volume of older adult patients who range from the very fit to the very frail, across inpatient and outpatient settings.

AGING

When working with the older adult, it is important to understand the concept of aging and the rationale behind the high variability and differences among older adults in the aging process. Usual aging, or typical changes in physiological functioning observed in older adults, represents a combination of normal (unavoidable) aging-related decline and modifiable factors associated with lifestyle such as physical activity, nutrition, and stress management. For many older adults, a substantial proportion of "usual" age-related decline in functional ability represents "deconditioning" as most older adults do not engage in sufficient physical activity and exercise to derive health benefits. This decline can be partially reversible with lifestyle modification.

Aging trajectories that go beyond typical aging have been described by a variety of terms such as *healthy aging*, *optimal aging*, *successful aging*, *active aging*, and *aging well*.[3] In 1997, Rowe and Kahn[4] provided a model of successful aging that includes the following components: (1) absence of disease and disability, (2) high cognitive and physical functioning, and (3) active engagement with life. Although helping older adults avoid disease and disease-related disability is a central consideration for all health care practitioners, the reality is that the majority of older adults do have at least one chronic health condition, and many, particularly among the very old, live with functional limitations and disabilities associated with the sequelae of one or more chronic health conditions. Brummel-Smith expanded the concepts of Rowe and Kahn in the depiction of optimal aging as a more inclusive term than successful aging. Brummel-Smith defines optimal aging as "the capacity to function across many domains—physical, functional, cognitive, emotional, social, and spiritual—to one's satisfaction and in spite of one's medical conditions."[5] This conceptualization recognizes the importance of optimizing functional capacity in older adults regardless of the presence or absence of a chronic health condition. Recently, the American Geriatrics Society published a *White Paper on Healthy Aging* in which they recommend that the definition of healthy aging include "concepts central to geriatrics, such as culture, function, engagement, resilience, meaning, dignity and autonomy, in addition to minimizing disease."[6]

HEALTH, FUNCTION, AND DISABLEMENT

The World Health Organization (WHO) defines *health* as a "state of complete physical, psychological, and social well-being, and not merely the absence of disease or infirmity."[7] According to this definition, "health" is best understood as an end point in the major domains of human existence: physical, psychological, and social. In contrast to assuming "complete health" as the expected end point of an episode of care, physical therapists work across the spectrum, from wellness to the end of life, to ensure outcomes associated with achieving the highest level of function possible wherever someone may be placed on that spectrum.

There have been several attempts to construct a model of health status that describes the relationship between health and function or, more precisely, describes the process of how individuals come to be disabled (disablement) and identifies factors, including therapeutic interventions, that can mitigate disablement (enablement process). The traditional medical model of disablement assumes a causal relationship between disease and illness. In this narrow perspective, disablement is primarily dependent on the characteristics of the individual (i.e., his or her pathology) that require an intervention to alleviate that can only be provided by a health care professional. The social model of disability fundamentally broadens the focus away from an exclusive concentration on the disease-related physical impairments of the individual to also include the individual's physical and social environments that can impose both disabling limitations and enabling mitigation of limitations.[8] Subsequent models of the twin processes of disablement and enablement have further explored the relationship of the environment to functional independence. In the 1960s, sociologist Saad Nagi characterized disablement as having four distinct components that evolve sequentially as an individual loses well-being: disease or pathology, impairments, functional limitations, and disability.[9,10] His work is associated with the biopsychosocial model, which recognizes the importance of psychological and social factors on the patient's experience of illness. In the late 1980s and early 1990s, Jette, Verbrugge, and Guccione began exploring the process of disablement as a framework to assist physical therapists to clarify the domains of practice.[11–15] They proposed a multifactorial disablement framework that included the influence of environmental demand and individual capabilities on disability (Fig. 1.1).

A further elaboration of Nagi's model was presented by Brandt and Pope in a 1997 report from the IOM.[16] This revised model introduced the concept of enablement that explicated the balance between inevitable and reversible disablement depending on the confluence of disabling and enabling factors at the interface of a person with the environment. If ramps were introduced to allow access to the home or therapeutic exercises implemented that improved functional performance, then the individual with a neuromuscular condition precluding his or her ability to negotiate stairs has experienced a "disabling–enabling process." The IOM model has three dimensions: the person, the environment, and the interaction between the person and the environment. Their conceptualization allows us to understand how two older adults presenting with similar impairments associated with a right cerebrovascular accident can have different levels of disability according to the uniqueness of each individual and the environment in which they live. Physical therapists can use this information to promote optimal aging in the older adult.

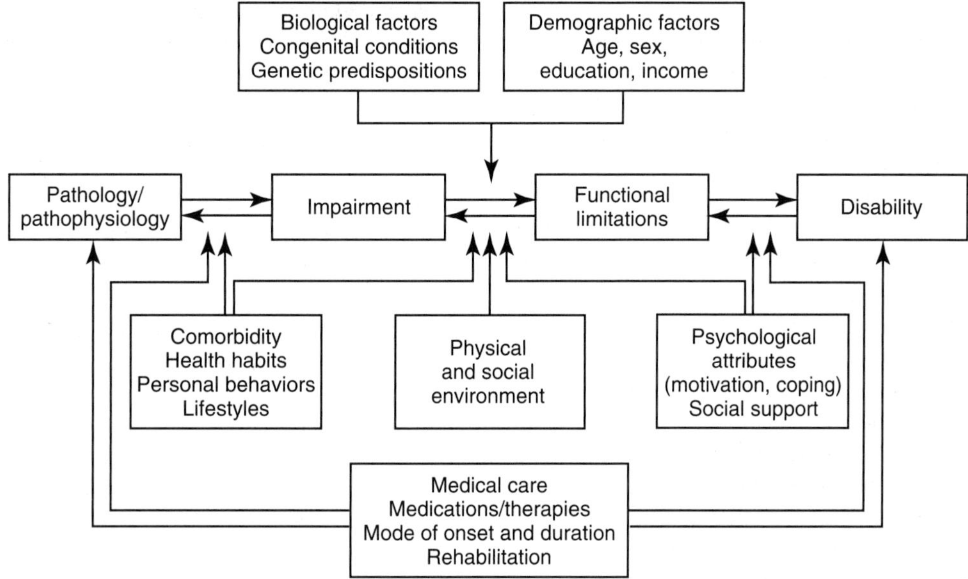

FIG. 1.1 An expanded disablement model. *(Adapted with permission from Guccione AA. Arthritis and the process of disablement. Phys Ther. 1994;74:410.)*

International Classification of Functioning, Disability, and Health

The WHO also independently took on the task of developing a conceptual framework for describing and classifying the consequences of diseases. In 1980, they presented the *International Classification of Impairments, Disabilities, and Handicaps* (ICIDH).[17] In response to concerns about the ICIDH, the WHO developed a substantially revised *International Classification of Functioning, Disability and Health* (ICF) in 2001 to "provide a unified and standard language and framework for the description of health and health-related states."[18] In 2007, the IOM endorsed the adoption of this framework "as a means of promoting clear communication and building a coherent base of national and international research findings to inform public and private decision making."[19] The 2008 House of Delegates for the American Physical Therapy Association also embraced terminology of the ICF and initiated the process of incorporating ICF language into all relevant association publications, documents, and communications (http://www.apta.org/uploadedFiles/APTAorg/About_Us/Policies/PracticeEndorsementICF.pdf#search=%22HOD%20P06-08%22. Accessed June 30, 2019).

The ICF model, illustrated in Fig. 1.2, employs a biopsychosocial approach that is compatible with many of the concepts from Nagi and the IOM's work on enablement and disablement. The ICF model is designed to encompass all aspects of health and include all situations that are associated with human functioning and its restrictions. Key operational definitions that allow interpretation and application of the ICF model are listed in Box 1.1. There are varying levels within the ICF's taxonomic classification schema of human functioning and disability. The first level consists of the broad categories of body functions, body structures, activities and participation, and environmental factors. Physical therapists will typically be most interested in the section that discusses activities and participation and the subsection on mobility that delineates actions associated with (1) changing and maintaining body position; (2) carrying, moving, and handling objects; (3) walking and moving; and (4) moving around using transportation. The ICF attempts to provide a common language to describe patients' behaviors and environmental situations that need to be taken into consideration when making clinical decisions, especially in regard to optimizing human performance in the older adult.

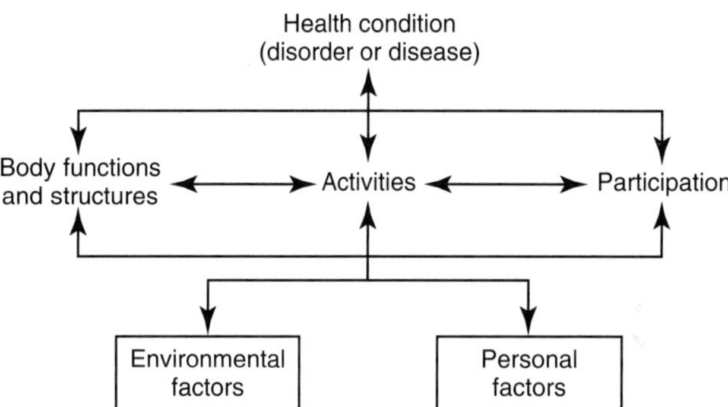

FIG. 1.2 International Classification of Functioning, Disability and Health (ICF) model. *(From the World Health Organization. International Classification of Functioning, Disability, and Health: ICF. Geneva, Switzerland: World Health Organization; 2001: 18.)*

Health Condition. In contrast to focusing on disease, health condition is an ongoing pathologic state that is delineated by a particular cluster of signs and symptoms. The ICF includes any health condition that takes the individual

BOX 1.1 International Classification of Functioning, Disability and Health (ICF) Definitions

Health Condition: umbrella term for disease (acute or chronic), disorder, injury, or trauma; may also include other circumstances such as pregnancy, aging, stress, congenital anomaly, or genetic predisposition; coded using *International Classification of Disease,* 11th revision

- *Body Functions*: the physiological functions of body systems, including psychological functions
- *Body Structures*: the structural or anatomic parts of the body such as organs, limbs, and their components classified according to body systems
- *Impairment*: a loss or abnormality in body structure or physiological function (including mental functions)
- *Activity*: the execution of a task or action by an individual; represents the individual perspective of functioning
- *Activity Limitation*: difficulties an individual may have in executing activities
- *Participation*: a person's involvement in a life situation; represents the societal perspective of functioning
- *Participation Restriction*: problems an individual may experience in involvement in life situations
- *Functioning*: umbrella term for body functions, body structures, activities, and participation; denotes the positive aspects of the interaction between an individual (with a health condition) and that individual's contextual factors (environmental and personal factors)
- *Disability*: umbrella term for impairments, activity limitations, and participation restrictions; denotes the negative aspects of the interaction between an individual (with a health condition) and that individual's contextual factors (environment and personal factors)
- *Contextual Factors*: factors that together constitute the complete context of an individual's life, and in particular the background against which health states are classified in the ICF; there are two components of contextual factors: environmental factors and personal factors
  - *Environmental Factors*: constitute a component of the ICF and refer to all aspects of the external or extrinsic world that form the context of an individual's life and as such have an impact on that person's functioning; they include the physical world and its features, the human-made physical world, other people in different relationships and roles, attitudes and values, social systems and services, and policies, rules, and laws
  - *Personal Factors*: contextual factors that relate to the individual such as age, gender, social status, life experience, and so on that are not currently classified in the ICF but which users may incorporate in their application of the classification

(From: World Health Organization. *International Classification of Functioning, Disability, and Health: ICF.* Geneva, Switzerland: World Health Organization; 2001.)

away from the "state of complete physical, psychological, and social well-being" and builds upon the evolving acceptance of wellness as an attainable goal.[18] The *International Classification of Disease,* 11th revision (ICD-11), also a product of the WHO, offers a classification schema that provides a comprehensive listing of health conditions.

Impairment of Body Structure or Function. Impairments, defined as alterations in anatomic, physiological, or psychological structures or functions, typically evolve as the consequence of disease, pathologic processes, or lesions, altering the person's normal health state and contributing to the individual's illness. For example, physical impairments, such as pain and decreased range of motion (ROM) in the shoulder, may be the overt manifestations (or symptoms and signs) of either temporary or permanent disease or pathologic processes for some, but not necessarily all, older adult patients. The genesis of an impairment can often be unclear. Poor posture, for example, is neither a disease nor a pathologic state, yet the resultant muscle shortening and capsular tightness may present as major impairments in a clinical examination. Thus, not all older adults are patients because they have a disease. Some individuals are treated by physical therapists because their impairments are a sufficient enough cause for intervention regardless of the presence (or absence) of disease or active pathology.

Given that much of physical therapy is directed toward remediating or minimizing impairments, additional elaboration of the concept of impairment is particularly useful in geriatric physical therapy. Schenkman and Butler have proposed that impairments can be classified in three ways: direct, indirect, and composite effect.[20] Direct impairments are the effect of a disease, syndrome, or lesion and are relatively confined to a single system. For example, they note that weakness can be classified as a neuromuscular impairment that is a direct effect of a peripheral motor neuropathy in the lower extremity. Indirect impairments are impairments in other systems that can "indirectly" affect the underlying problem. For example, ambulation training of a patient with a peripheral motor neuropathy may put excessive strain on joints and ligaments, resulting in new musculoskeletal impairments. The combination of weakness from the primary motor neuropathy and ligamentous strain from excessive forces on the joints may lead to a composite effect, the impairment of pain.

Using neurologic dysfunction as the vehicle, Schenkman and Butler described this three-category concept of impairment by categorizing clinical signs and symptoms into impairments that have a direct, indirect, or composite effect, thus bringing together into a cohesive relationship the diverse data of the medical history and the findings of the clinical examination. For example, consider a 79-year-old woman with severe peripheral vascular disease (PVD). Upon clinical examination, the physical therapist notes that this individual has lost sensation below the right knee. Sensory loss is an impairment that would be classified as a direct effect of PVD. As the individual is ambulating less and cannot sense full ankle ROM, loss of ROM may be an indirect effect of the patient's PVD on the musculoskeletal system. The combination of the direct impairment (sensory loss below the knee) and the indirect impairment (decreased ROM in the ankle) may help to explain another clinical finding, poor balance, which can be understood as a composite effect of other impairments. Piecing clinical data together in this fashion allows the therapist to uncover the interrelationships among a patient's PVD, loss of sensation, limited ROM, and balance deficits. Without a framework that sorts the patient's clinical data into relevant categories, the therapist might never comprehend how the patient's problems came to be and thus how to intervene. Treatment consisting of balance activities alone would be inappropriate, because the therapist must also address the loss in ROM as well as teach the patient to compensate for the sensory loss to remediate the impairments.

Activity Limitation. Although most of us anticipate that our body systems will deteriorate somewhat as we age, an inability to do for oneself from day to day perhaps most clearly identifies when adults are losing their health. Activity limitations result from impairments and consist of an individual's inability to perform his or her usual functions and tasks such as reaching for something on an overhead shelf or carrying a package. As measures of behaviors at the level of a person, and not anatomic or physiological conditions, limitations in the performance of activities should not be confused with diseases or impairments that encompass aberrations in specific tissues, organs, and systems that present clinically as the patient's signs and symptoms.

Although most older adults seeking care for a health condition are likely to carry at least two medical diagnoses, each of which will manifest itself in particular impairments of the cardiopulmonary, integumentary, musculoskeletal, or neuromuscular systems, impairment does not always entail activity limitations. One cannot assume that an individual will be unable to perform the actions and roles of usual daily living by virtue of having an impairment alone. For example, an adult with osteoarthritis (disease) may exhibit loss of ROM (impairment) and experience great difficulty in transferring from a bed to a chair (action). Another individual with osteoarthritis and equal loss of ROM may transfer from bed to chair easily by choosing to use an assistive device or by participating in a supervised muscle-strengthening program. Sometimes patients will overcome multiple, and even permanent, impairments by the sheer force of their motivation.

The degree to which limitations in physical functional activities may be linked to impairments has not been fully determined through research, and there is a critical need to update the epidemiology of impairment and action/function among older adults. The relatively few studies that have been reported in the literature support a generally linear but modest relationship between impairments such as strength and functional status, perhaps because functional status requires a relatively low level of strength and thus experiences a ceiling effect. Such data are essential to both (1) identifying relevant functional outcomes of an intervention and (2) establishing the dose–response relationship for an efficacious intervention that is known to remediate impairments to a particular degree or magnitude and is sufficient to produce a clinically important change in an individual's functional status.

Participation Restriction. In revising the ICIDH, the WHO rejected the term *handicap* and introduced an alternative concept, *participation*, which is associated with its specific definition of *activity* and *activity limitation*.[18] It is defined as "involvement in life situations" and is characterized by a person's performance of actions and tasks in that individual's actual environment. *Participation restriction* is characterized by discordance between the actual performance of an individual in a particular role and the expectations of the community for what is normal or typically expected behavior for an adult. Being unable to fulfill desired social roles is also associated with the term *disability*.[9] The meaning of disabled is taken from the community in which the individual lives and the criteria for normal within that social group. The term *disabled* connotes a particular status in society. Labeling a person as disabled requires a judgment, usually by a professional, that an individual's behaviors are somehow inadequate based on the professional's understanding of the expectations that the activity should be accomplished in ways that are typical for a person's age as well as cultural and social environment.

The ICF has redefined the term *disability* to reflect the summative negative aspects of the interaction between an individual who has a health condition and that individual's environment and personal factors. It encompasses impairment, activity limitations, and participation restrictions. Thus, *disability* is the broadest term in the ICF framework and harkens back to the IOM conceptualization that locates disability at the interface of a person's capabilities and abilities, personal factors, and the biopsychosocial environment.

The evidence suggests that activity limitations and participation restrictions in an older adult population change over time, and not all older adults exhibit functional decline. If we follow any cohort of older adults over time, there will be more activity limitations and subsequent restrictions in participation overall within the group, but some individuals will actually improve and others will maintain their functional level. Restricting the use of the term *disabled* to describe only long-term overall functional decline in older adult populations encourages us to understand a particular older adult's activity limitations and participation restrictions in a dynamic context subject to change, particularly after therapeutic intervention. Participation restrictions depend on both the capacities of the individual and the expectations that are imposed on the individual by those in the immediate social environment, most often the patient's family and caregivers. Physical therapists who apply a health status perspective to the assessment of patients draw on a broad appreciation of an older adult as a person living in a particular social context as well as having individual characteristics. Changing the expectations of a social context—for example, explaining to family members what level of assistance is appropriate to an older adult after a stroke—may help to diminish disability as much as supplying the patient with assistive devices or increasing the physical ability to use them.

KEY PRINCIPLES IN GERIATRIC PHYSICAL THERAPY

Role of Physical Activity and Exercise in Maximizing Optimal Aging

Lack of physical activity (sedentary lifestyle) is a major public health concern across age groups. In 2014, 26.9% of adults between 65 and 74 years and 35.3% aged ≥75 years reported participating in no leisure-time physical activity.[21] Sedentary lifestyle increases the rate of age-related functional decline and reduces capacity for exercise sustainability to regain physiological reserve following an injury or illness. It is critical that physical therapists overtly address sedentary behavior as part of the plan of care for their older adult patients.

Exercise may well be the most important tool a physical therapist has to positively affect function and increase physical activity in older adults.[22] Despite a well-defined body of evidence to guide decisions about optimal intensity, duration, and mode of exercise prescription, physical therapists often underutilize exercise, with a negative impact on the potential to achieve optimal outcomes in the least amount of time. Underutilization of appropriately constructed exercise prescriptions may be associated with such factors as age biases that lower expectations for high levels of function, lack of awareness of age-based functional norms that can be used to set goals and measure outcomes, and perceived as well as real restrictions imposed by third-party payers regarding number of visits or the types of interventions (e.g., prevention) that are covered and reimbursed under a person's insurance benefit. Physical therapists should take every opportunity to apply evidence-based recommendations for physical activity and exercise programs that encourage positive lifestyle changes and thus maximize healthy aging.

Slippery Slope of Aging

Closely linked to the concept of healthy aging is the concept of a "slippery slope" of aging (Fig. 1.3). The slope, originally proposed by Schwartz,[23] represents the general decline in overall physiological ability (that Schwartz expressed as "vigor") that is observed with increasing age. The curve is arbitrarily plotted by decade on the x-axis so the actual location of any individual along the y-axis—regardless of age—can be modified (in either a positive or negative direction) based on lifestyle factors and illness that influence physiological functioning.

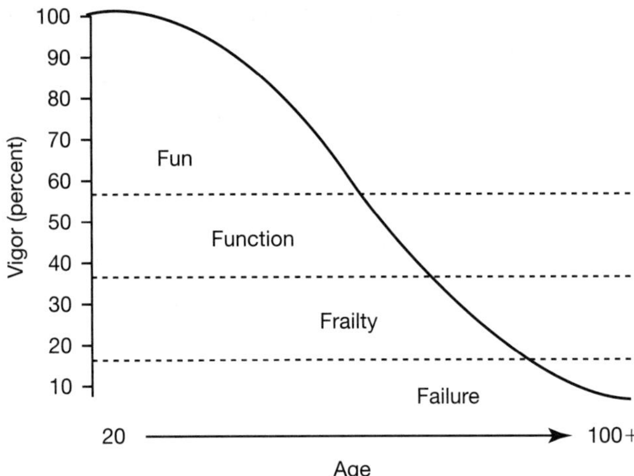

FIG. 1.3 Slippery slope of aging depicts the general decline in overall physiological ability observed with increasing age and its impact on function. *(Adapted from Schwartz RS. Sarcopenia and physical performance in old age: introduction. Muscle Nerve. 1997;20[Suppl 5]:S10-S12.)*

Schwartz has embedded functional status thresholds at various points along this slope. Conceptually, these thresholds represent key impact points where small changes in physiological ability can have a large impact on function, participation, and disability. These four distinctive functional levels are descriptively labeled fun, function, frailty, and failure. Fun, the highest level, represents a physiological state that allows unrestricted participation in work, home, and leisure activities. The person who crosses the threshold into function continues to accomplish most work and home activities but may need to modify performance and will substantially self-restrict or adapt leisure activities (fun) because of declining physiological capacity. Moving from function into frailty occurs when managing basic activities of daily living (BADLs; walking, bathing, toileting, eating, etc.) consumes a substantial portion of physiological capacity, with substantial limitations in ability to participate in community activities and requiring outside assistance to accomplish many home or work activities. The final threshold into failure is reached when an individual requires assistance with BADLs as well as instrumental daily activities and may be completely bedridden.

The concept of functional thresholds and the downward movement from fun to frailty helps explain the apparent disconnect that is often observed between the extent of change of physiological functions (impairments) and changes in functional status. For example, for a person who is teetering between the thresholds of function and frailty, a relatively small physiological challenge (a bout of influenza or a short hospitalization) is likely to drop him or her squarely into the level of "frailty," with its associated functional limitations. Once a person moves to a lower functional level (down the curve of the y-axis), it requires substantial effort and, typically, a longer time period to build physiological capacity to move back up to a higher level (back up the y-axis). Clegg et al., as depicted in Fig. 1.4, depicted this phenomenon around a comparable threshold descriptor of "functional dependency."[24] Lifestyle changes including increased exercise activities may enhance efforts for an upward movement along the slippery slope. Moreover, the further the person is able to move above a key threshold, the more physiological reserve is available for protection from an acute decline in a physiological system. A major role of physical therapy is to maximize the movement-related physiological ability (vigor) of older adult patients/clients to keep them at their optimal functional level and with the highest physiological reserve.

Ageism

The perception of someone as being old or geriatric is a social construct that can differ greatly among cultures and social groups. A Pew Foundation survey[25] found that, on average, a representative sample of the U.S. population perceives age 68 years as the age at which a person crosses the threshold to be classified as old. However, the age of the survey respondent influenced perceptions: Respondents under the age of 30 years identified old age as starting at 60 years; those between 30 and 64 years indicated 70 years as the beginning of old age; and those older than age 64 years indicated that old age starts at 74 years. The age of 65 years, which is the typical age when individuals in the United States become eligible for Medicare, is probably the most common age identified by medical researchers and social policy advocates when categorizing individuals as old.

In reality, perceiving a specific individual as old is often more associated with the person's physical appearance

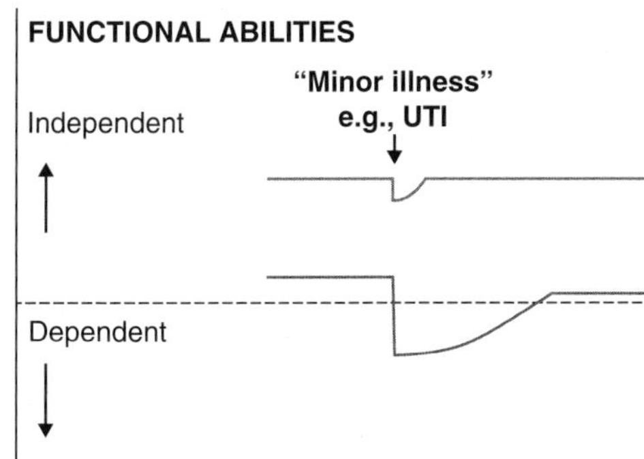

FIG. 1.4 Vulnerability of frail older people to a sudden change in health status following a minor illness. The green line represents a fit older person who, following a minor stress such as an infection, experiences a relatively small deterioration in function and then returns to homeostasis. The red line represents a frail older person who, following a similar stress, experiences a larger deterioration that may manifest as functional dependency and who does not return to baseline homeostasis. *UTI*, urinary tract infection. *Reprinted with permission from Elsevier (Clegg A, Young J, Iliffe S, Rikkert MO, Rockwood K. Frailty in elderly people. The Lancet. 2013;381(9868):752-762).*

and health status than his or her chronological age. An 80-year-old who is independent, fit, and healthy may not be described as old by those around her, whereas a 60-year-old who is unfit, has multiple chronic health problems, and needs help with daily activities that are physically challenging is likely to be perceived and described as old.

Ageism, stereotyping, and prejudice toward older adults, is prevalent in Western culture, including health care settings.[26] The subtle negative attitudes toward older adults that are often identified among health care practitioners become more obvious and influential when old age is combined with a perception of the patient as having low motivation, poor compliance, or poor prognosis. Ageism can result in disparate treatment for women as compared to men if they are viewed as being too frail and less encouragement of older patients to follow widely endorsed physical activity guidelines, and can lead to ineffective communication if the health condition is seen as just being associated with "old age."[27,28]

Many interactions with physical therapists occur at very vulnerable points in an older adult's life. For example, it is common to first evaluate an older adult in the midst of an acute hospitalization from a sudden and significant illness, in a skilled nursing facility for rehabilitation after hip fracture, or in the outpatient department during a disabling bout of back pain. When formulating a prognosis and making recommendations for the aggressiveness of interventions, it is easy to fall back on stereotypes suggesting old patients have low potential for improvement and low motivation for rehabilitation. It is true that some older adults enter physical therapy very low on the slippery slope of aging (frailty and failure stages). Rehabilitation may be particularly challenging given prior functional level, requiring the individual to make conscious decisions about where they want to place their efforts in the presence of substantially limited energy reserves, in which case goals not achievable through physical rehabilitation may guide their decisions. However, for most older patients, appropriately aggressive physical therapy can substantially affect functional ability and quality of life. Physical therapists who let ageist stereotypes influence their judgment are likely to make assumptions that underestimate prior functional ability of individuals and future potential for improvement. Do not let stereotypes cloud judgment about the capacity of older adults and the benefit to be achieved by appropriately aggressive rehabilitation.

Objectivity in Use of Outcome Tools

Older adults become increasingly dissimilar with increasing age. A similarly aged person can be frail and reside in a nursing home or be a senior athlete participating in a triathlon. Dissimilarities cannot be attributed to age alone and can challenge the therapist to set appropriate goals and expectations. Functional markers are useful to avoid inappropriate stereotyping and undershooting of an older adult's functional potential. Functional tests, especially those with normative values, can provide a more objective and universally understood description of actual performance relative to similarly aged older adults, serving as a common language and as a baseline for measuring progress. For example, describing an 82-year-old man in terms of gait speed (0.65 m/s), 6-minute walk test (175 m), Berg balance test (26/56), and timed five-repetition chair rise (0) provides a more accurate description than "an older man who requires mod assistance of two to transfer, walks 75 feet with a walker, and whose strength is WFL." Reliable, valid, and responsive tests, appropriate for a wide range of abilities, enhance practice, and provide valuable information for our patients and referral sources.

Evidence-Based Practice

Evidence-based practice is an approach to clinical decision making about the care of an individual patient that integrates three separate but equally important sources of information in making a clinical decision about the care of a patient. Fig. 1.5 illustrates these three information sources: (1) best available scientific evidence, (2) clinical experience and judgment of the practitioner, and (3) patient preferences and circumstances.[29] The term *evidence-based practice* sometimes misleads people into thinking that the scientific evidence is the only factor to be considered when using this approach to inform a patient-care decision. Although the scientific literature is an essential and substantive component of credible clinical decision making, it is only one of the three essential components. An alternative, and perhaps more accurate, label for this approach is evidence-informed practice.

The competent geriatric practitioner must have a good grasp of the current scientific literature and be able to interpret and apply this literature in the context of an individual patient situation. This practitioner must also have the clinical expertise to skillfully perform the appropriate tests and measures needed for diagnosis, interpret the findings in light of age-related and condition-specific characteristics of the patient, and then skillfully apply the appropriate interventions to best manage the problem.

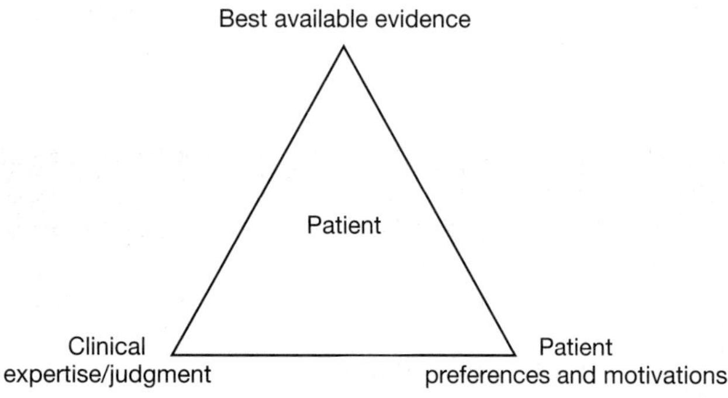

FIG. 1.5 Key elements of evidence-informed practice.

This is all done with clear and full communication with the patient to ensure the goals and preferences of the patient are a central component of the development of a plan of care.

Incorporation of best evidence into clinical decision making is an anchor of quality clinical practice. We live in an information age. For almost any topic, an overwhelming amount of information can be accessed in seconds with an Internet search. The challenge is to quickly identify and apply the best evidence. The best evidence is credible, clinically important, and applicable to the specific patient situation.

When faced with an unfamiliar clinical situation, a clinician reflects on past knowledge and experience, and may identify missing evidence needed to guide his or her decision making. A four-step process is typically used to locate and apply best evidence: (1) asking a searchable clinical question, (2) searching the literature and locating evidence, (3) critically assessing the evidence, and (4) determining the applicability of the evidence to a specific patient situation.

Sources of Evidence. Physical therapists must be competent in finding and assessing the quality, importance, and applicability of the many evidence sources available to them. As depicted in Box 1.2, each piece of evidence falls along a continuum from foundational concepts and theories to the aggregation of high-quality and clinically applicable empirical studies. On casual review of published studies, it is sometimes difficult to determine just where a specific type of evidence falls within the continuum of evidence and a closer review is often required.

The highest-quality research to answer a clinical question (i.e., providing the strongest evidence that offers the most certainty about the implications of the findings) is typically derived from the recommendations emerging from a valid systematic review that aggregates numerous high-quality studies directly focusing on the clinical question. However, only a very small proportion of evidence associated with the physical therapy management of older adults is well enough developed to support systematic reviews yielding definitive and strong recommendations. And the variety of factors that contribute to the health status of older adults makes it hard to aggregate across multiple studies or apply findings directly to your unique situation. More commonly, best evidence consists of the integration of the findings of one or several individual studies of varying quality by practitioners who then incorporate this evidence into their clinical judgments. The evidence-informed practitioner must be able to quickly locate, categorize, interpret, and synthesize the available evidence and also judge its relevance to the particular situation.

Finding Evidence. PubMed is generally the best database to search for biomedical evidence. PubMed is a product of the U.S. National Library of Medicine (NLM) at the National Institutes of Health (NIH) and thus is free to access. This database provides citations and abstracts

BOX 1.2 Continuum of Evidence: Studies Representing Early Foundational Concepts Through Integration of Findings Across Multiple Studies

Foundational Concepts and Theories →	Initial Testing of Foundational Concepts →	Definitive Testing of Clinical Applicability →	Aggregation of the Clinically Applicable Evidence
Descriptive studies Case reports Idea papers (based on theories and observations) "Bench research" (cellular or animal model research for initial testing of theories) Opinions of experts in the field (based on experience and review of literature)	Single-case design studies Testing on "normals" (no real clinical applicability) Small cohort studies (assessing safety and potential for benefit with real patients) Clinical trials,* phase I and II	Well-controlled studies with high internal validity and clearly identified external validity: • Diagnosis • Prognosis • Intervention • Outcomes • Clinical trials,* phase III and IV	Systematic review and meta-analysis Evidence-based clinical practice guideline

*Clinical trials:
Phase I: examines a small group of people to evaluate treatment safety, determine safe dosage range, and identify side effects.
Phase II: examines a somewhat larger group of people to evaluate treatment efficacy and safety.
Phase III: examines a large group of people to confirm treatment effectiveness, monitor side effects, compare it to commonly used treatments, and further examine safety.
Phase IV: postmarketing studies delineate additional information including the documented risks, benefits, and optimal use.

from an expansive list of biomedical journals, most in English, but also including major non-English biomedical journals. All journals indexed in PubMed must meet high-quality standards, thus providing a certain level of comfort about using PubMed-indexed journals as trusted sources. PubMed Central provides a link to all articles freely available full-text.

Cumulative Index of Nursing and Allied Health Literature (CINAHL) is a database that focuses specifically on nursing and allied health literature. You must either pay to subscribe to CINAHL or gain access through membership in a library or a professional organization such as the American Physical Therapy Association (APTA). The criteria for being indexed in CINAHL are less stringent than PubMed. Thus, although there is an overlap with many journals indexed in both databases, those indexed in CINAHL but not PubMed tend to be smaller journals containing studies more likely to be representing foundational concepts.

Finally, a simple Google search can be a reasonable initial starting place. It is easy to use, is familiar to most, and handles specific search terms that other search engines might find difficult. However, the reader must pay particular attention to the source of the evidence for quality and bias. Google Scholar, which limits the search to scholarly works, provides a simple way to broadly search the peer-reviewed literature. A disadvantage is that Scholar is not limited to medicine, so it may return a variety of results across disciplines; however, it links to full-text when available.

All health care practitioners should have a strategy to regularly review current evidence in their specialty area. A simple review of the table of contents of core journals in the topic area can be useful. Most journals will send you a list of the table of contents and newly published articles when you sign up to receive them. Core peer-reviewed journals in geriatrics and geriatric physical therapy are listed in Box 1.3. In addition, choose one or two core journals in a professionally applicable subspecialty area of your choice (stroke, arthritis, osteoporosis, etc.) and check table of contents regularly.

A second approach is to go to a site such as AMEDEO (http://www.amedeo.com), which is a free service providing regular e-mails aggregating article citations specific to any interest across a wide range of health care specialties. The citations are typically taken from ongoing searches of newly published issues of core journals in the specialty area (or a subset of these journals as requested) and pushed to you through an e-mail listing. PubMed also allows an individual to identify and save a specific search strategy within it, have the search automatically run periodically to identify any new citations, and have the new citations automatically forwarded via e-mail. The PubMed approach allows you to be the most specific about the characteristics of the studies of interest and searches across the widest variety of journals.

BOX 1.3 Key Journals Particularly Relevant to Geriatric Physical Therapy

Journal of the American Geriatric Society
Journals of Gerontology: Series A, Biological Sciences and Medical Sciences
Journal of Geriatric Physical Therapy
Physical Therapy

Evidence Translation Sources. Clinical practice guidelines, particularly those based on a systematic review of the literature and expert consensus in applying the evidence to clinical practice, can be efficient sources of evidence. When examining the practice guidelines, confirm the comprehensiveness and objective analysis of the literature on which the guideline is based. The strength of the evidence should be based on quality, consistency, and number of studies supporting the recommendation.

Patient Autonomy

The scientific evidence and the expertise of the practitioner are combined with the preferences and motivations of the patient to reach a shared and informed decision about goals and interventions. Patient autonomy is grounded in the principle that patients have the right to make their own decisions about their health care. There is a tendency for health care providers to behave paternalistically toward older adult patients, assuming these patients are less capable than younger adults to make decisions about their health and rehabilitation. The reality of clinical practice is that physical therapists encounter a wide variety of decision-making capabilities in their older adult patients. Physical therapists have a responsibility to ensure their patients (and family/caretakers, as appropriate) have all pertinent information needed to make therapy-related health care decisions, and that this information is shared in a manner that is understandable to the patient and free of clinician bias. The patient should understand the potential risks, benefits, and harms; amount of effort and compliance associated with the various options; and likely prognosis.

Patients should have the opportunity to express their preferences and be satisfied that the practitioner has heard them accurately and without bias. The goals and preferences of the older adult patient may be very different from what the physical therapist assumes (or believes he or she would want for him- or herself under similar circumstances). Part of the "art" of physical therapy is creatively addressing the patient's goals using appropriate evidence, clinical skills, and available resources.

THE PHYSICAL THERAPIST IN GERIATRICS

Geriatric Care Team

Physical therapists working with older adults must be prepared to serve as autonomous primary care practitioners and as consultants, educators (patient and community), clinical researchers (contributors and critical assessors), case managers, patient advocates, interdisciplinary team members, and practice managers.[30] Although none of these roles is unique to geriatric physical therapy, what is unique is the remarkable variability among older adult patients and the regularity with which the geriatric physical therapist encounters patients with particularly complex needs. Unlike the typical younger individual, older adults are likely to have several complicating comorbid conditions in addition to the condition that has brought them to physical therapy. Patients with similar medical diagnoses often demonstrate great variability in baseline functional status and may be simultaneously dealing with significant psychosocial stresses such as loss of a spouse, loss of an important aspect of independence, or a change in residence. Thus, issues such as depression, fear, reaction to change, and family issues can compound the physical aspects and provide an additive challenge to the physical therapist. The physical therapist must be creative, pay close attention to functional clues about underlying modifiable or accommodative impairments, and listen carefully to the patient to ensure goal setting truly represents mutually agreed-upon goals.

In addition, the older patient is likely to be followed by multiple health care providers, thus making the physical therapist a member of a team (whether that team is informally or formally identified). As such, the physical therapist must share information and consult with other team members, recognize signs and symptoms that suggest a need to refer out to other practitioners, coordinate services, provide education to the patient and caretaker/family, and advocate for the needs of patients and their families.

Geriatric Competencies

Following the 2008 IOM report on the critical need to "retool" the health care workforce,[1] 21 professional organizations representing 10 different health professions (including physical therapy) came together to develop a consensus document of core competencies applicable across health disciplines. The *Multidisciplinary Competencies in the Care of Older Adults at the Completion of the Entry-Level Health Professional Degree*[31] emerged and was subsequently endorsed by 31 professional organizations, including the APTA.

Six key competency domains emerged as critical to all professions when serving older adults: (1) health promotion and safety, (2) evaluation and assessment, (3) care planning and coordination across the care spectrum, (4) interdisciplinary and team care, (5) caregiver support, and (6) health care systems and benefits. Competency and subcompetency statements listed under each domain were specific enough to provide structure and direction for each profession to operationalize yet general enough to allow customizing to the needs of each profession. Each profession was encouraged to provide guidance statements that tailored the competencies to practitioners within their field.

Over the next several years, three different national task forces appointed by the Academy of Geriatric Physical Therapy, using the multidisciplinary competency document as a framework, customized the original document to three levels of practitioner within physical therapy[32]: completion of physical therapist entry-level program of study, completion of physical therapist assistant entry-level program of study, and physical therapist completion of a postprofessional program of study such as geriatric residency programs. The concepts and competencies embedded within each domain are captured across the various chapters of this book. A review of the competencies attests to the breadth and depth knowledge, skills, and attitudes needed for best practice as a geriatric physical therapist.

Expert Practice

Jensen and colleagues[33] provide compelling insights into the process of moving from novice to expert in physical therapy clinical practice. All experts, regardless of specialty area, were found to be highly motivated with a strong commitment to lifelong learning. Experts sought out mentors and could clearly describe the role each mentor had in their development, whether for enhanced decision making, professional responsibilities, personal values, or technical skill development. Experts had a deep knowledge of their specialty practice and used self-reflection regularly to identify strengths and weaknesses in their knowledge or thought processes to guide their ongoing self-improvement. The expert did not "blame the patient" if a treatment did not go as anticipated. Rather, the expert reflected deeply about what he or she could have done differently that would have allowed the patient to succeed.

The geriatric clinical specialists interviewed by Jensen and colleagues each provided reflections about how they progressed from novice to expert. In describing their path from new graduate generalist to geriatric clinical specialist, the geriatric experts noted that they did not start their careers anticipating specialization in geriatrics. They each sought a generalist practice experience as a new graduate and found themselves gradually gravitating toward the older adult patient as opportunities came their way. They came to recognize the talent they had for working with older adults and were called to action by their perceptions that many at-risk older adults were receiving inadequate care. They became firm believers in the principles of optimal aging and had a genuine high regard for the capabilities of older adults if given the opportunity to fully participate in rehabilitation. These specialists model clinical excellence by not settling for less than what the patient is capable of. Physical therapists are essential practitioners in geriatrics. The physical therapist must embrace this essential role—and recognize the positive challenge—of mastering the management of a complex and variable group of patients.

Physical therapists who find geriatrics particularly rewarding and exciting enjoy being creative and being challenged to guide patients through a complex maze to achieve their highest level of healthy aging. Navigating an effective solution in the midst of a complex set of patient issues is professionally affirming and rarely dull or routine.

Clinical Decision Making

The complexity of clinical decision making can be daunting because of the sheer volume of information and detailed considerations unique to the individual. However, physical therapists who make movement-related human performance the central focus of their decision-making process and approach each decision-making step systematically with a clear organizational strategy for gathering and utilizing information will find it easier to identify and apply pertinent information. Many approaches are organized around the five components of the *Guide to Physical Therapist Practice*'s Patient/Client Management Model (Fig. 1.6). Schenkman and Butler argue that task analysis in the environmental context is one of the skills that defines the physical therapist and is essential for effective decision making.[20] They also include the previously described enablement–disablement process as a fundamental organizing principle to formulate clinical hypotheses that guide the analysis, synthesis, and judgments made by physical therapists about the physical therapy management of their individual patients (Fig. 1.7).

Examination. Older adults typically enter physical therapy with a referral that may contain a few useful facts about the patient's medical history or the medical reason for the referral. In these circumstances the first question to ask oneself is, "Given the facts about the patient that are available before the examination, have any impairments or activity limitations been identified even before the patient is seen for the first time?" The collection of two kinds of clinical data should be integrated into the format for the first clinical encounter. First, as summarized in Box 1.4, there are a number of factors identified in the literature and reviewed elsewhere in this text that may influence the trajectory of a patient from disease to disability. Physical therapists should always account for these potentially enabling–disabling influences as part of the patient examination. Additional information that would assist in setting goals and designing intervention, and information from other disciplines can also be very helpful. Data on the individual's current medical conditions and medications, for example, are extremely relevant.

If the overall goal is to optimize patient function, then one of the first steps is to ascertain the patient's current level of function. Whenever the patient's communication ability is intact, the initial interview begins by allowing patients to identify what they see as the primary activity limitations that have prompted the need for physical therapy. In their formulation of a hypothetico-deductive

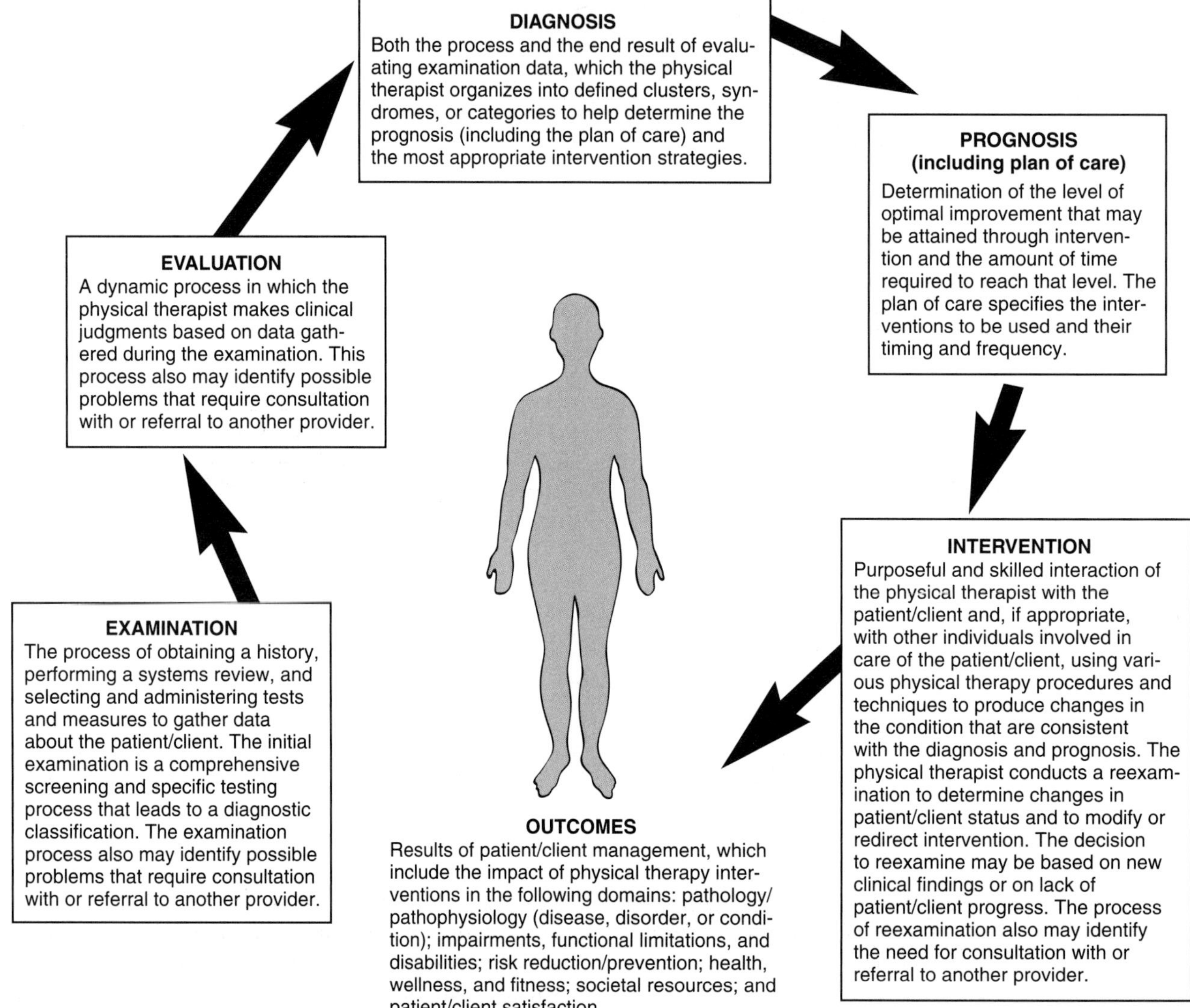

DIAGNOSIS
Both the process and the end result of evaluating examination data, which the physical therapist organizes into defined clusters, syndromes, or categories to help determine the prognosis (including the plan of care) and the most appropriate intervention strategies.
PROGNOSIS (including plan of care)
Determination of the level of optimal improvement that may be attained through intervention and the amount of time required to reach that level. The plan of care specifies the interventions to be used and their timing and frequency.
EVALUATION
A dynamic process in which the physical therapist makes clinical judgments based on data gathered during the examination. This process also may identify possible problems that require consultation with or referral to another provider.
INTERVENTION
Purposeful and skilled interaction of the physical therapist with the patient/client and, if appropriate, with other individuals involved in care of the patient/client, using various physical therapy procedures and techniques to produce changes in the condition that are consistent with the diagnosis and prognosis. The physical therapist conducts a reexamination to determine changes in patient/client status and to modify or redirect intervention. The decision to reexamine may be based on new clinical findings or on lack of patient/client progress. The process of reexamination also may identify the need for consultation with or referral to another provider.
EXAMINATION
The process of obtaining a history, performing a systems review, and selecting and administering tests and measures to gather data about the patient/client. The initial examination is a comprehensive screening and specific testing process that leads to a diagnostic classification. The examination process also may identify possible problems that require consultation with or referral to another provider.
OUTCOMES
Results of patient/client management, which include the impact of physical therapy interventions in the following domains: pathology/pathophysiology (disease, disorder, or condition); impairments, functional limitations, and disabilities; risk reduction/prevention; health, wellness, and fitness; societal resources; and patient/client satisfaction.

FIG. 1.6 The elements of patient/client management. *(Redrawn from the American Physical Therapy Association. Guide to Physical Therapist Practice. Alexandria, VA: American Physical Therapy Association; 2001: 32.)*

strategy for making clinical judgments, Rothstein and Echternach emphasize the value of listening as patients identify their problems and allowing the individuals to express the desired goal of treatment in their own terms.[34] By talking with the patient, the therapist begins to develop not only a professional rapport but also an appreciation of the patient's understanding of the situation. The input of the patient in terms of preferences, motivations, and goals are central pieces of "evidence" in an evidence-based approach to decision making.[35] This is especially pertinent to care provided to older individuals, who may find their ability to control their own personal destinies compromised by professional judgments made "in their best interests." When the patient is unable to communicate effectively, the therapist may turn to proxy information. The patient's family and friends may be able to give some insight as to what the patient would regard as the goals of intervention. The therapist may also hypothesize about a patient's functional deficits based on previous experience with similar patients.

Data from the history, as well as data on how the patient's problems have been treated in the past, allow the therapist to hypothesize that certain impairments or activity limitations might exist by virtue of the individual's medical condition(s) and sociodemographic and other personal characteristics. For example, suppose the physical therapist learns from the patient's history that the patient has a medical diagnosis of Parkinson disease, that she is 81 years old, and that she lives alone. The diagnosis of Parkinson disease suggests the possibility of the following impairments: loss of motor control and abnormal tone, ROM deficits, faulty posture, and decreased endurance for functional activities. Using epidemiologic research about what activity limitations are likely for women living alone, specific questions about independence in instrumental activities of daily living (IADLs),

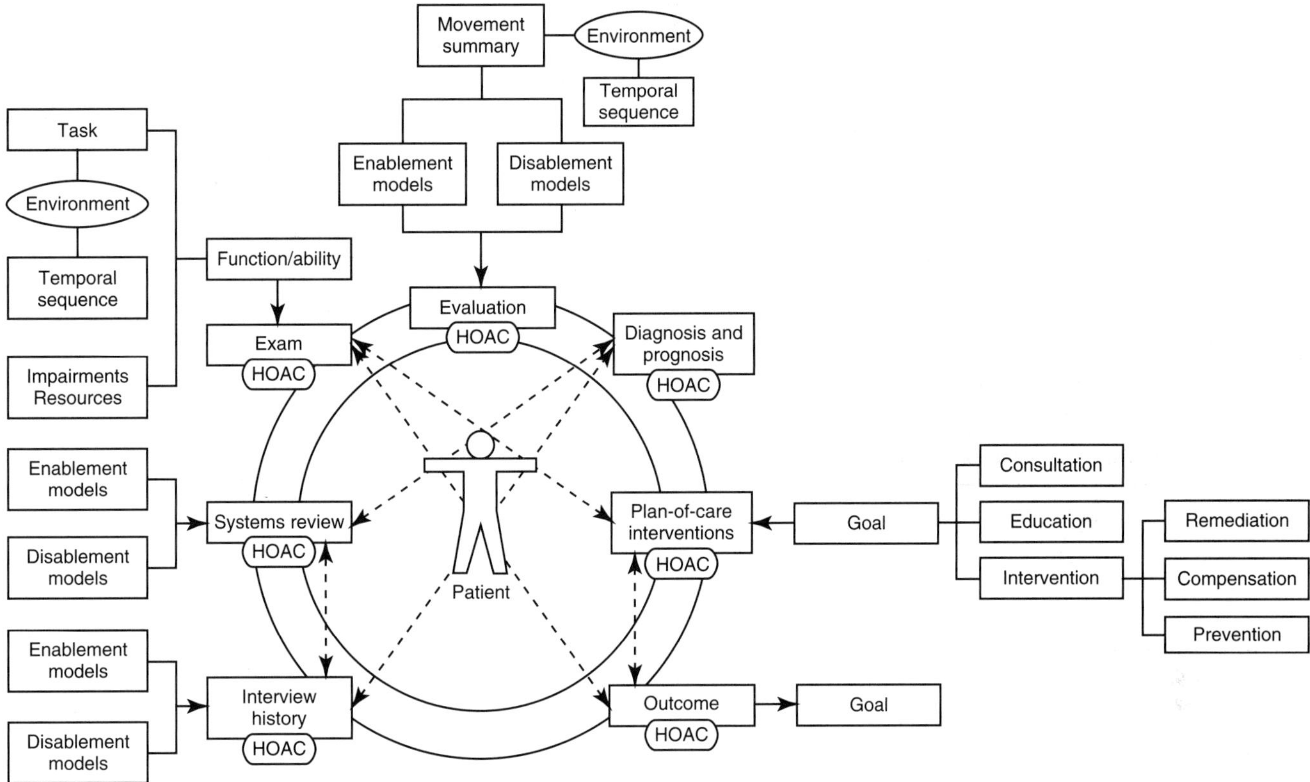

FIG. 1.7 Schenkman's model of integration and task analysis. *HOAC*, Hypothesis-Oriented Algorithm for Clinicians. *(Redrawn from Schenkman M, Duetsch JE, Gill-Body KM. An integrated framework for decision making in neurologic physical therapist practice. Phys Ther. 2006;86:1683.)*

BOX 1.4 Components of Patient History

HISTORY

Previous	Current
• Demographics	• Current conditions
• Social history	• Chief complaint
• Work/school/play	• Current function
• Living environment	• Activity level
• General health status	• Medications
• Health habits	• Clinical labs/tests
• Behavioral health	• Review of other systems
• Family history	
• Medical/surgical history	

with specific tests and measures as indicated, would be appropriate to include in the examination. Social isolation, for example, may lead to depression, which could further aggravate a person's functional difficulties.

Because there is a lot of variability (e.g., physical fitness, cognition, chronic conditions) in older adults, a screen of all systems is crucial to ensure that the physical therapist does not miss a critical finding. Screening begins with a thorough patient history as the physical therapist relies heavily on the clinical presentation of the patient and any signs or symptoms that indicate the need for specific screening tests or questions.[36] Therapists must recognize, for example, when integumentary signs may be indicative of systemic connective tissue disorders or oncologic disease, when the patient would concomitantly benefit from the services of other health care professionals, and when additional signs and symptoms may suggest other impairments that would benefit from physical therapy. The combination of the patient history and screening of systems leads to more focused tests and measures. As physical therapists strive to be efficient, they realize that performing all tests to rule in or out a potential diagnosis is time prohibitive. Expert clinicians rely on "pattern recognition" as well as early generation of hypotheses for interpreting collected data.[37] Concurrent with these observations and interim judgments, the physical therapist may reach a conclusion that the signs and symptoms are not consistent with any pattern of disease or illness that is in the scope of physical therapist practice and may refer the patient to another health care professional.

The therapist initially makes a working hypothesis regarding the underlying cause of any deficits noted during the history and systems review and then selects specific tests and measures that would most likely confirm his or her suspicions about a tentative diagnosis. The process of confirming or refuting clinical impressions is the substance of the examination. Without knowing what you are looking for, it is difficult to know when you find it.

Without this important list of possible conditions or issues, a therapist can get lost in the multitude of impairments and functional deficits that may be present. Thus, the clinical hypothesis (or hypotheses) provides focus for the examination.

During the examination, the therapist should begin by performing a detailed analysis of functional activities (e.g., transferring from the bed to a chair) that also takes into consideration the environment in which the task is being performed. Functional activities will inform impairments that are observed to affect function. Movement analysis is at the crux of establishing a diagnosis that can point to an intervention in the domain of physical therapist practice. Physical therapists are well prepared to identify dysfunction at the level of actions by examining the movement-oriented component of tasks. Specific tests and measures are used in the examination to clarify and characterize the nature and extent of activity limitations and further implicate impairments and other factors that impede performance. Is the inability to climb stairs in an older adult associated with knee and hip extensor weakness? What about balance deficits due to sensory loss in the feet and ankles? Thus, broadening the examination to focus on observing and critiquing the performance of actions and tasks is crucial to ensure a thorough evaluation of the patient's inability to perform specific goal-directed activities. The inability to perform movements needed to execute specific goal-directed activities is particularly relevant to physical therapist practice as they capture the complex integration of systems that permits an individual to maintain a posture, transition to other postures, or sustain safe and efficient movement.

Evaluation and Diagnosis. After the examination, the therapist evaluates the data by making clinical judgments about their meaning and their relevance to the patient's condition and to confirm or reject hypotheses posed during the examination. The therapist then hypothesizes which findings contribute to the patient's functional deficits and will be the focus of patient-related instruction and direct intervention.

It is not unusual for older patients to have multiple impairments and activity limitations, many of which can be identified by a physical therapist and treated using physical therapy procedures. However, the overall purpose of evaluation is twofold: (1) to indicate which deficiencies in functioning prevent a person from achieving optimal well-being and (2) to identify the actions and tasks that are most associated with the patient's current level of function and must be remediated for the patient to reach an optimal functional level. An element of assessing data on the patient's ability to perform functional activities is to determine whether the manner in which actions and tasks are done represents an important quantitative or qualitative deviation from the way in which most people of similar age would perform them. In the absence of norms for age-stratified functional performance, the therapist must bring previous experience with similar patients to bear on this judgment. Even if the therapist concludes that the patient's performance is other than "normal," this judgment does not imply that a person cannot meet socially imposed expectations of what it means to be independent or that an individual is permanently disabled. Furthermore, identifying the impairment alone may not fully explain the inability to perform an activity as the individual's motivation to perform the activity as well as the environment in which it is performed may affect goal achievement. Thus, the physical therapist must review activity limitations in light of other clinical findings that identify the patient's impairments and other psychological, social, and environmental factors that modify function in determining whether a patient will become disabled. Upon completion of the evaluation, physical therapists establish a prognosis and plan of care, if needed.

Physical therapists are encouraged to take an integrated approach to diagnosing deficits in human performance. Deconstructing movement in the context of human performance requires the examination of the complex interaction of sensoriperceptual, biomechanical, neuromotor, respiratory, and circulatory capabilities as well as the influence of personal motivation, cognition, behavior, and the environment on movement. Physical therapists must determine if the limitation in activity is at the level of task, action, and/or impairment. Ultimately, the physical therapist will pose a hypothesis or several hypotheses linking an inability to perform an action to a specific impairment or cluster of impairments. Consider, for example, the range of impairments that might explain the deficit in performing the required actions to accomplish the tasks that compose the activity limitation that is reported as "I can't get to my mailbox to get my mail." Furthermore, suppose that we know that individual has low vision, lives in a second-floor walk-up, is somewhat reluctant to go outside particularly in strong daylight, has osteoarthritis in one knee, and is currently on medication for early stages of congestive heart failure. Each component of this activity (getting the mail) involves a series of tasks to be accomplished (e.g., opening a door, descending stairs, negotiating terrain, handling latches) that require specific actions (e.g., standing, walking, stepping, turning, pulling, grasping, carrying). It is highly likely that several impairments such as decreased muscle strength, reduced joint mobility, limited dynamic balance, or diminished endurance will need to be hypothesized and confirmed to account for this activity limitation.

Prognosis and Plan of Care. The physical therapist uses the data gathered in the evaluation and diagnosis process to state a prognosis, which is a prediction about the optimal level of function that the patient will achieve and the time that will be required to reach that level. Having done that, the therapist and the patient can then mutually agree upon anticipated goals of treatment, which generally are related to expected outcomes of care. Therefore, the functional outcomes of treatment should be stated in patient-centered (behavioral) terms. On the basis of these anticipated goals and expected outcomes, the physical therapist then completes a plan of care that specifies the interventions to be implemented, including their frequency, intensity, and duration.

When the therapist's attention turns toward planning intervention, the key question is: Of the impairments that are hypothesized to be causal to the patient's activity limitations, which ones require a physical therapist intervention? Furthermore, if the patient's impairments cannot be remediated initially or even with extensive treatment, the physical therapist then seeks to determine how the patient may compensate by using other abilities to accomplish the action or task, and also how the task can be adapted so that the activity can be performed within the restrictions that the patient's condition imposes on the situation. The current evidence base for determining the optimal proportion, timing, and sequence of remediation, compensation, and adaptation of both initial and subsequent plans of care is shallow. Therefore, physical therapists must consider the balance among each of these three intervention approaches dynamically, depending on the persistence of deficits in structure or function, availability of compensatory resources without unintended negative consequences for other functioning, likelihood of full recovery with further remediation, and surmountability of environmental challenges. If it is decided that an individual's impairments and activity limitations are amenable to physical therapy intervention, the therapist should establish a schedule for evaluating the effectiveness of the intervention. If the patient achieves the anticipated goals for changes in impairments but does not also achieve the expected functional outcomes, this is an indication that the therapist has incorrectly hypothesized the relationship between the patient's impairments and functional status. In this instance, the therapist may reexamine the patient to modify the plan of care.

Although a host of procedures and techniques might be used to remediate an impairment or minimize an activity limitation, those that are most likely to promote the outcome and that consider cost-effectiveness should be chosen for inclusion in the plan of care. The combination of direct interventions used with any particular patient will vary according to the impairments and activity limitations that are addressed by the plan of care for that individual. Three patients may have the same activity limitation, for example, an inability to transfer independently from bed to chair, yet require entirely different programs of intervention. If the first individual lacked sufficient knee strength to come to a standing position, then the plan of care would incorporate strengthening exercises to remedy the impairment and improve the patient's function. If the second patient lacked sufficient ROM at the hip owing to flexion contractures to allow full upright standing, then intervention would focus on increasing ROM at the hip to improve function. The third individual may possess all the musculoskeletal and neuromuscular prerequisites to allow function but still require appropriate instruction to do it safely and with minimal exertion. Each individual may achieve a similar level of functional independence, yet none of the three would have received the exact same treatment to achieve the same outcome.

Most of the direct interventions used by physical therapists are aimed at remediating impairments that underlie activity limitations. Although physical therapists sometimes apply therapeutic exercise in the position of function (e.g., standing balance exercises) or try to simulate the environment in which the functional activity is performed (e.g., a staircase), the functional activity in and of itself should not be confused with the core elements of a physical therapist's plan of care, that is, therapeutic exercise and functional training. It is particularly helpful for the therapist working with older adult patients to appreciate that there are some impairments that will not change, no matter how much direct intervention is provided. This realization will diminish unnecessary treatment. In these instances, physical therapists may still achieve positive patient outcomes by teaching patients how to compensate for their permanent impairments by capitalizing on other capabilities or by modifying the environment to reduce the demands of the task. One of the beneficial consequences of a careful deconstruction of an activity limitation into tasks and actions is that this analysis indicates what kinds of outcomes are most suitable to demonstrating the success of the intervention. The most proximate outcomes of the remediation of impairments can be found in an improved ability to perform actions, somewhat irrespective of personal and environmental factors that are outside of the physical therapist's control. In comparison, activity limitations are typically measured with respect to broader outcome measures such as basic and instrumental activities of daily living. Relevant chapters of this book provide recommendations for valid and reliable functional measures to assess the outcomes of a physical therapy episode of care.

SUMMARY

The key principles underlying contemporary geriatric physical therapy practice described in this chapter are woven throughout the remainder of this book. The need is great and opportunities abound for talented physical therapists committed to optimal aging and ready to apply best evidence, to fully develop their clinical expertise, and work collaboratively with their patients and other health care providers. It is a time full of opportunity to be a geriatrically focused physical therapist. However, whether as a geriatrically focused physical therapist or a physical therapist who occasionally treats older patients, the number and complexity of the older adult patients among the caseload of all physical therapists will increase in the decades to come, emphasizing the clinical relevance of the material in this book.

REFERENCES

1. Institute of Medicine. *Retooling for an Aging America: Building the Health Care Workforce*. Washington, DC: National Academies Press; 2008.
2. Vespa J, Armstrong D, Medina L. Demographic Turning Points for the United States: Population Projections for 2020 to 2060. US Census Bureau. https://www.census.gov/content/dam/Census/library/publications/2018/demo/P25_1144.pdf. Published 2018. Accessed December 17, 2018.
3. Friedman SM, Mulhausen P, Cleveland ML, et al. Healthy aging: American Geriatrics Society white paper executive summary. *J Am Geriatr Soc*. 2019;67:17–20.
4. Rowe JW, Kahn RL. Successful aging. *Gerontologist*. 1997; 37(4): 433–440.
5. Brummel-Smith K. Optimal aging, part I: demographics and definitions. *Ann Long Term Care*. 2007;15(11):26–28.
6. Friedman SM, Mulhausen P, Cleveland ML, et al. *American Geriatrics Society White Paper on Healthy Aging*. https://geriatricscareonline.org/ProductAbstract/american-geriatrics-society-white-paper-on-healthy-aging/CL025/?param2=search. Published 2018. Accessed December 18, 2018.
7. World Health Organization. *Frequently Asked Questions*. http://www.who.int/suggestions/faq/en/. Accessed December 16, 2018.
8. Oliver M. *Understanding Disability: From Theory to Practice*. New York: St. Martin's Press; 1996.
9. Nagi S. Some conceptual issues in disability and rehabilitation. In: Sussman M, ed. *Sociology and Rehabilitation*. Washington, DC: American Sociological Association; 1965.
10. Nagi S. Disability concepts revisited: implications for prevention. In: Pope A, Tarlov A, eds. *Disability in America: Toward a National Agenda for Prevention*. Washington, DC: National Academies Press; 1991.
11. Jette AM. Diagnosis and classification by physical therapists: a special communication. *Phys Ther*. 1989;69(11):967–969.
12. Guccione AA. Physical therapy diagnosis and the relationship between impairments and function. *Phys Ther*. 1991;71(7): 499–503.
13. Guccione AA. Arthritis and the process of disablement. *Phys Ther*. 1994;74(5):408–414.
14. Jette AM. Physical disablement concepts for physical therapy research and practice. *Phys Ther*. 1994;74(5):380–386.
15. Verbrugge LM, Jette AM. The disablement process. *Soc Sci Med*. 1994;38(1):1–14.
16. Brandt E, Pope A. *Enabling America: Assessing the Role of Rehabilitation Science and Engineering*. Washington, DC: National Academies Press; 1997.
17. World Health Organization. *International Classification of Impairments, Disabilities, and Handicaps: A Manual of Classification Relating to the Consequences of Disease*. Geneva, Switzerland: World Health Organization; 1980. https://insights.ovid.com/crossref?an=00004356-198012000-00032. Accessed December 17, 2018.
18. World Health Organization. *International Classification of Functioning, Disability and Health*. Geneva, Switzerland: World Health Organization; 2001. http://www.who.int/classifications/icf/en/. Accessed December 17, 2018.
19. Institute of Medicine (US) Committee on Disability in America. In: Field MJ, Jette AM, eds. *The Future of Disability in America*. Washington, DC: National Academies Press; 2007. http://www.ncbi.nlm.nih.gov/books/NBK11434/. Accessed December 17, 2018.
20. Schenkman M, Butler R. A model for multisystem evaluation, interpretation, and treatment of individuals with neurologic dysfunction. *Phys Ther*. 1989;69(7):538–547.
21. Watson KB, Carlson S, Gunn J, et al. Physical inactivity among adults aged 50 years and older — United States, 2014. *MMWR*. 2016;65(36):954–958.
22. U.S. Department of Health and Human Services. *Physical Activity Guidelines for Americans*. 2nd ed. Washington, DC: U.S. Department of Health and Human Services; 2018.
23. Schwartz RS. Sarcopenia and physical performance in old age: introduction. *Muscle Nerve*. 1997;20(S5):10–12.
24. Clegg A, Young J, Iliffe S, Rikkert MO, Rockwood K. Frailty in elderly people. *Lancet*. 2013;381(9868):752–762.
25. Taylor P, Morin R, Parker K, Cohn D, Wang W. *Growing Old in America: Expectations vs. Reality*. Washington, DC: Pew Research Center; 2009. http://www.pewsocialtrends.org/2009/06/29/growing-old-in-america-expectations-vs-reality/. Accessed December 18, 2018.
26. Levy SR, Macdonald JL. Progress on understanding ageism. *J Soc Issues*. 2016;72(1):5–25.
27. Chrisler JC, Barney A, Palatino B. Ageism can be hazardous to women's health: ageism, sexism, and stereotypes of older women in the healthcare system. *J Soc Issues*. 2016;72(1): 86–104.
28. Austin S, Qu H, Shewchuk RM. Age bias in physicians' recommendations for physical activity: a behavioral model of healthcare utilization for adults with arthritis. *J Phys Act Health*. 2013;10(2):222–231.
29. Fetters L, Tilson J. *Evidence Based Physical Therapy*. 2nd ed. Philadelphia: FA Davis; 2019.
30. Avers D. Scope of practice in geriatric physical therapy. *Gerinotes*. 2006;13(5):14–17.
31. Semla T, Barr J, Beizer J, et al. *Multidisciplinary Competencies in the Care of Older Adults at the Completion of the Entry-Level Health Professional Degree* https://www.americangeriatrics.org/geriatrics-profession/core-competencies. Published 2018. Accessed January 13, 2019.
32. Academy of Geriatric Physical Therapy. *Essential Competencies in the Care of Older Adults at the Completion of a Physical Therapist Postprofessional Program of Study*. https://geriatricspt.org/essential-competencies/index.cfm. Published 2011. Accessed January 13, 2019.
33. Jensen G, Gwyer J, Hack LM, Shepard K. *Expertise in Physical Therapy Practice*. 2nd ed. Philadelphia: Saunders; 2007. https://evolve.elsevier.com/cs/product/9781416002147?role=student. Accessed December 19, 2018.
34. Rothstein JM, Echternach JL. Hypothesis-Oriented Algorithm for Clinicians. A method for evaluation and treatment planning. *Phys Ther*. 1986;66(9):1388–1394.
35. Sackett D, Haynes R, Tugwell P, Guyatt G. *Clinical Epidemiology: A Basic Science for Clinical Medicine*. 2nd ed. Boston: Lippincott Williams & Wilkins; 1991.
36. Goodman C, Heick J, Lazaro R. *Differential Diagnosis for Physical Therapists: Screening for Referral*. 6th ed. St. Louis: Saunders; 2018.
37. May BJ, Dennis JK. Expert decision making in physical therapy—a survey of practitioners. *Phys Ther*. 1991;71(3): 190–202. discussion 202–206.

CHAPTER 2

Aging Demographics and Trends

Dale Avers

OUTLINE

INTRODUCTION

The older adult population, most commonly referring to individuals 65 years and older, is a diverse group, so much so that it is impossible to describe an 82-year-old individual accurately. An 82-year-old could be scaling the most challenging rock faces,[1] running a marathon, regularly fast-speed walking, sedentary but independent, or frail and near death. What are the implications of this variability in how one ages on physical therapy practice? The purpose of this chapter is to review the sociodemographic characteristics of older adults in America, then relate these factors to mortality, morbidity, and function in this population. In doing so, we shall find that conflicting portrayals of older persons as active and healthy or as sick and frail are neither incorrect nor contradictory, but more appropriately applied to only some segments of an increasingly heterogeneous population.

Although physical therapists implement plans of care that are individualized, they also tend to categorize patients according to the various physical, psychological, and social characteristics they expect to encounter associated with these characteristics. Knowing that individuals with certain characteristics—for example, being a particular age or sex—are more likely to experience a particular health problem can assist physical therapists in anticipating some clinical presentations, placing an individual's progress in perspective, and even sometimes altering outcomes through preventive measures. It is also useful to know the prevalence of a particular condition (i.e., the number of cases of that condition in a population) and its incidence (the number of new cases of a condition in a population within a specified time period). Taken beyond examination of a single person, physical therapists can use this information to plan and develop services that will meet the needs of an aging society whose members span a continuum across health, infirmity, and death.

However, when considering a demographic such as the high prevalence of dementia in women over the age of 85 years, it is easy to stereotype all 85-year-old women as being confused or unmotivated. This stereotyping, albeit unintentional, is called ageism. Ageism is the negative stereotyping that leads to prejudice and therefore discriminatory practice[2] such as low expectations or inadequate exercise prescription. Although a study of demographics may appear to easily promote stereotyping because of the nature of population statistics, viewing these demographics from the perspective of the diversity of the older adult population will help decrease stereotyping and optimize person-centered care for each older adult.

There is one critical caveat to any of the inferences about aging or older persons that may be drawn from the data given later. Much of what we know in the United States about gerontology and geriatrics has been derived from two specific cohorts. Many of the first cohort, born between 1885 and 1920 and reaching age 65 between 1950 and 1985, came to America as impoverished child immigrants or were born into families recently arrived in

America. Thus, the initial emergence of gerontological research in the 1970s is based largely on these individuals, whose early health and vitality into adulthood were determined long before the medical advances and economic prosperity that marked the "American Century." Their children, born between 1910 and 1945 and turning age 65 between 1975 and 2010 and the parents of the baby boomers, make up the second cohort, whose experiences define our current-day understanding of aging. Geriatric and gerontological research in this group is contextually situated in the defining events of the first half of the 20th century: two world wars and the Great Depression. Therefore, whenever we analyze aging in terms of physical health or social well-being, we must appreciate that our understandings are based on a unique cohort and not necessarily what will be the norm in the future. A very different, third cohort of older adults, called the post–World War II "baby boom" generation, were born between 1946 and 1965. This cohort began to turn 65 years of age in 2011. Typical of this generation, we can expect that gerontological theories and geriatric practice—geriatric physical therapy included—will change markedly by the mid-21st century to accommodate new findings that emerge from scientific study of this third and markedly distinct cohort. Many "boomers" will be more active in their later years. They'll continue to bike, hike, swim, sail, and ski. They'll be more likely to relocate and go where the physical and intellectual action is. Boomers expect to work at least part time after retirement and will be adept with technology compared to their parents. These trends will be described in this chapter.

DEMOGRAPHY

Defining "Older" Adult

The first gerontological question is, how does a particular segment of a population come to be categorized as "older"? The chronological criterion that is presently used for identifying the older adult in America is strictly arbitrary and usually has been set at age 65 years. However, the onset of some "geriatric" health problems of older individuals may occur in the early 50s. And athletes over the age of 40 may be called "master athletes." As the mean age of the population increases and more individuals live into their 9th and 10th decades, we can expect that our notion of who is "older" will change.

Population Pyramids

Population pyramids are useful to view large trends of population in graphic form. From a population pyramid you can view the size of various age groups by year and sex and how they compare over several generations. Historically, as illustrated in the 1960 pyramid of Fig. 2.1, an

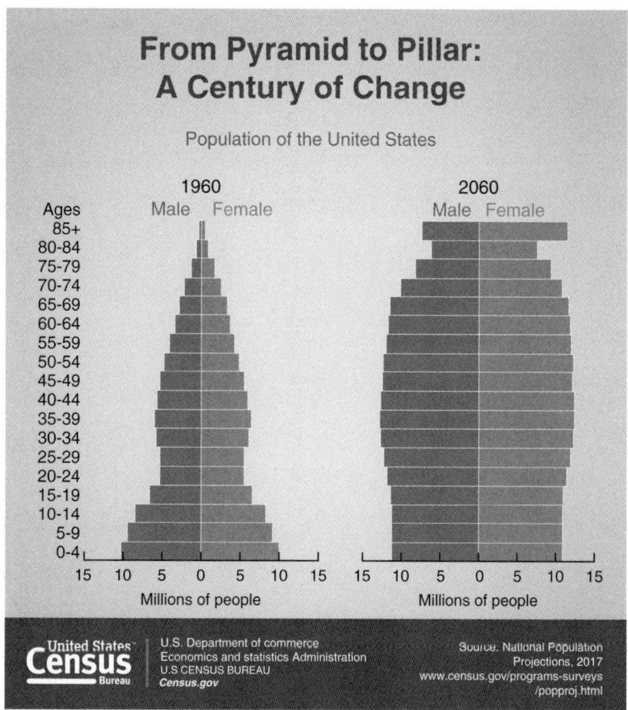

FIG. 2.1 1960 pyramid to 2060 pillar. *(From National Population Projections. 2017. http://www.census.gov/programs-surveys/popproj.html.)*

age–sex pyramid had the longest bars of the graph at the bottom of the pyramid, indicating a large population of infants and children, with declines toward the top due to death rate. However, the shape of this pyramid has gradually changed over time such that, by 2060, the pyramid is projected to reflect a more rectangular shape, indicating a very slow rate of population growth as shown in the 2060 pyramid of Fig. 2.1. This slow rate of growth reflects a lower birth rate for more recent years and longer lives for those born in earlier generations. For example, in the current pyramid of 2020 (Fig. 2.2) the sharper point reflects the last of the World War II generation and the majority of the pyramid is more rectangular, indicating, as in the 2060 pyramid, a slowing population growth (declining birth rate) and an aging population (declining death rate).

Another way to think about population structure is to examine dependency ratios. Dependency ratios provide an indicator of the *potential* burden on the working-age (i.e., tax-paying) population. Youth dependency is the ratio of the population under age 20 to the population aged 20 to 64, whereas old-age dependency is the ratio of the population age 65 and older to the population aged 20 to 64. Although the youth dependency ratio is projected to increase slightly between 2020 and 2040, indicating a slightly higher birth rate compared to those between ages 20 and 64, the old-age dependency ratio is projected to skyrocket, increasing by more than 50% by 2030.[3] Implications are that the labor force is reduced,

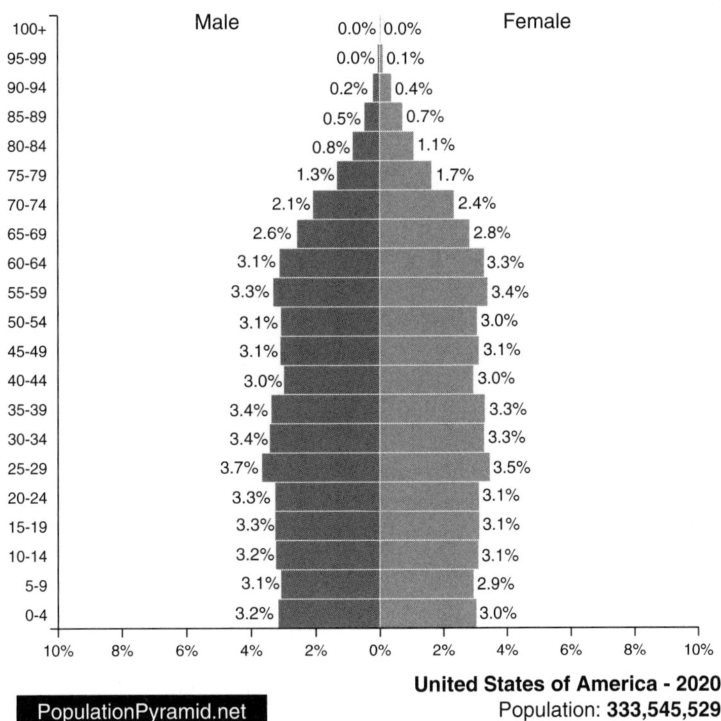

FIG. 2.2 2020 pyramid. *(From PopulationPyramid.net.)*

decreasing overall economic spending and tax revenues. At the same time there is increased government spending through payment of pensions and social security and in higher health care costs. This increased dependency on government services with fewer people contributing to the federal budget through the workforce will create budget issues and will drive policy. Although these implications can be viewed as an economic crisis, two factors can be seen as mitigating this potential crisis. Immigration may introduce more adults of younger, working age into the workforce, and children born in the 1980s and 1990s entering the workforce will partly offset the boomer exit. There is much debate about the meaning of the high old-age dependency ratio, a debate that will drive policy. But as will be mentioned many times throughout this chapter, physical therapists can positively impact the effects of this trend by helping older adults stay healthy and therefore less dependent.

U.S. Population Estimates and Age Structure

The number of Americans age 65 years and older continues to grow at an unprecedented rate. In 2015, the best available estimate of persons age 65 years or older was 47.8 million,[4] reflecting the major changes in the population structure of the United States in the past century. In 1900, individuals who had reached their 65th birthday accounted for only 4% of the total population. In 1940, they were 6.9% of the population, and by 1950, they were equal to 8.2%. Although they represented just fewer than 10% of the population in 1970, they currently account for nearly 15% of the U.S. population.[4] By 2020, for the first time in history, people age 65 and over will compose 20% of the population and will outnumber children under the age of 5.

Those individuals born between the years 1946 and 1965 (the baby boomer cohort) currently represent nearly 25% of the overall U.S. population. This boomer cohort will be responsible for the majority of the growth in the 65-and-older population between the years 2010 and 2030. By 2030, older adults are predicted to account for nearly 20% of the total U.S. population.[5] Fig. 2.3 illustrates the impact of the baby boomer generation on aging in the United States.

Despite the "young-old" baby-boomer group being the prime group responsible for the rapid increase in the overall older adult population, the segment within the older population that is growing the fastest is the "old-old" group, that is, individuals over 85 years of age. Individuals older than 85 years of age grew from just over 100,000 in 1900 to 6 million in 2014 and is projected to grow to 20 million by 2060 (Fig. 2.4).[6] In 2014, older women accounted for 66% of the population age 85 and older. Between 1980 and 2016, the centenarian population experienced a 44% growth, a larger percentage increase than in the total population. In 2016, there were 81,896 persons age 100 and over (0.2% of the total 65-and-over population), a number that is more than double the 1980 figure of 32,194.[7] More than 80% of centenarians were female.

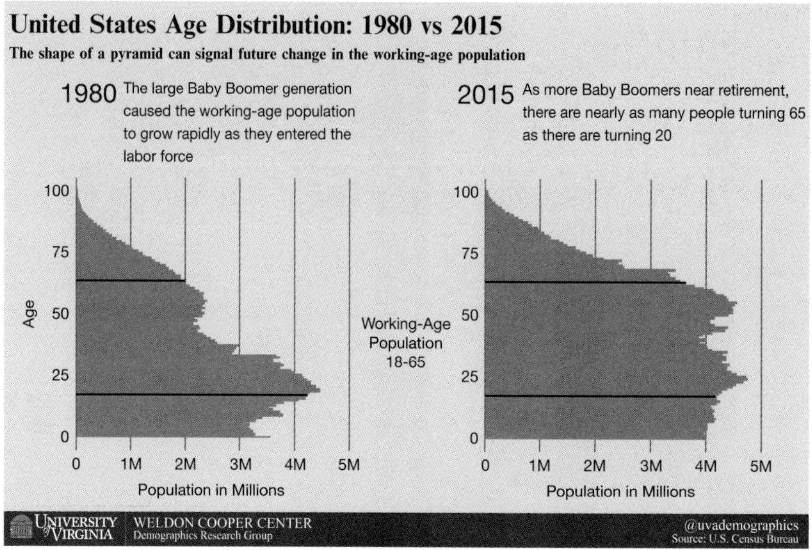

FIG. 2.3 Impact of the Baby Boomer generation on aging in the United States. *(From Weldon Cooper Center, Demographics Research Group @uvademographics. Source: U.S. Census Bureau. http://statchatva.org/2016/11/02/in-most-of-the-united-states-the-working-age-population-is-now-shrinking/.)*

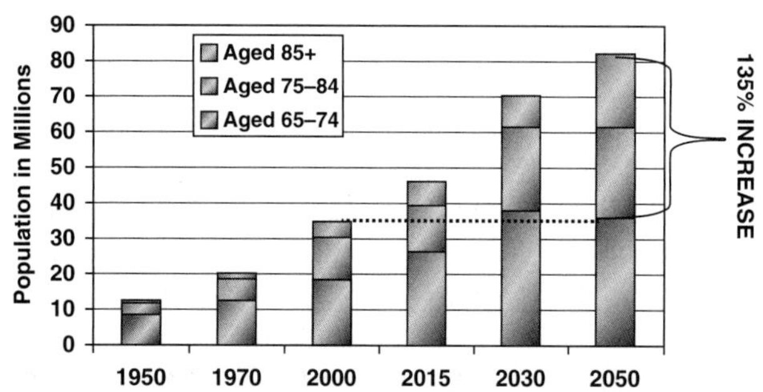

FIG. 2.4 Growth of populations over age 65 and over age 85. *(From https://www.ncbi.nlm.nih.gov/pmc/articles/PMC1464018/; Knickman JR, Snell EK. The 2030 problem: caring for aging baby boomers. Health Serv Res. 2002;37(4):849-884.)*

Life Expectancy

A child born in 2016 could expect to live 78.6 years, more than 30 years longer than a child born in 1900 (47.3 years). In the first half of the 20th century, mortality declined primarily as a result of advances in health at birth and younger ages, especially infant mortality. However, by 2000, the changes in life expectancy were primarily the result of reduced mortality at older ages, not the least of which was the dramatic increase in the number of adults who lived to age 80 years and beyond. In 1900, a person who lived until age 65 years might expect another 12 years of life. In 2016, additional life expectancy had grown to 19.4 years: 20.6 years for women and 18 years for men.[7] Female life expectancy continues to outpace male life expectancy, despite gains made for both sexes, although the gap has begun to decrease. There is some concern that because of a variety of factors (e.g., past smoking, current obesity levels, socioeconomic inequalities, and environmental issues), especially for women age 50 and over, life expectancy may begin to decrease rather than increase as evidenced in the decrease of life expectancy from birth, from 78.7 years in 2016 to 78.6 years in 2017, as illustrated in Fig. 2.5.[8,9]

Racial differences in life expectancy have been demonstrated. White women generally live the longest, whereas black women and white men live about the same as each other and black men have the lowest survivorship.[10] Table 2.1 illustrates the projections in life expectancy for the years 2012 and 2050 by sex, race, and Hispanic origin at birth, if one survives to age 65 and to age 85.[10]

Growth of Race and Ethnicity Populations

The United States' older population is becoming increasingly more racially and ethnically diverse as the overall minority population grows and experiences increased longevity and the shrinking of the non-Hispanic white-alone population.[11] Between 2016 and 2030, the white (non-Hispanic) population age 65 and over is projected to only increase by 39%, compared to 89% for older racial and ethnic minority populations.[7] Racial and ethnic minority populations have increased from 6.9 million in 2006 (19% of the older adult population) to 11.1 million in 2016 (23% of older adults) and are projected to increase to 21.1 million in 2030 (28% of older adults). Fig. 2.6 provides a breakdown of this growth by racial and ethnic group.[12]

One of the significant challenges facing the geriatric physical therapist will be the increasing diversity among older adults. From 2015 to 2060, the number of black

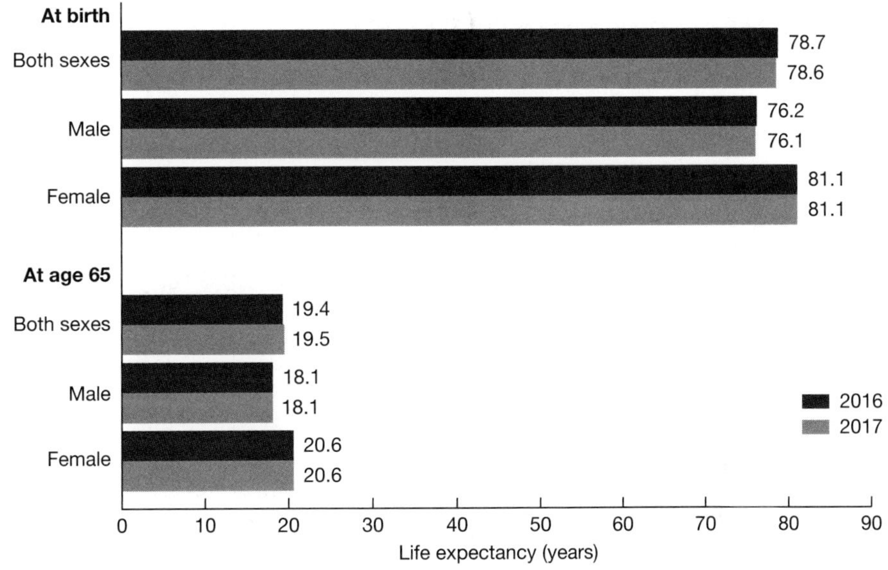

FIG. 2.5 Life expectancy for years 2016 and 2017. *(From https://www.cdc.gov/nchs/products/databriefs/db328.htm.)*

TABLE 2.1 Projections of Life Expectancy by Sex, Race, and Hispanic Origin at Ages 0, 65, and 85 Years

		Age 0		Age 65		Age 85	
		2012	2050	2012	2050	2012	2050
Race and Hispanic Origin	**Sex**			**Added Years**		**Added Years**	
Non-Hispanic white and Asian or Pacific Islander	M	77.1	82.2	18.1	20.6	6.0	7.0
	F	81.7	86.2	20.7	23.5	7.1	8.5
Non-Hispanic black and American Indian or Alaska Native	M	71.7	79.0	16.3	19.2	6.3	7.0
	F	78.0	83.5	19.5	22.3	7.4	8.4
Hispanic (of any race)	M	78.9	82.2	19.5	20.6	7.1	7.0
	F	83.7	86.2	22.1	23.5	8.0	8.5

Source: U.S. Census Bureau 2012 National Projections.

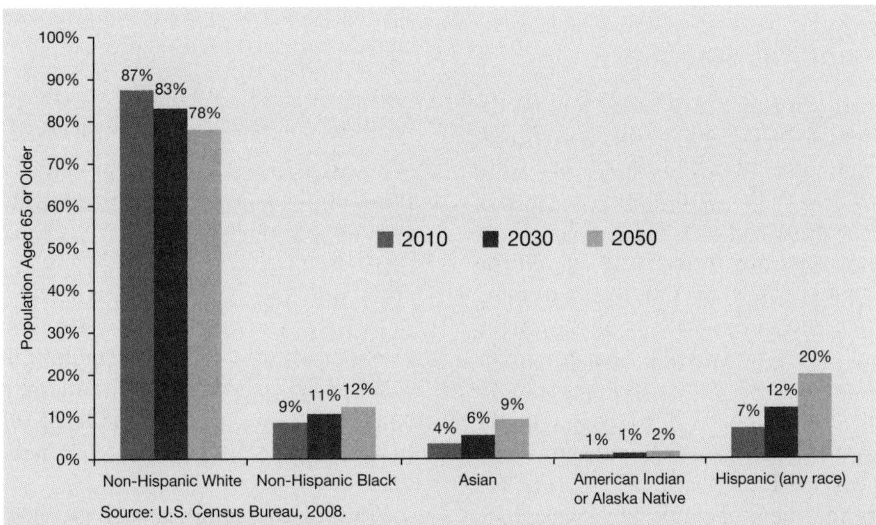

FIG. 2.6 U.S. population aged 65 years or older and diversity 2010–50. *(From Centers for Disease Control and Prevention. State of Aging and Health in America 2013. https://www.cdc.gov/aging/agingdata/data-portal/state-aging-health.html. Accessed February 9, 2019.)*

older adults in the United States will nearly triple and the number of Hispanic older adults will more than quintuple, whereas the number of whites will less than double. This increase is the result of both higher birth rates and immigration. Hispanics and Asians are changing the balance between majority and minority, just as Southern and Eastern European immigrants did a century ago when their numbers overtook those for immigrants from Northern and Western Europe. Immigration is driven largely by young people from Asia and Latin America drawn by economic opportunities, who themselves will become older someday.

While most foreign-born elders have been in the United States many years, the numbers of older newcomers, especially from Asia and Latin America, are increasing. Older immigrant arrivals are typically the parents of children who are US citizens; often, these children sponsor their parents' immigration so they can help with childcare and housework.[13] Newcomers differ from the elders who arrived earlier. They are less familiar with American customs and less fluent in English. On average, they are more socioeconomically disadvantaged than U.S.-born older adults or long-term immigrants. Without jobs, pensions, or government benefits, they often look to offspring for support.[13] Clearly, the geriatric physical therapist must be prepared to communicate in languages other than English and practice cultural humility,* especially in increasingly diverse areas. For example, approximately 60% of the residents of the District of Columbia are black and 60% of the residents of Hawaii are Asian/Pacific Islander. In New Mexico, California, and Texas—the states with the highest proportion of Hispanics—more than 30% of people age 65-plus are not white.[14] About one-third of older adults in California (35%), New Mexico (35%), and Hawaii (30%) spoke a language other than English at home in 2014. About one-fourth in Texas (26%) and New York (25%) were non–English speaking at home.[14]

Sex Distribution and Marital Status

The ratio of men to women changes over the human life span. For every 100 female births, 105 male births occur. As time passes, the number of males continues to exceed females until the third decade (ages 20 to 29). Because of life events such as war and accidents, from that age on, women increasingly outnumber men. For every 100 females in the 65 to 74 age group, we find only 86 males. Their number continues to drop to 72 for 100 females in the 75 to 84 age group. For the 85 and older age group, the sex ratio becomes even more pronounced, expanding to an astounding 49 men for every 100 women. Clearly, the oldest-old segment is dominated by women.

In 2017, a larger percentage of older men were married as compared with older women—70% of men, 46% of women. Widows accounted for 33% of all older women in 2017. There were more than three times as many widows (8.9 million) as widowers (2.5 million).[7] Divorce and separated rates have increased since 1980 when approximately 5.3% of the older population were divorced or separated/spouse absent compared with 15% in 2017.[7]

It has been long thought, based on one study, that married people (especially men) have a lower mortality at all ages than their unmarried peers.[15] However, closer scrutiny reveals that the study made an assumption that divorced or widowed individuals never were married, an obvious misrepresentation.[16] What is known is that two groups of people live the longest: those who got married and stayed married, and those who stayed single. This is true for both men and women. What seems to matter to longevity is consistency, not marriage.[16,17] However, women may do better than men when living alone, whereas men do relatively better when they live with other people, typically a wife.[17] This may be because of a greater freedom to pursue one's own interests if single and female and the positive effect of socialization. Men are less satisfied with the number of friends they have, whereas women are always more satisfied with the number of friends they have, regardless of living situation.[17] However, the male boomers are generally a more independent group, and thus, this trend may change.

In addition to the caregiving burdens and socioeconomic implications of being partnered, loss of a significant other brings its own set of psychosocial challenges to the individual in contemporary society. Any individual whose identity is linked to being a couple or part of a long-term relationship may experience a severe disruption of social roles when left alone. This disruption complicates the search for self-validation through the recognition, esteem, and affection of another who may have been present in a marital or partnered relationship.

Living Arrangements and Environments

As depicted in Fig. 2.7 illustrating 2017 data, 59% of community-dwelling older persons lived with their spouse or partner. The vast majority were men (72%), compared with 48% of older women. This proportion decreased with age, especially for women. Of women 75 years of age and older, 66% lived alone.[7]

Living arrangements differed by race and Hispanic origin for older adults. For example, older black and non-Hispanic white adults were most likely to live alone compared with Asian and Hispanic older adults (Fig. 2.8).[6] Additionally, older women of black and non-Hispanic white groups were almost twice as likely to live alone (43% black and 37% non-Hispanic white) as were Asian and Hispanic older women (20% Asian

*The reader is referred to the chapters on psychosocial principles and patient education within this text for discussions of cultural humility (see Chapters 4 and 11).

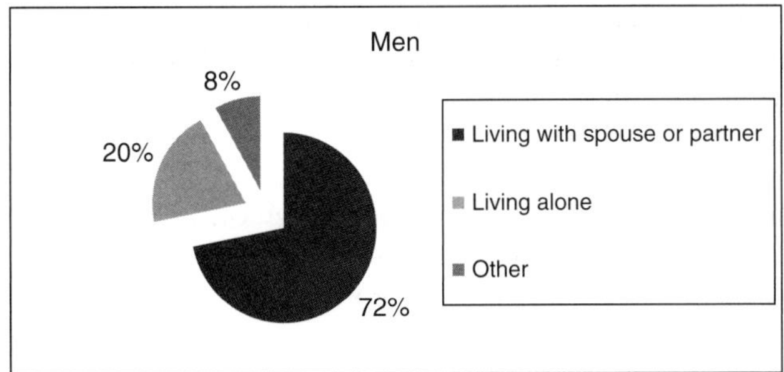

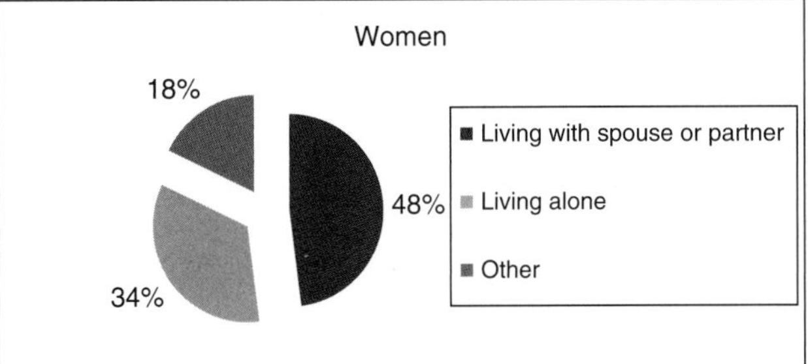

FIG. 2.7 Living arrangements by sex of persons 65 and older. *(Source: U.S. Census Bureau, Current Population Survey, Annual Social and Economic Supplement/U.S. Census Bureau, American Community Survey; Current Population Survey, Annual Social and Economic Supplement 1967 to present; Table AD3. Living arrangements of adults 65 to 74 years old, 1967 to present; Table AD3. Living arrangements of adults 75 and over, 1967 to present.)*

and 23% Hispanic). About 30% of older black men lived alone compared with 20% of non-Hispanic white men and just 10% of older Asian men.[6]

The Pew Research Center found that multigenerational family households were increasing, driven in part by the job losses and home foreclosures of recent years but also because of social factors including delayed marriage of children and the wave of immigration that has occurred since 1980.[18] Since 1990, the share of those aged 65 years and older who live in multigenerational family households has grown to 20%, compared with 17% in 1990.[18] Racial minorities and Hispanics were far more likely to live in multigenerational homes than non-Hispanic white older adults.[19] Of those older adults who live with children, 58% were the household head.

A majority of housing occupied by older adults (88%) in 2011–15 consisted of either detached single-family houses (68%) or apartments/condos (19%). Attached one-family houses (6%), mobile homes or trailers (6%), or boats, recreational vehicles, vans, and so forth (0.1%) made up the balance of older adult-occupied units.[19] Of the housing units occupied by older adults, 44% were built in 1969 or earlier, which has implications for the ability to age in place. Renovations and repairs are likely to be needed in older housing to make the housing safe and accessible. Twenty-four percent rented their housing. Approximately 44% of older householders spent more than one-third of their income on housing costs—36% for owners and 78% for renters.[7]

The vast majority of individuals aged 65 years and over (93%) live in traditional community settings as described previously but may receive help through informal care by family and friends, in-home support (e.g., meals), personal care assistants, adult day care, and senior

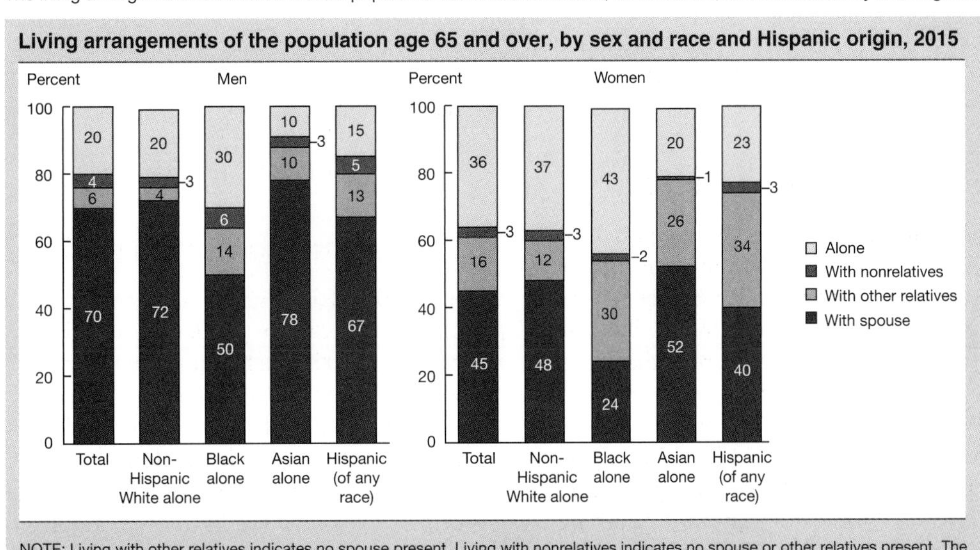

FIG. 2.8 Living arrangements by sex, race, and Hispanic origin. *(Source: U.S. Census Bureau, Current Population Survey, Annual Social and Economic Supplement.)*

living residences. Residential housing with services such as meals, medication assistance, household cleaning, and transportation provides an option for those who choose or cannot live independently. Approximately 3% live in residential housing with services such as assisted living.[6] Another 3.1% live in a long-term care setting (1.5 million), which has decreased since the year 2000 (5%). The percentage who reside in long-term care settings dramatically increases with age as shown in Fig. 2.9. Of those who reside in long-term care, only 1% are persons aged 65 to 74 years; 4% are persons aged 75 to 84 years and 15% are persons aged 85 years and above.[7] In addition, people with dementia and women were more likely to move into long-term care facilities during the last months of life.[20] The vast majority of long-term care residents are non-Hispanic white (76%, compared with 14% non-Hispanic black and 5.2% Hispanic).[21] Obviously physical therapists working in a short-term or long-term rehabilitation setting will be treating patients who are considered "old-old" and may be near the end of their life, a point of consideration and awareness.

The increasing number of older adults combined with the value of independency has pushed the industry to develop other residential options that provide non-health-related services. Of those aged 85 years and older, 15% live in community housing with non-health-related services.[6] In 2014, approximately 180,000 older adults received care in adult day service centers and 780,000 individuals aged 65 years and over lived in residential care communities such as assisted living centers.[6] However, 59% of the cost of residential options is covered by the public sector, with out-of-pocket expenses accounting for the other 41%.[22] As the pool of individuals aged 85 and over swells in 2030 and beyond, economists warn of the crisis that is looming in providing long-term care for all who may need it. Again, an opportunity for physical therapists is to create the expectation that older adults can age successfully and remain independent to age in place (as most older adults desire), and to assist them to do this. Projections from work done in the late 1990s suggest that reducing the rate of disability of 1.5% a year over the coming decades would maintain the current level of economic burden of long-term care.[23] In fact, there is some data that suggests that disability rates are declining at a 2.2% per annum rate (1999–2004), driven by improving health. However, concerns exist about whether these recent trends will be sustained owing to the obesity prevalence.[24]

Economic Status

The tendency to regard older adults as a homogeneous group biases any understanding of their economic status. The heterogeneity of this population group is perhaps best illustrated by considering who is financially well-off and who is economically disadvantaged among older adults. Overall, the entrance of the youngest stratum of older adults, who benefit from private and workers' pension programs, has improved the economic well-being of older adults as a whole, as the proportion of older adults living

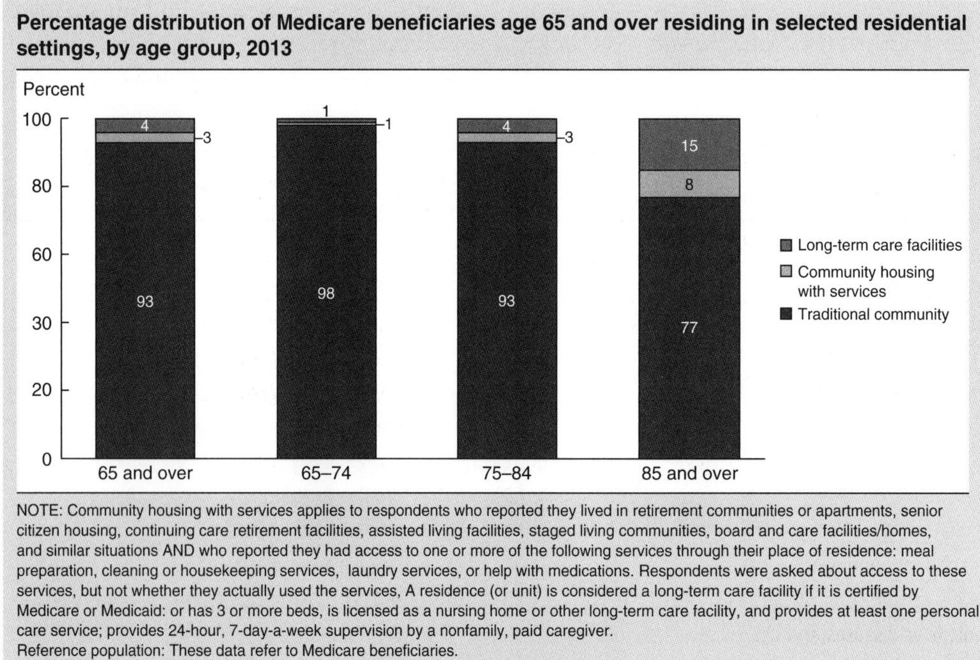

Percentage distribution of Medicare beneficiaries age 65 and over residing in selected residential settings, by age group, 2013
Percent
100
80
60
30
20
0
4
3
93
1
1
98
4
3
93
15
8
77
65 and over
65–74
75–84
85 and over
Long-term care facilities
Community housing with services
Traditional community
NOTE: Community housing with services applies to respondents who reported they lived in retirement communities or apartments, senior citizen housing, continuing care retirement facilities, assisted living facilities, staged living communities, board and care facilities/homes, and similar situations AND who reported they had access to one or more of the following services through their place of residence: meal preparation, cleaning or housekeeping services, laundry services, or help with medications. Respondents were asked about access to these services, but not whether they actually used the services, A residence (or unit) is considered a long-term care facility if it is certified by Medicare or Medicaid: or has 3 or more beds, is licensed as a nursing home or other long-term care facility, and provides at least one personal care service; provides 24-hour, 7-day-a-week supervision by a nonfamily, paid caregiver.
Reference population: These data refer to Medicare beneficiaries.
SOURCE: Centers for Medicare & Medicaid Services, Medicare Current Beneficiary Survey, Access to Care.

FIG. 2.9 Percentage distribution of Medicare beneficiaries aged 65 and over residing in selected residential settings, by age group, 2013. *(Source: Centers for Medicare & Medicaid Services, Medicare Current Beneficiary Survey, Access to Care. U.S. Department of Health and Human Services. Key Indicators of Well-Being | ACL Administration for Community Living. https://acl.gov/aging-and-disability-in-america/data-and-research/key-indicators-well-being. Published 2018. Accessed February 6, 2019.)*

in poverty has shrunk from 35% in 1959 to 9.3% in 2016.[7] Poverty increases after age 75 years, however, with women more often in poverty than men, and older Hispanics and older blacks experiencing greater economic deprivation than non-Hispanic whites.[7] Furthermore, although older adults may be less likely to enter into poverty than individuals younger than age 18 years, people age 65 years and older who do enter poverty are less likely to transition out than their younger counterparts.

Social security benefits accounted for 33% of the aggregate income of the older population and accounted for 90% or more of total income received by 33% of beneficiaries.[7] The four highest-budget items accounting for nearly 80% of an older adult's expenditures were for housing (33%), transportation (17%), food (12.6%), and health care expenditures, which increased with age from 12.2% for those aged 65 to 74 to 15.6% for those aged 75 years and older.[25] Health costs incurred on average by older consumers in 2016 consisted of $4159 (69%) for insurance, $913 (15%) for medical services, $715 (12%) for drugs, and $207 (3%) for medical supplies.[7]

MORTALITY

Causes of Death

As displayed in Table 2.2, heart disease and cancer are the leading causes of death for females and males over 65 years of all races and ethnicities, accounting for nearly half of all deaths in 2016.[26,27] Despite the position of heart disease as the leading cause of death since before 1980 and stroke as one of the top four causes of death, age-adjusted death rates in the United States from heart disease and stroke have declined in the past 35 years, most likely because of improvements in the detection and treatment of hypertension as well as improvements in emergency and critical care. However, death rates for both diabetes and respiratory diseases increased dramatically in the same period as shown in Table 2.2. Given the role of physical activity, exercise, and behavior change in primary and secondary prevention as well as rehabilitation of all of these conditions, physical therapists are able to make a major contribution to the well-being of the geriatric population.

MORBIDITY

Chronic Conditions

Chronic diseases are broadly defined as conditions that last 1 year or more and require ongoing medical attention or limit activities of daily living or both. Chronic disease health care management is responsible for over 90% of the $3.3 trillion annual health care costs in the United States (all ages) and account for most of the deaths in the United States.[28] Approximately 60% of adults (individuals 18 years and older) have at least one chronic disease/condition and 12% had five or more as illustrated in Fig. 2.10.[29] The risk of having a chronic condition increases with age. For example, based on 2012 data from community-dwelling Medicare beneficiaries, 63% of individuals aged 65 to 74 years had multiple chronic conditions, which increased to 78% for those aged 76 to 84 years and to 83% for those aged 85 years or older.[30] Specifically, Alzheimer disease (the fifth-leading cause of death for older people) and infectious diseases such as flu and pneumonia affect older adults at higher rates.[30] Individually, as the number of chronic conditions

TABLE 2.2 Leading Causes of Death and Numbers of Deaths for Those Aged 65 Years and Older, 1980 and 2016

	1980		2016	
Rank	Cause of Death	Deaths	Cause of Death	Deaths
1	Diseases of heart	595,406	Diseases of heart	507,118
2	Malignant neoplasms	258,389	Malignant neoplasms	422,927
3	Cerebrovascular diseases	146,417	Chronic lower respiratory diseases	131,002
4	Pneumonia and influenza	45,512	Cerebrovascular diseases	121,630
5	Chronic obstructive pulmonary diseases	43,578	Alzheimer disease	114,883
6	Atherosclerosis	28,081	Diabetes mellitus	56,452
7	Diabetes mellitus	24,844	Unintentional injuries	42,479
8	Unintentional injuries	24,844	Influenza and pneumonia	53,141
9	Nephritis, nephrotic syndrome, and nephrosis	12,968	Nephritis, nephrotic syndrome, and nephrosis	41,095
10	Chronic liver diseases and cirrhosis	9519	Septicemia	30,405
	Total	1,341,848	Total	2,003,458

Source: National Vital Statistics System. Vital Statistics for the United States, 1980. Volume II – Mortality, Part A. 1985; Public-Use 2016 Mortality File. Xu JQ, Murphy SL, Kochanek KD, Bastian B, Arias E. Deaths: final data for 2016. National Vital Statistics Reports. Hyattsville, MD: National Center for Health Statistics; 2018, vol. 67. Available from https://www.cdc.gov/nchs/products/nvsr.htm. See Appendix I, National Vital Statistics (NVSS).

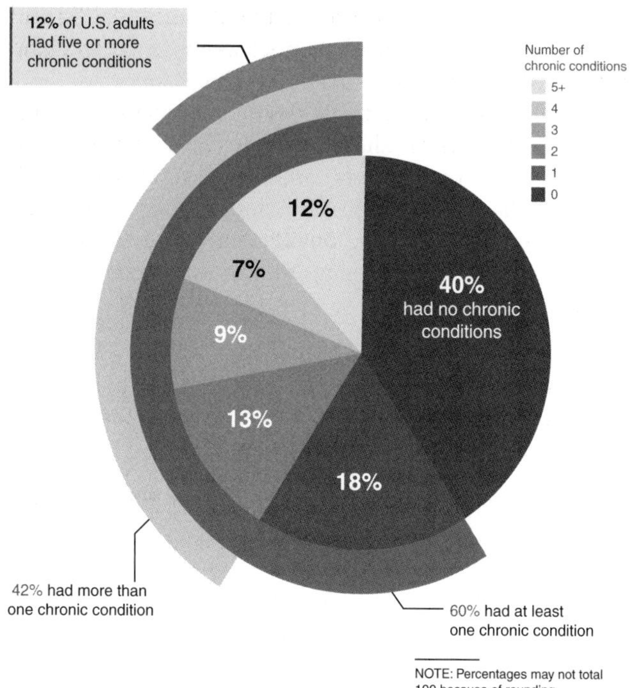

FIG. 2.10 Prevalence of chronic conditions. *(From Buttorff C, Ruder T, Bauman M. Multiple Chronic Conditions in the United States. Santa Monica, CA: Rand Corporation; 2017. https://www.rand.org/content/dam/rand/pubs/tools/TL200/TL221/RAND_TL221.pdf. To get permission: www.rand.org/pubs/permission.)*

TABLE 2.3 10 Most Common Chronic Diseases and Behaviors for Adults Aged 65 Years and Older

Disease	Percentage of Older Adults	Behaviors Causing Most Chronic Diseases*
Hypertension	58%	Tobacco use and exposure to second-hand smoke
Hyperlipidemia	47%	Poor nutrition, including diets low in fruits and vegetables and high in sodium and saturated fats
Arthritis	31%	Lack of physical activity
Ischemic heart disease	29%	Excessive alcohol use
Diabetes mellitus	27%	
Chronic kidney disease	18%	
Heart failure	14%	
Depression	14%	
Alzheimer disease and dementia	11%	
Chronic obstructive pulmonary disease	11%	

*From https://www.cdc.gov/chronicdisease/about/index.htm.
Adapted from https://www.ncoa.org/blog/10-common-chronic-diseases-prevention-tips/.

increases, the risk for dying prematurely, being hospitalized, and even receiving conflicting advice from health care providers increases. The most common chronic conditions for adults over age 65 years and the risk behaviors causing most chronic diseases are listed in Table 2.3.[31,32]

Besides being the cause of most deaths for older adults, chronic diseases/conditions often affect quality of life and ability to perform important and essential activities, both inside and outside the home. The physical limitations that so often accompany chronic conditions such as arthritis and stroke are of particular concern to physical therapy professionals. Loss of the ability to care for oneself can mean a loss of independence and lead to the need for a more restrictive environment such as residential care. The inability to perform daily activities can adversely affect an individual's engagement in life and enjoyment of family and friends. Social isolation and depression can result.

Much of the illness, disability, and premature death from these conditions can be prevented with healthier behaviors, more supportive environments, and better access to preventive health services. Efforts to prevent chronic disease and its sequalae will be a major focus of health care professionals and others in the years to come, offering physical therapists an opportunity to better the health of Americans for decades. However, much needs to be done to promote healthy lifestyles. The low rates of older adults engaging in even minimal physical activity, discussed next, is an area physical therapists must address.

Social Participation

The World Health Organization's *International Classification of Functioning, Disability and Health* (ICF) (Fig. 2.11) defines participation as involvement in a life situation at the societal level.[33] Participation includes activities and tasks within the social role. In this section, social participation will be discussed in terms of physical activity, work, and recreation.

Work. More older Americans are working, and working more, than ever before. The rate of labor force

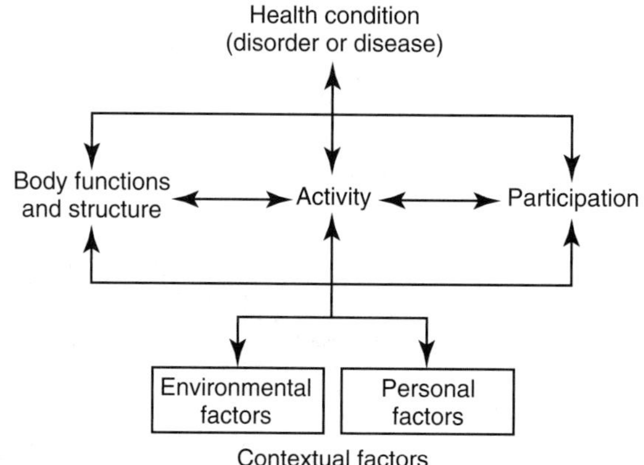

FIG. 2.11 The World Health Organization's International *Classification of Functioning, Disability and Health.*

participation for older Americans, as presented in Fig. 2.12, has grown steadily since 2002 and is projected to continue to grow[34] from the smallest segment of any age group to more than the labor force of the 16- to 24-year age group. Older workers now represent over 20% of the labor force. These numbers are increasing the most rapidly for older women as shown in Fig. 2.13.[7,35] Although the number of older workers working fewer than 35 hours per week has decreased since 2000, they still make up 40% of the part-time labor force, the highest percentage of any age group.[35] Older Asians (20.2%) and whites (19%) are somewhat more likely to be working after age 65 than older blacks (16.7%).[36]

People are working later in life for a number of reasons. They are healthier and have a longer life expectancy than previous generations. They are better educated, which increases their likelihood of staying in the labor force. Changes in federal regulations have raised the minimum age at which individuals may receive full Social Security benefits, and mandatory retirement at a specific age for

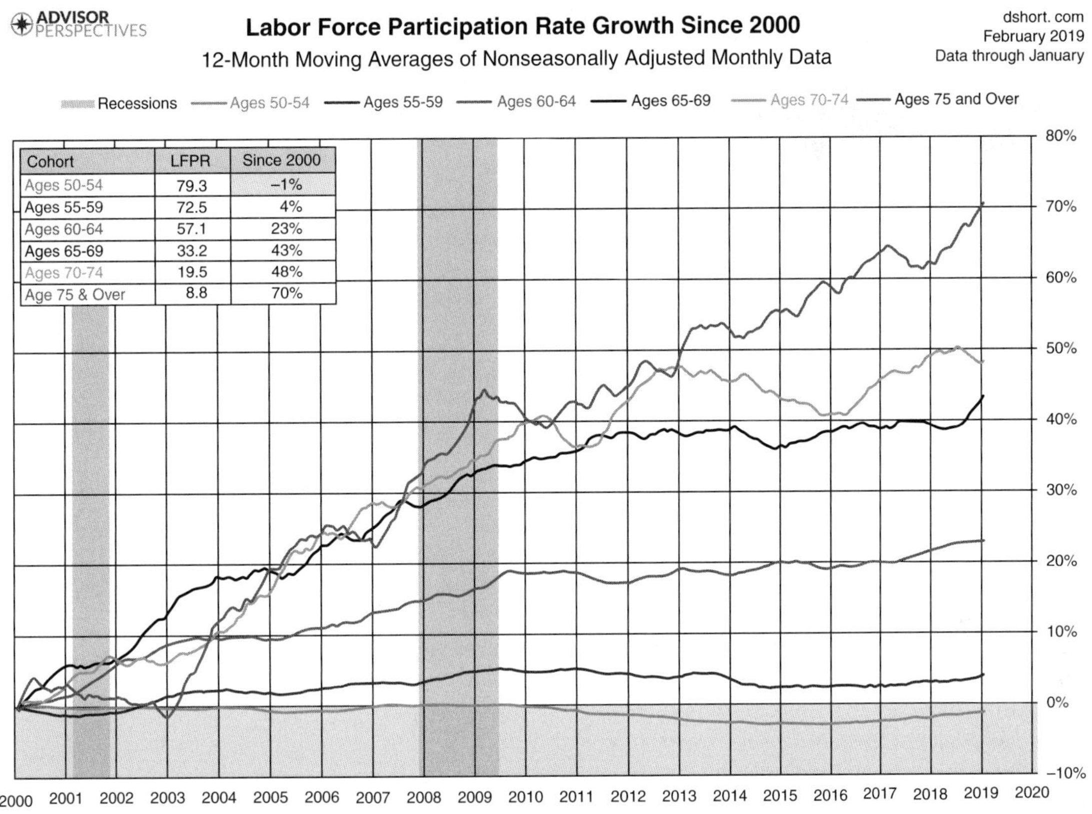

FIG. 2.12 Labor force participation rate (LFPR) growth since 2000, ages 50 to over 75 years. *(From https://www.advisorperspectives.com/dshort/updates/2019/02/05/demographic-trends-for-the-50-and-older-work-force.)*

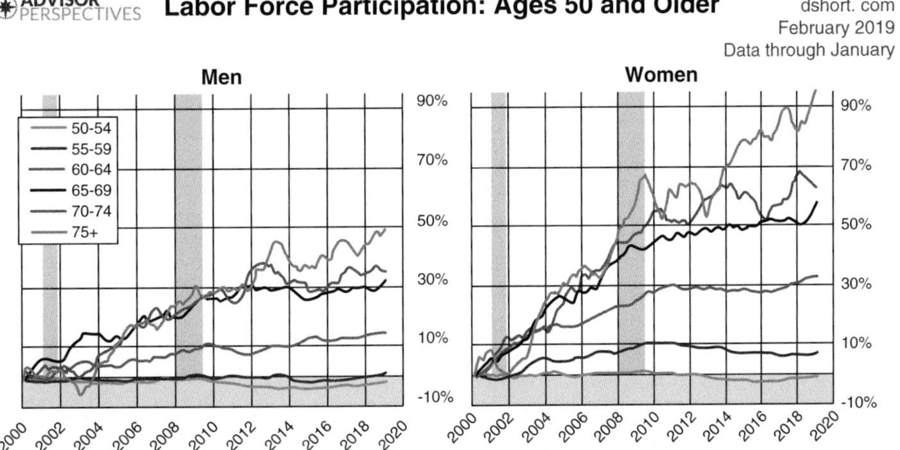

FIG. 2.13 Labor Force Growth Rates: Age 50 and Older. *(https://www.advisorperspectives.com/dshort/updates/2019/08/06/demographic-trends-for-the-50-and-older-work-force?utm_source=dshort_feed&utm_medium=rss&utm_campaign=item_link.)*

most occupations is not typically permitted. Therefore, older adults who want to, or need to, remain in the workforce may do so if they are physically able to perform the tasks of their employment. And it appears the Baby Boomer generation is working at older ages than previous generations, especially women. Fig. 2.13 illustrates that the rate of women in the labor force has risen about 96% since the turn of the century compared to men at 49%.[34]

The most frequently seen job type for older adults is management, professional, and community service–related jobs and least likely are computer and mathematical, food preparation, and construction-related occupations.[36] Interestingly, as depicted in Fig. 2.14, older adults have much higher rates of self-employment than younger workers.[35] Perhaps years of experience and knowledge of the industry better position older adults to be self-employed.

Volunteerism. Estimates to the extent to which older adults participate in volunteer activities vary, but it is generally accepted that approximately one-quarter of individuals over age 50 participate in some sort of volunteer activity; this figure is likely to increase as an anecdote to retirement. Volunteerism seems to be for the young-old, as the rate of volunteerism begins to drop after age 70. Individuals are likely to continue to volunteer as they age if the activity is professional or managerial, with a 74.8% retention. Women are somewhat more likely than men to say they expect to do volunteer work when they are older (83% women vs. 77% of men).[37] Individuals older than age 65 were slightly more likely to volunteer with secular groups compared with those aged 50 to 64 years, who were slightly more likely to volunteer with religious groups.[37]

Volunteerism affords many benefits to older adults and to society that physical therapists should be aware of. Volunteers tend to be more physically active, have a higher sense of self-esteem and personal control, experience increased socialization, and be more likely to practice good health behaviors.[38] Volunteerism can reduce the likelihood of frailty and falls and enhance physical activity.[39] Volunteerism is known to improve psychological well-being and therefore may reduce depressive symptoms and cognitive decline[40] and is even linked to living longer. Society benefits as well, although this has not been studied extensively. For example, improved academic performance was seen in an older adult volunteer program focused on K-6 schools.[41] In anticipation of the retirement wave of aging boomers, volunteerism may be a solution to unmet needs that are not filled by younger workers. Ideally, as the benefits of volunteerism become more apparent, further opportunities for those who are not as physically able will become a focus so that all older adults, no matter their physical abilities, can derive the benefits that come from volunteering and continued engagement.

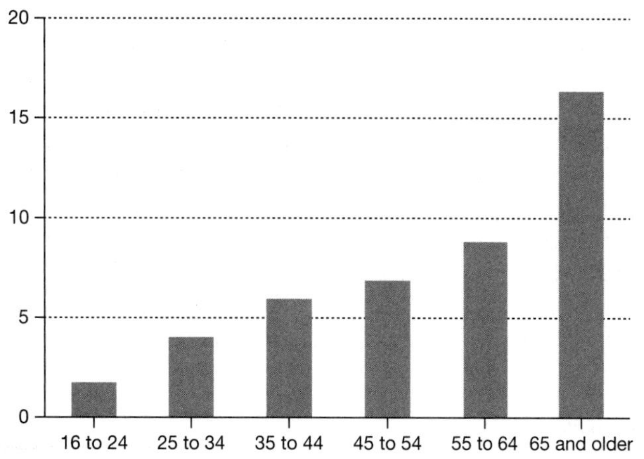

FIG. 2.14 Self-employment rates. *(Source: U.S. Bureau of Labor Statistics. https://www.bls.gov/careeroutlook/2017/article/older-workers.htm.)*

Caregiving. A significant role of older individuals is that of caregiving, whether caregiving for a spouse, a friend, or grandchildren. Although most informal caregivers were middle-aged, older spouses provided 31% of the total hours of informal care in 2011.[6] About two-thirds of older adults needing care receive *only* informal care provided by family or friends.[6,18] Grandparenting is another significant role for older individuals. Eighty percent of those age 65 and older have grandchildren. In 2016, approximately 1 million grandparents age 60 and over were responsible for the basic needs of one or more grandchildren under age 18 living with them. Of these caregivers, 58% were grandmothers and 42% were grandfathers[7] and they were more likely to be black and Hispanic than white. More older adults caring for grandchildren has occurred since 2007, when the economy took a significant downturn. But the sharpest increase since the recession has been among whites at a 9% increase, compared to an increase of just 2% among black grandparents and no change among Hispanic grandparents.[42] Older adults with children who have intellectual and developmental disabilities find themselves caring for them when they become adults. Twenty-four percent of these had caregivers aged 60 and over.[7] A take-home from these demographics is the importance of family involvement and the need for appropriate education regarding caregiving. Chapter 12 in this text provides a deeper look at the ramifications of providing intensive care in one's later years.

Leisure Activities. In 2014, older Americans spent, on average, more than one-quarter of their time in leisure activities. The amount of time spent in leisure activities increased with age, so that Americans over age 75 reported spending 33% of their time in leisure activities.[6] Leisure activities are preferred and enjoyable activities one participates in during free time and characterized as representing freedom and providing intrinsic satisfaction.[43] Leisure activities may provide social support, increase social participation, and help one adapt to potential

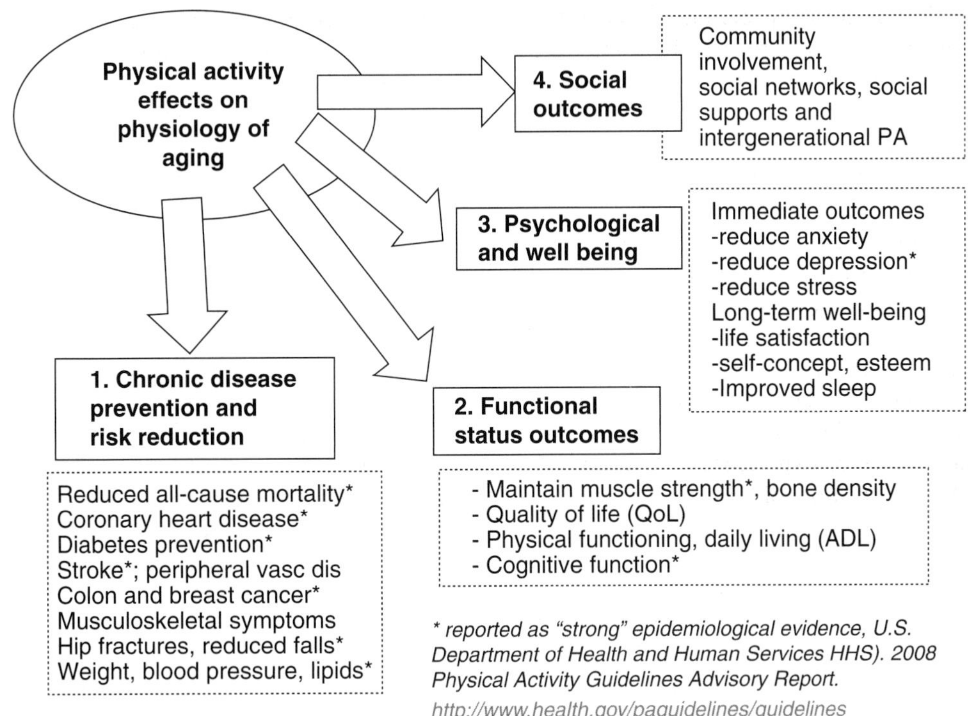

FIG. 2.15 A conceptual framework for the benefits of physical activity in older adults. *(From Updating the evidence for physical activity: summative reviews of the epidemiological evidence, prevalence, and interventions to promote "active aging." Gerontologist. 2016;56[Suppl 2]:S268-S280. https://doi.org/10.1093/geront/gnw031. Gerontologist | © The Author 2016. Published by Oxford University Press on behalf of the Gerontological Society of America. All rights reserved.)*

restrictions of chronic diseases and conditions, recover from stress, and overcome negative life events (e.g., losing a spouse).[43] Chang et al. found that leisure-time activities, particularly physical ones, had a positive effect on physical and psychosocial functioning.[43] However, most older adults engage in passive leisure-time activities. When asked how they engaged in specific leisure activities in the past 24 hours, 90% reported talking with family or friends, 83% reading, and 77% watching an hour or more of television.[44] Watching television made up over half (56%) of daily leisure time.[6] This is concerning, because sedentary habits, mobility disability, and cognitive deficits are linked to 4 to 5 or more hours of television viewing per day.[45–47]

Physical activities are no less important than work to maintain a sense of well-being. Clearly, more older men and women today are maintaining interests in recreational sports that they developed earlier in life. Others are discovering the pleasures of recreational sports as older adults as described in Chapter 28 on the senior athlete elsewhere in this text. Many adults enjoy dancing and gardening, which require a relatively high degree of balance, flexibility, and strength.[48] Even sedentary activities, such as stamp collecting or playing chess, require a certain degree of physical ability in the hand and upper extremity, and therefore may be functional measures of the outcomes of intervention for some older adults. Including participation in less passive leisure-time activities would be a worthy goal that physical therapists might encourage.

Physical Activity. Physical therapists are aware of the many benefits of engaging in physical activity listed in Fig. 2.15. Physical activity, comprising leisure-time aerobic and muscle-strengthening activities, is generally measured in terms of the 2008 federal physical activity guidelines of 150 minutes/week of moderately intense activity. Unfortunately, physical activity typically declines with age, and although the number of people reporting recommended levels has increased since 1998, Fig. 2.16 illustrates that only about 12% of people age 65 and over reported meeting this recommended amount.[6] Men are more likely to meet the guideline (15%) than women (9%). Non-Hispanic whites age 65 and over reported higher levels of physical activity than non-Hispanic black (9%) and Hispanic (7%) individuals.[6] When looking at aerobic and strengthening exercise separately, the picture improves. Thirty-seven percent of older adults reported participating in at least 150 minutes of aerobic exercise per week, and 17% reported engaging in muscle-strengthening activities at least twice per week.[6] Clearly these statistics have room for improvement with many benefits at the individual and societal level.

FUNCTION

Limitations in physical function and mobility have many consequences including reduced access to goods and services, which leads to poor health outcomes. For example, older adults with limited mobility are less

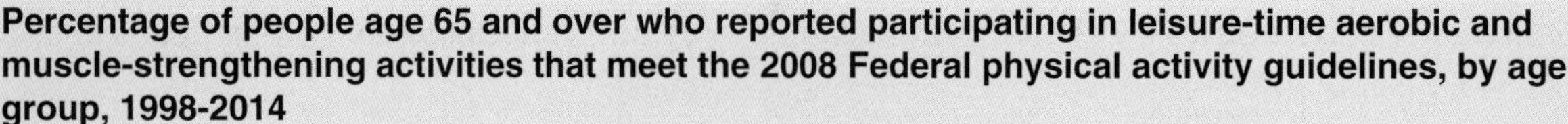
Percentage of people age 65 and over who reported participating in leisure-time aerobic and muscle-strengthening activities that meet the 2008 Federal physical activity guidelines, by age group, 1998-2014

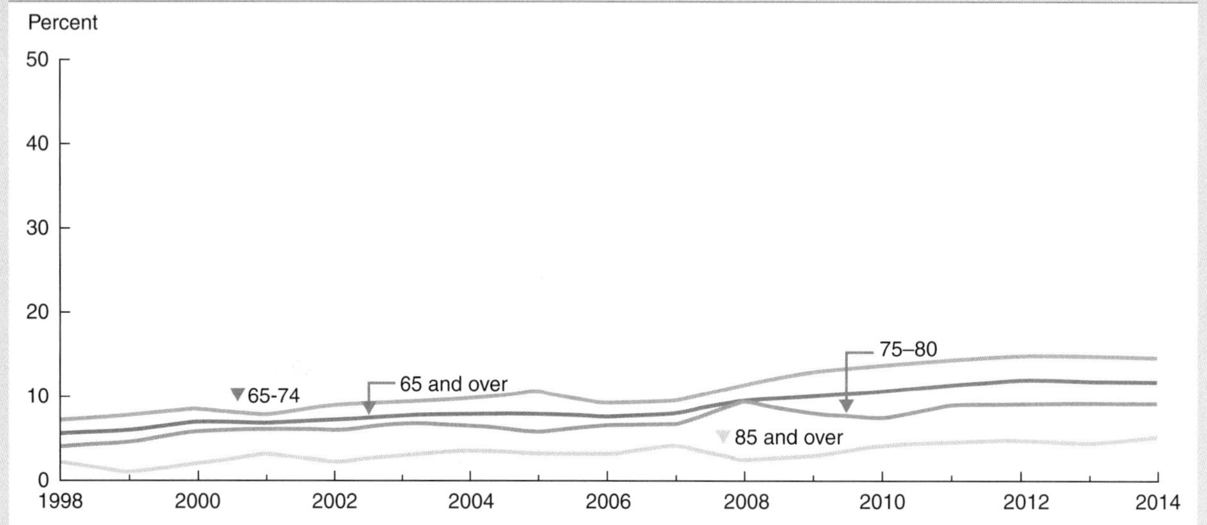

NOTE: This measure of physical activity reflects the 2008 federal physical activity guidelines for Americans (available from: http://www.health.gov/PAGuidelinesf/). The 2008 federal guidelines recommend that adults age 65 and over who are fit and have no limiting chronic conditions perform at least 150 minutes (2 hours and 30 minutes) a week of moderate-intensity, or 75 minutes (1 hour and 15 minutes) a week of vigorous-intensity aerobic physical activity or an equivalent combination of moderate- and vigorous-intensity aerobic activity. Aerobic activity should be performed in episodes of at least 10 minutes, and preferably, it should be spread throughout the week. In addition, they should perform muscle-strengthening activities that are moderate or high intensity and involve all major muscle groups on 2 or more days a week, because these activities provide additional health benefits. The measure shown here presents the percentage of people who fully met both the aerobic activity and muscle-strengthening guidelines, irrespective of their chronic condition status.
Reference population: These data refer to the civilian noninstitutionalized population.
SOURCE: Centers for Disease Control and Prevention, National Center for Health Statistics, National Health Interview Survey.

FIG. 2.16 Older Adults who meet the 2008 federal physical activity guideline by age group. *(From Edwards JJ, Khanna M, Jordan KP, et al. Older Americans 2016: key indicators of well-being.* Federal Interagency Forum on Aging-Related Statistics. *https://doi.org/10.1136/annrheumdis-2013-203913. Published 2016. Source: Centers for Disease Control and Prevention, National Center for Health Statistics, National Health Interview Survey.)*

able to access grocery stores and supermarkets, thus providing fewer nutritional options, which affects health outcomes.[49] Another consequence is the increased risk for injury and health problems related to sedentary activity. Consequences of injury and the sequelae of health problems can lead to residential and institutional living. Mobility disability, defined as difficulty walking one-quarter of a mile, climbing a flight of stairs, or standing for long periods of time, is associated with reduced socialization, depression, and frailty, which again has a cascade of undesired effects leading to a poor quality of life.[50] It is well established that the prevalence of functional limitations and disability is associated with aging.[51] To help mitigate these untoward effects, the physical therapist should recognize that much mobility disability and functional limitations can be addressed through lifestyle counseling and physical therapy services.

Physical Function and Disability

In general, independent physical function declines with age, and this decline is influenced by a host of biological, psychological, and social factors. Function is not a static phenomenon, and individual transitions in functional status are more the norm than the exception. Function is also a sociological phenomenon. Physical function activities can be subdivided into five areas: mobility, which includes transfers and ambulation; basic self-care and personal hygiene (activities of daily living [ADLs]); more complex activities essential to an adult's living in the community, known as instrumental ADLs (IADLs); work; and recreation.

Fig. 2.17 illustrates that, in 2014, 22% of community-dwelling people age 65 and older reported at least one disability as defined by limitations in vision, hearing, mobility, communication, cognition, and self-care. Of those, two-thirds had difficulty in walking or climbing stairs.[58] This same report documents that 42% of community-dwelling adults 85 years of age or older self-identified difficulty with mobility. Difficulty with independent living, such as visiting a doctor's office or shopping, was the second-most-cited disability, followed by serious difficulty in hearing, cognition, bathing or dressing, and vision.[52]

Lower education and economic levels adversely affected independence. For example, 13% of older adults with a disability lived in poverty, compared with 7% of those without a disability who lived in poverty.[52]

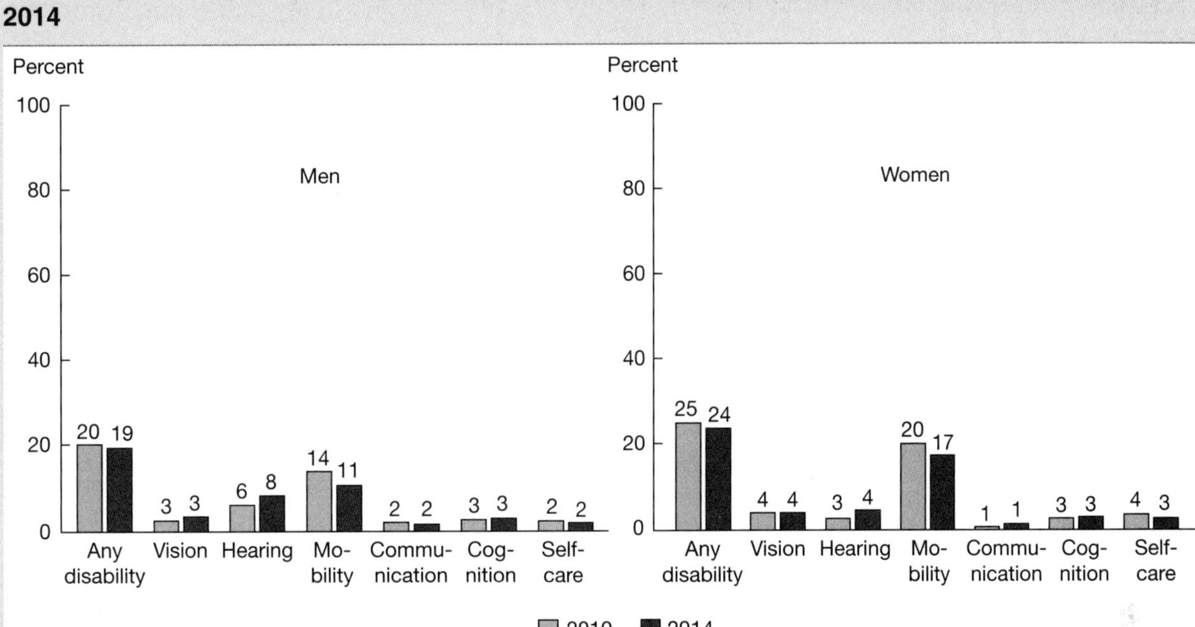
Percentage of people age 65 and over with a disability, by sex and functional domain, 2010 and 2014
Percent
100
80
60
40
20
0
Men
20 19
3 3
6 8
14 11
2 2
3 3
2 2
Any disability
Vision
Hearing
Mo-bility
Commu-nication
Cog-nition
Self-care
Women
25 24
4 4
3 4
20 17
1 1
3 3
4 3
2010
2014
NOTE: Disability is defined as "a lot" or "cannot do/unable to do" when asked about difficulty with seeing, even if wearing glasses (vision); hearing, even if wearing hearing aids (hearing); walking or climbing steps (mobility); communicating, for example, understanding or being understood by others (communication); remembering or concentrating (cognition); and self-care. such as washing all over or dressing (self-care). Any disability is defined as having difficulty with at least one of these activities. The data source and measures presented have changed from previous editions of Older Americans. Data labels in this chart are based on rounded values.
Reference population: These data refer to the civilian noninstitutionalized population.
SOURCE: Centers for Disease Control and Prevention, National Center for Health Statistics, National Health Interview Survey.

FIG. 2.17 Percentage of people age 65 and over with a disability, by sex and functional domain, 2010 and 2014. *(Source: Centers for Disease Control and Prevention, National Center for Health Statistics, National Health Interview Survey.)*

Likewise, women and those of racial and ethnic minority status were also more likely to report a disability.[52]

Activities of Daily Living

Basic Activities of Daily Living. Basic ADLs include all of the fundamental tasks and activities necessary for survival, hygiene, and self-care within the home. ADLs consist of eating, bathing, grooming, dressing, bed mobility, and transfers. As depicted in Fig. 2.18 and based on 2016 data, 20% of individuals 85 years of age and older required assistance with one or more ADLs, compared with 7% of those aged 75 to 84 and 3.4% of those aged 65 to 74. In 2013, about two-thirds of people who reported difficulty with one or more ADLs received personal assistance or used special equipment; 7% received personal assistance only, 35% used equipment only, and 25% used both.[6]

An inability to perform ADLs, especially toileting and bathing, often means a transition to some form of residential living as indicated by nearly 70% of older adults in residential care using assistance for ADLs.[53] The number of chronic conditions adversely affects the ability to perform ADLs as shown in Fig. 2.19, with ADL limitations increasing with the number of chronic conditions.

Instrumental Activities of Daily Living. Instrumental activities of daily living encompass eight areas of focus listed in Box 2.1. In 2013, 13.6% of those age 65 and over reported some limitation in IADLs. Increasing age adversely affected limitations, with 15.4% of those age 85 and over reporting limitations in IADLs compared with just 9.8% of those aged 65 to 74 years. The number of chronic conditions also adversely affects IADL limitations as shown in Fig. 2.20.

Relationship Between ADLs and IADLs. Most older adults living in the community are generally independent in both ADLs and IADLs. However, as the number of limitations grows, the risk for residential housing with services, including long-term care, grows. For example, as depicted in Fig. 2.21, 67% of those living in a long-term care facility had three or more limitations in ADLs, compared with only 17% living in other residential living facilities with services and 9% living in the community.[6] Limitations in IADLs frequently occur first, especially when cognitive issues are present. Poor self-rated health and depression were the strongest risk factors for needing assistance in one or more ADLs in a survey of a large sample of individuals aged 60 to 69 in Norway. Excessive sitting time, physical inactivity, and short or prolonged sleeping time were the most important lifestyle risk factors for ADL/IADL disability.[54] Again, the opportunity for physical therapists is clear.

Mobility. Those reporting no mobility limitation composed the majority of people over 65 years; however,

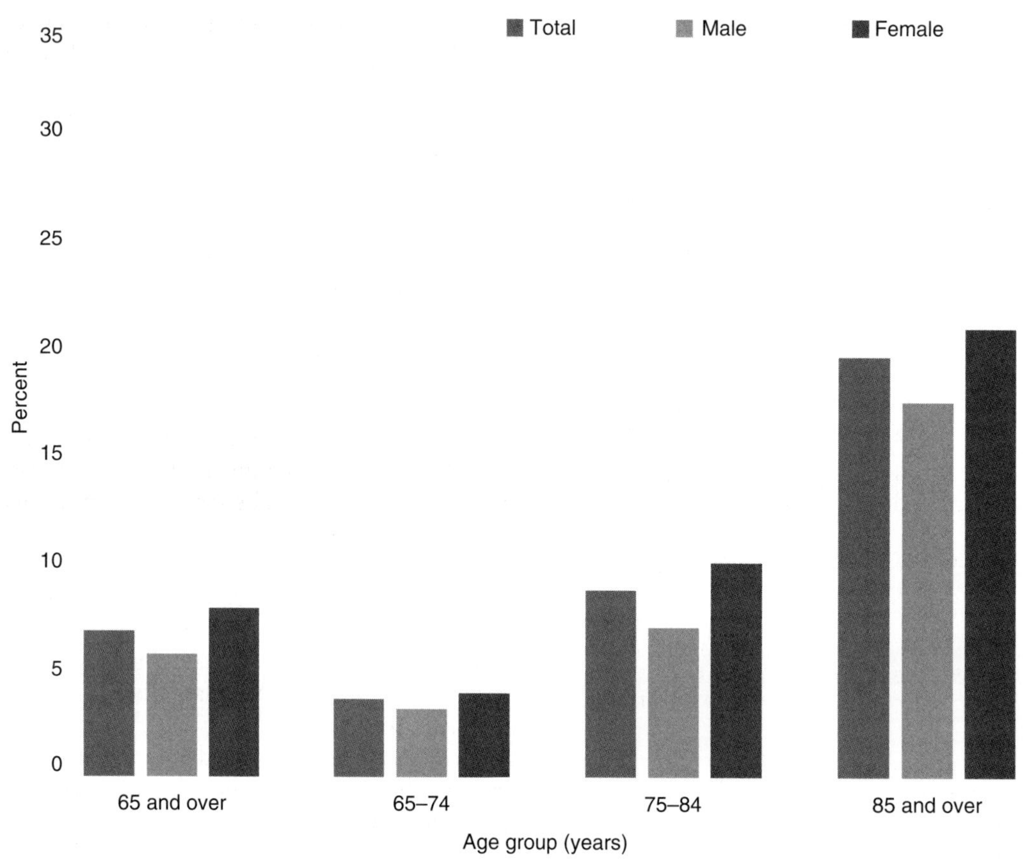

FIG. 2.18 Percentage of adults aged 65 and over who needed assistance with activities of daily living, January–June 2018. *(Source: National Center for Health Statistics, National Health Interview Survey, Family Care Component.)*

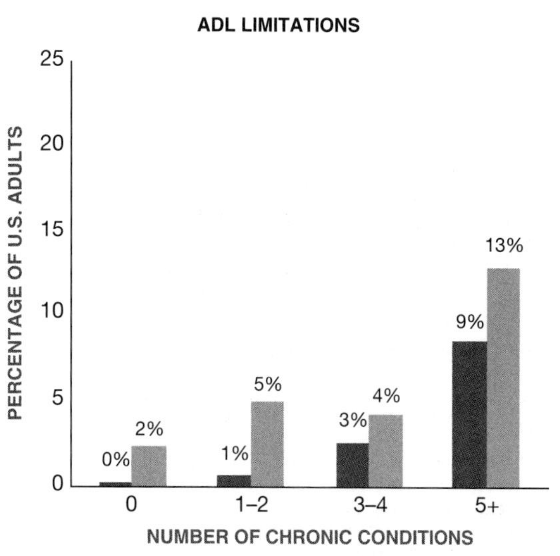

FIG. 2.19 Relationship of activities of daily living (ADL) limitations and number of chronic conditions. *(From Buttorff C, Ruder T, Bauman M. Multiple Chronic Conditions in the United States. Santa Monica, CA: Rand Corporation; 2017. https://www.rand.org/content/dam/rand/pubs/tools/TL200/TL221/RAND_TL221.pdf.)*

BOX 2.1 Instrumental Activities of Daily Living: Eight Focus Areas

Ability to use the telephone
Laundry and dressing
Shopping and running errands
Transportation
Meal preparation
Medication management
Housekeeping activities
Ability to manage finances

similar to those with ADL and IADL limitations, older age groups reported more difficulty with mobility. For example, only 26% of those aged 85 years and older reported no mobility limitations. And the majority of these older individuals also reported limitations in ADLs and IADLs (65.3% reported mobility, ADL, and IADL difficulties, compared with 25.5% of those aged 65 to 74).[55] Mobility limitations increased for residents of long-term care facilities, with a staggering 93.2% of 85-plus-year-olds reporting a combination

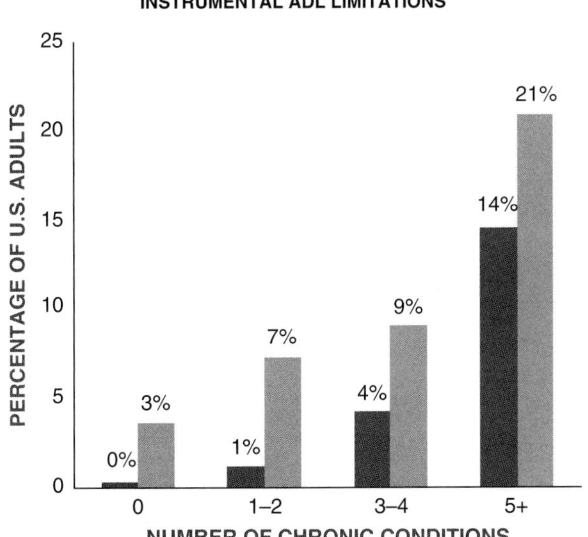

FIG. 2.20 Relationship of instrumental activities of daily living (ADL) limitations and number of chronic diseases. *(From Buttorff C, Ruder T, Bauman M. Multiple Chronic Conditions in the United States. Santa Monica, CA: Rand Corporation; 2017. https://www.rand.org/content/dam/rand/pubs/tools/TL200/TL221/RAND_TL221.pdf.)*

of mobility, ADL, and IADL limitations.[56] Black non-Hispanic and Hispanic older adults at any age were more likely to report mobility limitations.[56] Interestingly, one study found an association between less proximity to goods and services and barriers to walking difficulty, as these older individuals reported more mobility disability than other older adults,[57] which provides an opportunity to consider the impact of the environment on mobility.

HEALTH AND HEALTH CARE UTILIZATION

Self-Rating of Health

In 2017, though 45% of community-dwelling older people assessed their health as excellent or very good (compared to 64% for adults 18 to 64 years of age), non-Hispanic blacks and Hispanics were more likely to rate their health as fair or poor. About 31% of persons aged 60 and older reported height/weight combinations that placed them in the obese category. Only 9% reported they were current smokers and 8% reported excessive alcohol consumption.[7] Not surprisingly, those who were residents of long-term care facilities were far less likely to rate their health as very good or excellent (10.5%). In fact, the majority of individuals residing in a long-term care facility rated their health as fair or poor: 68% of individuals 65 to 74 years of age, 68.2% of individuals 75 to 84 years of age, and 60.2% of individuals 85 years of age and older.[56]

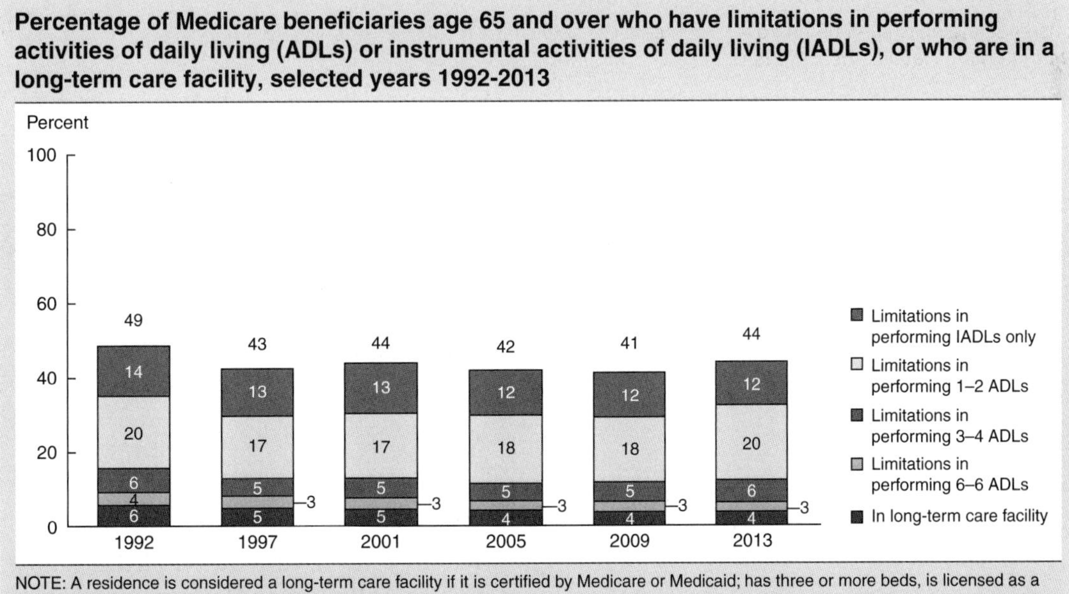

FIG. 2.21 Percentage of Medicare enrollees aged 65 and over who have limitations in activities of daily living (ADLs) or instrumental activities of daily living (IADLs) or who are in a long-term care facility. *(Source: Edwards JJ, Khanna M, Jordan KP, et al. Older Americans 2016: Key Indicators of Well-Being. Federal Interagency Forum on Aging-Related Statistics; https://acl.gov/aging-and-disability-in-america/data-and-research/key-indicators-well-being. Published 2018. Accessed February 6, 2019.)*

Utilization of Services and Expenditures

As illustrated in Fig. 2.22, health care costs increase with age, with the oldest-old (age 85 years and older) incurring higher costs than for any other group. In 2016, consumers age 65 and over averaged out-of-pocket expenditures of $5994, an increase of 38% since 2006 and considerably less than younger consumers ($4331). Older individuals account for 34% of all prescription medication use, with 48% of all older adults reporting taking a prescription drug, compared with 39% 10 years earlier.

Twenty percent of older individuals age 75 years and older reported 10 or more visits to a health care practitioner in the past year, compared with 13% of adults aged 45 to 64 years. The type of provider seen differs with age. The younger the person is, the more exclusively they saw a physician, whereas older adults were more likely to see nonphysician providers (e.g., nurse practitioner, physician assistant) (41.3%). Utilization of specialized services such as home health and hospice increase with age as shown by Fig. 2.23.[6]

The number of chronic conditions increases health care utilization and cost. For example, 14% of those with one to two chronic conditions visited the emergency department within a year compared with 32% of those with five or more chronic conditions.[29] Twice as many drugs on average are used by those with five or more chronic conditions/diseases compared with those with three or four conditions.[29] And people with five or more conditions averaged 20 doctor visits per year, compared with 12 visits for those with three or four conditions.[29] This greater utilization by those with more chronic diseases results in the staggering statistic that those with five or more chronic diseases account for 41% of total health care spending while making up only 12% of the population.[29]

Challenges and Future Possibilities

Changes in the demographic characteristics of the U.S. population represent a critical challenge to, and opportunity for, geriatric physical therapists. Two different cohorts will be aging simultaneously: the World War II and Great Depression cohort, who make up the old-old category, and the boomer cohort, who make up the young-old category. A flexible approach to deal with such different cohorts will be needed, with individualized expectations responsive to each older adult's vision for his or her own aging. Additionally, older adults are expected to live longer than ever before, but the quality of their lives in these added years is still a matter of conjecture. Aging with multiple chronic conditions/diseases and poor participation in physical activity and other healthy lifestyle behaviors further aggravates a propensity toward physical decline with advanced age. Function deficits are the expected outcomes of disease or permanent effects of an injury; in turn, functional limitations predict decreased social participation, increased utilization of services, further morbidity, and death. The physical therapy profession is uniquely positioned to add life to years as medical science adds years to life.

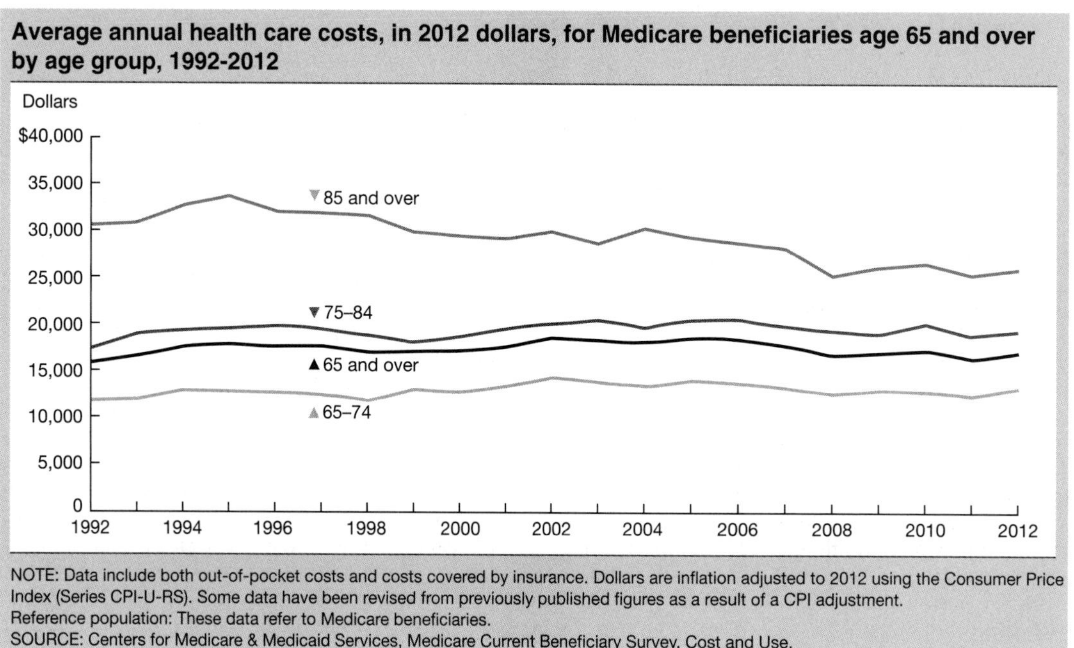
Average annual health care costs, in 2012 dollars, for Medicare beneficiaries age 65 and over by age group, 1992-2012
Dollars
$40,000
35,000
30,000
25,000
20,000
15,000
10,000
5,000
0
85 and over
75–84
65 and over
65–74
1992
1994
1996
1998
2000
2002
2004
2006
2008
2010
2012
NOTE: Data include both out-of-pocket costs and costs covered by insurance. Dollars are inflation adjusted to 2012 using the Consumer Price Index (Series CPI-U-RS). Some data have been revised from previously published figures as a result of a CPI adjustment.
Reference population: These data refer to Medicare beneficiaries.
SOURCE: Centers for Medicare & Medicaid Services, Medicare Current Beneficiary Survey, Cost and Use.

FIG. 2.22 Health care costs by age. *(Source: Centers for Medicare & Medicaid Services, Medicare Current Beneficiary Survey, Cost and Use. U.S. Department of Health and Human Services. Key Indicators of Well-Being | ACL Administration for Community Living. https://acl.gov/aging-and-disability-in-america/data-and-research/key-indicators-well-being. Published 2018. Accessed February 6, 2019.)*

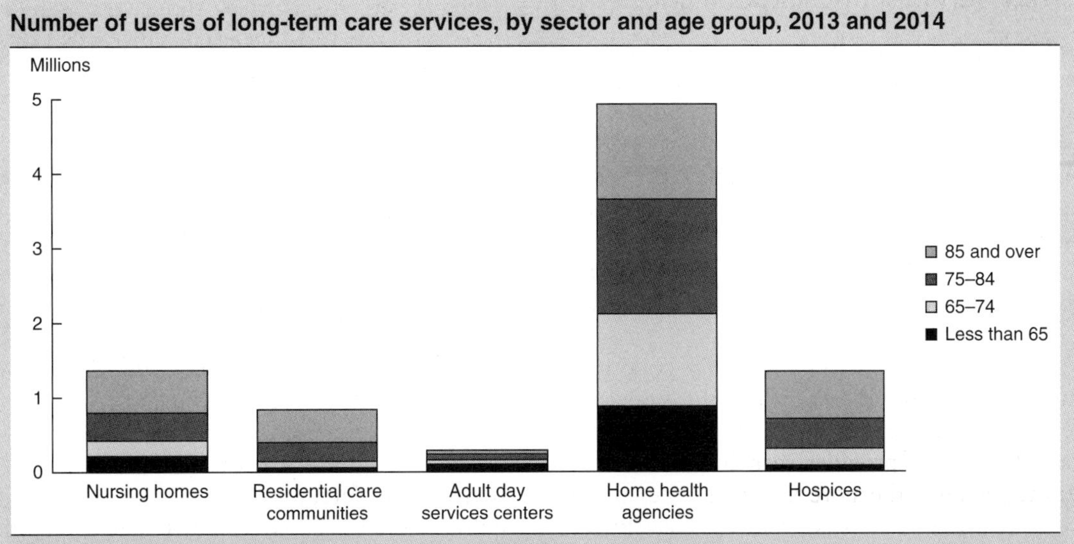
Number of users of long-term care services, by sector and age group, 2013 and 2014
Millions
5
4
3
2
1
0
Nursing homes
Residential care communities
Adult day services centers
Home health agencies
Hospices
85 and over
75–84
65–74
Less than 65
NOTE: Long-term care services are provided by paid, regulated providers. They comprise both health-care-related and non–health-care-related services, including postacute care and rehabilitation. People can receive more than one type of service. The estimated number of users of nursing homes, residential care communities, and adult day services centers represents participants or residents enrolled on the day of data collection in 2014. The estimated number of users of home health agencies represents patients who ended care (i.e., were discharged) in 2013. The estimated number of users of hospice represents patients who received care at any time in 2013. The number in each age group is calculated by applying the percentage distribution by age to the estimated total number of users. See http://www.cdc.gov/nchs/data/series/sr_03/sr03_038.pdf for definitions.
Reference population: These data refer to the resident population.
SOURCE: Centers for Disease Control and Prevention, National Center for Health Statistics, National Study of Long-Term Care Providers.

FIG. 2.23 Specialized service use by age. *(Source: Centers for Disease Control and Prevention, National Center for Health Statistics, National Study of Long-Term Care Providers.)*

REFERENCES

1. Climbing Staff. Forever: 80-years-old and still climbing. *Climbing Magazine*. https://www.climbing.com/videos/forever-80-years-old-and-still-climbing/. Published 2017. Accessed February 5, 2019.
2. Levy SR, Macdonald JL. Progress on understanding ageism. *J Soc Issues*. 2016;72(1):5–25. https://doi.org/10.1111/josi.12153.
3. Tippett R. Population Aging and Growing Dependency | StatChat. University of Virginia. http://statchatva.org/2012/11/20/population-aging-and-growing-dependency/. Published 2012. Accessed February 12, 2019.
4. U.S. Census Bureau. *Older Americans Month: May 2017*. https://www.census.gov/newsroom/facts-for-features/2017/cb17-ff08.html. Published 2017. Accessed February 5, 2019.
5. U.S. Census Bureau. *Nation's Older Population to Nearly Double*. https://www.census.gov/newsroom/press-releases/2014/cb14-84.html. Published 2014. Accessed February 5, 2019.
6. Edwards JJ, Khanna M, Jordan KP, et al. Older Americans 2016: key indicators of well-being. Federal Interagency Forum on Aging-Related Statistics. https://doi.org/10.1136/annrheumdis-2013-203913.
7. Administration on Aging, Administration for Community Living, U.S. Department of Health and Human Services. *A Profile of Older Americans: 2017*. Washington, DC; 2018. https://acl.gov/aging-and-disability-in-america/data-and-research/profile-older-americans. Accessed February 10, 2019.
8. Avendano M, Kawachi I. Why do Americans have shorter life expectancy and worse health than do people in other high-income countries? *Annu Rev Public Health*. 2014;35:307–325. https://doi.org/10.1146/annurev-publhealth-032013-182411.
9. Murphy SL, Xu J, Kochanek KD, Arias E. Mortality in the United States, 2017. CDC/National Center for Health Statistics. https://www.cdc.gov/nchs/products/databriefs/db328.htm. Published 2018. Accessed February 7, 2019.
10. Ortman JM, Velkoff VA, Hogan H. An Aging Nation: The Older Population in the United States. https://www.census.gov/library/publications/2014/demo/p25-1140.html. Published 2014. Accessed February 11, 2019.
11. U.S. Census Bureau. Older People Projected to Outnumber Children. Newsroom. https://www.census.gov/newsroom/press-releases/2018/cb18-41-population-projections.html. Published 2018. Accessed February 6, 2019.
12. Centers for Disease Control and Prevention. *State of Aging and Health in America 2013*. Centers for Disease Control and Prevention, U.S. Department of Health and Human Services. https://www.cdc.gov/aging/agingdata/data-portal/state-aging-health.html. Published 2013. Accessed February 9, 2019.
13. O'Neil K, Tienda M. Age at immigration and the incomes of older immigrants, 1994–2010. *J Gerontol Ser B Psychol Sci Soc Sci*. 2015;70(2):291–302. https://doi.org/10.1093/geronb/gbu075.
14. Fox-Grange W. AARP Blog - The Growing Racial and Ethnic Diversity of Older Adults. Thinking Policy. https://blog.aarp.org/2016/04/18/the-growing-racial-and-ethnic-diversity-of-older-adults/. Published 2016. Accessed February 6, 2019.
15. Rand Corporation. *Health, Marriage, and Longer Life for Men*. RAND: Santa Monica, CA; 1998. https://www.rand.org/pubs/research_briefs/RB5018/index1.html. Accessed 6 February 2019.
16. dePaulo B. No, Getting Married Does Not Make You Live Longer. *Psychology Today*. https://www.psychologytoday.com/us/blog/living-single/200902/no-getting-married-does-not-make-you-live-longer. Published 2009. Accessed February 6, 2019.
17. dePaulo B. Is It True That Single Women and Married Men Do Best? *Psychology Today*. https://www.psychologytoday.com/us/blog/living-single/201701/is-it-true-single-women-and-married-men-do-best. Published 2017. Accessed February 6, 2019.
18. Pew Research Center. The Return of the Multi-Generational Family Household. Social & Demographic Trends. http://www.pewsocialtrends.org/2010/03/18/the-return-of-the-multi-

generational-family-household/. Published 2010. Accessed February 7, 2019.

19. Johnson JH, Appold SJ. *Older U.S. Adults: Demographics, Living Arrangements, and Barriers to Aging in Place.* Kenan Institute White Paper. 2017. www.kenaninstitute.unc.edu/wp-content/uploads/2017/AgingInPlace_06092017.pdf.
20. Aaltonen M, Forma L, Pulkki J, Raitanen J, Rissanen P, Jylha M. Changes in older people's care profiles during the last 2 years of life, 1996-1998 and 2011-2013: a retrospective nationwide study in Finland. *BMJ Open.* 2017;7(11): e015130. https://doi.org/10.1136/bmjopen-2016-015130.
21. Harris-Kojetin L, Sengupta M, Park-Lee E, et al. Long-term care providers and services users in the United States: data from the National Study of Long-Term Care Providers, 2013–2014. *Vital Health Stat.* 2016;3(38):x–xii, 1–105. https://www.cdc.gov/nchs/data/series/sr_03/sr03_038.pdf.
22. Knickman JR, Snell EK. The 2030 problem: caring for aging baby boomers. *Health Serv Res.* 2002;37(4):849–884. https://doi.org/10.1034/J.1600-0560.2002.56.X.
23. Singer BH, Manton KG. The effects of health changes on projections of health service needs for the elderly population of the United States. *Proc Natl Acad Sci USA.* 1998; 95(26):15618–15622. http://www.ncbi.nlm.nih.gov/pubmed/9861019. Accessed 11 February 2019.
24. Manton KG. Recent declines in chronic disability in the elderly U.S. population: risk factors and future dynamics. *Annu Rev Public Health.* 2008;29(1):91–113. https://doi.org/10.1146/annurev.publhealth.29.020907.090812.
25. Foster AC. A closer look at spending patterns of older Americans: beyond the numbers: U.S. Bureau of Labor Statistics. *Beyond Numbers Pricing Spend.* 2016;5(4). https://www.bls.gov/opub/btn/volume-5/spending-patterns-of-older-americans.htm. Accessed 7 February 2019.
26. Centers for Disease Control and Prevention/National Center for Health Statistics. FastStats - Older Persons Health. https://www.cdc.gov/nchs/fastats/older-american-health.htm. Published 2017. Accessed February 7, 2019.
27. Centers for Disease Control and Prevention. LCOD by Race/Ethnicity All Males 2015 - Health Equity. https://www.cdc.gov/healthequity/lcod/men/2015/race-ethnicity/index.htm. Published 2015. Accessed February 7, 2019.
28. Centers for Disease Control and Prevention. Health and Economic Costs of Chronic Disease. National Center for Chronic Disease Prevention and Health Promotion. https://www.cdc.gov/chronicdisease/about/costs/index.htm. Published 2018. Accessed February 8, 2019.
29. Buttorff C, Ruder T, Bauman M. Multiple chronic conditions in the united states. Santa Monica; Rand Corporation: 2017. https://www.rand.org/content/dam/rand/pubs/tools/TL200/TL221/RAND_TL221.pdf.
30. Centers for Disease Control and Prevention. Healthy Aging | At a Glance Reports | Publications | Chronic Disease Prevention and Health Promotion. National Center for Chronic Disease Prevention and Health Promotion. https://www.cdc.gov/chronicdisease/resources/publications/aag/healthy-aging.htm. Published 2016. Accessed February 8, 2019.
31. National Aging Team. 10 Most Common Chronic Diseases [Infographic] - Healthy Aging Blog | NCOA. NCOA Blog Healthy Living. https://www.ncoa.org/blog/10-common-chronic-diseases-prevention-tips/. Published 2017. Accessed February 8, 2019.
32. Centers for Disease Control and Prevention. About Chronic Diseases. National Center for Chronic Disease Prevention and Health Promotion. https://www.cdc.gov/chronicdisease/about/index.htm. Published 2018. Accessed February 8, 2019.
33. Theis KA, Murphy L, Hootman JM, Wilkie R. Social participation restriction among US adults with arthritis: a population-based study using the International Classification of Functioning, Disability and Health. *Arthritis Care Res.* 2013;65(7):1059–1069. https://doi.org/10.1002/acr.21977.
34. Mislinski J. Demographic Trends for the 50-and-Older Work Force - dshort. Advisor Perspectives. https://www.advisorperspectives.com/dshort/updates/2019/02/05/demographic-trends-for-the-50-and-older-work-force. Published 2019. Accessed February 9, 2019.
35. Toosi M, Torpey E. Older workers: labor force trends and career options: career outlook. Bureau of Labor Statistics. https://www.bls.gov/careeroutlook/2017/article/older-workers.htm. Published 2017. Accessed February 9, 2019.
36. Desilver D. More older Americans are working than in recent years. Pew Research Center. http://www.pewresearch.org/fact-tank/2016/06/20/more-older-americans-are-working-and-working-more-than-they-used-to/. Published 2016. Accessed February 9, 2019.
37. Cohen B. Trends in Volunteerism Among Older Adults: Fact Sheet 03 - Sloan Center on Aging and Work at Boston College. Center on Aging and Work. https://www.bc.edu/research/agingandwork/archive_pubs/FS03.html. Published 2010. Accessed February 9, 2019.
38. Fried LP, Carlson MC, Freedman M, et al. A social model for health promotion for an aging population: initial evidence on the Experience Corps model. *J Urban Health.* 2004;81(1):64–78. https://doi.org/10.1093/jurban/jth094.
39. Fried LP, Carlson MC, McGill S, et al. Experience Corps: a dual trial to promote the health of older adults and children's academic success. *Contemp Clin Trials.* 2013;36(1):1–13. https://doi.org/10.1016/j.cct.2013.05.003.
40. Piliavin JA, Siegl E. Health benefits of volunteering in the Wisconsin longitudinal study. *J Health Soc Behav.* 2007;48(4):450–464. https://doi.org/10.1177/002214650704800408.
41. Morrow-Howell N, Hinterlong J, Rozario PA, Tang F. Effects of volunteering on the well-being of older adults. *J Gerontol B, Psychol Sci Soc Sci.* 2003;58(3):S137–S145.
42. Livingston G, Parker K. Since the start of the great recession, more children raised by grandparents. *Pew Res Cent Publ.* 2010;7. http://pewresearch.org/pubs/1724/sharp-increase-children-with-grandparent-caregivers.
43. Chang P-J, Wray L, Lin Y. Social relationships, leisure activity, and health in older adults. *Health Psychol.* 2014;33(6):516–523. https://doi.org/10.1037/hea0000051.
44. Taylor P, Morin R, Parker K, Cohn D, Wang W. Growing Old in America: Expectations vs. Reality. http://www.pewresearch.org/wp-content/uploads/sites/3/2010/10/Getting-Old-in-America.pdf. Published 2009.
45. Owen N, Healy GN, Matthews CE, Dunstan DW. Too much sitting: the population health science of sedentary behavior. *Exerc Sport Sci Rev.* 2010;38(3):105–113. https://doi.org/10.1097/JES.0b013e3181e373a2.
46. Lindstrom HA, Fritsch T, Petot G, et al. The relationships between television viewing in midlife and the development of Alzheimer's disease in a case-control study. *Brain Cogn.* 2005; 58(2):157–165. https://doi.org/10.1016/j.bandc.2004.09.020.
47. García-Esquinas E, Andrade E, Martínez-Gómez D, Caballero FF, López-García E, Rodríguez-Artalejo F. Television viewing time as a risk factor for frailty and functional limitations in older adults: results from 2 European prospective cohorts. *Int J Behav Nutr Phys Act.* 2017;14(1):54. https://doi.org/10.1186/s12966-017-0511-1.
48. Singh B, Kiran U. Recreational activities for senior citizens. *Int J Humanit Soc Sci.* 2014;19(4):2279–2837.
49. Satariano WA, Guralnik JM, Jackson RJ, Marottoli RA, Phelan EA, Prohaska TR. Mobility and aging: new directions for public health action. *Am J Public Health.* 2012;102(8):1508–1515. https://doi.org/10.2105/AJPH.2011.300631.
50. Fried LP, Guralnik JM. Disability in older adults: evidence regarding significance, etiology, and risk. *J Am Geriatr Soc.* 1997;45(1):92–100.

51. Palazzo C, Ravaud JF, Papelard A, Ravaud P, Poiraudeau S. The burden of musculoskeletal conditions. *PLoS One*. 2014; 9(3):e90633, https://doi.org/10.1371/journal.pone.0090633.
52. U.S. Census Bureau. Mobility Is Most Common Disability Among Older Americans. Newsroom. https://www.census.gov/newsroom/press-releases/2014/cb14-218.html. Published 2014. Accessed February 10, 2019.
53. Khatutsky G, Catherine O, Wiener JM, et al. Residential care communities and their residents in 2010: a national portrait. DHHS Publication No. 2016-1041. *Natl Cent Heal Stat*. 2016.
54. Storeng SH, Sund ER, Krokstad S. Factors associated with basic and instrumental activities of daily living in elderly participants of a population-based survey: the Nord-Trøndelag Health Study, Norway. *BMJ Open*. 2018;8(3):e018942. https://doi.org/10.1136/BMJOPEN-2017-018942.
55. Gennuso KP, Matthews CE, Colbert LH. Reliability and validity of 2 self-report measures to assess sedentary behavior in older adults. *J Phys Act Health*. 2015;12(5):727–732. https://doi.org/10.1123/jpah.2013-0546.
56. Centers for Medicare & Medicaid Services. Health and Health Care of the Medicare Beneficiary Survey. https://www.cms.gov/Research-Statistics-Data-and-Systems/Research/MCBS/Data-Tables-Items/2013HHC.html?DLPage=1&DLEntries=10&DLSort=0&DLSortDir=descending; 2013. Published 2013. Accessed February 10, 2019.
57. Satariano WA, Kealey M, Hubbard A, et al. Mobility disability in older adults: at the intersection of people and places. *Gerontologist*. 2016;56(3):525–534. https://doi.org/10.1093/geront/gnu094.

CHAPTER

3

Age-Related Physiological Changes: An Overview

Carol Sames

OUTLINE

INTRODUCTION

Aging is a fundamental process that affects all of our systems and tissues by causing numerous alterations and damage within molecular pathways. The rate and magnitude of change in each system may differ from person to person, but decline across multiple body systems is an inevitable part of life. As such, aging is the most significant risk factor for most noncommunicable diseases, including cardiovascular disease, cancer, diabetes, and neurologic diseases.[1]

Although there are a multitude of theories that describe proposed mechanisms for the aging process, there is no singular unifying theory that satisfactorily accounts for all the changes the body undergoes. Proposed mechanisms include oxidative stress, mitochondrial changes, DNA damage/repair, telomere length, and genotoxicity that interact with genetics, lifestyle choices, and environment to impact biological aging. Although enormous strides have been made in our understanding of the aging process, there is still much to discover about the science of age-related decline. The recognition that whole-body inflammation is an important contributor to age-related decline is a significant shift from concepts such as wear and tear and the biological clock based on genetic programming. In addition, research with identical twins has identified that depending on the outcome variable, 25% to 50% of the decline with age has a genetic basis, which becomes stronger with greater longevity.[2] Most age-related change is the consequence of lifestyle choices, such as inadequate nutrient intake, excess body weight (which puts stress on tissues, increases inflammation, and predisposes toward disease), and variables such as smoking and excessive alcohol intake and a sedentary lifestyle. The lack of physical activity may have the most impact on successful aging.[3–8]

Even though age-related decline may result in the loss of strength, power, aerobic endurance, bone mass, and vital capacity, we have enough tissue reserve in each of our systems to get through 80 to 90 years without infirmity. For example, master athletes (>40 years old) who compete in endurance and ultra-endurance events (>6 hours) demonstrate improvement in their endurance performance at a faster rate than their younger counterparts in swimming, cycling, and running.[9]

Because so much of the decline with aging is lifestyle related, physical therapists are uniquely positioned to intervene along the way, with successful results likely at any age. Indeed, there is a growing body of evidence indicating that exercise is a powerful modifier of inactivity-related decline, even for sarcopenia, the age-related wasting of muscle.[3–5,8,10,11] Loss of skeletal muscle mass and force is inevitable with aging and can be further exacerbated by a host of variables, such as nutrition and disease; however, sedentary lifestyle is likely to take the greatest toll.[4,5,10,11] In the latest position stand on exercise and physical activity for older adults, the American College of Sports Medicine (ACSM) states that although no amount of physical activity can stop the biological aging process, there is strong evidence that regular exercise can minimize the physiological effects of an otherwise sedentary lifestyle and increase active life expectancy by limiting the development and progression of chronic disease and disabling conditions.[12] By and large, men and women who include physical activity in their daily routine should have sufficient muscle mass and force to achieve all of the fundamental activities of daily living throughout their life span.

Aging and longevity are controlled by multiple cellular and subcellular changes within all tissues that interact with lifestyle and environmental choices and factors. The intent of this chapter is to describe what occurs in selected systems for the purpose of understanding the functional consequences of aging as they present to the physical therapist clinically. For example, the natural decline in bone mineral content may predispose patients to osteoporosis through cellular and hormonal changes that can be exacerbated with lifestyle choices such as a sedentary lifestyle and poor nutrition. It is not uncommon for those with osteoporosis to manifest postural changes that affect balance, diminish lung capacity and strength, and shorten step and stride length. Once cellular changes are described, other inactivity- and lifestyle-related events that further contribute to systemic decline will be addressed. Thus, to develop an effective treatment plan, physical therapists must consider all the sequelae of health disorders.

Although there is not a single tissue or system that does not undergo age-related changes, only those systems that physical therapists treat directly or affect the ability to render optimal care are the focus of this chapter. Gastrointestinal or genitourinary systems, for example, will not be discussed in detail. Skeletal muscle, cognitive changes with aging, and exercise interventions to improve function in older adults are covered in later chapters. This chapter is an overview of the aging process in specific systems and will start with a discussion of the decline in homeostasis and demographics on functional loss and ability with aging. Next, changes with aging in the musculoskeletal system, collagenous tissues, and cardiovascular, nervous, somatosensory, immune, and endocrine systems will be introduced. Lastly, research on exercise for reversing decline and preventing disease will be presented in addition to the consequences of adopting a sedentary lifestyle. A comprehensive discussion of impaired muscle performance, motor performance, cognition, exercise, and physical fitness for older adults and wellness for the aging adult will be covered in subsequent chapters.

AGING: A DECLINE IN HOMEOSTASIS

Homeostasis refers to the physiological processes that maintain a stable internal environment of the body and is a critical element in the aging process. The extent to which the body can adapt to physiological stressors and maintain homeostasis will influence susceptibility to illness and injury and is known as adaptive homeostasis. As individuals age, the expansive ability of the adaptive homeostatic range diminishes, and this decline has been suggested to contribute to the higher incidence of disease development among older populations.[13] With increasing age, the capacity to tolerate stressors decreases but remains partially modifiable with lifestyle adaptations. The physical stress theory (PST) proposed by Mueller and Maluf[14] captures the essence of homeostasis. The basic premise of the PST is that changes in the relative level of physical stress cause a predictable adaptive response in all biological tissue.[14] Fig. 3.1 illustrates the relationship between various levels of physical stress and the adaptive responses of tissue. Fig. 3.2 provides a conceptual picture of the relationship of successful and unsuccessful aging to a tolerance for challenges to homeostasis and the effect of varying levels of challenge on homeostasis.

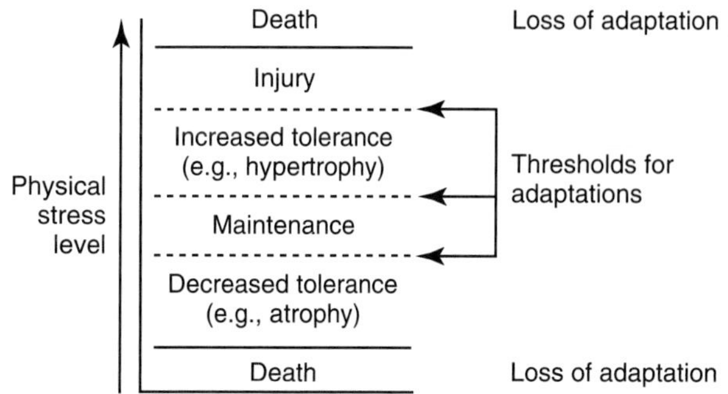

FIG. 3.1 Effect of varying levels of physical stress (inadequately low to excessively high) on tissue's ability to adapt and to maintain homeostasis. *(Reprinted with permission from Muellér MJ, Maluf KS: Tissue adaptation to physical stress: a proposed "Physical Stress Theory" to guide physical therapist practice, education, and research. Phys Ther 82(4):383–403, 2002.)*

The successfully aging older adult maintains a high capacity to tolerate physiological stress, whereas the person who is aging unsuccessfully generally has a low tolerance to physiological stressors that challenge the aging body's homeostasis. The ability to improve tolerance for physiological stress and, thus, provide a wider homeostasis window is possible using principles incorporated in the PST. Tolerance range increases in response to exercise and decreases with the addition of chronic disease and greater inactivity. The older individual with very low tolerance to physiological stressors is highly susceptible to illness and has low capacity to combat the effects of the illness: A bout of influenza may kill.

When a person is in homeostasis, exercise results in robust positive changes with systemic adaptation. Strength and balance can increase, as can aerobic and muscle endurance. When the inactive older adult with stable chronic disease engages in exercise, positive changes also occur, albeit not at the same magnitude as their active counterparts. Under both sets of circumstances, a widening of the window of homeostasis occurs, providing greater tolerance to physiological stress, thus reducing the possibility of moving from homeostasis into illness and disease. The wider the window of homeostasis is, the greater the chance of survival and of maintaining

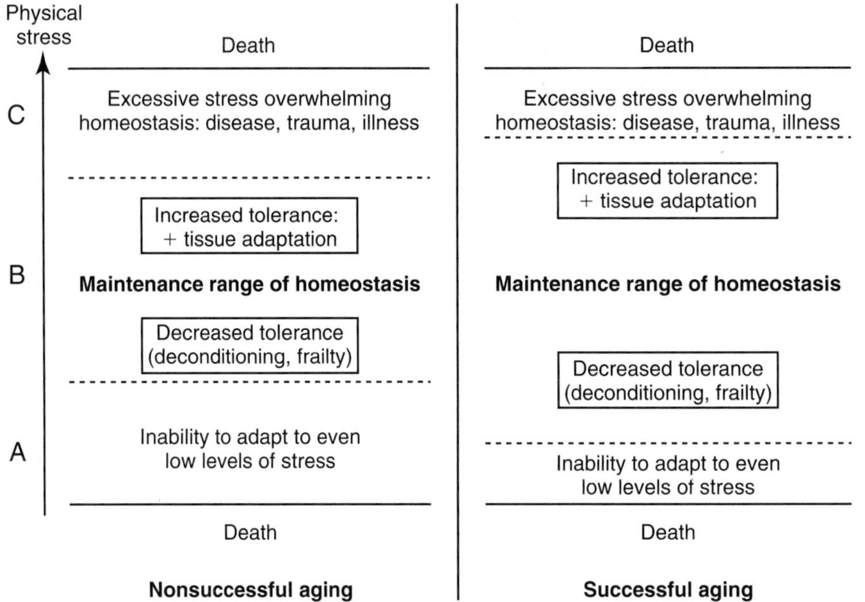

FIG. 3.2 A depiction of the differences in range of homeostasis tolerance and ability to adapt to stress in individuals who have aged nonsuccessfully and those who have aged successfully. The dotted lines represent the limits of homeostasis centered around the range of physical stress that maintains tissue at physiological equilibrium and the effect of increased or decreased stress on tolerance to challenges to homeostasis. **A,** Inadequate ability to adapt (maintain tissue homeostasis) against even small stresses. **B,** Level of stress that maintains homeostasis tolerance at the same level. **C,** Level of stress that overwhelms the tissue's ability to maintain homeostasis.

independence in physical function, and the greater the physical reserve as well as resilience—the capacity of the body to draw on a "well" of immune function, strength, and endurance among other resources to meet the demands of life. One of the biggest challenges of physical therapy practice is to promote and maintain enough physiological reserve to maintain homeostasis even in the presence of large stressors. Thus, physical therapists should promote wellness and enhance quality of life as part of every episode of care.

When discussing physiological changes with aging, it is important to define several terms. *Cachexia* typically refers to an inexorable decline in muscle (and body) wasting that cannot be arrested nutritionally.[15,16] Cachexia is rapid and relentless muscle wasting that frequently occurs before death and is associated with end-stage cancer, chronic obstructive pulmonary disease (COPD), congestive heart failure (CHF), and certain infectious diseases as a response to one or more pathologies that overwhelm the body. Although some young adults with more "reserve" may recover from a cachectic state, most people do not, and rarely do older adults recover from cachexia. The cachexia of old age typically precedes death, and even though the cause of cachexia is not well defined, it is believed to be the consequence of a massive increase in inflammatory cytokines, which will be discussed later in this chapter.[17,18]

The other term that must be defined is *sarcopenia*, which is the muscle wasting of old age.[19] First described by Rosenberg in 1989 as the progressive decrease in muscle mass and strength during aging, there is currently not a universally accepted definition; however, an expansion of the definition now includes a decline in muscle strength, power, and functional quality.[16,20] Sarcopenia is present if muscle mass, as determined by dual-energy x-ray absorptiometry, is two or more standard deviations below values obtained for young adults.[15,20] It has been estimated that between 22% and 33% of community-dwelling older adults have sarcopenia, and for those older than age 80 years that number approaches 50%, with a higher percentage for men than women.[21–23] Because the underlying pathophysiology of cachexia and sarcopenia is different, it is not surprising that they respond differently to strength training. Indeed, sarcopenic muscle is capable of responding to strength-training exercise, with significant increases in muscle mass and strength. There is strong evidence that progressive resistance training has a profound effect on virtually all of the physiological mechanisms in the nervous and muscular system in older individuals, including those with mobility issues.[24–26] In contrast, cachexic muscle does not respond to progressive resistance training, and physical therapy treatment to improve strength with this condition is generally unwarranted.

Sarcopenia is frequently the hallmark of increasing disability in aging adults. In Western society as many as 42% of individuals over 60 years of age have difficulty performing activities of daily living; 15% to 30% report being unable to lift or carry 10 pounds; and >30% have some type of physical disability.[27] Because sarcopenia is associated with increasing disability in aging adults, the increasing number of aging adults with decreasing functional ability provides limitless opportunities for positive impact through physical therapy. A detailed discussion of sarcopenia is included elsewhere in this text. Physical changes occur in all systems in the aging adult. The age-related changes in the systems most applicable to physical therapy are presented in the following sections. The potential for enhanced tissue and organ function through physical therapy is also discussed.

MUSCULOSKELETAL SYSTEM

Skeletal Tissue

Skeletal tissue is remarkably susceptible to change in response to nutritional status, activity/inactivity, weight bearing, hormones, and medications.[28] Peak bone mass is reached at skeletal maturity (20 to 30 years of age) and is followed by a progressive and slow decline (Fig. 3.3). In postmenopausal women this loss is more severe, with an increased rate of bone resorption immediately after menopause clearly indicating a hormonal influence on bone density in women.[29] The most likely explanation for this increased resorption is the drop in ovarian estrogen production that accompanies menopause.[29] Bone loss begins to accelerate approximately 2 to 3 years before the last menses, and this acceleration ends 3 to 4 years after menopause. For an interval of a few years around menopause, women lose 2% of bone annually.[30] Afterward, bone loss slows to about 1% to 1.5% per year in women unless there is an underlying condition or immobilization that increases the rate.[31] Men also lose bone mass with age, but their bone loss acceleration begins after the age of 75.[32]

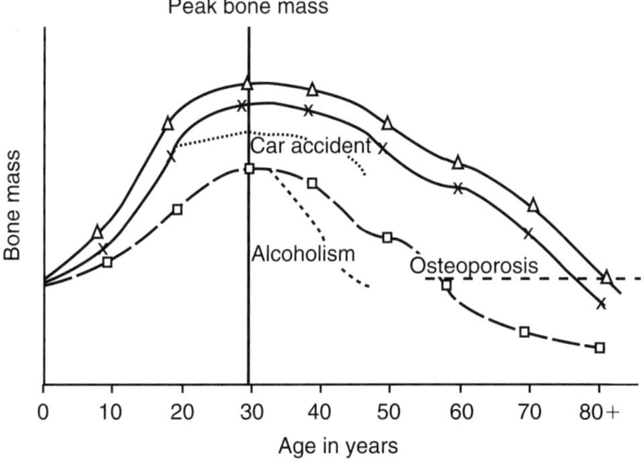

FIG. 3.3 Bone mass profiles of three women throughout the course of a lifetime. The *top line* (Δ) represents usual lifestyle, including adequate nutrition including calcium, occasional or no weight-bearing exercise, some outdoor time (vitamin D exposure), minimal inactivity-related diseases including obesity, modest alcohol intake, and no drugs that diminish bone. The *middle line* (X) reflects optimal bone mass in a woman who embraced a healthy lifestyle over the course of her lifetime. Healthy lifestyle includes adequate nutrition including protein and calcium intake, a regular weight-bearing exercise program, routine exposure to sunshine, minimal disease burden, modest alcohol consumption, and no drugs that diminish bone. The *bottom line* (□) reflects one of several possibilities: inadequate calcium during the teenage years and/or amenorrhea as a teen or early adult stage of life, or anorexia as a teenager with inadequate calcium and protein intake. Anorexia often results in low estrogen values as well. Major points: Calcium intake during adolescence is critical; loss of normal serum estrogen results in accelerated bone loss with age or failure to maximize bone stock in youth; poor lifestyle choices (e.g., alcoholism, sedentary lifestyle, poor nutrition) diminish bone at all ages; and serious physical compromise (e.g., car accident with prolonged bed rest) has lifelong consequences.

Bone is composed of three cell types: the osteoclast, which breaks down bone; the osteoblast, which produces and increases bone mineral; and the osteocyte, which maintains bone. These three cell types form the basic metabolic unit (BMU) of bone as suggested by Frost.[33] In normal bone remodeling there is a balance between osteoblast and osteoclast activity. With aging, there are alterations in the maturation and function of the osteoblast and the osteoclast, which results in greater bone removal than replacement. Thus, with advancing age, the BMU favors bone catabolism rather than bone anabolism. With the onset of menopause, the rate of bone remodeling increases, which magnifies the impact of bone loss.[34] The loss of bone tissue leads to a disordered skeletal architecture and an increase in fracture risk.[34]

Factors other than aging may affect the bone health of men and women throughout the life span and account for more decline in bone mass than aging alone. Some of these factors are nonmodifiable, but many factors affecting bone mass are modifiable with lifestyle. Factors that are modifiable with lifestyle and those that are not modifiable are summarized in Box 3.1. It is important to realize that estrogen is critical for the maintenance of bone mass in

BOX 3.1 Nonmodifiable and Modifiable Risk Factors for Bone Loss

Nonmodifiable Risk Factors for Bone Loss

Genetics: women with small frames
Caucasian race
Hispanic women
Age: female older than age 50 years
Family history of osteoporosis
Premature at birth
Low estrogen: menopause
Childhood malabsorption disease
Seizure disorder—using Dilantin
Age-associated loss of muscle mass

Modifiable Risk Factors

Calcium intake: 1200 mg/day or more is required
Excessive alcohol intake: maximum allowable is not defined
Smoking cigarettes
Low body mass index (<18.5)
Low estrogen: amenorrhea, anorexia
Low estrogen: ovariohysterectomy
Inactivity, immobilization
Substituting soda for milk, especially among children
Insufficient protein at all ages
Inadequate vitamin D
Hyperthyroidism
Prednisone and cortisone use, hyperparathyroidism

both men and women. Recently, it has become evident that testosterone and estrogen are independent mediators of bone health in men.[35,36] Thus, any condition affecting sex hormones (e.g., prostate cancer, breast cancer) automatically affects skeletal health in both sexes.

Osteoporosis has traditionally been diagnosed based on T-scores less than −2.5 in the lumbar spine, total hip, and femoral neck and/or a 33% radius. The American Association of Clinical Endocrinologists and American College of Endocrinology (AACE/ACE) has recently agreed with the proposed new clinical diagnosis by the National Bone Health Alliance that osteoporosis may also be diagnosed in patients with osteopenia (T-scores between −1.0 and −2.5) and increased risk using the Fracture Risk Assessment Tool (FRAX).[28] Wright and colleagues estimate that 10 million Americans have osteoporosis and that 2 million osteoporosis-related fractures occur yearly, with more than 70% of these occurring in women.[37] Given the smaller bone size of women compared to men, women are much more susceptible to developing osteoporosis after menopause.

The fact that tomorrow's osteoporotic women are being created among the youth of today gravely concerns the Centers for Disease Control and Prevention (CDC).[38] Young women are not drinking milk, are highly sedentary, are not using their muscles, are not going outside routinely for sun exposure, and are eating nutritionally poor foods without adequate calcium, protein, and vitamin D. Each day spent without the building blocks of bone robs the skeletal system of more mineral.[38] During the teenage years, bone mass increases tremendously and it is during the ages of 12 to 18 that the ultimate skeletal profile is determined. Thus, if a teenager doesn't meet minimum dietary recommendations for calcium, vitamin D, and protein; exercise regularly; and get adequate sun exposure, chances increase that these adolescents will emerge from their teens with a skeletal profile of an older adult. At the other end of the age spectrum are older, sedentary postmenopausal women who have a high risk for fracture, becoming more osteoporotic and frail, and falling.[33,37] A recent retrospective analysis demonstrated that the annual cost associated with osteoporotic fractures exceeds the costs of breast cancer, myocardial infarction, or stroke in women aged 55 years and older.[39]

Exercise is critical to the health and prevention of osteoporosis. The force applied by contracting muscles places tension on bone and helps maintain bone mineral density; inactivity deprives bone of a critical stimulus for osteoblastic activity. The impact of bone loss that occurs during the extreme unloading of space has been estimated at 0.5% to 1.0% *per day* because muscle contractions are not producing any demand on bone, further highlighting the importance of weight bearing and resistance training in bone health.[40] The AACE/ACE Clinical Practice Guidelines recommend that regular exercise (e.g., walking 30 to 40 minutes/session; resistance training 2 to 3 days/week) should be advocated throughout life.[33] Progressive resistance training is a strong stimulus for improving and maintaining bone mass during the aging process.[41] The best BMD improvements occur through high-intensity resistance training with three sessions per week and two to three sets per session.[41] A recent meta-analysis concluded that the exercise-induced improvements in lumbar spine and femoral neck BMD would reduce osteoporotic fracture risk by approximately 10%.[42] Using data from the Longitudinal Aging Study, Furrer and colleagues concluded that higher handgrip strength and physical performance was related to high bone quality and reduced fracture risk in men, whereas in women, a moderate to high level of physical activity was associated with reduced fracture risk.[43]

Several studies have indicated that exercise combined with hormone replacement therapy (dehydroepiandrosterone [DHEA], testosterone, estrogen, or estrogen/progesterone combined) can add bone mineral density to the osteopenic framework of older men and women. Villareal et al. demonstrated that frail older women (older than age 75 years) on hormone replacement therapy (HRT) also had significant increases of approximately 3.5% in lumbar spine BMD with 9 months of resistance and aerobic exercise training.[44,45] In one of the few studies that included men, DHEA was given for 2 years to subjects of both sexes aged 65 to 75 years. Women on DHEA increased spine BMD by 1.7% in the first year and by 3.6% after 2 years of supplementation. No increases in bone were observed for men.[46] Given the current trend of increasing osteoporosis in men, successful therapies are needed. A further discussion of pharmacological intervention is discussed elsewhere in this text.

Muscle Tissue

Muscle tissue undergoes a number of physiological changes with aging including changes in muscle fiber atrophy, muscle fiber type, contractile function, muscle structure, and composition that ultimately impact physical performance, velocity, force, and strength of movement, potentially leading to functional disability.[47] There is about a 20% to 40% decrease in muscle mass by the age of 70 years.[48] The median decline in muscle mass throughout the life span is 0.37% per year in women and 0.47% in men, accelerating in individuals aged 75 years or older at a rate of 0.64% to 0.70% per year in women and 0.80% to 0.98% per year in men.[49] At the cellular level, studies have reported a significant decrease in muscle fiber size in aging adults.[50] Muscle fiber composition also appears to be impacted by the aging process. Type I or slow-twitch fibers are considered oxidative or more aerobic in nature, whereas type II or fast-twitch fibers are glycolytic and are used under anaerobic conditions. A 10% to 40% reduction in type II fibers has been observed in aging adults.[51] Loss of type II fibers in older adults can be problematic because those fibers are related to muscle strength and power, which is needed to rise from a chair or lift heavy loads. Aging is also associated with a decrease in absolute and relative contractile skeletal muscle content in both males and females, which reduces the force per unit area of skeletal muscle and is observed at the single-fiber and whole-muscle level.[52,53] Muscle structure changes that occur with aging include higher levels of intermuscular adipose tissue, which is associated with a decrease in physical performance and limited mobility in older adults.[54,55] The age-related low-grade chronic inflammation is associated with pathological remodeling of skeletal muscle, which contributes to reduced muscle function.[56] Higher cytokine levels are associated with lower muscle mass and overall strength and physical decline among older adults.[57,58] Changes in excitation–contraction coupling, calcium release from the sarcoplasmic reticulum, and a reduction in the number of mitochondria, mitochondrial DNA, and muscle protein synthesis with aging also can reduce muscle performance.[54,59–61]

As with bone health, exercise has a significant positive effect on muscle performance and physical function. Higher-intensity exercise is demonstrated to be an effective intervention for improving physical functioning in older adults, including improving strength (hypertrophy) and the performance of some simple and complex activities such as rising from a chair.[62] In two meta-analyses, Peterson and colleagues identified two important aspects of resistance training to promote positive adaptations: The first is that higher-intensity training is associated with greater improvements in muscle strength and the second is that higher training volume (total number of sets per session) is associated with greater improvements in lean body mass (LBM) after controlling for confounders such as age, training duration, gender, training intensity, and frequency.[63,64] A detailed discussion of aging changes in muscle and exercise recommendations can be found elsewhere in this text.

Body Composition

There is a gradual shift in body composition with aging such that lean mass decreases and fat mass proportionately increases (Fig. 3.4). The loss of LBM and gain of fat mass contribute to a decrease in resting metabolic rate of 1% to 2% per decade after 20 years of age.[65] Because LBM is more metabolically active (energy wise) than fat mass, the resting metabolic rate (RMR) decreases. Therefore, a loss of LBM causes a reduction in RMR with fewer total calories utilized at rest, which unbalances the energy equation, predisposing an individual to gain weight over time without a change in caloric intake. From 2011 to 2014 in the United States, the prevalence of adult obesity was 36.5%, with a higher percentage for women than men.[66] Since 1999–2000 the prevalence of adult obesity has increased from 30.5% to 37.7% in 2013–2014.[66] Although obesity ultimately results from an energy imbalance, many factors contribute to its development

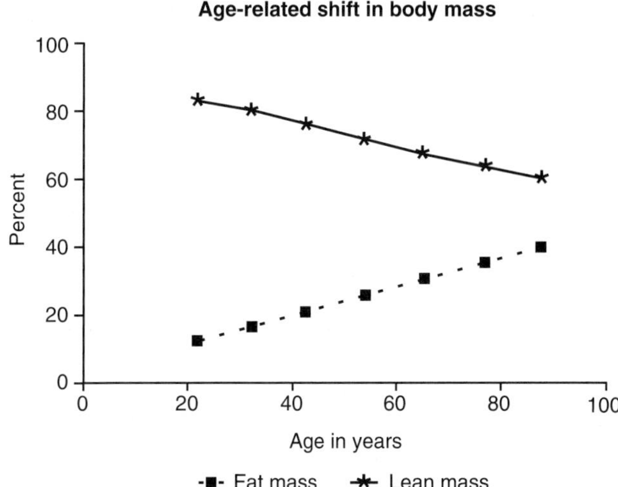

FIG. 3.4 Typical shift in fat and lean mass in an aging male. Lean mass, which is mostly muscle, declines continuously after the 3rd decade. Fat mass increases concomitantly. In this individual, body weight has not changed over the 60 years that are represented.

including genetics, metabolism behavior, environment, culture, socioeconomic status, and certain medical conditions such as thyroid disorder, Cushing syndrome, and polycystic ovarian syndrome, in addition to certain medications.[67]

The presence of intra-abdominal adipose tissue (visceral fat) is a normal aspect of aging and is an independent predictor of cardiovascular disease, associated risk factors, and all-cause mortality. Visceral fat secretes proinflammatory cytokines and C-reactive protein, which promote and sustain low-grade chronic inflammation beyond the aging process.[68,69] The increase in intra-abdominal fat is also believed to predispose older individuals, particularly women, to elevated lipids and prediabetes.[70] Increased visceral fat also increases the risk for hypertension, triglycerides, metabolic syndrome, type 2 diabetes, gallbladder disease, and certain types of cancer.[67] Women are particularly vulnerable to these diseases after menopause as the protective effects of estrogen are reduced and women have more total fat mass than men at all ages.[45] Exercise plays an important role in controlling intra-abdominal fat.[71] When the heart rate increases in response to aerobic exercise and muscles are engaged with resistance training, the metabolic rate increases and fat is burned as fuel. Men and women of all ages who are consistently active do not add intra-abdominal fat to the same extent as those who are sedentary.[69–71] Consequently, active men and women have less whole-body inflammation and less obesity-related disease.[70–73]

Osteosarcopenic obesity syndrome is a recent term describing the triad of osteopenia, obesity, and sarcopenia.[57,74] Previously it was believed that obesity had a protective role on bone and muscle by providing mechanical load for both; however, it is now recognized that adipose tissue, particularly visceral fat, secretes proinflammatory cytokines that promote and sustain low-grade chronic inflammation (LGCI) beyond the aging process.[68,69] The mechanisms of LGCI cause changes in all three tissues simultaneously and propagate more fat deposition, maintaining decreased bone and muscle mass and increased adipose tissue as fat infiltrates muscle and bone tissue.[57,58]

Connective Tissue and Collagen

Connective tissue is probably the most ubiquitous tissue type in the body, found in bone, muscle, blood vessels, skin, tendons, ligaments, fascia, cartilage, and other body tissues. Subtle change occurs in all collagenous tissues with aging, but only three of these changes will be discussed here: loss of water from the extracellular matrix, increase in collagen crosslinks, and loss of elastin fibers.[75–77]

Connective tissues are composed of collagen, which provides substantial tensile strength, and a surrounding semiliquid extracellular matrix, which binds water and permits collagen fibers to easily glide past one another. Extracellular matrix composition changes over the years such that water content decreases considerably. The most obvious consequence of decreased water content in connective tissue is the height loss that occurs when water is lost from the intervertebral discs.[78] Articular cartilage also loses water with age and becomes more susceptible to breakdown (osteoarthritis). Simultaneously a reduction in the rate of collagen turnover occurs, which is associated with an increase in the formation of crosslinks between collagen molecules.[77] The increase of collagen crosslinks and loss of water alter biomechanical function with two observable clinical changes apparent: a decreased range of motion and an increase in stiffness and loss of ability to absorb shock.[77]

Loss of elastin, which is another connective tissue protein that functions with collagen to return structures to their original shape after deformation, occurs with aging.[79] A reduction of elastin is abundantly evident in aging skin, which no longer has its turgor and tends to hang or wrinkle. Aging tendons, ligaments, and muscles also demonstrate a reduction in functioning elastin, further contributing to change in function.[79] As inconceivable as it is to regard 35-year-old baseball or basketball players as "too old" for their sport, age-related changes in connective tissue are one of the major contributors to injury and decreased performance in athletics. In addition to tendons and muscles, internal organs are no longer held in place as well and age-related changes in connective tissues contribute to the tendency for uterine prolapse, bladder issues, constipation, and hernia in aging adults. Box 3.2 summarizes the three major age-related changes in collagenous tissues: decreased water content from the extracellular matrix, increase in number of collagen crosslinks, and loss of elastin.

From an exercise standpoint, working toward end range becomes more and more important with advancing age to prevent range-of-motion losses from limiting function. Even though joint end range is diminished with advancing years, range should still be sufficient to accomplish all activities of daily living, including reaching into high cupboards and down to the floor. Range loss should *not* preclude accomplishing any basic activities—it merely reduces the potential for extremes. Stiffness, on the other hand, has several clinical implications. From a biomechanical perspective, stiffness implies a lack of "give" that translates, for example, to a greater likelihood of tendon avulsion rather than rupture. Stiffness also means that the passive tension within tissues is increased. Stated another way, the proportion of total tension (i.e., total muscle tension as the sum of active and passive tension) that can be attributed to passive stiffness is increased with age. Couple the increase in passive "drag" with the decline in muscle force that occurs with aging, and the consequence is greater muscular effort required for movement. Increased tissue stiffness is one factor contributing to less muscle endurance with age.

When water loss becomes excessive, such as in the presence of osteoarthritis, exercises may need to limit high-impact/force activities such as jumping from high surfaces. Although plyometric exercises are recommended as an excellent stimulus to increase bone mass and muscle power, care should be taken to choose exercises that balance the stimulus to bone and the ability of the joint surface and muscle to absorb high-force impact.

BOX 3.2 Major Age-Related Changes in Collagenous Tissues and Associated Clinical Consequences

Age-Related Change	Clinical Consequence
Loss of water from the matrix	Shrinkage of articular cartilage, vertebral discs Decreased ability to absorb shock Reduced range of motion
Increase in number of collagen cross-links	"Stiffer" tissues, greater passive tension within tissues More effort required to move Loss of end range of motion
Loss of elastic fibers	Sagging skin and organs Less "give" to tendons, ligaments, fascia

Cardiovascular System

Fundamental functional changes in the cardiovascular system that occur with aging are summarized in Box 3.3. These age-associated cardiovascular changes lower the threshold for changes that manifest as increased cardiovascular disease (CVD) and cardiovascular morbidity and mortality.[80] The prevalence of CVD increases in people older than 65 years of age, especially in those over 80 years old, and is anticipated to increase approximately 10% by 2020.[81]

BOX 3.3 Major Age-Related Changes in Cardiovascular Tissues and Associated Clinical Consequences

Anatomic/Physiological Change with Age	Clinical Consequences
Decline in maximum heart rate	Smaller aerobic workload possible
Decline in $\dot{V}o_2$max	Smaller aerobic workload possible
Stiffer, less compliant vascular tissues	Higher blood pressure Slower ventricle filling time with reduced cardiac output
Loss of cells from the sinoatrial node	Slower heart rate Lower maximum heart rate
Reduced contractility of the vascular walls	Slower heart rate Lower $\dot{V}o_2$max Smaller aerobic workload possible
Thickened basement membrane in capillary	Reduced arteriovenous O_2 uptake

Probably the most notable and clinically important change is the decline in maximum heart rate (HR), which directly impacts maximal aerobic capacity represented by peak exercise oxygen capacity.[82] The commonly used formula of 220 minus age developed by Fox and colleagues provides a relative guideline for an expected change in maximum HR but has been demonstrated to underestimate maximum HR in older populations.[83,84] The magnitude of the age-associated reduction in maximal exercise HR has been estimated to be about 30% between 20 and 85 years of age.[85]

Does participation in lifelong exercise prevent the decline in maximum HR? At this juncture, research has not supported this contention and scientists do not fully understand what causes the decline in maximum HR, although factors contributing to the process have been identified including increased stiffness of the heart with slower filling of the left ventricle, reduced sensitivity to sympathetic stimulation, and an age-related decrease in the number of cells in the sinoatrial (SA) node.[86,87]

The decline in maximal aerobic capacity, which is represented by maximum or peak exercise oxygen capacity (peak VO_2), is a hallmark of aging and is the universally accepted measure of cardiorespiratory fitness.[88] Coupled with the decline in maximum HR is a concomitant and related decline in peak VO_2. The age-associated decrease in maximal aerobic capacity increases progressively from 3% to 6% in the third and fourth decades of life to >20% per decade after age 70.[89] The presence of vascular and cardiovascular disease, however, can decrease maximal aerobic capacity even further. Later-life decreases in aerobic capacity have been demonstrated to be more rapid in men than in women, suggesting a difference in age-associated changes in cardiac morphology.[90]

Maximal cardiac output reflects peak VO_2 and consequently maximal aerobic capacity. Cardiac output is the amount of blood pumped by the heart during 1 minute and is expressed as HR multiplied by stroke volume (SV). Stroke volume also decreases with age, reflecting changes in ventricular functioning. Therefore, maximal cardiac output during exercise is reduced with aging because both HR and SV decline with age. This reduction in cardiac output during exercise reflects changes that impact the delivery of oxygen to the working muscles and the ability of the muscles to use the available oxygen in addition to reductions in HR and SV.

There is also a correlation between muscle mass and peak VO_2, which is the primary reason men have higher maximum peak VO_2 values than women.[89,90] The higher the lean mass at any age is, the higher the maximal aerobic capacity.[89] Those who are sarcopenic have very low aerobic capacity.[49,50,91] Hypothetically, adding muscle mass to the sarcopenic individual will enhance adaptation to aerobic exercise, which is another compelling reason for frail older adults with sarcopenia to participate in resistance training.

Physical therapists regularly treat older adults who have a long history of inactivity and periodic bouts of disease- or illness-related bed rest. Thus, it is quite common for patients older than age 60 years to have peak VO_2 values in the 13 to 18 mL O_2/kg/min range, which translates to an inability to climb a flight of stairs without resting and inability to walk a quarter of a mile. Most physical therapists have faced the challenge of the deconditioned older adult with comorbidities, further imposing inactivity-related decline on a body with minimal cardiovascular capacity and who reaches a high percentage of maximum HR just getting from the bed to the bathroom. This scenario, reflecting enormous loss in cardiovascular reserve, is one major contributor to loss in homeostasis, frailty, and loss of functional capacity.

Because of the fundamental changes in connective tissues, increased cross-linking of collagen, altered matrix composition, and loss of elastin, the entire vascular system, including the heart and peripheral vessels, is stiffer and less compliant.[75–77] Cross-sectional and longitudinal studies have demonstrated that central elastic arteries dilate with age, leading to an increase in lumen size with their walls becoming thickened.[92] Most noticeable is the increase in systolic blood pressure that occurs with age, the consequence of vascular stiffening in large arteries while diastolic pressure decreases.[92] The decrease in diastolic pressure reduces the drive for coronary perfusion that occurs when the heart is "resting."[92] The combination of increased systolic pressure and decreased diastolic pressure that occurs with age can be problematic during exercise when oxygen supply is decreased while oxygen demand is augmented. Increased elevation of systolic blood pressure with age increases left ventricular afterload and, combined with increased stiffness of the aorta, causes the heart to pump harder against more resistance, leading to left ventricular hypertrophy. Contractility of the left ventricle is reduced with aging, which results in a reduction of cardiac output, one of the major components of peak VO_2 and aerobic capacity. In the author's experience most clients older than age 70 years seen in physical therapy are medicated for hypertension. Consequently, from the standpoint of exercise safety, the physical therapist must watch for blood pressure increases that are unacceptably high. It is imperative that older adults perform warm-ups prior to intense aerobic exercise to accommodate for the slower arteriovenous oxygen exchange, stiffer vascular tissues, reduction in sympathetic nervous system output, and lower aerobic capacity associated with older age.

Perhaps as a consequence of connective tissue changes, endothelial dysfunction, and loss of vasodilatory nitric oxide, the basement membrane in the capillary wall thickens with age, reducing efficient oxygen extraction.[92,93] Thus, the exchange of oxygen and nutrients from the vasculature to working tissues occurs more slowly. The difference between arterial and mixed venous blood oxygen content (a–VO_2 difference) represents the amount of oxygen used by the body and increases with exercise owing to the metabolic demands of working muscle. Because tissue perfusion occurs more slowly in older adults, the "burn" or increase in lactate produced by the working muscles takes longer to subside during the initial phases of exercise, necessitating a warm-up longer than the usual requisite 3 minutes prior to more vigorous activity. Whether membrane thickening occurs at older ages in men and women with a lifetime history of exercise is not known. Diseases of the peripheral vasculature such as diabetes and peripheral vascular disease (PVD) further increase basement membrane thickness, which can result in reduced aerobic capacity and lack of oxygen perfusion to skin tissues for breakdown and nonhealing of ulcers.

Peripheral to the discussion of age-related decline in the cardiovascular system is an issue of enormous importance to physical therapy: anesthesia. Men and women of all ages are affected by inhalation anesthesia, but the effects are most noticeable in older adults who have already lost a significant amount of cardiovascular reserve. Although the mechanism is unknown, inhalation anesthesia obliterates mitochondria, and thus, the ability to deliver ATP during exercise is severely compromised.[94] Thus, after surgery with inhalation anesthesia, muscular and cardiovascular endurance is severely compromised.[94] Physical therapists often see patients the day of total joint replacement surgery and surgical repair of a fractured hip even when patients become exhausted with minimal effort. It is no surprise that spontaneous improvement begins to manifest 2 months after surgery, long after physical therapy has ended as the effects of the inhalation anesthesia dissipate. The initial phase of physical therapy following lower extremity surgery is effective for teaching patients the essentials: transfers, walker use, home exercise, proper gait pattern, and mobility strategies; however, evidence strongly suggests that therapy aimed at strengthening and endurance adaptations given to patients in the days immediately following surgery for hip fracture is ineffectual.[95] The enormous devastation to the energy delivery system, coupled with bed rest, the trauma of surgery, and inactivity, indicates that perhaps physical therapy intervention would be more effective 2 to 3 months after hospital discharge. As a profession, physical therapists need to reevaluate intervention effectiveness under these treatment conditions.

One aspect of cardiovascular aging needs to be emphasized. Even though maximum heart rate, stroke volume, cardiac output, and aerobic capacity are reduced, there is no reason that exercise in healthy older adults should be restricted to a low-intensity level for fear of a heart attack or stroke. In fact, prospective evidence from the Physicians' Health Study and the Nurses' Health Study suggests that sudden cardiac death (SCD) occurs every 1.5 million episodes of vigorous exertion in men and every 36.5 million hours of moderate to vigorous exertion in women, which is low risk for vigorous intensity.[96,97] The risk of SCD or anterior wall myocardial infarction (AMI) is higher in middle-aged and older adults than in younger individuals owing to the higher prevalence of CVD in older populations and also is higher in sedentary versus active individuals regardless of age.[98] The relative risk of SCD and AMI during vigorous to near-maximal intensity exercise is directly related to the presence of CVD and/or exertional symptoms and is inversely related to the habitual level of physical activity, implicating inactivity as a much greater risk factor for SCD than physical activity.[96,98,99]

Nervous System

There are fundamental changes with aging in the central and peripheral nervous systems that have significant importance for function. Slowing of the nervous system is an inherent aspect of aging, and nerve conduction studies of older adults have found lower conduction velocities in the peripheral nervous system in older adults.[100,101] The motor unit is the basic functional unit in the neuromuscular system that allows production of muscular force and ultimately movement performance. The motor unit consists of the alpha motor neuron and the muscle fibers it innervates. With aging, there is a loss of motor units, changes in morphology and properties of motor units, and altered input from the nervous system, which impact power, strength, and muscular endurance. In addition to loss of motor neurons, there is denervation and reinnervation of muscle fibers and this process occurs primarily after 60 years of age.[102] The process of denervation and reinnervation leads to fewer but larger surviving motor units, which impacts motor unit recruitment and decreases performance involving fine motor control in aging adults.[103] Aging also reduces rate coding (i.e., action potential firing rates at which motor units fire), which alters power production and muscle contraction speed. The duration of twitch contraction of the tibialis anterior during maximal voluntary contraction was found to be 23% longer, and the maximal rate of force production was found to be lower in older adults than in younger controls.[104]

Slowing of movement speed is one of the major clinical manifestations of a slowing nervous system. Wojcik and colleagues identified that men and women in the young-old category (65 to 74 years) are already at heightened risk for falling as response time to an induced fall was too slow for recovery.[105] In this study, subjects were leaning forward into a harness that was preventing them from falling forward, but when the harness was released and subjects were allowed to stumble and fall, most of the young-old healthy adults could not get their legs back underneath their body quickly enough and step appropriately to prevent a fall.[105] Sensorimotor changes with aging that decreased motor strength, slowed reaction time, and diminished reflexes contribute to balance difficulty and slower, more deliberate movements that are frequently seen in older adults.[106]

Slowing of reflex responses is also a hallmark of aging in peripheral and afferent axon action potential conduction velocity, which is related to declines in the density of unmyelinated and myelinated neurons. Most of the slowing occurs centrally, but sloughing of myelin has been demonstrated anatomically in peripheral nerves, which will certainly slow conduction velocity. It should be emphasized that most studies on changes in movement speed were performed on healthy individuals, not those with disease that would further affect movement speed. In addition, the potential blunting effects of many drugs have not been considered.

Although the aging of muscle is covered thoroughly elsewhere, it should be emphasized that another facet of age-related decline is neuronal atrophy throughout the central nervous system with a reduction of approximately 40% in the volume/size by 80 years of age.[107] Recent evidence suggests that age-related muscle weakness is not entirely explained by muscle atrophy but rather that the communication between the brain and skeletal muscles is impaired with advancing age.[108] Many neurologic changes associated with aging are mechanistically linked to impaired skeletal muscle function, and therefore, neuronal atrophy and axonal degeneration impact muscle loss and performance in aging adults.[108] Indeed, muscle is not the only tissue that experiences loss of innervation; innervation declines in all tissues, with far-reaching outcomes that affect the sympathetic, parasympathetic, sensory, and motor systems.

Before age-related decline begins, the reciprocal relationship of the parasympathetic and sympathetic nervous systems is delicately balanced and poised to participate in flight or fight, or rest and digest. With age, the balance of the parasympathetic and sympathetic nervous system output is altered (although poorly defined) and impacts the slowing of gastric motility (along with the enteric nervous system), possible issues with bladder control, hypertension and hypotension, and deficits in control of blood flow to and from the periphery.[109]

One of the most complex and poorly understood phenomena with aging is altered somatic sensory input.[110] It is common for vague symptoms of pain in one area of the body to represent a totally unrelated event. It is a tremendous challenge for physical therapists to discern if and when something is wrong with an older patient based on vague somatic complaints. Abdominal pain could reflect a host of possible issues ranging from simple indigestion to pancreatitis, cancer, intestinal obstruction, peritonitis, impending heart attack, or inguinal hernia. Back pain could reflect a simple muscle or joint irritation but could also reflect an abdominal aortic aneurysm, appendicitis, bladder infection, and cancer. Carefully noting these complaints is important, particularly if complaints are coupled with sudden change in function and sensorium, the emergence of fever, or an increase or sharpening of symptoms.

Box 3.4 summarizes physiological changes of the nervous system and impact on function.

Sensory Function

Peripheral sensory systems including the visual, proprioceptive, auditory, olfactory, tactile, and vestibular systems provide feedback from the environment that augments interaction with the external world. These sensory systems become impaired with age regardless of the presence of vascular disease or neuropathy, which can contribute to increased isolation and inability to connect with the outside world. Age-related reductions in visual function, including visual acuity, field of view, and contrast sensitivity, are universal in older individuals. Hearing is also well known to decline with age, with presbycusis a widespread phenomenon among individuals aged 80 and above.[111] Research has suggested that the loss in sensory function is a critical component of health and quality of life in aging adults. Visual impairment is correlated with depression,

BOX 3.4 Major Age-Related Changes in the Nervous System and Associated Clinical Consequences

Anatomic/ Physiological Changes	Clinical Consequences
Sloughing/loss of myelin	Slowed nerve conduction
Axonal loss	Fewer muscle fibers Loss of fine sensation
Autonomic nervous system dysfunction	Slower systemic function (e.g., cardiovascular, gastrointestinal) with altered sensory input
Loss of sensory neurons	Reduced ability to discern hot/cold, pain
Slowed response time (speed of reaction)	Increased risk of falls

poor quality of life, cognitive decline, and mortality.[112] In addition, hearing loss is associated with slower gait speed, poor cognition, and mortality.[113,114] Tactile perception declines with age owing to decreased nerve conduction velocity, change in specific types of corpuscles, and changes in the central nervous system, and is associated with cognitive decline.[115] Cross-sectional analysis of the Baltimore Longitudinal Study of Aging (BLSA) participants revealed that multiple sensory impairments reduced physical performance among individuals in middle-old age (ages 70 to 79).[116] Correia and associates used data from the National Social Life, Health, and Aging Project (NSHAP), a longitudinal population-based study of adults aged 57 to 85 years old, and found that multisensory impairment was prevalent in older U.S. adults, with 66% of individuals having two of more sensory deficits, 27% having one sensory impairment, and 6% having no sensory impairments.[117] These same investigators using the NSHAP database developed an integrated measure of sensory dysfunction called the Global Sensory Impairment and found that it predicted impaired physical function, cognitive dysfunction, significant weight loss, and mortality 5 years later in older adults. The authors concluded that multisensory evaluation may identify vulnerable older adults, offering the opportunity for early intervention to mitigate adverse outcomes.[118] It is important for physical therapists to identify sensory changes when working with older adults to understand how these changes impact physical function, quality of life, and their ability to interact in their environment so that adaptations can be made to maximize health outcomes. The reader is referred to elsewhere in this text for a more thorough discussion of the sensory changes with aging.

The Immune System

There are myriad theories postulated to explain the biology of aging. These theories are divided into two main groups: extrinsic or stochastic theories that propose that aging is caused by random damage to cell molecules such as DNA mutations, mitochondrial DNA, DNA repair mechanisms, free radical damage, oxidative stress, and overall wear and tear, and nonstochastic theories that focus on developmental-genetic theories such as replication of fibroblasts, telomerase enzymes, and genes that are associated with the reduction or increase of certain diseases. In reality, evidence suggests that both environmental factors and genetics impact the process of aging.[119] Although many of the current theories are likely to have some veracity, few of the current theories significantly impact physical therapy practice. Recently, however, one aspect of age-related decline emerged as a major contributor to the loss of muscle and organ reserve that has considerable importance for physical therapy. It is now evident that with advancing age, there is an increase in systemic inflammation because of changes in the immune system. Major increases in known proinflammatory cytokines such as interleukin 1, 6, and 10 (IL-1, IL-6, IL-10); C-reactive protein (CRP); and tumor necrosis factor–α (TNF-α) occur with advancing age, which is significantly associated with muscle wasting, obesity, and loss of physical function.[5,7,17,56,57,120,121] Not only do increased inflammatory cytokines result in muscle wasting, but also they diminish the function of other organ systems, which reduces reserve and shrinks the window of homeostasis. The increase in inflammatory cytokines is also associated with metabolic syndrome, which is a major risk factor for CVD.[122]

The increase in systemic inflammation is also an underlying factor in the development of age-related diseases such as Alzheimer disease, atherosclerosis, cancer, and diabetes.[18,120,123] Thus, it is hypothesized that controlling inflammatory status may allow for more successful aging.[8,124,125]

Four main approaches to the management of increased systemic inflammation have been considered: anti-inflammatory drugs, use of antioxidants through diet, caloric restriction, and exercise is far superior to the minimal impact noted from anti-inflammatory drugs and antioxidants.[18,126,127] One exercise bout results in a significant reduction in markers of inflammation such as IL-1, IL-6, and TNF-α and an increase in brain-derived neurotrophic factor (BDNF).[121,123,126] Cumulative exercise sessions further reduce inflammation, which should enable chronic exercisers to resist fatal infections and aggressive pathogens.[128] Men and women who are habitually physically active have less systemic inflammation than those who are sedentary, which may be the major reason for the enhanced well-being of exercisers, who also have a wider window of homeostasis. Because visceral fat secretes proinflammatory cytokines such as IL-1, IL-6, IL-10, CRP, and TNF-α, consistent physical activity can help reduce visceral fat accumulation, thereby reducing the inflammatory process, which impacts bone, muscle, and cardiovascular health.

These current findings suggest that physical therapy can play an important role in the management of systemic inflammation, enhancing systemic "reserve," reducing risk for disease, and delaying functional decline through the use of exercise. A prospective study of 19,000 participants in the Cooper Institute Aerobic Center in Dallas, Texas, found that higher midlife fitness levels were associated with lower hazards of developing all-cause dementia later in life (70 to 85 years old). The magnitude and direction of the association were similar with or without previous stroke, suggesting that higher fitness levels earlier in life may lower risk for dementia later in life, independent of cerebrovascular disease.[129]

The Hormonal Axis

One of the realities of aging is altered function of endocrine glands, decrease in hormone production, a loss in responsiveness of hormone target tissues, or multiple combinations.[130–132] The hypothalamic–pituitary–gonadal axis is a central endocrine gland regulator impacting body temperature, nutrient intake and energy balance, sleep/wakefulness cycles, sexual behavior, productive cycles, water and electrolyte balance, stress adaptation, and circadian cycles.[133] As a result, the hypothalamus is the master regulator of homeostasis as well as the source and target of continual regulatory adjustments during aging.[133] In women, alterations in stimulating hormones from the hypothalamus and anterior pituitary gland decrease ovarian estradiol output, which initiates the cessation of menses (menopause). Changes in males occur more slowly than in women with decreases in total and free testosterone (andropause).

Aging of the hypothalamic–pituitary–gonadal axis has clinical importance because a reduction in sex hormones negatively affects muscle and bone mass, visceral adipose tissue accumulation, insulin sensitivity, low-density lipoprotein (LDL) metabolism, libido, and cognition.[134] The loss of sex hormones has been determined to be a contributor to the reduction in muscle mass and, in particular, muscle strength.[135,136] Indeed, older hypogonadal men given testosterone replacement gain a significant amount of lean mass, although data suggest that the increase in mass is not accompanied by much strength change unless resistance exercise and testosterone are given together.[132]

Sipila and colleagues investigated 187 women aged 75 years old and determined that higher serum estradiol concentration and greater muscle strength were independently associated with a low incidence of fall-related limb fractures even after adjustment for bone density.[137] A recent study of postmenopausal twins, one of whom was on HRT while the other was not, has further substantiated estrogen effectiveness. The women taking HRT were between 5 and 15 years postmenopausal. Vertical jump height, fast gait, and grip strength were higher in the twin taking hormones. Curiously, knee extension strength was not greater.[136] HRT has been linked to clear cardiovascular benefits. A significant reduction in rates of CHD by 18% to 54% and an increase in life expectancy by 12% to 38% have been reported.[138]

Hormonal changes also impact water balance in aging adults, making them susceptible to dehydration. Vasopressin (antidiuretic hormone) secretion is increased, but the action in the collecting ducts is subnormal in the older adult, leading to increased urine flow rate, which, combined with decreased thirst, leads to an impaired ability to conserve water and reduction of plasma volme.[139] Aging also impacts the thyroid gland in addition to the amount of iodine intake in the diet. When the thyroid gland is underactive, fewer hormones are produced, which can reduce metabolism and cause symptoms such as weakness, fatigue, and weight gain. When the thyroid gland is overactive, there is an increase in cardiac arrhythmias and weight loss.

Replacement of one hormone may not be sufficient to overcome a specific deficit as hormones tend to work synergistically with each other. For example, testosterone has been shown to increase insulin-like growth factor-I (IGF-I), which stimulates protein synthesis in muscle.[135] If IGF-I levels are already low, however, then perhaps the utility of testosterone is limited. One investigator has recommended hormone replacement, particularly for men, as they lose muscle mass at a more rapid rate than women. His conclusion was that perhaps in future studies multiple hormones should be administered simultaneously as low values in one hormone are likely to reflect deficiencies in other hormones.[140] Hormone supplementation is still an evolving science, and future understanding of how hormones can influence health and well-being is expected in the future.

From a rehabilitative perspective, it is important to understand that the endocrine system undergoes significant alterations during aging that, combined with physiological changes in tissues and systems, impact function and subsequent treatment plans. Of particular note is the loss of muscle and bone mass that affects strength, power, and endurance; body temperature regulation; water and solute regulation; fatigue; and development of comorbidities such as diabetes, CVD, and increased adiposity.

EXERCISE FOR REVERSING DECLINE/PREVENTING DISEASE AND SEDENTARY LIFESTYLE

It is becoming evident that a lifestyle that includes consistent exercise/physical activity can be extremely influential in preventing physical decline and disease. Those who exercise regularly have fewer incidences of cardiovascular disease, osteoarthritis, diabetes, vascular disease, metabolic syndrome, and Alzheimer disease.[141] The exceptional strength of regular physical activity to improve health can be seen in individuals with established CVD. A recent meta-analysis confirmed the results of previous meta-analyses that exercise-based cardiac rehabilitation reduces cardiovascular mortality, reduces hospital admissions, and improves health-related quality of life.[142] Master athletes and habitual older exercisers represent a unique example of exceptional aging to maintain physical performance and function.

In the past three decades, there has been an increase in the number of master athletes (>40 years old) in endurance and ultra-endurance (>6 hours) events that has been accompanied by an improvement in their performance at a faster rate than younger athletes.[143] Although age-related declines in endurance performance have been well described in the literature, the improvement in the performance of master athletes has been steadily increasing and most impressive in the oldest age group categories (>60 years). Lee and associates compared runners and nonrunners and in the subset over 50 years old found significant reduction in adjusted risk of all-cause and cardiovascular mortality even in those individuals who ran 5 to 10 min/day at slow speeds <6 mph.[144] The Master Athletes Model represents a unique insight into viewing peak endurance performance and physiological functioning with increasing age.

Despite the plethora of benefits associated with regular physical activity (PA), only 41% of American adults achieve the minimum guidelines established by the American College of Sports Medicine (ACSM).[145] Individuals aged 55 years and older are more sedentary than their younger counterparts even when walking is considered, which is an activity that is popular among, and easily accessible for, older adults, with activity levels dropping lower with each subsequent aging decade.[146] Current ACSM guidelines recommend 150 minutes of moderate PA or 75 minutes of vigorous PA per week in bouts of 10 minutes; resistance exercise of major muscle groups two to three times per week; and flexibility exercise two to three times per week.[88] The research evidence underlying many of these recommendations demonstrates primary and secondary prevention of cardiovascular disease; reduction in all-cause mortality; reduction in breast and colon cancer; weight loss; improved bone, joint, and muscular fitness; reduction in the risk of falls and injuries, and prevention or mitigation of functional limitations in older adults with and without chronic disease.[88] No combinations of medications available today can replicate the benefits associated with consistent physical activity, prompting the ACSM to develop an initiative entitled "Exercise Is Medicine."

Occurring concurrently with decreased activity levels in adults is the increased time spent in sedentary activity, which has been demonstrated to be a risk factor for cardiovascular disease, type 2 diabetes mellitus, and all-cause mortality.[147,148] In developed economies, modern lifestyles are characterized by increased opportunities to be sedentary during work, commuting, and domestic life.[149] A recent systematic review and meta-analysis has demonstrated that increased sedentary time, *independent of physical activity,* is associated with an increased risk of CVD, all-cause mortality, type 2 diabetes mellitus, cancer incidence, and mortality.[150] The same authors also suggest that the "deleterious outcome effects associated with sedentary time generally decreased in magnitude among individuals who participated in higher levels of physical activity compared with lower levels."[150]

Is there a threshold for physical activity that is protective? Evidence suggests a dose–response benefit aspect for both resistance and cardiovascular training frequency, intensity, and duration (volume). For example, it is possible to gain strength with a stimulus that is 50% of one-repetition maximum (1RM); however, more strength is gained if the load is higher.[151] The same holds true for cardiovascular training; additional health benefits are gained with higher intensity, frequency, and duration. Several large-scale epidemiology studies have documented a dose–response relationship between cardiovascular training and risk of CVD, and premature mortality in both men and women.[152,153] The meta-analysis of Biswas found that the deleterious outcome effects associated with sedentary time decreased in magnitude among persons who participated in higher levels of physical activity compared with lower levels.[150] In all likelihood, there is a threshold of activity that is protective, but it differs from individual to individual based on genetics, natural endowment of muscle mass and cardiovascular capability, predisposition to disease based on family history, self-efficacy, soft-tissue integrity, and a host of other physiological and behavioral factors.

As movement specialists, it is important to understand that meeting the ACSM activity guidelines *and* decreasing sedentary time need to be viewed as separate but related interventions. This is especially important when working with lower-functioning individuals who already have decreased activity levels and are even more susceptible to the negative consequences of a sedentary lifestyle.

SUMMARY

Aging is an inevitable process and decline occurs across all tissues and systems. Nonetheless, with a thoughtful lifestyle approach, it is possible to prevent or attenuate the severity of some diseases and delay (possibly avoid) functional decline and frailty. Indeed, physical activity is the most potent tool of physical therapists to optimize function throughout the entire life span. Inactivity should be considered as much a contributor to impairments and loss of function as pathology or disease. Physical therapists can utilize the principles espoused in the physical stress theory to help guide the modulation of exercise for older adults to the appropriate level to achieve positive gains in tissue functioning and homeostasis, while avoiding both the tissue damages of excessively high stress and the physiological decline of inadequately low stress. It is appropriate for physical therapists to consider the impact of age-related changes on the rehabilitation and wellness plan for their older adult patients. However, physical therapists must take care not to underutilize active rehabilitation; rather, they need to adjust the rehabilitation to meet the unique needs of the older patient. Physical therapists should use their understanding of age- and disease-related changes in tissue functioning to focus a rehabilitation and wellness plan. This plan should be based on a careful examination of the specific impairments, tasks, and activities affecting function; an integration of all evaluation data (including patient goals and preferences) to inform prognosis; then careful targeting of the structures and tasks that can provide greatest functional gain; and finally determination of the intensity of the intervention to optimize positive adaptation to stress.

REFERENCES

1. Wagner KH, Cameron-Smith D, Wessner B, Franzke B. Biomarkers of aging: from function to molecular biology. *Nutrients*. 2016;8(6):338.
2. Scheike TH, Holst KK, Hjelmborg JB. Measuring early or late dependence for bivariate lifetimes of twins. *Lifetime Data Anal*. 2015;21(2):280–299.
3. Chakravarty EF, Hubert HB, Lingala VB, Fries JF. Reduced disability and mortality among aging runners: a 21-year longitudinal study. *Arch Intern Med*. 2008;168(15): 1638–1646.
4. Faulkner JA, Davis CS, Mendias CL, Brooks SV. The aging of elite male athletes: age-related changes in performance and skeletal muscle structure and function. *Clin J Sport Med*. 2008;18(6):501–507.
5. Buford TW, Cooke MB, Manini TM, et al. Effects of age and sedentary lifestyle on skeletal muscle NF-kappaB signaling in men. *J Gerontol A Biol Sci Med Sci*. 2010;65(5):532–537.
6. Lightfoot JT, De Geus JC, Booth FW, et al. Biological/genetic regulation of physical activity level: consensus from GenBioPac. *Med Sci Sports Exerc*. 2018;50(4):863–873.
7. Hsu FC, Kritchevsky SB, Liu Y, et al. Association between inflammatory components and physical function in the health, aging, and body composition study: a principal component analysis approach. *J Gerontol A Biol Sci Med Sci*. 2009;64(5):581–589.
8. Marzetti E, Lees HA, Wohlgelmuth SE, Leeuwenburgh C. Sarcopenia of aging: underlying cellular mechanisms and protection by caloric restriction. *Exp Gerontol*. 2010;45:138–148.
9. Lepers R, Stapley PJ. Master athletes are extending the limits of human endurance. *Front Phys*. 2016;7:613.
10. Binder EF, Yarasheski KE, Steger-May K, et al. Effects of progressive resistance training on body composition in frail older adults: results of a randomized, controlled trial. *J Gerontol A Biol Sci Med Sci*. 2005;60(11):1425–1431.
11. Bean JF, Kiely DK, LaRose S, et al. Increased velocity exercise specific to task training versus the National Institute on Aging's strength training program: changes in limb power and mobility. *J Gerontol A Biol Sci Med Sci*. 2009;64(9): 983–991.
12. Chodzko-Zajko WJ, Proctor DN, Fiatarone Singh MA, et al. Exercise and physical activity for older adults. *Med Sci Sports Exerc*. 2009;44(7):1510–1530.
13. Lomeli N, Bota DA, Davies KJA. Diminished stress resistance and defective adaptive homeostasis in age-related diseases. *Clin Sci*. 2017;131:2573–2599.
14. Mueller MJ, Maluf KS. Tissue adaptation to physical stress: a proposed "Physical Stress Theory" to guide physical therapist practice, education, and research. *Phys Ther*. 2002;82(4): 383–403.
15. Evans WJ. Skeletal muscle loss: cachexia, sarcopenia, and inactivity. *Am J Clin Nutr*. 2010;91(4):1123S–1127S.
16. Morley JE. Anorexia of ageing: a key component in the pathogenesis of both sarcopenia and cachexia. *J Cachexia Sarcopenia Muscle*. 2017;8:523–526.
17. Michaud M, Balardy L, Moulis G, et al. Proinflammatory cytokines, aging, and age-related diseases. *J Am Med Dir Assoc*. 2013;14:877–882.
18. Schaap LA, Pluijm SM, Deeg DJ, et al. Higher inflammatory marker levels in older persons: associations with 5-year change in muscle mass and muscle strength. *J Gerontol A Biol Sci Med Sci*. 2009;64(11):1183–1189.
19. Cruz-Jentoft AJ, Baeyens JP, Bauer JM, et al. Sarcopenia: European consensus on definition and diagnosis: report of the European Working Group on Sarcopenia in Older People. *Age Ageing*. 2010;39(4):412–423.
20. Baumgartner RN, Koehler KM, Gallagher D, et al. Epidemiology of sarcopenia among the elderly in New Mexico. *Am J Epidemiol*. 1998;147(8):755–763.
21. Patel HP, Syddall HE, Jameson K, et al. Prevalence of sarcopenia in community dwelling older people in the UK using the European Working Group on Sarcopenia in Older People definition: findings from the Hertfordshire cohort study (HCS). *Age Ageing*. 2013;42(3):378–384.
22. Cruz-Jentoft AJ, Landi F, Schneider SM, et al. Prevalence of and interventions for sarcopenia in ageing adults: a systematic review. Report of the International Sarcopenia Initiative, *Age Ageing*. 2014;43(6):748–759.
23. Lang T, Streeper T, Cawthon P, et al. Sarcopenia: etiology, clinical consequences, intervention, and assessment. *Osteoporos Int*. 2010;21(4):543–559.
24. Burton LA, Sumukadas D. Optimal management of sarcopenia. *Clin Interven*. 2010;5:217–228.
25. Russ DW, Gregg-Cornell K, Conaway MJ, Clark BC. Evolving concepts on the age-related changes in "muscle quality". *J Cachexia Sarcopenia Muscle*. 2012;3:95–109.
26. Chale A, Choutier GJ, Hau C, Phillips EM, Dallal GE, Fielding RA. Efficacy of whey protein supplementation on resistance exercise-induced changes in lean mass, muscle strength, and physical function in mobility-limited older adults. *J Gerontol A Biol Sci Med Sci*. 2013;68(6):682–690.
27. Centers for Disease Control and Prevention. Adults with disabilities: physical activity is for everybody. CDC Vital Signs. Atlanta: Centers for Disease Control and Prevention; 2014. https://www.cdc.gov/ncbddd/disabilityandhealth/pa.html. Accessed March 29, 2018.
28. Camacho PM, Petak SM, Binkley N, et al. American Association of Clinical Endocrinologists and American College of Endocrinology clinical practice guidelines for the diagnosis and treatment of postmenopausal osteoporosis. *Endocr Pract*. 2016;22(Suppl 4):1–42.
29. Management of osteoporosis in postmenopausal women. 2010 position statement of the North American Menopause Society. *Menopause*. 2010;17(1):25–54.
30. Recker RR, Lappe J, Davies K, Heaney R. Characterization of peri-menopausal bone loss: a prospective study. *J Bone Miner Res*. 2000;15:1965–1973.
31. Pouilles JM, Tremollieres F, Ribot C. Vertebral bone loss in peri-menopause: results of a 7-year longitudinal study. *Presse Med*. 1996;25:277–280.
32. Riggs BL, Melton LJ, Robb RA, et al. A population-based assessment of rates of bone loss at multiple skeletal sites: evidence for substantial trabecular bone loss in young adult women and men. *J Bone Miner Res*. 2008;23(2):205–214.
33. Frost HM. An approach to estimating bone and joint loads and muscle strength in living subjects and skeletal remains. *Am J Hum Biol*. 1999;11(4):437–455.
34. Cosman F, deBeur SJ, LeBoff MS, et al. Clinician's guide to prevention and treatment of osteoporosis. *Osteoporos Int*. 2014;25:2359–2381.
35. Khosla S. Update in male osteoporosis. *J Clin Endocrinol Metab*. 2010;95(1):3–10.
36. Vandenput L, Ohlsson C. Estrogens as regulators of bone health in men. *Nat Rev Endocrinol*. 2009;5(8):437–443.
37. Wright NC, Looker AC, Saag KG, et al. The recent prevalence of osteoporosis and low bone mass in the United States based on bone mineral density at the femoral neck or lumbar spine. *J Bone Min Res*. 2014;29(11):2520–2526.
38. Faulkner RA, Bailey DA. Osteoporosis: a pediatric concern. *Med Sport Sci* 2007;51:1–12.
39. Singer A, Exuzides A, Spangler L, et al. Burden of illness for osteoporotic fractures compared with other serious diseases among postmenopausal women in the United States. *Mayo Clin Proc*. 2015;90:53–62.

40. Sibonga JD, Evans HJ, Sung HG, et al. Recovery of spaceflight-induced bone loss: bone mineral density after long-duration missions as fitted with an exponential function. *Bone.* 2007;41(6):973–978.
41. Gomez-Cabello A, Ara I, Gonsalez-Aguero A, et al. Effects of training on bone mass in older adults: a systematic review. *Sports Med.* 2012;42(4):301–325.
42. Kelly GA, Kelly KS, Kohrt WM. Effects of ground and joint reaction force exercise on lumbar spine and femoral neck bone mineral density in postmenopausal women: a meta-analysis of randomized controlled trials. *BMC Musculoskelet Disord.* 2012;13:177.
43. Furrer R, van Schoor NM, de Haan A, Lips P, de Jongh RT. Gender-specific associations between physical functioning, bone quality, and fracture risk in older people. *Calcif Tissue Int.* 2014;94:522–530.
44. Villareal DT, Steger-May K, Schechtman K, et al. Effects of exercise training on bone mineral density in frail older women and men: a randomised controlled trial. *Age Ageing.* 2004;33(3):309–312.
45. Villareal DT, Binder EF, Yarasheski KE, et al. Effects of exercise training added to ongoing hormone replacement therapy on bone mineral density in frail elderly women. *J Am Geriatr Soc.* 2003;51(7):985–990.
46. Weiss EP, Shah K, Fontana L, et al. Dehydroepiandrosterone replacement therapy in older adults: 1– and 2–y effects on bone. *Am J Clin Nutr.* 2009;89(5):1459–1467.
47. Reid KF, Fielding RA. Skeletal muscle power: a critical determinant of physical functioning in older adults. *Exerc Sport Sci Rev.* 2012;40:4–12.
48. Kalyani RR, Corriere M, Ferrucci L. Age-related and disease-related muscle loss: the effects of diabetes, obesity, and other diseases. *Lancet.* 2014;2:819–829.
49. Mitchell WK, Williams J, Atherton P, Lavin M, Lund J, Narici M. Sarcopenia, dynapenia, and the impact of advancing age on human skeletal muscle size and strength; a quantitative review. *Front Physiol.* 2012;3:260.
50. Goodpaster BH, Parks SW, Harris TB, et al. The loss of skeletal muscle strength, mass and quality in older adults: the health, aging and body composition study. *J Gerontol A Biol Sci Med Sci.* 2006;61:1059–1064.
51. Nilwik R, Snijders T, Leenders M, et al. The decline in skeletal muscle mass with aging is mainly attributed to a reduction in type II muscle fiber size. *Exp Gerontol.* 2013;48:492–498.
52. Kent-Braun JA, Ng AV, Young K. Skeletal muscle contractile and noncontractile components in young and older women and men. *J Appl Physiol.* 2000;88:662–668.
53. Russ DW, Gregg-Cornell K, Conaway MJ, Clark BC. Evolving concepts on the age-related changes in "muscle quality". *J Cachexia Sarcopenia Muscle.* 2012;3:95–109.
54. Kragstrup TW, Kjaer M, Mackey AL. Structural, biochemical, cellular, and functional changes in skeletal muscle extracellular matrix with aging. *Scand J Med Sci Sports.* 2011;21:749–757.
55. Delmonico MJ, Harris TB, Visser M, et al. Longitudinal study of muscle strength, quality, and adipose tissue infiltration. *Am J Clin Nutr.* 2009;90:1579–1585.
56. Schaap LA, Pluijm SM, Deeg DJ, Visser M. Inflammatory markers and loss of muscle mass and strength. *Am J Med.* 2006;119:526.e9–526.e17.
57. Ilich JZ, Kelly OJ, Inglis JE, et al. Interrelationship among muscle, fat, and bone: connecting the dots on cellular, hormonal, and whole body levels. *Ageing Res Rev.* 2014;15:51–60.
58. Zhang P, Peterson M, Su GL, Wang SC. Visceral adiposity is negatively associated with bone density and muscle attenuation. *Am J Clin Nutr.* 2015;101:337–343.
59. Payne AM, Jimenez-Moreno R, Wang ZM, Messi ML, Delbono O. Role of Ca2+, membrane excitability, and Ca2+ stores in failing muscle contraction with aging. *Exp Gerontol.* 2009;44:261–273.
60. Conley KE, Jubrias SA, Esselman PC. Oxidative capacity and ageing in human muscle. *J Physiol.* 2000;526(Part1): 203–210.
61. Short KR, Bigelow ML, Kahl J, Singh R, Coenen-Schimke J. Decline in skeletal muscle mitochondrial function with aging in humans. *PNAS.* 2005;102:5618–5623.
62. Liu CJ, Latham NK. Progressive resistance strength training for improving physical function in older adults. *Cochrane Database Sys Rev.* 2009;3:CD002759.
63. Peterson MD, Rhea MR, Sen A, Gordon PM. Resistance exercise for muscular strength in older adults: a meta-analysis. *Ageing Res Rev.* 2010;9(3):226–237.
64. Peterson MD, Sen A, Gordon PM. Influence of resistance exercise on lean body mass in aging adults: a meta-analysis. *Med Sci Sport Exerc.* 2011;43(2):249–258.
65. Elia M, Ritz P, Stubbs RJ. Total energy expenditure in the elderly. *Eur J Clin Nutr.* 2000;54(Suppl 3):S92–S103.
66. Ogden CL, Carroll MD, Fryar CD, Flegal KM. Prevalence of obesity among adults and youth: United States 2011-2014. NCSH Data Brief. No. 219; November 2015. https://www.cdc.gov/nchs/data/databriefs/db219.pdf. Accessed April 13, 2018.
67. Centers for Disease Control and Prevention. Division of Nutrition, Physical Activity, Evaluation and Treatment of Overweight and Obesity in Adults. http://www.cdc.gov/obesity/causes/index.html. Accessed April 13, 2018.
68. Ilich JZ, Kelly OJ, Kim Y, Spicer MT. Low-grade chronic inflammation perpetuated by modern diet as a promoter of obesity and osteoporosis. *Arch Indust Hygiene Toxicol.* 2014;65:139–148.
69. Liu P-Y, Hornbuckle LM, Panton LB, Kim J-S, Ilich JZ. Evidence for the association between abdominal fat and cardiovascular risk factors in overweight and obese African American women. *J Am Coll Nutri.* 2012;31:126–132.
70. Racette SB, Evans EM, Weiss EP, et al. Abdominal adiposity is a stronger predictor of insulin resistance than fitness among 50–95 year olds. *Diabetes Care.* 2006;29(3):673–678.
71. Pratley RE, Hagberg JM, Dengel DR, et al. Aerobic exercise training-induced reductions in abdominal fat and glucose-stimulated insulin responses in middle-aged and older men. *J Am Geriatr Soc.* 2000;48(9):1055–1061.
72. Hurley BF, Hanson ED, Sheaff AK. Strength training as a countermeasure to aging muscle and chronic disease. *Sports Med.* 2011;41(4):289–306.
73. Kelly GA, Kelly KS. Impact of progressive resistance training on lipids and lipoproteins in adults: a meta-analysis of randomized controlled trials. *Prev Med.* 2009;48(1):9–19.
74. JafaiNasablan P, Inglis JE, Reilly W, Kelly OJ, Ilich JZ. Aging human body: changes in bone, muscle and body fat with consequent changes in nutrient intake. *J Endocrine.* 2017;234:R37–R51.
75. Vaughan-Thomas A, Dudhia J, Bayliss MT, et al. Modification of the composition of articular cartilage collagen fibrils with increasing age. *Connect Tissue Res.* 2008;49(5):374–382.
76. Hall DA. The ageing of connective tissue. *Exp Gerontol.* 1968;3 (2):77–89.
77. Freemont AJ, Hoyland JA. Morphology, mechanisms and pathology of musculoskeletal ageing. *J Pathol.* 2007;211:252–259.
78. Frobin W, Brinckmann P, Kramer M, et al. Height of lumbar discs measured from radiographs compared with degeneration and height classified from MR images. *Eur Radiol.* 2001;11:263–269.
79. Barros EM, Rodrigues CJ, Rodrigues NR, et al. Aging of the elastic and collagen fibers in the human cervical interspinous ligaments. *Spine J.* 2002;2:57–62.

80. North BJ, Sinclair DA. The intersection between aging and cardiovascular disease. *Circ Res.* 2012;110:1097–1108.
81. Heidenreich PA, Trogdon JG, Khavjou OA, et al. Forecasting the future of cardiovascular disease in the United States: a policy statement from the American Heart Association. *Circulation.* 2011;123:933–944.
82. Huang G, Gibson CA, Tran ZV, Osness WH. Controlled endurance exercise training and Vo2max changes in older adults: a meta-analysis. *Prev Cardiol.* 2005;8(4):217–225.
83. Gellis RL, Goslin BR, Olson RE. Longitudinal modeling of the relationship between age and maximal heart rate. *Med Sci Sports Exerc.* 2007;39(5):822–829.
84. Zhu N, Suarez-Lopez JR, Sidney S, et al. Longitudinal examination of age-predicted symptom-limited exercise maximum HR. *Med Sci Sports Exerc.* 2010;42(8): 1519–1527.
85. Goldspink DF, George KP, Chantler PD, et al. A study of presbycardia, with gender differences favoring ageing women. *Int J Cardiol.* 2009;137(3):236–245.
86. Vaitkevicius PV, Fleg JL, Engel JH, et al. Effects of age and aerobic capacity on arterial stiffness in healthy adults. *Circulation.* 1993;88(4 Pt 1):1456–1462.
87. Lakatta EG, Levy D. Arterial and cardiac aging: major stakeholders in cardiovascular disease enterprises: part II: the aging heart: links to heart disease. *Circulation.* 2003;107 (2):346–354.
88. Riebe D. *ACSM's Guidelines for Exercise Testing and Prescription.* 10th ed. Philadelphia: Wolters-Kluwer; 2018: 81,162,168,171,5–8.
89. Fleg JL, Morrell CH, Bos AG, et al. Accelerated longitudinal decline of aerobic capacity in healthy adults. *Circulation.* 2005;112(5):674–682.
90. Weiss EP, Spina RJ, Holloszy JO, Ehsani AA. Gender differences in the decline in aerobic capacity and its physiological determinants during the later decades of life. *J Appl Physiol.* 2006;101(3):938–944.
91. Steffl M, Bohannon RW, Sontakova L, Tufano JJ, Shiells K, Holmerova I. Relationship between sarcopenia and physical activity in older people: a systematic review and meta-analysis. *Clin Inter Aging.* 2017;12:835–845.
92. Lakatta EG, Levy D. Arterial and cardiac aging: major shareholders in cardiovascular disease enterprises: part I: aging arteries: a "set-up" for vascular disease. *Circulation.* 2003;107(1):139–146.
93. Franzoni F, Galetta F, Morizzo C, et al. Effects of age and physical fitness on microcirculatory function. *Clin Sci (Lond).* 2004;106(3):329–335.
94. Miro O, Barrientos A, Alonso JR, et al. Effects of general anaesthetic procedures on mitochondrial function of human skeletal muscle. *Eur J Clin Pharmacol.* 1999;55(1):35–41.
95. Magaziner J, Hawkes W, Hebel JR, et al. Recovery from hip fracture in eight areas of function. *J Gerontol A Biol Sci Med Sci.* 2000;55(9):M498–M507.
96. Albert CM, Mittleman MA, Chae CU, Lee IM, Hennekens CH, Manson JE. Triggering of sudden death from cardiac causes by vigorous exertion. *Med Sci Sports Exerc.* 2000;32(Suppl 9):1355–1361.
97. Whang W, Manson JE, Hu FB, et al. Physical exertion, exercise, and sudden cardiac death in women. *JAMA.* 2006;295 (12):1399–1403.
98. American College of Sports Medicine, American Heart Association. Exercise and acute cardiovascular events: placing the risks into perspective. *Med Sci Sports Exerc.* 2007;39 (5):886–897.
99. Franklin BA, McCullough P. Cardiorespiratory fitness: an independent and additive marker of risk stratification and health outcomes. *Mayo Clin Proc.* 2009;84(9):776–779.
100. Verdu E, Ceballos D, Vilches JJ, Navarro X. Influence of aging on peripheral nerve function and regeneration. *J Peripher Nerv Syst.* 2005;5:191–208.
101. Rivner MH, Swift TR, Malik K. Influence of age and height on nerve conduction. *Muscle Nerve.* 2001;24:1134–1141.
102. Brown WF, Strong MJ, Snow R. Methods for estimating number of motor units in biceps-brachialis muscles and losses of motor units with aging. *Muscle Nerve.* 1988;11:423–432.
103. Reid KF, Fielding RA. Skeletal muscle power: a critical determinant of physical functioning in older adults. *Exerc Sport Sci Rev.* 2012;40:4–12.
104. Connelly DM, Rice CL, Roos MR, Vandervoort AA. Motor unit firing rates and contractile properties in tibialis anterior of young and old men. *J Appl Physiol.* 1999;1999 (87):843–852.
105. Wojcik LA, Thelen DG, Schultz AB, et al. Age and gender differences in single-step recovery from a forward fall. *J Gerontol A Biol Sci Med Sci.* 1999;54(1):M44–M50.
106. Tarawneh R, Galvin JE. Neurologic signs in the elderly. In: Fillit HM, Rockwood K, Woodhouse K, eds. *Brocklehurst's Textbook of Geriatric Medicine and Gerontology.* 7th ed. Philadelphia: Saunders; 2010:101–105.
107. Ward NS. Compensatory mechanisms in the aging motor system. *Ageing Res Rev.* 2006;5:239–254.
108. Manini TM, Hong SL, Clark BC. Aging and muscle: a neuron's perspective. *Curr Opin Nutr Metab Care.* 2013;16:21–26.
109. Phillips RJ, Walter GC, Powley TL. Age-related changes in vagal afferents innervating the gastrointestinal tract. *Auton Neurosci.* 2010;153(1–2):90–98.
110. Yun AJ, Lee PY, Bazar KA. Many diseases may reflect dysfunctions of autonomic balance attributable to evolutionary displacement. *Med Hypotheses.* 2004;62 (6):847–851.
111. Lin FR, Niparko JK, Ferrucci L. Hearing loss prevalence in the United States. *Arch Intern Med.* 2011;171(20):1851–1852.
112. Wang JJ, Mitchell P, Simpson JM, et al. Visual impairment, age-related cataract, and mortality. *Arch Ophthalol.* 2001;119:1186–1190.
113. Li L, Simonsick EM, Ferrucci L, et al. Hearing loss and gait speed among older adults in the United States. *Gait Posture.* 2013;38:25–29.
114. Genther DJ, Betz J, Pratt S, et al. Association of hearing impairment and mortality in older adults. *J Gerontol Ser A Biol Sci Med Sci.* 2014;70A:85–90.
115. Yang J, Ogasa T, Ohta Y, et al. Decline of human tactile angle discrimination in patients with mild cognitive impairment and Alzheimer's disease. *J Alzheimer's Dis.* 2010;22:225–234.
116. Gadkaree SK, Sun DQ, Li C, et al. Does sensory function decline independently or concomitantly with age? Data from the Baltimore Longitudinal Study of Aging. *J Aging Res.* 2016;2016:1–8.
117. Correia C, Lopez KJ, Wroblewski KE, et al. Global sensory impairment in older adults in the United States. *J Am Geriatr Soc.* 2016;64:306–313.
118. Pinto JM, Wroblewski KE, Huisingh-Scheetz M, et al. Global sensory impairment predicts morbidity and mortality in older U.S. adults. *J Am Geriatr Soc.* 2017;65:2587–2595.
119. Lange J, Grossman S. Theories of aging. In: Mauk KL, ed. *Gerontological Nursing Competencies for Care.* 2nd ed. Sudbury, MA: Janes & Bartlett; 2009:50–73.
120. Kalogeropoulos A, Georgiopoulou V, Psaty BM, et al. Inflammatory markers and incident heart failure risk in older adults: the Health ABC (Health, Aging, and Body Composition) study. *J Am Coll Cardiol.* 2010;55(19): 2129–2137.

121. Freund A, Orjalo AV, Desprez PY, Campisi J. Inflammatory networks during cellular senescence: causes and consequences. *Trends Mol Med.* 2010;16(5):238–246.
122. Licastro F, Candore G, Lio D, et al. Innate immunity and inflammation in ageing: a key for understanding age-related diseases. *Immun Ageing.* 2005;2:8.
123. Chung HY, Cesari M, Anton S, et al. Molecular inflammation: underpinnings of aging and age-related diseases. *Ageing Res Rev.* 2009;8(1):18–30.
124. Opalach K, Rangaraju S, Madorsky I, et al. Lifelong calorie restriction alleviates age-related oxidative damage in peripheral nerves. *Rejuvenation Res.* 2010;13(1):65–74.
125. Dirks Naylor AJ, Leeuwenburgh C. Sarcopenia: the role of apoptosis and modulation by caloric restriction. *Exerc Sport Sci Rev.* 2008;36(1):19–24.
126. Zoico E, Rossi A, Di Francesco V, et al. Adipose tissue infiltration in skeletal muscle of healthy elderly men: relationships with body composition, insulin resistance, and inflammation at the systemic and tissue level. *J Gerontol A Biol Sci Med Sci.* 2010;65(3):295–299.
127. Calvani R, Miccheli A, Landi F, et al. Current nutritional recommendations and novel dietary strategies to manage sarcopenia. *J Frailty Aging.* 2013;2:38–53.
128. Witkowski S, Hagberg JM. Progenitor cells and age: can we fight aging with exercise? *J Appl Physiol.* 2007;102 (3):834–835.
129. DeFina LF, Willis BL, Radford NB, et al. The association between midlife cardiorespiratory fitness levels and later life dementia. *Ann Intern Med.* 2013;158:162–168.
130. Roubenoff R. Physical activity, inflammation, and muscle loss. *Nutr Rev.* 2007;65(12 Pt 2):S208–S212.
131. Roddam AW, Appleby P, Neale R, et al. Association between endogenous plasma hormone concentrations and fracture risk in men and women: the EPIC-Oxford prospective cohort study. *J Bone Miner Metab.* 2009;27 (4):485–493.
132. Sattler FR, Castaneda-Sceppa C, Binder EF, et al. Testosterone and growth hormone improve body composition and muscle performance in older men. *J Clin Endocrinol Metab.* 2009;94(6):1991–2001.
133. Diamanti-Kandarakis E, Dattilo M, Macut D, et al. Aging and anti-aging: a combo-endocrinology overview. *Eur J Endocr.* 2017;176:R283–R308.
134. Faubion SS, Kuhle CL, Shuster LT, Rocca WA. Long-term health consequences of premature or early menopause and considerations of premature or early menopause and considerations for management. *Climacteric.* 2015;18: 483–491.
135. Bhasin S. The brave new world of function-promoting anabolic therapies: testosterone and frailty. *J Clin Endocrinol Metab.* 2010;95(2):509–511.
136. Ronkainen PH, Kovanen V, Alen M, et al. Postmenopausal hormone replacement therapy modifies skeletal muscle composition and function: a study with monozygotic twin pairs. *J Appl Physiol.* 2009;107(1):25–33.
137. Sipila S, Heikkinen E, Cheng S, et al. Endogenous hormones, muscle strength, and risk of fall-related fractures in older women. *J Gerontol A Biol Sci Med Sci.* 2006;61(1):92–96.
138. Mikkola TS, Tuomikoski P, Lyytinen H, et al. Estradiol-based postmenopausal hormone therapy and risk of cardiovascular and all-cause mortality. *Menopause.* 2015;22:976–983.
139. Tian Y, Serino R, Verbalis JG. Downregulation of renal vasopressin V2 receptor and aquaporin-2 expression parallels age-associated defects in urine concentration. *Am J Physiol Renal Physiol.* 2004;287:F797–F805.
140. Morley JE. Developing novel therapeutic approaches to frailty. *Curr Pharm Des.* 2009;15(29):3384–3395.
141. Physical Activity Guidelines Advisory Committee. Physical Activity Guidelines Advisory Committee Report. Washington. DC: U.S. Department of Health and Human Services; 2008.
142. Anderson L, Oldridge N, Thompson DR, et al. Exercise-based cardiac rehabilitation for coronary heart disease. *J Am Coll Cardiol.* 2016;67:1–12.
143. Zaryski C, Smith DJ. Training principles and issues for ultra-endurance athletes. *Curr Sports Med Rep.* 2005;43:165–170.
144. Lee DC, Pate RR, Lavie CJ, et al. Leisure-time running reduces all-cause and cardiovascular mortality risk. *J Am Coll Cardiol.* 2014;64:472–481.
145. Zhao G, Li C, Ford ES. Leisure-time aerobic physical activity, muscle-strengthening activity and mortality risks among US adults: the NHANES linked mortality study. *Br J Sports Med.* 2014;48:244–249.
146. Centers for Disease Control and Prevention. Vital signs: walking among adults—United States, 2005 and 2010. *Morb Mortal Wkly Rep.* 2012;61:595–601.
147. Dunstan DW, Barr ELM, Healy GN, et al. Television viewing time and mortality: the AusDiab Study. *Circulation.* 2010;121:384–391.
148. Grontved A, Hu F. Television viewing and risk of type 2 diabetes, cardiovascular disease, and all-cause mortality: a meta-analysis. *JAMA.* 2011;305:2448–2455.
149. Stamatakis E, Hamer M, Dunstan DW. Screen-based entertainment time, all-cause mortality and cardiovascular events: population-based study with ongoing mortality and hospital events follow up. *J Am Coll Cardiol.* 2011;57:292–299.
150. Biswas A, Oh PI, Faulkner GE, et al. Sedentary time and its association with risk for disease incidence, mortality, and hospitalization in adults. *Ann Intern Med.* 2015;162: 123–132.
151. Bamman MM. The exercise dose response: key lessons from the past. *Am J Physiol Endocrinol Metab.* 2008;294(2): E230–E231.
152. Naci H, Ioannidis J. Comparative effectiveness of exercise and drug interventions on mortality outcomes: meta-epidemiological study. *BMJ.* 2013;347:f5577.
153. Yu S, Yarnell JW, Sweetman PM, Murray L. What level of physical activity protects against premature death? The Caerphilly study. *Heart.* 2003;89(5):502–506.

CHAPTER

4

Psychosocial Aspects of Aging

Susan Wenker, PT, PhD, Daniel Liebzeit, PhD, RN

OUTLINE

INTRODUCTION

An older adult's psychosocial context can affect the care received by health care providers, specifically physical therapists. Physical therapists are better positioned to provide quality interventions when the "whole" person is assessed, not just the physical impairments and limitations in activities alone. This chapter addresses several psychosocial considerations for the aging adult that can inform the therapist about the psychosocial context of the individual.

PSYCHOSOCIAL THEORIES

Historical Perspective

Carl Jung's work on aging during the 1920s and 1930s may be viewed as the most significant forerunner of modern gerontological thinking.[1] He identified late life as a process of psychologically turning inward. Two contrasting theories existed in the 1960s: activity theory[2] and disengagement theory.[3]

Activity theory stated that aging successfully meant maintaining middle-aged activities and attitudes into later adulthood, which seemed to capture the desire of aging individuals.[2] Disengagement theory, on the other hand, meant that a person aging successfully would want, over time, to disengage from an active life.[3] These two theories, which remained popular until recently, were followed by Neugarten's theory, which postulates that personality is the element that predicts successful aging.[4,5] Coping style, prior ability to adapt, and expectations of life as well as income, health, social interactions, freedoms, and constraints were all seen as part of the coalescence of personality and thus played into the complexity of successful aging.[6]

More recently, Rowe and Kahn developed their three-factor model. which added social adjustment and engagement to health and cognitive functioning, to define successful aging.[7,8] Erickson's[9] seventh stage of the life span, generativity versus stagnation, proposes that challenges involve successful mastery of work life, creative activity, and raising a family, all involving contributions to the next generation. The eighth and final stage, integrity versus despair, involves an evaluation of one's life as having been fulfilling and satisfying. Ego despair results when one views his or her life as a failure or unproductive, causing depression, anger, and finding fault with oneself and the surrounding world.[10]

Another influential theory often associated with Erickson's is Robert Peck's tasks of ego integrity.[11] This theory is about ego differentiation, body transcendence, and ego transcendence, which involves overcoming physical limitations and emphasizing compensating rewards of one's cognitive, social, and emotional life. It refers to the positive anticipation of death through legacy building and coping with life's challenges in a positive and constructive manner. Baltes and Baltes recognized human choice and agency,[12] as did Kahana and Kahana in their proactivity theory.[13] Similarly, Tornstam's developmental theory of positive aging, termed *gerotranscendence*, focuses on legacy building and existential concerns and counteracts erroneous projection of midlife values, activity patterns, and expectations into old age.[14]

The socioemotional selectivity theory of Carstensen and associates applies to models of successful aging.[15] This theory suggests that older adults prioritize emotional goals and adjust emotional regulation and social interaction to maximize positive experiences as they confront increasingly limited time left in life. Baltes and Baltes in their selective optimization with compensation theory describe how personal goals are flexibly adjusted in reaction to age-related losses.[12]

Another relevant theory is the terror management theory, which argues that an awareness of one's eventual death creates existential terror; one way to manage this terror is by affirming cultural worldviews.[16] In doing so, one achieves some immortality, which is consistent with the belief that a person's spirit will remain in the same culture after death. Old age can be viewed as where future time is perceived as more limited and/or mortality is made salient, but one can derive emotional meaning from life through affirming and internalizing the values of one's culture.[17]

Mainstream Theory

The life course theory is the mainstream theory of today[18] and is often used interchangeably with terms such as *life span*, *life history*, and *life cycle*.[19] However, distinct features of the life course exist. The theory contextualizes aging based on birth cohort, major social events, and personal factors. Experiences include macro-level or societal situations and micro-level or personal situations. Macro-level societal experiences include historical events and situations that broadly influenced society. These events, such as the Great Depression, World War II, the women's movement, and the Twin Tower bombing on September 11, 2001 (9/11), affect impressionable younger children differently than adults, called a cohort effect. For example, the millennials who experienced the effects of 9/11 may place their trust more in the government to keep them safe, as opposed to the baby boomer cohort, who developed a mistrust of the government in response to the Vietnam War.

Another example of the effect of history on aging is the sociopolitical context of the gay movement. This era created a social stigma for lesbian, gay, or bisexual (LGB) identity and a lack of equal legal rights for same-sex couples and LGB individuals. These constraints have limited the actions of older LGB adults over their life course.[19,20] Additionally, lesbian, gay, bisexual, or transgender (LGBT) people who grew up in the McCarthy era, when homosexuality was severely stigmatized and when the *Diagnostic and Statistical Manual of Mental Disorders* (DSM) labeled homosexuality a sociopathic personality disorder (later removed in 1973), have a different viewpoint when compared with LGBT people who aged during the late 1960s and 1970s when society started to demonstrate an increased level of openness for people who are different than mainstream.[21]

Micro-level situations include the family unit and social constructs occurring within each family. For example, in earlier generations, parents died when their children were young adults or teenagers. Yet today many older adults are living well into their 80s and possibly into their 90s. Therefore, families experience longer relationships, positive and negative, between children, grandchildren, and parents. These relationships can create purpose for the older adult, perhaps as a caregiver while contributing to the family unit. However, older adults vary in the degree to which they are capable of meeting additional emotional, financial, and social distress brought about by these extended familial relationships (Box 4.1).

Applying the life course theory to patient care provides insights into patients' backgrounds, social determinants of health, and life course. Physical therapists can improve patient-centered care with this knowledge. The history portion of the exam may enlighten the therapist to the

BOX 4.1 Life Transition Example

Take the case of Betty and Rachel. Betty is moving from a home where she raised her family to an assisted living setting secondary to failing health related to chronic obstructive pulmonary disorder (COPD). Betty has her two adult children and grandchildren living in the area and they visit her at least once a week. Betty has survived two major life events: her husband's deployment and the death of a child in a motor vehicle accident (MVA). Betty is saddened about moving but feels supported by her family.

Rachel is experiencing this same move but is grieving the loss of the family home. Rachel had one child who lives in a different state and now is unable to see her grandchildren because of her health. Additionally, she has experienced very few negative life events and was raised in a financially secure, upper-middle class family. She has become isolated secondary to the COPD and inability to get outside of her home, thus limiting her social support systems. The loss of her home and independence contribute to loneliness. Rachel feels a mix of emotions including anger and sadness as a result of these changes.

A few months pass, and Betty falls at the assisted living center. Betty's family visits her in the hospital, assists with her return to the assisted living facility, and facilitates the provision of physical therapy in the home. Rachel also falls at the center but relies on the community and hospital social worker to facilitate her admission to the hospital and discharge back to the assisted living facility. Betty is excited for physical therapy as she will return to visiting her friends and family. Rachel, on the other hand, lacks interest in receiving physical therapy as she is uncertain of the benefits, fearing she will fall again. The lack of social support predominates Rachel's rehabilitation and contributes to her disengagement from rehabilitation.

struggles and successes each patient has experienced. An appreciation for the patient's experiences, support networks, personality, and preexisting and potential mental health conditions can facilitate the appropriate administration of physical therapy interventions and appropriate referral to a social worker or other mental health specialist should one be needed and desired.

SUCCESSFUL AGING

Therapists' and older adults' concepts of successful aging are informed by the aforementioned theories. Older adults' conceptualization of successful aging impacts their expectations and perceptions in receiving care. Thus, it is important to understand how philosophers/scientists and patients think about and define successful aging.

The concept of successful aging has intrigued philosophers and scientists for many years.[6] The term was first introduced in the scientific literature in 1961 by Robert J. Havinghurst, in which he states that the science of gerontology has the practical purpose of "adding life to the years," with the goal of increasing enjoyment and satisfaction during the latter stages of an individual's life span.[22] Since then, many models and definitions have emerged, and the most relevant to physical therapists are discussed next.

In the biopsychosocial model, biological and psychosocial concepts are integrated. For example, one of the most widely accepted and applied models is the Rowe and Kahn model of successful aging, defined as avoiding disease and disability, and maintaining high cognitive and physical function and engagement with life.[7] However, many do not experience all aspects of a positive aging process. Many people age "successfully" by adapting to adverse health conditions. Additionally, the biopsychosocial model does not take the individual's perspective into consideration, which becomes increasingly important in those nearing 100 years of age.[23] Expanding on Rowe and Kahn's three domains of successful aging, Baltes and Baltes highlighted the importance of psychological and behavioral strategies and presented successful aging as an adaptive process of selection, optimization, and compensation strategies.[12] It encompasses subjective and objective criteria, explicitly recognizing individual and cultural variation.[12] Kahana and Kahana's theory of proactivity acknowledges that older adults are likely to face normative stressors of chronic illness, social losses, and lack of person–environment fit.[13] However, maintenance of a good quality of life, according to this theory, is possible when elders call upon internal coping resources and external social resources.[10] Proactive behavioral adaptations can include health promotion, helping others, and planning ahead along with marshaling support, role substitution, and environmental modifications. Therefore, successful aging can be viewed as both an outcome and a process with subjective and objective elements.[10]

Definitions of successful aging have drawn criticism when values of older people are not taken into consideration. For example, three themes consistently emerged (good health, satisfaction/happiness, and keeping active) in a study of older Canadian men.[24] In this same study, 83% of the participants felt that they had aged successfully.[24] In a study of centenarians, self-ratings demonstrated that 46.5% of older adults felt successful and reported either having good, very good, or excellent health, despite not being objectively considered as so.[23,25] In a study by Cho et al., about half of all centenarians in the Georgia Centenarian Study could be classified as successful agers if definitions of subjective health, perceived happiness, and better-perceived economic status were used in definitions of successful aging.[26] In contrast, none of the centenarians would be classified as "successful" when Rowe and Kahn's criteria were used. The aforementioned studies demonstrate the need to consider individuals' values and perception of their aging as well as objective criteria. It has been otherwise stated that "Healthy centenarians do not exist, but autonomous centenarians do."[27]

Although the biopsychological definition that incorporates both a subjective and an economic component is popular, there is no simple, agreed-upon definition of successful aging. The inclusion of subjective information (e.g., perceived quality of life and happiness) seems to be especially valuable for long-lived individuals who often have declines in physical health. Adaptation and resilience appear to be relevant, yet underappreciated, aspects of successful aging. Perhaps successful aging should ultimately be about what older adults value, rather than idealizing health based on levels of physical and physiologic function observed in younger individuals.[28] For instance, a survey of 53 older adult men from New Jersey revealed that social relationships and supports, positive life satisfaction, and perceived good health may also be important aspects of successful aging, in addition to physical activity and health.[29]

Further, successful aging includes the capacity to function across many domains (physical, functional, cognitive, emotional, social, and spiritual) to one's satisfaction and in spite of one's medical conditions. Thus, successful aging requires adaptation to changes (e.g., illness and life events such as relocation) throughout life. These experiences contribute to development of resiliency. Successful aging is influenced by an individual's personality, attitudes, self-determination, and resilience. Having realistic yet optimistic expectations of aging as a younger person also contributes to successful aging. A person is more likely to embrace the changes that accompany aging if a positive attitude about aging is cultivated as a younger person. As an example, optimism predicted better success before, during, and after heart surgery in the elderly.[30]

Although successful aging is an individually perceived state, research has identified five factors that interact to produce successful aging: life satisfaction (a sense of having a rewarding life with few regrets), a social support system, good physical and mental health, financial security, and control over one's life. Those who feel well supported by others will demonstrate more positive health behaviors including exercising, better nutritional habits, and decreased risky behaviors such as smoking and alcohol use.[31,32] Alternatively, depressive symptoms are associated with having smaller social networks, less social support, and fewer close relationships.[33,34] A certain amount of financial security provides a sense of peace and lack of worry that an uncertain financial situation can bring. Lastly, personal control that allows some independence and dignity can produce a sense of self-worth that contributes to successful aging and can predict longevity.[35–37] Considering the psychosocial factors of an individual when providing physical therapy may help to maximize therapeutic outcomes and relationships. For the purposes of this chapter, we consider successful aging a framework from which physical therapists can assess psychosocial aspects of the older patient.

Cultural Influences

An additional element for consideration when defining successful aging is the influence of culture (Box 4.2). Individual cultures have unique understandings within each community and interact in different ways to promote or detract from the concept of aging successfully.[38] For example, individuals in more independent cultures learn to value personal autonomy and uniqueness from birth, whereas individuals in more interdependent cultures learn to see themselves embedded within social units and to prioritize the needs of the group over their own.[17] Eastern countries may be characterized by family and social relations that promote open-mindedness and tolerance, whereas in Western countries, activity, engagement, and vitality are more likely to be associated with successful aging.[38] Consistent with life span developmental theories, Fung posits that as people age, they shape their world in ways that maximize their well-being, but do so within the confines and definitions of their respective cultures.[17]

In a multicultural study on successful aging, Fry found commonalities as well as differences across cultures, with declining health and functionality emerging as the singular most important factor detracting from aging well.[38] However, comparative research has also revealed the importance of compensatory mechanisms for age-related functional decline, such as control of wealth, people, and knowledge, and how these factors facilitate well-being later in life. These characteristics take on more or less importance in different cultures.

Individual variation also plays into cultural values. For example, one set of immigrant grandparents may refuse to speak with their American-born grandchildren in their original language in order to help them learn English. Another set of immigrant grandparents may immerse their American-born grandchildren in their home culture by only speaking their original language or through culturally related meals and rituals.

The influence of culture is particularly relevant with the increase of diversity across the United States. African Americans, Native Americans, Asian Americans and Pacific Islanders, and Hispanics make up the four standard major groups, with the largest migration occurring from Latin America and Asia.[21] Immigrants tend to be of a younger age, and aging immigrants tend to live with their children because of limited financial resources, because of a preference to live with an aging loved one, and to assist in caring for older adults as they age.[39] In general, compared to 1965, the number of older immigrants (65 + years old) is decreasing.[40] Yet, younger immigrants are aging and, upon becoming U.S. citizens, bringing their aged parents to the United States to live with them. This relationship is often beneficial to both groups as older adults provide care for grandchildren and, at times, assist with financial concerns.[41]

BOX 4.2 Examples of Cultural Influences

An understanding of basic cultural tendencies or predispositions, along with an appreciation for each patient's and family's individuality, can make communication with patients and families more effective and respectful. The following are specific examples of cultural tendencies and predispositions that can inform the most effective communication and care.

One example is that of patients from China. They may perceive that a person's behavior is a reflection on the family.[251] Thus, the patient may be very compliant with the exercises to avoid disgracing the family, even though the patient may be disinterested in exercise. A second example is that of older individuals in Asian cultures. Most elders believe it is the duty of the child to take care for the elder in return for the years of the elder taking care of the child. Patients from India and Pakistan may resist diagnoses of severe emotional distress or cognitive impairments because it reflects badly on the family (perhaps affecting the odds of other family members getting married). Patient cultural humility,[251] awareness that one can learn from another, can be enhanced by asking questions and researching the literature to increase understanding of cultural backgrounds.

Personality

Personality has been considered as a potential explanatory mechanism for longevity and a healthy aging process.[42] Personality is often described in terms of the big five personalities: extraversion, agreeableness, conscientiousness, neuroticism, and openness to experience. Personality changes can be categorized through the completion of personality profiles. These profiles may use a variety of methods to characterize a person's personality. A common personality profile is the Myers-Briggs Type Indicator.[43,44] Except for neuroticism, the four Myers-Briggs categories correlate with the big five personalities. Table 4.1 provides a summary of the big five personalities and a comparison to the Myers-Briggs Personality

TABLE 4.1 Summary of the Big Five Personality Traits[43,44]

Trait	Characteristic	Myers-Briggs Type Indicator
Extraversion	Energetic approach toward social interactions; likely to seek leadership roles and have positive emotions	Extraversion–introversion
Agreeableness	Altruistic, trusting, works better in groups, higher risk for interpersonal problems	Thinking–feeling
Conscientiousness	Thinks before acts, delayed gratification, arrives early or on time for appointments	Thinking–feeling and judging–perceiving
Neuroticism	Feels anxious, sad and tense, experiences job burnout yet feels committed to work	N/A
Openness	Learns something just for the joy of learning, has many years of education, conservative attitudes	Extraversion–introversion Thinking–feeling Judging–perceiving Sensing–intuitive

Indicators. For example, a person with an extroverted personality tends to be more outgoing and seek leadership roles, whereas someone with higher neuroticism tends to feel more anxious and less optimistic.

Personality can be assessed several ways: mean-level change, rank-order consistency, structural consistency, and individual differences.[45,46] When focusing on mean-level changes and individual differences, personality tends to change in midadulthood, but older adults maintain this personality change into older age.[45,46] For example, conscientiousness tends to increase in middle adulthood, perhaps because of the demands of child-rearing, but then levels off after age 40.[43] Findings regarding personality changes may vary depending on the way in which they are assessed.

Physical health affects personality, specifically in adults older than 80.[45] Older adults who are more active demonstrate less pronounced changes in consciousness, extraversion, and openness.[47] Alternatively, poor physical health predicts declines in the degree of extraversion and openness in later life.[48] Presence of chronic disease can lead to a decrease in emotional stability, extraversion, consciousness, and openness to experiences; additional presence of disease processes accelerates these personality changes.

Older adults who disengage from culturally accepted social events (e.g., playing cards, going to a movie) also experience an accelerated decrease in openness to experiences.[49] Physical therapists are well positioned to educate patients, families, and caregivers about the relationships between physical well-being, social isolation, and personality changes. Educational interventions that assist the patient in connecting physical health with mental health can increase patient adherence. For example, integrating a walk with a friend, neighbor, or partner can improve both mental and physical health.

Eugenic and pathological age-related changes can affect the way aging adults view and participate in their physical and social environments. Eugenic aging includes physiologic and sensory changes that occur naturally with age, differentiating between pathological changes and changes due to poor nutrition, decreased physical activity, and so forth.[50] Hearing impairments, as a result of eugenic aging, were the only sensory change older adults experienced that increased isolation and resulted in a decline in extraversion and openness to experiences.[51] Pathological changes such as Alzheimer disease contribute to a substantial increase in neuroticism and decline in extraversion.[52] One study found that the characteristics of low openness to experience and high neuroticism distinguished those who committed suicide and those who died from natural causes.[53]

Resilience

Resilience is a personality trait that moderates the effects of stress, enhances adaptation, and is linked to successful aging.[54,55] Resilience has been proposed to help older adults adjust to changes and challenges that may come with aging.[56] Resilient individuals tend to manifest adaptive behaviors, especially with regard to social functioning, morale, and physical health.[57] Some research has found that older adults have higher levels of resilience, especially related to emotional regulation and problem solving, compared to young adults.[58] Stronger family networks, higher household incomes, and good mental and physical health status have been identified as potential predictors of higher resilience in older adults.[56]

Resilience, a component of an individual's personality, develops and changes over time through ongoing experiences with the physical and social environment.[59,60] Resilience, unlike basic personality factors, may be more of a dynamic process influenced by life events and challenges.[61–63] One study found that the presence of mental or physical illness or dysfunction may actually promote higher levels of resilience in older adults, especially when related to social support.[58] With chronic illness in particular, individuals must learn to accommodate and make adjustments in their daily lives, which could, in turn, increase their sense of resilience.[64]

Wisdom

Wisdom, when discussed relative to aging, is a social decision-making and pragmatic knowledge about life and value relativism (tolerance for another person's or culture's value systems).[65,66] Age alone does not constitute a person being wise. Theories about wisdom vary[67] yet have consistent elements. Wisdom includes adapting and adjusting to life, developing value-permeated life, and acknowledging and accepting human limitations.[67]

Wisdom is an important consideration given that wisdom is a sign of successful aging[66] and relies on experiences, coping skills, and resilience. Early-career physical therapists may not fully appreciate the breadth and depth of experiences an older adult has faced. Integrating an older adult's experience and respecting their wisdom may improve outcomes. For example, older adult patients may be in the best position to decide which therapies or strategies may work best for their recovery, based on their experiences and goals for the future. They may have lived with multiple chronic illnesses or conditions for many years and spoken with numerous health care providers, so they may likely value having a provider listen to their ideas and preferences for care.[68,69] Older adults' knowledge of their ability to adapt to changes in health or physical condition, and knowledge of their own limitations, can help inform more appropriate plans of care.

Loss

Frequently, loss is associated with death and dying. However, aging adults experience loss in a variety of ways, including loss of others, loss of control, and loss of function and engagement in their social environments. Loss involves making adjustments, coping, and identifying and applying strategies. These strategies can have either positive or negative outcomes relative to the individual's psychosocial well-being.

Older adults often experience loss of others. Loss of others may involve death of a partner. Following the death of a partner, older adults often struggle with finding meaning of both that loss and their ongoing life.[70] Factors such as their ability to predict the loss and the quality of the social connections following the loss can impact their coping and feelings of loneliness.[71] Loss of a partner has been linked to suicide risk in older adults, especially older men.[72] However, there is variation in the length of grief after loss of a partner, which can lead to either positive adjustment after loss or negative outcomes including lower quality of life or death.[73] It is important to identify those with chronic grief and help them find additional support.[73]

Loss of others is not limited to death of a partner but also includes death of other family and friends. Further, loss of others can manifest with relocation away from family or friends. In general, having several close and high-quality social supports appears to be protective for older adults against negative consequences including suicidal ideation, depression, functional decline, and declining physical and cognitive health.

Older adults may also experience loss of control, such as over medical decision making. Older adults report feelings of being disempowered when receiving medical attention and an inability to control their care and health outcomes.[74] One study found that older patients' goals are often mal-aligned with goals of physicians and caregivers, representing a need for shared decision making and an appreciation of patient preferences.[75]

More recently, function has also been looked at in terms of space of movement outside the home.[76–78] Those with greater space of movement outside the home report slower rates of cognitive decline and better survival.[76,78] On the other hand, inability to drive places outside the home often means a further decrease in interactions within their social environments.[77] Early recognition of any signs of loss of function (higher-level engagement in their social environments or more basic physical functions) and seeking opportunities to support engagement in normal activities inside and outside the home are important in promoting healthy aging and higher quality of life in older adults.

Loneliness

Loneliness is a subjective, negative feeling related to a lack of social interactions and internal factors such as personality and self-efficacy.[79] Loneliness occurs more often among rural-dwelling older adults than urban-dwelling elders, and is associated with older age, living alone, widowhood, low level of education, and poor income.[80] Loss can contribute to loneliness, such as loss of function, ranging from vision and hearing to mobility and death of a spouse.[80] Older adults also report that declines in health or lack of friends contribute to feelings of loneliness.[80]

Negative social connections may actually worsen older adults' physical and mental health. For example, women experienced worse mental health conditions if an increase in social supports also created increased obligations to support others.[80] Identification of both positive and negative social supports is important as negative social supports are predictive of both worsening psychological well-being and increased distress.[81] The quality of the social supports is as important as the quantity of supports.

Loneliness can lead to major negative health outcomes and has been linked with an increased risk of cardiovascular disease,[82] elevated blood pressure,[82–84] an increased response to stress along with higher levels of cortisol,[85] and modifications in pathways linked to glucocorticoid and inflammatory processes.[86] Loneliness is a major factor contributing to depression, suicide, and suicide attempts.[79] Additionally, loneliness is associated with poor psychological development and dissatisfaction with family, friends, and social acquaintances.[34,87] Moreover, loneliness is associated with increased functional decline and mortality.[88]

Loneliness can develop when a loss of a spouse or relative or a decline in health inhibits the continuation or development of new relationships.[89] Limited engagement in typical activities (e.g., work, leisure, social activities) may also contribute to demoralization and depression. However, therapists cannot assume an older person is lonely or depressed. Depression is only associated with mortality in the oldest-old when feelings of loneliness are present.[90] Therefore, physical therapists may want to check their own assumptions and actively listen to the patient to identify patient needs and provide appropriate patient interventions.

How social supports provide protective effects varies across societal groups.[91] In Chinese cultures, elders seek support within a close, inner circle (spouse and children) and then move to external circles (friends).[87] Fiori et al. found social isolation to be related to lower well-being among older adults in the United States, but this finding was not confirmed in older adults in Japan.[33] Perhaps other cultural factors moderate a potential relationship between social isolation and well-being.

Moreover, social supports may differ by gender identity. Tobiasz-Adamczyk et al. identified several differences between women and men.[81] In the old-old group (age 80+), the size of social supports and their effect on subjective well-being were more significant for women. In the 65- to 79-year-old age group, a similar increase in the degree of participation in social activities led to a higher degree of positive health-related measures in women. However, the relationship between health outcomes and loneliness was not moderated by gender.[81]

Physical therapists may find benefit in identifying older adults' sources of social support. Identification of both positive and negative social supports can facilitate an appreciation of the needs of the patient. Some needs may be outside of the scope of physical therapy and result in collaborations with other health care providers. Ultimately, collaborative, interprofessional care can improve care and patient outcomes.

Grief

Grief can be an outcome of loss at any age. Many health care providers are familiar with the stages of grief identified by Kubler-Ross et al.[92] Yet this theory has limitations: stages occur out of sequence or are skipped altogether. Older adults who experience loss of a partner are more prone to experience long-term or chronic grief than other types of loss, but grief can vary based on circumstances such as readiness for the loss or nature of the loss.[73] Given the possibility of long-term or chronic grief in older adults, therapists who feel comfortable speaking with older patients about grief can explore coping strategies. In many cases, an individual's grief may go unmitigated or be minimized as certain cultures and social groups can promote a more stoic demeanor. Yet the physical therapist can advocate for the patient and consult with other health care providers or trusted persons in the community (e.g., clergy).

Health care providers can monitor the duration of the grieving process to help prevent prolonged grief. An overextended period of grief following a loss can be detrimental to a person's well-being. Some sleep disturbances and anxiety are expected. Yet symptoms lasting longer than 2 months, feelings of guilt unrelated to the loss, thoughts of death unrelated to survivorship, a morbid preoccupation with worthlessness, and hallucinations other than hearing and seeing the deceased are all signs of prolonged grief.[93] Physical therapists can recognize these signs and consult with other health care professionals to provide the patient with additional coping resources.

The psychological ramifications of any type of loss can have lasting effects that also include physical functioning. A loss of a spouse or other significant other can lead to traumatic stress, anxiety, and depression.[94] Prolonged grieving can also contribute to diminished memory and executive functioning.[95] Loss of more basic functions, such as urinary or fecal incontinence, can lead to feelings of worthlessness, helplessness, and shame; loss of self-esteem; and social isolation.[96] Aged survivors of widespread catastrophic events also experience an increased risk of erosion of social cohesion, creating an additional risk for depression.[97] Increased age, financial struggles, poorer general health, and social isolation can further complicate healing from a loss and lead to limitations in performance of activities of daily living (ADLs).[94]

MOTIVATION AND ENGAGEMENT

Motivation is an important factor in the older adult's ability and willingness to participate in functional activities and engage in healthy behaviors such as exercise. Yet therapists frequently encounter older adult patients who seem uninterested or reluctant to engage in the physical therapy plan of care. Their lack of engagement affects outcomes and can have the unintended consequences of producing ethical conflicts when the therapist tries to persuade or even force the patient to participate. Lack of engagement also can affect reimbursement, which may deprive the older adult of needed rehabilitation. Box 4.3 lists the various ethical principles present in a typical patient encounter. Box 4.4 describes ethical dilemmas that can occur

BOX 4.3 Ethical Principles Related to Patient Motivation

Autonomy—allowing refusal
Justice—early mobilization as a way of being efficient with a hospital's resources or insurance limitations
Duty—to do one's best
Beneficence—providing treatments that are of benefit
Nonmalfeasance—no harm

BOX 4.4	Ethical Dilemmas when Attempting to Motivate a Patient
Persuasion	
Inducements	
Interpersonal leverage	
Threats	

when trying to engage a patient who is reluctant to participate.[98] Persuasion is the least problematic as it shows respect for the person's autonomy, but inducements, interpersonal leverage, and threats are all ethically problematic in greater degrees.

Understanding the complex dynamic of motivation and engagement and effective strategies to utilize may help achieve the patient's desired outcomes. Recognizing the difference between the terms *motivation*, *compliance*, *engagement*, and *empowerment* is a beginning to achieving desired outcomes. Table 4.2 describes these terms.

Motivation may only become a factor when the older individual is not doing the desired behavior, in other words, not complying with the therapist's desires or intentions. It is at this time that the patient is labeled as unmotivated or noncompliant. Too often the term *unmotivated* is evoked when the patient is at odds with the therapist's plan.

As discussed in Chapter 11, older adults tend to possess an internal self-regulation that guides behavior, which contrasts with children and younger adults, who are generally influenced more by external reinforcements. Older adults also tend to be more optimistic and focus on the positive. Thus, although there is a tendency to use motivational strategies that focus on losses (e.g., if you do not go to therapy you will not be able to get back home, independently ambulate, or be able to walk without an assistive device), older adults respond better to emphasizing the positive outcomes of engaging in a behavior, avoiding regret, and maximizing satisfaction associated with a behavior.[99] Specifically, older individuals are interested in the immediate benefits of behaviors such as improved functional ability, improved mood, overall sense of well-being, or improved strength and ability to carry grocery bags or laundry. In contrast, they do not respond well to long-term benefits such as the possibility of decreased evidence of cardiovascular disease. In addition, older individuals tend to be more focused on positive rather than negative emotions.[100] Therefore, disappointments following behavior change (e.g., slower improvements in strength) are less likely to undermine the new behavior than they are for younger people.

Self-efficacy and outcome expectations are dynamic and are both appraised and enhanced by four sources of information[101]: (1) enactive mastery experience, or successful performance of the activity of interest; (2) verbal persuasion, or verbal encouragement given by a credible source that the individual is capable of performing the activity of interest; (3) vicarious experience, or seeing like individuals perform a specific activity; and (4) physiological and affective states such as pain, fatigue, or anxiety associated with a given activity. The theory of self-efficacy suggests that the stronger the individual's self-efficacy and outcome expectations are, the more likely he or she will be to initiate and persist with a given activity.

Beliefs, both in relationship to outcomes (outcome expectations) and with regard to what older adults believe they are capable of doing (self-efficacy expectations), have been noted to influence motivation to engage in health-promoting behaviors[102] (behavior change). Physical sensations associated with a treatment plan, such as pain, fear of falling or exacerbating underlying medical problems, or medication side effects, influence beliefs and actual behavior. Some older adults believe, for example, that exercise will exacerbate arthritis pain and therefore will not engage in a regular exercise program. These unpleasant sensations, and their beliefs about them, must be addressed and eliminated to facilitate motivation.

TABLE 4.2 Terms Central to the Psychology of Patient Care

Term	Definition
Motivation	Inner urge that moves or prompts a person to action. Refers to the need, drive, or desire to act in a certain way to achieve a certain end
Compliance	Doing what others want or ask rather than being driven by an inner desire
Engagement	Psychological presence. Individuals feel a vested interest in the success of the task and/or effort
Empowerment	A process of recognizing, promoting, and enhancing people's ability to meet their own needs, solve their own problems, and mobilize the necessary resources to feel in control of their own lives

Personalization

Individualized or person-centered care and demonstrating caring have an important influence on older adults' motivation to perform a given activity. Individualized care includes recognizing individual differences and needs, using kindness and humor, empowering older adults to take an active part in their care, providing gentle verbal persuasion to perform an activity, and using positive reinforcement after performance of an activity.[103] An essential component of individualized care is letting individuals know *exactly* what it is that you recommend they perform. This may be simple written instructions about what exercise program to engage in or what medication to take, why it is important, and exactly how the activity should be done or how the medication should be taken. At each care interaction, it is critical to reevaluate how the individual is doing with the behavior of interest as it demonstrates caring and remembering. Individualized care is, in part, effective because the older adult simply wants to reciprocate for the care given to him or her by doing what the therapist requests (e.g., doing a certain exercise or a home revision such as getting a grab bar). Once the behavior is initiated, however, it is likely that the older individual will experience the benefit(s) associated with the behavior and thus continue to adhere for reasons beyond initial reciprocity for care received.

Demonstrations of caring and confidence in the skills necessary to help the individual (e.g., providing assistance with transfers) are central to motivating older adults in this area. Care can be demonstrated by behaviors and activities perceived by the individual as expressions of love, attention, concern, respect, and support. Another important aspect of caring is setting some guidelines or limits with regard to behaviors. This does not relate to punishment or threats. Rather, it is focused on being firm and informing individuals of the activity they need to do and why they need to do it. For example, an older individual may need to get up and walk to the bathroom to prevent skin breakdown, optimize continence, and regain strength and function. In addition, individualized care includes recognizing individual differences and needs, using kindness and humor, empowering older adults to take an active part in their care, providing gentle verbal persuasion to perform an activity, and using positive reinforcement after performance, or even attempts at performance.[104]

Social Support

Social support networks including family, friends, peers, and health care providers are important determinants of behavior.[105,106] Repeatedly, motivation to exercise has been found to be influenced by the social milieu of the individual and/or the care setting. These social interactions can alter recovery trajectories by disrupting the progression of functional limitations to disability. The influence of any member of the individual's social network can be positive or negative depending on his or her philosophy and beliefs related to exercise. Social supports can directly serve as powerful external motivators by (1) providing encouragement, (2) helping the older adult feel cared for and cared about, and (3) helping to establish goals such as regaining self-care abilities and being able to return home alone. Social supports can also indirectly affect motivation by strengthening the individual's beliefs in his or her ability to participate in rehabilitation activities, for example, or engaging in a regular exercise program.

Patient-Centered Goals

The ability to develop personal goals and evaluate one's performance toward that goal can influence motivation to engage in a given behavior.[101] Articulated goals give older adults something to work toward and help motivate them to adhere to a specific health-promoting activity. First and foremost, it is critical to establish whose motives are being addressed in the motivational interaction. If goals are established without the input of the older individual, it is not likely he or she will be willing to participate in the activities needed to achieve the goal. Findings show that patients involved in structured goal setting such as is described in Table 4.3 experienced greater autonomy and perceived relevance than those whose goals were set by the therapist. For individuals who are cognitively impaired and cannot articulate goals, it is useful to review old records and speak with families, friends, and caregivers who have known the individual previously. Goals can then be developed based on their prior life and accomplishments.[107] However, input from therapists is important to goal development and motivation as the goal delineates for the individual what others believe he or she is capable of doing in a particular functional area, for example. Articulated goals should be short and long term. Short-term goals should provide the older individual with exactly what he or she should do on a daily basis (e.g., walk for 20 minutes; do 10 sit-to-stands). Long-term goals should focus more on ultimate goals that the individual wants to achieve, such as being able to ambulate without an assistive device, care for oneself, walk to the grocery store, or go on a trip. Goals are most effective when they are (1) related to a specific behavior, (2) challenging but realistically attainable, and (3) achievable in the near future.[101] Two strategies in how to use patient-centered goals are described in Table 4.3. The goals clarification process centers around concerns clarification. Concerns clarification is a multifaceted process that includes the patient identifying personal functional, disabling problems caused by his or her pathology and/or impairments, ranking those problems as to importance, and specifying the elements to accomplish that goal.[108] The Enhanced Medical Rehabilitation (EMR) model is a structured plan to apply the science of behavioral change and the principles of rehabilitation intensity to a patient's therapeutic encounter.[109] The aim is to engage patients in rehabilitation to work harder and therefore achieve better results. The three principles are listed in Table 4.3. In the EMR model, feedback is always linked to the goal, including graphs of progress.

Personality

Lastly, the individual's personality, self-determination, and resilience have an important influence on motivation. Older adults report that it is their own personality, that is, determination, and their own firm resolutions and adherence to those resolutions that motivate them to perform specific tasks.[110]

Older adults are a heterogeneous group with very rich and diverse life experiences. Consequently, the factors that facilitate motivation in one may not work as effectively for another individual. As noted previously, the model of motivation can be used to explore the many

TABLE 4.3 Models to Enhance Engagement Through Patient-Centered Goals

	Ozer-Payton-Nelson Goals Clarification Method	Enhanced Medical Rehabilitation
Principle	Increased patient participation in goal setting and treatment planning improves outcomes and patient satisfaction.	1. Link activities to goals 2. Patient as boss 3. Optimize intensity
Goal-setting process	Through a patient-centered interview, elicit patient concerns and goals with objective to stay at the highest level possible. Move down only with permission of the patient.	Interview patient to identify enjoyable, everyday activities that represent the life he or she most wants to restore.
	Five levels of patient participation 1. Open-ended/free choice ("What would you like to be able to do?") 2. Multiple choice (e.g., "Would you like to walk faster or climb stairs?") 3. Confirmed choice (e.g., "Would you like me to offer you a suggestion or recommendation?") 4. Forced choice (e.g., "Is it OK if I tell you what to do?") 5. Prescription (no choice)	Once goals are established, self-efficacy and outcome expectations play influential roles. Outcome expectations are particularly relevant to older adults.
	Integrate personal goals into the therapeutic encounter.	Provide photos of patient's home to guide adaptations and problem solving by the patient. Frequently incorporate patient's goal into therapeutic conversation—for example, "You're building strength to get back to climbing stairs." Link progress to patient's goal.

factors that influence motivation and behavior in older adults. In so doing, interventions can be developed to specifically address identified areas that may be negatively influencing the individual's motivation to engage in a certain activity.

Effective Strategies to Help Motivate the Older Adult

The theoretical guidance for motivational interventions with older adults is extremely important for ensuring a successful outcome for any intervention geared toward increasing physical or functional activity. Appreciating the techniques that can be used in the development of theory-based interventions is likewise helpful. Table 4.4 describes specific interventions that have been used successfully in the past and can be considered useful building blocks for more comprehensive motivational interventions.

Examining the setting in which motivational interventions are occurring, although basic, is important to ensuring successful interactions. If the older adult cannot see or hear what a therapist is telling him or her to do, for example, he or she will not perform the activity and thus be labeled noncompliant or unmotivated. Simple interventions such as eliminating background noise and speaking slowly, in a low tone, and loudly can greatly help these situations. For profound hearing loss, or if the therapist is soft spoken, an external device that amplifies sound can be used. In addition, establish an environment in which the older individual does not feel stressed that he or she has to move quickly. If stressed in this manner, it is likely the individual will freeze and not be able to perform at all.

Lastly, recognizing and appreciating the heterogeneity of older adults and the fact that what is effective in motivating one individual may or may not be useful when working with a different individual is important. Moreover, multiple interventions (e.g., individualized care, setting goals, providing verbal encouragement, and ensuring mastery experiences) may be necessary to optimally motivate the older individual.

Overcoming Fear. Fear of falling is common among older adults and occurs in 42% to 73% of those who have fallen.[111] Fear of falling is associated with reduced physical activity, decreased participation in functional activities, lower perceived physical health status, and lower quality of life and life satisfaction.[111] When trying to increase participation in functional activities and time spent in physical activity, it is important to decrease or eliminate fear of falling. Most of the research that has been done to address fear has focused on fear of back pain. The interventions utilized for fear of experiencing back pain, however, are theoretically based and may be effective if translated to fear of falling.

Interventions to decrease fear of back pain are based on cognitive–behavioral therapy and include either Graded Activity or Graded Exposure treatment.[112] Graded Activity starts by finding out how much activity each patient can do before pain occurs. Then the patient is enrolled in a program that starts with that level of exercise or activity. The therapist guides the patient in building tolerance by slowly increasing the duration, intensity, and

TABLE 4.4 Interventions to Strengthen Motivation

Components of Motivation	Specific Interventions to Improve Motivation
Beliefs	Interventions to strengthen efficacy beliefs: 1. Verbal encouragement of capability to perform 2. Expose older adult to role models (similar others who successfully perform the activity) 3. Decrease unpleasant sensations associated with the activity 4. Encourage actual performance/practice of the activity 5. Educate about the benefits of the behavior, and reinforce and underline those benefits
Unpleasant physical sensations (pain, fear)	1. Facilitate appropriate use of pain medications to relieve discomfort 2. Use alternative measures such as heat/ice to relieve pain associated with the activity 3. Cognitive–behavioral therapy: • Explore thoughts and feelings related to sensations • Help patient develop a more realistic attitude to the pain—i.e., pain will not cause further bone damage • Relaxation and distraction techniques • Graded exposure to overcome fear of falling
Individualized care	1. Demonstrating kindness and caring to the patient 2. Use of humor 3. Positive reinforcement following a desired behavior 4. Recognition of individual needs and differences, such as setting a rest period or providing a favorite snack 5. Clearly and simply writing out/informing patient of what activity is recommended
Social support	1. Evaluate the presence and adequacy of social network 2. Teach significant other(s) to verbally encourage/reinforce the desired behavior 3. Use social supports as a source of goal identification
Goal identification	1. Develop appropriate realistic goals with the older adult 2. Set goals that can be met in a short time frame—daily or weekly—as well as a long-range goal to work toward 3. Set goals that are challenging but attainable 4. Set goals that are clear and specific

frequency of the exercise or activity that was noted to cause pain. Educational strategies are incorporated into the intervention to teach the patient that pain is not harmful in terms of his or her underlying back problems and that the exercise/activity recommended is beneficial in spite of the pain that may occur. Positive reinforcement is provided as the individual works toward achieving success and overcoming fear associated with the activity.

In contrast, Graded Exposure treatment involves presenting the participant with anxiety-producing material (e.g., having him or her engage in an activity that causes pain) for a long enough time to decrease the intensity of his or her emotional reaction. Ultimately, the feared situation no longer results in the individual becoming anxious or avoiding the activity. Exposure treatment can be carried out in real-life situations, which is called in vivo exposure; or it can be done through imagination, which is called imaginal exposure. The Graded Exposure intervention starts by looking at which activities cause fear (e.g., walking, stair climbing, twisting) and then having the individual engage in that activity repeatedly. As fear associated with the activity decreases, the frequency, intensity, and duration of the activity are increased.

Other interventions to decrease fear of falling have included exercise activities (walking, strengthening, balance activities, Tai Chi), educational programs, and use of hip protectors. There was some, albeit limited, evidence for the effectiveness of these interventions in decreasing fear of falling.[113,114] Outcomes are better when interventions are combined, such as when a behavior program is combined with an exercise program.

Motivation in older adults is a complex multidimensional factor that must be evaluated on an individual basis. The evaluation should include intrapersonal, interpersonal, environmental, and larger social policy implications of motivation. Interventions can then be individualized based on where challenges are identified. Assessing motivation and intervening is an ongoing process, and persistence and determination to overcome motivational problems are needed on the part of the health care providers and lay caregivers. Working together, motivation can be treated and improved with regard to function and physical activity. In so doing, the individual will be able to obtain and maintain his or her highest level of function and optimal quality of life.

LIFE TRANSITIONS

Social supports may be most important when older adults transition through various stages of their life. Transitions occur when they adopt and adjust to new life roles. Examples of life transitions include retirement or loss of job, parent to grandparent, and relocation.

Retirement or Loss of Job

Work can often become a part of an individual's identity. Role theory suggests people will experience a decline in their psychosocial well-being when they move on from a job because an occupation provides a sense of purpose and identity.[115] A loss of this role can lead to increased financial burdens, which has been related to lower life satisfaction, lower subjective well-being, and a decrease in social contacts. At these times, the disadvantages of retirement can be more evident and include a loss of identity, decrease in financial status, and depression should isolation occur.

Yet many older adults adjust to the transition out of the workforce positively. A large multinational study found evidence of overall positive psychosocial well-being following voluntary retirement in both men and women.[116] Older adults who choose to retire may perceive more control over their decision and thus have more positive outcomes.

Retirement or loss of a job is often the first major life transition for older adults, and many choose to continue to work in some capacity.[93] The decision to remain in the workforce, even to a lesser extent or in a different role, may offer physical and mental health benefits.[117] Some older adults may find volunteering as a way of regaining identity and sense of purpose after leaving their prior work, increasing their psychological well-being.[118]

Additionally, physical therapists may be able to better prescribe interventions by recognizing that following retirement, a "sugar rush" may be experienced by the retiree.[117] A sugar rush occurs when retirees are satisfied with their lives immediately following retirement and then experience a sharp decline in happiness. This sharp decline can be the result of several psychological effects including partial identity disruption, diminished self-trust, and a search for meaningful engagement in society.[93] This may assist the physical therapist in understanding why the patient's behaviors and adherence to an exercise prescription may change. The physical therapist may need to adjust the program in a way that seems counterintuitive relative to the patient's prior level of engagement. Yet the patient may drop out of therapy altogether if the therapist overprescribes the intervention while the patient experiences this sharp decline.[116]

In others, the way one leaves the workforce can affect how an individual experiences retirement. An unplanned or forced retirement owing to downsizing, job elimination, or poor health is related to lower satisfaction following retirement. Lower satisfaction may be secondary to financial hardships, stress, decreased self-image, and being "off time" (meaning they are not experiencing the same cultural normative transitions as their peers).[119] Mosca and Barrett analyzed data from the Irish Longitudinal Study on Ageing and determined that forced retirements lead to a decline in mental health, with increased risk for depression for people aged 50 and older.[120] Mandal and Roe analyzed data from the Health and Retirement Study and noted similar findings, and that a return to another job decreased the negative effect of a forced retirement.[121] Physical therapists are in a position to assist retirees through this transition by identifying potential psychological effects and providing appropriate guidance.

For example, recognition that retirement can create a sense of either peace, joy, and optimism or anxiety, boredom, and loss can inform a therapist's communications with the patient and how to tailor his or her care.[122] The therapist may also be able to connect the retiree to community organizations and groups that may support his or her current interests or engage the patient in a new skill. In any case, older adults will experience a more positive outcome following retirement if they find continued meaning in their lives.

From Parent to Grandparent

Another life transition occurs when older adults have grandchildren and assume new responsibilities such as parenting during anticipated years of retirement. Parenting grandchildren may not be a choice; it may be forced upon older adults owing to their child(ren)'s inability to care for the grandchild. The number of grandparents assuming the role of primary guardian is increasing. In 2005, 2.5 million grandparents were assuming parental responsibilities to raise their grandchildren.[123] Stress can occur when an older adult who used to support a family through the workforce moves to providing childcare for a grandchild.

Raising a young child brings a host of psychological stressors and benefits. Stressors include limited legal custody, as securing full custody means they must take their own child to court. A decision to gain full custody adds an emotional stress related to increased financial burden because state or federal government funds may be required to move through the legal process, yet funds may be limited. Grandparents may have additional emotional stress, leading to depression and isolation from friends.[124]

A depressed state can lead to decreased energy to care for themselves. Eating healthy foods and exercising may be limited and thus spiral into decreased activity and overall mobility.[123,124] In addition to depression, grandparents can experience alcohol and drug abuse and an uptick in other medical conditions, including heart disease secondary to the added emotional stress when parenting grandchildren.[124]

Despite potential challenges, many older adults will also experience benefits when raising grandchildren. Grandparents and grandchildren demonstrate increased warmth and appreciation and a more positive sense of value for each other. Intimate involvement with grandchildren can provide a social network of younger friends. Additionally, grandparents may have a sense of gratification from being able to provide for their grandchildren.[124]

The negative physical and emotional effects observed in some grandparents vary across societal groups. Therapists who create an environment of trust and respect with the patient will better understand how to meet the patient where he or she is in terms of time and resources for physical therapy. For example, a strong sense of familial care is part of Chinese culture and only one in five Chinese Americans report caregiving burden, pressure, or negative effects of health.[125] Instead, Chinese caregivers reported lower levels of depressive symptoms, anxiety, stress, and loneliness. These findings contrast with African American grandparents living in southern rural areas, who often become grandparents in their mid-20s to late 30s.[126] Physical therapists who integrate the patient's context into care will have a better understanding of the appropriate exercise dose to prescribe the patient. Frequency and duration of therapy may be modified based on patients' additional priorities and resources as they may be placing their grandchildren's needs before their own.

Relocation

With loss of function and health, among other losses, many older adults eventually deal with relocation as a major life transition.[127] Relocation often involves moving out of the homes they remained in for much of their adulthood. In some cases, older adults must move to increasingly supportive environments, such as a retirement community or nursing home.[128] More frequently, they move within the community to places that are more accessible given their current state of health and function.[128] Data suggest that older adults' preferences for living and care arrangements vary, but they are often not matched with their current living arrangement.[129] Some older adults may choose to relocate, or rationalize being relocated, because they can no longer function independently in their current environment, they do not want to be a burden on their family and friends, or they have health challenges.[127] Others may be less involved in the decision of where they live and receive care.

Although their new environment may support their level of health or function, older adults can struggle with increased feelings of disconnectedness, loss of autonomy, and independence upon relocation.[127] Further, older adults can struggle with moving out of the home in which they had familiarity and memories, as well as a sense of control.[130] Avoiding relocation out of the home may provide a source of motivation for older adults to work to improve their health or physical function. Thus, discussing realistic goals that relate to the patients' preferences may help them improve their health and functioning and stay independent at home longer.[131–134] Even in the case of relocation, maintenance of physical function and health, as well as helping them maintain a sense of choice in their new environment, can help older adults maintain a sense of autonomy through the life transition.[127]

The scenario of Jean provides an example of transitions and the effect they may have on a person's well-being. Jean has wanted to age in place in her home of 50 years, but when a fall resulting in a fractured ankle required inpatient rehabilitation, her children decided it was unsafe for her to return home. Without much interaction with their mother, the two adult children, who lived in a different state, made arrangements for their mother to move into assisted living. They disregarded the neighborhood Jean was leaving or moving into, access to religious services, or that she would lose contact with her bridge group.

Dependent on others for transportation, Jean became isolated because of the new living situation. She was naturally an introvert and did not make friends easily. She also had an independent spirit and resisted receiving help. Jean's limited family and social supports along with limited participation in making decisions contributed to anxiety and depression. This example provides insight into the snowball effect a life transition can have into loss and the long-term impact on an older adult's well-being.

GENDER AND SEXUAL IDENTITY

A patient's sexuality and gender identity may play a role in the provision of physical therapy. A dearth of information exists regarding elders who identify as LGBT. A review of the literature indicates that few older LGB adults have been included as study participants, with the least amount of information on elders who identify as transgender.[135]

Intersectionality is an important consideration when treating LGBT older adults, which is minimally discussed in the literature. Research reveals concerns of aging homosexual men about prejudices that may be exhibited to them in their later life, more because they were homosexual rather than because they were "old."[136] Another example is that an older African American female who identifies as transgender can have confounding factors of high blood pressure, macro and micro aggressions, and a lower income based on birth sex, gender identification, and race.

Literature varies in regard to life satisfaction of LGBT elders. Existing literature suggests that a large portion of adults who identify as LGBT report a high degree of life satisfaction, yet 55% of LGBT adults report a lack of companionship and 53% feel isolated. Additionally, more than 50% of individuals in a national health study on LGBT elders were diagnosed with depression by a health care provider and 39% reported having suicidal ideations.[137]

Predictors of positive psyche include accepting and managing a gay or lesbian identity, living with a partner, and being openly gay or lesbian.[138] Many older adults face negative factors affecting psychosocial well-being; however, the LGBT community also has additional negative factors of internalized homophobia, stigma, and victimization based on sexual orientation along with a history of discrimination.[138] Negative factors affecting psychosocial well-being can be moderated by a high degree of resilience, quality and number of social supports, and successful coping skills.[138,139]

Similar to other groups of older adults, resiliency can contribute to a higher degree of successful aging in LGBT elders. Resilient older adults manage their stress levels better and have lower levels of depression.[139] LGBT older adults experience more isolation relative to heterosexual and cisgender counterparts. LGBT elders do not marry as frequently as their counterparts and tend to live alone,[139] which contributes to isolation and loneliness. Fear of macro and micro aggressions can prevent LGBT elders from connecting with and finding others within their community. Additionally, caregiving support is often provided by friends or "families of choice" (composed of close friends) because many LGBT older adults do not have children.[140]

A challenge facing physical therapists who treat older adults identifying as LGBT is a limited understanding of contextual factors that vary among cohorts. Because older adults may have survived severe discrimination, many older LGBT adults have spent a majority of their lives "in the closet," or masking their sexual orientation. This lack of knowledge combined with the limited training therapists receive in the delivery of care for patients identifying as LGBT or queer creates a vacuum of awareness. Self-reflective physical therapists will identify their biases and positionality. Recognizing areas of growth promotes openness and a sense of empathy. Therapists can also develop empathy by increasing their awareness about the LGBT community, appreciating that the "family" unit may look different than the traditional nuclear family, and having community resources available for patients. Table 4.5 provides additional competencies and guidelines to providing services to LGBT older adults.[141]

TABLE 4.5 Summary of 10 Competencies and Strategies When Treating LGBT Older Adults

Self-reflect on personal and professional bias, and educate yourself on how culture, media, and health systems influence decisions.
Describe ways that societal and cultural contexts may historically, negatively influence care of LGBT older adults.
Compare and contrast differences within LGBT older adults along with the intersecting identities.
Relate current theories and up-to-date social health perspectives to engage in a culturally sensitive practice.
Integrate the effect the larger social context, environment, and structures may have on a person when completing an assessment.
Demonstrate empathy and sensitivity when completing the history portion of the exam, being mindful to use appropriate language.
Describe the ways in which current policy (organizational and societal) may marginalize LGBT older adults.
Advocate for LGBT elders.
Facilitate connecting LGBT elders, caregivers, and families to the community.
Provide LGBT older adults, their caregivers, and their families the tools to be supported in the community and navigate aging and social and health services.

LGBT, lesbian, gay, bisexual, and transgender.
Data from Center for Sexual Health Promotion. Center for Sexual Health Promotion. https://sexualhealth.indiana.edu/index.html. Accessed January 11, 2019.

SEX AND INTIMACY

Sex

Regardless of negative stereotypes, people of any age need to feel love and experience intimate relationships. The Center for Sexual Health Promotion indicates that 46% of men and 33% of women over age 70 report that they masturbate and 43% of men and 22% of women in the same age bracket say they engage in sexual intercourse.[142] The act of sex is complex and involves the body, mind, and emotions.[143] Sex is the physical and emotional response to sexual stimuli and allows general affirmation of life and joy.

Physical therapists who appreciate that sexuality is a core dimension of life throughout the life span will be more comfortable discussing sex as it relates to the patient's activity restrictions. Physiological changes such as dryer vaginal tissues and impotence, as well as loss of a loved one, can create a sense of grief and a need to reconnect with others in different ways. The physical therapist can serve multiple roles when discussing sex with a patient that extend beyond sexual positions for injury prevention (e.g., a joint) or postsurgical procedure. The physical therapist can assist the older adult with identifying resources and a safe place to have these discussions.

Intimacy

Intimacy is being in a close, familiar, and usually affectionate or loving personal relationship with another group or person.[144] Five types of intimacy are possible.[145,146] Emotional intimacy is when people confide in and connect with others. They share stories, fears, joy, and pain. Intellectual intimacy is concerned with ideas you think and care about, for example, sharing a favorite song, place, or hobby. Physical intimacy is about physical touch. Experiential intimacy is about activities that people have shared together such as biking, hiking, or a vacation. Lastly, spiritual intimacy consists of those moments when you feel connected to another person with minimal interaction, perhaps as in attending a prayer service or yoga session.

Older adults' intimate relationships may change over time depending on if they are in a relationship with a partner, if their partner has passed away, if they are reconnecting again after a loss, and the quality of close friends. However, the desire for intimacy does not decrease with age.[145] The death of a significant other, children and grandchildren moving a longer distance away, chronic medical conditions, age-related changes such as decreased sex hormones, a lack of privacy, and alcohol and drug abuse can affect an intimate relationship. Additionally, illness, pain and suffering, a state of frailty, and recurrent thoughts of death can lead to a decrease in spontaneously showing affection. Decreased affection and intimacy among people can lead to isolation, loneliness, and depression.[143]

Older adults need to reconcile with being alone and still feeling the capacity to give love and be loved. Dowrick suggests that older adults will need to find intimacy within themselves first before being able to honestly and openly communicate intimately with others.[147] Therapists may be the first health care provider to identify that a person's loss of a loved one has affected his or her functional activities. Interprofessional collaborations become more valuable when psychosocial needs are addressed before or in conjunction with physical therapy.

The case of Tom is an example of improved outcomes owing to a physical therapist's collaboration with other health care providers. Tom is a 79-year-old male, recently immigrated to the United States. He has a limited social network, does not speak English, and relies on an interpreter for verbal communication. The interpreter is persistent that Tom requires a full-back massage to help him walk farther, yet the team (consisting of a nurse, nurse practitioner, and physical therapist) feel strongly that a therapy consult is a better option. Following the examination, the physical therapist cannot identify limitations in impairments that would relate to a decline in his ability to ambulate. The physical therapist returns to the team and shares the examination and evaluation findings. The team determines that a referral to a massage therapist may be the next step in his care as they have also discovered that his wife had died prior to his immigration to the United States. The team recognized that Tom may be grieving the loss of his wife and home country, resulting in feelings of isolation and experiencing a lack of intimacy. This isolation could contribute to depression, which would further complicate his health. Tom completed two sessions with the massage therapist and continued to meet with the team regarding his physical and mental health needs. Following these interventions, Tom returned to his prior level of function without physical therapy interventions. Tom's case highlights the benefits of collaborative care, a team approach.

Physical therapists working in assisted living and other communal environments can benefit from recognizing that older adults may be living apart yet are together. A unique set of barriers exist for older adults residing in communal settings in achieving physical and emotional intimacy. Adult children may not want their parent to become intimate with another resident for several reasons. Potentially, the child is grieving the loss of the deceased parent or the parent in the communal setting has dementia and does not remember the living parent. Children can also be fearful of financial shifting of inheritance. In any case, effectively communicating the concerns at hand with the appropriate persons provides space for open conversations that will minimize stress.

In addition to newly formed intimate relationships, older adults may also lack private spaces to demonstrate physical intimacy. Cognitive impairments in some older adults can make it challenging for staff to decide if the demonstration of intimacy is consensual. Lastly, newly intimate older adults may not want to get married, yet can provide insights into medical conditions of their loved ones. However, the medical insights may not be welcomed by adult children, which can create friction among the family and intimate partners. When part of the team, physical therapists can facilitate effective communication strategies and assist in educating and learning from others how to best make the patient feel comfortable and safe.

SPIRITUALITY

The definition of spirituality has changed over time from a deep religious connection to a general state of well-being.[148–150] Some consider spirituality as a component of successful aging,[151] and older adults may, in some cases, become more faith based with age.[150,152] Spirituality has been related to positive physical and mental health outcomes.[148] Spirituality tends to improve patients' coping skills, promote healthy lifestyles, contribute to an increased interest in preventative programs (e.g., blood pressure and falls risk screens), and encourage the seeking out of nutritional information through support groups and programming. A strong faith has positive effects on quality of life and end-of-life issues because it has been correlated with more positive attitude and self-enhancing behaviors.[151]

Research supports the benefits of spirituality in mitigating mental health issues.[148] The benefits are observed across a diverse group of older adults including elders from different races, disease states, and genders. Older adults with a strong spiritual connection experience a decrease in stress and an improvement in overall emotional well-being and higher self-esteem. Additionally, elders with a spiritual connection will demonstrate less paranoia and a lower rate of depression and anxiety.

Physical therapists frequently limit discussions about spirituality during sessions. However, identifying patients' spiritual needs will assist in providing optimal care for the aging adult. For example, patients may be less engaged in the session if they believe that a higher power controls their destiny. Patients with this belief may appear less motivated, yet they are following the path their faith is guiding them down. By respecting their beliefs, the physical therapist can then determine what strategies they may find beneficial.

TRAUMA-INFORMED CARE AND MENTAL HEALTH CONDITIONS

Mental health conditions are not unique to aging adults. However, the length of time they have managed the condition can vary significantly. Frequently, older patients have coped with their mental health condition for a significant period of their lives. On the other hand, mental health conditions may occur later in life, such as after repeated traumas (e.g., fires, hurricanes, abuse). Patients can benefit when therapists have a heightened awareness to collaborate with other health care providers when developing the plan of care based on the patient's life experiences. Moreover, clinicians' knowledge of the signs and symptoms of mental health conditions in the aging adult, as well as most appropriate management of conditions, can improve health and related outcomes for the patient.

The following sections discuss mental health conditions that follow a person into old age or that occur in mid- to late life. Signs and symptoms, common pharmacological therapies and psychological interventions, and the effect the condition may have on physical therapy are discussed.

Trauma-Informed Care

The phrase *trauma informed care* (TIC) has been around since 2004; however, increased usage and awareness of the phrase has been noted since 2011.[153] Therapists may first think of posttraumatic stress disorder (PTSD) in regard to TIC.[154] However, to understand what TIC is and how to provide it, we must first define trauma. The word *trauma* holds a variety of meanings. The National Institute of General Medical Sciences defines trauma as a serious injury to the body, either by a blunt force or penetrating injury.[155] The National Association of State Mental Health Program Directors (NASMHPD) defines trauma as the experience of violence and victimization including severe neglect, sexual abuse, physical abuse, domestic violence, and/or the witnessing of violence.[156] This experience leaves the person with an intense fear, horror, and helplessness,[157] which produces extreme stress and can overwhelm the person's capacity to cope. Therapists who are cognizant that patients treated for mental health conditions may have sustained repeated traumas that were interpersonal in nature, intentional, and prolonged, and that occurred in childhood, adolescence, or adulthood, may have more empathy for the patient's situation.[158] These definitions, along with the awareness of how deeply rooted the experience may be, have implications for physical therapists and physical therapist assistants.

Older adults may experience trauma in many ways. Elders may have suffered mental or physical assaults as a young child or during an adult relationship. Other examples include weather-related trauma, such as surviving tornadoes, hurricanes, floods, and fires. Lastly, older adults may live in unsafe neighborhoods where muggings, burglaries, and gunshots are common occurrences. These events, even when indirectly affecting the person, can create trauma-induced mental health issues.

Each person experiences an event and responds differently. A similar trauma or series of traumas will exhibit different outcomes in each person. Therefore, therapists should demonstrate unconditional positive regard when listening to a patient's story. Patients with a history of trauma may have problems that affect their psychosocial and physical health, creating a complexity that extends beyond neuromuscular and musculoskeletal concerns that physical therapists are specifically trained in. For example, patients may be treated for mental health conditions, addictions, and physical health, or may be perpetrators of crimes.[156]

Accessing resources about the various interventions will best support the patient and provide TIC. For example, the model by Harris and Fallot uses five guiding principles: safety, trustworthiness, choice, collaboration, and empowerment.[159] Physical therapists and physical therapist assistants may not receive formal training yet need to be aware of signs and symptoms and know when to involve other health care providers. According to the NASMHPD, TIC starts with an understanding of the neurologic, biological, psychological, and social effects trauma has on an individual.[158]

General guidelines for practicing TIC are provided in Table 4.6. The integration of guidelines in Box 4.5 can prove helpful in the management of TIC. The U.S. Preventive Services indicates that a reliable screening tool to identify abuse of elderly or vulnerable adults in the primary care setting has yet to be identified.[175] Integrating TIC guidelines into daily sessions will promote trust and lead to better patient outcomes. Physical therapists can find additional resources on the National Center for Trauma Informed Care website (https://www.nasmhpd.org/content/national-center-trauma-informed-care-nctic-0). A thorough discussion about elder abuse is included in Chapter 12 of this text.

TABLE 4.6 General Guidelines for Providing Trauma Informed Care[159]
Recognition of high prevalence of trauma
Assess for traumatic histories and symptoms
Recognition of culture and practices that are retraumatizing
Collaborative care with caregivers/supporters
Educate staff to understand function of behavior (rage, repetition-compulsion, self-injury)
Use neutral language when developing objectives

BOX 4.5 Example of Trauma-Informed Care Integrated into Practice

The following scenario provides a concrete example of how therapy providers can integrate trauma-informed care (TIC) into their practice.

Deana is a physical therapist who has worked with aging adults for the past 25 years. She is familiar with the high prevalence of elder abuse, specifically emotional and financial abuse. Deana is evaluating Mrs. Harmon for left hip pain. Mrs. Harmon's chart indicates she is living with her grandson, Joe, who is 40 years old and works the third shift. Mrs. Harmon has lived with Joe for the past 10 years, as she does not have any living children, and Joe is her only grandchild in the area. Joe is present with Mrs. Harmon today and Deana discovers that Joe has taken away Mrs. Harmon's car, so she can't drive, and he has gradually assumed responsibility for her finances. Deana attempts to discover the reasons, but Joe interrupts and indicates it is best for his grandma.

Joe leaves the room for the examination and Deana takes the opportunity to ask Mrs. Harmon if she feels safe. Mrs. Harmon says yes, but also indicates that she never has any spending money and misses her friends. She can no longer dine with them because she can't drive, and her grandson won't take her. Deana asks if Mrs. Harmon would be comfortable if Deana contacted a community social worker to assist her in reconnecting with friends by taxi or other means. Additionally, Deana inquires why Joe is managing her finances, and Mrs. Harmon indicates she is unsure. She states that the transition happened over time. Deana suggests that a community social worker can also assist her with determining if she needs this assistance, as it seems Joe may be limiting her social activities. Mrs. Harmon is agreeable to this plan.

This scenario aligns with the TIC guidelines in that the therapist does not make assumptions about the situation. The physical therapist uses her knowledge of TIC to ask appropriate questions, determine the patient's needs and interests, and then provide additional resources. The physical therapist remained objective, avoiding assumptions that the patient and the caregiver were in an abusive relationship.

Depression

The connection between depression, frailty, and failure to thrive is often overlooked. Frequently, medical professionals correlate failure to thrive with poor nutritional intake and a decline in function. Yet frailty and failure to thrive are complex and involve physical, functional, social, and psychological aspects of health.[160] Depression, even though not a normal part of aging, is common in older adults.

Depression is the most common mental health condition of adults aged 65 and older worldwide. The prevalence of depression ranges from 11% to 16% in the overall older adult population and 1% to 2% percent of those living in the community[161] and is more prevalent in ages 50 to 64 (19.3%) relative to ages 65+ years (10.5%).[162] This difference may be related to stress during the preretirement years. Gender differences also exist among men and women over the age of 50; 19.1% of women and 11.7% of men have lifetime depression.[162]

Prevalence of depression also varies across race and health care environments. The prevalence of depression by race has been 6.4% for non-Hispanic whites, 4.2% for African Americans, 7.2% for Hispanics, and 3.8% for others.[18] Prevalence of depression in various health care environments ranges between 0% and 45% for elders hospitalized, and 30% and 44% for those who receive health care at communal living facilities.[163–165]

Depression rates among older adults demonstrate that significant racial/ethnic differences exist.[163] Reasons for these disparities include an income less than 150% of the federal poverty line for a two-person income, financial cost barriers to medications and health care, limited access to health care, and cultural beliefs. For example, African Americans are more likely to believe that symptoms will improve over time without interventions, and the risk of stigma and shame from their communities prevents them from seeking help.

Factors Contributing to Depression. The cause of depression is unknown. According the Centers for Disease Control and Prevention, several factors may increase the likelihood of a person becoming depressed, such as having a blood relative that has depression, going through a major life change, or suffering from a recent trauma or chronic medical problem. Any medical diagnosis can contribute to depression. However, the literature points out some specific conditions that may contribute to depression, including cancer, stroke, and chronic pain. Table 4.7 provides a list of other conditions contributing to depression.[166,167] Less considered diseases, such as dry eye disease (DED), have also been associated with depressive symptoms and an increased risk for severe psychological distress and anxiety.[168,169] Moreover, certain personality types have been linked to depression: extraversion, neuroticism, and conscientiousness. Comorbid conditions, being female, perceived social isolation, and social disconnectedness are also associated with depression.[170–172]

TABLE 4.7 Specific Medical Conditions Contributing to Depression[167,168]

• Cancer
• Stroke
• Chronic pain
• Rheumatoid arthritis
• Low thyroid activity
• Chronic obstructive pulmonary disease
• Diabetes
• Vitamin B_{12} deficiency
• Dementias
• Lupus
• Multiple sclerosis
• Dry eye disease

Lastly, life events, transitions, and the responses to them can contribute to depression. A change in a living situation may create a sense of isolation and loneliness. Unplanned retirement or loss of a job can lead to a reduced sense of purpose. Loss of family members and close friends can lead to extended duration of bereavement.[164] These events may naturally result in a worsened mood and, when undetected and unmitigated, can contribute to depression.

Negative Outcomes of Depression. Negative effects of depression are far-reaching. Depression can further complicate existing conditions common among older adults, including congestive heart failure,[170–172] diabetes,[173,174] and arthritis. Moreover, depression can lead to a decline in quality of life secondary to falls, isolation, mortality, and impaired cognition.[161,174–176] Depression may also increase the risk of developing liver and lung cancer and increase the risk of hip fractures.[177–179] Depression is one of the priority conditions covered by the World Health Organization's mental health Gap Action Programme (mhGAP).[180] The mhGAP aims to increase services for people with mental, neurologic, and substance use disorders through care provided by health workers who are not specialists in mental health. The World Health Organization also led a 2-year global campaign on depression.

Depression can also affect caregivers and their health. Emotional stress reported by caregivers has been associated with a higher likelihood of the care receiver reporting depressive symptoms. Caregivers who exhibit characteristics of resentfulness, discourteousness, reluctance, and criticism led to additional negative reactions by the care recipient.[181] Therefore, it is important to consider what support systems are in place for aging adults with depression and provide resources for them as needed to minimize their stress levels.

Diagnosis of Depression. Diagnosis of depression should be done by a physician or physician's representative. Generally, diagnosing and treating depression in older adults can be challenging secondary to preexisting conditions, underreporting of depressive symptoms, dementia, and bereavement. Additionally, many older adults are resistant to the notion of having mental health issues and don't readily admit to needing help. Health care providers can dismiss signs and symptoms of depression in the elderly secondary to multiple comorbidities and the effects of medication, complicating the diagnosis of depression. Table 4.8 provides a summary of the signs and symptoms of depression in the older adult including a sense of sadness, irritability, and reduced concentration.[182]

Similar challenges are present when treating depression. Depression is often difficult to treat because of lower perceived need of treatment, resulting in a lower rate of treatment-seeking behaviors and poorer prognosis for older patients with major depressive disorder.[183] The DSM-5 provides several diagnostic categories involving depression.[184] Physical therapists may encounter patients with various diagnoses, including major depressive order, adjustment disorder with or without anxiety, or depressed mood.[185] Depression should always be suspected before considering dementia because of the significant impact a diagnosis of dementia can have on a patient's life. Additionally, depression can coexist with dementia, especially early dementia, and symptoms may improve when the depression is treated.

TABLE 4.8 Common Signs and Symptoms of Depression in Older Adults
A sense of sadness
Irritability
Somatic and cognitive alterations affecting function
Decreased self-esteem
Decreased appetite
Decreased energy
Feelings of worthlessness
Loss of interest or joy
Reduced concentration
Anxiety

Data from Hajjar R, Nardelli GG, Gaudenci EM, Santos A da S. Depressive symptoms and associated factors in elderly people in the primary health care. *Rev Rede Enferm Nordeste*. 2018;18(6):727–733.

Depression Scales. Three depression scales are widely used for the screening of depression and are frequently reported on in the literature: the Geriatric Depression Scale (GDS) (30- and 15-item versions),[186,187] the Center for Epidemiologic Studies Depression Scale (CES-D),[188,189] and the SelfCARE(D).[187,189,190] Table 4.9 provides a summary of these tools.

Generally, the scales make statements about feelings or situations, and the respondent indicates how frequently each item occurs. The GDS[191] and the CES-D scales deemphasize somatic signs of depression. Although each measure has a unique scoring system, higher scores reflect more severe symptoms. All measures have a statistically predetermined cutoff score at which depressive symptoms are significant and demand further referral. Caution should be taken when testing individuals with cognitive impairments, as the results may not be reflective of depression.[192]

Treatment of Depression. In general, use of multiple interventions is more effective to buffer or assist in the management of depression. These interventions include medication management and psychotherapy, along with physical activity and prescribed exercise. Social supports are also critical in buffering negative effects of depression while minimizing declines in function.[192,193] Table 4.10 provides a summary of alternative treatments for depression.[194]

Pharmacologic Interventions. Despite previous reports of undertreatment of depression in older adults, a study by Ivanova et al. suggests that physicians prescribe

TABLE 4.9 Common Depression Scales[186–191]

Scale	No. of Items	Total Score	Diagnostic Accuracy	How Scored	Sample Item
Geriatric Depression Scale (GDS)	15 (short) or 30 (long)	30	GDS-30 produced a sensitivity of 84% and specificity of 95% with a cutoff score of 11/12; a cutoff of 14/15 decreased the sensitivity rate to 80% but increased specificity to 100%* In a sample of age >85 years and a cutoff point of 3 to 4 of 15, the sensitivity and specificity of the GDS-15 were 88% and 76%, respectively†	Scored yes/no	"Do you feel that your life is empty?"
Center for Epidemiological Studies Depression Scale (CES-D)	10 or 20	60	The CES-D revealed a sensitivity of 40% and specificity of 82% for detecting minor depression‡ Sensitivity, 97%–100% with a cutoff score of 16 Specificity, 84%–93%	Scored for frequency A cutoff score of 16 has been suggested to differentiate patients with mild depression from normal subjects, with a score of 23 and higher indicating significant depression	"I felt that I could not shake off the blues even with help from my friends and family."
SelfCARE(D)	12	5 for outpatient care	Outpatient: sensitivity of 77% and specificity of 98%† General practice and home care: sensitivity in the 90% range, but the specificity in home care was 53% vs. 86% in general practice¶	Self-administered scale using a Likert scale	

*Yesavage JA, Brink TL, Rose TL, et al. (1982). Development and validation of a geriatric depression screening scale: a preliminary report. J Psychiatr Res 17:37–49.
†de Craen AJ, Heeren TJ, Gussekloo, J (2003). Accuracy of the 15-item geriatric depression scale (GDS-15) in a community sample of the oldest old. Int J Geriatr Psychiatry, 18(1), 63–66.
‡Lyness JM, Noel TK, Cox C, et al. (1997). Screening for depression in elderly primary care patients. A comparison of the Center for Epidemiologic Studies-Depression Scale and the Geriatric Depression Scale. Arch Intern Med, 157(4), 449–454.
¶Williams LS, Brizendine EJ, Plue L, et al. (2005). Performance of the PHQ-9 as a screening tool for depression after stroke. Stroke, 36(3), 635–638.

TABLE 4.10 Alternative Interventions to Mitigate Depression

Consistent exercise
Surrounding and engaging in positive social supports
Mind-body meditation
High quality sleep hygiene (e.g. establish a bed time routine, limit the use of screen time, maintain regular wake times, use the bed for sleep and sex only)
Interactions with nature
Repeating positive affirmations in the morning
Reflecting on positive attributes in your life (journaling, diary, sharing with another person)
Interacting with pets

antidepressants to the majority of older patients with depression.[195] However, Cochrane reviews identified very little evidence as to the benefits of antidepressants in older adults; the majority of findings relate to middle-aged adults.[196] Adverse drug effects are common with drugs that are used to treat anxiety and depression. Patients may choose to forego medications, owing to refusal to accept diagnosis/treatment and noncompliance, as approximately 40% of older patients who were recommended new antidepressant therapy did not fill an antidepressant prescription.[195] Therapists should be aware that some patients may respond fairly rapidly to the antidepressant effects of these drugs; that is, some patients receiving selective serotonin reuptake inhibitors experience beneficial effects within 1 week after beginning drug treatment. Other patients, however, may take 6 or more weeks from the onset of drug therapy until an improvement occurs in the depressive symptoms. This substantial time lag is critical because the patient may actually become more depressed before mood begins to improve. Therapists should therefore look for signs that depression is worsening, especially during the first few weeks of antidepressant drug therapy. A suspected increase in depressive symptoms should be brought to the attention of the appropriate member of the health care team (e.g., physician or psychologist). An in-depth discussion of pharmacology for depression occurs in Chapter 6 within in this text.

Psychotherapy. Psychotherapy for older adults with depression is beneficial in managing depression and often used in combination with pharmacologic therapy.[197] Cognitive therapy has shown success in remediation of symptoms when combined with continued pharmacologic therapy.[197,198] Psychotherapy is particularly useful in older adults who are diagnosed with late-life depression in the context of comorbidities. Patients diagnosed with chronic conditions such as chronic obstructive pulmonary disease (COPD), heart failure, Parkinson disease, stroke, cognitive impairment, and suicidal ideations have demonstrated decreased depressive symptoms with psychotherapy.[167]

A variety of psychotherapies are available as interventions. Cognitive–behavioral therapy (CBT) combines elements of behavioral and cognitive approaches. CBT involves the challenging of pessimistic and negative thoughts by rewarding activities and thoughts that are engaging and positive. Inclusion of CBT in fall prevention programs is likely to enhance the effects of exercise programs on both falls and fear of falling.[199] Psychodynamic therapy focuses on personality characteristics common in depression. Problem-solving therapy has proven to be particularly effective when treating depression in older adults, whereas interpersonal therapies have mixed results in the treatment of depression.[200,201]

Physical Therapy. Because of the nature of depression, older persons with depression may have a reduced functional capacity.[202] The link between severity of depression and functional decline has been consistent across ethnic groups. Additionally, a decline in instrumental activities of daily living (IADLs) is associated with the severity of depression.[195] The relationship between depression and disability is likely bidirectional, with depression being an independent risk factor for disability and disability being a risk factor for depression.[193,203]

Symptoms such as apathy, loss of pleasure in activities, and psychomotor slowness reduce the aging individual's capacity to participate in everyday activities and even perform IADLs. The deconditioning effects of age and illness combine with depression to result in a greater perceived effort for minor, everyday tasks. Moreover, depressive symptoms have been linked to a slower recovery the first 6 months following a hip fracture. In general, patients experience a poorer functional recovery in rehabilitation when they have depression and exacerbated pain symptoms.[204,205] Recognizing that both physical and affective impairments can affect rehabilitation outcomes[206–209] will facilitate the physical therapist in asking pertinent questions and prescribing appropriate interventions.

Researchers indicate a positive effect of exercise/activity on the reduction of depressive symptoms in older persons. Exercise may increase self-mastery and self-efficacy beliefs; it may also provide distraction from negative thoughts. Increases in endorphin and monoamine transmitters in the brain as a result of exercise may also reduce depression. Exercise/activity has been shown to have a comparable reduction in depression compared to antidepressant medication.[210,211]

Improvement in depressive symptoms may be required prior to the start of exercise.[212] Barriers to participation in exercise programs by older persons with depression include accessibility to services, level of energy available to exercise, and a 20% chance of dropping out of the exercise program,[213] during or after symptoms are mitigated.[214] However, "being" on antidepressants does not mitigate the 20% dropout rate.[213]

Despite the benefits of exercise, the dosing of exercises while considering interactions with standard treatments (e.g., antidepressants) is poorly understood.[215] Studies vary in their findings and, for the most part, apply exercises designed for the general population. According to Dunn et al., general public health exercise recommendations are beneficial for people who are depressed and diagnosed with major depressive symptoms.[216] Initially, exercises may need to be prescribed within 10-minute blocks of time and progress to a longer duration. However, Legrand and Heuze suggest that moderate-to-vigorous cardiovascular activities performed at least three to five times per week were more effective in reducing moderate clinical depression than light exercise at a lower frequency.[217] Self-selected intensity of aerobic exercise was shown to have superior psychological benefits, but these results are controversial.[218] Dosing is an important principle determined with consideration of the patients' contextual and medical factors.

Aerobic exercise is consistently recommended in the literature.[219,220] Recommended modes of activity include indoor or outdoor walking, stationary cycling, or cross-trainer exercises. Intensity recommendations vary from moderate intensity to vigorous intensity, depending on individual needs and comorbidities. Frequency of exercises ranges from three to four sessions per week, between 20 and 40 minutes per session, for 8 to 14 weeks. As with any exercise prescription, the more tailored it is to the patient's needs, the more effective the intervention will be.[220,221] Specific recommendations may be appropriate when treating a person with major depression and diurnal changes. The patient should be informed that, in rare cases, bodily sensations relating to exercise-induced changes may trigger panic attacks, to support the patient and decrease the risk of dropping out.[222] See Box 4.6 for other recommendations for exercise and activity programs for older persons with depression.

BOX 4.6 Recommendations for Exercise/Activity Programs for Older Persons with Depression

- Screen for possible medical conditions that might limit exercise participation.
- Provide multiple choices for exercise/activity so that the individual can pick enjoyable activities for himself or herself.
- Recognize possible barriers such as issues of accessibility and low energy levels.

Working with the Depressed Older Patient. Depression can affect many aspects of physical therapy treatment. The person with depression may have more difficulty with fatigue and may express negative or self-critical thoughts. The course of therapy may be longer, because the apathy that may be present and extra energy required necessitates more time to accomplish goals. Goal setting may be more difficult with the older adult who is depressed, but once individual goals are identified, the physical therapist can help the patient see relevance in the treatment plan and recognize progress. Managing the patient with depression may be psychologically difficult for the therapist. Research has shown that most people respond negatively and interact less with persons who exhibit depressed behaviors.[223] Health care professionals are not immune from these natural responses. It is important to remember that for patients suffering from depression, large amounts of energy may be required to accomplish even simple tasks.

Physical therapists may need to have flexible approaches when working with an older person who is depressed. Experts agree that a matter-of-fact approach that emphasizes the patient's feelings of mastery is more effective than one of forced cheerfulness to combat the depressed affect. Therapists can be more helpful by discouraging the patient's negative self-perception and place emphasis on achievement and promote self-efficacy.[224] Encouragement and acknowledgment of the patient's efforts should be frequent. The person with depression may have difficulty visualizing goals far into the future, so physical therapists need to establish realistic goals in achievable steps. Achievement of short-term goals may enhance the person's sense of mastery and improve motivation. Furthermore, persons with depression may need assistance and training to improve their interactive skills in order to maximize the effectiveness of their support networks.[223]

Apathy. Apathy, or a lack of interest, concern, or emotion, has been conceptualized as the opposite of motivation.[225] Although apathy is commonly noted in those with dementia and depression, it can occur independent of either of those two conditions.[225] Unfortunately, the presence of apathy is associated with a decrease in functional and physical activities in older adults and has adverse effects on rehabilitation outcomes.[226]

Medication management for apathy may be a useful, even necessary, first step in engaging older adults with apathy. Numerous pharmacologic interventions have been used to decrease apathy and improve participation in rehabilitation activities with some positive effects. The best results for people with dementia and apathy occur with acetylcholinesterase inhibitors.[227] There was some evidence of efficacy for memantine but less evidence for stimulants, calcium antagonists, and antipsychotics. There was no evidence to support the use of antidepressants or anticonvulsants.[227]

Behavioral interventions, however, should likewise be initiated. Behavioral interventions focus on structure and stimulation such that the individual is encouraged to engage in activities that he or she can easily do successfully. New and different activities such as participating in a visiting pet program or a Tai Chi class generally tend to be good sources of stimulation and motivation. Individuals with apathy will likely say no to participating in any of the activities that are recommended or that they are invited to attend. In situations in which the apathy is profound and persistent, it may be necessary to ignore the "no" and engage the individual—if only for a short period of time—in the activity. This can sometimes be done by walking with the individual to the activity and sitting with him or her for a period of time. The course of therapy may be longer, because the apathy that may be present and extra energy required necessitate more time to accomplish goals. Persistent and regular encouragement to participate in activities in the community or within a facility, or encouragement to participate in simple bathing and dressing activities, is critical. All too often, health care providers and lay caregivers stop asking apathetic older individuals to engage in activities and thus propagate the disease.

Anxiety

The literature has debated the prevalence of anxiety in older adults, yet late-life anxiety disorders are twice as prevalent as dementia among older adults and four to eight times more prevalent than major depressive disorders.[224] The Anxiety and Depression Association of American (ADAA) indicates that anxiety is as common in aging adults as it is in younger populations and older adults are often diagnosed with an anxiety disorder in their youth.[228] Diagnosing anxiety later in life can be difficult secondary to comorbidities, especially depression.[224] Although not a formally recognized disorder, a coexistence of anxiety and depression is referred to as "anxious depression."[229]

Generalized anxiety disorder (GAD) is the most common form of anxiety in older adults and, when combined with depression, requires 50% more time to respond to treatment and decreases the chance of a full recovery.[230] Table 4.11 provides a summary of the symptoms of GAD, such as worrying for extended time periods that

TABLE 4.11 Symptoms of General Anxiety Disorder
Excessive worry about health, family, money, and work
Worries contribute to disruption of social activities and interfere with work, school, or family
Restlessness or feeling keyed up or on edge
Being easily fatigued
Difficulty concentrating or mind going blank
Irritability
Muscle tension
Sleep disturbance (difficulty falling or staying asleep, or restless, unsatisfying sleep)

Data from Stanley MA, Wilson NL, Novy DM, et al. Cognitive behavior therapy for generalized anxiety disorder among older adults in primary care: a randomized clinical trial. *JAMA*. 2009;301(14):1460–1467.

TABLE 4.12 Interview Questions to Identify Anxiety in Older Adults
Do you frequently worry?
Do you focus on the "what ifs" in life?
Do you have a hard time stopping the worry?
Is your sleep interrupted or do you have difficulties falling asleep at night?
Do you experience headaches, body aches, or tension because of your worry?

Geriatrics & Aging journal (Cassidy K-L, Rector NA. The Silent Geriatric Giant: Anxiety Disorders in Late Life. *Geriatrics & Aging*. 2008;11(3):150–56.)

affects patients' daily lives. Older adults with GAD may also have symptoms that overlap with depression, such as restlessness, difficulty concentrating, and irritability.

When anxiety is expected, asking appropriate questions during the interview will facilitate the identification of contributing factors. Many factors increase the risk of anxiety in older adults, including frailty, medical illness, and losses during the later years of their lives. Lack of high-quality social supports, a recent traumatic event, side effects of medications, and poor self-rated health also contribute to anxiety in older adults.[231] Table 4.12 provides specific questions to ask patients during the interview. Collaborating with other health professionals will optimize care as all will have a common, patient-centric goal.

Multiple options are available to manage anxiety disorders. CBT and acceptance commitment therapy (ACT) help the person change the relationship with his or her symptoms and make better choices. Pharmacologic approaches may include selective serotonin reuptake inhibitors; however, concerns exist owing to side effects in older, frail, or medically ill patients.[232,233] Alternative therapies include meditation, yoga, and exercise. Physical therapists are able to prescribe exercises that are specific to the patient. For example, if a person has diurnal changes, then exercises should be incorporated later in the day.[215]

Collaboration with community members will assist patients in maximizing their ability to be active. In general, patients of any age with anxiety and depression tend to adhere to exercises better when physical therapists collaborate with other health professions. Patients with severe anxiety and depression may require treatment of mental health symptoms prior to initiating physical therapy. Therefore, treatment of comorbidities, along with educating family and caregivers and collaborating with other health care providers, will improve patient outcomes relative to mental and physical health.[232]

Bipolar Disorder

Bipolar disorder affects approximately 0.1% of people over the age of 64.[234] As with other mental health conditions, diagnosing bipolar disorder in older adults is challenging because they do not exhibit typical signs of feeling elated or demonstrating risky behaviors.[234] Instead, symptoms may include agitation, irritability, confusion, psychosis, and hyperactivity. Older adults often cycle more quickly between depression and mania and can experience both at the same time. Elders may exhibit problems with memory, impaired perception and judgment, and difficulties solving problems.

The first onset of mania can occur in early or late life. Mania can be triggered by any one of several situations[235]: traumatic life events such as the death of a significant loved one, significant loss of sleep over time,[236] and events surrounding the achievement of goals.[237] Older adults with bipolar disorder can fall into one of two subgroups.[237–239] The first group is diagnosed with mania in middle age and symptoms may be latent for up to 15 years with repeated depressive symptoms. This group tends to have first-generation relatives with affective disorders. The second group experiences the first onset in late life. This group has a lower genetic propensity along with a higher prevalence of co-occurring neurologic disorders. People diagnosed with mania later in life have a 34% to 50% higher mortality rate within 3 to 5 years after diagnosis than individuals diagnosed earlier.

Not only do older adults present with different symptoms relative to younger people who experience bipolar disorder, but also the symptoms may mimic those of dementia. Symptoms of bipolar disease may also be related to negative side effects of medications.[238] Bipolar conditions may be differentiated from dementia, given that the mania lasts approximately 1 week and is not explained by a medical condition, an ataxic gait may be present, a positive family history for mood disorders is present, and the person is alert and may exhibit any of the two symptoms presented in Table 4.13. Additionally, the person may be easily distractible and tend to report decreased sleep.[238]

Treatment options include pharmacotherapy for mood and convulsions, electroconvulsive therapy (ECT), and psychotherapy. However, medications used in younger adults carry a higher risk of adverse effects in the aging population. For example, lithium has an increased serum level and longer half-life in older adults. Electroconvulsive therapy is used when the disease does not respond to medications, or in those who require relief of symptoms

TABLE 4.13 Cognitive Symptoms with Bipolar Disorder in the Older Adult
Grandiosity
Pressured speech
Psychomotor agitation
Flight of ideas
Increased goal-directed activity
Excessive behaviors

Data from Bipolar Disorder in the Elderly: Differential Diagnosis and Treatment | Psychiatric Times. http://www.psychiatrictimes.com/addiction/bipolar-disorder-elderly-differential-diagnosis-and-treatment. Published January 2, 2019. Accessed January 2, 2019.

quickly owing to danger to themselves or others, or malnutrition. In general, lithium and ECT should not be used together owing to increased confusion. The benefits of psychotherapy have been reported in younger populations but are less established in older patients. People who have managed mania over their lifetime can become resistant to pharmacologic therapies, demonstrate a higher psychopathology, and may be vulnerable to relapses.[239]

Physical therapists will not diagnose bipolar disorder, but being aware of the signs and symptoms, along with recognizing comorbidities, will contribute to optimal care for the aging patient. The physical therapist may not be able to prescribe interventions until the patient's condition is medically managed. However, the physical therapist can provide the patient and family with activity guidelines and community resources to assist them in decreasing stress, improving sleep, and decreasing the risk for depression.

Suicide

Even though young and middle-aged adults have a higher suicide rate than older adults, suicide is the 17th-leading cause of death among people aged 65 and older.[240,241] Suicide rates tend to increase over time, and risk of suicide tends to follow birth cohorts. For example, since 2007, baby boomers have had the highest suicide rate.[242] Historically, this age group has had the lowest rate, and more concerning is that this trend will continue into old age. Additionally, white older males have a seven times higher suicide rate than women.[243] White males aged 85 and older have a four times higher rate of suicide than the nation's overall rate.[241,243–245] Compared to younger populations, older adults tend to be more deliberate in their planning of suicide, with the top three means of committing suicide in persons aged 50 and older being firearms (67%), suffocation (14%), and poisoning (12%).[246,247] Although older adults attempt suicide less often, they are more successful, with a ratio of four attempts per completed suicide compared with 200 attempts to one death in younger age groups.[240]

Asking patients if they are thinking of suicide and getting a response can be as challenging as seeking answers about potential abuse. This statement is supported by the data that suggests that 77% of older individuals who commit suicide have visited their primary care doctor within that same year and 45% of older adults visited a primary care doctor within the month they committed suicide.[248] Physical therapists may see the patient before the patient sees his or her primary care physician, especially with direct access. Therefore, physical therapists need to be diligent in recognizing the signs and symptoms of suicide, and have knowledge about patient resources and the roles of other health care professionals.

Risk Factors. Risk factors for suicide among older persons differ from those among the young. In addition to a higher prevalence of depression, suicidal risk factors in older persons include social isolation, stressful life events, family discord, insufficient social supports, loneliness, loss of a significant loved one, and multiple medical conditions that significantly limit their function or life expectancy.[247,249,250] Additionally, older adults more frequently use highly lethal methods and have made prior suicide attempts.[247] Older adults who are suicidal tend to be frailer, have a well-developed plan, and are more determined to succeed than younger adults. The confluence of these factors contributes to the importance of recognizing the signs early and initiating an aggressive treatment and multiple-level interventions.

Using common language to describe three tiers of prevention will assist physical therapists in discussing patient risk factors with other health care providers. Universal prevention focuses on the entire population. Examples of universal prevention strategies include depression screenings and provision of educational materials. Selective prevention focuses on people with risk factors yet who do not display suicidal thoughts or behaviors. Examples of selective prevention strategies include improving function and caregiver awareness of losses that may affect the aged person (e.g., loss of driver's license, vision, mobility). Indicated prevention focuses on older adults who have attempted suicide or are at high risk for suicide. These interventions include policy implementation at the organizational level to identify and manage suicide in later life and strategies to assist a high-risk person.

Physical therapists can identify risk factors and inquire if the patient feels down or is having suicidal thoughts. A patient who responds yes to the question "In the last 2 weeks have you had any thoughts of hurting or killing yourself?" should be asked additional follow-up questions regarding past suicide attempts. If a suicide plan has been developed, the perceived likelihood of the person to carry out the plan and what preventative factors, if any, may prevent the person from carrying out the plan, should be determined.[246] The physical therapist, physician, and other health care providers can work collaboratively to provide prevention interventions as early as possible.

SUMMARY

Physical therapists will improve the ability to provide patient-centered care when they can help address the psychosocial and physical needs of the patient. An appreciation and positive regard toward patients' psychosocial factors will lead to improved patient relationships, collaborative care, and the ability to meet patients where they are in their rehabilitative process. The cases and tips provided in this chapter will assist clinicians in recognizing areas to consider should patients be deemed "noncompliant," and instead the therapist may find that patients' needs could be more fully understood and integrated into their care.

REFERENCES

1. Jung C. *Modern Man in Search of a Soul (WS Dell, CF Baynes, trans.)*. New York: A Harvest Book; 1933.
2. Havighurst RJ. Successful aging. *Process Aging Soc Psychol Perspect.* 1963;1:299–320.
3. Cumming E, Henry WE. *Growing Old, the Process of Disengagement.* New York, NY: Basic Books; 1961.
4. Neugarten BL. Adult personality: toward a psychology of the life cycle. In: *Middle Age Aging*; 1968:137–147.
5. Havinghurst RJ. Personality and patterns of aging. *Gerontologist.* 1968;8(1):20–23.
6. Martin P, Kelly N, Kahana B, et al. Defining successful aging: a tangible or elusive concept? *Gerontologist.* 2014;55 (1):14–25.
7. Rowe JW, Kahn RL. Successful aging. *Gerontologist.* 1997;37 (4):20–23.
8. Rowe JW, Kahn RL. Human aging: usual and successful. *Science.* 1987;237(4811):143–149.
9. Erikson EH, Erikson JM. *The Life Cycle Completed (Extended Version).* New York, NY: WW Norton & Company; 1998:143–149.
10. Snyman S, van Zyl M, Müller J, Geldenhuys M. International Classification of Functioning, Disability and Health: catalyst for interprofessional education and collaborative practice. In: *Leading Research and Evaluation in Interprofessional Education and Collaborative Practice.* New York, NY: Springer; 2016: 285–328.
11. Peck RF, Berkowitz H. Personality and adjustment in middle age. In BL Neugarten (Ed) *Personality in Middle and Late Life.* New York, NY: Empirical Studies; 1964.
12. Baltes PB, Baltes MM. Psychological perspectives on successful aging: the model of selective optimization with compensation. *Success Aging Perspect Behav Sci.* 1990;1(1):1–34.
13. Kahana E, Kahana B. Conceptual and empirical advances in understanding aging well through proactive adaptation. In VL Bengtson (Ed.), *Adulthood and aging: Research on continuities and discontinuities.* New York, NY: Springer Publishing; 1996:18–40.
14. Tornstam L. *Gerotranscendence: A Developmental Theory of Positive Aging.* New York, NY: Springer Publishing Company; 2005.
15. Carstensen LL, Fung HH, Charles ST. Socioemotional selectivity theory and the regulation of emotion in the second half of life. *Motiv Emot.* 2003;27(2):103–123.
16. McCoy SK, Pyszczynski T, Solomon S, Greenberg J. Transcending the self: a terror management perspective on successful aging. *Death Attitudes Older Adult.* 2000; 37–63.
17. Fung HH. Aging in culture. *Gerontologist.* 2013;53(3): 369–377.
18. Stowe JD, Cooney TM. Examining Rowe and Kahn's concept of successful aging: importance of taking a life course perspective. *Gerontologist.* 2014;55(1):43–50.
19. Mortimer JT, Shanahan MJ. *Handbook of the Life Course.* New York, NY: Springer Science & Business Media; 2007.
20. Fredriksen-Goldsen KI, Muraco A. Aging and sexual orientation: a 25-year review of the literature. *Res Aging.* 2010;32 (3):372–413. https://doi.org/10.1177/0164027509360355.
21. Grieco EM, Trevelyan E, Larsen L, Acosta YD, Gambino C. The size, place of birth, and geographic distribution of the foreign-born population in the United States: 1960 to 2010. Population Division Working Paper No. 96. Washington, D.C.: U.S. Census Bureau; 2012. https://www, census.gov/library/working-papers/2012/demo/POP-twps0096. html. Accessed July 2, 2019.
22. Psychosocial Disorders. TheFreeDictionary.com. https://medical-dictionary.thefreedictionary.com/Psychosocial+Disorders. Published January 2, 2019. Accessed January 2, 2019.
23. Araújo L, Ribeiro O, Teixeira L, Paúl C. Successful aging at 100 years: the relevance of subjectivity and psychological resources. *Int Psychogeriatr.* 2016;28(2):179–188.
24. Tate RB, Lah L, Cuddy TE. Definition of successful aging by elderly Canadian males: the Manitoba follow-up study. *Gerontologist.* 2003;43(5):735–744.
25. Araujo L, Teixeira L, Ribeiro O, Paul C. Looking at objective and subjective health in centenarians: always in agreement? *Innov Aging.* 2018;2(Suppl 1):691. https://doi.org/10.1093/geroni/igy023.2570.
26. Cho J, Martin P, Poon LW. The older they are, the less successful they become? Findings from the Georgia Centenarian Study. *J Aging Res.* 2012;2012:695854.
27. Andersen-Ranberg K, Schroll M, Jeune B. Healthy centenarians do not exist, but autonomous centenarians do: a population-based study of morbidity among Danish centenarians. *J Am Geriatr Soc.* 2001;49(7):900–908.
28. Glass TA. Assessing the success of successful aging. Part 1. *Ann Intern Med.* 2003;139(5):382–383.
29. Ferri C, James I, Pruchno R. Successful aging: definitions and subjective assessment according to older adults. *Clin Gerontol.* 2009;32(4):379–388.
30. Giltay EJ, Geleijnse JM, Zitman FG, Hoekstra T, Schouten EG. Dispositional optimism and all-cause and cardiovascular mortality in a prospective cohort of elderly Dutch men and women. *Arch Gen Psychiatry.* 2004;61(11):1126–1135. https://doi.org/10.1001/archpsyc.61.11.1126.
31. Uchino BN. Social support and health: a review of physiological processes potentially underlying links to disease outcomes. *J Behav Med.* 2006;29(4):377–387. https://doi.org/10.1007/s10865-006-9056-5.
32. Uchino BN. Understanding the links between social support and physical health: a life-span perspective with emphasis on the separability of perceived and received support. *Perspect Psychol Sci.* 2009;4(3):236–255.
33. Fiori KL, Antonucci TC, Cortina KS. Social network typologies and mental health among older adults. *J Gerontol Ser B.* 2006;61(1):P25–P32. https://doi.org/10.1093/geronb/61.1.P25.
34. Kawachi I, Berkman LF. Social ties and mental health. *J Urban Health.* 2001;78(3):458–467. https://doi.org/10.1093/jurban/78.3.458.
35. Curtis RG, Windsor TD, Luszcz MA. Perceived control moderates the effects of functional limitation on older adults' social activity: findings from the Australian Longitudinal Study of Ageing. *J Gerontol B Psychol Sci Soc Sci.* 2015;72 (4): 571–581.
36. DeVellis BM, DeVellis RF. Self-efficacy and health. *Handb Health Psychol.* 2001;235–247.
37. Levy BR, Slade MD, Kasl SV, Kunkel SR. Longevity increased by positive self-perceptions of aging. *J Pers Soc Psychol.* 2002;83(2):261–270.
38. Fry C, Dickerson-Putman J, Draper C, et al. Culture and the meaning of a good age. In: Sokolovsky J. *The Cultural Context of Aging: Worldwide Perspectives.* Westport, CT: Praeger; 2009: 99–115. https://www.researchgate.net/publication/232425845_Culture_and_the_Meaning_of_a_Good_Old_Age. Accessed January 16, 2019.
39. Angel JL, Angel RJ, Markides KS. Late-life immigration, changes in living arrangements, and headship status among older Mexican-origin individuals. *Soc Sci Q.* 2000;81(1): 389–403.
40. Batalova JBJ. Senior immigrants in the United States. migrationpolicy.org. https://www.migrationpolicy.org/article/senior-immigrants-united-states. Published May 30, 2012. Accessed January 2, 2019.
41. How culture influences health beliefs. https://www.euromedinfo.eu/how-culture-influences-health-beliefs.html/. Published January 2, 2019. Accessed January 2, 2019.

42. Arnold J, Dai J, Nahapetyan L, et al. Predicting successful aging in a population-based sample of Georgia centenarians. *Curr Gerontol Geriatr Res.* 2010;989315:1–9. https://doi.org/10.1155/2010/989315.
43. Furnham A. The big five versus the big four: the relationship between the Myers-Briggs Type Indicator (MBTI) and NEO-PI five factor model of personality. *Personal Individ Differ.* 1996;21(2):303–307. https://doi.org/10.1016/0191-8869(96)00033-5.
44. The Myers & Briggs Foundation. https://www.myersbriggs.org/home.htm?bhcp=1. Published January 1, 2019. Accessed January 1, 2019.
45. John OP, Robins RW, Pervin LA. *Handbook of Personality: Theory and Research.* 3rd ed. New York, NY: Guilford Press; 2008.
46. Roberts BW, Mroczek D. Personality trait change in adulthood. *Curr Dir Psychol Sci.* 2008;17(1):31–35.
47. Luchetti M, Barkley JM, Stephan Y, Terracciano A, Sutin AR. Five-factor model personality traits and inflammatory markers: new data and a meta-analysis. *Psychoneuroendocrinology.* 2014;50:181–193. https://doi.org/10.1016/j.psyneuen.2014.08.014.
48. Wagner J, Ram N, Smith J, Gerstorf D. Personality trait development at the end of life: antecedents and correlates of mean-level trajectories. *J Pers Soc Psychol.* 2016;111(3):411.
49. Schwaba T, Bleidorn W. Individual differences in personality change across the adult life span. *J Pers.* 2018;86(3):450–464.
50. Lewis CB, Bottomley JM. *Geriatric Rehabilitation: A Clinical Approach.* 3rd ed. Upper Saddle River, NJ: Pearson Education Inc.: 2008. https://www.pearson.com/us/higher-education/program/Lewis-Geriatric-Rehabilitation-A-Clinical-Approach-3rd-Edition/PGM320089.html. Accessed January 17, 2019.
51. Berg AI, Johansson B. Personality change in the oldest-old: is it a matter of compromised health and functioning? *J Pers.* 2014;82(1):25–31. https://doi.org/10.1111/jopy.12030.
52. Wahlin T-BR, Byrne GJ. Personality changes in Alzheimer's disease: a systematic review. *Int J Geriatr Psychiatry.* 2011;26(10):1019–1029. https://doi.org/10.1002/gps.2655.
53. Duberstein PR. Openness to experience and completed suicide across the second half of life. *Int Psychogeriatr.* 1995;7(2):183–198.
54. Rowe JW, Kahn RL. Successful aging and disease prevention. *Adv Chronic Kidney Dis.* 2000;7(1):70–77.
55. Wagnild G. Resilience and successful aging: comparison among low and high income older adults. *J Gerontol Nurs.* 2003;29(12): 42–49.
56. Wells M. Resilience in older adults living in rural, suburban, and urban areas. *Online J Rural Nurs Health Care.* 2012;10(2): 45–54.
57. Lee TY, Cheung CK, Kwong WM. Resilience as a positive youth development construct: a conceptual review. *Sci World J.* 2012;2012:390450. doi:https://doi.org/10.1100/2012/390450 (web archive link).
58. Gooding P, Hurst A, Johnson J, Tarrier N. Psychological resilience in young and older adults. *Int J Geriatr Psychiatry.* 2012;27(3):262–270.
59. Lee H-S, Brown SL, Mitchell MM, Schiraldi GR. Correlates of resilience in the face of adversity for Korean women immigrating to the US. *J Immigr Minor Health.* 2008;10(5): 415–422. https://doi.org/10.1007/s10903-007-9104-4.
60. Hegney DG, Buikstra E, Baker P, et al. Individual resilience in rural people: a Queensland study, Australia. *Rural Remote Health.* 2007;7(4):620.
61. Grotberg EH. *Resilience for Today: Gaining Strength from Adversity.* Westport, CT: Greenwood Publishing Group; 2003.
62. Hardy SE, Concato J, Gill TM. Resilience of community-dwelling older persons. *J Am Geriatr Soc.* 2004;52(2):257–262. https://doi.org/10.1111/j.1532-5415.2004.52065.x.
63. Hardy SE, Concato J, Gill TM. Stressful life events among community-living older persons. *J Gen Intern Med.* 2002;17(11):841–847. https://doi.org/10.1046/j.1525-1497.2002.20105.x.
64. Charmaz K. *Good Days, Bad Days: The Self in Chronic Illness and Time.* New Brunswick, NJ: Rutgers University Press; 1993.
65. Lim KTK, Yu R. Aging and wisdom: age-related changes in economic and social decision making. *Front Aging Neurosci.* 2015;7:120. https://doi.org/10.3389/fnagi.2015.00120.
66. Parisi JM, Rebok GW, Carlson MC, et al. Can the wisdom of aging be activated and make a difference societally? *Educ Gerontol.* 2009;35(10):867–879. https://doi.org/10.1080/03601270902782453.
67. Brugman GM. Twenty - wisdom and aging. In: Birren JE, Schaie KW, Abeles RP, Gatz M, Salthouse TA, eds. *Handbook of the Psychology of Aging.* 6th ed. Burlington, VT: Academic Press; 2006:445–476. https://doi.org/10.1016/B978-012101264-9/50023-9.
68. Alejandro R-SO, Ariadna G-ES, Lorenzo R-CJ, David C-MR. Preferences and expectations of the older adult care. *Arch Gen Intern Med.* 2017;1(3):1–2. http://www.alliedacademies.org/abstract/. Accessed 10 January 2019.
69. Etkind SN, Bone AE, Lovell N, Higginson IJ, Murtagh FEM. Influences on care preferences of older people with advanced illness: a systematic review and thematic synthesis. *J Am Geriatr Soc.* 2018;66(5):1031–1039. https://doi.org/10.1111/jgs.15272.
70. Golsworthy R, Coyle A. Spiritual beliefs and the search for meaning among older adults following partner loss. *Mortality.* 1999;4(1):21–40.
71. Van Baarsen B, Smit JH, Snijders TA, Knipscheer KP. Do personal conditions and circumstances surrounding partner loss explain loneliness in newly bereaved older adults? *Ageing Soc.* 1999;19(4):441–469.
72. Erlangsen A, Jeune B, Bille-Brahe U, Vaupel JW. Loss of partner and suicide risks among oldest old: a population-based register study. *Age Ageing.* 2004;33(4):378–383.
73. Ott CH, Lueger RJ, Kelber ST, Prigerson HG. Spousal bereavement in older adults: common, resilient, and chronic grief with defining characteristics. *J Nerv Ment Dis.* 2007;195(4):332–341.
74. Walker R, Johns J, Halliday D. How older people cope with frailty within the context of transition care in Australia: implications for improving service delivery. *Health Soc Care Community.* 2015;23(2):216–224. https://doi.org/10.1111/hsc.12142.
75. Kuluski K, Gill A, Naganathan G, Upshur R, Jaakkimainen RL, Wodchis WP. A qualitative descriptive study on the alignment of care goals between older persons with multi-morbidities, their family physicians and informal caregivers. *BMC Fam Pract.* 2013;14(1):133.
76. Jacobs JM, Hammerman-Rozenberg A, Stessman J. Frequency of leaving the house and mortality from age 70 to 95. *J Am Geriatr Soc.* 2018;66(1):106–112.
77. Pristavec T. Social participation in later years: the role of driving mobility. *J Gerontol B Psychol Sci Soc Sci.* 2018;73(8):1457–1469.
78. Silberschmidt S, Kumar A, Raji MM, Markides K, Ottenbacher KJ, Al Snih S. Life-space mobility and cognitive decline among Mexican Americans aged 75 years and older. *J Am Geriatr Soc.* 2017;65(7):1514–1520.
79. Singh A, Misra N. Loneliness, depression and sociability in old age. *Ind Psychiatry J.* 2009;18(1):51–55. https://doi.org/10.4103/0972-6748.57861.

80. Savikko N, Routasalo P, Tilvis RS, Strandberg TE, Pitkälä KH. Predictors and subjective causes of loneliness in an aged population. *Arch Gerontol Geriatr.* 2005;41(3): 223–233.
81. Tobiasz-Adamczyk B, Galas A, Zawisza K, et al. Gender-related differences in the multi-pathway effect of social determinants on quality of life in older age—the COURAGE in Europe project. *Qual Life Res.* 2017;26(7):1865–1878.
82. Thurston RC, Kubzansky LD. Women, loneliness, and incident coronary heart disease. *Psychosom Med.* 2009;71(8):836–842. https://doi.org/10.1097/PSY.0b013e3181b40efc.
83. Hawkley LC, Thisted RA, Masi CM, Cacioppo JT. Loneliness predicts increased blood pressure: five-year cross-lagged analyses in middle-aged and older adults. *Psychol Aging.* 2010;25(1):132–141. https://doi.org/10.1037/a0017805.
84. Steptoe A, Shankar A, Demakakos P, Wardle J. Social isolation, loneliness, and all-cause mortality in older men and women. *Proc Natl Acad Sci.* 2013;110(15):5797–5801. https://doi.org/10.1073/pnas.1219686110.
85. Doane LD, Adam EK. Loneliness and cortisol: momentary, day-to-day, and trait associations. *Psychoneuroendocrinology.* 2010;35(3):430–441. https://doi.org/10.1016/j.psyneuen.2009.08.005.
86. Hackett RA, Hamer M, Endrighi R, Brydon L, Steptoe A. Loneliness and stress-related inflammatory and neuroendocrine responses in older men and women. *Psychoneuro-endocrinology.* 2012;37(11):1801–1809. https://doi.org/10.1016/j.psyneuen.2012.03.016.
87. Li H, Ji Y, Chen T. The roles of different sources of social support on emotional well-being among Chinese elderly. *PLOS ONE.* 2014;9(3):e90051. https://doi.org/10.1371/journal.pone.0090051.
88. Perissinotto CM, Cenzer IS, Covinsky KE. Loneliness in older persons: a predictor of functional decline and death. *Arch Intern Med.* 2012;172(14):1078–1084. https://doi.org/10.1001/archinternmed.2012.1993.
89. Holmén K, Furukawa H. Loneliness, health and social network among elderly people—a follow-up study. *Arch Gerontol Geriatr.* 2002;35(3):261–274.
90. Stek ML, Vinkers DJ, Gussekloo J, Beekman ATF, van der Mast RC, Westendorp RGJ. Is depression in old age fatal only when people feel lonely? *Am J Psychiatry.* 2005;162(1):178–180. https://doi.org/10.1176/appi.ajp.162.1.178.
91. Gierveld J de J, Havens B. Cross-national comparisons of social isolation and loneliness: introduction and overview. *Can J Aging Rev Can Vieil.* 2004;23(2):109–113. https://doi.org/10.1353/cja.2004.0021.
92. Kübler-Ross E, Wessler S, Avioli LV. On death and dying. *JAMA.* 1972;221(2):174–179.
93. *Effects of Life Transitions on the Elderly - Geriatrics.* Merck Manuals Professional Edition. https://www.merckmanuals.com/professional/geriatrics/social-issues-in-the-elderly/effects-of-life-transitions-on-the-elderly. Published January 1, 2019. Accessed January 1, 2019.
94. Bui E, Chad-Friedman E, Wieman S, et al. Patient and provider perspectives on a mind–body program for grieving older adults. *Am J Hosp Palliat Med.* 2018;35(6):858–865. https://doi.org/10.1177/1049909117743956.
95. Pérez HCS, Ikram MA, Direk N, Tiemeier H. Prolonged grief and cognitive decline: a prospective population-based study in middle-aged and older persons. *Am J Geriatr Psychiatry.* 2018;26(4):451–460. https://doi.org/10.1016/j.jagp.2017.12.003.
96. Farage MA, Miller KW, Berardesca E, Maibach HI. Psychosocial and societal burden of incontinence in the aged population: a review. *Arch Gynecol Obstet.* 2008;277(4):285–290. https://doi.org/10.1007/s00404-007-0505-3.
97. Lê F, Tracy M, Norris FH, Galea S. Displacement, county social cohesion, and depression after a large-scale traumatic event. *Soc Psychiatry Psychiatr Epidemiol.* 2013;48(11):1729–1741. https://doi.org/10.1007/s00127-013-0698-7.
98. Anderson L, Delany C. From persuasion to coercion: responding to the reluctant patient in rehabilitation. *Phys Ther.* 2016;96(8):1234–1240.
99. Courtney MR, Spivey C, Daniel KM. Helping patients make better decisions: how to apply behavioral economics in clinical practice. *Patient Prefer Adherence.* 2014;8:1503.
100. With age comes happiness: here's why. *Scientific American.* https://www.scientificamerican.com/article/with-age-comes-happiness-here-s-why/. Accessed January 30, 2019.
101. Bandura A, Freeman W, Lightsey R. *Self-efficacy: The exercise of control.* New York, NY: W H Freeman/Times Books/Henry Holt & Co. 1997.
102. McAuley E, Szabo A, Gothe N, Olson EA. Self-efficacy: implications for physical activity, function, and functional limitations in older adults. *Am J Lifestyle Med.* 2011;5(4):361–369.
103. Resnick B, Vogel A, Luisi D. Motivating minority older adults to exercise. *Cultur Divers Ethnic Minor Psychol.* 2006;12(1):17.
104. American Geriatrics Society Expert Panel on Person-Centered Care, Brummel-Smith K, Butler D, et al. Person-centered care: a definition and essential elements. *J Am Geriatr Soc.* 2016;64(1):15–18.
105. Resnick B, Orwig D, Magaziner J, Wynne C. The effect of social support on exercise behavior in older adults. *Clin Nurs Res.* 2002;11(1):52–70.
106. Jackson T. Relationships between perceived close social support and health practices within community samples of American women and men. *J Psychol.* 2006;140(3):229–246.
107. Galik EM, Resnick B, Pretzer-Aboff I. "Knowing what makes them tick": motivating cognitively impaired older adults to participate in restorative care. *Int J Nurs Pract.* 2009;15(1):48–55.
108. Tripicchio B, Bykerk K, Wegner C, Wegner J. Increasing patient participation: the effects of training physical and occupational therapists to involve geriatric patients in the concerns-clarification and goal-setting processes. *J Phys Ther Educ.* 2009;23(1):55–63.
109. Lenze EJ, Host HH, Hildebrand MW, et al. Enhanced medical rehabilitation increases therapy intensity and engagement and improves functional outcomes in postacute rehabilitation of older adults: a randomized-controlled trial. *J Am Med Dir Assoc.* 2012;13(8):708–712.
110. Judge TA, Ilies R. Relationship of personality to performance motivation: a meta-analytic review. *J Appl Psychol.* 2002;87(4):797.
111. Deshpande N, Metter EJ, Bandinelli S, Lauretani F, Windham BG, Ferrucci L. Psychological, physical and sensory correlates of fear of falling and consequent activity restriction in the elderly: the InCHIANTI Study. *Am J Phys Med Rehabil Acad Physiatr.* 2008;87(5):354.
112. George SZ, Zeppieri Jr G, Cere AL, et al. A randomized trial of behavioral physical therapy interventions for acute and sub-acute low back pain (NCT00373867). *Pain* 2008;140(1):145–157.
113. Whipple MO, Hamel AV, Talley KM. Fear of falling among community-dwelling older adults: a scoping review to identify effective evidence-based interventions. *Geriatr Nur (Lond).* 2018;39(2):170–177.
114. Zijlstra GR, Van Haastregt JC, Van Rossum E, Van Eijk JTM, Yardley L, Kempen GI. Interventions to reduce fear of falling in community-living older people: a systematic review. *J Am Geriatr Soc.* 2007;55(4):603–615.
115. Hardy ME, Conway ME. *Role Theory: Perspectives for Health Professionals.* Norwalk, CT: Appleton & Lange; 1988.

116. Asenova A. The effect of retirement on mental health and social inclusion of the elderly. Paper. http://www.econ.msu.edu/seminars/docs/AsenovaPaper.pdf. Accessed July 2, 2019.
117. Retiring minds want to know. http://www.apa.org/monitor/2014/01/retiring-minds.aspx. Published January 2, 2019. Accessed January 2, 2019.
118. Greenfield EA, Marks NF. Formal volunteering as a protective factor for older adults' psychological well-being. *J Gerontol B Psychol Sci Soc Sci.* 2004;59(5):S258–S264.
119. Hershey DA, Henkens K. Impact of different types of retirement transitions on perceived satisfaction with life. *Gerontologist.* 2014;54(2):232–244. https://doi.org/10.1093/geront/gnt006.
120. Mosca I, Barrett A. The impact of voluntary and involuntary retirement on mental health: evidence from older Irish adults. *J Ment Health Policy Econ.* 2016;19(1):33–44.
121. Mandal B, Roe B. Job loss, retirement and the mental health of older Americans. *J Ment Health Policy Econ.* 2008;11(4):167–176.
122. Osborne JW. Psychological effects of the transition to retirement. Canadian Journal of Counselling and Psychotherapy. 2012;46(1):45–58.
123. Brandon Gaille. 23 Statistics on Grandparents Raising Grandchildren. https://brandongaille.com/21-statistics-on-grandparents-raising-grandchildren/. Published May 2017. Accessed January 2, 2019.
124. Hayslip B, Kaminski PL. Grandparents raising their grandchildren: a review of the literature and suggestions for practice. *Gerontologist.* 2005;45(2):262–269. https://doi.org/10.1093/geront/45.2.262.
125. Tang F, Xu L, Chi I, Dong X. Psychological well-being of grandparents caring for grandchildren among older Chinese Americans: burden or blessing? *J Am Geriatr Soc.* 2016;64(11):2356–2361. https://doi.org/10.1111/jgs.14455.
126. Clottey E, Scott A, Alfonso M. Grandparent caregiving among rural African Americans in a community in the American South: challenges to health and wellbeing. *Rural Remote Health.* 2015;15(3):3313.
127. Jungers CM. Leaving home: an examination of late-life relocation among older adults. *J Couns Dev.* 2010;88(4):416–423.
128. Granbom M, Perrin N, Szanton S, Cudjoe T, Gitlin LN. Household accessibility and residential relocation in older adults. *J Gerontol Ser B.* 2018; [ahead of print].
129. Kasper JD, Wolff JL, Skehan M. Care arrangements of older adults: what they prefer, what they have, and implications for quality of life. *Gerontologist.* 2018; [ahead of print] https://doi.org/10.1093/geront/gny127.
130. Golant SM. The quest for residential normalcy by older adults: Relocation but one pathway. *J Aging Stud.* 2011;25(3):193–205.
131. Boltz M, Resnick B, Chippendale T, Galvin J. Testing a family-centered intervention to promote functional and cognitive recovery in hospitalized older adults. *J Am Geriatr Soc.* 2014;62(12):2398–2407.
132. Gill TM, Gahbauer EA, Han L, Allore HG. Functional trajectories in older persons admitted to a nursing home with disability after an acute hospitalization. *J Am Geriatr Soc.* 2009;57(2):195–201. https://doi.org/10.1111/j.1532-5415.2008.02107.x.
133. Harris-Kojetin L, Sengupta M, Park-Lee E, Valverde R. Long-term care services in the United States: 2013 overview. *Vital Health Stat 3.* 2013;(37):1–107.
134. Wu HY, Sahadevan S, Ding YY. Factors associated with functional decline of hospitalised older persons following discharge from an acute geriatric unit. *Ann Acad Med Singap.* 2006;35(1):17–23.
135. Choi SK, Meyer IH. LGBT Aging: A Review of Research Findings, Needs, and Policy Implications. https://escholarship.org/uc/item/03r9x8t3. Published August 2016. Accessed January 2, 2019.
136. Kushner B, Neville S, Adams J. Perceptions of ageing as an older gay man: a qualitative study. *J Clin Nurs.* 2013;22(23–24):3388–3395.
137. Cameron K. Top 3 Health Issues in LGBT Seniors - Healthy Aging Blog. NCOA. https://www.ncoa.org/blog/top-3-health-issues-lgbt-seniors/. Published June 15, 2017. Accessed January 2, 2019.
138. Fredriksen-Goldsen KI, Emlet CA, Kim H-J, et al. The physical and mental health of lesbian, gay male, and bisexual (LGB) older adults: the role of key health indicators and risk and protective factors. *Gerontologist.* 2013;53(4):664–675. https://doi.org/10.1093/geront/gns123.
139. Fredriksen-Goldsen K, Kim H-J, Emlet C, et al. The aging and health report: disparities and resilience among lesbian, gay, bisexual, and transgender older adults. *Seattle Inst Multigenerational Health.* https://digitalcommons.tacoma.uw.edu/socialwork_pub/117. Published November 2011.
140. Grossman AH, D'Augelli AR, Hershberger SL. Social support networks of lesbian, gay, and bisexual adults 60 years of age and older. *J Gerontol Ser B.* 2000;55(3):P171–P179. https://doi.org/10.1093/geronb/55.3.P171.
141. Fredriksen-Goldsen KI, Hoy-Ellis CP, Goldsen J, Emlet CA, Hooyman NR. Creating a vision for the future: key competencies and strategies for culturally competent practice with lesbian, gay, bisexual, and transgender (LGBT) older adults in the health and human services. *J Gerontol Soc Work.* 2014;57(2–4):80–107. https://doi.org/10.1080/01634372.2014.890690.
142. Center for Sexual Health Promotion. https://sexualhealth.indiana.edu/index.html. Accessed January 11, 2019.
143. Sexuality in Later Life. National Institute on Aging. https://www.nia.nih.gov/health/sexuality-later-life. Published January 2, 2019. Accessed January 2, 2019.
144. Definition of intimacy. https://www.dictionary.com/browse/intimacy. Published January 2, 2019. Accessed January 2, 2019.
145. *Intimacy and Older People - Older People's Health Issues.* Merck Manuals Consumer Version. https://www.merckmanuals.com/home/older-people%E2%80%99s-health-issues/social-issues-affecting-older-people/intimacy-and-older-people. Accessed January 11, 2019.
146. Guest Editor's Message: Addressing the Elephant in the Room: Dealing with Matters of Sexuality and Sexual Orientation in Care Management Practice – Aging Life Care Association. https://www.aginglifecarejournal.org/guest-editors-message-addressing-the-elephant-in-the-room-dealing-with-matters-of-sexuality-and-sexual-orientation-in-care-management-practice/. Accessed January 17, 2019.
147. Dowrick S. *The Almost Perfect Marriage: One Minute Relationship Skills.* Crows Nest, NSW, Australia: Allen & Unwin; 2013.
148. Hill PC, Pargament KI. Advances in the conceptualization and measurement of religion and spirituality: implications for physical and mental health research. *Am Psychol.* 2003;58(1):64–74. https://doi.org/10.1037/0003-066X.58.1.64.
149. Ortiz LPA, Langer N. Assessment of spirituality and religion in later life. *J Gerontol Soc Work.* 2002;37(2):5–21. https://doi.org/10.1300/J083v37n02_02.
150. Lavretsky H. Spirituality and aging. *Aging Health.* 2010;6:749–769. https://doi.org/10.2217/ahe.10.70.
151. Crowther MR, Parker MW, Achenbaum WA, Larimore WL, Koenig HG. Rowe and Kahn's model of successful aging revisited positive spirituality—the forgotten factor. *Gerontologist.* 2002;42(5):613–620. https://doi.org/10.1093/geront/42.5.613.
152. Seifert LS. Toward a psychology of religion, spirituality, meaning-search, and aging: past research and a practical application. *J Adult Dev.* 2002;9(1):61–70. https://doi.org/10.1023/A:1013829318213.

153. Becker-Blease KA. As the world becomes trauma–informed, work to do. *J Trauma Dissociation.* 2017;18(2):131–138. https://doi.org/10.1080/15299732.2017.1253401.
154. Jones E, Wessely S. A paradigm shift in the conceptualization of psychological trauma in the 20th century. *J Anxiety Disord.* 2007;21(2):164–175. https://doi.org/10.1016/j.janxdis.2006.09.009.
155. Physical Trauma. https://www.nigms.nih.gov/education/pages/Factsheet_Trauma.aspx. Published January 2, 2019. Accessed January 2, 2019.
156. National Association of State Mental Health Program Directors. Center for Innovation in Trauma-Informed Approaches. https://www.nasmhpd.org/content/national-center-trauma-informed-care-nctic-0. Accessed January 13, 2019.
157. American Psychiatric Association. *Diagnostic and Statistical Manual of Mental Disorders (DSM-5®).* Washington, DC: American Psychiatric Publishing; 2013.
158. Jennings A. Models for developing trauma-informed behavioral health systems and trauma-specific services. Alexandria, VA: National Technical Center for State Mental Health Planning (NTAC); 2004. www.theannainstitute.org/MDT.pdf. Accessed June 29,2019.
159. Harris ME, Fallot RD. *Using Trauma Theory to Design Service Systems.* San Francisco, CA: Jossey-Bass; 2001.
160. Rocchiccioli JT, Sanford JT. Revisiting geriatric failure to thrive: a complex and compelling clinical condition. *J Gerontol Nurs.* 2009;35(1):18–24. https://doi.org/10.3928/00989134-20090101-08.
161. Babatsikou F, Konsolaki E, Notara V, Kouri M, Zyga S, Koutis C. Depression in the elderly: a descriptive study of urban and semi-urban Greek population. International Journal of Caring Sciences. 2017;10(3):1286. www.internationaljournalofcaringsciences.org/docs/19_bbatsikou_original_10_3.pdf.
162. Benson WF. CDC promotes public health approach to address depression among older adults. Accessed at: https://www.cdc.gov/aging/pdf/cib_mental_health.pdf.
163. Andrade L, Caraveo-Anduaga JJ, Berglund P, et al. The epidemiology of major depressive episodes: results from the International Consortium of Psychiatric Epidemiology (ICPE) surveys. *Int J Methods Psychiatr Res.* 2003;12(1):3–21. https://doi.org/10.1002/mpr.138.
164. Mojtabai R, Olfson M. Major depression in community-dwelling middle-aged and older adults: prevalence and 2- and 4-year follow-up symptoms. *Psychol Med.* 2004;34(4):623–634. https://doi.org/10.1017/S0033291703001764.
165. Waugh CE, Fredrickson BL. Nice to know you: positive emotions, self–other overlap, and complex understanding in the formation of a new relationship. *J Posit Psychol.* 2006;1(2):93–106. https://doi.org/10.1080/17439760500510569.
166. Depression in Older Adults - HelpGuide.org. https://www.helpguide.org/articles/depression/depression-in-older-adults.htm. Published November 2018. Accessed January 2, 2019.
167. Raue PJ, McGovern AR, Kiosses DN, Sirey JA. Advances in psychotherapy for depressed older adults. *Curr Psychiatry Rep.* 2017;19(9):57. https://doi.org/10.1007/s11920-017-0812-8.
168. Kim KW, Han SB, Han ER, et al. Association between depression and dry eye disease in an elderly population. *Invest Ophthalmol Vis Sci.* 2011;52(11):7954–7958. https://doi.org/10.1167/iovs.11-8050.
169. Na K-S, Han K, Park Y-G, Na C, Joo C-K. Depression, stress, quality of life, and dry eye disease in Korean women: a population-based study. *Cornea.* 2015;34(7):733. https://doi.org/10.1097/ICO.0000000000000464.
170. Barkow K, Maier W, Üstün TB, Gänsicke M, Wittchen H-U, Heun R. Risk factors for depression at 12-month follow-up in adult primary health care patients with major depression: an international prospective study. *J Affect Disord.* 2003;76(1):157–169. https://doi.org/10.1016/S0165-0327(02)00081-2.
171. Cole MG, Dendukuri N. Risk factors for depression among elderly community subjects: a systematic review and meta-analysis. *Am J Psychiatry.* 2003;160(6):1147–1156. https://doi.org/10.1176/appi.ajp.160.6.1147.
172. Strine TW, Mokdad AH, Balluz LS, et al. Depression and anxiety in the United States: findings from the 2006 Behavioral Risk Factor Surveillance System. *Psychiatr Serv.* 2008;59(12):1383–1390. https://doi.org/10.1176/ps.2008.59.12.1383.
173. Frasure-Smith N, Lespérance F, Talajic M. Depression following myocardial infarction: impact on 6-month survival. *JAMA.* 1993;270(15):1819–1825. https://doi.org/10.1001/jama.1993.03510150053029.
174. Romanelli J, Fauerbach JA, Bush DE, Ziegelstein RC. The significance of depression in older patients after myocardial infarction. *J Am Geriatr Soc.* 2002;50(5):817–822. https://doi.org/10.1046/j.1532-5415.2002.50205.x.
175. Lebowitz BD. The future of clinical research in mental disorders of late life. *Schizophr Res.* 1997;27(2):261–267. https://doi.org/10.1016/S0920-9964(97)00064-9.
176. Sutcliffe C, Burns A, Challis D, et al. Depressed mood, cognitive impairment, and survival in older people admitted to care homes in England. *Am J Geriatr Psychiatry.* 2007;15(8):708–715. https://doi.org/10.1097/JGP.0b013e3180381537.
177. Bakken MS, Engeland A, Engesæter LB, Ranhoff AH, Hunskaar S, Ruths S. Increased risk of hip fracture among older people using antidepressant drugs: data from the Norwegian Prescription Database and the Norwegian Hip Fracture Registry. Age Ageing. 2013;42(4):514–520.
178. Cheng B-H, Chen P-C, Yang Y-H, Lee C-P, Huang K-E, Chen VC. Effects of depression and antidepressant medications on hip fracture. *Medicine (Baltimore).* 2016;95(36). https://doi.org/10.1097/MD.0000000000004655.
179. Jia Y, Li F, Liu YF, Zhao JP, Leng MM, Chen L. Depression and cancer risk: a systematic review and meta-analysis. *Public Health.* 2017;149:138–148. https://doi.org/10.1016/j.puhe.2017.04.026.
180. World Health Organization. Depression. http://www.who.int/mental_health/management/depression/en/. Accessed January 30, 2019.
181. Ejem DB, Drentea P, Clay OJ. The effects of caregiver emotional stress on the depressive symptomatology of the care recipient. *Aging Ment Health.* 2015;19(1):55–62. https://doi.org/10.1080/13607863.2014.915919.
182. Hajjar R, Nardelli GG, Gaudenci EM, Santos Á da S. Depressive symptoms and associated factors in elderly people in the primary health care. *Rev Rede Enferm Nordeste.* 2018;18(6):727–733. https://doi.org/10.15253/2175-6783.2017000600004.
183. Manetti A, Hoertel N, Le Strat Y, Schuster J-P, Lemogne C, Limosin F. Comorbidity of late-life depression in the United States: a population-based study. *Am J Geriatr Psychiatry.* 2014;22(11):1292–1306. https://doi.org/10.1016/j.jagp.2013.05.001.
184. Major Depressive Disorder. https://www.coursehero.com/file/30383538/DSM5-DiagnosticCriteria-MajorDepressiveDisorderpdf/. Published January 2, 2019. Accessed January 2, 2019.
185. HealthyPlace. Adjustment Disorder DSM-5 Criteria. https://www.healthyplace.com/ptsd-and-stress-disorders/adjustment-disorder/adjustment-disorder-dsm-5-criteria. Published January 2, 2019. Accessed January 2, 2019.
186. Yesavage JA, Brink TL, Rose TL, et al. Development and validation of a geriatric depression screening scale: a preliminary report. *J Psychiatr Res.* 1982;17(1):37–49. https://doi.org/10.1016/0022-3956(82)90033-4.

187. Watson LC, Pignone MP. Screening accuracy for late-life depression in primary care: a systematic review. *J Fam Pract.* 2003;52(12):956.
188. Radloff LS. The CES-D Scale: a self-report depression scale for research in the general population. *Appl Psychol Meas.* 1977;1(3):385–401. https://doi.org/10.1177/014662167700100306.
189. Upadhyaya AK, Stanley I. Detection of depression in primary care: comparison of two self-administered scales. *Int J Geriatr Psychiatry.* 1997;12(1):35–37. https://doi.org/10.1002/(SICI)1099-1166(199701)12:1<35::AID-GPS447>3.0.CO;2-H.
190. Banerjee S, Shamash K, Macdonald AJD, Mann AH. The use of the selfCARE(D) as a screening tool for depression in the clients of local authority home care services—a preliminary study. *Int J Geriatr Psychiatry.* 1998;13(10):695–699. https://doi.org/10.1002/(SICI)1099-1166(1998100)13:10<695::AID-GPS850>3.0.CO;2-7.
191. Wancata J, Alexandrowicz R, Marquart B, Weiss M, Friedrich F. The criterion validity of the Geriatric Depression Scale: a systematic review. *Acta Psychiatr Scand.* 2006;114(6):398–410.
192. Bosworth HB, Hays JC, George LK, Steffens DC. Psychosocial and clinical predictors of unipolar depression outcome in older adults. *Int J Geriatr Psychiatry.* 2002;17(3):238–246. https://doi.org/10.1002/gps.590.
193. Hays JC, Steffens DC, Flint EP, Bosworth HB, George LK. Does social support buffer functional decline in elderly patients with unipolar depression? *Am J Psychiatry.* 2001;158(11):1850–1855. https://doi.org/10.1176/appi.ajp.158.11.1850.
194. Johnstone M. I Had a Black Dog: His Name Was Depression. Literary Ames. https://literaryames.wordpress.com/2015/03/01/i-had-a-black-dog-his-name-was-depression-by-matthew-johnstone/. Published March 1, 2015. Accessed January 2, 2019.
195. Ivanova JI, Bienfait-Beuzon C, Birnbaum HG, Connolly C, Emani S, Sheehy M. Physicians' decisions to prescribe antidepressant therapy in older patients with depression in a US managed care plan. *Drugs Aging.* 2011;28(1):51–62. https://doi.org/10.2165/11539900-000000000-00000.
196. Arroll B, Elley CR, Fishman T, et al. Antidepressants versus placebo for depression in primary care. *Cochrane Database Syst Rev.* 2009;3:CD007954. https://doi.org/10.1002/14651858.CD007954.
197. Mottram PG, Wilson K, Scally L, Vassilas C. Psychotherapeutic treatments for older depressed people. *Cochrane Database Syst Rev.* 2000;4:CD007954. https://doi.org/10.1002/14651858.CD004853.
198. Mann JJ. The medical management of depression. *N Engl J Med.* 2005;353(17):1819–1834. https://doi.org/10.1056/NEJMra050730.
199. Zijlstra GR, Van Haastregt JC, Ambergen T, et al. Effects of a multicomponent cognitive behavioral group intervention on fear of falling and activity avoidance in community-dwelling older adults: results of a randomized controlled trial. *J Am Geriatr Soc.* 2009;57(11):2020–2028.
200. Kiosses DN, Alexopoulos GS. Problem-solving therapy in the elderly. *Curr Treat Options Psychiatry.* 2014;1(1):15–26. https://doi.org/10.1007/s40501-013-0003-0.
201. Kiosses DN, Leon AC, Areán PA. Psychosocial interventions for the acute treatment of late-life major depression: a systematic review of evidence-based treatments, predictors of treatment outcomes and moderators of treatment effects. *Psychiatr Clin North Am.* 2011;34(2):377–401. https://doi.org/10.1016/j.psc.2011.03.001.
202. Huang BY, Cornoni-Huntley J, Hays JC, Huntley RR, Galanos AN, Blazer DG. Impact of depressive symptoms on hospitalization risk in community-dwelling older persons. *J Am Geriatr Soc.* 2000;48(10):1279–1284.
203. Lenze EJ, Rogers JC, Martire LM, et al. The association of late-life depression and anxiety with physical disability: a review of the literature and prospectus for future research. *Am J Geriatr Psychiatry.* 2001;9(2):113–135. https://doi.org/10.1097/00019442-200105000-00004.
204. Morrison RS, Magaziner J, McLaughlin MA, et al. The impact of post-operative pain on outcomes following hip fracture. *Pain.* 2003;103(3):303–311. https://doi.org/10.1016/S0304-3959(02)00458-X.
205. Williams CS, Tinetti ME, Kasl SV, Peduzzi PN. The role of pain in the recovery of instrumental and social functioning after hip fracture. *J Aging Health.* 2006;18(5):743–762. https://doi.org/10.1177/0898264306293268.
206. Cully JA, Gfeller JD, Heise RA, Ross MJ, Teal CR, Kunik ME. Geriatric depression, medical diagnosis, and functional recovery during acute rehabilitation. *Arch Phys Med Rehabil.* 2005;86(12):2256–2260. https://doi.org/10.1016/j.apmr.2005.07.292.
207. Hama S, Yamashita H, Shigenobu M, et al. Depression or apathy and functional recovery after stroke. *Int J Geriatr Psychiatry.* 2007;22(10):1046–1051. https://doi.org/10. 1002/gps.1866.
208. Lieberman D, Friger M, Lieberman D. Inpatient rehabilitation outcome after hip fracture surgery in elderly patients: a prospective cohort study of 946 patients. *Arch Phys Med Rehabil.* 2006;87(2):167–171. https://doi.org/10.1016/j.apmr.2005.10.002.
209. Patrick L, Knoefel F, Gaskowski P, Rexroth D. Medical comorbidity and rehabilitation efficiency in geriatric inpatients. *J Am Geriatr Soc.* 2001;49(11):1471–1477. https://doi.org/10.1046/j.1532-5415.2001.4911239.x.
210. Krogh J, Nordentoft M, Sterne JA, Lawlor DA. The effect of exercise in clinically depressed adults: systematic review and meta-analysis of randomized controlled trials. *J Clin Psychiatry.* 2011;72(4):529.
211. Schuch FB, Vancampfort D, Richards J, Rosenbaum S, Ward PB, Stubbs B. Exercise as a treatment for depression: a meta-analysis adjusting for publication bias. *J Psychiatr Res.* 2016;77:42–51. https://doi.org/10.1016/j.jpsychires.2016.02.023.
212. Otto MW, Church TS, Craft LL, Greer TL, Smits JAJ, Trivedi MH. Exercise for mood and anxiety disorders. *Prim Care Companion J Clin Psychiatry.* 2007;9(4):287–294.
213. MacGillivray S, Arroll B, Hatcher S, et al. Efficacy and tolerability of selective serotonin reuptake inhibitors compared with tricyclic antidepressants in depression treated in primary care: systematic review and meta-analysis. *BMJ.* 2003;326(7397):1014.
214. Stathopoulou G, Powers MB, Berry AC, Smits JA, Otto MW. *Exercise Interventions for Mental Health: A Quantitative and Qualitative Review.* Centre for Reviews and Dissemination. https://www.ncbi.nlm.nih.gov/books/NBK73406/. Published 2006. Accessed January 2, 2019.
215. Ströhle A. Physical activity, exercise, depression and anxiety disorders. *J Neural Transm.* 2008;116(6):777. https://doi.org/10.1007/s00702-008-0092-x.
216. Dunn AL, Trivedi MH, Kampert JB, Clark CG, Chambliss HO. Exercise treatment for depression: efficacy and dose response. *Am J Prev Med.* 2005;28(1):1–8. https://doi.org/10.1016/j.amepre.2004.09.003.
217. Legrand F, Heuze JP. Antidepressant effects associated with different exercise conditions in participants with depression: a pilot study. *J Sport Exerc Psychol.* 2007;29(3):348–364. https://doi.org/10.1123/jsep.29.3.348.
218. Ekkekakis P. Let them roam free? *Sports Med.* 2009;39(10):857–888.
219. Stanton R, Reaburn P. Exercise and the treatment of depression: a review of the exercise program variables. *J Sci*

Med Sport. 2014;17(2):177–182. https://doi.org/10.1016/j.jsams.2013.03.010.
220. Strecher V, Wang C, Derry H, Wildenhaus K, Johnson C. Tailored interventions for multiple risk behaviors. *Health Educ Res*. 2002;17(5):619–626.
221. Segar M, Jayaratne T, Hanlon J, Richardson CR. Fitting fitness into women's lives: effects of a gender-tailored physical activity intervention. *Womens Health Issues*. 2002;12(6):338–347. https://doi.org/10.1016/S1049-3867(02)00156-1.
222. Ströhle A, Feller C, Onken M, Godemann F, Heinz A, Dimeo F. The acute antipanic activity of aerobic exercise. *Am J Psychiatry*. 2005;162(12):2376–2378. https://doi.org/10.1176/appi.ajp.162.12.2376.
223. Gilbert P, Procter S. Compassionate mind training for people with high shame and self-criticism: overview and pilot study of a group therapy approach. *Clin Psychol Psychother*. 2006;13(6):353–379. https://doi.org/10.1002/cpp.507.
224. Blazer DG. Self-efficacy and depression in late life: a primary prevention proposal. *Aging Ment Health*. 2002;6(4):315–324. https://doi.org/10.1080/1360786021000006938.
225. Marin RS. Apathy: a neuropsychiatric syndrome. *J Neuropsychiatry Clin Neurosci*. 1991;3(3):243–254.
226. Lenze EJ, Munin MC, Dew MA, et al. Apathy after hip fracture: a potential target for intervention to improve functional outcomes. *J Neuropsychiatry Clin Neurosci*. 2009;21(3):271–278.
227. Berman K, Brodaty H, Withall A, Seeher K. Pharmacologic treatment of apathy in dementia. *Am J Geriatr Psychiatry*. 2012;20(2):104–122.
228. Anxiety and Depression Association of America. Older Adults. https://adaa.org/living-with-anxiety/older-adults. Accessed January 2, 2019.
229. Silverstone PH, von Studnitz E. Defining anxious depression: going beyond comorbidity. *Can J Psychiatry*. 2003;48(10):675–680.
230. Stanley MA, Wilson NL, Novy DM, et al. Cognitive behavior therapy for generalized anxiety disorder among older adults in primary care: a randomized clinical trial. *JAMA*. 2009;301(14):1460–1467.
231. Cassidy K-L, Rector NA. The silent geriatric giant: anxiety disorders in late life. *Geriatr Aging*. 2008;11(3):150–156.
232. Mulsant BH, Whyte E, Lenze EJ, et al. Achieving long-term optimal outcomes in geriatric depression and anxiety. *CNS Spectr*. 2003;8(S3):27–34. https://doi.org/10.1017/S1092852900008257.
233. Anxiety and Depression Association of America. Symptoms. https://adaa.org/understanding-anxiety/generalized-anxiety-disorder-gad/symptoms. Published April 2018. Accessed January 2, 2019.
234. Lives TB. Bipolar Disorder and Seniors. *Bipolar Lives*. https://www.bipolar-lives.com/bipolar-disorder-and-seniors.html. Accessed January 2, 2019.
235. Johnson SL, Cueller AK, Ruggero C, et al. Life events as predictors of mania and depression in bipolar I disorder. *J Abnorm Psychol*. 2008;117(2):268–277. https://doi.org/10.1037/0021-843X.117.2.268.
236. Malkoff-Schwartz S, Frank E, Anderson BP, et al. Social rhythm disruption and stressful life events in the onset of bipolar and unipolar episodes. *Psychol Med*. 2000;30(5):1005–1016.
237. Nusslock R, Alloy LB, Abramson LY, Harmon-Jones E, Hogan ME. Impairment in the achievement domain in bipolar spectrum disorders: role of behavioral approach system hypersensitivity and impulsivity. *Minerva Pediatr*. 2008;60(1):41–50.
238. Trinh N, Forester BP. Bipolar disorder in the elderly: differential diagnosis and treatment. *Psychiatric Times*. http://www.psychiatrictimes.com/addiction/bipolar-disorder-elderly-differential-diagnosis-and-treatment. Published December 1, 2007. Accessed January 2, 2019.
239. Diagnostic Considerations in Geriatric Bipolar Disorder. http://imaging.ubmmedica.com/CME/pt/content/2007/0712/table1_Trinh.gif. Published January 2, 2019. Accessed January 2, 2019.
240. Conwell Y, Van Orden K, Caine ED. Suicide in older adults. *Psychiatr Clin North Am*. 2011;34(2):451–468. https://doi.org/10.1016/j.psc.2011.02.002.
241. Centers for Disease Control and Prevention. WISQARS (Web-based Injury Statistics Query and Reporting System). Injury Center. https://www.cdc.gov/injury/wisqars/index.html. Published December 3, 2018. Accessed January 2, 2019.
242. Baby Boomer Suicide Rate Rising, May Go Higher with Age. Healthline. https://www.healthline.com/health-news/baby-boomer-suicide-rate-rising-031515. Published March 13, 2015. Accessed January 17, 2019.
243. SAMHSA and AOA. Older Americans Behavioral Health Issue Brief 4: Preventing Suicide in Older Adults. 2012. https://www.sprc.org/resources-programs/older-americans-behavioral-health-issue-brief-4-preventing-suicide-older-adults. Accessed June 29, 2019.
244. Mental Health America. Preventing Suicide in Older Adults. http://www.mentalhealthamerica.net/preventing-suicide-older-adults. Published April 28, 2015. Accessed January 2, 2019.
245. NIMH. Suicide. https://www.nimh.nih.gov/health/statistics/suicide.shtml. Published April 2019. Accessed January 2, 2019.
246. Dombrovski AY, Szanto K, Siegle GJ, et al. Lethal forethought: delayed reward discounting differentiates high- and low-lethality suicide attempts in old age. *Biol Psychiatry*. 2011;70(2):138–144. https://doi.org/10.1016/j.biopsych.2010.12.025.
247. SAMHSA. Promoting Emotional Health and Preventing Suicide. https://store.samhsa.gov/product/Promoting-Emotional-Health-and-Preventing-Suicide/SMA15-4416. Published August 2015. Accessed January 2, 2019.
248. Nelson JC. Diagnosing and treating depression in the elderly. *J Clin Psychiatry*. 2001;62(Suppl 24):18–22.
249. Conwell Y, Duberstein PR, Hirsch JK, Conner KR, Eberly S, Caine ED. Health status and suicide in the second half of life. *Int J Geriatr Psychiatry J Psychiatry Late Life Allied Sci*. 2010;25(4):371–379.
250. Van Orden KA, Stone DM, Rowe J, McIntosh WL, Podgorski C, Conwell Y. The Senior connection: design and rationale of a randomized trial of peer companionship to reduce suicide risk in later life. *Contemp Clin Trials*. 2013;35(1):117–126.
251. Chang E, Simon M, Dong X. Integrating cultural humility into health care professional education and training. *Adv Health Sci Educ*. 2012;17(2):269–278. https://doi.org/10.1007/s10459-010-9264-1.

CHAPTER 5

Environmental Design

Accommodating Sensory Changes and Mobility Limitations in the Older Adult

Moira Gannon Denson, MA, ASID, IDEC, IIDA, LEED AP, and Rita Wong, EdD, PT, FAPTA

OUTLINE

INTRODUCTION

According to Sanford and Hernandez, "consumers of all ages and abilities want to live, work, and play in healthy, supportive environments that are well designed, function for their needs and abilities and enhance well-being."[1] Physical therapists often view environmental modifications only through the lens of accommodating movement impairments and disabilities. Although this is an important lens, accommodating sensory deficits (vision, hearing, smell, and touch) may be just as important.

Physical therapists can promote continued independent functioning, well-being, and improved quality of life of older adults by ensuring that their systems review, assessment, treatment interventions, referral recommendations, and outcome goals consider sensory changes and options to accommodate these changes. The therapist should recognize the relationship between sensory changes and common environmental challenges, be aware of potential adaptations to accommodate these challenges, recognize when and how to seek recommendations from other health and environmental design professionals, and educate the patient and/or caregivers in basic environmental and functional modifications to minimize the risk of injury and increase independence.

This chapter will focus predominantly on sensory deficits that impact older adults' interaction and functioning in their home and community, and suggest commonly available environmental adaptations to accommodate the sensory deficits of vision, hearing, smell, and touch. The chapter begins with a general overview of the principles of design and theories that guide a designer's approach to environmental design, continues with a description of sensory changes with aging and general strategies to accommodate these changes, then provides suggestions for basic environmental modifications to accommodate mobility limitations, and ends with suggestions for environmental design in senior living and residential facilities and physical therapy clinic spaces that are "age friendly."

GENERAL PRINCIPLES OF DESIGN

Environmental designs can enhance independence and the overall health of older individuals when they accommodate age-related changes in sensation and physical functioning. The ideal environment will vary according to the needs of individuals but should be supportive of sensory and physical changes while promoting satisfaction, safety, security, and well-being.

Environmental press refers to the extent to which an environment demands a behavioral response. *Competence*, as a design term, refers to the ability of the individual to respond adaptively to challenges to functional health, social roles, sensory-motor and perceptual functions, and cognition. As the demands of the physical environment begin to overcome the competence of the aging individual to respond to the demands, issues of safety, self-image, stress, and interactions with others may be adversely affected. In high-environmental-demand circumstances, individuals with high competence levels will withstand greater levels of press, whereas individuals with low capabilities likely will exhibit maladaptive behavior. Individuals in such situations must either improve their competence (i.e., improving physical, psychological, or emotional functioning) or alter their physical environment to adequately respond to the demand. Often, an approach that combines both rehabilitation strategies and environmental adaptations is the best option to maximize independence and well-being. Simple environmental changes, such as increased lighting, providing easily identifiable landmarks for cuing, or decreased background noise, can foster meaningful changes in behavior and interaction within the environment.[2,3]

Environmental adaptations are applicable to all aspects of personal/living space and to community settings: senior living and long-term care residences, physical therapy clinics, workspaces, retail and grocery stores, libraries, restaurants, fitness centers, gardens, and environmental components such as stairs, escalators, moving walkways, elevators, and driving. Special considerations must be addressed for adapting an environment for individuals with dementia.

GENERAL THEORIES OF ENVIRONMENTAL DESIGN

The development of age-related environmental design research provides an increased variety of environmental design approaches and philosophies (theories) to help support the independent functioning of older individuals. Being aware of these different approaches can help physical therapists guide patients and their families in recognizing the different options available among designers, architects, or builders when considering age-friendly environmental designs.

Aging in place and *universal design* are unique philosophies with thoughtful applications for residential design targeting specific functional accessibility and usability needs.[1,4] In the past, aging in place was the end goal and now universal design is the more widely accepted philosophy with its broader goal to improve design for all age groups and ability levels through specific general principles. That is, universal design is intended to be more inclusive.

The Certified Aging-in-Place Specialist (CAPS) is a designation program by the National Association of Home Builders (NAHB) in partnership with the American Association of Retired Persons (AARP). Individuals holding the CAPS designation have received training on how to guide end-users through a kit of parts (or tools) to support renovating a living space for aging. Additionally, interior designers and architects often receive advanced education in design for aging, complete degree programs with modules on universal design, or receive continuing education credits (CEUs) as part of ongoing licensure with updates on innovative design solutions that can improve the quality of the build environment for individuals with and without disabilities. Research centers, such as the Center for Inclusive Design and Environmental Access (IDeA) at the University of Buffalo,[5,6] are resources for information on universal design strategies.

User-centered theories such as *empathic design* and *human-centered design* not only put the user at the center of the design process to improve function but also further suggest that understanding the emotional needs of the user is paramount to overall health.[7] Human-centered design (HCD) begins with the users and includes them in the planning for the spaces they will inhabit.[7] Empathic design is practiced by designers who seek deep understanding of the user's experience. They do this by immersing themselves in the user experience (through behavioral observation studies) while also giving the user ownership (through participatory design strategies). The designer, therefore, stays engaged in the design process.

SENSORY CHANGES IMPACTING INDEPENDENCE AND WELL-BEING WITHIN THE ENVIRONMENT

Age-related decline in acuity of sensory systems is a normal part of aging. The extent and age of onset of normal age-related decline is variable. Some senses may experience change as early as 40 years of age, whereas others, including vision and smell, may not begin to decline until age 50 or 60. Environmental factors, such as prolonged exposure to loud music or excessive ultraviolet B sun exposure, impact the trajectory of age-related decline in hearing or vision, respectively. Typically, the declines occur gradually and may go unnoticed until the individual or a family member notes substantial challenges to independent functioning within the environment. Multisensory deficits can further compound the challenge. For example, as vision becomes impaired, individuals tend to depend more on their sense of hearing and touch to move through the environment. Substantial declines across multiple senses decrease the ability to accommodate losses.

Throughout life, individuals rely on sensory cues to perceive and interpret information from their surroundings and then respond appropriately. As one ages, a decline in sensory acuity occurs along with a slowing of the reception, integration, and response to sensory stimuli.[8,9] Consequently, older persons may miss environmental cues they would have noticed when younger, may misinterpret cues from the environment, or may experience sensory deprivation, resulting in a loss of independence, safety concerns, or diminished quality of life. Individuals with sensory impairments may need higher thresholds of stimulation to continue to function in the environment. Table 5.1 provides examples of accommodations to enhance functioning in the presence of sensory loss, further described in the following sections.

Vision

Vision is important in identifying environmental cues, distinguishing environmental hazards, maintaining upright balance, and communicating. As people age, declines in vision and visual perception may lead to missing visual cues or misinterpretation of visual cues that negatively impact functional independence. Because of the gradual decline in most sensory loss, the older individual may not be aware of the impact of the decline until an adverse circumstance such as a fall or accident occurs. Both normal age-related visual changes and pathologic conditions of the eye and visual system occur more frequently with increasing age and contribute to impaired vision in older adults.[10] Table 5.2 describes the four most common pathological conditions affecting vision in older adults. Changes at three broad levels of visual functioning can each impact overall vision: (1) anatomical changes that impact the projection of light through the lens and onto the retina, (2) structures in the retina that respond to visual impulses and transmit these impulses to the brain, and (3) the perceptual processing of visual information for interpretation in higher cortical centers.[11] Adapting to visual impairments typically involves the use of visual aids, environmental modifications, and behavioral changes to minimize the functional impact of these impairments.

Visual Field. Some reduction of one's visual field is typically associated with age-related anatomical changes such as decreased pupil size, which lowers the amount of light reaching the peripheral retina; diminished retinal metabolism; relaxation of the upper eyelid; and loss of

TABLE 5.1 Examples of Accommodations to Enhance Functioning for Older Individuals Experiencing Sensory Loss

Sensory Change	Examples of Accommodations
Vision	
Visual field	Lower height for directional and informational signs
Acuity	Visual aids (glasses, contact lenses); magnifiers; large-print books and devices; large-print computer software
Illumination	UV-absorbing lenses; increased task illumination; gooseneck lamps; 200- to 300-watt light bulbs
Glare	Lamp shades, curtains, or blinds to soften light; cove lighting to conceal light source, indirect lighting to bounce off ceiling before redirecting into the room; nonglare wax on vinyl floors; carpeting; wallpaper or flat paints; avoid shiny materials such as glass or plastic furniture and metal fixtures
Dark adaptation	Nightlights with red bulbs; pocket flashlights; automatic light timers; light switches at point of entry to a room; lights under stairs and cabinets
Color	Bright, warm colors (reds, oranges, yellows); avoid pastel hues; avoid monotones
Contrast	Bright detail on dark backgrounds (white lettering/black background); warm colors to highlight handrails, steps; place mats or table coverings that contrast with plates, floor
Depth perception	Avoid patterned floor surfaces; toilet seat and counter surfaces in bathrooms should contrast to floor
Hearing	
	Hearing aids; pocket amplifiers; increasing bass and turning down treble on radios, televisions; smoke alarms, telephones, and doorbells with visual cues such as flashing lights; insulating acoustic materials to minimize background noise. Acoustically absorbent window sheers help with glare but also now have acoustical noise reduction properties
Taste and Smell	
Taste	Color to increase perceived flavor intensity; use of spices, herbs, and flavorings to enhance foods; feel for bulges in canned goods to detect spoilage; check date stored of frozen foods
Smell	Adapt smoke detectors with loud buzzers; safety-spring caps for gas jets on stoves; vent kitchens in institutions to allow residents to experience cooking aromas; place flowers in living areas
Touch	
Tactile sensitivity	Introduce texture into the environment through wall hangings, carpet, textured upholstery; use soft blankets and textured clothing
Thermal sensitivity	Avoid temperature extremes from air conditioning, hot bathwater, heating pads

TABLE 5.2 Pathologic Visual Conditions Common to the Older Adult

Condition	Symptoms	Accommodations
Cataracts	Vision becomes cloudy, blurred, or dim. Harder to see at night. Sensitivity to glare and light. Halos may be seen around lights. Fading or yellowing of colors	Bright light on object of focus Limit night driving
Macular degeneration	Blind spot in the center of the visual field Printed words and images may appear to be distorted or blurred in the center of vision Colors are washed out or dull Haziness to visual field Difficulty transitioning from low-light to bright-light conditions Side vision is not affected May only affect one eye	Bright light on object of focus
Glaucoma	Blind spots develop in visual field with a gradual loss of side vision Increased sensitivity to light and glare Difficulty discriminating between shades of color Reduced night vision Affects both eyes	Low visual aids (e.g., magnifiers or telescopes, visors, filters, reading slits, stands, etc.) Long cane Signature guides Computer screen enlargement software
Diabetic retinopathy	Spots (floaters) in vision Blurred vision Fluctuating vision Impaired color vision Dark or empty areas in vision Usually affects both eyes	Monitor and maintain blood sugar levels

retrobulbar fat, which causes the eyes to sink more deeply into their orbits.[10] Decreased peripheral vision (the ability to detect motion, form, or color on either side of the head while looking straight ahead) impacts the ability to detect people or objects in the lateral visual fields. This is especially true with glaucoma. During gait activities, the therapist may want to avoid standing to the side and rather stand more in front to allow visual cueing. A decrease in the upper visual field may cause an individual to miss traffic and street signs, wayfinding signage, or environmental hazards such as hanging tree limbs that are in this upper visual field area. A decrease in lower peripheral vision may lead to an increased risk of falling from decreased awareness of tripping hazards in the lower visual fields.[12] Older drivers with significant overall visual field limitations or with limitations in either the lower visual fields or left visual fields are more likely to be involved in a traffic accident than comparable drivers with a normal visual field.[13]

Visual Acuity. Visual acuity, the capacity of the eyes to discriminate fine details of objects in the visual field, including words and letters, generally declines with age, although the extent of the decline is quite variable. A gradual decline of visual acuity occurs between the ages of 50 and 70 years, with a greater rate of decline after age 70. Factors responsible for decreased visual acuity include decreased transparency of both the cornea and the lens with aging, loss of flexibility of the lens of the eye, and impaired ability of the iris to change width to accommodate both dim and bright light. These changes affect the amount of light allowed to reach the retina and the ability of the eyes to adapt their focus on the retina independent of object distance (near and far objects) and to adapt vision under various illumination conditions. However, it is likely that optical factors alone are insufficient to account fully for acuity loss and that age-related changes in the retina and brain are also contributing factors. These include such factors as a loss of photoreceptors and ganglion cells in the retina as well as metabolic changes, condensation of the vitreous gel, and anatomical or functional changes in visual neural pathways.[14]

Functionally, the inability to focus clearly over a range of distances occurs gradually and affects near vision first (presbyopia). Visual aids can be beneficial in improving visual acuity for older adults. Reading glasses improve near-vision acuity but must be removed to see clearly at a distance. Progressive lenses (bifocal and trifocal), available both as glasses and as contact lenses, allow for acuity improvement in both near and far vision as well as "computer distance" for trifocals. Progressive lenses can present a hazard to stair negotiation, however, as will be explored later in this chapter. Simple handheld or table-stand magnifiers that enlarge small print are often beneficial as loss of acuity becomes more pronounced. Illuminated magnifiers that hang from the neck can be useful when a person is sewing or performing close work. Many everyday household, office, and recreational devices (e.g., measuring cups, timekeeping devices, playing cards) are available in large print for purchase through local agencies for the blind.

Low-vision technologies are advancing rapidly with improved ability to enlarge print, enhance background lighting, and decrease glare. As technology has advanced, many computers, tablets, and smartphones either have been adapted or have adaptations available to better magnify or otherwise improve the visual display of text and objects on their screens. Although low-vision technologies are increasingly available, most currently published studies of older adults caution that many older adults do not have the same level of familiarity and comfort with computer and smartphone devices as younger adults.[15] However, as baby boomers become today's older adults, they are much more likely to have substantial work and home experience with computers and smart technology than prior generations. As these individuals begin to experience age-related visual changes, consumer pressure for older-adult-friendly devices that are affordable and easy to use will undoubtedly spur innovation. We can anticipate continued enhancements to image clarity and text magnification, decreased glare, improved contrast, high-quality speech-to-text microphone features, and screen-reader-to-text options. Smart systems that more easily accommodate visual, hearing, or tactile limitations common in older adults as well as individuals with cognitive impairments will continue to grow and improve.

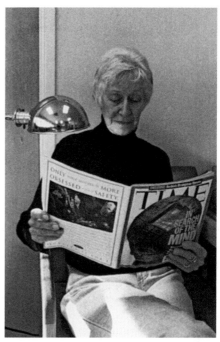

FIG. 5.1 Use of a gooseneck lamp to increase effective task lighting without increasing light bulb wattage. *(From Melore GG. Visual function changes in the geriatric patient and environmental modifications. In Melore GG, ed. Treating Vision Problems in the Older Adult. St. Louis, MO: Mosby; 1997. Used with permission.)*

Illumination. Illumination levels are classified as either (1) photopic, reasonably bright-light conditions equivalent to normal daylight; (2) scotopic, low-light conditions similar to dusk; or (3) mesotopic, vision in very low light similar to being outside at night with only the moon and the stars as light sources. Vision under photopic conditions tends to remain the least affected by age-related visual changes, absent disease processes. Declining visual acuity is particularly noticeable under low-illumination (scotopic) situations and is prevalent in people with cataracts. By age 60, anatomical changes in eye structures (such as thickening of lenses, loss of flexibility of associated structure, pupillary miosis) can result in only 20% of environmental light transmitted through the eye, thus making vision under low-light conditions particularly challenging. As a result of these changes, older individuals require as much as two to four times more light than their younger counterparts.[3] Increased environmental illumination is a key strategy to accommodate declining visual acuity.

Wall-mounted light fixtures and peripheral lighting from floor lamps are superior to a central ceiling source because they do not foster the formation of shadows on critical corner and furniture areas. Background lighting should not be as bright as that in the area on which we direct attention. Lighting that focuses directly on the task, rather than overhead lighting, is recommended to meet the needs of older individuals for reading, task performance, and other close work. Using reading lamps that allow you to increase the wattage of the light bulb is one of the simplest ways to provide adequate task illumination. Another way to modify the necessary amount of illumination independent of light-bulb wattage is to simply move the light source closer to the task material, because the effective amount of illumination is inversely proportional to the distance of the light source to the surface. Gooseneck lamps (Fig. 5.1) or small, high-intensity lamps with three-way switches are helpful in achieving the proper ratio of background-to-task lighting.

Glare. Increasing illumination runs the risk of increasing glare, which can also inhibit clear vision. Glare results from diffuse light scattering on the retina as it passes through mildly opaque refractive media, reducing the contrast of the retinal image.[3] Degenerative changes that take place in the cornea can also contribute to glare. Direct glare occurs when light reaches the eye directly from its source. An example of direct glare is uncontrolled natural light that enters a darkened room through a window or excessive light from exposed light bulbs. Indirect glare can be the result of light reflecting off another surface such as reflections off of highly glossed paper, polished floor surfaces or plastic coverings on furniture, or highly polished building exterior surfaces and high-gloss wayfinding signage.

Modifying light sources lessens glare. Diffuse, soft lighting is preferable to single-light sources. Lamp shades should be used to soften the light. Glare from windows can be minimized by the use of sheer curtains, Venetian blinds, tinted-glass windows, or drapes. Wall-mounted valance or cove lighting that conceals the light source is also recommended. Fluorescent fixtures can be used to reduce glare, but they must be checked to ensure that they do not create another hazard for older individuals in the form of flickering. Also, "white" fluorescent lights are recommended because they make it possible to choose a "cool" light to eliminate the harshness and minimize accentuation of the blues, greens, and yellows created by older-style fluorescent lights.

Another method of controlling glare is reducing the number of reflective surfaces. Positioning light sources to avoid reflection from shiny surfaces, such as waxed floors, is helpful. Use of carpeting, wallpaper, flat paints, and paneling is preferable to use of high-gloss paints. Glass, plastic, and glossy furniture should be avoided or covered with textured surfaces to minimize the effects of glare. Therapists can suggest that builders replace gleaming metal fixtures with low-reflective options. Assistive devices, including grab bars and walkers, should not be constructed of shiny materials.

Awareness of the adverse impacts of glare in public areas can lead to enhanced design. For example, architects and designers could cover mall directories and bus signs with nonglare materials rather than highly reflective plastics. Grocery stores and drugstores could refrain from displaying products wrapped in plastic. Name tags, street signs, and publicity materials for older individuals could be prepared on nongloss surfaces to minimize glare.

Outdoor areas are also vulnerable to glare, especially with bright sunlight or with wet, shiny surfaces on rainy or snowy days. Sunscreens and adequate shade from trees are recommended to limit glare from direct sunlight. If it is not possible to provide adequate control for glare, older individuals should be encouraged to use sunglasses, visors, brimmed hats, or umbrellas. Many older individuals find the glare that occurs at dusk particularly troublesome as poorly illuminated objects are set against a bright, post-sunset sky. Night glare that occurs from oncoming headlights can also be hazardous. Use of well-lit routes and divided highways can minimize this hazard for older individuals.[13,16]

Dark Adaptation. Older adults require more time for their eyes to adapt (become more visually sensitive) when moving from high- to low-light environments. For an individual in his or her 70s, it can take the eyes 10 minutes longer to adapt than an individual in their 20s.[17] Many factors contribute to these changes. Traditional thought is that structural and metabolic changes in the lens and pupil are the major factors. More recent research suggests that biochemical changes, particularly the time needed to regenerate rhodopsin, a pigment-containing sensory protein found in the rods of the retina, contribute substantially to the delay in adaptation to low-light environments.[17] Older persons have particular difficulty adapting to abrupt and extreme changes in light, such as when leaving a darkened theater in the middle of a bright day.[8,9] Donning sunglasses before exiting may help the adaptation.

Use of a nightlight is recommended to assist in overcoming the decreased ability for the eyes to adapt to the dark. Red light stimulates the cones but not the rods, allowing improved night vision to an older person functioning in the dark and reducing the time required for adaptation to the dark. Older individuals should carry a pocket flashlight such as what is included on a smartphone to aid in the transition to dimly lit environments. Improving the lighting at the point of entry to an area, through light switches near the entrance to a room, voice-activated light switches, or motion detection activation, is also recommended. Automatic timers or keeping a light on at all times in dimly lit areas can help in adaptation to darkened environments.

Color. The ability to perceive, differentiate, and distinguish colors declines with aging as a result of changes in retinal cones, the retinal bipolar and ganglion cells, and the visual pathways that terminate in the occipital cortex. Thickening and yellowing of the lens with age lead to decreased sensitivity to light and, thus, more difficulty distinguishing between colors that have shorter wavelengths such as blues, greens, and violets, often described as cool colors. Hue and saturation levels are particularly affected by aging. However, brightness appears to be spared. Colors with longer wavelengths such as reds, oranges, and yellows, often described as warm colors, are easier to differentiate and, therefore, good choices as focal points against sharply contrasting backgrounds. With aging, in addition to the loss of color discrimination at the blue end of the color spectrum, there is a loss of sensitivity to color discrimination over the entire spectrum. As a result, light pastel colors may be difficult to distinguish from each other and monotones may blend into shadows, leading to difficulty negotiating around dark furniture and dark floor surfaces when these come together. Optimal lighting or higher color contrast is needed to minimize this hazard.

Both cool and warm colors can be included in a color scheme when designing living environments for older individuals. Even though cool colors are more difficult to distinguish, they have soothing effects that may be particularly beneficial for agitated persons. These cool colors are particularly suited for bedrooms because they promote calm and peacefulness. However, bright, warm colors are seen better, and their use should be encouraged for sensory stimulation. They are considered to be welcoming and uplifting and are suitable for entrances, dayrooms, and dining rooms, particularly in residential care facilities. Contrasting bright yellows, reds, and oranges with cool blue, green, and violet colors may help minimize difficulties associated with loss of depth perception. The goal with the use of color is to use contrast to assist older individuals in distinguishing objects from their backgrounds.[16–18] It is also important that the use of color be aesthetically pleasing.[19,20]

Contrast. The ability to discriminate among degrees of brightness appears to decrease with age. In particular, contrast sensitivity to medium- and high-spatial frequencies declines progressively with age, and contrast sensitivity to low-spatial frequencies remains unchanged.[11] Typically, older individuals have difficulty seeing objects that have low contrast. Older persons require more than two times as much light to see low-contrasting objects with the same degree of clarity as younger people. Earlier studies attributed this decreased ability to an increase in light scatter secondary to age-related eye changes. More recent studies indicate that changes in the retina, neural pathways, and brain also contribute.[10]

Use of sharp contrast enhances the visual performance of older individuals. Bright detail on dark backgrounds is easier to distinguish than low contrast or dark detail on a light background. Use of warm colors—reds, oranges, and yellows—is recommended to highlight important visual targets such as handrails, steps, intersections, and traffic signs. Floors and rugs should contrast with woodwork and walls. In those with significant visual loss, high contrast can be used to enhance independence in daily activities. Sharply contrasting colored rims on dishes and glasses helps identify the edges of the eating and drinking surfaces. Using a table covering that contrasts sharply with the floor enhances the ability to see the edges of the table, thus helping to prevent bumps and falls. The use of tone is another way to improve the contrast in the environment. An example of contrasting tones is pairing a lighter shade against a darker shade. Therapists and designers should apply this principle in any area where the older individual needs a sensory cue to navigate safely such as doors, door handles, handrails, and furniture coverings.[19,21]

Depth Perception. The ability to discriminate colors and the convergence of input from binocular vision (visual input from both eyes) are major contributors to depth perception and spatial integration of objects. Binocular vision contributes to our ability to build a 3-D construction of the environment.[10] Depth perception allows a person to accurately construct spatial relationships that contribute to the ability to estimate, for example, the relative distance between objects or the height of curbs and steps or to discriminate among objects on a shelf.[11] Individuals functioning primarily with monocular vision (visual input from one eye only) will have impairments of depth cues. Related to depth perception is "figure–ground," the ability to visually separate the object of focus from a diffuse background. With increasing age, the ability to recognize a simple visual figure embedded in a complex figure background declines. Using complex patterns on a floor surface may create a hazard if individuals perceive differing figure–ground patterns as changes in surface height or as objects. Furniture with different horizontal and vertical surfaces that contrast with the floor and walls can improve safety in visualizing surfaces when transferring from one furniture piece to another (or wheelchair to the furniture).

Hearing

An individual's hearing provides a primary link that allows him or her to identify with the environment and communicate effectively. Presbycusis, age-related hearing loss, is the most common cause of sensorineural hearing loss in older adults. Presbycusis results in decreasing sensitivity to sound, decreased ability to discriminate words in a noisy environment, slowing of the processing and interpretation of sounds, and difficulty localizing sound.[22,23] Tu and Friedman[24] report that presbycusis is independently associated with cognitive decline, dementia, depression, and loneliness. This loss can lead to decreased awareness of environmental cues, poor communication skills, and, ultimately, social isolation. With aging, there are both physiological and functional changes in the auditory system. Both the peripheral auditory system, which includes the structures of the ear itself, and the central nervous system, which integrates and gives meaning to sound, are affected. High-tone frequencies are generally affected before low-tone frequencies.[23] Scientists attribute the age-related hearing loss to three factors: conductive loss, sensorineural loss, and combined conductive and sensorineural loss.

Conductive hearing loss results from dysfunction of the external ear, the middle ear, or both that results in decreased transmission of sound wave vibration into the inner ear. The inner ear can receive and analyze the sound that reaches it. Thus, increasing the intensity of the signal through louder speech or mechanical amplification, such as a hearing aid, may help restore the ability to hear.

With a conductive loss, hearing impairment occurs across all sound frequencies. An appropriate intervention when speaking to older individuals with conductive hearing loss is to increase the speaker's volume to enable the person to hear the signal more clearly and to understand the speech. For individuals with profound hearing loss, an appropriate strategy may be to speak directly into the individual's ear. Devices such as timers, alarm clocks, smoke detectors, and doorbells can be modified or changed so that the signal is within the hearing range of older persons or to add a visual cue such as a flashing light.

Sensorineural hearing loss occurs when there is damage to the cochlea or the eighth cranial nerve. Presbycusis is the most common type of sensorineural hearing loss. Presbycusis can be associated with a number of changes in the inner ear cochlear structures: degenerative changes in nerve fibers, arteriosclerotic vascular changes in the stria vascularis, loss of elasticity in the basement membranes, or loss of ganglion hair along the auditory pathway. A person with presbycusis continues to hear tone but cannot understand what is heard, particularly in loud settings. Amplifications may be of limited benefit because these devices can amplify unintelligible sounds. High-pitched consonants such as *s*, *t*, *f*, and *g* are increasingly difficult to understand, especially in the presence of background noise, which masks the weak consonant sounds, or those rapidly articulated.[22]

Amplification technologies that allow frequency-selective amplification may be of some benefit. Some assistive listening devices, such as pocket amplifiers with external earphones and microphones, may also be beneficial. Many public venues now offer wireless voice amplification systems that a hearing-impaired individual can insert (as a Bluetooth-type device) in the ear. The speaker then uses an adapted microphone that amplifies the sound directly to the listener's Bluetooth device. Using lower frequency and pitch of signals from the television, stereo systems, or radio, which can be achieved by tuning the bass up and the treble down, can assist in compensating for the loss of high frequency.

Individuals with severe to profound bilateral sensorineural hearing loss may be candidates for cochlear implants if they are unable to benefit from conventional amplification. With these implants, the level of speech perception is predicted by the duration of deafness, duration of implant use, and hearing ability before implantation. As the technology for implants improves, better outcomes are achieved, including improved ability to detect sound at lower intensities, improved word recognition, and higher health-related quality-of-life scores.[25,26]

Therapists or designers may minimize the environmental background noise that competes with the older person's ability to hear by the use of acoustic materials such as drapes, upholstered furniture, and carpets, which absorb noise. Insulating sheet rock in noisy areas such as kitchens or community dining areas also helps improve individuals' hearing. Tight window seals can minimize exterior noise. In institutions and public buildings, attention should be paid to eliminating extraneous noise from commonly used devices such as motors associated with dishwashers, air conditioners, or heaters; fluorescent lighting that creates a buzzing sound; and loud background music. Interestingly, recent research using mice found that exercise had a protective effect on hearing loss, hypothesized as related to protective effects of exercise on arteriosclerotic vascular changes.[27] Further research with humans is needed to assess the potential impact of exercise to delay the onset of hearing loss and decrease the extent of hearing loss in older adults.

Specific strategies to use when communicating with an older adult with hearing loss are listed in Box 5.1.

BOX 5.1 Strategies to Use When Communicating with an Older Individual with Hearing Loss

- Face patient; make eye contact
- Say the person's name before beginning a conversation
- Talk clearly, at a normal pace, when in front of the patient
- Slightly project voice, as in speaking to a group
- Incorporate visual aids
- Change hearing aid batteries on a regular schedule (~2-week intervals)
- Avoid chewing gum or covering mouth when speaking, to allow the individual to use visual cues
- Do not speak into the person's ear
- Eliminate background noise or visual distractions
- Use rephrasing if repeating isn't effective
- When giving specific directions (such as an appointment), write it down
- Minimize side conversations

Smell

The sensation of smell declines gradually with age as well as in response to exposure to environmental pollutants or smoking.[28] A decline in the sense of smell can also be associated with respiratory system diseases and may be an early indication of a neurologic disorder such as Parkinson or Alzheimer disease.[29,30] The gradual nature of the loss of smell with advancing age might result in an older individual being unaware of the extent of the loss, which may place the person at risk of injury from undetected fire, fumes, or spoiled food.[31]

It is critically important that older persons who experience a decline in the ability to smell and live alone employ environmental adaptations such as smoke detectors with loud buzzers and safety-spring caps for gas jets on a stove. If the sensory loss is profound, switching from gas to electrical appliances may be indicated.

Touch

The sense of touch involves many separate processes labeled collectively as somatesthetic senses: touch and pressure, temperature, pain, and limb movement. People employ touch for awareness and protective responses. Our somatesthetic senses are used to interact with the environment and perceive multiple characteristics of an object.[22] For example, a surface may feel smooth or rough, soft or hard, warm or cold.

Evidence suggests that touch sensation decreases with age and varies from individual to individual. Many of the losses in touch sensitivity are the result of diseases such as diabetes or stenotic neuropathies that occur with greater frequency in older persons rather than as a result of the normal aging process. Increased thresholds for touch, especially textures, temperature, and limb movement, have implications for the older individual's ability to obtain important sensory input from the environment.

Decreased touch acuity can affect the ability of older individuals to localize stimuli. As a result, older individuals may have problems differentiating or manipulating small objects. The decrease in the speed of reaction to tactile stimulation can cause harm to an older person who takes longer to become aware of harmful or noxious stimuli such as temperature extremes, chemical irritants, or pressure from a stone in a shoe. Introducing texture into the environment can be valuable in assisting the independent functioning of older individuals, especially if there is impairment in other senses. Use of texture on handrails, doorknobs, and wall surfaces can give environmental cues and enhance safety.

Thermal Sensitivity. Changes in vascular circulation and loss of subcutaneous tissue as normal aging-related changes in older adults may result in changes in thermal sensitivity and impaired ability to cope with extreme environmental temperatures. One consequence is that older persons may feel cold and uncomfortable, even on a day that seems warm to a younger person. Air conditioning may not be tolerated, especially in the institutional environment. However, older adults have less ability to adapt their thermoregulatory system to adapt to heat exposure.[32]

Also, extremes in hot temperatures, for example, from hot bathwater or a heating pad, may not be readily detected by older individuals. As a consequence, individuals may experience a burn from the inability to react quickly to the temperature extreme. To accommodate the sensory decline in perceiving temperatures, having sensors on fixture controls and pressure balance features that prevent hot and cold surges are recommended.[33,34] As well, mounting the p-trap to the back wall provides space for wheelchair accessibility and helps prevent burns if used with extra insulated pipes. Fig. 5.2 illustrates wall-mounted p-trap plumbing with extra insulated pipes. For comfort, designers can suggest the installation of radiant heating beneath cold floorings such as under tiles or wood.

IMPACT OF SENSORY CHANGES ON DRIVING

Driving is a symbol of independence for most older adults and a necessity for many to commute to work and leisure activities and attend to instrumental activities of daily living. Age-related sensory changes impact driving performance as well as slowed reflexes and motor responses. Poor vision does not necessarily result in unsafe driving as many older adults self-restrict their driving to times of the day when light conditions are favorable. Nevertheless, several studies link specific visual impairments with accident-causing behaviors. These studies have found positive relationships between driver skills and visual acuity, depth perception, and contrast sensitivity.[13,35,36]

Age-related decline in visual acuity is highly individualistic, and deterioration in static acuity under optimal illumination, reduced illumination, and glare is generally not significant before age 60 years. Older drivers should recognize the importance of adequate visual correction with glasses or contact lenses and may need to modify driving patterns in low-light conditions.

Dynamic visual acuity, or the ability to detect a moving object, is a more complex task than static visual acuity. Deterioration in this ability begins at an earlier age and accelerates with increasing age. Studies have demonstrated a significant relationship between dynamic visual acuity and the amount of driving and accident involvement. Another skill that is conceptually critical to safe driving is motion perception. The driver's ability to detect movement in the environment relative to him- or herself is critical to detecting imminently dangerous situations. Visual changes discussed earlier, such as sensitivity to glare, reduced visual field, and the ability to discriminate foreground and background figures, increase the challenge of driving, especially in adverse conditions such as when raining, nighttime, and in bright, sunny times of the day. The declining visual field is another factor to

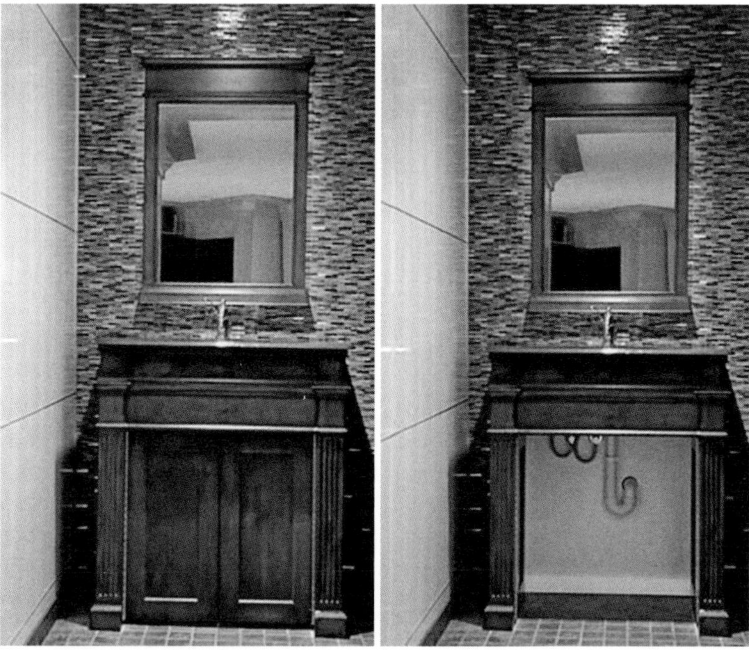

FIG. 5.2 Kohler vanity remodeled to clear the space for wheelchair users. Wall-mounted p-trap for the sink (to clear the knee space) with horizontal pipe and extra insulation. *(Courtesy of Cynthia Leibrock)*

consider. Older individuals must be aware of pedestrians or vehicles in the lateral field. Individuals who experience declines in peripheral vision must be taught to compensate by turning their heads or by using car mirrors. However, dissociating the hands on the steering wheel from vision is important as many older individuals will turn the steering wheel in the direction of the visual gaze. Similarly, drivers who have experienced loss in the upper visual field must be alerted to the need to look upward to avoid missing overhead road signs and traffic signals.

Depth perception is also known to decline with age and is additionally affected by increased susceptibility to glare, loss of visual acuity, dark adaptation, changing needs for illumination and contrast, and altered color perception. Older drivers need the ability to judge distances between their vehicle and other moving or stationary objects, which is critical for judging distances from oncoming cars, maintaining appropriate distances, safely passing other vehicles, merging onto a highway, or braking before reaching an intersection. Older drivers who experience difficulty with depth perception and are unable to compensate for this loss should be strongly cautioned to avoid driving.

Because older individuals have problems with dark adaptation, they may experience difficulty with changes in illumination coming from oncoming headlights or streetlights. As a result, night driving may pose a safety hazard, and older individuals may need to confine driving to daylight hours. Also, older drivers may be limited in night driving by glare intolerance. They should be instructed to compensate for this by avoiding looking at oncoming headlights, traveling on divided highways, or traveling on well-lit roads. Vehicle-design modifications introduced beginning with 1986 models have proved beneficial for older drivers who experience decreased night vision and difficulty with glare. These include changes in headlights, rear lights, and directional signals that are on the side of the vehicle. They also include design concepts that result in a reduction in windshield and dashboard glare and installation of rear-window defrosters and wipers.[13,36]

The impact of diminished color discrimination on driving is questionable. However, some suggest that it may take some older drivers twice as long as younger drivers to detect the flash of a brake light because red colors may appear dimmer as individuals age. The high-mounted rear brake light introduced in 1986 vehicle models may serve as an accommodation for older drivers.

In addition to the visual loss, older drivers may experience difficulty because of age-related changes in hearing. Specifically, they may be unable to hear horns from other motorists warning of oncoming hazards, or they may be unable to localize the source of such signals. Vehicle malfunction warnings, such as brake sensors, may also go undetected with diminished hearing. Older drivers can compensate for this loss by adhering to a strict vehicle maintenance schedule.

The final deterrents to safe driving for older individuals that safety experts consider are hazards specific to the road environment itself, for example, poorly placed and poorly designed road signs. Signs should be of sufficient size and should provide adequate color contrast for older drivers to see them. Traffic lights pose another difficulty. Hazards regarding traffic light changes at intersections occur when older drivers react slowly to light changes from green to red. Because night drivers rely on median and roadside delineator lines as visual cues, some experts believe that increasing the width of these markers from 4 to 8 inches would benefit older night drivers. Older drivers with visual deficits may have difficulty on two-lane highways and older highways that have closely placed on-ramps and off-ramps. Newer highway design that includes four-lane highways with wide separation and better delineation of on-ramps and off-ramps should prove valuable for older drivers.[36] Driving safety programs and online assessment of driving ability, specifically tailored for the older driver, are now readily available in both online and face-to-face formats. Two examples are provided in the references.[37,38]

ADAPTING LIVING ENVIRONMENTS TO ACCOMMODATE SENSORY CHANGES

Residential Facilities

Residential facilities designed using traditional concepts derived from the medical model may fail to meet the needs of the older population with multiple chronic conditions and sensory impairments. To enhance the quality of life for these individuals, architects and administrators are challenged to incorporate design principles that create environments to support age-related changes and enhance the functional performance of individuals with sensory losses.

Appropriate lighting can support greater independence and enhance the safety of older individuals with visual deficits. Although direct, incandescent lighting adds warmth, it may not provide adequate illumination and may also create light pools and shadows. Therefore, experts do not recommend direct lighting for use in corridors. It is, however, appropriate as supplemental task lighting. Instead, caregivers and administrators should provide desk lamps and table lamps by chairs for reading and close work. Indirect "white" fluorescent lighting is recommended for use in corridors because this type of lighting provides adequate and even illumination while minimizing glare. Experts suggest warm white bulbs that provide a softer tint. Minimize flickering, which can be a hazard, through a regular schedule for checking ballasts on fluorescent lights and replacing worn-out bulbs.

Choose window treatments to minimize the effect of glare. Allowing sufficient light through windows while minimizing glare is the goal. Using sheer draperies with a plain weave provides translucency without glare.

Draperies can also serve to absorb extraneous background noise.

Ceilings and wall coverings in residential facilities should be chosen to support the sensory deficits of older residents. Ceilings covered with acoustic tile are specially designed to absorb noise and extraneous sounds that interfere with speech discrimination. Designers recommend the use of these materials in corridors, dining rooms, and other areas where background noise is prevalent. Wall coverings can be chosen to serve multiple purposes. Color can be used for resident orientation and cuing. Choosing paint or fabric of different colors for various areas within the facility can provide meaning, especially for residents with cognitive deficits. Use of contrast on door frames can serve as added landmarks and assist residents in locating their personal room. The color contrast between walls and floors can provide valuable sensory information to minimize falls. Textured wall coverings that are soft to the touch have the added benefit of providing tactile cues for older individuals and for visually impaired residents. Repetitive, random, and vivid patterns that create visual illusions and unstable figure–ground relationships should be avoided, especially on stairs.

Floor coverings should be selected to enhance the mobility of older residents. Vinyl or linoleum is popular because it is easy to clean and provides little resistance to wheelchair mobility. Vinyl surfaces can, however, be a major source of glare, which designers suggest controlling through the use of nonglare wax. An alternative to vinyl is the use of carpet, which administrators often avoid because of concerns about stains and odor. Newer designs, including solution-dyed fibers and liquid-barrier backing, has minimized these problems. Low-looped pile very tightly woven can minimize friction, thus making it an acceptable option for individuals using wheelchairs for mobility.

In one study of the impact of carpeting versus vinyl floors in hospitals on older adult falls with injury, 17% of subjects who fell on carpeting sustained an injury versus 46% of individuals who fell on vinyl flooring, which represented a statistically significant difference.[39] Results of this study support the hypothesis that individuals who fall on a more compliant surface are less likely to be injured than those who fall on a noncompliant surface (vinyl flooring). However, there are also concerns that exceptionally high-compliant surfaces (plush carpeting) can be a destabilizing force on balance, thus increasing the risk of a fall. Recent studies of compliant floor covering (more compliant than vinyl but not carpeting) demonstrate a decreased risk of fall-related injuries without having a negative effect on balance.[40,41] Despite this important benefit, this type of flooring has been slow to be accepted because of concerns about installation costs and unknown features of longevity and maintenance.[40]

Furniture selected for residential facilities should be functional and, at the same time, supportive of sensory changes. Use of fabric upholstery can provide tactile cues and eliminate problems of glare created by vinyl upholstery. Choosing a color that contrasts with flooring can serve as a valuable visual cue for residents with visual deficits. Repetitive and illusionary patterns should be avoided. Administrators should avoid purchasing furniture that is subject to tipping such as lightweight chairs and tables.

Glare can be an unanticipated problem in bathrooms that tend to have strong lighting but also highly reflective surfaces such as vinyl flooring; porcelain sinks, bathtubs, and toilets; and chrome towel bars and grab bars. Suggestions to minimize glare include use of colored fixtures that can provide additional contrast with the floor and wall coverings. These are aesthetically pleasing and can serve as an important safety feature for older individuals with visual deficits who may experience difficulty in judging distance and differentiating surfaces when the toilet, bathtub, or grab bar are of the same color as the floor.

Communal dining areas can pose several design challenges in residential facilities. In addition to the usual problems with lighting and control of glare, there is the added problem of noise control. Because architects commonly locate dining areas adjacent to the kitchen, background noise from dishwashers and food processors can contribute to the difficulty hearing-impaired residents may have and can cause further social isolation of these individuals. Use of good insulating materials or locating dining areas away from kitchens is recommended to minimize this problem. Administrators can further reduce background noise through the use of tablecloths and placement of paper pads between cups and saucers.

For the older person living in a residential nursing facility, unpleasant odors from cleaning equipment, sanitizing sprays, and substances designed to mask offensive odors abound. Institutional administrators and others too often ignore pleasant odors associated with positive life experiences. The absence of "good" smells adversely affects the quality of life for these individuals. Opportunities should be created to stimulate positive life experiences with pleasant smells. Flowers with light fragrant scents, or diffusers with subtle smells of essential oils designed to calm or stimulate, can be placed in living areas to enhance the older person's sensory experience.

Physical Therapy Clinics

If older adults are to receive maximum benefit from physical therapy intervention, it is crucial that architects and designers incorporate previously discussed recommendations to accommodate the sensory losses that occur with aging when they renovate or build new facilities. These recommendations include controlling light sources; minimizing glare; and choosing appropriate ceilings, wall coverings, and floor coverings, as mentioned earlier. The materials covering mat tables and treatment tables should provide contrast to floor coverings so that older clients receive a specific visual cue that will enhance safety in transfers.

One significant problem in many physical therapy clinics is background noise. Suggestions to minimize this noise include confining equipment that produces substantial noise (such as whirlpools) to separate rooms insulated with acoustic material. Another recommendation is to provide individual treatment rooms rather than sectioning treatment areas with curtains. Not only will this afford privacy for older individuals, but also it will serve as a means of limiting background noise. Background music from radios and use of intercom devices should be discouraged because they serve as further distracters for the older persons with hearing loss. Low-pile carpeting or compliant noncarpet flooring should be considered to enhance ambulation, absorb sound, increase safety, and minimize glare.

Stairs

Stairs are one area within the environment that require special consideration because they are common sites of accidents leading to injury, hospitalization, and even death. Safe negotiation of stairs requires integration of visual, touch, and kinesthetic senses in combination with the conditions of the stairs—especially critical for the descent, which is generally more hazardous than the ascent. Successful stair negotiation requires that individuals make a transition from free-form movement on level surfaces to the highly specific foot placement required on stairs. Visual feedback is used initially to judge the position of the stair treads and maximize the accuracy of foot placement. Visual inspection of the steps allows the user to scan for hazards, including broken treads, irregularities, or obstacles on the stairs. Individuals then rely on their kinesthetic and touch sensations to obtain a feel of the treads and railings to ensure accurate foot placement. In older individuals, visual distractions that draw the user's attention away from the stair-climbing task and the presence of visually deceptive design of stair placement or depth are the leading causes of stair accidents (Fig. 5.3). The most critical piece of visual information for successful descent of stairs for the visually impaired is a singular and unambiguous indication of the edge of each step on the set of stairs. Optical illusions created by patterned carpeting or high-pile carpeting that masks tread edges can overpower the ability of individuals to detect tread edges and create a significant hazard.

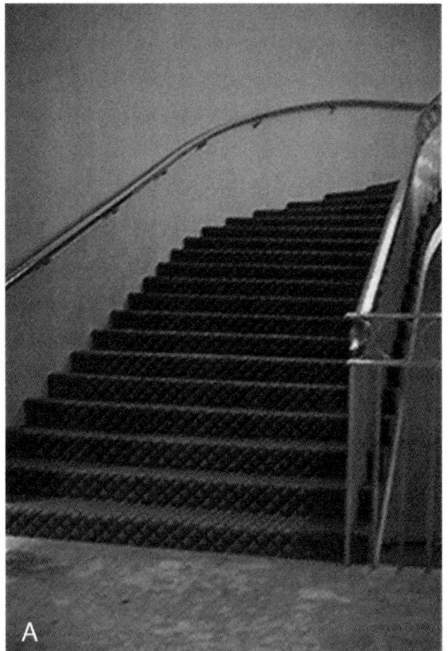

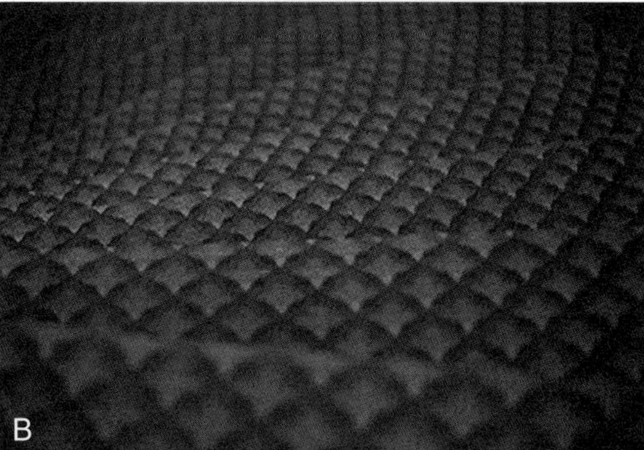

FIG. 5.3 Visual deception created by the design of the staircase carpeting: **(A)** depicting the overall **visual distraction** created from the carpet's embedded figure background and **(B)** providing a close up illustration of how the patterned carpeting can create a potential **challenge to depth perception and figure-ground discrimination**, making visualization of individual stair treads particularly difficult.

Other environmental considerations on stairs include the use of adequate lighting to enhance visual feedback, which includes placing light switches at both the top and bottom of the flight of steps, using nightlights located near the first and last steps to provide cuing during darkness, controlling glare from windows located near stairs with use of window coverings, and avoiding exposed light bulbs. LED strip lights mounted under the nose of each step, as depicted in Fig. 5.4, can be a low-cost option for providing even lighting. Kinesthetic feedback can be increased with the use of low-pile carpeting or ribbed vinyl or rubber stair nosing. The edges of noncarpeted stairs can be identified by a strip of paint or tape in a contrasting color that enhances the detection of the edge of the step.

Multifocal glasses (bifocals, trifocals, and progressive lenses) may contribute to the inability of older individuals to deal with challenges in the environment, especially on stairs. These multifocal glasses require the wearer to view the environment through the lower lenses when looking down, which have a typical focal length of 0.6 m. Normally, people view the environment at a distance approximating two steps ahead, at a critical focal distance of 1.5 to 2 m, which is the focal distance needed for detecting and discriminating floor-level objects. As a result, vision may blur and contrast sensitivity and depth perception may be adversely affected by individuals wearing multifocal glasses, thereby increasing the risk of falling.[42,43] One study verified that wearers of the multifocal lens had

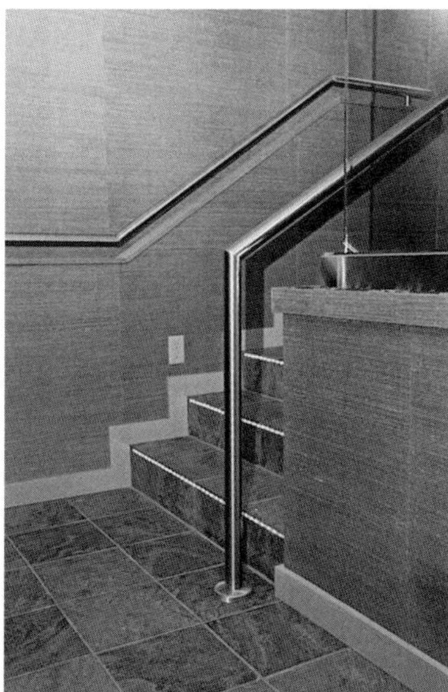

FIG. 5.4 Example of staircase modifications to enhance safety: LED lighting strips at nose of stairs, good lighting, extensions on the handrails to support balance after the last step, and textured wall surface that offers traction when leaning on the wall to prevent slips and falls. *(Photo courtesy of docktorpaul@mac.com.)*

significantly greater odds of falling than non-multifocal lens wearers. In this study, the falls were more likely to occur outside the home and when the individuals were walking up or down stairs.[42]

Personal/Living Space

All of the recommendations identified for residential or clinic spaces can be applied to the home on a more individualized level. Because the home is the hub of most activity for older individuals, creating an environment to support sensory loss and enhance maximum functional independence and well-being is critical. Incorporating the design principles and accommodative strategies for losses in vision, hearing, smell, and touch will not only facilitate independence but also may minimize the occurrence of accidents leading to disability or death. Adhering to these design principles will facilitate aging in place when constructing new dwellings or retrofitting existing residences. Additional recommendations for the home are identified next. References to useful materials to guide basic universal design home renovation and safety guidelines are provided in Box 5.2.

Environmental adaptations to support mobility limitations can range from high-priced structural changes to low-cost safety modifications. For example, widening doors to 36 inches to allow for wheelchair passage and providing a clearance space of 60 inches for adequate turning radius for a wheelchair may each involve major expenses, depending on the existing home layout. By contrast, adding bathroom grab bars and reinforcing existing grab bars by placing wood blocking between studs or the plywood are low-cost modifications with high safety value.

BOX 5.2 Aging in Place and Universal Design Resources and Checklists

American Association of Retired Persons (AARP): https://assets.aarp.org/www.aarp.org_/articles/families/HousingOptions/200590_HomeFit_rev011108.pdf

National Association of Home Builders: https://www.nahb.org/en/learn/designations/certified-aging-in-place-specialist/related-resources/aging-in-place-remodeling-checklist.aspx

AgingCare: https://www.agingcare.com/articles/grab-bar-safety-tips-139130.htm

The radius of grab bars should be appropriate for a good grip and sufficient clearance from the wall, but not too much clearance where the arm can become wedged between the gap if the hand slips off the bar. Some grab bars are made with textured materials to minimize slippage.

In the foyer/entry, a low-cost option is to add a seat for a person to sit on while donning or doffing outdoor clothing. Storage in this area should allow placement of bags and keys on the counter or console or even on wheelchairs when entering or leaving. Such an area should include visual access to outdoors to see guests arriving and judging the weather to decide what garments are appropriate for the weather.

There are options for kitchen cabinetry that allow accessibility for older persons with disabilities or from a wheelchair. The ideal (albeit expensive) solution is to provide adjustable-height cabinetry or cabinetry at varying heights. A not-too-expensive solution is to install adjustable-lift shelf hinges for appliances such as blenders and to use transparent storage containers (glass fronts with lights) to increase the visibility of objects. Homeowners should switch base cabinets into drawers that are not too deep or too low to be inaccessible. Using drawer and cabinet pulls instead of knobs can allow for minimal physical effort. Self-closing kitchen drawers and cabinets minimize hazards from open drawers and cabinets. Consideration of accommodations for wheelchair clearance around objects is needed to ensure sufficient space to maneuver around the kitchen.

In the bathroom, fixtures should be accessible from a seated position. The bathroom p-trap plumbing fixture should be turned and tucked into the wall to allow for clearance under the sink (Fig. 5.2). A shower with a "no lip transition" into and out of the shower is ideal for the individual in a wheelchair or an individual with significant balance impairments for which standing on one leg to transition over the side of a bathtub is a safety risk. A lower shower caddy should be available for individuals using a shower seat while showering. The shower space ideally would have sufficient room to accommodate a shower seat and allow for a second person to assist the individual, as needed.

There should be minimal transitions and an absence of thresholds between rooms. If the changes of materials on the floors between rooms requires a transition threshold, employ a beveled transition. If a step transition between rooms cannot be avoided, then a railing or secure grab bar should be provided. Additionally, the step transition should include a contrasting material change or a tape of a contrasting color. A flight of stairs should, preferably, have hand railings on both sides. Hand railings on outside steps are particularly important. In the absence of hand rails, lighting or color material contrasts are particularly important.

In the bedroom, individuals need adequate storage space for medicine or necessities at the sides of beds as well as adequate space and seating for family members. Throw rugs, while looking pleasant, may be hazardous and should not be used. Adequate overhead and task lighting will enhance mobility and safety and improve individuals' ability to engage in activities.

Special Considerations for Individuals with Dementia

Alzheimer disease and related dementias significantly alter the ability to perceive and interpret the environment. The extent of the changes is highly individual and depends on multiple factors, including neuropathologic changes, sensory loss, time of day, medications, and the social and physical environment. Some changes are consistent with normal age-related changes in sensory systems and common disease processes (cataracts or macular degeneration). Other changes relate to cognitive decline that affects the person's ability to perceive, process, and interpret sensory input.

Establishing a community as a "dementia-friendly community" was a concept first introduced by Alzheimer's Disease International and then adopted by organizations and communities across the world. The goal of a dementia-friendly community is to establish environments that minimize social isolation and foster participation and independence of individuals with dementia.[44] These environments may be at home, in the wider community, or in a residential living facility. Advocates of environmental modifications to create dementia-friendly communities remind us that the modifications that support independence and social connectedness for individuals with dementia are consistent with universal design principles that benefit all individuals with impaired sensory systems, regardless of the underlying cause.

For individuals with dementia, both under- and overstimulation can lead to confusion, illusions, frustration, and agitation. Wayfinding (finding your way from one place to another) can be problematic in individuals with dementia. Wayfinding when walking requires the person to first perceive directional information/landmarks in the environment, process the information, interpret the information, and encode the information to memory for future use (cognitive mapping).[18,45] Individuals with dementia benefit from a well-planned environment with uncomplicated designs that provide applicable—but not overwhelming—visual and auditory cues.

Studies[43,45,47] demonstrate that the physical layout of space in residential living communities impacts wayfinding. Decreasing environmental press can help accommodate declining cognitive competence and improve wayfinding. An ideal layout minimizes the number of directional choice points the individual needs to navigate. Ideally, key destinations are located along one straight or circular hallway, thus limiting the number of side hallways and turns. The more hallways and options for turns, the more difficult the wayfinding. Hallways should provide clearly identifiable landmark cues that are present regardless of the direction from which a person approaches the choice point. The landmark could be an object or picture that is easily recognizable to most people, such as a large and easily identifiable picture of a bird or flower. An abstract figure or drawing that is not easily linked to a concrete object should be avoided. Wayfinding landmarks should be brightly colored and placed at a height that most older adults will easily see while walking. Identifying specific rooms with specific and distinct colors on the doors and walls as you approach the room can help wayfinding. A clearly visible picture of the resident at a younger age can help the individual identify his or her own room. Brightly colored doors against a neutral background can be cues to guide individuals into and out of spaces that require opening doors. In contrast, doors that do not lead to common spaces for residents can be painted a color that blends in with the surrounding walls and thus are harder to perceive.

The combination of normal age-related sensory changes experienced by all older adults in concert with added difficulty in interpreting sensory input in the presence of dementia requires well-thought-out accommodations. Visual misperceptions where individuals with dementia have difficulty differentiating reality from representation may contribute to agitation. They may perceive framed photographs as family members watching them or perceive television shows as reality. Reflected glare may contribute to illusions and misperceptions. Taking care to minimize or control glare and avoiding use of highly patterned floor and wall coverings may reduce these misperceptions. Increasing light levels during activities may be effective in reducing agitation levels.

Some individuals with dementia experience auditory hallucinations and "static-like" noise. Further, noise can be an additional stressor. Suggestions to decrease background noise include using sound-absorbing fabrics such as drapes, carpeting, and wall hangings; using placemats on dining tables; choosing upholstered furniture; and eliminating or minimizing the use of overhead call systems in institutional environments. Introducing music and pleasant sounds, along with music therapy, is considered therapeutic and is known to help decrease agitation in individuals with dementia.[46] However, care must be exercised to ensure that content and volume are appropriate and the sounds are soothing.

Many residential facilities provide outdoor spaces or courtyards where older adults with dementia can "wander" on their own. These are carefully designed spaces that allow safe and free walking within a confined area. Walking and enjoying "outdoor" or brightly lit indoor garden/courtyard spaces can decrease agitation and enhance quality of life for individuals with dementia.

Touch is important and can have a therapeutic effect for individuals with dementia. Hand massages, the warm touch from a hug, and the presence of pets can have a positive effect on individuals with dementia. Related to the sensation of touch is thermoregulation. It is important to consider comfort levels, especially during activities of daily living. Use of heat lamps, sweat suits, layered clothing, and warming blankets can increase comfort level. One situation often causing agitation is discomfort associated with the perception of being cold during bathing. Suggestions to avoid this associated agitation are reducing chill by use of terrycloth robes, exposing a minimal amount of the body at any one time, and incorporating pleasant sensory stimulation to reduce the trauma of bathing. Specific suggestions are to control light levels in the bathing area with dimmer switches; to use rich apricot, yellow, or blue tones on bathroom walls; to add a fragrance to bathwater; and to play soothing, favorite music.

Because individuals with dementia experience sensory declines in taste and smell, it is important to enhance nutrition with flavor-enhanced food and to design the dining environment to maximize sensory cues to eating such as ensuring adequate lighting, minimizing distracting noise, enhancing pleasant smells of food, choosing tables and tableware that allow color and contrast between the tabletop and dinnerware, and using placemats and tablecloths with plain patterns to enhance contrast but avoid figure–ground confusion.[48–50]

TEACHING/CONSULTING STRATEGIES

Physical therapists working with the older adult are challenged to incorporate teaching strategies to accommodate sensory loss into treatment programs. Their unique knowledge of sensory changes that accompany aging, coupled with knowledge of appropriate interventions, will maximize the rehabilitation experience and afford older people an opportunity to use newly acquired skills in an environment that maintains reasonable control over functional ability and enhances the quality of their life.

Physical therapists should support and encourage referral to appropriate specialists for evaluation of specific deficits and prescription of needed devices, and encourage the use of adaptive equipment and assistive technology to compensate for the specific sensory loss. The therapists should also be knowledgeable about service agencies within the community that specialize in assistive technologies and resources for patients to identify and contact these resources.

Physical therapists can use their knowledge and skills related to movement dysfunction and ergonomics to further enhance the functional independence of older individuals who require accommodations for sensory changes. For example, physical therapists can be particularly helpful in providing positional recommendations to enhance comfort for older individuals who use accommodations for low vision that require maintenance of a specific focal distance. Identifying the best ergonomic positioning to maintain the focal distance while maintaining correct line of sight, head tilt, back position, and body posture for comfort and efficiency can be an essential component of utilizing low-vision systems.

Therapists should make similar suggestions for computer users who are visually impaired. Also, therapists may serve a valuable role in recommending adaptations to prescribed devices that address concurrent problems often experienced by older, visually impaired patients. These may include the use of adjustable reading stands to hold large-print reading material or special stands, clamps, or headbands to position magnifying devices for individuals with arthritis, stroke, or Parkinson disease, who may otherwise have difficulty using the prescribed device.

Specific teaching strategies that incorporate instruction in techniques to strengthen the sensory stimulus should be part of the physical therapy intervention for older individuals with sensory impairment. Examples might include adjustments to volume and tone of radios and televisions for hearing-impaired individuals or use of large-print books for the visually impaired. Another technique is to teach older individuals to compensate with other senses. For example, individuals with a diminished sense of smell can be taught to inspect food visually for signs of spoilage, or individuals with visual impairments can be encouraged to use auditory substitutions, including talking books and other talking products. The final strategy is to teach older individuals to modify their behavior. One example is to pause when entering a darkened room from a bright, outdoor environment.

Because of their knowledge of age-related sensory change, functional mobility, and environmental modifications, physical therapists should assume active roles as consultants. Applying this knowledge as a resource to architects and designers can foster designs that provide safer access of older individuals into a wide range of buildings, hospitals, outpatient clinics, and senior community centers. Physical therapists can also contribute to design planning to maximize independence of individuals in retirement complexes, senior housing, and long-term care facilities during new construction or renovation of existing facilities.

Encouraging architects and builders to incorporate universal design and aging-in-place concepts and design considerations to allow adaptability of structures to accommodate sensory changes related to age and disability may allow older individuals to remain in their own homes, and may be more economically feasible than renovating structures that do not incorporate such principles. Also, therapists should take an active role in the purchase of supplies for existing facilities. Therapists can maximize the quality of life for older residents by selecting such items as furniture, wall and floor coverings, and window treatments that enhance, rather than impede, functional performance. Finally, physical therapists can encourage the development of appropriate products to meet the needs of older individuals with a sensory loss by serving as consultants to companies that design and manufacture these devices.

SUMMARY

It is important for physical therapists who work with older adults to recognize sensory changes that occur with aging and to understand the effects that these changes have on the ability of older individuals to function in the environment. Knowledge of adaptations within the environment to accommodate and support losses that occur in vision, hearing, taste, smell, and touch can maximize the rehabilitation experience, promote optimal functional independence, and enhance the quality of life.

Physical therapists should be able to apply this information concerning sensory losses and environmental adaptations to general principles of design to create meaningful environments for older persons. Therapists should consider all aspects of the environment in which older individuals function. These include personal living space and long-term care residencies. They should give specific attention to architectural design of physical therapy departments and of all community spaces. Facilitating environmental design adaptations emphasizes the role of physical therapists as consultants. Physical therapists have unique knowledge of the needs of aging individuals, and they should be encouraged to share this knowledge with architects, designers, administrators, and others who deal with facilities and products used by older individuals.

REFERENCES

1. Sanford JA, Corry Hernandez S. Universal design, design for aging in place, and rehabilitative design in residential environments. In: Kopec D, ed. *Health and Well-Being for Interior Architecture*. New York: Routledge; 2017:137–147.
2. Chaudhury H, Cooke HA, Cowie H, Razaghi L. The influence of the physical environment on residents with dementia in long-term care settings: a review of the empirical literature. *Gerontologist*. 2018;58(5):e325–e337.
3. Nylen P, Favero F, Glimne S, Fahnehjelm KT, Eklund J. Vision, light and aging: a literature overview on older-age workers. *Work (Reading, Mass)*. 2014;47(3):399. http://kipublications.ki.se/Default.aspx?queryparsed=id:128538405.
4. Leibrock C, Terry JE. *Beautiful Universal Design*. New York: John Wiley & Sons; 1999.
5. University of Buffalo. *School of Architecture and Planning*. http://ap.buffalo.edu/research/research-centers/center-for-inclusive-design-and-environmental-access.html. Accessed March 24, 2019.
6. Safescore.org. https://safescore.org/checklists. Accessed March 24, 2019.
7. Denson MG. Empathic design matters. In: Kopec D, ed. *Health and Well-Being for Interior Architecture*. New York: Routledge; 2017:148–158.
8. Guest D, Howard CJ, Brown LA, Gleeson H. Aging and the rate of visual information processing. *J Vis*. 2015;15(14):10. https://doi.org/10.1167/15.14.10.
9. Cid-Fernández S, Lindín M, Díaz F. Information processing becomes slower and predominantly serial in aging: characterization of response-related brain potentials in an auditory-visual distraction-attention task. *Biol Psychol*. 2016; 113:12–23. https://doi.org/10.1016/j.biopsycho.2015.11.002.
10. Saftari LN, Kwon O. Ageing vision and falls: a review. *J Physiol Anthropol*. 2018;37(1):11–14. https://www.ncbi.nlm.nih.gov/pubmed/29685171. https://doi.org/10.1186/s40101-018-0170-1.
11. Andersen GJ. Aging and vision: changes in function and performance from optics to perception. *Wiley Interdisc Rev Cogn Sci*. 2012;3(3):403–410. https://doi.org/10.1002/wcs.1167. https://onlinelibrary.wiley.com/doi/abs/10.1002/wcs.1167.
12. Black AA, Wood JM, Lovie-Kitchin JE. Inferior field loss increases rate of falls in older adults with glaucoma. *Optom Vis Sci*. 2011;88:1275–1282.
13. Huisingh C, McGwin G Jr, Wood J, Owsley C. The driving visual field and a history of motor vehicle collision involvement in older drivers: a population-based examination. *Invest Ophthalmol Vis Sci*. 2014;56(1):132–138. https://www.ncbi.nlm.nih.gov/pubmed/25395488. https://doi.org/10.1167/iovs.14-15194.
14. Akpek E, Smith RA. *Overview of age-related ocular conditions*. https://www.ajmc.com/journals/supplement/2013/ace011_13may_agingeye/ace011_13may_agingeye_akpek?p=3. Published 2013.
15. Gell NM, Rosenberg DE, Demiris G, LaCroix AZ, Patel KV. Patterns of technology use among older adults with and without disabilities. *Gerontologist*. 2015;55(3):412–421. https://www.ncbi.nlm.nih.gov/pubmed/24379019. https://doi.org/10.1093/geront/gnt166.
16. McKendrick AM, Chan YM, Nguyen BN. Spatial vision in older adults: perceptual changes and neural bases. *Ophthal Physiol Optics*. 2018;38(4):363–375. https://onlinelibrary.wiley.com/doi/abs/10.1111/opo.12565. https://doi.org/10.1111/opo.12565.
17. Owsley C. Aging and vision. *Vision Res*. 2011;51(13):1610–1622. https://doi.org/10.1016/j.visres.2010.10.020.
18. Davis R, Weisbeck C. Creating a supportive environment using cues for wayfinding in dementia. *J Gerontol Nurs*. 2016;42(3):36–44.
19. Cooper BA, Ward M, Gowland CA, McIntosh JM. The use of the Lanthony New Color Test in determining the effects of aging on color vision. *J Gerontol*. 1991;46:320–324.
20. Green M. Using colour to improve care environments. *Nurs Residential Care*. 2005;7:510–512.
21. Swann J. Visual impairments: environmental considerations. *Nurs Residential Care*. 2008;10:90–92.
22. Linton AD. Age-related changes in the special senses. In: Linton AD, Lach HW, eds. *Matteson & McConnell's gerontological nursing: concepts and practice*. 3rd ed. Philadelphia: Saunders/Elsevier; 2007.
23. Yang CH, Schrepfer T, Schacht J. Age-related hearing impairment and the triad of acquired hearing loss. *Front Cell Neurosci*. 2015;9. https://doi.org/10.3389/fncel.2015.00276.
24. Tu NC, Friedman RA. Age-related hearing loss: unraveling the pieces. *Laryngoscope Investig Otolaryngol*. 2018;3(2):68–72. https://doi.org/10.1002/lio2.134.

25. Tang L, Thompson CB, Clark JH, et al. Rehabilitation and psychosocial determinants of cochlear implant outcomes in older adults. *Ear Hear.* 33017;38(6):663–671.
26. Sladen DP, Peterson A, Schmitt M, et al. Health-related quality of life outcomes following adult cochlear implantation: a prospective cohort study. *Cochlear Implants Int.* 2017;18(3):130–135.
27. Han C, Ding D, Lopez MC, et al. Effects of long-term exercise on age-related hearing loss in mice. *J Neurosci.* 2016;36(44):11308–11319. https://doi.org/10.1523/JNEUROSCI.2493-16.2016.
28. Hummel T, Kobal G, Gudziol H, Mackay-Sim A. Normative data for the "sniffin' sticks" including tests of odor identification, odor discrimination, and olfactory thresholds: an upgrade based on a group of more than 3,000 subjects. *Eur Arch Otorhinolaryngol.* 2007;264(3):237–243.
29. White TL, Sadikot AF, Djordjevic J. Metacognitive knowledge of olfactory dysfunction in Parkinson's disease. *Brain Cogn.* 2016;104:1–6.
30. Doty RL. Measurement of chemosensory function. *World J Otorhinolaryngol Head Neck Surg.* 2018;4(1):11–28.
31. White TI, Kurtz DB. The relationship between metacognitive awareness of olfactory ability and age in people reporting chemosensory disturbances. *Am J Psychol.* 200;116:99–110.
32. Kenny GP, Yardley J, Brown C, Sigal RJ, Jay O. Heat stress in older individuals and patients with common chronic diseases. *CMAJ.* 2010;182(10):1053–1060.
33. Leibrock C, Harris D. *Design Details for Health Making the Most of Design's Healing Potential.* 2nd ed. Hoboken, NJ: John Wiley & Sons; 2011.
34. Kopec D. *Environmental Psychology for Design.* 2nd ed. New York: Bloomsbury Publishing; 2012.
35. Pitts BJ, Sarter N. What you don't notice can harm you: age-related differences in detecting concurrent visual, auditory, and tactile cues. *Hum Factors.* 2018;60(4):445–464. https://doi.org/10.1177/0018720818759102.
36. Shinar D, Schieber F. Visual requirements for safety and mobility of older drivers. *Hum Factors.* 1991;33:507–519.
37. District of Columbia, Department of Motor Vehicles. Online Driving Assessment. http://onlinedrivingassessment.dmv.dc.gov/. Accessed July 3, 2019.
38. Driving Assessment for Elderly Drivers. The Drive Safety Team. July 28, 2017. https://drivesafety.com/how-to-assess-the-driving-fitness-of-the-elderly/
39. Healey F. Does flooring type affect risk of injury in older in-patients? *Nurs Times.* 1994;90:40–41.
40. Lachance CC, Jurkowski MP, Dymarz AC, et al. Compliant flooring to prevent fall-related injuries in older adults: a scoping review of biomechanical efficacy, clinical effectiveness, cost-effectiveness, and workplace safety. *PLoS ONE.* 2017;12(2):e0171652.
41. Wright AD, Heckman GA, McIlroy WE, Laing AC. Novel safety floors do not influence early compensatory balance reactions in older adults. *Gait Posture.* 2014;40(1):160–165. https://doi.org/10.1016/j.gaitpost.2014.03.015.
42. Lord, SR. Visual risk factors for falls in older people. *Age Ageing.* 2006;35(Suppl 2):ii42–ii45.
43. Lord SR, Smith ST, Menant JC. Vision and falls in older people: risk factors and intervention strategies. *Clin Geriatr Med.* 2010;26(4):569–581.
44. Shannon K, Bail K, Neville S. Dementia-friendly community initiatives: an integrative review. *J Clin Nurs.* 2019;28(11–12):2035–2045.
45. O'Malley M, Innes A, Wiener JM. Decreasing spatial disorientation in care-home settings: how psychology can guide the development of dementia friendly design guidelines. *Dementia.* 2017;16(3):315–328.
46. Abraha I, Rimland JM, Trotta FM, et al. Systematic review of systematic reviews of nonpharmacological interventions to treat behavioural disturbances in older patients with dementia. The SENATOR-OnTop series. *BMJ Open.* 2017;7. https://doi.org/10.1136/bmjopen-201601275. e012759.
47. Habell M. Specialised design for dementia. *Perspect Public Health.* 2013;133(3):151–157.
48. Bakker R. Sensory loss, dementia, and environments. *Generations.* 2003;27:46–51.
49. Brush JA, Calkins MP. Environmental interventions and dementia. *ASHA Leader.* 2008;13:24–25.
50. Burke TJ. Significance of tonal contrast in dementia accommodation. *Geriatrician.* 2003;21:11–15.

CHAPTER 6

Geriatric Pharmacology

Charles D. Ciccone

OUTLINE

INTRODUCTION

Physical therapists working with any patient population must be aware of the drug regimen used in each patient. Therapists must have a basic understanding of the beneficial and adverse effects of each medication and must be cognizant of how specific drugs can interact with various rehabilitation procedures. This idea seems especially true for geriatric patients receiving physical therapy. Older adults are generally more sensitive to the adverse effects of drug therapy, and many adverse drug reactions (ADRs) impede the patient's progress and ability to participate in rehabilitation procedures. An adequate understanding of the patient's drug regimen, however, can help physical therapists recognize and deal with these adverse effects as well as capitalize on the beneficial effects of drug therapy in their geriatric patients.

The purpose of this chapter is to discuss some of the pertinent aspects of geriatric pharmacology with specific emphasis on how drug therapy can affect older individuals receiving physical therapy. This chapter begins by describing the pharmacologic profile of the geriatric patient, with emphasis on why ADRs tend to occur more commonly in older adults. Specific ADRs that commonly occur in the older adult are then discussed. Finally, the beneficial and adverse effects of specific medications are examined, along with how these medications can have an impact on the rehabilitation of older adults.

Older adults are more likely than younger adults to experience an ADR, and these adverse reactions are typically more severe in older adults.[1] The increased incidence of adverse drug effects in older adults is influenced by two principal factors: the pattern of drug use that occurs in a geriatric population and the altered response to drug therapy in older adults.[2,3] A number of other contributing factors, such as multiple disease states, lack of proper drug testing, and problems with drug education and compliance, also increase the likelihood of adverse effects in older adults. The influence of each of these factors on drug response in older adults is discussed briefly here.

PATTERN OF DRUG USE IN OLDER ADULTS: PROBLEMS OF POLYPHARMACY

Older adults consume a disproportionately large number of drugs relative to younger people.[1] Adults older than age 65 years, for example, currently compose about 15% of the U.S. population,[2] but they purchase over 30% of all prescription drugs.[3] Given that more and more of the population is reaching advanced age, it seems certain that older adults will continue to receive a disproportionate share of drugs over the next several decades.[4]

A logical explanation for this disproportionate drug use is that older adults take more drugs because they suffer more illnesses.[5] Indeed, more than 80% of individuals older than age 65 years suffer from one or more chronic conditions, and approximately 36% of adults aged 65 and older living in the United States take at least five medications.[7] Likewise, older subpopulations such as nursing home residents and frail older patients often receive multiple drugs, with an increased likelihood of ADRs.[6,7] Use of nonprescription (over-the-counter) products is also an important factor in geriatric pharmacology, especially among the community-dwelling older adults who have greater access to these products.[8] Over-the-counter analgesics, cough/cold preparations, antacids, laxatives, and other nonprescription medications are often self-administered by older adults to help resolve various symptoms. In addition, older adults often seek out herbal preparations, vitamins, minerals, and other nutritional supplements, with the belief that such products can help promote optimal health.

Older adults therefore rely heavily on various prescription and nonprescription products, and medications are often essential in helping resolve or alleviate some of the illnesses and other medical complications that occur commonly in older adults. A distinction must be made, however, between the reasonable and appropriate use of drugs and the phenomenon of polypharmacy. Although sources may vary somewhat in exactly how they define this term, *polypharmacy* typically refers to the excessive or inappropriate use of medications.[9,10] Owing to the extensive use of medications in this population, older adults are often at high risk for polypharmacy.[4,11]

Polypharmacy can be distinguished from a more reasonable drug regimen by the criteria listed in Table 6.1. Of these criteria, the use of drugs to treat ADRs is especially important. The administration of drugs to treat drug-related reactions often creates a vicious cycle in which additional drugs are used to treat ADRs, thus creating more adverse effects, thereby initiating the use of more drugs, and so on (Fig. 6.1).[9] This cycle, known also as a "medication cascade effect," can rapidly accelerate until the patient is receiving a dozen or more medications.

In addition to the risk of creating the vicious cycle seen in Fig. 6.1, there are several obvious drawbacks to polypharmacy in older adults. Because each drug will inevitably produce some adverse effects when used alone, the number of adverse effects will begin to accumulate when several agents are used concurrently.[9,11] More importantly, the interaction of one drug with another (drug–drug interaction) increases the risk of an untoward reaction because of the ability of one agent to modify the effects and metabolism of another drug. If many drugs are administered simultaneously, the risk of ADRs increases exponentially.[11] Other negative aspects of polypharmacy are the risk of decreased patient adherence to

TABLE 6.1 Characteristics of Polypharmacy in Older Adults

Characteristic	Example
Use of medications for no apparent reason	Digoxin use in patients who do not exhibit heart failure
Use of duplicate medications	Simultaneous use of two or three laxatives
Concurrent use of interacting medications	Simultaneous use of a laxative and an antidiarrheal agent
Use of contraindicated medications	Use of aspirin in bleeding ulcers
Use of inappropriate dosage	Failure to use a lower dose of a benzodiazepine sedative-hypnotic
Use of drug therapy to treat adverse drug reactions	Use of antacids to treat aspirin-induced gastric irritation
Patient improves when medications are discontinued	Withdrawal of a sedative-hypnotic results in clearer sensorium

(Adapted from Simonson W. *Medications and the Elderly: A Guide for Promoting Proper Use.* Rockville, MD: Aspen Publications; 1984.)

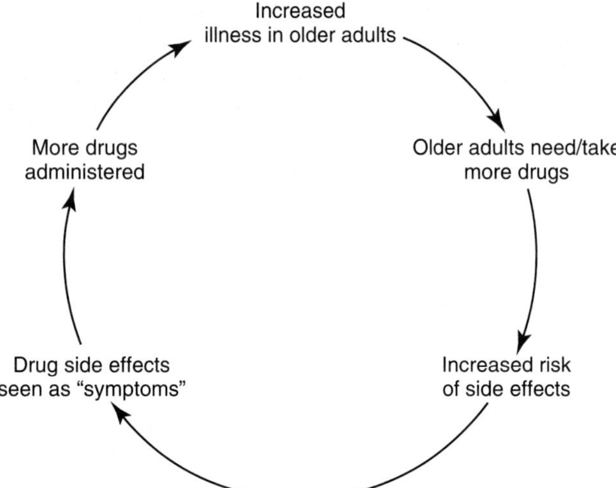

FIG. 6.1 Vicious cycle of drug administration that can lead to polypharmacy in the older adult.

the drug regimen[11,12] and the increased financial burden of using large numbers of unnecessary drugs.[10]

Polypharmacy can occur in older adults for a number of reasons. In particular, physicians may rely on drug therapy to accomplish goals that could be achieved through nonpharmacologic methods; that is, it is often relatively easy to prescribe a medication to resolve a problem in the older adult even though other methods that do not require drugs could be used. For instance, the patient who naps throughout the day will probably not be sleepy at bedtime. It is much easier to administer a sedative-hypnotic agent at bedtime rather than institute activities that keep the patient awake during the day and allow nocturnal sleep to occur naturally.

In some cases, the patient may also play a contributing role toward polypharmacy. Patients may obtain prescriptions from various practitioners, thus accumulating a formidable list of prescription medications. Older individuals may receive medications from friends and family members who want to "share" the benefits of their prescription drugs. Some older adults may also use over-the-counter and self-help remedies to such an extent that these agents interact with one another and with their prescription medications.

Polypharmacy can be prevented if the patient's drug regimen is reviewed periodically and any unnecessary or harmful drugs are discontinued.[13] Also, new medications should only be administered if a thorough patient evaluation indicates that the drug is truly needed in that patient.[14,15] When several physicians are dealing with the same patient, these practitioners should make sure that they communicate with one another regarding the patient's drug regimen.[10] Physical therapists can play a role in preventing polypharmacy by recognizing any changes in the patient's response to drug therapy and helping to correctly identify these changes as drug reactions rather than disease "symptoms." In this way, therapists may help prevent the formation of the vicious cycle illustrated in Fig. 6.1.

ALTERED RESPONSE TO DRUGS

There is little doubt that the response to many drugs is affected by age and that the therapeutic and toxic effects of any medication will be different in an older adult than in a younger individual. Alterations in drug response in older adults can be attributed to differences in the way the body handles the drug (pharmacokinetic changes) as well as differences in the way the drug affects the body (pharmacodynamic changes).[16,17] The effects of aging on drug pharmacokinetics and pharmacodynamics are discussed briefly here.

Pharmacokinetic Changes

Pharmacokinetics is the study of how the body handles a drug, including how the drug is absorbed, distributed, metabolized, and excreted. Several changes in physiological function occur as a result of aging that alter pharmacokinetic variables in older adults. The principal pharmacokinetic changes associated with aging are summarized in Fig. 6.2 and are discussed briefly here. The effects of aging on pharmacokinetics has been the subject of extensive research, and the reader is referred to several excellent reviews for more information on this topic.[17,18]

Drug Absorption. Several well-documented changes occur in gastrointestinal (GI) function in the older adult that could potentially affect the way drugs are absorbed from the GI tract. Such changes include decreased gastric acid production, decreased gastric emptying, decreased GI blood flow, diminished area of the absorptive surface, and decreased intestinal motility.[19,20] The effect of these changes on drug absorption, however, is often

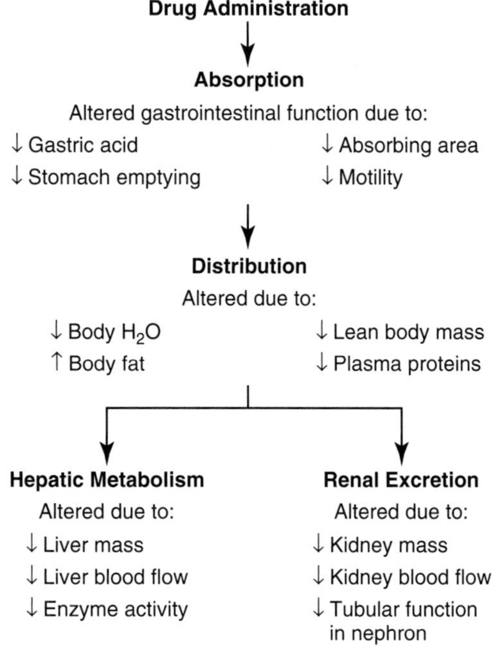

FIG. 6.2 Summary of the physiological effects of aging that may alter pharmacokinetics in older adults.

inconsistent; that is, aging does not appear to significantly alter the absorption of most orally administered drugs. This may be due in part to the fact that the aforementioned changes may offset one another. For instance, factors that tend to decrease absorption (e.g., decreased GI blood flow, decreased absorptive surface area) could be counterbalanced by factors that allow the drug to remain in the gut for longer periods (decreased GI motility), thus allowing more time for absorption. Hence, altered drug absorption does not appear to be a major factor in determining pharmacokinetic changes in older adults.

Drug Distribution. After a drug is absorbed into the body, it undergoes distribution to various tissues and body fluid compartments (e.g., vascular system, intracellular fluid, and so forth). Drug distribution may be altered in older adults because of several physiological changes such as decreased total body water, decreased lean body mass, increased percentage body fat, and decreased plasma protein concentrations.[21,22] Depending on the specific drug, these changes can affect how the drug is distributed in the body, thus potentially changing the response to the drug. For instance, drugs that bind to plasma proteins (e.g., aspirin, warfarin) may produce a greater response because there will be less drug bound to plasma proteins and more of the drug will be free to reach the target tissue. Drugs that are soluble in water (e.g., alcohol, morphine) will be relatively more concentrated in the body because there is less body water in which to dissolve the drug. Increased percentages of body fat can act as a reservoir for lipid-soluble drugs, and problems related to drug storage may occur with these agents. Hence, these potential problems in drug distribution must be anticipated, and dosages must be adjusted accordingly in older individuals.

Drug Metabolism. The principal role of drug metabolism (biotransformation) is to inactivate drugs and create water-soluble by-products (metabolites) that can be excreted by the kidneys. Although some degree of drug metabolism can occur in tissues throughout the body, the liver is the primary site for metabolism of most medications. Several distinct changes in liver function occur with aging that affect hepatic drug metabolism. The total drug-metabolizing capacity of the liver decreases with age because of a reduction in liver mass, a decline in hepatic blood flow, and decreased activity of drug-metabolizing enzymes.[23,24] As a result, drugs that undergo inactivation in the liver will remain active for longer periods because of the general decrease in the hepatic metabolizing capacity seen in older adults.

Drug Excretion. The kidneys are the primary routes for drug excretion from the body. Drugs reach the kidney in either their active form or as a drug metabolite after biotransformation in the liver. In either case, it is the kidney's responsibility to filter the drug from the circulation and excrete it from the body via the urine. With aging, declines in renal blood flow, renal mass, and function of renal tubules result in a reduced ability of the kidneys to excrete drugs and their metabolites.[25,26] These changes in renal function tend to be some of the most important factors affecting drug pharmacokinetics in older adults, and reduced renal function should be taken into account whenever drugs are prescribed to these individuals.[27,28]

The cumulative effect of the pharmacokinetic changes associated with aging is that drugs and drug metabolites often remain active for longer periods, thus prolonging drug effects and increasing the risk for toxic side effects. This is evidenced by the fact that drug half-life (the time required to eliminate 50% of the drug remaining in the body) is often substantially longer in an older individual versus a younger adult.[17] For example, the half-life of certain medications such as the benzodiazepines (e.g., diazepam [Valium], chlordiazepoxide [Librium]) can be increased as much as fourfold in older adults.[29] Obviously, this represents a dramatic change in the way the older adult's body deals with certain pharmacologic agents. Altered pharmacokinetics in older adults must be anticipated by evaluating changes in body composition (e.g., decreased body water, increased percentages of body fat) and monitoring changes in organ function (e.g., decreased hepatic and renal function) so that drug dosages can be adjusted and ADRs minimized in older individuals.[17]

Finally, it should be noted that the age-related pharmacokinetic changes described here vary considerably from person to person within the geriatric population.[17,30] These changes are, however, considered part of the "normal" aging process. Any disease or illness that affects drug distribution, metabolism, or excretion will cause an additional change in pharmacokinetic variables, thus further increasing the risk of ADRs in older adults.[16,31]

Pharmacodynamic Changes

Pharmacodynamics is the study of how drugs affect the body, including systemic drug effects as well as cellular and biochemical mechanisms of drug action. Changes in the control of different physiological systems can influence the systemic response to various drugs in older adults.[16,32] For instance, deficits in the homeostatic control of circulation (e.g., decreased baroreceptor sensitivity, decreased vascular compliance) may change the response of older adults to cardiovascular medications. Other age-related changes, such as impaired postural control, decreased visceral muscle function, altered thermoregulatory responses, and declines in cognitive ability, can alter the pharmacotherapeutic response as well as the potential side effects that may occur when various agents are administered to the older adult.[18,33] The degree to which systemic drug response is altered will vary depending on the magnitude of these physiological changes in each individual.

In addition to these systemic changes, the way a drug affects tissues on a cellular level may be different in the older adult. Most drugs exert their effects by first binding to a receptor that is located on or within specific target

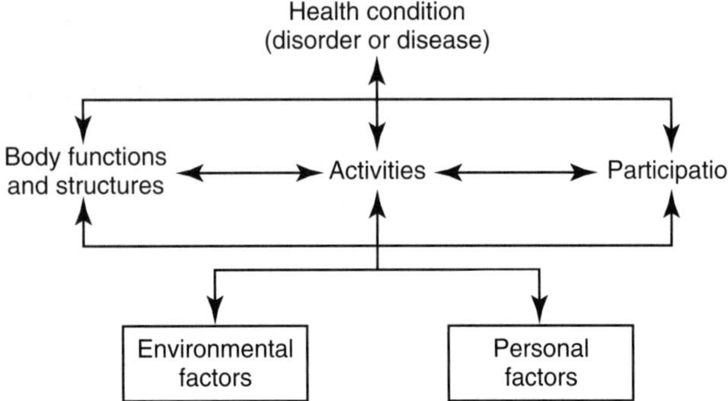

FIG. 6.3 Potential sites for altered cellular responses in older adults. Changes may occur (1) in drug–receptor affinity, (2) in the coupling of the receptor to an intracellular biochemical event, and (3) in the cell's ability to generate a specific biochemical response.

cells that are influenced by each type of drug. This receptor is usually coupled in some way to the biochemical "machinery" of the target cell, so that when the drug binds to the receptor, a biochemical event occurs that changes cell function in a predictable way (Fig. 6.3). For instance, binding of epinephrine (adrenaline) to β1-receptors on myocardial cells causes an increase in the activity of certain intracellular enzymes, which in turn causes an increase in heart rate and contractile force. Similar mechanisms can be described for other drugs and their respective cellular receptors. The altered response to certain drugs seen in older adults may be caused by one or more of the cellular changes depicted in Fig. 6.3. For instance, alterations in the drug–receptor attraction (affinity) could help explain an increase or decrease in the sensitivity of the older adult to various medications.[28,34] Likewise, changes in the way the receptor is linked or coupled to the cell's internal biochemistry have been noted in certain tissues as a function of aging.[32,35] Finally, the actual biochemical response within the cell may be blunted because of changes in subcellular structure and function that occur with aging.[36] Age-related declines in mitochondrial function, for example, could influence how the cell responds to various medications.[37]

Changes in cellular activity, however, vary according to the tissue and the drugs that affect that tissue. Although some tissues might be more sensitive to certain drugs (e.g., increased sensitivity of central nervous system [CNS] tissues to psychotropics and opioids), other tissues may be less responsive (e.g., decreased sensitivity of the cardiovascular system to β-adrenergic agents).[35] Age-related changes in cellular response must therefore be considered according to each tissue and the specific drugs that affect that tissue.

Consequently, pharmacodynamics may be altered in older adults as a result of systemic physiological changes acting in combination with changes in drug responsiveness that occur on a cellular or even subcellular level. These pharmacodynamic changes along with the pharmacokinetic changes discussed earlier help explain why the response of a geriatric individual to drug therapy often differs from the analogous response in a younger individual.

OTHER FACTORS THAT INCREASE THE RISK OF ADVERSE DRUG REACTIONS IN OLDER ADULTS

In addition to the pattern of drug use and the altered response to drugs seen in older adults, several other factors may contribute to the increased incidence of ADRs seen in these individuals. Several of these additional factors are presented here.

Presence of Multiple Disease States

The fact that older people often suffer from several chronic conditions greatly increases the risk of ADRs.[5,38] The presence of more than one disease (comorbidity) often necessitates the use of several drugs, thus increasing the risk of drug–drug interactions. Even more important is the fact that various diseases and illnesses usually alter the pharmacokinetic and pharmacodynamic variables discussed earlier. For instance, the age-related changes in hepatic metabolism and renal excretion of drugs are affected to an even greater extent if liver or kidney disease is present. Many older patients suffer from diseases that further decrease function in both of these organs as well as cause diminished function in other physiological systems. The involvement of several organ systems, combined with the presence of several different drugs, makes the chance of an ADR almost inevitable in older adult patients with multiple disease states.

Lack of Proper Drug Testing and Regulation

The Food and Drug Administration (FDA) is responsible for monitoring the safety and efficacy of all drugs marketed in the United States. The FDA requires all drugs to undergo extensive preclinical (animal) and clinical (human) trials before they receive approval. With regard to older adults, some question has been raised about the evaluation of drugs in geriatric individuals prior to FDA approval. It has been recognized that an adequate number of patients older than age 65 years should be included at various stages of the clinical testing, especially for drugs that are targeted for problems that occur primarily in older adults (e.g., dementia, Parkinson disease, and so forth).[39,40] It is unclear, however, whether efforts to increase drug testing in geriatric subjects have been successful in providing improved information about drug safety in older adults.[39] Clinical trials, for example, may lack adequate numbers of older subjects, especially subjects who are older than age 75 years.[40] Additional efforts on the part of the FDA and the drug manufacturing companies may be necessary to help reduce the risk of adverse effects through better drug testing.

There also has been concern that many drugs are overprescribed and misused in older adults. This concern seems especially true for certain classes of psychotropic agents (e.g., antipsychotics, sedative-hypnotic agents).[41] Fortunately, efforts have been made to institute government regulations and guidelines that limit the use of these medications.[42] It is hoped that enforcement of existing regulations and development of guidelines for other types of drugs will reduce the incidence of inappropriate drug use in older adults.

Problems with Patient Education and Nonadherence to Drug Therapy

Even the most appropriate and well-planned drug regimen will be useless if the drugs are not taken as directed. Patients may experience an increase in adverse side effects, especially if drugs are taken in excessive doses or for the wrong reason.[43,44] Conversely, older patients may stop taking their medications, resulting in a lack of therapeutic effects and a possible increase in disease symptoms. The fact that older patients often neglect to take their medications is one of the most common types of drug nonadherence.[45,46]

Many factors can disrupt the older individual's adherence (compliance) to drug therapy. A decline in cognitive function, for example, may impair the older person's ability to understand instructions given by the physician, nurse practitioner, or pharmacist. This can hamper the ability of the geriatric patient to take drugs according to the proper dosing schedule, especially if several medications are being administered, with a different dosing schedule for each medication.[45] Other factors such as poor eyesight may limit the older person's ability to distinguish one pill from another, and arthritic changes may make it difficult to open certain "childproof" containers.

Some patients may fail to adhere to drug therapy because they feel that their medications are simply not effective; that is, they fail to see any obvious benefit from the drugs.[43] The older adult may also stop taking a medication because of an annoying but unavoidable side effect.[46,47] For instance, older patients with hypertension may refuse to take a diuretic because this particular medication increases urinary output and may necessitate several trips to the bathroom in the middle of the night. To encourage patient self-adherence, it must be realized that these annoying side effects are not trivial and can represent a major source of concern to the patient. Hence, health care professionals should not dismiss these complaints but should make an extra effort to help the patient understand the importance of adhering to the drug regimen whenever such unavoidable side effects are present.

Use of Inappropriate Medications

Because of the physiological changes described earlier, certain medications pose an especially high risk for ADRs in older adults. To identify these medications, an expert panel developed criteria and compiled a specific list of medications that should probably be avoided in people older than age 65 years.[15,48] These criteria and the related list are known commonly as the Beers criteria (or Beers list) because they were created originally by geriatrician Mark Beers. The Beers criteria/list has been updated periodically to indicate medications that should be avoided and thus help improve geriatric prescribing.[7,48] For a current listing of Beers criteria, the reader is directed to https://www.guidelinecentral.com/summaries/american-geriatrics-society-2015-updated-beers-criteria-for-potentially-inappropriate-medication-use-in-older-adults/#section-420. Other guidelines such as the Screening Tool of Older Persons Prescriptions (STOPP) and the Screening Tool to Alert for Right Treatment (START) provide specific criteria that can help determine appropriate versus inappropriate use of medications in older adults.[15,49,50] Physicians and pharmacists can refer to these criteria to avoid the use of certain drugs in older adults, thereby reducing the risk of serious adverse effects in this population.

Additional Factors

Other factors, including poor diet, excessive use of over-the-counter products, cigarette smoking, and consumption of various other substances (e.g., caffeine, alcohol), may help contribute to the increased risk of adverse drug effects in older adults.[51–54] These factors must be taken into consideration when a prescription drug program is implemented for older individuals. For instance, it must be realized that the older adult with a protein-deficient diet may have extremely low plasma protein levels, thus further altering drug pharmacokinetics and increasing the risk of an adverse drug effect. It is therefore important to consider all aspects of the lifestyle and environment of the older adult that may affect drug therapy in these individuals.

COMMON ADVERSE DRUG REACTIONS

An ADR is any unwanted and potentially harmful effect caused by a drug when the drug is given at the recommended dosage.[1] Listed here are some of the more common ADRs that may occur in older adults. Of course, this is not a complete list of all the potential ADRs, but these are some of the responses that physical therapists should be aware of when dealing with geriatric patients in a rehabilitation setting.

Gastrointestinal Symptoms

Gastrointestinal problems such as nausea, vomiting, diarrhea, and constipation are among the most commonly occurring adverse drug reactions in older adults.[55] These reactions can occur with virtually any medication, and GI symptoms are especially prevalent with certain medications such as the opioid (narcotic) and nonopioid (nonsteroidal anti-inflammatory drugs [NSAIDs]) analgesics. Although these symptoms are sometimes mild and transient in younger patients, older individuals often require adjustments in the type and dosage of specific medications that cause gastrointestinal problems.

Sedation

Older adults seem especially susceptible to drowsiness and sleepiness as a side effect of many medications. In particular, drugs that produce sedation as a primary effect (e.g., sedative-hypnotics) as well as drugs with sedative side effects (e.g., opioid analgesics, antipsychotics) will often produce excessive drowsiness in older adults.

Confusion

Various degrees of confusion ranging from mild disorientation to delirium may occur with a number of medications, such as antidepressants, narcotic analgesics, and drugs with anticholinergic activity.[56,57] Confusion can also indicate that certain drugs, such as lithium and digoxin, are accumulating and reaching toxic levels in the body. Older individuals who are already somewhat confused may be more susceptible to drugs that tend to further increase confusion.

Depression

Symptoms of depression (e.g., intense sadness and apathy, as described elsewhere in this text) may be induced in older adults by certain medications. Drugs such as barbiturates, antipsychotics, alcohol, and several antihypertensive agents (e.g., clonidine, reserpine, propranolol) have been implicated in producing depression as an ADR in older adults.[47,58,59]

Orthostatic Hypotension

Orthostatic (postural) hypotension is typically described as a 20-mmHg or greater decline in systolic blood pressure or a 10-mmHg or greater decline in diastolic blood pressure that occurs within 3 minutes after an individual assumes a more upright posture (e.g., moving from lying to sitting or from sitting to standing).[60] Owing to the fact that many older adults are relatively sedentary and have diminished cardiovascular function, these individuals tend to be more susceptible to episodes of orthostatic hypotension, even without the influence of drug therapy.[60,61] A number of medications, however, augment the incidence and severity of this blood pressure decline.[62] In particular, drugs that tend to lower blood pressure (e.g., antihypertensives, antianginal medications) are a common cause of orthostatic hypotension in older adults. Orthostatic hypotension often leads to dizziness and syncope, because blood pressure is too low to provide adequate cerebral perfusion and oxygen delivery to the brain. Hence, orthostatic hypotension may precipitate falls and subsequent injury (e.g., hip fractures, other trauma) in older individuals.[63,64] Because older patients are especially susceptible to episodes of orthostatic hypotension during certain rehabilitation procedures (e.g., gait training, functional activities), physical therapists should be especially alert for this ADR.

Fatigue and Weakness

Strength loss and muscular weakness may occur for a number of reasons in response to drug therapy. Some agents, such as the skeletal muscle relaxants, may directly decrease muscle contraction strength, whereas other drugs, such as the diuretics, may affect muscle strength by altering fluid and electrolyte balance. Prolonged used of anti-inflammatory steroids (glucocorticoids) can cause muscle breakdown, and muscle pain and weakness can be induced in certain patients taking statin drugs to control hyperlipidemia. Older individuals who are already debilitated will be more susceptible to strength loss as an ADR.

Dizziness and Falls

Drug-induced dizziness can be especially detrimental in older adults because of the increased risk of loss of balance and falling. Problems with dizziness result from drugs that produce sedation or from agents that directly affect vestibular function. Examples of such agents include sedatives, antipsychotics, opioid analgesics, antiepileptics, and antihistamine drugs.[65,66] Dizziness may also occur secondary to drugs that cause orthostatic hypotension (see previous discussion). Anticholinergic drugs (see the next section) are also notorious for causing dizziness and slowed postural reflexes that lead to falls. Drug-induced dizziness and increased risk of falling may be especially prevalent in older adults who already exhibit balance problems, and physical therapists should be especially alert for these ADRs in these individuals.

Anticholinergic Effects

Acetylcholine is an important neurotransmitter that controls function in the CNS and also affects peripheral organs such as the heart, lungs, and GI tract. A number of drugs exhibit anticholinergic side effects, meaning that these agents tend to diminish the response of various tissues to acetylcholine. In particular, antihistamines, antidepressants, and certain antipsychotics tend to exhibit anticholinergic side effects. Acetylcholine affects several diverse physiological systems throughout the body, and drugs with anticholinergic effects are therefore associated with a wide range of ADRs. Drugs with anticholinergic effects may produce CNS effects, such as confusion, nervousness, drowsiness, and dizziness. Peripheral anticholinergic effects include dry mouth, constipation, urinary retention, tachycardia, and blurred vision. Older adults seem to be more sensitive to anticholinergic effects, possibly because the acetylcholine influence has already started to diminish as a result of the aging process. In any event, physical therapists should be aware that a rather diverse array of potentially serious ADRs may arise from drugs with anticholinergic properties.

Extrapyramidal Symptoms

Drugs that produce side effects that mimic extrapyramidal tract lesions are said to exhibit extrapyramidal symptoms. Such symptoms include tardive dyskinesia, pseudoparkinsonism, akathisia, and other dystonias. Antipsychotic medications are commonly associated with an increased risk of extrapyramidal symptoms. The problem of extrapyramidal symptoms as an antipsychotic ADR is presented in more detail later in this chapter.

DRUG CLASSES COMMONLY USED IN OLDER ADULTS

This section provides a brief overview of drug therapy in older adults. Included are some of the more common groups of drugs that are prescribed to older adults. For each group, the principal clinical indication or indications are listed, along with a brief description of the mechanism of action of each type of drug. The primary adverse effects and any specific concerns for physical therapy in older patients receiving these drugs are also discussed. Examples of typical drugs found in each of the major groups are indicated in several tables in this section. For additional information about specific agents listed here, the reader can refer to one of the sources listed at the end of this chapter.[67–69]

Psychotropic Medications

Psychotropic drugs include a variety of agents that affect mood, behavior, and other aspects of mental function. As a group, older adults exhibit a high incidence of psychiatric disorders.[70,71] Psychotropic drugs are therefore commonly used in older individuals and are also associated with a high incidence of adverse effects that can have an impact on rehabilitation.[29,71] The major groups of psychotropic drugs are listed in Table 6.2, and pertinent aspects of each group are discussed here.

Sedative-Hypnotic and Antianxiety Agents. Sedative-hypnotic drugs are used to relax the patient and promote a relatively normal state of sleep. Antianxiety drugs are intended to decrease anxiety without producing excessive sedation. Insomnia and disordered sleep may occur in older individuals concomitant to normal aging or in response to medical problems and lifestyle changes that occur with advanced age.[72,73] Likewise, medical illness, depression, and other aspects of aging may result in increased feelings of fear and apprehension in older adults.[70] Hence, use of sedative-hypnotic and antianxiety drugs is commonly encountered in older adults.

Historically, a group of agents known as the benzodiazepines have been the primary drugs used to promote sleep and decrease anxiety in older adults (see Table 6.2).[74] Benzodiazepines exert their beneficial effects by increasing the central inhibitory effect of the neurotransmitter γ-aminobutyric acid (GABA).[75] This increase in GABA-mediated inhibition seems to account for the decreased anxiety and increased sleepiness associated with these drugs.

TABLE 6.2 Psychotropic Drug Groups

Group	Common Examples: Generic Name	Common Examples: Trade Name
Sedative-Hypnotic Agents		
Benzodiazepines	Estazolam	ProSom
	Flurazepam	Dalmane
	Temazepam	Restoril
	Triazolam	Halcion
Others	Eszopiclone	Lunesta
	Ramelteon	Rozerem
	Suvorexant	Belsomra
	Zaleplon	Sonata
	Zolpidem	Ambien, others
Antianxiety Agents		
Benzodiazepines	Chlordiazepoxide	Librium, others
	Diazepam	Valium
	Lorazepam	Ativan
Azapirones	Buspirone	BuSpar, Vanspar
Antidepressants		
Tricyclics	Amitriptyline	Elavil, Endep, Vanatrip
	Imipramine	Tofranil
	Nortriptyline	Aventyl, Pamelor
	Trimipramine	Surmontil
MAO inhibitors	Isocarboxazid	Marplan
	Phenelzine	Nardil
Selective serotonin reuptake inhibitors	Citalopram	Celexa
	Escitalopram	Lexapro
	Fluoxetine	Prozac
	Fluvoxamine	Luvox
	Paroxetine	Paxil
	Sertraline	Zoloft
Serotonin–norepinephrine reuptake inhibitors	Desvenlafaxine	Khedezla, Pristiq
	Duloxetine	Cymbalta, Irenka
	Venlafaxine	Effexor
Other antidepressants	Bupropion	Wellbutrin
	Maprotiline	Ludiomil
	Mirtazapine	Remeron
	Nefazodone	Serzone
	Trazodone	Oleptro, Desyrel
Antipsychotics		
Conventional agents	Chlorpromazine	Ormazine, Thorazine
	Haloperidol	Haldol
	Loxapine	Loxitane
	Molindone	Moban
	Prochlorperazine	Compazine
	Thioridazine	Mellaril
Second generation (atypical antipsychotics)	Aripiprazole	Abilify
	Clozapine	Clozaril, Versacloz
	Iloperidone	Fanapt
	Lurasidone	Latuda
	Olanzapine	Zyprexa
	Paliperidone	Invega
	Quetiapine	Seroquel
	Risperidone	Risperdal
	Ziprasidone	Geodon

MAO, monoamine oxidase.

There is considerable debate, however, over whether benzodiazepines should be administered to older adults. These drugs tend to have long half-lives, which can lead to prolonged effects, especially in older adults, who have decreased elimination of these drugs.[29] Older patients also seem to be more sensitive to their adverse effects, and problems such as dizziness, confusion, delirium, and falls are especially problematic.[76] Although a causal link has not been established, there is concern that these drugs can predispose older adults to dementia, including Alzheimer disease.[77,78] Long-term use can also lead to tolerance and dependence, which could be problematic if the drug is suddenly discontinued.[76]

Despite these concerns, benzodiazepine use in older adults remains relatively high, with many patients receiving an inappropriate drug, dose, or duration of treatment.[74,76] Perhaps benzodiazepines can help the older patient cope with occasional sleep disturbances or acute anxiety, but these drugs should be used at the lowest possible dose and for only short periods while trying to find nonpharmacologic methods (e.g., counseling and decreased caffeine use) to deal with the patient's insomnia or anxiety.[72,74]

To treat insomnia and anxiety more effectively in older adults, several newer strategies have been explored. Regarding sleep disorders, nonbenzodiazepine agents such as eszopiclone, zolpidem, and zaleplon are now available (see Table 6.2).[79–81] Although these newer drugs also affect the GABA receptor, they appear to bind somewhat more selectively to this receptor than the benzodiazepines, and these drugs may have more favorable elimination characteristics than the benzodiazepines.[82] Another option is suvorexant (Belsomra), which blocks orexin receptors in the brain, thereby reducing the ability of orexin neuropeptides to promote wakefulness.[83] Additionally, ramelteon (Rozerem) is a drug that stimulates CNS melatonin receptors, and this drug may also be effective in promoting sleep in older adults with less risk of residual effects and addiction.[84,85] Given the important role that endogenous melatonin plays in promoting sleep, it follows that melatonin can also be given directly as a drug to help improve sleep and reduce insomnia.[84] Therapeutic doses of melatonin have therefore gained acceptance as a viable treatment for sleep disorders in certain older patients.[86]

Regarding treatment of anxiety, agents known as the azapirones (e.g., buspirone) can be used as an alternative to benzodiazepines.[87] These agents appear to decrease anxiety by directly stimulating serotonin receptors in certain parts of the brain (dorsal raphe nucleus) rather than by increasing GABA-mediated inhibition like the benzodiazepines.[87] More importantly, azapirones such as buspirone do not cause sedation, do not impair cognition and psychomotor function, and appear to have a much lower potential for the patient developing tolerance and physical dependence than traditional agents such as the benzodiazepines.[88] The primary shortcoming is that buspirone does not take effect very quickly, and is not as effective in treating more sudden, severe episodes of anxiety.

Likewise, certain antidepressants are currently regarded as effective treatments for anxiety disorders in older adults. In particular, antidepressants such as escitalopram and paroxetine selectively affect serotonin activity (see later), and these drugs may also be effective in treating anxiety.[88] Certain patients have symptoms of depression combined with anxiety, and these drugs certainly seem like a good option for these patients. It appears, however, that these antidepressants may also be effective in treating anxiety even in the absence of depression.[89] Other options for treating anxiety include antipsychotic drugs such as quetiapine (Seroquel) and antiseizure drugs such as pregabalin (Lyrica).[90] These agents will be discussed later with respect to their primary indications.

Hence, several nonbenzodiazepine options are now available to treat sleep disorders and anxiety in older adults, and these drugs may provide a safer and better-tolerated alternative to the more traditional benzodiazepines.

Antidepressants. Depression is the most common form of mental illness in the general population as well as the most commonly observed mental disorder in older adults.[71,91] Feelings of intense sadness, hopelessness, and other symptoms may occur in older adults after a specific event (e.g., loss of a spouse, acute illness) or in response to the gradual decline in health and functional status often associated with aging. Drug therapy may be instituted to help resolve these symptoms, along with other nonpharmacologic methods, such as counseling and behavioral therapy.

There are several distinct groups of antidepressant medications: tricyclics, monoamine oxidase (MAO) inhibitors, and the newer "second generation" drugs (see Table 6.2). All antidepressant drugs share a common goal—to increase synaptic transmission in central neural pathways that use amine neurotransmitters such as norepinephrine, dopamine, or 5-hydroxytryptamine (serotonin). Antidepressants, however, vary in their ability to affect specific amine neurotransmitters. For example, tricyclic antidepressants (TCAs) and MAO inhibitors tend to affect all three neurotransmitters, whereas selective serotonin reuptake inhibitors (SSRIs) are more selective for serotonin than norepinephrine or dopamine. Other second-generation drugs can also have specific effects on certain neurotransmitters as indicated in Table 6.2.

Although their effect on amine neurotransmitters is well documented, it is not exactly clear how this change in neurotransmitter function might ultimately improve mood and reduce symptoms of depression. It is currently believed that antidepressants increase amine neurotransmitter influence, which in turn increases the synthesis and effects of other brain chemicals such as brain-derived neurotrophic factor (BDNF).[92] The increase in BDNF is then thought to increase signaling and synaptic growth in the hippocampus and other areas of the brain that affect mood.[93,94] Researchers continue to investigate exactly how antidepressants affect brain neurochemistry and how BDNF and other factors affect mood and behavior.

A primary focus in treating depression in older adults has been identifying which agents produce the best effects with the least side effects.[91,95] Although most studies indicate that antidepressant drugs are more effective than placebo, it does not appear that any specific type of antidepressant will be uniformly more effective than another when treating depression in older adults.[91,96] Drug selection is often based on potential side effects and the relative risk of adverse effects in a given patient.[97] For example, tricyclic antidepressants should be avoided in patients at risk for cardiac arrhythmias, and SSRIs can increase the risk of abnormal bleeding.[98,99] Hence, there is agreement that early detection and intervention is important,[95] but selection of a particular drug remains unclear.

Antidepressants produce various side effects, depending on the particular type of drug. Tricyclic antidepressants produce anticholinergic effects and may cause dry mouth, constipation, urinary retention, and CNS symptoms such as confusion, cognitive impairment, and delirium. Tricyclics also cause sedation and orthostatic hypotension, and these drugs can produce serious cardiotoxic effects after overdose.[99] Monoamine oxidase inhibitors also produce orthostatic hypotension and tend to cause insomnia. Side effects associated with the second-generation drugs vary depending on the specific agent. Certain effects that are particularly troublesome in older adults (i.e., sedation, anticholinergic effects, orthostatic hypotension) tend to occur less frequently with the SSRIs. SSRIs, however, have a greater tendency to cause other bothersome effects, such as GI irritation and upper GI bleeding.[97,98]

Physical therapists should be aware that antidepressants may help improve the patient's mood and increase the patient's interest in physical therapy. Certain side effects, however, such as sedation and confusion, may impair the patient's cognitive ability and make it difficult for some older patients to participate actively in rehabilitation procedures. Hence, selection of drugs that minimize these effects may be especially helpful. Therapists should also be aware that some patients may respond fairly rapidly to the antidepressant effects of these drugs; that is, some patients receiving SSRIs experience beneficial effects within 1 week after beginning drug treatment.[100] Other patients, however, may take 6 or more weeks from the onset of drug therapy until an improvement occurs in the depressive symptoms. This substantial time lag is critical because the patient may actually become more depressed before mood begins to improve. Therapists should therefore look for signs that depression is worsening, especially during the first few weeks of antidepressant drug therapy. A suspected increase in depressive symptoms should be brought to the attention of the appropriate member of the health care team (e.g., physician or psychologist).

Treatment of Bipolar Disorder. Bipolar disorder, known also as manic depression, is a form of mental illness characterized by mood swings from an excited, hyperactive state (mania) to periods of apathy and dysphoria (depression). Although the cause of bipolar disorder is unknown, this condition responds fairly well to the drug lithium.[101] It is not exactly clear how lithium prevents episodes of manic depression, but this drug may prevent the excitable, or manic, phase of this disorder, thus stabilizing disposition and preventing the mood swings characteristic of this disease.[102]

It is important to be aware of older patients taking lithium to treat manic depression because this drug can rapidly accumulate to toxic levels in these individuals.[103] Lithium is an element and cannot be degraded in the body to an inactive form. The body must therefore rely solely on renal excretion to eliminate this drug. Because renal function is reduced in older adults, the elimination of this drug is often impaired. Accumulation of lithium beyond a certain level results in lithium toxicity.[104] Symptoms of mild lithium toxicity include a metallic taste in the mouth, fine hand tremor, nausea, and muscular weakness and fatigue. These symptoms increase as toxicity reaches moderate levels, and other CNS signs such as blurred vision and incoordination may appear. Severe lithium toxicity may cause irreversible cerebellar damage, and prolonged lithium neurotoxicity can lead to coma and even death.[104]

Hence, physical therapists working with older patients who are taking lithium must continually be alert for any signs of lithium toxicity. This idea is especially important if there is any change in the patient's health or activity level that might cause an additional compromise in lithium excretion.

In addition to lithium, several other medications can be used to help treat bipolar disorder. In particular, antipsychotic medications such as aripiprazole, quetiapine, and olanzapine can help stabilize mood, especially during the acute manic phase of this disorder.[101,105] The neurochemistry of antipsychotic medications is addressed in the next section. Finally, certain antiseizure medications (carbamazepine, gabapentin, lamotrigine, valproate) and traditional antidepressants (fluoxetine, paroxetine, imipramine) can be used as an alternative if lithium is poorly tolerated or contraindicated.[101]

Antipsychotics

Antipsychotic medications are often used to help normalize behavior in older adults. *Psychosis* is the term used to describe the more severe forms of mental illness that are characterized by marked thought disturbances and altered perceptions of reality.[106] Aggressive, disordered behavior may also accompany symptoms of psychosis. In older adults, psychotic-like behavior may occur because of actual psychotic syndromes (e.g., schizophrenia, severe paranoid disorders) or may be associated with various forms of dementia.[107] In any event, antipsychotic drugs may be helpful in improving behavior and compliance in older patients.

Further, antipsychotic drugs are often characterized as either first-generation (conventional) or second-generation (atypical) agents (see Table 6.2). Conventional agents have been on the market for some time, and they tend to produce different side effects than the newer, second-generation antipsychotic drugs (see later). Regardless of their classification, these drugs all share a common mechanism in that they impair synaptic transmission to some extent in central dopamine pathways.[108,109] It is theorized that psychosis may be due to increased central dopamine influence in cortical and limbic system pathways. Antipsychotic drugs are believed to reduce this dopaminergic influence, thus helping to decrease psychotic-like behavior. Second-generation antipsychotics also appear to affect certain serotonin receptors, with a more moderate effect on dopamine receptors.[110,111] Their effect on serotonin receptors, however, is complex, with possible stimulation of the 5-HT1A receptor subtype, and simultaneous blockade of the 5-HT2 receptor subtype.[111] These complex effects on serotonin and dopamine pathways may explain why these second-generation agents are preferable in terms of controlling psychosis with relatively fewer side effects than the first-generation drugs. There is also evidence that second-generation drugs may have other positive effects such as neuroprotection and increased synaptic growth (neurogenesis) in the hippocampus, and researchers continue to investigate the effects of these drugs on CNS function.[111]

Antipsychotic drugs are associated with several annoying but fairly minor side effects, such as sedation and anticholinergic effects (e.g., dry mouth, constipation). Orthostatic hypotension may also occur, especially within the first few days after drug treatment is initiated. A more serious concern with antipsychotic drugs is the possibility of extrapyramidal side effects.[112] As discussed earlier in this chapter, motor symptoms that mimic lesions in the extrapyramidal tracts are a common ADR associated with these medications, especially in older adults.[113] For instance, patients may exhibit involuntary movements of the face, jaw, and extremities (tardive dyskinesia), symptoms that resemble Parkinson disease (pseudoparkinsonism), extreme restlessness (akathisia), or other problems with involuntary muscle movements (dystonias).[113] Early recognition of these extrapyramidal signs is important because they may persist long after the antipsychotic drug is discontinued, or these signs may even remain permanently. This fact seems especially true for drug-induced tardive dyskinesia, which may be irreversible if antipsychotic drug therapy is not altered when these symptoms first appear.[114]

Hence, patients taking antipsychotic drugs should be monitored closely for any motor abnormalities that may indicate drug-induced extrapyramidal side effects. The risk of these effects is somewhat lower with second-generation antipsychotics compared to first-generation agents (see Table 6.2).[115] Nonetheless, tardive dyskinesia and other motor side effects can still occur with second-generation antipsychotics, especially when these drugs are used for prolonged periods at higher doses.[116] Second-generation antipsychotics can also produce other serious problems such as cardiovascular toxicity, weight gain, and metabolic disturbances that resemble diabetes mellitus.[112,117]

The use of antipsychotic drugs may have beneficial effects on rehabilitation outcomes because patients may become more cooperative and less agitated during physical therapy. Therapists should be especially alert for the onset of any extrapyramidal symptoms because of the potential that these symptoms may result in long-term or permanent motor side effects. Therapists should realize, however, that antipsychotics may sometimes be used inappropriately in older adults.[118,119] These medications are approved to help control certain psychotic-related symptoms, including behavioral problems such as aggression and severe agitation. They must be used carefully, however, and preferably for only short periods of time in older adults because of the increased risk of adverse cardiovascular events such as stroke.[120] Likewise, these drugs should not be used indiscriminately as "tranquilizers" to control all unwanted behaviors in older adults. As indicated earlier, government regulations have been instituted to help decrease the inappropriate and unnecessary use of these medications in older adults.[118]

Treatment of Dementia. *Dementia* is a term used to describe a fairly global decline in intellectual function, with marked impairments in cognition, speech, personality, and other skills.[121] Some forms of dementia may be due to specific factors such as an infection, a metabolic disorder, or an adverse reaction to drugs that have psychoactive side effects.[122] These so-called reversible dementias are often resolved if the precipitating factor is identified and corrected. Irreversible dementia is typically associated with progressive degenerative changes in cortical structure and function, such as those occurring in Alzheimer disease. Drug treatment of irreversible dementia follows two primary strategies: improving cognitive function and treating behavioral symptoms. These strategies are discussed briefly here.

The drugs most commonly used to treat Alzheimer disease attempt to increase acetylcholine function in the brain.[123] It is known that acetylcholine influence in the brain begins to diminish because of the neuronal degeneration inherent to Alzheimer disease. Therefore, drugs that increase cholinergic activity may help improve intellectual and cognitive function in persons with Alzheimer-type dementia. As a result, agents such as tacrine (Cognex) and donepezil (Aricept), galantamine (Reminyl), and rivastigmine (Exelon) have been developed to specifically improve cognition and behavioral function in persons with Alzheimer disease.[124,125] These drugs inhibit the acetylcholinesterase enzyme, thus decreasing acetylcholine breakdown and prolonging the activity of this neurotransmitter in the brain.

Regrettably, cholinergic stimulants provide only moderate benefits in patients who are in the relatively early stages of this disease[125]; that is, these drugs may help patients retain more cognitive and intellectual function during the mild to moderate stages of Alzheimer disease, but these benefits are eventually lost as the disease progresses.[126] Likewise, side effects such as GI distress and liver toxicity may limit the use of these drugs in some patients.[127] Still, these agents may help sustain cognitive function during the early course of Alzheimer disease, thus enabling patients to continue to participate in various activities, including physical therapy.

A second pharmacotherapeutic option for treating Alzheimer disease is memantine (Namenda). This drug blocks the *N*-methyl-D-aspartate (NMDA) receptor in the brain.[128] This receptor normally responds to glutamate, an amino acid neurotransmitter that is important in memory and learning.[129] Evidently, glutamate overstimulation of the NMDA receptor can contribute to the neurodegenerative changes associated with Alzheimer disease. By reducing this glutamate activity, memantine may help improve memory and cognition and reduce symptoms of agitation and aggression.[127] Moreover, this drug may offer some protection for CNS neurons and thus help decrease the progression of Alzheimer disease.[128] Hence, memantine offers an additional therapeutic option, and use of this drug alone or in combination with cholinesterase inhibitors may help improve symptoms in people with Alzheimer disease.[130] Likewise, other pharmacologic strategies that enhance cognition or delay the degenerative changes in Alzheimer disease are currently being explored, and these strategies may help provide more long-lasting effects in the future.[131]

Finally, other drugs already discussed in this chapter may be used to help normalize and control behavior in patients with Alzheimer disease and other forms of dementia. In particular, antipsychotic drugs may help improve certain aspects of behavior, such as decreased hallucinations and diminished feelings of hostility and suspiciousness.[132,133] Response to these drugs, however, is highly variable, and side effects can be problematic when these drugs are given to older people.[118,120]

As noted earlier, efforts are also being made to decrease the indiscriminate use of antipsychotics in persons with Alzheimer disease. For example, nonpharmacologic interventions such as therapeutic activities, environmental modification, and caregiver support/education should be considered before resorting to drug therapy.[134–136] If drug therapy is required, choice of a specific medication should be based on the specific symptoms exhibited by each patient.[133] For example, the severely anxious patient may respond better to an antianxiety drug, the depressed patient may respond to an antidepressant, and so on.[137] Antipsychotics should not be considered as a panacea for all dementia-like symptoms, and the use of alternative interventions may decrease the incidence of polypharmacy and antipsychotic-related side effects.

Neurologic Agents

In addition to the drugs that affect mood and behavior, there are specific agents that are important in controlling certain neurologic conditions in older adults. Drug treatment of two of these conditions, Parkinson disease and seizure disorders, is discussed here.

Drugs Used for Parkinson Disease. Parkinson disease is one of the more prevalent disorders in older adults, with more than 1% of the population older than age 60 years being afflicted.[138] This disease is caused by the degeneration of dopamine-secreting neurons located in the basal ganglia.[139,140] Loss of dopaminergic influence initiates an imbalance in other neurotransmitters, including an increase in acetylcholine influence. This disruption in transmitter activity ultimately results in the typical parkinsonian motor symptoms of rigidity, bradykinesia, and resting tremor.[138]

Drug treatment of Parkinson disease usually focuses on restoring the balance of neurotransmitters in the basal ganglia.[141] The most common way of achieving this is to administer 3,4-dihydroxyphenylalanine (dopa), which is the immediate precursor to dopamine. Dopamine itself will not cross the blood–brain barrier, meaning that dopamine will not move from the bloodstream into the brain, where it is ultimately needed. However, levodopa (the L-isomer of dopa) will pass easily from the bloodstream into the brain, where it can then be transformed into dopamine and help restore the influence of this neurotransmitter in the basal ganglia.

Levodopa is often administered orally with a drug known as carbidopa. Carbidopa inhibits the enzyme that transforms levodopa to dopamine in the peripheral circulation, thus allowing levodopa to cross into the brain before it is finally converted to dopamine. If levodopa is converted to dopamine before reaching the brain, the dopamine will be useless in Parkinson disease because it becomes trapped in the peripheral circulation. The simultaneous use of carbidopa and levodopa allows smaller doses of levodopa to be administered, because less of the levodopa will be wasted as a result of the premature conversion to dopamine in the periphery.

Levodopa therapy often produces dramatic beneficial effects, especially during the mild to moderate stages of Parkinson disease. Nonetheless, levodopa is associated with several troublesome side effects.[140,142] In particular, levodopa may cause GI distress (e.g., nausea, vomiting) and cardiovascular problems (e.g., arrhythmias, orthostatic hypotension), especially for the first few days after drug therapy is initiated. Neuropsychiatric problems (e.g., confusion, depression, anxiety, hallucinations, impulse control disorders) and problems with involuntary movements (e.g., dyskinesia) have also been noted in patients on levodopa therapy.[142,143] Perhaps the most frustrating problem, however, is the tendency for the effectiveness of levodopa to diminish after 4 or 5 years of continuous use.[142] The reason for this diminished response is not fully understood but may be related to the fact that levodopa replacement simply cannot adequately restore neurotransmitter dysfunction in the final stages of this disease; that is, levodopa therapy may help supplement endogenous dopamine production in early to moderate Parkinson disease, but this effect is eventually lost when the substantia nigra neurons degenerate beyond a certain point. Other fluctuations in the response to levodopa have been noted with long-term use.[142,144] These fluctuations include a spontaneous decrease in levodopa effectiveness in the middle of a dose interval (on–off phenomenon) or loss of drug effects toward the end of a dose cycle (end-of-dose akinesia). The reasons for these fluctuations are poorly understood but may be related to problems in the absorption and metabolism of levodopa in the later stages of Parkinson disease.

Fortunately, several other agents are currently available to help alleviate the motor symptoms associated with Parkinson disease (Table 6.3).[144,145] Drugs such as bromocriptine (Parlodel), pergolide (Permax), and other dopamine agonists mimic the effects of dopamine and can be used to replace the deficient neurotransmitter. Anticholinergic drugs (e.g., biperiden, ethopropazine) act to decrease acetylcholine influence in the brain and can attenuate the increased effects of acetylcholine that occur when dopamine influence is diminished. Amantadine (Symmetrel) is actually an antiviral drug that also exerts antiparkinson effects, presumably by blocking the NMDA receptor and decreasing the excitatory effects of CNS amino acids. Selegiline (Eldepryl) and rasagiline (Azilect) inhibit the MAO enzyme that degrades dopamine, thus prolonging the effects of any dopamine that exists in the basal ganglia. Finally, drugs such as entacapone (Comtan) and tolcapone (Tasmar) inhibit the catechol-O-methyltransferase enzyme, thereby preventing premature destruction of levodopa in the bloodstream and allowing more levodopa to reach the brain.

Consequently, levodopa therapy is still the cornerstone of treatment in persons with Parkinson disease, but several other agents are now available that can be used in combination with, or instead of, levodopa to create an optimal drug regimen for each patient.[145,146] Nonetheless, current pharmacotherapy of Parkinson disease has some considerable shortcomings, and treatment of patients is often limited by inadequate effects or toxic side effects, especially during the advanced stages of this disease. Additional drug treatments are being considered that may actually help delay the neurodegenerative changes inherent to Parkinson disease.[147] If proven effective, these treatments would offer substantial benefits because they would help slow the progression of this disease rather than merely treat the parkinsonian symptoms.

Physical therapists working with patients with Parkinson disease should attempt to coordinate rehabilitation sessions with the peak effects of drug therapy whenever possible. For instance, scheduling physical therapy when levodopa and other antiparkinson drugs reach peak effects (usually 1 hour after oral administration) will often maximize the patient's ability to actively participate in exercise programs and functional training. Therapists should also be cognizant of the potential side effects of levodopa, including the tendency for responses to fluctuate or diminish with prolonged use. Physical therapists

TABLE 6.3 Neurologic Drug Groups

	Generic Name	Trade Name
Drugs Used in Parkinson Disease		
Dopamine precursors	Levodopa	Sinemet*
Dopamine agonists	Bromocriptine	Parlodel
	Pergolide	Permax
	Pramipexole	Mirapex
	Ropinirole	Requip
Anticholinergic drugs	Benztropine	Cogentin
	Biperiden	Akineton
	Diphenhydramine	Benadryl, others
	Procyclidine	Kemadrin
	Trihexyphenidyl	Artane
COMT inhibitors	Entacapone	Comtan
	Tolcapone	Tasmar
Others	Amantadine	Symmetrel
	Rasagiline	Azilect
	Selegiline	Eldepryl, Zelapar
Drugs Used in Seizure Disorders		
Barbiturates	Phenobarbital	Luminal, Solfoton
	Primidone	Mysoline
Benzodiazepines	Clonazepam	Klonopin
	Clorazepate	Tranxene
Carboxylic acids	Divalproex	Depakote
Hydantoins	Ethotoin	Peganone
	Mephenytoin	Mesantoin
	Phenytoin	Dilantin, Phenytek
Succinimides	Ethosuximide	Zarontin
	Methsuximide	Celontin
Iminostilbenes	Carbamazepine	Carbatrol, Tegretol, others
	Oxcarbazepine	Oxtellar, Trileptal
Second-generation agents	Felbamate	Felbatol
	Gabapentin	Gabarone, Neurontin, others
	Lacosamide	Vimpat
	Lamotrigine	Lamictal, others
	Levetiracetam	Keppra, Roweepra, others
	Pregabalin	Lyrica
	Tiagabine	Gabatril
	Topiramate	Topamax, Topiragen, others
	Vigabatrin	Sabril
	Zonisamide	Zonegran

*Indicates trade name for levodopa combined with carbidopa, a peripheral decarboxylase inhibitor.
COMT, catechol-*O*-methyltransferase.

may also play an important role in documenting any decline or alteration in drug effectiveness while working closely with patients with Parkinson disease.

Drugs Used to Control Seizures. Seizure disorders such as epilepsy are characterized by the sudden, uncontrolled firing of a group of cerebral neurons.[148] This uncontrolled neuronal excitation is manifested in various ways, depending on the location and extent of the neuronal involvement, and seizures are classified according to the motor and sensory symptoms that occur during a seizure. In the general population, the exact cause of the seizure disorder is often unknown. In older adults, however, seizure activity may be attributed to a fairly well-defined cause such as a previous CNS injury (e.g., stroke, trauma), tumor, or degenerative brain disease.[149,150] If the cause cannot be treated by surgical or other means, pharmacologic management remains the primary method of preventing recurrent seizures.

The primary goal of antiseizure drugs is to normalize the excitation threshold in the group of hyperexcitable neurons that initiate the seizure.[151] Ideally, this can be accomplished without suppressing the general excitation level within the brain. Several groups of chemically distinct antiseizure drugs are currently in use, and each group uses a different biochemical mechanism to selectively decrease excitability in the seizure-prone neurons (see Table 6.3). The selection of a particular antiseizure drug depends primarily on the type of seizure present in each patient.[151]

Sedation is the most common side effect that physical therapists should be aware of when working with older patients who are taking seizure medications.[152,153] Other annoying side effects include GI distress, headache, dizziness, incoordination, and dermatologic reactions (e.g., rashes). More serious problems, such as liver toxicity and blood dyscrasias (aplastic anemia), may occur in some patients. In addition to monitoring for these side effects, physical therapists can play an important role in helping assess the effectiveness of the antiseizure medications by observing and documenting any seizures that may occur during the rehabilitation session.

Treatment of Pain and Inflammation

Pharmacologic treatment of pain and inflammation is used in older adults to help resolve symptoms of chronic conditions (e.g., rheumatoid arthritis and osteoarthritis) as well as acute problems resulting from trauma and surgery.[154] Drugs used for analgesic and anti-inflammatory purposes include the opioid analgesics, nonopioid analgesics, and glucocorticoids (Table 6.4). These medications are discussed briefly here.

Opioid Analgesics. Opioid analgesics compose the group of drugs used to treat relatively severe, constant pain. These agents, also known as *narcotics*, are commonly used to reduce pain in older patients after surgery or trauma, or in more chronic situations such as cancer.[33] Opioids vary in terms of their relative analgesic strength, with drugs such as morphine and meperidine (Demerol) having strong analgesic properties, and drugs such as

TABLE 6.4 Analgesic and Anti-inflammatory Drugs Groups

	Common Examples	
Category	**Generic Name**	**Trade Name**
Opioid Analgesics		
	Codeine	Many trade names
	Meperidine	Demerol
	Morphine	Many trade names
	Oxycodone	OxyContin, Roxicodone, others
	Propoxyphene	Darvon, others
Nonopioid Analgesics		
NSAIDs	Aspirin	Many trade names
	Ibuprofen	Advil, Motrin, others
	Ketoprofen	Orudis, others
	Naproxen	Aleve, Naprosyn, others
	Piroxicam	Feldene
	Sulindac	Clinoril
COX-2 inhibitor	Celecoxib	Celebrex
Acetaminophen	—	Tylenol, Panadol
Corticosteroids	Betamethasone	Celestone, others
	Cortisone	Cortone
	Hydrocortisone	Cortef, Hydrocortone, others
	Prednisone	Rayos, Sterapred
Disease-Modifying Antirheumatic Drugs*		
Gold compounds	Auranofin	Ridaura
	Gold sodium thiomalate	Myochrysine
Antimalarials	Chloroquine	Aralen
	Hydroxychloroquine	Plaquenil, Quineprox
Tumor necrosis factor inhibitors	Adalimumab	Humira, others
	Certolizumab	Cimzia
	Etanercept	Enbrel, others
	Golimumab	Simponi
	Infliximab	Inflectra, Remicade, Renflexis
Interleukin inhibitors	Anakinra	Kineret
	Sarilumab	Kevzara
	Tocilizumab	Actemra
	Usterkinumab	Stelara
Others	Abatacept	Orencia
	Azathioprine	Azasan, Imuran
	Cyclosporine	Gengraf, Neoral, Sandimmune
	Leflunomide	Arava
	Methotrexate	Rheumatrex, others
	Penicillamine	Cuprimine, Depen
	Rituximab	Rituxan
	Sulfasalazine	Asulfidine, Sulfazine
	Tofacitinib	Xeljanz

*Drugs used to slow the progression of rheumatoid arthritis.
COX, cyclooxygenase; *NSAIDs,* nonsteroidal anti-inflammatory drugs.

codeine having a more moderate ability to decrease pain. These drugs exert their beneficial effects by binding to opioid receptors in the brain and spinal cord, thereby altering synaptic transmission in pain-mediating pathways.[155] Opioid analgesics are often characterized by their ability to alter pain perception rather than completely eliminating painful sensations. This effect allows the patient to focus on other things rather than being continually preoccupied by the painful stimuli.

Physical therapists should be aware that opioid analgesics cause many side effects that can influence the patient's participation in rehabilitation.[156,157] Adverse side effects such as sedation, mood changes (e.g., euphoria or dysphoria), and GI problems (e.g., nausea, vomiting, constipation) are quite common. Orthostatic hypotension and respiratory depression are also common side effects, especially for the first few days after opioid analgesic therapy is started. Confusion may be a problem, particularly in older adults. Finally, prolonged or excessive opioid administration can cause tolerance and physical dependence, and may also lead to addiction in susceptible individuals. Recent increases in opioid addiction and opioid-related deaths have raised concerns about overreliance on these drugs when managing pain.[158] Hence, opioids are still very useful in managing acute and chronic pain, but there is consensus that these drugs must be used carefully at the lowest effective dose for the shortest period of time.[157] Alternatives to opioids should therefore be explored to avoid possible adverse effects, especially when these drugs are administered to older adults.[159,160]

Nonopioid Analgesics. Treatment of mild to moderate pain is often accomplished by the use of two types of nonopioid agents: NSAIDs and acetaminophen. NSAIDs compose a group of drugs that are therapeutically similar to aspirin (see Table 6.4). These aspirin-like drugs produce four therapeutic effects: analgesia, decreased inflammation, decreased fever (antipyresis), and decreased platelet aggregation (anticoagulant effects). Acetaminophen appears to have analgesic and antipyretic properties similar to the NSAIDs, but acetaminophen lacks any significant anti-inflammatory or anticoagulation effects. NSAIDs and acetaminophen exert most, if not all, of their beneficial effects by inhibiting the synthesis of a group of compounds known as the *prostaglandins*. Prostaglandins are produced locally by many cells and are involved in mediating certain aspects of pain and inflammation.[161] Aspirin and other NSAIDs inhibit the cyclooxygenase (COX) enzyme that synthesizes prostaglandins in the central nervous system as well as peripheral tissues, thus diminishing the painful and inflammatory effects of these compounds throughout the body.[162] Acetaminophen also inhibits prostaglandin biosynthesis, but this inhibition may only occur in the central nervous system, thus accounting for the differences in acetaminophen and NSAID effects.[161]

Because certain prostaglandins produce beneficial or cytoprotective effects in the body, efforts were made to produce a type of NSAID that impaired the production of only the harmful prostaglandins. These efforts lead to the development of COX-2 inhibitors such as celecoxib (Celebrex). These drugs are so named because they tend to inhibit the COX-2 form of the enzyme that synthesizes prostaglandins that cause pain and inflammation while sparing the production of the beneficial prostaglandins produced by the COX-1 enzyme.[163] Indeed, COX-2 inhibitors can reduce pain and inflammation in some patients with less chance of adverse effects such as gastric irritation.[164] These benefits, however, are not universal and some patients experience serious gastric toxicity from COX-2 drugs.[163] Moreover, COX-2 inhibitors were linked to potentially serious cardiovascular problems in some people, including myocardial infarction and stroke.[165,166] These adverse effects were the primary reason that certain COX-2 drugs such as rofecoxib (Vioxx) and valdecoxib (Bextra) were removed from the market.

The risk of cardiovascular problems, however, may not be limited to just the COX-2 drugs. Traditional NSAIDs that inhibit both COX-1 and COX-2 may also increase the risk of heart attack and stroke in susceptible patients.[167,168] Although the reasons are complex, inhibition of certain prostaglandins may affect platelet activity, and therefore lead to increased infarction in coronary and carotid arteries that are partially occluded by atherosclerotic plaques. Inhibition of prostaglandin synthesis can also increase blood pressure, especially in patients who are hypertensive.[169] Hence, patients should be screened carefully before using traditional NSAIDs and COX-2 selective drugs, and these drugs should be probably avoided in patients with risk factors for cardiovascular disease.[167]

Nonetheless, many older patients can use NSAIDs safely and effectively when these drugs are used in moderate doses for short periods.[154] The most common side effect is gastrointestinal irritation, and problems ranging from minor stomach upset to serious gastric ulceration can occur in older adults.[166] Renal and hepatic toxicity may also occur, especially if higher doses are used for prolonged periods or in patients with preexisting kidney or liver disease.[166] As mentioned earlier, traditional NSAIDs and COX-2 selective drugs can cause cardiovascular problems in patients at risk for infarction, hypertension, and heart failure.[167] NSAIDs impair platelet function, and the risk of bleeding is increased especially in older adults taking other anticlotting drugs (discussed later).[170] Some studies suggest that NSAIDs can impair bone healing and that they should probably be avoided after fractures and certain surgeries such as spinal fusions.[171,172] Other problems that may occur in older patients include allergic reactions (e.g., skin rashes) and possible CNS toxicity (e.g., confusion, hearing problems). In particular, tinnitus (a ringing or buzzing sound in the ears) may develop with prolonged aspirin use, and this side effect may be especially annoying and distressing to older adults.

Acetaminophen does not produce any appreciable gastric irritation and may be taken preferentially by older patients for that reason.[161] It should be noted, however, that acetaminophen lacks anti-inflammatory effects and may be inferior to NSAIDs if pain and inflammation are present. Acetaminophen may also be more hepatotoxic than the NSAIDs in cases of overdose or in persons who are dehydrated, consume excessive amounts of alcohol, and so forth.

Glucocorticoids. Glucocorticoids are steroids produced by the adrenal cortex that have a number of physiological effects, including a potent ability to decrease inflammation.[161] Synthetic derivatives of endogenously produced glucocorticoids can be administered pharmacologically to capitalize on the powerful anti-inflammatory effects of these compounds. These agents are used to treat rheumatoid arthritis and a variety of other disorders that have an inflammatory component. Glucocorticoids exert their anti-inflammatory effects through several complex mechanisms, including the ability to suppress leukocyte function and to inhibit the production of proinflammatory substances, such as cytokines, prostaglandins, and leukotrienes, at the site of inflammation.[173,174]

The powerful anti-inflammatory effects of glucocorticoids must be balanced against the risk of several serious adverse effects. In particular, physical therapists should be aware that these drugs produce a general catabolic effect on supporting tissues throughout the body.[175,176] Breakdown of bones, ligaments, tendons, skin, and muscle can occur after prolonged systemic administration of glucocorticoids. This breakdown can be especially devastating in older adult patients who already have some degree of osteoporosis or muscle wasting.[175,176] Glucocorticoids also produce other serious adverse effects, including hypertension, peptic ulcer, aggravation of diabetes mellitus, glaucoma, increased risk of infection, and suppression of normal corticosteroid production by the adrenal cortex. Adrenocortical suppression can have devastating or even fatal results if the exogenous (drug) form of the glucocorticoid is suddenly withdrawn because the body is temporarily incapable of synthesizing adequate amounts of these important compounds. Hence, these drugs should not be suddenly discontinued after prolonged use, but should be tapered off gradually under close medical supervision. Finally, it should be realized that glucocorticoids often treat a disease manifestation (inflammation) without resolving the underlying cause of the disease. For instance, older patients with rheumatoid arthritis may appear quite healthy as a result of this "masking" effect of glucocorticoids, whereas other sequelae of this disease (e.g., bone erosion, joint destruction) continue to worsen.

Other Drugs Used in Inflammatory Disease: Disease-Modifying Agents. Because NSAIDs and other anti-inflammatory drugs do not usually slow the disease process in rheumatoid arthritis, efforts have been made to develop drugs that try to curb the progression of this disease.[177,178] These so-called disease-modifying antirheumatic drugs (DMARDs) include an assortment of agents with different chemical and pharmacodynamic properties (see Table 6.4).[177,179] In general, these agents have immunosuppressive effects that blunt the autoimmune response that is believed to underlie rheumatic joint disease. Some drugs in this category, such as methotrexate, produce a fairly nonselective effect on the immune system and attempt to slow the proliferation of lymphocytes and reduce the production of various chemicals that promote autoimmune destruction of joint tissues.[177] Several strategies have also been developed to limit a specific component in the immune response. Etanercept (Enbrel), for example, selectively inhibits the effects of tumor necrosis factor-α, and anakinra (Humira) inhibits the effects of interleukin-1.[180,181] These agents and similar biologic response modifiers (see Table 6.4) may help slow the progression of rheumatoid arthritis when used alone or in combination with other DMARDs.[178,180]

Disease-modifying antirheumatic drugs have therefore been successful in arresting or even reversing some of the arthritic changes in certain patients with this disease.[182,183] Hence, DMARDs should be used fairly early in the course of rheumatoid arthritis so that these drugs can help prevent some of the severe joint destruction associated with this disease.[182] Regrettably, use of these DMARDs is limited in some patients because of toxic effects such as GI distress and renal impairment, and these drugs will increase the risk of infection because of their immunosuppressive effects.[179,184,185] Research continues to determine which DMARDs, or combinations of these agents, will provide optimal benefits in people with rheumatoid arthritis.[183,186]

Cardiovascular Drugs

Cardiovascular disease is one of the leading causes of morbidity and mortality in older individuals. Various drugs are therefore used to prevent and treat cardiovascular problems in older adults, and many of these medications can directly affect rehabilitation of older adults. Cardiovascular drugs are often categorized according to the types of diseases they are used to treat. The pharmacotherapeutic management of some common cardiovascular problems seen in older adults is presented to follow, and drugs used to treat these problems are also summarized in Table 6.5.

Drugs Used in Geriatric Hypertension. An increase in blood pressure is commonly observed in older adults, and this increase is believed to be due to changes in cardiovascular function (e.g., decreased compliance of vascular tissues, decreased baroreceptor sensitivity) and diminished renal function (e.g., decreased ability to excrete water and sodium) that normally occur with aging.[187] A mild increase in blood pressure may not necessarily

TABLE 6.5 Cardiovascular Drug Groups

Drug Group	Primary Indications	Common Examples: Generic Name	Common Examples: Trade Name
α-Blockers	Hypertension	Phenoxybenzamine Prazosin	Dibenzyline Minipress
Angiotensin-converting enzyme inhibitors	Hypertension, CHF	Captopril Enalapril Quinapril Other drugs with generic names that end with "-pril"	Capoten Epaned, Vasotec Accupril
Angiotensin II receptor blockers	Hypertension, CHF	Irbesartan Losartan Valsartan Other drugs with generic names that end with "-sartan"	Avapro Cozaar Diovan
Anticoagulants	Overactive clotting	Heparin* Warfarin Argatroban Bivalirudin Dabigatran Desirudin Lepirudin Apixaban Fondaparinux Rivaroxaban	Fragmin, Lovenox, others Coumadin, Jantoven Acova Angiomax Pradaxa Iprivask Refludan Eliquis Arixtra Xarelto
β-Blockers	Hypertension Angina Arrhythmias	Atenolol Metoprolol Propranolol Other drugs with generic names that end with "-olol"	Tenormin Lopressor, Toprol Inderal, others
Calcium channel blockers	Hypertension Angina Arrhythmias	Diltiazem Nifedipine Verapamil Other drugs with generic names that end with "-ipine"	Cardizem, others Adalat, Procardia Calan, Isoptin
Centrally acting sympatholytics	Hypertension	Clonidine Methyldopa	Catapres, Kapvay Aldomet
Digitalis glycosides	CHF	Digoxin	Lanoxin, others
Diuretics	Hypertension, CHF	Chlorothiazide Furosemide Spironolactone	Diuril Lasix, others Aldactone, CaroSpir
Drugs that prolong repolarization	Arrhythmias	Amiodarone Bretylium	Cordarone, Pacerone Bretylol
Organic nitrates	Angina	Nitroglycerin	Nitrostat, others
Presynaptic adrenergic depleters	Hypertension	Guanethidine Reserpine	Ismelin —
Sodium channel blockers	Arrhythmias	Quinidine Tocainide	Cardioquin, others Tonocard
Statins	Hyperlipidemia	Atorvastatin Rosuvastatin Simvastatin Other drugs with generic names that end with "-statin"	Lipitor Crestor Zocor
Vasodilators	Hypertension	Hydralazine Minoxidil	Apresoline Loniten

*Trade names refer to low-molecular-weight heparins.
CHF, congestive heart failure.

be harmful in the older adult and may in fact have a protective effect in maintaining adequate blood flow to the brain and other organs.[188] It is clear, however, that an excessive increase in blood pressure is associated with various cardiovascular problems such as stroke, coronary artery disease, and heart failure, and that efforts should be made to keep blood pressure within an acceptable range.[187,188]

Nonetheless, there has been considerable debate about which blood pressure values are optimal in older adults. Many experts believe that systolic and diastolic values in older adults should be less than 140 and 90 mmHg, respectively, or less than 130/80 mmHg in older adults with comorbidities such as chronic renal insufficiency or diabetes mellitus.[189,190] Results from some studies, however, suggest that more aggressive antihypertensive management will further reduce the risk of cardiovascular problems, especially if systolic values are 120 mmHg or less.[190,191] Guidelines for blood pressure management in older adults continue to be revised, and future studies will hopefully clarify target blood pressure values in specific subgroups of older adults.

Fortunately, a large and diverse array of antihypertensive agents is available for treating older adults with hypertension (see Table 6.5). Diuretic agents act on the kidneys to increase the excretion of water and sodium, thereby diminishing blood pressure by reducing the volume of fluid in the vascular system. Sympatholytic agents (e.g., β-blockers, α-blockers) work in various ways to interrupt sympathetic stimulation of the heart and peripheral vasculature. Vasodilators reduce peripheral vascular resistance by directly relaxing vascular smooth muscle. Angiotensin-converting enzyme (ACE) inhibitors block the formation of angiotensin II, a potent vasoconstrictor that also produces adverse structural changes in vascular tissues. Likewise, angiotensin receptor blockers (ARBs) prevent angiotensin II from reaching vascular tissues, thereby reducing the harmful effects of angiotensin II on the heart and vasculature. Finally, calcium channel blockers inhibit the entry of calcium into cardiac muscle cells and vascular smooth muscle cells, thus reducing contractility in these tissues.

Which antihypertensive agent or agents will be used in a given older patient depends on several factors, such as the magnitude of the hypertension and any other medical problems existing in that patient. Often, two or more drugs are combined to provide optimal effects.[192,193] Common drug combinations used as initial treatment in older adults include an ACE inhibitor or ARB combined with a calcium channel blocker or diuretic.[192,194] In some situations, two antihypertensive drugs can be combined in the same pill to make it easier and more convenient to administer, and thus improve patient adherence.[195] Other antihypertensive drugs can be added or substituted based on the individual needs of each patient.[196] Regardless of which agents are used initially, a successful antihypertensive drug regimen should be designed specifically for each patient and should incorporate the "low and slow" philosophy of starting with low doses of each drug and slowly increasing dosages as needed.

The various drugs that could be used to manage hypertension are all associated with specific side effects. A common concern, however, is that blood pressure will be reduced pharmacologically to the point where symptoms of hypotension become a problem. Therapists should always be aware that dizziness and syncope may occur as a result of low blood pressure when the patient is stationary and especially when the patient stands (orthostatic hypotension). Also, any physical therapy intervention that causes an additional decrease in blood pressure should be used very cautiously in geriatric patients who are taking antihypertensive drugs. Treatments such as systemic heat (e.g., large whirlpool, Hubbard tank) and exercise using large muscle groups may cause peripheral vasodilation that exaggerates the effects of the antihypertensive drugs to produce a profound and potentially serious decrease in blood pressure.

Drugs Used in Congestive Heart Failure. Congestive heart failure is a common disorder in older adults and is characterized by a progressive decline in cardiac pumping ability.[197] As the pumping ability of the heart diminishes, fluid often collects in the lungs and extremities (hence the term *congestive heart failure*). Treatment of this disorder focuses primarily on reducing excessive stress on the heart by the renin–angiotensin system and the sympathetic nervous system. As such, drugs that reduce renin–angiotensin activity (ACE inhibitors, ARBs, direct renin inhibitors) and sympatholytics (β-blockers) have become a mainstay in treating heart failure.[198,199] Diuretics and vasodilators can also be added to help reduce fluid volume and vascular resistance, respectively.[198,199] Finally, digitalis glycosides may be used in specific patients to increase myocardial pumping ability by a complex biochemical mechanism that increases the calcium concentration in myocardial cells.[200]

Each drug category used to treat heart failure is associated with specific adverse effects. Diuretics, for example, can cause fluid and electrolyte imbalances if too much water, sodium, or potassium is excreted by the kidneys. β-Blockers and nitrates can cause hypotension, thus leading to dizziness and syncope. These adverse effects, however, are typically dose related and the agents are relatively safe at doses used to treat heart failure in older adults. Likewise, ACE inhibitors and ARBs are often tolerated fairly well in older adults, although hypotension and orthostatic hypotension may occur when these drugs are first administered to older individuals. On the other hand, digoxin and similar drugs are often associated with some common and potentially serious adverse effects. These agents can accumulate rapidly in the bloodstream of an older patient, resulting in digitalis toxicity.[200,201] Digitalis toxicity is characterized by gastrointestinal symptoms (e.g., nausea, vomiting, diarrhea), CNS disturbances (e.g., confusion, blurred vision, sedation), and cardiac arrhythmias. Arrhythmias can be quite severe and may be fatal if digitalis toxicity is not quickly rectified. Physical therapists should be alert for signs of digitalis toxicity because early recognition is essential in preventing the more serious and potentially fatal side effects of these drugs.

Treatment of Cardiac Arrhythmias. Disturbances in cardiac rhythm—that is, a heart rate that is too slow, too fast, or irregular—may occur in older adults for various reasons.[202] Although some cardiac arrhythmias are asymptomatic and do not require any intervention, certain rhythm disturbances such as atrial fibrillation and complex ventricular arrhythmias should be treated to decrease the risk of stroke and sudden cardiac death in older adults.[203,204] A variety of different drugs can be used to stabilize heart rate and normalize cardiac rhythm, and these agents are typically grouped into four categories.[205] Sodium channel blockers (lidocaine, quinidine) control myocardial excitability by stabilizing the opening and closing of membrane sodium channels. β-Blockers (metoprolol, propranolol) normalize heart rate by blocking the effects of cardio-acceleratory substances such as norepinephrine and epinephrine. Drugs that prolong cardiac repolarization (amiodarone) stabilize heart rate by prolonging the refractory period of cardiac action potentials. Calcium channel blockers (diltiazem, verapamil) decrease myocardial excitability and conduction of action potentials by limiting the entry of calcium into cardiac muscle cells. Although different antiarrhythmic drugs have various side effects, the most common adverse reaction is an increased risk of cardiac arrhythmias[205,206]; that is, drugs used to treat one type of arrhythmia may inadvertently cause a different type of rhythm disturbance. Physical therapists should be alert for changes in cardiac rhythm by monitoring heart rate in older patients who are taking antiarrhythmic drugs.

Treatment of Angina Pectoris. Older adults often develop chest pain (angina pectoris) as a symptom of coronary artery disease. Organic nitrates such as nitroglycerin are the primary drugs used to prevent episodes of angina pectoris.[207] Angina typically occurs when myocardial oxygen demand exceeds myocardial oxygen supply. Nitroglycerin decreases myocardial oxygen demand by vasodilating the peripheral vasculature.[208] Peripheral vasodilation causes a decrease in the amount of blood returning to the heart (cardiac preload) as well as the amount of pressure in the vascular system that the heart must pump against (cardiac afterload). Consequently, cardiac workload and oxygen demand are temporarily reduced, thus allowing the anginal attack to subside.[208]

Nitrates can be administered at the onset of an anginal attack by placing the drug under the tongue (sublingually). These drugs can also be administered transdermally using drug-impregnated patches that allow slow, steady absorption of nitrate into the bloodstream. The use of nitrate patches has gained favor because the continuous administration of small amounts of drug may help prevent the onset or reduce the severity of anginal attacks.[209]

Several other drug strategies can also be used to reduce cardiac workload and prevent the onset of angina pectoris. These strategies include β-blockers, calcium channel blockers, and drugs that moderate the renin–angiotensin system (ACE inhibitors, ARBs).[207,210] Likewise, use of low-dose aspirin therapy or other platelet inhibitors can help prevent angina attacks from progressing to myocardial infarction.[210] It must be realized, however, that drug therapy often treats the symptoms of coronary artery disease (i.e., angina pectoris) but does not necessarily resolve the underlying issues that created an imbalance in the supply and utilization of oxygen in the heart (e.g., coronary artery atherosclerosis). Hence, drug therapy should always be combined with exercise and lifestyle changes that help restore a more normal balance between myocardial oxygen supply and demand.[207]

The primary adverse effects that may affect physical therapy are related to the peripheral vasodilating effects of the nitrates. Blood pressure may decrease in patients taking nitroglycerin, and dizziness due to hypotension is a common problem. Likewise, orthostatic hypotension may occur if the patient stands suddenly. Headache may also occur owing to vasodilation of meningeal vessels. These side effects are most common immediately after the patient takes a rapid-acting sublingual dose. Hence, therapists should be especially concerned about hypotensive effects from the first minutes to 1 hour after a patient self-administers a sublingual dose of nitrates. Continuous nitrate administration via patches can also cause tolerance, resulting in loss of the drug's therapeutic effects.[209] Hence, patients using nitrate patches often alternate between wearing the patch for several hours each day and nitrate-free intervals where the patch is removed for several hours.[209] Finally, patients who take nitrates sublingually must be sure to bring their medications with them to physical therapy so that they can self-administer the nitrate if anginal symptoms occur during the rehabilitation session.

Treatment of Hyperlipidemia. Older adults may have high cholesterol levels and other plasma lipid disorders that can lead to atherosclerotic lesions and cardiovascular disease.[211,212] Hence, drug therapy should be combined with dietary changes to help improve plasma lipid profiles and reduce the risk of myocardial infarction and stroke.[213] Statins are the primary drug group used to manage lipid disorders[214] (see Table 6.5). These drugs, known also as hydroxymethylglutarate coenzyme A (HMG/Co-A) reductase inhibitors, block a key enzyme responsible for cholesterol biosynthesis in the liver.[215] Reduced cholesterol production can help lower total cholesterol and produce other beneficial effects on plasma lipids such as reduced low-density lipoproteins and increased high-density lipoproteins. These agents may also produce a number of other favorable effects such as improving function of the vascular endothelium and stabilizing atherosclerotic plaques within the vascular wall.[216]

Statins are generally well tolerated, but some patients may develop serious muscle pain and inflammation (myopathy) when taking these drugs.[217,218] Although the exact reason for these myopathic changes is not clear, these drugs may impair skeletal muscle mitochondrial function and energy production in susceptible individuals.[219] Clinicians should therefore be alert for any muscle pain and weakness in patients taking statin drugs. Patients with these symptoms should be referred back to the physician immediately to consider whether these myopathic changes are drug induced and if drug therapy needs to be changed or discontinued. There is also controversy about whether statins should be administered to adults after they progress beyond a certain age.[211] That is, some experts question whether these drugs continue to provide cardiovascular benefits in those older than 75 years, given that the risk of muscle damage seems more likely in these individuals.[214] Much of this controversy arises from the relative lack of randomized trials of these drugs in the very old population.[211] Future research will hopefully clarify whether the benefits of statins are worth the risks when these drugs are used in adults beyond a certain age.

Drugs Used in Coagulation Disorders. Excessive hemostasis, or a tendency for the blood to clot too rapidly, is a common and serious problem in older adults.[220,221] Formation of blood clots may result in thrombophlebitis and thromboembolism. These problems are especially important in the older patient after surgery and prolonged bed rest, which can increase the risk of venous thromboembolism and subsequent pulmonary embolism.[222,223] The use of two anticoagulants, heparin and warfarin, is a mainstay in preventing excessive hemostasis.[224,225] These agents work by different mechanisms to prolong and normalize the clotting time of the blood.[224] Although warfarin is taken orally, heparins must be administered by parenteral (nonoral) routes. The traditional or "unfractionated" form of heparin is usually administered via intravenous injection, whereas "low molecular weight" heparins such as enoxaparin (Lovenox) and dalteparin (Fragmin) can be administered by subcutaneous injection. Low-molecular-weight heparins are also safer than the traditional forms, thus offering a more convenient route of administration as well as decreased risk of adverse effects such as hemorrhage.

Traditionally, anticoagulant treatment started with parenteral heparin to achieve a rapid decrease in blood clotting, followed by long-term management of excessive coagulation through oral warfarin administration. However, several other oral anticoagulant therapies have been developed, including drugs that directly inhibit clotting factor X (e.g., fondaparinux, rivaroxaban) and drugs that directly inhibit thrombin (e.g., bivalirudin, dabigatran) (see Table 6.5).[226,227] These drugs offer certain advantages to warfarin, including less need to periodically monitor clotting time, fewer interactions with other drugs, and no dietary restrictions (patients taking warfarin must be careful about ingesting foods that contain vitamin K).[228,229] Hence, these newer oral drugs provide an alternative to warfarin and can be incorporated into anticoagulant regimens in older adults following joint replacement surgeries and other situations where thrombosis must be controlled.

The most common problem with anticoagulant drug therapy is an increased tendency for hemorrhage.[230,231] Although the risk will depend on the specific drug, all anticoagulants delay blood clotting to some extent, and excessive bleeding can occur. Physical therapists should be cautious when dealing with open wounds or procedures that potentially induce tissue trauma (e.g., chest percussion, vigorous massage) because of the increased risk for hemorrhage. On the other hand, clinicians should encourage their patients to continue to take anticoagulant drugs as directed to maintain normal hemostasis. Problems or adverse effects should certainly be brought to the attention of the physician, but patients should not independently decide to stop taking these drugs because it could lead to serious thrombogenesis.

Respiratory and Gastrointestinal Drugs

Drugs Used in Respiratory Disorders. Older adults may take drugs to treat fairly simple respiratory conditions associated with the common cold and seasonal allergies. Such drugs include cough medications (antitussives), decongestants, antihistamines, and drugs that help loosen and raise respiratory secretions (mucolytics and expectorants). Drugs may also be taken for more chronic, serious problems such as chronic obstructive pulmonary disease (COPD) and bronchial asthma.[232,233] Drug therapy for asthma and COPD includes bronchodilators such as β-adrenergic agonists (albuterol, epinephrine), xanthine derivatives (aminophylline, theophylline), and anticholinergic drugs (ipratropium, tiotropium).[234] Corticosteroids may also be given to treat inflammation in the respiratory tracts that is often present in these chronic respiratory problems.[235,236] Certain respiratory drugs also work synergistically when combined with one another. In particular, combining a β-adrenergic agonist with a corticosteroid can help control bronchoconstriction and airway inflammation, respectively, thus providing optimal control for many patients with COPD or asthma.[234,235]

These respiratory drugs are associated with various side effects that may affect physical therapy of the older adult. In particular, older adults may be more susceptible to sedative side effects of drugs such as antihistamines and cough suppressants. For some of the prescription medications, side effects are often reduced if the medication can be applied directly to the respiratory tissues by inhalation.[237,238] For instance, even corticosteroids can be used fairly safely in older adults if these drugs are inhaled rather than administered orally and distributed into the systemic circulation. Inhaled forms of respiratory medications, however, can cause systemic side effects, especially when applied in higher doses or when used excessively.[237,239] Likewise, when these medications are administered systemically, lower doses of the prescription bronchodilators may be necessary in older adults. This fact is especially true in older patients with reduced liver or kidney function, because metabolism and elimination of the active form of the drug will be impaired. Finally, some older patients may use excessive amounts of certain over-the-counter products. Physical therapists should question the extent to which their geriatric patients routinely take large doses of cough suppressants, antihistamines, and other over-the-counter respiratory drugs. Clinicians should inform their patients that these drugs are intended to be used at the recommended dose for short-term relief of respiratory symptoms but that prolonged or excessive use is not healthy. Chronic problems that do not respond to these over-the-counter products should be brought to the attention of the physician.

Drugs Used in Gastrointestinal Disorders. Gastrointestinal drugs such as antacids and laxatives are among the most commonly used medications in older adults.[55,240] Antacids typically consist of a base that neutralizes hydrochloric acid, thus helping to alleviate stomach discomfort caused by excess gastric acid secretion. Other drugs that decrease gastric acid secretion include the H_2 blockers (e.g., cimetidine, ranitidine), which work by blocking certain histamine receptors (H_2 receptors) that are located in the gastric mucosa, and proton pump inhibitors (esomeprazole, omeprazole), which decrease formation of hydrochloric acid in the stomach by inhibiting transport of H^+ ions across the gastric lining. Laxatives stimulate bowel evacuation and defecation by a number of different methods depending on the drug used. Drugs used to treat diarrhea are also commonly taken by older patients. These drugs consist of agents such as opioids (diphenoxylate, loperamide) that help decrease GI motility and products such as the adsorbents (e.g., kaolin, pectin) that help sequester toxins and irritants in the GI tract that may cause diarrhea.

The major concern for GI drug use in older adults is the potential for inappropriate and excessive use of these agents.[241] Most of these drugs are readily available as over-the-counter products. Older individuals may self-administer these agents to the extent that normal GI activity is compromised. For instance, the older person who relies on daily laxative use (or possibly even several laxatives each day) may experience a decline in the normal regulation of bowel evacuation. Drugs may also be used as a substitute for proper eating habits. Antacids, for example, may be taken routinely to disguise the irritant effects of certain foods that are not tolerated well by the older adult. Antacids, however, should not be used indiscriminately for the long-term management of problems such as gastroesophageal reflux disease (GERD). Physical therapists can advise their geriatric patients that most over-the-counter GI drugs are meant to be used for only brief episodes of GI discomfort, and that GERD and other chronic GI disorders should be brought to the attention of the physician. Therapists can also encourage their patients to consult nutritionists and dieticians so that proper nutrition and eating habits might serve as a safer and healthier alternative than prolonged use of GI drugs.

Hormonal Agents

General Strategy: Use of Hormones as Replacement Therapy. The endocrine glands synthesize and release hormones that travel through the blood to regulate the physiological function of various tissues and organs. If hormonal production is interrupted, natural or synthetic versions of these hormones can be administered pharmacologically to restore and maintain normal endocrine function. This replacement therapy is commonly used in older adults when endocrine function is diminished because of age-related factors (e.g., loss of ovarian hormones after menopause) or if endocrine function is lost after disease or surgery.[242,243] Some of the more common hormonal agents used in older adults are listed in Table 6.6 and are discussed here.

Estrogen Replacement. The primary female hormones—estrogen and progesterone—are normally produced by the ovaries from puberty until approximately the 5th or 6th decade when menopause occurs. Loss of these hormones is associated with a number of problems, including vasomotor symptoms (hot flashes), atrophic vaginitis, and atrophic dystrophy of the vulva. Replacement of the ovarian hormones, especially estrogen, can help resolve all these symptoms.[244] In addition, estrogen replacement can substantially reduce the risk of osteoporosis in postmenopausal women.[245] The effects of estrogen replacement on other physiological systems, however, are less clear. Some studies, for example, suggest that estrogen replacement can improve the plasma lipid profile and might therefore reduce the risk of coronary heart disease when relatively low doses of estrogen are administered fairly soon after the onset of menopause.[245] Many studies, however, discovered an increased risk of stroke and venous thromboembolism, especially when higher doses were administered to older women (mid-60s).[245,246] Likewise, the effects of estrogen on cognitive function in older women remain unclear. Observational data suggest that estrogen may reduce the risk of Alzheimer disease if initiated soon after menopause but that estrogen replacement may increase the risk of dementia when initiated in women over 65 years of age.[247]

Estrogen replacement is therefore associated with certain beneficial effects, but there is concern that estrogen therapy may increase the risk of stroke and venous thromboembolic disease. Estrogen replacement may also increase the risk of some forms of cancer, including breast and endometrial cancer.[245,246] However, the exact relationship between estrogen replacement and the risk of cancer and cardiovascular disease remains uncertain.[244,245] The risks of these problems vary substantially

TABLE 6.6 Endocrine Drugs Groups

Category	Indication	Common Examples	
		Generic Name	Trade Name
Androgens	Androgen deficiency	Methyltestosterone Testosterone	Android, others AndroGel, others
Estrogens	Osteoporosis Severe postmenopausal symptoms Some cancers	Conjugated estrogens Estradiol	Premarin, others Estrace, others
Insulin	Diabetes mellitus	—	Humulin, Novolin, others
Antihyperglycemics	Diabetes mellitus (type 2)	Acarbose Chlorpropamide Glipizide Liragluride Metformin Repaglinide Rosiglitazone Sitagliptin Tolbutamide	Precose Diabinese Glucotrol Saxenda, Victoza Glucophage, others Prandin Avandia Januvia Orinase
Antithyroid agents	Hyperthyroidism	Methimazole Propylthiouracil	Tapazole —
Thyroid hormones	Hypothyroidism	Levothyroxine (T_4) Liothyronine (T_3)	Synthroid, others Cytomel, Triostat

from person to person, and other variables such as estrogen dose, route of administration, and combining estrogen with progesterone may greatly influence the adverse effects of estrogen replacement.[244,248] In addition, a key variable seems to be the timing of estrogen replacement relative to onset of menopause, with a better risk–benefit ratio observed if replacement is initiated within 10 years after menopause occurs.[245,247]

At the present time, there is consensus that estrogen replacement therapy is not indicated for every woman after menopause, but that the risk–benefit ratio should be considered individually for each woman.[249,250] A woman with severe postmenopausal symptoms who is also at high risk for developing osteoporosis, for example, may be a good candidate for short-term (preferably 5 years or less) estrogen replacement. This intervention, of course, should only be considered if she does not have other risk factors that predispose to cancer or cardiovascular disease.[244,250] Likewise, newer estrogen-like compounds such as raloxifene and tamoxifen are an option for certain women. These agents, known also as selective estrogen-receptor modulators (SERMs), stimulate estrogen receptors on bone and certain cardiovascular tissues while blocking estrogen receptors on breast and uterine tissues.[250,251] This selectivity may provide beneficial effects on bone and postmenopausal symptoms while decreasing the risk of breast cancer.[251] Efforts continue to develop effective and safer hormonal strategies for women who require estrogen replacement.

Androgen Replacement. In a situation analogous to postmenopausal women, certain older men may have reduced production of male hormones (androgens) such as testosterone. Testosterone production slowly declines with aging, but in certain men it may decline faster than normal.[252] Inadequate testosterone production is associated with several problems, including decreased lean body mass, increased body fat, decreased bone density, lack of energy, and decreased libido.[253] It therefore makes sense to identify men who might benefit from androgen and provide small doses of testosterone-like drugs.[253]

Research suggests that androgen replacement can indeed reduce muscle loss associated with aging (sarcopenia), increase bone density, and provide other improvements in mood, libido, and quality of life in older men who lack adequate endogenous testosterone production.[252,253] The primary concern, of course, is that androgen replacement may stimulate prostate growth and perhaps lead to prostate cancer. This risk, however, seems to be acceptable if specific, low-dose androgens are used to treat testosterone deficiencies in older men.[254,255] Originally, there was also concern that androgen replacement might increase the risk of cardiovascular events such as heart attack and stroke in susceptible men.[256] This concern has been refuted by more recent studies, and there is reasonable evidence that appropriate testosterone levels may actually decrease the risk of cardiovascular disease in older men.[255,256] Future research will continue to clarify how testosterone replacement can provide optimal health benefits in older men.

Diabetes Mellitus. Insulin is normally synthesized by pancreatic β cells, and this hormone regulates the metabolism of glucose and other energy substrates. Diabetes mellitus is a complex metabolic disorder caused by inadequate insulin production, decreased peripheral effects of insulin, or a combination of inadequate insulin production and decreased insulin effects. Diabetes mellitus consists of two principal types: type 1 and type 2 (known formerly as insulin-dependent and non-insulin-dependent diabetes mellitus, respectively). The onset of type 1 diabetes mellitus is commonly associated with younger individuals, whereas type 2 diabetes mellitus occurs quite commonly in older adults.[257,258] Likewise, type 2 diabetes often occurs in older adults as part of a "metabolic syndrome" that consists of impaired glucose metabolism, obesity, hyperlipidemia, and hypertension.[259] If diabetes mellitus is not managed appropriately, acute effects (e.g., impaired glucose metabolism, ketoacidosis) and chronic effects (e.g., neuropathy, renal disease, blindness, poor wound healing) may occur.

Ideally, type 2 diabetes mellitus in older adults is managed successfully through diet, exercise, and maintenance of proper body weight.[259,260] When drug therapy is required, it is usually in the form of noninsulin drugs that lower blood glucose and are often referred to as *antihyperglycemics* (see Table 6.6).[261–263] Depending on the exact agent, these drugs help improve glucose metabolism by enhancing the release of insulin from the pancreas, increasing the sensitivity of peripheral tissues to insulin, stabilizing hepatic glucose output, delaying absorption of glucose from the GI tract, or increasing urinary glucose excretion. In some people with type 2 diabetes, insulin can also be added to the drug regimen to provide optimal glucose control, especially in patients who are unable to achieve target glucose values with the oral drugs.[264]

The principal problem associated with drug therapy in older diabetic patients is that the blood glucose level may be reduced too much, resulting in symptoms of hypoglycemia.[262] Physical therapists should be alert for signs of a low blood glucose level, such as headache, dizziness, confusion, fatigue, nausea, and sweating.

Thyroid Disorders. The thyroid gland normally produces two hormones: thyroxine and triiodothyronine. These hormones affect a wide variety of tissues and are primarily responsible for regulating basal metabolic rate and other aspects of systemic metabolism. Thyroid dysfunction is quite common in older adults and can be manifested as either increased or decreased production of thyroid hormones.[265,266] Excess thyroid hormone production (hyperthyroidism, thyrotoxicosis) produces symptoms such as nervousness, weight loss, muscle wasting, and tachycardia. Inadequate production of the thyroid hormones (hypothyroidism) is characterized by weight gain, lethargy, sleepiness, bradycardia, and other features consistent with a slow body metabolism.

Hyperthyroidism can be managed with drugs that inhibit thyroid hormone biosynthesis, such as propylthiouracil, methimazole, or high doses of iodide.[267,268] The primary problems associated with these drugs are transient allergic reactions (e.g., skin rashes) and blood dyscrasias such as aplastic anemia and agranulocytosis. A more permanent treatment of hyperthyroidism can be accomplished by surgical thyroidectomy, or by administering radioactive iodine.[267] The radioactive iodine is taken up by the thyroid gland, where it selectively destroys the overactive thyroid tissues.

Hypothyroidism is usually managed quite successfully by replacement therapy using natural and synthetic versions of one or both of the thyroid hormones.[269] The most significant problem associated with thyroid hormone replacement in older patients is that older adults require smaller doses of these hormones than younger individuals.[242] Replacement doses that are too high evoke symptoms of hyperthyroidism, such as nervousness, weight loss, and tachycardia. Physical therapists should be alert for these symptoms when working with older patients who are receiving thyroid hormone replacement therapy.

Treatment of Infections

Various microorganisms such as bacteria, viruses, fungi, and protozoa can invade and proliferate in older individuals. Often the immune system is able to combat these microorganisms successfully, thus preventing infection. Occasionally, however, drugs must be used to supplement the body's normal immune response in combating infection caused by pathogenic microorganisms. Older adults are often susceptible to such infections, especially if their immune system has already been compromised by previous illness, a general state of debilitation, or prolonged use of immunosuppressant drugs such as the glucocorticoids. These agents can also be administered prophylactically prior to joint replacement and other surgeries to reduce the chance of infections in older adults. Two of the more common types of infections, bacterial and viral, are presented along with a brief description of the related drug therapy.

Antibacterial Drugs. Although some bacteria exist in the body in a helpful or symbiotic state, infiltration of pathogenic bacteria may result in infection. If the immune system is unable to contain or destroy these bacteria, antibacterial drugs must be administered. Some of the principal groups of antibacterial drugs are shown in Table 6.7. These agents are often grouped according to how they inhibit or kill bacterial cells. For instance, certain drugs (e.g., penicillins, cephalosporins) act by inhibiting bacterial cell-wall synthesis. Other drugs (e.g., aminoglycosides, tetracyclines) specifically inhibit the synthesis of bacterial proteins. Drugs such as the fluoroquinolones (e.g., ciprofloxacin) and sulfonamides (e.g., sulfadiazine) work by selectively inhibiting the synthesis and function of bacterial DNA and RNA. The selection of a specific agent from one of these groups is based primarily on the type of bacterial infection present in each patient.

The side effects that tend to occur with these agents vary from drug to drug, and it is not possible in this limited space to discuss all the potential antibacterial ADRs. With

TABLE 6.7 Infection Drug Groups

	Common Examples	
	Generic Name	Trade Name
Antibacterial Drugs		
Major Groups		
Aminoglycosides	Gentamicin	Garamycin, others
	Streptomycin	—
Cephalosporins	Cefaclor	Ceclor, Raniclor
	Cephalexin	Daxbia, Keflex
Erythromycins	Erythromycin	Many trade names
Fluoroquinolones	Ciprofloxacin	Cipro, Proquin
	Norfloxacin	Noroxin
Penicillins	Penicillin G	Bicillin, many others
	Amoxicillin	Moxatag, many others
	Ampicillin	Principen, many others
Sulfonamides	Sulfadiazine	Silvadene
	Sulfisoxazole	Gantrisin, Truxazole
Tetracyclines	Doxycycline	Vibramycin, many others
	Tetracycline	Panmycin, others
Antiviral Drugs		
Principal Indication		
Herpesviruses	Acyclovir	Sitavig, Zovirax
	Docosanol	Abreva
Cytomegalovirus	Foscarnet	Foscavir
	Ganciclovir	Cytovene
Influenza	Amantadine	Gocovri, Symmetrel
	Oseltamivir	Tamiflu
Human immunodeficiency virus (HIV)	Delavirdine	Rescriptor
	Didanosine	Videx
	Efavirenz	Sustiva
	Enfuvirtide	Fuzeon
	Nelfinavir	Viracept
	Raltegravir	Isentress
	Ritonavir	Norvir
	Saquinavir	Fortovase, Invirase
	Zidovudine (AZT)	Retrovir

regard to their use in older patients, many of the precautions discussed earlier tend to apply. For instance, ADRs tend to occur more frequently because of the decreased renal clearance of antibacterial drugs in older adults.[26,270] Hence, physical therapists should be alert for any suspicious reactions such as severe GI symptoms (vomiting, diarrhea), CNS signs (seizures, vertigo), and hypersensitivity reactions (rashes, difficulty breathing). Such reactions are especially prevalent if renal function is already somewhat compromised. Resistance to antibacterial drugs is also a major concern in all age groups, including older adults.[271,272] Overuse and improper use of these agents have enabled certain bacterial strains to develop antidrug mechanisms, thus rendering these drugs ineffective against these "superbug" bacterial infections. Physical therapists should be aware of the need to prevent the spread of bacterial infections through the use of frequent handwashing, regular equipment wipedowns, and other universal precautions.

Antiviral Drugs. Viruses are small microorganisms that can invade human (host) cells and use the biochemical machinery of the host cell to produce more viruses. As a result, the virus often disrupts or destroys the function of the host cell, causing specific symptoms that are indicative of viral infection. Viral infections can cause disease syndromes ranging from the common cold to serious conditions such as acquired immunodeficiency syndrome (AIDS). Because the viral invader usually functions and coexists within the host cell, it is often difficult to administer a drug that will kill the virus without simultaneously destroying the host cell. The number of antiviral agents is therefore limited (see Table 6.7), and these drugs often attenuate viral replication rather than actually destroy a virus that already exists in the body.

Because of the relatively limited number of effective antiviral agents, pharmacologic management of viral disease often focuses on preventing viral infection through the use of vaccines. Vaccines are usually a modified, inactive form of the virus that stimulates the patient's immune system to produce specific antiviral antibodies. When exposed to an active form of the virus, these antibodies help destroy the viral invader before an infection is established.

Physical therapists should realize that the antiviral agents shown in Table 6.7 are often poorly tolerated and produce a number of adverse side effects, especially in older or debilitated patients.[273,274] Hence, prevention of viral infection through the use of vaccines is especially important in older adults. For instance, influenza vaccines are often advocated for older individuals before annual seasonal outbreaks of the "flu,"[275] and a vaccine for pneumococcal pneumonia is advocated for all adults age 65 or older (see Centers for Disease Control and Prevention at http://www.cdc.gov/vaccines/vpd/pneumo/public/index.html). Of course, some vaccines are not always completely effective in preventing viral infections, and an appropriate vaccine has yet to be developed for certain viral diseases such as AIDS. Still, vaccines represent the most effective method of preventing viral infections in older individuals.

Cancer Chemotherapy

Cancer is the term used to describe diseases that are characterized by a rapid, uncontrolled cell proliferation and conversion of these cells to a more primitive and less functional state. Cancer is often treated aggressively through the use of a combination of several different techniques, such as surgery, radiation, and one or more cancer chemotherapeutic agents.

Older adults represent the majority of patients who will ultimately require some form of anticancer medication.[276]

In general, the cancer chemotherapy regimens in older adults are similar to those used in younger individuals, with the exception that dosages are adjusted according to changes in liver and kidney function or other changes that affect drug pharmacokinetics.[27] The results of cancer chemotherapy in the older patient also parallel those seen in the younger individual, with the possible exception that some hematologic malignancies (certain leukemias) do not appear to respond as well to drug therapy in older adults.[277,278] The principal chemotherapeutic strategies and types of anticancer agents are presented here.

Basic Strategy of Cancer Chemotherapy. Traditional anticancer drugs work by inhibiting the synthesis and function of DNA and RNA. This action impairs the proliferation of cancer cells because they must rely on the rapid replication of genetic material to synthesize new cancer cells. Of course, DNA and RNA function is also impaired to some extent in healthy noncancerous cells, and this accounts for the many severe side effects and high level of toxicity associated with traditional cancer chemotherapeutic agents.[279,280] Cancer cells, however, should suffer to a relatively greater degree because these cells typically have a greater need to replicate their genetic material to sustain a high rate of cell reproduction. Recently, however, several "targeted" drug strategies have been developed to better focus the effects of certain anticancer drugs on the malignant cells while sparing normal human tissues.[281,282] Some of the general drug strategies used in cancer chemotherapy are outlined here.

Types of Anticancer Drugs. Anticancer medications are classified according to their biochemical characteristics and mechanism of action (Table 6.8).[283] For example, alkylating agents form strong bonds between nucleic acids in the DNA double helix so that the DNA strands within the helix are unable to unwind and allow replication of the cell's genetic code. Antimetabolites impair the normal biosynthesis of nucleic acids and other important cellular metabolic components necessary for cell function. Antimitotic agents directly inhibit the mitotic apparatus that is responsible for controlling the actual division of one cell into two identical cells (mitosis). Certain antibiotics are effective as anticancer agents because they become inserted (intercalated) directly into the DNA double helix and either inhibit DNA function or cause the helix to break at the point where the drug is inserted. Hormones and drugs that block hormonal effects (antiestrogens, antiandrogens) are often used to attenuate the growth of hormone-sensitive tumors such as breast cancer and prostate cancer. Certain agents such as interferons, interleukin-2, and monoclonal antibodies are classified as biologic response modifiers because these drugs enhance the immune system's ability to destroy cancerous cells, or they selectively inhibit mechanisms within the cancer cells that cause proliferation of the cancer. Finally, several other "targeted" strategies such as angiogenesis inhibitors and tyrosine kinase inhibitors attempt to inhibit a specific biochemical trait of the cancer cell or tumor, thus focusing the drug's effect on the cancer cell with less harm to normal cells.

TABLE 6.8 Cancer Drug Groups

	Common Examples	
Major Groups	**Generic Name**	**Trade Name**
Alkylating agents	Busulfan Carmustine Cyclophosphamide Mechlorethamine	Myleran, others BiCNU, Gliadel Cytoxan, Neosar Mustargen
Antimetabolites	Cytarabine Floxuridine Fluorouracil Methotrexate	Cytosar-U, others FUDR Adrucil Trexall, Xatmep, others
Antimicrotubule agents	Paclitaxel Vinblastine Vincristine	Taxol, Onxol Velban Oncovin, Vincasar
Antineoplastic antibiotics	Daunorubicin Doxorubicin Idarubicin	Cerubidine Adriamycin, others Idamycin
Hormones		
Estrogens	Conjugated estrogens Estradiol	Premarin, others Estrace, others
Antiestrogens	Tamoxifen	Soltamox
Androgens	Testosterone	Many trade names
Antiandrogens	Flutamide	Eulexin
Targeted and Biological Therapies		
Interferons	Aldesleukin Interferon α-2a Interferon α-2b	Proleukin Roferon-A Intron A
Monoclonal antibodies	Bevacizumab Panitumumab Rituximab Traztuzumab	Avastin, Mvasi Vectibix Rituxan Herceptin
Tyrosine kinase inhibitors	Imatinib Gefitinib	Gleevec Iressa

Anticancer drugs therefore inhibit replication and function of the cancer cell through one of the mechanisms just described. Likewise, several different drugs are often used simultaneously to achieve a synergistic effect between the antiproliferative actions of each drug.

Adverse Effects and Concerns for Rehabilitation. As mentioned, patients receiving cancer chemotherapy typically experience a number of severe adverse drug effects. Side effects such as GI distress (e.g., anorexia, vomiting), skin reactions (e.g., hair loss, rashes), and toxicity of various organs are extremely common. Older patients receiving cancer chemotherapy are especially prone to certain adverse effects such as cardiotoxicity, neurotoxicity, and blood disorders (e.g., anemia, thrombocytopenia).[27,284,285] Unfortunately, these adverse effects must be tolerated because of the serious nature of cancer and the fact that death will ensue if these drugs are not used. In terms of rehabilitation of older patients, physical therapists must recognize that these adverse effects will inevitably interfere with rehabilitation procedures. There will be some days that the patient is simply unable to participate in any aspect of physical therapy. Still, the therapist can provide valuable and timely support for older adults receiving cancer chemotherapy and reassure the patient that these drug-related effects are often unavoidable because of the cytotoxic nature of the drugs.

Drugs Used to Treat Urinary and Fecal Incontinence

The treatment of bladder and bowel dysfunction is understandably a complex and difficult task. The lower urinary tract and bowel are controlled by the complex interaction of the autonomic and somatic nervous systems, and there are many issues that can impair the ability of these systems to regulate bowel and bladder function.[286] It follows that many older adults have problems related to urinary or fecal incontinence, and drug therapy is often used to help control these problems.

Urinary incontinence is often categorized according to the cause of the problem or the factors that initiate inadvertent urination.[287,288] Overactive bladder, for example, describes feelings of increased urinary frequency; that is, a person senses the need to urinate much more often than usual. Stress incontinence typically describes a small amount of urinary leakage during sneezing, coughing, or exercise. Leakage of larger amounts of urine without warning is described as urge incontinence, and inability to completely empty the bladder can lead to overflow incontinence. Functional incontinence occurs whenever a person cannot get to a toilet in time because of physical restrictions (unable to get to the toilet from the bed, chair, or wheelchair) or simply an inability to communicate the need to urinate (e.g., people with dementia). Urinary incontinence may also be temporary, such as transient incontinence due to urinary tract infections. Finally, two or more types of incontinence may occur simultaneously, resulting in mixed incontinence.

Some of the drugs used to treat urinary problems are listed in Table 6.9. Several of the more commonly used drugs attempt to relax the bladder by blocking the excitatory effects of acetylcholine (anticholinergic drugs)[289,290] or by stimulating specific β-adrenergic (β3) receptors that cause inhibition of bladder smooth muscle cells (Mirabegron [Mirbetriq]).[291,292] Estrogen may also help strengthen pelvic floor muscles in women after menopause,[293,294] and certain antidepressants can improve

TABLE 6.9 Drugs Used To Treat Urinary Incontinence

Drug	Mechanism of Action	Primary Indications	Primary Side Effects
Anticholinergics Darifenacin (Enablex) Fesoterodine (Toviaz) Oxybutynin (Ditropan, Urotrol) Solifenacin (Vesicare) Tolterodine (Detrol) Trospium (Sanctura)	Inhibit bladder spasms by blocking muscarinic acetylcholine receptors on bladder smooth muscle	OAB; urge incontinence	Dry mouth, constipation, urinary retention, nausea, dizziness, drowsiness; may also increase confusion in patients with dementia
Antidepressants Duloxetine (Cymbalta) Imipramine (Tofranil)	Inhibit reuptake and prolong effects of CNS serotonin and norepinephrine (antidepressant effects); may also cause relaxation of urethral sphincter, thus allowing more complete emptying and less urinary retention	Stress incontinence	Suicidal thoughts, fatigue, sleep disturbances, nausea, dry mouth, constipation
Estrogen	Can help restore strength and tone in pelvic floor muscles and other tissues supporting the bladder and urethra	Stress incontinence (postmenopausal)	Relatively few side effects if applied locally via vaginal cream or ring
Mirabegron (Mirbetriq)	Relaxes bladder by stimulating specific β-adrenergic (β3) receptors on detrusor muscle; allows bladder to fill more completely without increased urge to urinate	OAB, urge incontinence, overflow incontinence	Headache, dizziness, nausea, diarrhea, constipation, increased blood pressure
Onabotulinumtoxin type A (Botox)	Inhibits release of acetylcholine at the neuromuscular junction in detrusor muscle; causes relaxation and partial paralysis of bladder	OAB	Few side effects when injected directly into bladder; systemic reactions (muscle weakness, difficulty speaking/swallowing) may indicate overdose or spread to the systemic circulation

CNS, central nervous system; *OAB*, overactive bladder.

the control of urethral sphincter muscles, thus resulting in more normal urinary retention and bladder emptying.[295] If these drugs are not effective, injection of botulinum toxin into bladder smooth muscle can be used to inhibit acetylcholine release at the neuromuscular junction of cholinergic synapses in the bladder.[296,297]

As indicated in Table 6.9, there is considerable variation in the clinical pharmacology and related side effects of drugs used for urinary incontinence. Likewise, certain drugs can be more effective in specific types of urinary problems, and drug therapy must therefore be individualized for each patient.[286] In addition, patient adherence to drug therapy is often problematic, with many patients failing to follow the recommended drug regimen. There are, however, several nonpharmacologic interventions that may help decrease urinary incontinence, including physical therapy interventions that strengthen the pelvic floor musculature and improve bladder control.[293,298] Hence, a comprehensive program of drug therapy combined with physical therapy might ultimately provide the best results for patients with urinary incontinence.

Regarding fecal incontinence, there are many physiological reasons for this problem such as diarrhea, constipation, weakness of sphincter muscles, and damage to nerves that control defecation. In addition, patients with dementia may simply lack awareness of their bowel function and be unable to communicate the need to use the toilet properly.

Drugs used to help control fecal incontinence typically attempt to correct problems in GI motility.[299,300] That is, antidiarrheal medications are used to slow down excessive movement through the lower GI tract, and laxatives are used to treat constipation. These drugs were addressed earlier in this chapter. Direct application of specific drugs (phenylephrine, valproate) to the anal sphincter muscles may help increase sphincter tone, but the success of these treatments may be limited to certain patients with loose stools.[300] Otherwise, there are not any medications that can directly decrease the incidence of fecal incontinence. Certain medications can, of course, indirectly improve the patient's awareness and ability to communicate the need to use the toilet. For example, an antipsychotic medication or antidementia medication can improve the patient's ability to control his or her bowels more effectively and to avoid episodes of incontinence.[301] The success of these indirect methods is highly variable from one person to another and may not be very successful in people with advanced dementia.

GENERAL STRATEGIES FOR COORDINATING PHYSICAL THERAPY WITH DRUG TREATMENT IN OLDER ADULTS

Based on the preceding discussion, it is clear that various medications can produce beneficial and adverse effects that may affect physical therapy of older adults in many different ways. There are, however, some basic strategies that therapists can use to help maximize the beneficial aspects of drug therapy and minimize the detrimental drug effects when working with geriatric individuals. These general strategies are summarized here.

Distinguishing Drug Effects from Symptoms

When evaluating a geriatric patient, therapists must try to account for the subjective and objective findings that may be due to ADRs rather than true disease sequelae and the effects of aging. For instance, the patient who appears confused and disoriented during the initial physical therapy evaluation may actually be experiencing an adverse reaction to a psychotropic drug, cardiovascular medication, or some other agent. The correct distinction of true symptoms from ADRs allows better treatment planning and clinical decision making.

As discussed earlier, therapists can also take steps to prevent inappropriate drug use and polypharmacy by helping distinguish ADRs from true disease symptoms. Distinguishing drug-related signs from true patient symptoms may require careful observation and consultation with family members or other health care professionals to see whether these signs tend to increase after each dosage. Periodic reevaluation should also take into account any changes in drug therapy, especially if new medications are added to the patient's regimen. Finally, the medical staff should be alerted to any change in the patient's response that may indicate an ADR.

Scheduling Physical Therapy Sessions Around Dosage Schedule

Physical therapy should be coordinated with peak drug effects if the patient's active participation will be enhanced by drug treatment. For instance, drugs that improve motor performance (e.g., antiparkinson agents), improve mood and behavior (e.g., antidepressants, antipsychotics), and decrease pain (e.g., analgesics) may increase the older patient's ability to take part in various rehabilitation procedures. Conversely, physical therapy should be scheduled when drug effects are at a minimum for older patients receiving drugs that produce excessive sedation, dizziness, or other adverse effects that may impair the patient's cognitive or motor abilities. Unfortunately, there is often a tradeoff between desirable effects and adverse effects with the same drug, such as the opioid analgesic that also produces sedation. In these cases, it may take some trial and error in each patient to find a treatment time that capitalizes on the drug's benefits with minimum interference from the adverse effects.

Promoting Synergistic Effects of Physical Therapy Procedures with Drug Therapy

One must not lose sight of the fact that many of the rehabilitation procedures used with geriatric clients may augment drug therapy. For instance, the patient with Parkinson disease may experience an optimal improvement in motor function through a combination of physical therapy and antiparkinson drugs. In some cases, drug therapy may be reduced through the contribution of physical therapy procedures (e.g., reduction of pain medications through the simultaneous use of transcutaneous electrical nerve stimulation, physical agents, and so forth). This synergistic relationship between drug therapy and physical therapy can help achieve better results than if either intervention is used alone.

Avoiding Potentially Harmful Interactions Between Physical Therapy Procedures and Drug Effects

Some physical therapy interventions used in older adults could potentially have a negative interaction with some medications. For instance, the use of rehabilitation procedures that cause extensive peripheral vasodilation (e.g., large whirlpool, some exercises) may produce severe hypotension in the patient receiving certain antihypertensive medications. These negative interactions must be anticipated and avoided when working with geriatric patients.

Improving Education and Compliance with Drug Therapy in Older Adults

Proper adherence to drug therapy is one area where physical therapists can have a direct impact. Therapists can reinforce the need for adhering to the prescribed regimen, and therapists can help monitor whether drugs have been taken as directed. Therapists can also help educate their geriatric patients and their families as to why specific drugs are indicated and what side effects should be expected and tolerated as opposed to side effects that may indicate drug toxicity.

Facilitating Medication Discussions with the Physician

Physical therapists are often in an ideal position to alert physicians about any untoward and potentially harmful drug effects in their geriatric patients. Critical or life-threatening events such as severe cardiovascular problems (uncontrolled hypertension, certain ventricular dysrhythmias), CNS disorders (seizures, unresponsiveness), severe hypoglycemia, and anaphylactic reactions are medical emergencies that must be brought immediately to the attention of the physician.

There are, however, less serious problems that impair the patient's progress and ability to participate in physical rehabilitation. It is incumbent for the physical therapist to discuss these issues with the physician whenever the therapist suspects that these problems might be related to a certain drug.

Certain ethical and professional boundaries should not be crossed, however. It is inappropriate for a therapist to tell a physician that he or she is administering the wrong drug or that the dose is too high. A more productive strategy is for the therapist to carefully monitor the patient's progress and objectively document any failure to improve or a decline in the patient's progress.

The physical therapist should approach the physician with the idea that the lack of successful rehabilitation outcomes is the problem, rather than an incorrect or inappropriate drug. The therapist can then tactfully and respectfully raise the question of whether an adverse drug effect might be impairing the patient's progress or limiting the patient's ability to participate in physical therapy. In other words, the therapist can broach the issue of whether a drug might be contributing to the lack of progress by focusing on the rehabilitation outcomes, rather than questioning whether the drug should or should not be prescribed. This strategy will hopefully help the therapist maintain a good professional relationship with the physician while facilitating optimal outcomes of the patient.

Box 6.1 provides a list of websites that are useful references for updated information about specific medications.

BOX 6.1 Websites for Medication Updates

Drugs.com: http://www.drugs.com
Features:
Search box
News
Drugs A–Z
Drugs by condition
Pill identifier
Interactions checker

Epocrates*: http://online.epocrates.com/home
Features:
Search box
Alphabetical drug list
Drugs by class/subclass
Check drug interactions
Pill identifier

FDA website: http://www.fda.gov
Click on DRUGS
Features:
Spotlight (on current issues)
Recalls and alerts
Approvals and clearances
News and announcements
Drug safety
Search drugs box
Others

Continued

BOX 6.1 Websites for Medication Updates—cont'd

PubMed: http://www.ncbi.nlm.nih.gov/PubMed

National Library of Medicine's computerized bibliographic database; 3000+ peer-reviewed journals; covered since 1966

Features:

Search articles by topic, author, or journals

Combine search terms (AND, OR, etc.) and use "limits" feature to refine search

WebMD: http://www.webmd.com

Click on DRUGS & SUPPLEMENTS

Features:

Find a drug

Pill identifier

Drug news

Mobile drug information (downloads to certain handheld devices)

Vitamins and supplements

Others

*Note: This site offers other features including an option to download drug information to handheld devices. Some options require a subscription and fee to access.

REFERENCES

1. Oscanoa TJ, Lizaraso F, Carvajal A. Hospital admissions due to adverse drug reactions in the elderly. A meta-analysis. *Eur J Clin Pharmacol.* 2017;73:759–770.
2. U.S. Census Bureau. https://www.census.gov/quickfacts/fact/table/US/PST045217. Accessed May 17, 2018.
3. Medical Expenditure Panel Survey. https://meps.ahrq.gov/data_files/publications/st245/stat245.pdf. Accessed May 17, 2018.
4. Kim J, Parish AL. Polypharmacy and medication management in older adults. *Nurs Clin North Am.* 2017;52:457–468.
5. Sánchez-Fidalgo S, Guzmán-Ramos MI, Galván-Banqueri M, et al. Prevalence of drug interactions in elderly patients with multimorbidity in primary care. *Int J Clin Pharm.* 2017;39:343–353.
6. Morin L, Laroche ML, Texier G, Johnell K. Prevalence of potentially inappropriate medication use in older adults living in nursing homes: a systematic review. *J Am Med Dir Assoc.* 2016;17. 862.e1–9.
7. Storms H, Marquet K, Aertgeerts B, Claes N. Prevalence of inappropriate medication use in residential long-term care facilities for the elderly: a systematic review. *Eur J Gen Pract.* 2017;23:69–77.
8. Qato DM, Wilder J, Schumm LP, et al. Changes in prescription and over-the-counter medication and dietary supplement use among older adults in the United States, 2005 vs 2011. *JAMA Intern Med.* 2016;176:473–482.
9. Wallace J, Paauw DS. Appropriate prescribing and important drug interactions in older adults. *Med Clin North Am.* 2015;99:295–310.
10. Stefanacci RG, Khan T. Can managed care manage polypharmacy? *Clin Geriatr Med.* 2017;33:241–255.
11. Stewart D, Mair A, Wilson M. SIMPATHY Consortium. Guidance to manage inappropriate polypharmacy in older people: systematic review and future developments. *Expert Opin Drug Saf.* 2017;16:203–213.
12. Wimmer BC, Cross AJ, Jokanovic N, et al. Clinical outcomes associated with medication regimen complexity in older people: a systematic review. *J Am Geriatr Soc.* 2017;65:747–753.
13. Thomas RE. Assessing medication problems in those ≥ 65 using the STOPP and START criteria. *Curr Aging Sci.* 2016;9:150–158.
14. Cadogan CA, Ryan C, Hughes CM. Appropriate polypharmacy and medicine safety: when many is not too many. *Drug Saf.* 2016;39:109–116.
15. Vrdoljak D, Borovac JA. Medication in the elderly - considerations and therapy prescription guidelines. *Acta Med Acad.* 2015;44:159–168.
16. Reeve E, Trenaman SC, Rockwood K, Hilmer SN. Pharmacokinetic and pharmacodynamic alterations in older people with dementia. *Expert Opin Drug Metab Toxicol.* 2017;13:651–668.
17. Schlender JF, Meyer M, Thelen K, et al. Development of a whole-body physiologically based pharmacokinetic approach to assess the pharmacokinetics of drugs in elderly individuals. *Clin Pharmacokinet.* 2016;55:1573–1589.
18. Lucas C, Byles J, Martin JH. Medicines optimisation in older people: taking age and sex into account. *Maturitas.* 2016;93:114–120.
19. Merchant HA, Liu F, Orlu Gul M, Basit AW. Age-mediated changes in the gastrointestinal tract. *Int J Pharm.* 2016;512:382–395.
20. Soenen S, Rayner CK, Jones KL, Horowitz M. The ageing gastrointestinal tract. *Curr Opin Clin Nutr Metab Care.* 2016;19:12–18.
21. Buch A, Carmeli E, Boker LK, et al. Muscle function and fat content in relation to sarcopenia, obesity and frailty of old age—an overview. *Exp Gerontol.* 2016;76:25–32.
22. Gérard S, Bréchemier D, Lefort A, et al. Body composition and anti-neoplastic treatment in adult and older subjects - a systematic review. *J Nutr Health Aging.* 2016;20:878–888.
23. Chan AW, Patel YA, Choi S. Aging of the liver: what this means for patients with HIV. *Curr HIV/AIDS Rep.* 2016;13:309–317.
24. Tajiri K, Shimizu Y. Liver physiology and liver diseases in the elderly. *World J Gastroenterol.* 2013;19:8459–8467.
25. Bitzer M, Wiggins J. Aging biology in the kidney. *Adv Chronic Kidney Dis.* 2016;23:12–18.
26. Gekle M. Kidney and aging - a narrative review. *Exp Gerontol.* 2017;87(Pt B):153–155.
27. Korc-Grodzicki B, Boparai MK, Lichtman SM. Prescribing for older patients with cancer. *Clin Adv Hematol Oncol.* 2014;12:309–318.
28. Ponticelli C, Sala G, Glassock RJ. Drug management in the elderly adult with chronic kidney disease: a review for the primary care physician. *Mayo Clin Proc.* 2015;90:633–645.
29. de Vries OJ, Peeters G, Elders P, et al. The elimination half-life of benzodiazepines and fall risk: two prospective observational studies. *Age Ageing.* 2013;42:764–770.
30. Waring RH, Harris RM, Mitchell SC. Drug metabolism in the elderly: a multifactorial problem? *Maturitas.* 2017;100:27–32.
31. Sobamowo H, Prabhakar SS. The kidney in aging: physiological changes and pathological implications. *Prog Mol Biol Transl Sci.* 2017;146:303–340.
32. Baker SE, Limberg JK, Ranadive SM, Joyner MJ. Neurovascular control of blood pressure is influenced by aging, sex, and sex hormones. *Am J Physiol Regul Integr Comp Physiol.* 2016;311:R1271–R1275.
33. Naples JG, Gellad WF, Hanlon JT. The role of opioid analgesics in geriatric pain management. *Clin Geriatr Med.* 2016;32:725–735.
34. Janssens J, Lu D, Ni B, et al. Development of precision small-molecule proneurotrophic therapies for neurodegenerative diseases. *Vitam Horm.* 2017;104:263–311.

35. Spadari RC, Cavadas C, de Carvalho AETS, et al. Role of beta-adrenergic receptors and sirtuin signaling in the heart during aging, heart failure, and adaptation to stress. *Cell Mol Neurobiol.* 2018;38:109–120.
36. Vatner SF, Park M, Yan L, et al. Adenylyl cyclase type 5 in cardiac disease, metabolism, and aging. *Am J Physiol Heart Circ Physiol.* 2013;305:H1–H8.
37. Yin F, Sancheti H, Liu Z, Cadenas E. Mitochondrial function in ageing: coordination with signalling and transcriptional pathways. *J Physiol.* 2016;594:2025–2042.
38. Zhou L, Rupa AP. Categorization and association analysis of risk factors for adverse drug events. *Eur J Clin Pharmacol.* 2018;74:389–404.
39. Banzi R, Camaioni P, Tettamanti M, et al. Older patients are still under-represented in clinical trials of Alzheimer's disease. *Alzheimers Res Ther.* 2016;8:32.
40. Shenoy P, Harugeri A. Elderly patients' participation in clinical trials. *Perspect Clin Res.* 2015;6:184–189.
41. Lapeyre-Mestre M. A review of adverse outcomes associated with psychoactive drug use in nursing home residents with dementia. *Drugs Aging.* 2016;33:865–888.
42. Hoyle DJ, Bindoff IK, Clinnick LM, et al. Clinical and economic outcomes of interventions to reduce antipsychotic and benzodiazepine use within nursing homes: a systematic review. *Drugs Aging.* 2018;35:123–134.
43. Kvarnström K, Airaksinen M, Liira H. Barriers and facilitators to medication adherence: a qualitative study with general practitioners. *BMJ Open.* 2018;8. e015332.
44. Mira JJ, Lorenzo S, Guilabert M, et al. A systematic review of patient medication error on self-administering medication at home. *Expert Opin Drug Saf.* 2015;14:815–838.
45. Costa E, Giardini A, Savin M, et al. Interventional tools to improve medication adherence: review of literature. *Patient Prefer Adherence.* 2015;9:1303–1914.
46. Leporini C, De Sarro G, Russo E. Adherence to therapy and adverse drug reactions: is there a link? *Expert Opin Drug Saf.* 2014;13(Suppl 1):S41–S55.
47. Dharmarajan TS, Dharmarajan L. Tolerability of antihypertensive medications in older adults. *Drugs Aging.* 2015;32:773–796.
48. Fick DM, Semla TP, Beizer J, et al. American Geriatrics Society 2015 Updated Beers criteria for potentially inappropriate medication use in older adults. *J Am Geriatr Soc.* 2015;63:2227–2246.
49. Blanco-Reina E, Ariza-Zafra G, Ocaña-Riola R, León-Ortiz M. 2012 American Geriatrics Society Beers criteria: enhanced applicability for detecting potentially inappropriate medications in European older adults? A comparison with the Screening Tool of Older Person's Potentially Inappropriate Prescriptions. *J Am Geriatr Soc.* 2014;62:1217–1223.
50. Lavan AH, Gallagher PF, O'Mahony D. Methods to reduce prescribing errors in elderly patients with multimorbidity. *Clin Interv Aging.* 2016;11:857–866.
51. Cruz-Jentoft AJ, Kiesswetter E, Drey M, Sieber CC. Nutrition, frailty, and sarcopenia. *Aging Clin Exp Res.* 2017;29:43–48.
52. Holton AE, Gallagher P, Fahey T, Cousins G. Concurrent use of alcohol interactive medications and alcohol in older adults: a systematic review of prevalence and associated adverse outcomes. *BMC Geriatr.* 2017;17:148.
53. Kinsey JD, Nykamp D. Dangers of nonprescription medicines: educating and counseling older adults. *Consult Pharm.* 2017;32:269–280.
54. Stine JG, Chalasani NP. Drug hepatotoxicity: environmental factors. *Clin Liver Dis.* 2017;21:103–113.
55. Baker NR, Blakely KK. Gastrointestinal disturbances in the elderly. *Nurs Clin North Am.* 2017;52:419–431.
56. Salahudeen MS, Duffull SB, Nishtala PS. Anticholinergic burden quantified by anticholinergic risk scales and adverse outcomes in older people: a systematic review. *BMC Geriatr.* 2015;15:31.
57. Swart LM, van der Zanden V, Spies PE, et al. The comparative risk of delirium with different opioids: a systematic review. *Drugs Aging.* 2017;34:437–443.
58. Rehm J, Anderson P, Manthey J, et al. Alcohol use disorders in primary health care: what do we know and where do we go? *Alcohol Alcohol.* 2016;51:422–427.
59. Ringoir L, Pedersen SS, Widdershoven JW, et al. Beta-blockers and depression in elderly hypertension patients in primary care. *Fam Med.* 2014;46:447–453.
60. Arnold AC, Raj SR. Orthostatic hypotension: a practical approach to investigation and management. *Can J Cardiol.* 2017;33:1725–1728.
61. Frith J, Parry SW. New Horizons in orthostatic hypotension. *Age Ageing.* 2017;46:168–174.
62. Butt DA, Harvey PJ. Benefits and risks of antihypertensive medications in the elderly. *J Intern Med.* 2015;278:599–626.
63. Hartog LC, Schrijnders D, Landman GWD, et al. Is orthostatic hypotension related to falling? A meta-analysis of individual patient data of prospective observational studies. *Age Ageing.* 2017;46:568–575.
64. Shaw BH, Claydon VE. The relationship between orthostatic hypotension and falling in older adults. *Clin Auton Res.* 2014;24:3–13.
65. Hamed SA. The auditory and vestibular toxicities induced by antiepileptic drugs. *Expert Opin Drug Saf.* 2017;16: 1281–1294.
66. Jahn K, Kressig RW, Bridenbaugh SA, et al. Dizziness and unstable gait in old age: etiology, diagnosis and treatment. *Dtsch Arztebl Int.* 2015;112:387–393.
67. Brunton LL, Hilal-Dandan R, Knollmann BC, eds. *The Pharmacological Basis of Therapeutics.* 13th ed. New York: McGraw-Hill; 2018.
68. Ciccone CD. *Pharmacology in Rehabilitation.* 5th ed. Philadelphia: FA Davis; 2016.
69. DiPiro JT, Talbert RL, Yee GC, et al, eds. *Pharmacotherapy: A Pathophysiologic Approach.* 10th ed New York: McGraw-Hill; 2017.
70. Kennedy GJ, Castro J, Chang M, et al. Psychiatric and medical comorbidity in the primary care geriatric patient-an update. *Curr Psychiatry Rep.* 2016;18:62.
71. Kok RM, Reynolds CF. Management of depression in older adults: a review. *JAMA.* 2017;317:2114–2122.
72. Lam S, Macina LO. Therapy update for insomnia in the elderly. *Consult Pharm.* 2017;32:610–622.
73. Nguyen-Michel VH, Vecchierini MF. Exploration of sleep disorders in the elderly: which particularities? *Geriatr Psychol Neuropsychiatr Vieil.* 2016;14:429–437.
74. Markota M, Rummans TA, Bostwick JM, Lapid MI. Benzodiazepine use in older adults: dangers, management, and alternative therapies. *Mayo Clin Proc.* 2016;91: 1632–1639.
75. Chua HC, Chebib M. GABA(A) receptors and the diversity in their structure and pharmacology. *Adv Pharmacol.* 2017;79: 1–34.
76. Airagnes G, Pelissolo A, Lavallée M, et al. Benzodiazepine misuse in the elderly: risk factors, consequences, and management. *Curr Psychiatry Rep.* 2016;18:89.
77. Billioti de Gage S, Pariente A, Bégaud B. Is there really a link between benzodiazepine use and the risk of dementia? *Expert Opin Drug Saf.* 2015;14:733–747.
78. Pariente A, de Gage SB, Moore N, Bégaud B. The benzodiazepine-dementia disorders link: current state of knowledge. *CNS Drugs.* 2016;30:1–7.

79. Burman D. Sleep disorders: insomnia. *FP Essent.* 2017;460:22–28.
80. Matheson E, Hainer BL. Insomnia: pharmacologic therapy. *Am Fam Physician.* 2017;96:29–35.
81. Pollmann AS, Murphy AL, Bergman JC, Gardner DM. Deprescribing benzodiazepines and Z-drugs in community-dwelling adults: a scoping review. *BMC Pharmacol Toxicol.* 2015;16:19.
82. Fitzgerald AC, Wright BT, Heldt SA. The behavioral pharmacology of zolpidem: evidence for the functional significance of α1-containing GABA(A) receptors. *Psychopharmacology.* 2014;231:1865–1896.
83. Wilt TJ, MacDonald R, Brasure M, et al. Pharmacologic treatment of insomnia disorder: an evidence report for a clinical practice guideline by the American College of Physicians. *Ann Intern Med.* 2016;165:103–112.
84. Liu J, Clough SJ, Hutchinson AJ, et al. MT1 and MT2 melatonin receptors: a therapeutic perspective. *Annu Rev Pharmacol Toxicol.* 2016;56:361–383.
85. Spadoni G, Bedini A, Lucarini S, et al. Pharmacokinetic and pharmacodynamic evaluation of ramelteon: an insomnia therapy. *Expert Opin Drug Metab Toxicol.* 2015;11: 1145–1156.
86. Cardinali DP, Golombek DA, Rosenstein RE, et al. Assessing the efficacy of melatonin to curtail benzodiazepine/Z drug abuse. *Pharmacol Res.* 2016;109:12–23.
87. Howland RH. Buspirone: back to the future. *J Psychosoc Nurs Ment Health Serv.* 2015;53:21–24.
88. Bandelow B, Michaelis S, Wedekind D. Treatment of anxiety disorders. *Dialogues Clin Neurosci.* 2017;19:93–107.
89. Driot D, Bismuth M, Maurel A, et al. Management of first depression or generalized anxiety disorder episode in adults in primary care: a systematic metareview. *Presse Med.* 2017;46(Pt 1):1124–1138.
90. Perna G, Alciati A, Riva A, et al. Long-term pharmacological treatments of anxiety disorders: an updated systematic review. *Curr Psychiatry Rep.* 2016;18:23.
91. Tham A, Jonsson U, Andersson G, et al. Efficacy and tolerability of antidepressants in people aged 65 years or older with major depressive disorder - a systematic review and a meta-analysis. *J Affect Disord.* 2016;205:1–12.
92. Björkholm C, Monteggia LM. BDNF - a key transducer of antidepressant effects. *Neuropharmacology.* 2016;102:72–79.
93. Castrén E, Kojima M. Brain-derived neurotrophic factor in mood disorders and antidepressant treatments. *Neurobiol Dis.* 2017;97(Pt B):119–126.
94. Leal G, Bramham CR, Duarte CB. BDNF and hippocampal synaptic plasticity. *Vitam Horm.* 2017;104:153–195.
95. Habert J, Katzman MA, Oluboka OJ, et al. Functional recovery in major depressive disorder: focus on early optimized treatment. *Prim Care Companion CNS Disord.* 2016;18:5.
96. Patel K, Abdool PS, Rajji TK, Mulsant BH. Pharmacotherapy of major depression in late life: what is the role of new agents? *Expert Opin Pharmacother.* 2017;18:599–609.
97. Carvalho AF, Sharma MS, Brunoni AR, et al. The safety, tolerability and risks associated with the use of newer generation antidepressant drugs: a critical review of the literature. *Psychother Psychosom.* 2016;85:270–288.
98. Andrade C, Sharma E. Serotonin reuptake inhibitors and risk of abnormal bleeding. *Psychiatr Clin North Am.* 2016;39: 413–426.
99. Sultana J, Spina E, Trifirò G. Antidepressant use in the elderly: the role of pharmacodynamics and pharmacokinetics in drug safety. *Expert Opin Drug Metab Toxicol.* 2015;11:883–892.
100. Taylor MJ, Freemantle N, Geddes JR, Bhagwagar Z. Early onset of selective serotonin reuptake inhibitor antidepressant action: systematic review and meta-analysis. *Arch Gen Psychiatry.* 2006;63:1217–1223.
101. Sani G, Perugi G, Tondo L. Treatment of bipolar disorder in a lifetime perspective: is lithium still the best choice? *Clin Drug Investig.* 2017;37:713–727.
102. Richardson T, Macaluso M. Clinically relevant treatment considerations regarding lithium use in bipolar disorder. *Expert Opin Drug Metab Toxicol.* 2017;13:1105–1113.
103. Oruch R, Elderbi MA, Khattab HA, et al. Lithium: a review of pharmacology, clinical uses, and toxicity. *Eur J Pharmacol.* 2014;740:464–473.
104. Baird-Gunning J, Lea-Henry T, Hoegberg LCG, et al. Lithium poisoning. *J Intensive Care Med.* 2017;32:249–263.
105. Aggarwal A, Schrimpf L, Lauriello J. Aripiprazole long-acting injectable for maintenance treatment of bipolar I disorder in adults. *Clin Schizophr Relat Psychoses.* 2018;11:221–223.
106. Gaebel W, Zielasek J. Focus on psychosis. *Dialogues Clin Neurosci.* 2015;17:9–18.
107. Morgan S. Psychotic and bipolar disorders: behavioral disorders in dementia. *FP Essent.* 2017;455:18–22.
108. Abi-Dargham A. Schizophrenia: overview and dopamine dysfunction. *J Clin Psychiatry.* 2014;75:e31.
109. Rao NP, Remington G. Targeting the dopamine receptor in schizophrenia: investigational drugs in Phase III trials. *Expert Opin Pharmacother.* 2014;15:373–383.
110. Amato D. Serotonin in antipsychotic drugs action. *Behav Brain Res.* 2015;277:125–135.
111. Kusumi I, Boku S, Takahashi Y. Psychopharmacology of atypical antipsychotic drugs: from the receptor binding profile to neuroprotection and neurogenesis. *Psychiatry Clin Neurosci.* 2015;69:243–258.
112. Holder SD, Edmunds AL, Morgan S. Psychotic and bipolar disorders: antipsychotic drugs. *FP Essent.* 2017;455:23–29.
113. Caroff SN, Campbell EC. Drug-induced extrapyramidal syndromes: implications for contemporary practice. *Psychiatr Clin North Am.* 2016;39:391–411.
114. Lanning RK, Zai CC, Müller DJ. Pharmacogenetics of tardive dyskinesia: an updated review of the literature. *Pharmacogenomics.* 2016;17:1339–1351.
115. Divac N, Prostran M, Jakovcevski I, Cerovac N. Second-generation antipsychotics and extrapyramidal adverse effects. *Biomed Res Int.* 2014;. 656370.
116. Correll CU, Kane JM, Citrome LL. Epidemiology, prevention, and assessment of tardive dyskinesia and advances in treatment. *J Clin Psychiatry.* 2017;78:1136–1147.
117. Orsolini L, Tomasetti C, Valchera A, et al. An update of safety of clinically used atypical antipsychotics. *Expert Opin Drug Saf.* 2016;15:1329–1347.
118. Kirkham J, Sherman C, Velkers C, et al. Antipsychotic use in dementia. *Can J Psychiatry.* 2017;62:170–181.
119. Thompson Coon J, Abbott R, Rogers M, et al. Interventions to reduce inappropriate prescribing of antipsychotic medications in people with dementia resident in care homes: a systematic review. *J Am Med Dir Assoc.* 2014;15:706–718.
120. Salzman C, Jeste DV, Meyer RE, et al. Elderly patients with dementia-related symptoms of severe agitation and aggression: consensus statement on treatment options, clinical trials methodology, and policy. *J Clin Psychiatry.* 2008;69:889–898.
121. Palm R, Jünger S, Reuther S, et al. People with dementia in nursing home research: a methodological review of the definition and identification of the study population. *BMC Geriatr.* 2016;16:78.
122. Day GS, Tang-Wai DF. When dementia progresses quickly: a practical approach to the diagnosis and management of rapidly progressive dementia. *Neurodegener Dis Manag.* 2014;4:41–56.

123. Khoury R, Patel K, Gold J, et al. Recent progress in the pharmacotherapy of Alzheimer's disease. *Drugs Aging.* 2017;34:811–820.
124. Deardorff WJ, Feen E, Grossberg GT. The use of cholinesterase inhibitors across all stages of Alzheimer's disease. *Drugs Aging.* 2015;32:537–547.
125. Mohammad D, Chan P, Bradley J, et al. Acetylcholinesterase inhibitors for treating dementia symptoms - a safety evaluation. *Expert Opin Drug Saf.* 2017;16:1009–1019.
126. Glynn-Servedio BE, Ranola TS. AChE inhibitors and NMDA receptor antagonists in advanced Alzheimer's disease. *Consult Pharm.* 2017;32:511–518.
127. Buckley JS, Salpeter SR. A risk-benefit assessment of dementia medications: systematic review of the evidence. *Drugs Aging.* 2015;32:453–467.
128. Wang R, Reddy PH. Role of glutamate and NMDA receptors in Alzheimer's disease. *J Alzheimers Dis.* 2017;57:1041–1048.
129. Zádori D, Veres G, Szalárdy L, et al. Glutamatergic dysfunctioning in Alzheimer's disease and related therapeutic targets. *J Alzheimers Dis.* 2014;42(Suppl 3): S177–S187.
130. Owen RT. Memantine and donepezil: a fixed drug combination for the treatment of moderate to severe Alzheimer's dementia. *Drugs Today.* 2016;52:239–248.
131. Amirrad F, Bousoik E, Shamloo K, et al. Alzheimer's disease: dawn of a new era? *J Pharm Pharm Sci.* 2017;20:184–225.
132. Kales HC, Gitlin LN, Lyketsos CG. Assessment and management of behavioral and psychological symptoms of dementia. *BMJ.* 2015;350:h369.
133. Porsteinsson AP, Antonsdottir IM. An update on the advancements in the treatment of agitation in Alzheimer's disease. *Expert Opin Pharmacother.* 2017;18:611–620.
134. Abraha I, Rimland JM, Trotta FM, et al. Systematic review of systematic reviews of non-pharmacological interventions to treat behavioural disturbances in older patients with dementia. The SENATOR-OnTop series. *BMJ Open.* 2017;7. e012759.
135. Fakhoury N, Wilhelm N, Sobota KF, Kroustos KR. Impact of music therapy on dementia behaviors: a literature review. *Consult Pharm.* 2017;32:623–628.
136. Millán-Calenti JC, Lorenzo-López L, Alonso-Búa B, et al. Optimal nonpharmacological management of agitation in Alzheimer's disease: challenges and solutions. *Clin Interv Aging.* 2016;11:175–184.
137. Ford AH. Neuropsychiatric aspects of dementia. *Maturitas.* 2014;79:209–215.
138. Tysnes OB, Storstein A. Epidemiology of Parkinson's disease. *J Neural Transm.* 2017;124:901–905.
139. Jagadeesan AJ, Murugesan R, Vimala Devi S, et al. Current trends in etiology, prognosis and therapeutic aspects of Parkinson's disease: a review. *Acta Biomed.* 2017;88: 249–262.
140. Kakkar AK, Dahiya N. Management of Parkinson's disease: current and future pharmacotherapy. *Eur J Pharmacol.* 2015;750:74–81.
141. Devos D, Moreau C, Dujardin K, et al. New pharmacological options for treating advanced Parkinson's disease. *Clin Ther.* 2013;35:1640–1652.
142. Aquino CC, Fox SH. Clinical spectrum of levodopa-induced complications. *Mov Disord.* 2015;30:80–89.
143. Voon V, Napier TC, Frank MJ, et al. Impulse control disorders and levodopa-induced dyskinesias in Parkinson's disease: an update. *Lancet Neurol.* 2017;16:238–250.
144. Ramirez-Zamora A, Molho E. Treatment of motor fluctuations in Parkinson's disease: recent developments and future directions. *Expert Rev Neurother.* 2014;14:93–103.
145. Reichmann H. Modern treatment in Parkinson's disease, a personal approach. *J Neural Transm.* 2016;123:73–80.
146. Marsili L, Marconi R, Colosimo C. Treatment strategies in early Parkinson's disease. *Int Rev Neurobiol.* 2017;132: 345–360.
147. Lindholm D, Mäkelä J, Di Liberto V, et al. Current disease modifying approaches to treat Parkinson's disease. *Cell Mol Life Sci.* 2016;73:1365–1379.
148. Jefferys JG. Are changes in synaptic function that underlie hyperexcitability responsible for seizure activity? *Adv Exp Med Biol.* 2014;813:185–194.
149. Born HA. Seizures in Alzheimer's disease. *Neuroscience.* 2015;286:251–263.
150. Wang JZ, Vyas MV, Saposnik G, Burneo JG. Incidence and management of seizures after ischemic stroke: systematic review and meta-analysis. *Neurology.* 2017;89: 1220–1228.
151. Liu G, Slater N, Perkins A. Epilepsy: treatment options. *Am Fam Physician.* 2017;96:87–96.
152. Brodie MJ. Tolerability and safety of commonly used antiepileptic drugs in adolescents and adults: a clinician's overview. *CNS Drugs.* 2017;31:135–147.
153. Motika PV, Spencer DC. Treatment of epilepsy in the elderly. *Curr Neurol Neurosci Rep.* 2016;16:96.
154. Horgas AL. Pain management in older adults. *Nurs Clin North Am.* 2017;52:e1–e7.
155. Stein C. Opioid Receptors. *Annu Rev Med.* 2016;67:433–451.
156. Chan HCS, McCarthy D, Li J, et al. Designing safer analgesics via μ-opioid receptor pathways. *Trends Pharmacol Sci.* 2017;38:1016–1037.
157. Harned M, Sloan P. Safety concerns with long-term opioid use. *Expert Opin Drug Saf.* 2016;15:955–962.
158. Ballantyne JC. Opioids for the treatment of chronic pain: mistakes made, lessons learned, and future directions. *Anesth Analg.* 2017;125:1769–1778.
159. Kumar K, Kirksey MA, Duong S, Wu CL. A review of opioid-sparing modalities in perioperative pain management: methods to decrease opioid use postoperatively. *Anesth Analg.* 2017;125:1749–1760.
160. Nicol AL, Hurley RW, Benzon HT. Alternatives to opioids in the pharmacologic management of chronic pain syndromes: a narrative review of randomized, controlled, and blinded clinical trials. *Anesth Analg.* 2017;125:1682–1703.
161. Candido KD, Perozo OJ, Knezevic NN. Pharmacology of acetaminophen, nonsteroidal antiinflammatory drugs, and steroid medications: implications for anesthesia or unique associated risks. *Anesthesiol Clin.* 2017;35:e145–e162.
162. Brouwers H, von Hegedus J, Toes R, et al. Lipid mediators of inflammation in rheumatoid arthritis and osteoarthritis. *Best Pract Res Clin Rheumatol.* 2015;29:741–755.
163. Rayar AM, Lagarde N, Ferroud C, et al. Update on COX-2 selective inhibitors: chemical classification, side effects and their use in cancers and neuronal diseases. *Curr Top Med Chem.* 2017;17:2935–2956.
164. Patrignani P, Patrono C. Cyclooxygenase inhibitors: from pharmacology to clinical read-outs. *Biochim Biophys Acta.* 2015;1851:422–432.
165. Patrono C. Cardiovascular effects of cyclooxygenase-2 inhibitors: a mechanistic and clinical perspective. *Br J Clin Pharmacol.* 2016;82:957–964.
166. Pereira-Leite C, Nunes C, Jamal SK, et al. Nonsteroidal anti-inflammatory therapy: a journey toward safety. *Med Res Rev.* 2017;37:802–859.
167. Tacconelli S, Bruno A, Grande R, et al. Nonsteroidal anti-inflammatory drugs and cardiovascular safety - translating pharmacological data into clinical readouts. *Expert Opin Drug Saf.* 2017;16:791–807.
168. Walker C, Biasucci LM. Cardiovascular safety of non-steroidal anti-inflammatory drugs revisited. *Postgrad Med.* 2018;130:55–71.

169. Patrono C. Cardiovascular effects of nonsteroidal anti-inflammatory drugs. *Curr Cardiol Rep*. 2016;18:25.
170. Ross SJ, Elgendy IY, Bavry AA. Cardiovascular safety and bleeding risk associated with nonsteroidal anti-inflammatory medications in patients with cardiovascular disease. *Curr Cardiol Rep*. 2017;19:8.
171. Giannoudis PV, Hak D, Sanders D, et al. Inflammation, bone healing, and anti-inflammatory drugs: an update. *J Orthop Trauma*. 2015;29(Suppl 12):S6–S9.
172. Marquez-Lara A, Hutchinson ID, Nuñez F, et al. Nonsteroidal anti-inflammatory drugs and bone-healing: a systematic review of research quality. *JBJS Rev*. 2016;4.
173. Ingawale DK, Mandlik SK, Patel SS. An emphasis on molecular mechanisms of anti-inflammatory effects and glucocorticoid resistance. *J Complement Integr Med*. 2015;12:1–13.
174. Petta I, Dejager L, Ballegeer M, et al. The interactome of the glucocorticoid receptor and its influence on the actions of glucocorticoids in combatting inflammatory and infectious diseases. *Microbiol Mol Biol Rev*. 2016;80:495–522.
175. Bodine SC, Furlow JD. Glucocorticoids and skeletal muscle. *Adv Exp Med Biol*. 2015;872:145–176.
176. Seibel MJ, Cooper MS, Zhou H. Glucocorticoid-induced osteoporosis: mechanisms, management, and future perspectives. *Lancet Diabetes Endocrinol*. 2013;1:59–70.
177. Biehl AJ, Katz JD. Pharmacotherapy pearls for the geriatrician: focus on oral disease-modifying antirheumatic drugs including newer agents. *Clin Geriatr Med*. 2017;33:1–15.
178. Smolen JS, Landewé R, Bijlsma J, et al. EULAR recommendations for the management of rheumatoid arthritis with synthetic and biological disease-modifying antirheumatic drugs: 2016 update. *Ann Rheum Dis*. 2017;76:960–977.
179. Ishchenko A, Lories RJ. Safety and efficacy of biological disease-modifying antirheumatic drugs in older rheumatoid arthritis patients: staying the distance. *Drugs Aging*. 2016;33:387–398.
180. Nam JL, Takase-Minegishi K, Ramiro S, et al. Efficacy of biological disease-modifying antirheumatic drugs: a systematic literature review informing the 2016 update of the EULAR recommendations for the management of rheumatoid arthritis. *Ann Rheum Dis*. 2017;76:1113–1136.
181. Wells AF, Curtis JR, Betts KA, et al. Systematic literature review and meta-analysis of tumor necrosis factor-alpha experienced rheumatoid arthritis. *Clin Ther*. 2017;39:1680–1694.
182. Negoescu A, Ostör AJ. Early recognition improves prognosis in elderly onset RA. *Practitioner*. 2014;258:11–14.
183. Zampeli E, Vlachoyiannopoulos PG, Tzioufas AG. Treatment of rheumatoid arthritis: unraveling the conundrum. *J Autoimmun*. 2015;65:1–18.
184. Hernández MV, Sanmartí R, Cañete JD. The safety of tumor necrosis factor-alpha inhibitors in the treatment of rheumatoid arthritis. *Expert Opin Drug Saf*. 2016;15:613–624.
185. Ramiro S, Sepriano A, Chatzidionysiou K, et al. Safety of synthetic and biological DMARDs: a systematic literature review informing the 2016 update of the EULAR recommendations for management of rheumatoid arthritis. *Ann Rheum Dis*. 2017;76:1101–1136.
186. Vashisht P, O'dell J. Not all TNF inhibitors in rheumatoid arthritis are created equal: important clinical differences. *Expert Opin Biol Ther*. 2017;17:989–999.
187. Kithas PA, Supiano MA. Hypertension in the geriatric population: a patient-centered approach. *Med Clin North Am*. 2015;99:379–389.
188. Chrysant SG. Aggressive systolic blood pressure control in older subjects: benefits and risks. *Postgrad Med*. 2018;130:159–165.
189. Garrison SR, Kolber MR, Korownyk CS, et al. Blood pressure targets for hypertension in older adults. *Cochrane Database Syst Rev*. 2017;(8):CD011575.
190. Jarraya F. Treatment of hypertension: which goal for which patient? *Adv Exp Med Biol*. 2017;956:117–127.
191. Aronow WS. Managing hypertension in the elderly: what is different, what is the same? *Curr Hypertens Rep*. 2017;19:67.
192. Ferdinand KC, Nasser SA. Management of essential hypertension. *Cardiol Clin*. 2017;35:231–246.
193. Mancia G, Rea F, Cuspidi C, et al. Blood pressure control in hypertension. Pros and cons of available treatment strategies. *J Hypertens*. 2017;35:225–233.
194. Sato N, Saijo Y, Sasagawa Y. CAMUI Investigators. Visit-to-visit variability and seasonal variation in blood pressure: Combination of Antihypertensive Therapy in the Elderly, Multicenter Investigation (CAMUI) Trial subanalysis. *Clin Exp Hypertens*. 2015;37:411–419.
195. Burnier M. Antihypertensive combination treatment: state of the art. *Curr Hypertens Rep*. 2015;17:51.
196. Yannoutsos A, Kheder-Elfekih R, Halimi JM, et al. Should blood pressure goal be individualized in hypertensive patients? *Pharmacol Res*. 2017;118:53–63.
197. Dharmarajan K, Rich MW. Epidemiology, pathophysiology, and prognosis of heart failure in older adults. *Heart Fail Clin*. 2017;13:417–426.
198. Chavey WE, Hogikyan RV, Van Harrison R, Nicklas JM. Heart failure due to reduced ejection fraction: medical management. *Am Fam Physician*. 2017;95:13–20.
199. Wojnowich K, Korabathina R. Heart failure update: outpatient management. *FP Essent*. 2016;442:18–25.
200. Albert CL, Kamdar F, Hanna M. Contemporary controversies in digoxin use in systolic heart failure. *Curr Heart Fail Rep*. 2016;13:197–206.
201. See I, Shehab N, Kegler SR, et al. Emergency department visits and hospitalizations for digoxin toxicity: United States, 2005 to 2010. *Circ Heart Fail*. 2014;7:28–34.
202. Lee HC, Tl Huang K, Shen WK. Use of antiarrhythmic drugs in elderly patients. *J Geriatr Cardiol*. 2011;8:184–194.
203. Desai Y, El-Chami MF, Leon AR, Merchant FM. Management of atrial fibrillation in elderly adults. *J Am Geriatr Soc*. 2017;65:185–193.
204. Jacobson JT, Iwai S, Aronow WS. Treatment of ventricular arrhythmias and use of implantable cardioverter-defibrillators to improve survival in older adult patients with cardiac disease. *Heart Fail Clin*. 2017;13:589–605.
205. Malhotra S, Das MK. Delayed and indirect effects of antiarrhythmic drugs in reducing sudden cardiac death. *Future Cardiol*. 2011;7:203–217.
206. Camm AJ. Hopes and disappointments with antiarrhythmic drugs. *Int J Cardiol*. 2017;237:71–74.
207. Kloner RA, Chaitman B. Angina and its management. *J Cardiovasc Pharmacol Ther*. 2017;22:199–209.
208. Boden WE, Padala SK, Cabral KP, et al. Role of short-acting nitroglycerin in the management of ischemic heart disease. *Drug Des Devel Ther*. 2015;9:4793–4805.
209. Thadani U. Challenges with nitrate therapy and nitrate tolerance: prevalence, prevention, and clinical relevance. *Am J Cardiovasc Drugs*. 2014;14:287–301.
210. Chong CR, Ong GJ, Horowitz JD. Emerging drugs for the treatment of angina pectoris. *Expert Opin Emerg Drugs*. 2016;21:365–376.
211. Hamilton-Craig I, Colquhoun D, Kostner K, et al. Lipid-modifying therapy in the elderly. *Vasc Health Risk Manag*. 2015;11:251–263.
212. Katsiki N, Kolovou G, Perez-Martinez P, Mikhailidis DP. Dyslipidaemia in the elderly: to treat or not to treat? *Expert Rev Clin Pharmacol*. 2018;11:259–278.

213. Anagnostis P, Paschou SA, Goulis DG, et al. Dietary management of dyslipidaemias. Is there any evidence for cardiovascular benefit? *Maturitas*. 2018;108:45–52.
214. Kazi DS, Penko JM, Bibbins-Domingo K. Statins for primary prevention of cardiovascular disease: review of evidence and recommendations for clinical practice. *Med Clin North Am*. 2017;101:689–699.
215. Oliveira EF, Santos-Martins D, Ribeiro AM, et al. HMG-CoA Reductase inhibitors: an updated review of patents of novel compounds and formulations (2011-2015). *Expert Opin Ther Pat*. 2016;26:1257–1272.
216. Bedi O, Dhawan V, Sharma PL, Kumar P. Pleiotropic effects of statins: new therapeutic targets in drug design. *Naunyn Schmiedebergs Arch Pharmacol*. 2016;389:695–712.
217. Fernandes V, Santos MJ, Pérez A. Statin-related myotoxicity. *Endocrinol Nutr*. 2016;63:239–249.
218. Thompson PD, Panza G, Zaleski A, Taylor B. Statin-associated side effects. *J Am Coll Cardiol*. 2016;67: 2395–2410.
219. Apostolopoulou M, Corsini A, Roden M. The role of mitochondria in statin-induced myopathy. *Eur J Clin Invest*. 2015;45:745–754.
220. Bochenek ML, Schütz E, Schäfer K. Endothelial cell senescence and thrombosis: ageing clots. *Thromb Res*. 2016;147:36–45.
221. Byrnes JR, Wolberg AS. New findings on venous thrombogenesis. *Hamostaseologie*. 2017;37:25–35.
222. Schlaudecker J, Becker R. Inflammatory response and thrombosis in older individuals. *Semin Thromb Hemost*. 2014;40:669–674.
223. Sepúlveda C, Palomo I, Fuentes E. Mechanisms of endothelial dysfunction during aging: predisposition to thrombosis. *Mech Ageing Dev*. 2017;164:91–99.
224. Boey JP, Gallus A. Drug treatment of venous thromboembolism in the elderly. *Drugs Aging*. 2016;33:475–490.
225. Harter K, Levine M, Henderson SO. Anticoagulation drug therapy: a review. *West J Emerg Med*. 2015;16:11–17.
226. Smith M, Wakam G, Wakefield T, Obi A. New trends in anticoagulation therapy. *Surg Clin North Am*. 2018;98: 219–238.
227. Weitz JI, Harenberg J. New developments in anticoagulants: past, present and future. *Thromb Haemost*. 2017;117: 1283–1288.
228. Brandao GM, Junqueira DR, Rollo HA, Sobreira ML. Pentasaccharides for the treatment of deep vein thrombosis. *Cochrane Database Syst Rev*. 2017;(12):CD011782.
229. Thakkar RN, Rathbun SW, Wright SM. Role of direct oral anticoagulants in the management of anticoagulation. *South Med J*. 2017;110:293–299.
230. Hellenbart EL, Faulkenberg KD, Finks SW. Evaluation of bleeding in patients receiving direct oral anticoagulants. *Vasc Health Risk Manag*. 2017;13:325–342.
231. Hur M, Park SK, Koo CH, et al. Comparative efficacy and safety of anticoagulants for prevention of venous thromboembolism after hip and knee arthroplasty. *Acta Orthop*. 2017;88:634–641.
232. Fragoso CA. Epidemiology of chronic obstructive pulmonary disease (COPD) in aging populations. *COPD*. 2016;13: 125–129.
233. Yawn BP, Han MK. Practical considerations for the diagnosis and management of asthma in older adults. *Mayo Clin Proc*. 2017;92:1697–1705.
234. Miravitlles M, Anzueto A, Jardim JR. Optimizing bronchodilation in the prevention of COPD exacerbations. *Respir Res*. 2017;18:125.
235. Castiglia D, Battaglia S, Benfante A, et al. Pharmacological management of elderly patients with asthma-chronic obstructive pulmonary disease overlap syndrome: room for speculation? *Drugs Aging*. 2016;33:375–385.
236. Melani AS. Management of asthma in the elderly patient. *Clin Interv Aging*. 2013;8:913–922.
237. Hajian B, De Backer J, Vos W, et al. Efficacy of inhaled medications in asthma and COPD related to disease severity. *Expert Opin Drug Deliv*. 2016;13:1719–1727.
238. Lexmond A, Forbes B. Drug delivery devices for inhaled medicines. *Handb Exp Pharmacol*. 2017;237:265–280.
239. Pasha MA, Sundquist B, Townley R. Asthma pathogenesis, diagnosis, and management in the elderly. *Allergy Asthma Proc*. 2017;38:184–191.
240. Vazquez Roque M, Bouras EP. Epidemiology and management of chronic constipation in elderly patients. *Clin Interv Aging*. 2015;10:919–930.
241. Serrano-Falcón B, Rey E. The safety of available treatments for chronic constipation. *Expert Opin Drug Saf*. 2017;16: 1243–1253.
242. Curtò L, Trimarchi F. Hypopituitarism in the elderly: a narrative review on clinical management of hypothalamic-pituitary-gonadal, hypothalamic-pituitary-thyroid and hypothalamic-pituitary-adrenal axes dysfunction. *J Endocrinol Invest*. 2016;39:1115–1124.
243. Jones CM, Boelaert K. The endocrinology of ageing: a mini-review. *Gerontology*. 2015;61:291–300.
244. Roberts H, Hickey M. Managing the menopause: an update. *Maturitas*. 2016;86:53–58.
245. Parish SJ, Gillespie JA. The evolving role of oral hormonal therapies and review of conjugated estrogens/bazedoxifene for the management of menopausal symptoms. *Postgrad Med*. 2017;129:340–351.
246. Boardman HM, Hartley L, Eisinga A, et al. Hormone therapy for preventing cardiovascular disease in post-menopausal women. *Cochrane Database Syst Rev*. 2015;(3):CD002229.
247. Henderson VW. Alzheimer's disease: review of hormone therapy trials and implications for treatment and prevention after menopause. *J Steroid Biochem Mol Biol*. 2014;142: 99–106.
248. Canonico M. Hormone therapy and risk of venous thromboembolism among postmenopausal women. *Maturitas*. 2015;82:304–307.
249. Kaunitz AM, Manson JE. Management of menopausal symptoms. *Obstet Gynecol*. 2015;126:859–876.
250. Santen RJ, Kagan R, Altomare CJ, et al. Current and evolving approaches to individualizing estrogen receptor-based therapy for menopausal women. *J Clin Endocrinol Metab*. 2014;99:733–747.
251. Mirkin S, Pickar JH. Selective estrogen receptor modulators (SERMs): a review of clinical data. *Maturitas*. 2015;80:52–57.
252. Corona G, Rastrelli G, Reisman Y, et al. The safety of available treatments of male hypogonadism in organic and functional hypogonadism. *Expert Opin Drug Saf*. 2018;17:277–292.
253. Sandher RK, Aning J. Diagnosing and managing androgen deficiency in men. *Practitioner*. 2017;261:19–22.
254. Kaplan AL, Hu JC, Morgentaler A, et al. Testosterone therapy in men with prostate cancer. *Eur Urol*. 2016;69: 894–903.
255. Traish A. Testosterone therapy in men with testosterone deficiency: are we beyond the point of no return? *Investig Clin Urol*. 2016;57:384–400.
256. Chrysant SG, Chrysant GS. Cardiovascular benefits and risks of testosterone replacement therapy in older men with low testosterone. *Hosp Pract*. 2018;46:47–55.
257. Lee PG, Halter JB. The pathophysiology of hyperglycemia in older adults: clinical considerations. *Diabetes Care*. 2017;40:444–452.
258. Mitrakou A, Katsiki N, Lalic NM. Type 2 diabetes mellitus and the elderly: an update on drugs used to treat glycaemia. *Curr Vasc Pharmacol*. 2017;15:19–29.

259. Dominguez LJ, Barbagallo M. The biology of the metabolic syndrome and aging. *Curr Opin Clin Nutr Metab Care.* 2016;19:5–11.
260. Ferriolli E, Pessanha FP, Marchesi JC. Diabetes and exercise in the elderly. *Med Sport Sci.* 2014;60:122–129.
261. Choby B. Diabetes update: new pharmacotherapy for type 2 diabetes. *FP Essent.* 2017;456:27–35.
262. Thrasher J. Pharmacologic management of type 2 diabetes mellitus: available therapies. *Am J Cardiol.* 2017;120:S4–S16.
263. Varghese S. Noninsulin diabetes medications. *Nurs Clin North Am.* 2017;52:523–537.
264. Davoren P. Glucose-lowering medicines for type 2 diabetes. *Aust Fam Physician.* 2015;44:176–179.
265. Hennessey JV, Espaillat R. Diagnosis and management of subclinical hypothyroidism in elderly adults: a review of the literature. *J Am Geriatr Soc.* 2015;63:1663–1673.
266. Tabatabaie V, Surks MI. The aging thyroid. *Curr Opin Endocrinol Diabetes Obes.* 2013;20:455–459.
267. Kravets I. Hyperthyroidism: diagnosis and treatment. *Am Fam Physician.* 2016;93:363–370.
268. Okosieme OE, Lazarus JH. Current trends in antithyroid drug treatment of Graves' disease. *Expert Opin Pharmacother.* 2016;17:2005–2017.
269. Walsh JP. Managing thyroid disease in general practice. *Med J Aust.* 2016;205:179–184.
270. Barber KE, Bell AM, Stover KR, Wagner JL. Intravenous vancomycin dosing in the elderly: a focus on clinical issues and practical application. *Drugs Aging.* 2016;33: 845–854.
271. Katz MJ, Roghmann MC. Healthcare-associated infections in the elderly: what's new. *Curr Opin Infect Dis.* 2016;29: 388–393.
272. Mitchell SL, Shaffer ML, Loeb MB, et al. Infection management and multidrug-resistant organisms in nursing home residents with advanced dementia. *JAMA Intern Med.* 2014;174:1660–1667.
273. Saab S, Rheem J, Sundaram V. Hepatitis C infection in the elderly. *Dig Dis Sci.* 2015;60:3170–3180.
274. Vespasiani-Gentilucci U, Galati G, Gallo P, et al. Hepatitis C treatment in the elderly: new possibilities and controversies towards interferon-free regimens. *World J Gastroenterol.* 2015;21:7412–7426.
275. Uyeki TM. Influenza. *Ann Intern Med.* 2017;167: ITC33–ITC48.
276. Li D, Soto-Perez-de-Celis E, Hurria A. Geriatric assessment and tools for predicting treatment toxicity in older adults with cancer. *Cancer J.* 2017;23:206–210.
277. Krug U, Gale RP, Berdel WE, et al. Therapy of older persons with acute myeloid leukaemia. *Leuk Res.* 2017;60:1–10.
278. Thomas X. The management and treatment of acute leukemias in the elderly population. *Expert Rev Hematol.* 2017;10:975–985.
279. Rycenga HB, Long DT. The evolving role of DNA inter-strand crosslinks in chemotherapy. *Curr Opin Pharmacol.* 2018;41: 20–26.
280. van Vuuren RJ, Visagie MH, Theron AE, Joubert AM. Antimitotic drugs in the treatment of cancer. *Cancer Chemother Pharmacol.* 2015;76:1101–1112.
281. Kanesvaran R, Roy Chowdhury A, Krishna L. Practice pearls in the management of lung cancer in the elderly. *J Geriatr Oncol.* 2016;7:362–367.
282. Tapia Rico G, Townsend AR, Broadbridge V, Price TJ. Targeted therapies in elderly patients with metastatic colorectal cancer: a review of the evidence. *Drugs Aging.* 2017;34:173–189.
283. Wellstein A. General principles in the pharmacotherapy of cancer. In: Brunton LL, Hilal-Dandan R, Knollmann BC, eds. *The Pharmacological Basis of Therapeutics.* 13th ed. New York: McGraw-Hill; 2018.
284. Accordino MK, Neugut AI, Hershman DL. Cardiac effects of anticancer therapy in the elderly. *J Clin Oncol.* 2014;32. 2654-2561.
285. Staff NP, Grisold A, Grisold W, Windebank AJ. Chemotherapy-induced peripheral neuropathy: a current review. *Ann Neurol.* 2017;81:772–781.
286. Abraham N, Goldman HB. An update on the pharmacotherapy for lower urinary tract dysfunction. *Expert Opin Pharmacother.* 2015;16:79–93.
287. Khandelwal C, Kistler C. Diagnosis of urinary incontinence. *Am Fam Physician.* 2013;87:543–550.
288. Parker WP, Griebling TL. Nonsurgical treatment of urinary incontinence in elderly women. *Clin Geriatr Med.* 2015;31: 471–485.
289. Orme S, Morris V, Gibson W, Wagg A. Managing urinary incontinence in patients with dementia: pharmacological treatment options and considerations. *Drugs Aging.* 2015;32:559–567.
290. Samuelsson E, Odeberg J, Stenzelius K, et al. Effect of pharmacological treatment for urinary incontinence in the elderly and frail elderly: a systematic review. *Geriatr Gerontol Int.* 2015;15:521–534.
291. Thiagamoorthy G, Cardozo L, Robinson D. Current and future pharmacotherapy for treating overactive bladder. *Expert Opin Pharmacother.* 2016;17:1317–1325.
292. Wu T, Duan X, Cao CX, et al. The role of mirabegron in overactive bladder: a systematic review and meta-analysis. *Urol Int.* 2014;93:326–337.
293. Faubion SS, Sood R, Kapoor E. Genitourinary syndrome of menopause: management strategies for the clinician. *Mayo Clin Proc.* 2017;92:1842–1849.
294. Tzur T, Yohai D, Weintraub AY. The role of local estrogen therapy in the management of pelvic floor disorders. *Climacteric.* 2016;19:162–171.
295. Malallah MA, Al-Shaiji TF. Pharmacological treatment of pure stress urinary incontinence: a narrative review. *Int Urogynecol J.* 2015;26:477–485.
296. Drake MJ, Nitti VW, Ginsberg DA, et al. Comparative assessment of the efficacy of onabotulinumtoxinA and oral therapies (anticholinergics and mirabegron) for overactive bladder: a systematic review and network meta-analysis. *BJU Int.* 2017;120:611–622.
297. Jhang JF, Kuo HC. Botulinum toxin A and lower urinary tract dysfunction: pathophysiology and mechanisms of action. *Toxins.* 2016;8:120.
298. Olivera CK, Meriwether K, El-Nashar S, et al. Nonantimuscarinic treatment for overactive bladder: a systematic review. *Am J Obstet Gynecol.* 2016;215:34–57.
299. Alavi K, Chan S, Wise P, et al. Fecal incontinence: etiology, diagnosis, and management. *J Gastrointest Surg.* 2015;19: 1910–1921.
300. Omar MI, Alexander CE. Drug treatment for faecal incontinence in adults. *Cochrane Database Syst Rev.* 2013;. CD002116.
301. Buswell M, Goodman C, Roe B, et al. What works to improve and manage fecal incontinence in care home residents living with dementia? A realist synthesis of the evidence. *J Am Med Dir Assoc.* 2017;18:752–760.

CHAPTER

7

Functional Performance Measures and Assessment for Older Adults

Dale Avers

"Many would say the quality of life in later years depends to a large degree on being able to continue to do what you want, without pain, for as long as possible."

Jones CJ & Rikli RE 2002

OUTLINE

INTRODUCTION

Function is a major focus of physical therapist assessment and intervention. Traditionally, therapists have assessed function through observation of the individual's performance, making a subjective assessment of the quantity, quality, and outcome of the functional movement or task. The use of performance measures has been driven by evidence-based practice and globalization, in particular the universal perspective of health, known as the World Health Organization's International Classification of Functioning, Disability, and Health (ICF). Measuring

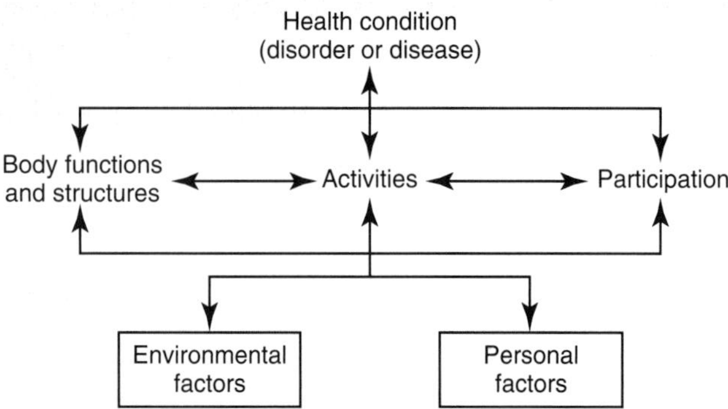

FIG. 7.1 World Health Organization's International Classification of Functioning, Disability, and Health (ICF) model. *(From the World Health Organization. International Classification of Functioning, Disability, and Health: ICF. Geneva, Switzerland: World Health Organization; 2001:18.)*

health and disability through the framework of the ICF model (Fig. 7.1) requires valid and reliable measures of both function and quality of life.[1]

Physical therapist interventions focus on functional deficits and the related impairments. Function is measured through performance testing. Although some might suggest that treating function as a whole is sufficient, others believe that analyzing the functional deficit or problem is necessary to identify the most relevant impairments to drive interventions. The latter would require the skills of a physical therapist; the former, perhaps not. This synthesis of information from physical performance testing is referred to as functional performance testing.[2] Functional performance testing captures the multiple dimensions of function described by the ICF model. Disability is defined as the inability to complete the tasks necessary for one's life role. Disability is the consequence of altered functional and impairment ability. Objectively testing the impairment and functional levels of an individual is the focus of this chapter.

Observing the performance of an older individual is one of the first elements in any examination by a geriatric physical therapist. This observation reveals the willingness and ability to move, quality of movement, safety and judgment issues, and effort. Additionally, observation is important because older adults are known to overestimate their abilities to do tasks, especially tasks they have modified or do infrequently. Thus, self-report measures, discussed later, may overestimate a person's abilities. Observation also reveals when and how task modifications are made and the significance of eliminating task modifications. For example, Marko et al. found that the presence of task modifications during performance strongly predicted future mobility disability.[3] Individuals who modified tasks exhibited less strength, and this strength deficit directly related to task modification.

PURPOSES OF MEASURING FUNCTIONAL PERFORMANCE

Functional performance measures (FPMs) serve many purposes and advantages across the patient care model, which are briefly described next.

Objective, Accurate Record. Functional performance measures are recorded using measurement scales, most often in ordinal or ratio measures, which can be more objective than qualitative words such as fair, good, or excellent. Reliable and valid FPMs have gone through rigorous scientific analysis for objectivity to help eliminate examiner bias and subjectivity. FPMs can provide feedback at regular intervals, providing an objective record of the individual's longitudinal performance.

Measures What is Important to the Individual. Individuals are interested in meaningful changes in task performance, rather than changes of specific impairments. FPMs can be used to measure a specific outcome the patient desires, thus giving accurate feedback on an important outcome.

Informs Impairments. Although impairments may not be as meaningful to the patient as functional performance, impairments are important to physical therapists as they can provide a gateway to improving functional performance. A task analysis of a specific performance, such as stair climbing, will help identify problematic areas (e.g., knee flexion or hip stability) that become the impairments to address in a therapeutic session. To maximize effectiveness, the therapist should specifically address only those impairments affecting the functional task, rather than taking a random approach to any impairment identified because multiple impairments are common in older adults.

Informs Goal Setting. Patient-centered goal setting is key to optimal therapy outcomes.[4] As mentioned earlier, FPMs can provide feedback about what is meaningful to the patient, which then can be used to measure a relevant and meaningful goal. For example, a patient may have the desire to walk quickly enough to keep up with his wife. Gait speed becomes the FPM to assess achievement of the specific goal equal to the patient's wife's gait speed. Similarly, a patient may offer a vague goal of "I want to return home," which can be further explored to identify specific functional tasks required to go home, such as stair climbing or moving through a narrow doorway. Goals using FPMs that are irrelevant to the patient will not provide meaningful feedback. For example, an FPM goal of improving gait speed by 0.10 m/s is not going to be relevant to the patient unless written in patient-specific terms.

Comparison with Age-based Normative Data. An advantage of FPMs in older age groups is the many collections of normative data that exist. This data can be used to compare an individual's performance to other similarly aged individuals, which may help identify those at risk of decline and those who are highly fit. For example, a 78-year-old woman may be able to perform seven sit to stands in 30 seconds. In determining the significance of her performance, the therapist can compare her performance against a normative data set such as the Senior Fitness Test.[5] From those norms, seven sit to stands is in the fifth percentile for women her age. Sharing quantitative data with the patient, without commentary from the therapist, can be a motivating factor for many individuals and may lead to improved performance.[6] Where community standards of functional tasks are available (e.g., gait speed), an individual's performance can be compared with the standard. For example, 1.2 m/s is the walking speed required to cross many streets.[7,8] Therefore, if the individual has a goal of walking to the library that necessitates crossing a street, achieving a walking speed of 1.2 m/s may be important and necessary. A patient-centered goal could then be written thusly: "Patient to achieve a community walking speed of 1.2 m/s required to cross a street near the patient's home to enable the patient to walk to the library."

Prognostic. Much research has been performed on prognostic indicators of FPMs. For example, walking speed is considered the most robust predictor of adverse health events such as mobility disability and hospitalization.[9] Diagnostic accuracy, a type of validity, is an indicator of the value of the prognostic ability of the FPM and should be considered before making decisions based on the outcome of a specific tool. This is particularly relevant when using an FPM to determine fall risk, which is discussed later in this chapter.

RELATIONSHIP BETWEEN FUNCTION AND IMPAIRMENTS

The direct relationship between function/activities and impairments (body functions/structures) influences activity (function) and participation[2] as illustrated by the ICF model (Fig. 7.1). For example, Puthoff and Nielsen[10] determined that lower extremity power and strength were related to lower extremity function such as climbing stairs. Therefore, task analysis is invaluable in addressing functional performance to note adaptations that are used to accomplish the tasks. Some of these adaptations are clever and useful, whereas some may be maladaptive and indicative of impending mobility disability. For example, the older adult who swings his jacket over his head to avoid painful or limited shoulder range may be satisfied with the task performance and not feel the need to address his shoulder issues. However, the older adult who is unable to get off the floor and limits mobility to avoid this task may require further assessment because of the consequences of self-limiting activity.

Strength testing of specific muscles (manual muscle testing) is a fundamental skill to physical therapists. However, as summarized in Box 7.1, muscle testing has major limitations, especially in lower extremity testing. Knowing these limitations will prevent the therapist from incorrectly grading strength as adequate in the presence of functional performance deficits. For example, the standing heel-raise test was developed because of the inherent strength of the gastrocnemius–soleus group.[11] When an older adult cannot lift the body weight on a single leg, the therapist should recognize the implications of this grade 2 (poor) performance[12] as insufficient strength to

BOX 7.1 Limitations of Manual Muscle Testing for Strength Assessment in Older Adults

1. Grade 5 (excellent) encompasses a wide range of dynamometer values leading to overestimation (ceiling effect) of available strength.*
2. Make test allows patient to determine how much resistance the therapist provides, leading to inaccurate assessment of available strength.
3. Break test can seem aggressive, especially when testing frail individuals, causing the tester to not elicit a maximum contraction, leading to an overestimation or underestimation of available strength.
4. Subjective term of "good" can bias the testing therapist toward an assessment of satisfactory strength, especially when functional performance testing is not done.
5. Patient's lassitude, ability to understand directions, range-of-motion limitations, willingness or ability to generate a maximum contraction, presence of pain, and/or fear may affect the ability to generate full effort, leading to an underestimation of available strength.
6. Muscle test positions may not reflect the way a muscle is used in functional performance (e.g., open-chain muscle testing position of the quad is not reflective of a closed-chain position of ambulation, transfers, or stair climbing).

(Modified from Avers D, Brown M. *Daniels and Worthingham's Muscle Testing.* 10th ed. St. Louis: Elsevier; 2019.)

*Bohannon RW, Corrigan D. A broad range of forces is encompassed by the maximum manual muscle test grade of five. *Percept Mot Ski.* 2000; 90(3 Pt 1):747–750.

push off during gait resulting in an adapted flat-footed stride with associated slowing of gait speed.[13] Similarly, the person who tests the quadriceps as a grade 4 (good) on a manual muscle test will be unlikely to rise from a chair without using the arms.[14,15] Evaluating strength accurately is important in light of the loss of muscle strength and power with aging.[16] Therefore, in light of the age-related loss of strength and prevalence of sedentary behavior, assessing an 80-year-old's initial strength as "normal" (5/5) or even "good" (4/5) should be considered the exception, rather than the norm. In light of the limitation of manual muscle testing, functional performance testing becomes an alternative and accurate way of measuring strength and performance, especially for the lower extremity. In fact, the timed sit-to-stand test is known to be a surrogate for lower limb strength.[17,18]

Impairments are typically anatomical (e.g., sensation), physiological (e.g., vital signs), or cognitive (e.g., Stroop test) abnormalities. Current practice reflects a shift from a focus on impairments to a focus on function as there is little evidence to support functional improvement through interventions focused on impairments. If, through an analysis of function performance, it is determined that an impairment should be addressed to improve the functional performance, several objective and reliable tests can be used. For example, leg press norms are established for groups aged 60 and over.[19]

TYPES OF FUNCTIONAL OUTCOME MEASURES

Self-Report

Self-report measures, also known as patient-reported outcomes, are common means of collecting the patient's perception of his or her impairments, function/activities, and even quality of life. They are often preferred owing to time, cost, and ease of administration. For example, a patient can complete a self-report measure while waiting to see the therapist. Self-report measures are valuable in defining the patient's perspective of change but are known to be affected by pain and may not relate to actual performance.[2] For example, a patient's perception of decreased pain following knee arthroplasty does not predict functional performance, which is often found to be worse following surgery.[20] In fact, functional performance is often inflated in the presence of decreased pain.[2] The numerical pain analog scale is a popular example of a self-assessment at the impairment level. The Short Form-36 is an example of a self-report assessment at the function/activities and participation level.[21]

Older individuals were more likely to self-report lower performance than the younger age category.[22] But even with lower self-reported performance, one study showed that of the majority of women who self-reported maximum scores on function, only 7% achieved maximum scores when assessed by the Physical Performance Test and only 30% achieved a maximum score for walking speed.[23] These results indicate that self-report measures of physical ability may not capture preclinical disability as self-report measures capture an individual's *perception* of ability rather than actual ability. The authors suggest that inquiring about whether task modifications were made reveals more information than asking whether the task can be accomplished at all. Self-report of functional performance can be influenced by the perceived effort involved in performing the task, as demonstrated by the underreporting of women who were overweight (body mass index [BMI] = 33.0), used an assistive device, and had multiple chronic conditions.

Patient Outcome Measures

Patient outcome measures are those questionnaires such as the Center for Epidemiological Studies Depression Scale (CES-D), Knee Injury and Osteoarthritis Outcome Score (KOOS), and Disabilities of the Arm, Shoulder, and Hand Questionnaire (DASH) that ask the patient about the impact of a condition on specific activities and roles in life. Although this chapter is focused on functional performance measures, patient outcome measures are useful to ascertain the patient's perception of the impact of a condition on specific activities and social roles. Table 7.1 lists outcome measures relevant to the older adult that are freely available from the Internet.

TABLE 7.1 Patient-Reported Outcome Measures

Name of Tool	Purpose
Physical Activity Scale for the Elderly (PASE)	Physical activity levels
Center for Epidemiological Studies Depression Scale (CES-D)	Depression
Sickness Impact Profile	Behavior, social relationships
Disabilities of the Arm, Shoulder, and Hand Questionnaire (DASH)	Shoulder impairment impact
Knee Injury and Osteoarthritis Outcome Score (KOOS)	Impact of knee impairment
Pelvic Floor Distress Inventory-20	Impact of incontinence
Dizziness Handicap Inventory	Impact of balance and vestibular concerns
Oswestry Disability Index	Impact of back pain
Pelvic Floor Impact Questionnaire	Impact of incontinence
Outcome Expectations for Exercise Scale	Assesses the outlook of older adults on the benefits of exercise
History of Falls Questionnaire	Assesses the circumstances surrounding a fall
Modified Gait Efficacy Scale	Addresses the older adult's perception of level of confidence in walking during challenging circumstances
Self-Efficacy for Exercise Scale	Assesses factors that influence adherence to a walking program for older adults
Short Form 12-item Health Survey (SF-12)	Generic assessment of health-related quality of life
Vestibular Disorders Activities of Daily Living Scale	Impact of vestibular impairment
Western Ontario and McMaster Universities Osteoarthritis Index (WOMAC)	Impact of pain, stiffness, and function from osteoarthritis of the hip or knee
Patient-Specific Functional Scale	Perception of ability to complete individualized specific activities to which goals are derived
Falls Efficacy Scale	Perception of balance and stability during activities of daily living and fear of falling
Geriatric Depression Scale (GDS)	Assesses depression and suicidal ideation in older adults
Stroke Impact Scale	Impact of stroke on health status
Activities-Specific Balance Confidence Scale (ABC)	Balance confidence in performing various activities
Functional Assessment of Chronic Illness – Fatigue (FACIT)	Assesses impact of fatigue on functional activities

Measures are freely available on the web.

Observer-Rated Measures

Observer measures, true to their title, are those measures that are observed, usually by the clinician, and usually physical in nature. Physical performance measures may be measures of impairments (e.g., range of motion or muscle strength), movement quality, or the ability to perform particular tasks.[24] Observer-rated measures may be subjective (personal judgment involved such as when observing edema or pain) or more objective by using time and/or quality of performance according to an ordinal or ratio rubric. No performance-based tool can be totally objective, but minimizing the clinician's subjective judgment as much as is possible is ideal. The clinician should be aware of influences on performance such as motivation and the ability to understand instructions to name a few.[24]

Physiological Measures

Measures of single biological entities such as cognitive ability and rate of perceived exertion or pain are referred to as physiological measures. The Mini-Mental Cognitive Index, St. Louis University Mental Status Examination (SLUMS),[25] and pain analog scale are examples of physiological measures. These measures are not traditionally thought of as functional performance measures, however, and are discussed throughout the text in relevant chapters.

SELECTION OF FUNCTIONAL PERFORMANCE MEASURES

The geriatric physical therapist has a plethora of measurement tools to select from. However, all measurement tools have different characteristics that affect the applicability of the results. The next section describes several characteristics of physical performance measurement tools that should be considered when selecting a specific tool. Only those tests that are freely available and have known reliability and validity are included in this chapter. Additionally, an effort is made to choose tests with known normative data to better interpret the test.

Safety

First and foremost, a performance-based measurement tool must be safe for the patient. For example, a patient who cannot safely walk without a contact guard should not be asked to perform tests that require independence in performance, such as balance tests. The clinician should be aware of the influence of physical touch and even close guarding on the patient's confidence and performance, and recognize that the objective of the performance test is to observe the patient's *actual* performance under realistic conditions. Safety is a clinical judgment issue.

Validity and Reliability

To be worthwhile, the measurement must be reliable and valid. Reliability is the extent to which a measurement is consistent and free from error. Validity assures the user that the test is measuring what it purports to measure. There are several types of validity, and the reader is encouraged to review these types. Definitions are provided in Box 7.2.[26] The tests included in this chapter have known validity and reliability.

Diagnostic Accuracy

Diagnostic accuracy is indicated by values of sensitivity (Sn) and specificity (Sp). Sn and Sp are used to calculate likelihood ratios that will inform the probability of the outcome of the test occurring. Likelihood ratios are calculated from the pretest probability (PrTP), combined with the result of the test, and the use of a nomogram to determine the posttest probability (PoTP). Likelihood values and their meaning are provided in Table 7.2. Many functional performance tests have insufficient diagnostic accuracy to change the clinician's pretest probability. Tests with insufficient diagnostic accuracy may not inform the probability but may provide other qualitative information, such as amount of sway, speed, and confidence.

Determining fall risk is a popular focus of many of the FPMs used by physical therapy clinicians. However, few individual measures have sufficient diagnostic accuracy to be used as a single measure to determine fall risk.[27,28] The multifactorial basis of balance and falls may account for this poor diagnostic accuracy of a single tool. Administering two tools that balance the values of Sn and Sp (e.g., the Berg Balance Scale and Timed Up and Go test) may improve the diagnostic accuracy.[28]Box 7.3 summarizes an extensive review by Lusardi et al. that evaluated the diagnostic accuracy of tools used to measure fall risk based on a pretest probability of 30% (incidence of falls from literature).[27] The authors found that of 56 measures evaluated, 5 medical history questions, 2-self-report measures, and 5 FPMs had sufficiently high-quality evidence to be considered. Fig. 7.2 lists the clinical indicators found to best predict the risk of one or more falls based on a 30% pretest probability.[27] When there is insufficient diagnostic accuracy of a test to be used individually to determine fall risk, values of diagnostic accuracy are not provided.

Floor and Ceiling Effects

For an FPM to demonstrate true change (responsiveness), it must reflect a range of tasks with increasing difficulty. An FPM is considered to have a floor effect when most of the subjects tested were at the lower end of the scale, indicating the FPM did not reflect a range of the lowest abilities.

A ceiling effect is exhibited when an FPM does not have a range of tasks that are challenging enough, and many individuals attain a maximum score. The Berg Balance Scale (BBS) is an example of a test with a ceiling effect

BOX 7.2 Definitions of Clinimetric Properties of Functional Performance Measures

Property	Definition
Validity	The degree to which a test tests what it purports to test. There are many kinds of validity including content, construct, concurrent, criterion, convergent, and predictive.
Intrarater reliability	Stability of data by one individual across two or more trials
Test–retest reliability	Consistency of the measure with repeated test administrations
Relative reliability	Measured by the intraclass correlation coefficient (ICC)
Floor and ceiling effects	The number of respondents who achieved the lowest or highest possible score
Minimal detectable change (MDC)	The amount of change that must be detected to demonstrate a true difference; the smallest amount of difference that passes the threshold of error with a 90% or 95% confidence interval. This is also known as absolute reliability and is computed from the standard error of measurement (SEM), which quantifies measurement error in the same units as the original measurement. It is also referred to as minimal detectable difference (MDD). It can be considered a conservative estimate of a patient's progress, identifying the smallest amount of change that could be considered as any improvement
Responsiveness	Ability to detect minimal change over time
Minimal clinically important difference (MCID)	Smallest difference in a measured variable that signifies an important rather than trivial difference in the patient's condition. It is also defined as the smallest difference *a patient* would perceive as beneficial.
Sensitivity (Sn)	Ability of the test to obtain a positive test when the target condition is really present, or a true-positive rate. A value of the proportion of individuals who test positive and actually have the condition. A test with high Sn is a good screening test as it captures more people with the condition. A negative test with high Sn would rule out the condition (SnNout).
Specificity (Sp)	Ability of the test to obtain a negative test when the condition is really absent, or the true-negative rate. A value of the proportion of individuals who test negative for the condition out of all those who are truly normal, i.e., do not have the target condition. A positive outcome for a test with high specificity rules in the diagnosis (SpPin).
Positive likelihood ratio	Utilizes Sn and Sp to calculate a value of how many times more likely a positive test will be seen in those with the disorder than those without the disorder. A good test will have a very high likelihood ratio.
Negative likelihood ratio	Utilizes Sn and Sp to calculate a value of how many times more likely a negative test will be seen in those with the disorder than in those without the disorder. A good test will have a very low likelihood ratio.
Pretest probability	A clinician's estimate and judgment of how likely a condition is present. Can be formed from epidemiology data (e.g., frequency of falls in older adults) or from clinical judgment (e.g., presentation of imbalance and need for assistance with walking indicating fall risk)
Posttest probability	Revised pretest probability based on the outcome of a test

TABLE 7.2 Likelihood Ratio Interpretation

(+) Likelihood Ratio (+LR)	(−) Likelihood Ratio (−LR)	Probability Interpretation
>10	<0.1	Generates large and often conclusive shifts in probability
5–10	0.1–0.2	Generates moderate shifts in probability
2–5	0.2–0.5	Generates small, but sometimes important, shifts in probability
1–2	0.5–1	Alters probability to a small, and rarely important, degree

when used to assess high-functioning individuals, as it tests relatively low-challenge balance skills. More challenging tasks such as jumping, walking, and turning one's head would be needed to assess balance at these higher challenge levels. The choice of the appropriate test is made with consideration of floor and ceiling effects to obtain the most accurate picture of relevant function. Some tests are more appropriate for lower-functioning individuals (e.g., Postural Assessment of Stroke Scale [PASS] or BBS), whereas others (e.g., Fullerton Activities Balance [FAB] test and Community Balance and Mobility Scale) are more appropriate for higher-functioning individuals. Walking speed, in part because of its ratio measure, does not exhibit floor or ceiling effects.

Relevance

Relevance to the patient is an important characteristic of a performance tool. Relevance enhances patient buy-in and therefore will affect performance. Generally, patients are more concerned with functional performance, rather than impairments such as strength, so identifying performance tests that require outcomes important to the patient can be important.

Sequence of Tests

The sequence of tests can determine success or failure in testing. Generally, the least fatiguing tests are performed first and those tests that require greater amounts of

BOX 7.3 Diagnostic Accuracy of Functional Performance Measures to Determine Fall Risk

Lusardi et al.[27] recommend that an effective screening strategy should combine the answers to the medical history questions (cited below) with the ability to maintain the single-leg stance (SLS) for at least 6.5 s and to walk at a speed of at least 1.0 m/s. The authors also found:

- No medical history questions achieved both high sensitivity (Sn) and specificity (Sp) for fall risk, with questions typically being more specific than sensitive. The questions about previous falls, use of psychoactive medications, need for assistance with activities of daily living, a yes response to the question "Are you concerned that you might fall?" and routine use of a cane or walker all increase the probability of falling.
- No single self-report measure is a strong predictor of falls.
- Performance-based measures generally have higher specificity than sensitivity, indicating greater usefulness for ruling in the risk of future falls than ruling them out.
- The Berg Balance Scale (BBS) increased posttest probability (PoTP) more than any other performance measure. A cut score of 50 points provides a PoTP of 59% for those who score 50 or less (a positive test).
- The single-task Timed Up and Go (TUG) at 12 seconds or more provides a PoTP of 47% (positive test).
- SLS with a score of <6.5 s (positive test) yielded a PoTP of 45%.
- Five Times Sit to Stand with a score of 12 s or more (positive test) yielded a PoTP of 41%.
- Performance-Oriented Mobility Assessment (POMA) with a score of <25 points (out of 28) (positive test) yielded a PoTP of 42%.
- The BBS is more useful than the POMA in determining risk of future falls.
- Self-selected walking speed (SSWS) <1.0 m/s (positive test) resulted in a PoTP of 39%. A cut score of 0.6 m/s yielded a PoTP of 61%.
- Combining tests increases PoTP. For example, the following test results increased the PoTP to 80%:
  - SLS (<6.5 s) (PoTP = 45%) with SSWS (<1.0 m/s) yielded a cumulative PoTP of 55%, adding the history question of previous falls increased the cumulative PoTP to 69%, adding the self-reported fear of falling increased the cumulative PoTP to 76%, and adding the routine use an assistive device created a total cumulative PoTP of 80%, which presented a more accurate picture of fall risk.

Category	Measure	Cut Point	+LR	−LR	PoTP, % If +Test	PoTP, % If −Test
Medical history questions	Any previous falls	Yes/no	1.8	0.8	44	26
	Psychoactive medication	Yes/no	1.4	0.8	38	26
	Requiring any ADL assistance	Yes/no	1.4	0.8	38	26
	Self-report fear of falling	Yes/no	1.4	0.9	38	28
	Ambulatory assistive device use	Yes/no	1.3	0.9	36	26
Self-report measures	Geriatric Depression Scale-15	<6 points	1.9	0.9	45	28
	Falls Efficacy Scale International	>24 points	1.7	0.6	42	20
Performance-based functional measures	Berg Balance Scale	<50 points	3.4	0.7	59	23
	Timed Up and Go Test	>11 s	2.1	0.8	47	25
	Single-limb stance eyes open	<6.5 s	1.9	0.9	45	28
	Five Times Sit-to-Stand Test	>12 s	1.6	0.7	41	20
	Self-selected walking speed	<1.0 m/s	1.5	0.6	39	20

Abbreviations: +LR, positive likelihood ratio; −LR, negative likelihood ratio; PoTP, posttest probability; PrTP, pretest probability; ADL, activities of daily living; +, test positive test result; −, test negative test result. [a]To the extent that tests are independent (unrelated) the PoTP of 1 positive test can be used as a new PrTP for the next positive test, etc., to develop a cumulative individualized risk estimate. Because the degree of relationship among tests is not clearly understood at this time, this strategy may inflate the cumulative risk estimate. Online resources such as www.easycalculation.com/statistics/post-test-probability.php can assist clinicians in quickly determining cumulative PoTP risk values.

FIG. 7.2 Summary of useful clinical indicators of risk of one or more future falls based on pretest probability of 30%. *(From Lusardi MM, Fritz S, Middleton A, et al. Determining risk of falls in community dwelling older adults. J Geriatr Phys Ther. 2017;40[1]:1–36. https://doi.org/10.1519/JPT.0000000000000099.)*

exertion last. For example, gait speed or the TUG might be done first, with a timed sit to stand or floor transfer done last. Endurance testing preceding tests requiring strength appears to significantly decrease strength test scores.[29] However, if the individual has a high fatigue level (tires easily and quickly), the test that will yield the most information might be administered first. Subsequent tests may be administered after sufficient rest or in subsequent visits.

FUNCTIONAL PERFORMANCE MEASURES

The following section will describe the applicability of each performance-based measure, provide a brief description of its administration, and provide useful clinimetric information. The reader should be aware of the plethora of freely available videos and websites containing summary information and test administration descriptions for FPMs such as the Shirley Ryan AbilityLab (formerly

RIC),[30] the American Physical Therapy Associations PTnow (available to members),[31]and physio-pedia.com.[32]

Self-Report Measures

Activities-Specific Balance Confidence Scale. The Activities-Specific Balance Confidence Scale (ABC) is a self-report measure of balance confidence in performing various activities without losing balance or experiencing a sense of unsteadiness. It is a 16-item self-report measure that prompts the question "How confident are you that you will not lose your balance or become unsteady when you…" to a variety of basic and community-related tasks of increasing difficulty. Items are rated on a Likert scale of 0 to 10 with 10 being the most confident. The sum of the responses is divided by the number of items to form a percentage. Higher scores are indicative of more balance confidence. The ABC has been examined on individuals with a variety of neurological conditions and fallers. It is a reliable and valid test for older individuals showing good internal consistency, construct, and criterion validity with the TUG, gait speed, and activity restrictions.[33,34]

Directions. The questionnaire and instructions are freely available on the web. Although the test is designed for people to read and answer themselves, it may be helpful to read the questions to the individual to get more accurate information. The test takes approximately 10 minutes to complete, depending on the individual.

Interpretation. A mean score of 80 was found in a group of community-dwelling older adults.[33] The developers of the test established a score of ≥80 to indicate high-functioning elders, 50 to 80 to indicate a moderate level of balance confidence characteristic of elders in retirement homes and persons with chronic health conditions, and <50 to indicate a low level of physical functioning characteristic of home care clients.[35] A cut off score of <67% indicates a risk for falling, accurately classifying people who fall 84% of the time.[36] A score of <85% indicates difficulty walking outside and climbing stairs (Sn = 0.73; Sp = 0.70; high positive likelihood ratio [+LR] = 2.43; very low likelihood ratio [−LR] = 0.04).[37] A minimal detectable change (MDC) of 15 points was found during a Rasch analysis.[38]

Falls Efficacy Scale-International. The Falls Efficacy Scale-International (FES-I) was developed to expand on the original FES. It assesses the concern about falling during activities of daily living. It is a 16-item questionnaire about the individual's confidence in performing daily tasks without falling, with a social component added to the original 10-item FES. Each item is rated from 1 ("very confident') to 4 ("not confident at all") and the item scores are summed for a total possible score of 64. The higher the score is, the more concern and greater fear of falling exist. The FES-I has been validated on many different international populations and in individuals with multiple conditions.[39] It is also reliable[40] and responsive.[41]

A shortened version of the FES-I was developed to increase the tool's feasibility. The shortened version contains 7 items rated on an ordinal scale of 0 to 4 with a total score of 28. The higher the score is, the more concern about falling. It is highly correlated with the FES-I and without ceiling effects and may assess fear better than the FES-I.[42]

Directions. The FES-I and short form are freely available from the web. The FES-I and short form are designed to be administered as a self-report questionnaire, but it may be helpful for the clinician to read the questions to the individual. The test takes approximately 10 minutes to complete.

Interpretation. FES-I scores >23 and short version scores >10 indicate high concern for falling.[43] A mean score for 70- to 79-year-olds was 26.7 on the FES-I and 11.8 on the short FES.[42] For those 80+ years of age, a mean score of 33 for the FES-I and 14.4 for the short FES was obtained.[42] Those with low fall self-efficacy (FES score of ≤75) have an increased risk of falling and greater declines in ability to perform activities of daily living (ADLs).[44]

Single-Test Mobility Measures

Although therapists are not administering FPM to perform research, the consistency and adherence to published procedures is the only way test results can inform accurate interpretations. An FPM's reliability and validity are established from specific procedures described by the authors. Their conclusions regarding reliability, diagnostic accuracy, and normative values are based on the published procedures. Therefore, administering the FPM in the same way will enable the therapist to make accurate interpretations with confidence of the FPM's reliability. However, many tests have differing procedures of administration, such as the walking speed, described next. When those differences exist, they are listed as variables in the test's administration. Variable administration procedures will negatively impact an FPM's accuracy. Where they exist, recommendations of the preferred procedures are described. Importantly, the clinician should be consistent in test administration. For example, if an assistive device is used at the baseline test, the same assistive device should be used for each subsequent test. Similarly, if the clinician chose to deviate from the published procedures, these deviations should be noted in documentation and test interpretation must be considered in light of these deviations.

Walking (Gait) Speed. Walking speed is so widely applicable to older adults and yields so much prognostic and functional ability information that it is considered the sixth vital sign. It is suitable to administer for all settings and has high interrater and intrarater reliability across settings.[45,46] Validity and responsiveness were demonstrated in multiple studies across settings and diagnoses.[47]

Decreased self-selected (usual, comfortable, habitual, or preferred) walking speed is a consistent risk factor for disability, cognitive impairment, institutionalization, falls, and mortality in men.[48,49] Walking speed correlates well with functional ability, future health status, and even confidence in balance. A decline in gait speed predicts cognitive impairments.[50] Walking speed predicts the need for rehabilitation, dependence in ADLs,[51] risk of adverse medical outcomes,[48] mobility disability, hospitalization, and risk of mortality.[51]

In one cross-sectional study of women aged 18 to 89, decline in walking velocity started at approximately age 65 years and became more pronounced after age 71 years. The estimated model showed that with each subsequent year in age, walking speed decreases by 0.03 m/s on average. After age 71 years, walking velocity decreased by 0.18 m/s per year, on average. The average walking velocity of women over the age of 71 years of 1.15 m/s is 7.8% less than a decade earlier.[52]

Maximum or fast walking speed provides information about abilities to walk in the community. Being able to increase walking speed in response to environmental demands, such as catching a bus, is an important aspect of functional mobility and safety, and is regarded as a more accurate measure of the person's community mobility.[53] Fast walking speed is dependent on the neuromuscular activation and force production of the triceps surae muscle group (soleus and gastrocnemius muscles), with ankle plantar flexion power as the largest contributor of energy to the gait cycle.[54,55]

Directions. Protocols differ for the amount of distance tested and starting time from a moving start or static start. Distances of 4 m or less have reduced accuracy and therefore are not recommended.[47] Using a straight path of 5 to 10 m without turns is ideal (Fig. 7.3).[56] If it is not possible to mark the distance with tape, using a precut rope of the distance desired is an easy and portable way of measuring out the distance.[56] Although acceleration is not necessary to enhance accuracy or reliability in the clinic,[57,58] the use of a 2.5- to 3-m acceleration and deacceleration distance decreases variability and may improve accuracy more so than a static start. A walking start on average increased walking speed by 0.17m/s compared with a standing start.[214] Self-selected and maximum walking speed may be tested. The use of an assistive device is permitted as necessary. Begin time at the first foot fall that crosses the starting line and finish line. The result is velocity, calculated by dividing the time of the walk into the length of the walk, typically in meters (meters/seconds). There are many online calculators and apps that can time walking speed. Instructions should be consistent and may need to be task based, especially for patients with neurological conditions.[56]

Interpretation. Normative walking speed ranges for community-dwelling older adults are listed in Table 7.3.[57,59] Changes in gait speed of 0.10 to 0.20 m/s may be important across multiple patient groups.[57] Accelerated decline of fast walking speed was associated with

TABLE 7.3 Normative Data for Walking Speed in Community-Dwelling Older Adults

	Men		Women	
Ages	Self-Selected	Maximum	Self-Selected	Maximum
60–69	1.59* 1.34†	2.05	1.44 1.24	1.87
70–79	1.38 1.26	1.83	1.33 1.13	1.71
80–89	1.21 96.8	1.65	1.15 94.3	1.59

Both used acceleration and deceleration distances.
*Steffen (2002)[146] distance of 10 meters.
†Bohannon (2011)[57]: included distances from 3 to 20 meters.

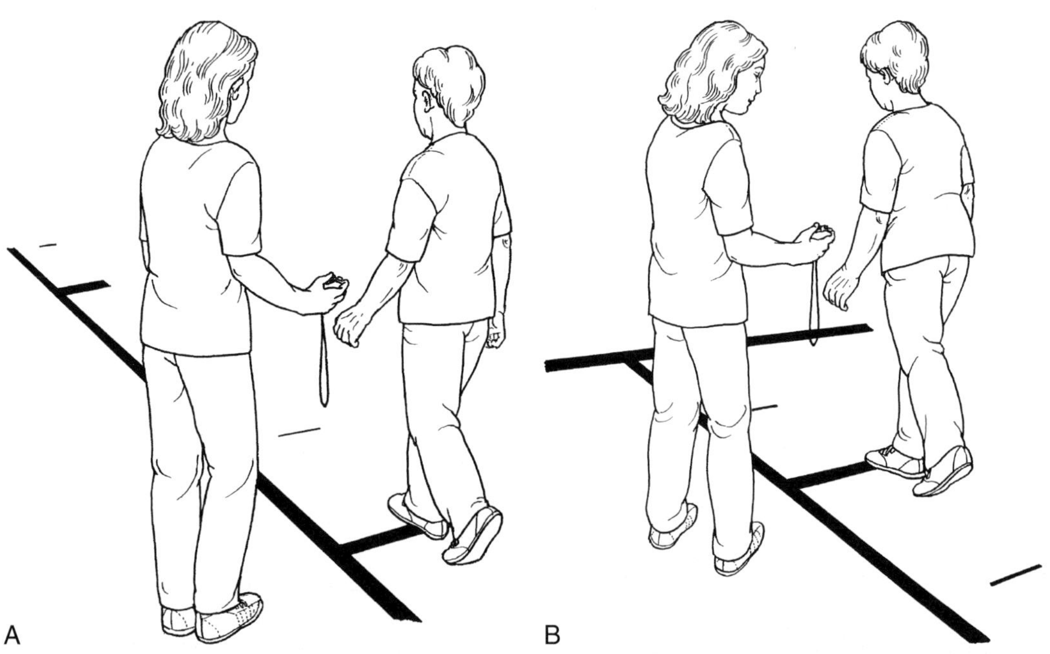

FIG. 7.3 Measuring walking speed. *(From Avers D and Brown M: Daniels and Worthingham's Muscle Testing, ed 10, St. Louis, 2019, Elsevier.)*

disability independent of baseline fast gait speed, implying that testing at regular intervals may help to detect declining mobility.[60] A walking speed of $\leq$0.8 m/s is a predictor of poor clinical outcomes.[48] Not surprisingly, lower gait speeds are reported in clinical settings (acute care: 0.46 m/s; subacute care: 0.53 m/s; ambulatory care: 0.74 m/s).[47] Higher gait speeds (0.35 to 0.37 m/s) upon admission to a transitional care setting demonstrated better functional outcomes, shorter rehabilitation stay, and discharge to the community than those with admitting gait speeds of 0.26 to 0.30 m/s.[61]

Sit-to-Stand (Chair Stand) Test. The sit-to-stand (STS) test is a measure of mobility and ability to rise from a chair and to sit back down, one component of a transfer skill. It specifically targets the force production of the leg muscles.[62] The two most widely used versions of the STS test are the time it takes to go from sit to stand five times (5TSTS)[63] or the number of chair stand repetitions possible in a 30-second period.[64] A 1-minute STS test is used to quantify exercise capacity.[65] Both shorter STS versions can serve as a proxy for lower extremity strength[66] and power.[17] The inability to complete 5TSTS chair stands indicates a physical performance limitation.[63] For example, 51% of home care clients were unable to complete the 5TSTS test.[67] The 30-second STS is suitable to measure physical performance in more physically fit older adults.[68]

The STS tests have been used as outcome measures following hip and knee arthroplasty[69] and for assessing outcomes following physical therapy[70,71] The 30-second version is part of the Fullerton Activities Balance Test (discussed in the balance section) and the timed five-repetition version is part of the Short Physical Performance Battery discussed in the mobility section. All STS versions have excellent test–retest reliability, validity, and responsiveness across numerous diagnoses.[72–75]

Directions. 30-second STS test: Individuals are required to stand from a standard chair (~43 cm) to a fully extended position as many times as possible with their arms folded across their chest. The number of completed repetitions achieved in 30 seconds is the score.[64] If a person cannot complete one STS, the score is zero.

5TSTS: The length of time for the individual to stand from a 43-cm-high chair five times. The time is the score. Arms should be folded across the chest.

The chair should be placed against the wall for safety reasons. The individual's back should not be against the back of the chair for the start of the test and should not have to touch the back of the chair for each repetition. The manner in which the individual stands should be monitored to avoid exacerbation of knee or hip pain. Typical problems are inability to avoid knee valgus during the rising and sitting portions (indicative of weakness in the gluteus medius), and rocking or extending the arms, which may indicate the need to use momentum to rise in the presence of leg weakness or inability to move the center of gravity enough forward to rise, implicating motor control issues or foot placement too far forward. Fig. 7.4 demonstrates difficulty in rising, necessitating the use of arms to drive momentum.

Interpretation. Normative scores for both versions of the STS for community-dwelling older adults and for senior athletes (defined as someone over age 60 who participates in any sport competition) are listed in Table 7.4.[76–78] An MDC for the 5TSTS was 2.5 to

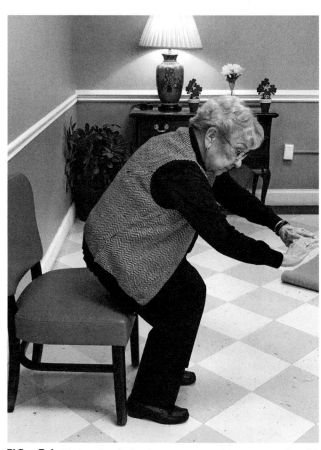

FIG. 7.4 Chair stand (patient was unable to stand with crossed arms).

TABLE 7.4 Chair Stand Norms for 30-Second STS and 5TSTS

Age	30-Second STS[78]		5TSTS[76]	5TSTS for Senior Athletes*
Test	Men	Women	Men and Women	Men and Women
60–64	16.4	14.5	11.4 s	7.26 s
65–69	15.2	13.5		
70–74	14.5	12.9	12.6 s	8.11 s
75–79	14.0	12.5		
80–84	12.4	11.3	12.7 s	9.18 s
85–89	11.1	10.3		
90–94	9.7	8.0		10.39 s

5TSTS, = 5 times Sit to Stand; *STS*, Sit to Stand.
*From Jorde B, Schweinie W, Beacom K, Graphenteen V, Ladwig, A. The five times Sit to Stand test in senior athletes. *JGPT.* 2013;1:47–50.

4.3s.[63,79] Eight or fewer STSs in 30 seconds is related to the risk of developing mobility disability and frailty.[80,81] Sarcopenia and prefrailty are indicated if the 5TSTS takes 13 seconds or more (Sn = 0.86; Sp = 0.53; +LR = 1.83; −LR = 0.62).[82,83] Tiedemann found that a score of ≥12 on the 30-second STS in individuals older than 74 identified the need of further assessment for fall risk.[73] A score of >15 s predicted multiple falls (Sn = 0.55; Sp = 0.65; +LR = 1.57; −LR = 0.15).[84] The inability to complete the 5TSTS test was a marginal predictor of falls (odds ratio [OR] = 4.22) and a significant predictor of ADL- (OR = 24.70) and instrumental activities of daily living (IADL)-related disability (OR = 17.10) at 3-year follow-up.[85] Finally, ≥10 s to complete the 5TSTS predicted risk of disability (Sn = 0.49; Sp = 0.78; +LR = 2.23; −LR = 0.37).[86]

Floor Transfer. Rising from the floor is a necessary skill for any older adult. The inability to get up from the floor following a noninjurious fall is responsible for a significant number of calls to emergency services,[87] and almost half of those who fall and are not injured are unable to rise from the floor without assistance.[88] The inability to rise from the floor may be the most significant predictor of injurious falls (primarily hip fractures).[89] It is considered a rigorous test and thus may be one of the earliest performance tests to indicate mobility disability.[90] An inability to rise from the floor is associated with increasing age, more comorbidities, and lower functional capacity.[91] The test is reliable[92] and valid for functional independence or dependence.[91]

Directions. As yet, there is not an agreed-upon protocol. Some authors begin with the person standing and record the time it takes to get onto the floor and into supine, then return to standing, whereas others only record the time it takes for the person to rise from the floor. Furthermore, the position on the floor is not standardized, with some authors starting in long sitting, whereas others require 75% contact with the floor. Regardless of the tester's preference, a chair should be placed nearby. We recommend recording the time it takes to return to standing from a supine position. The timing of the transfer starts on the command "Go!" The patient should then rise from the floor into a standing position that is stable, whereupon the timing stops. It is valuable to document the strategy the patient uses and if any help was needed. The score (amount of time) should include any help that was needed (i.e., the chair or another person). If the tester desires to time the person both getting onto the floor and rising, the patient starts in a standing position, with the start of timing on the command "Go!" Demonstration of how to get onto the floor and the desired supine position is helpful but should not dictate how a person chooses to get up. Many people will need reassurance that help is available, should it be needed, before they agree to the test. In the author's opinion the transition from sitting to quadruped as shown in Fig. 7.5 is the most difficult motor planning aspect of the floor rise test.

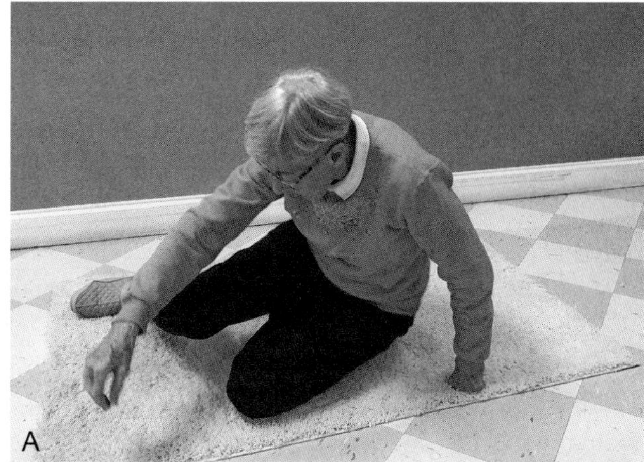

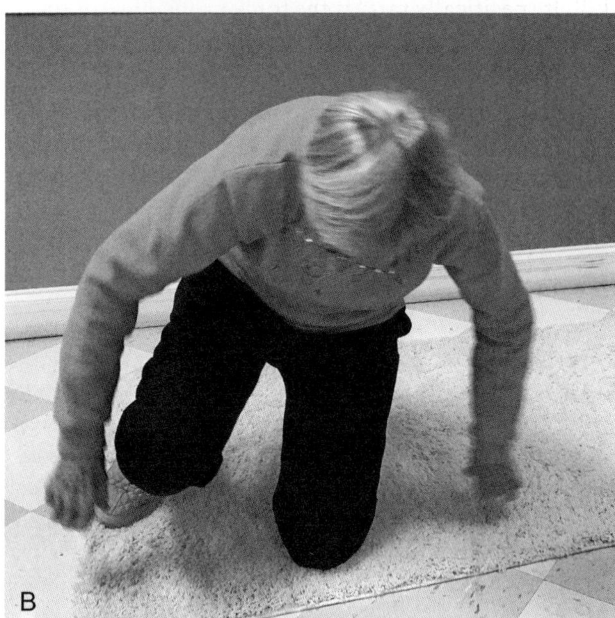

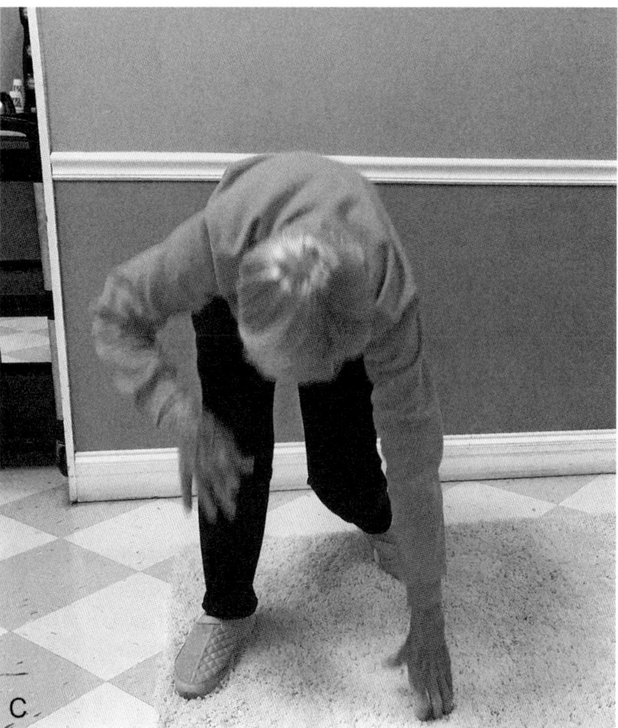

FIG. 7.5 Floor rise transition from supine (**A**) to quadruped (**B**) to standing (**C**).

Interpretation. There are no normative data for this test. A mean score of 8.8 seconds was taken to get onto the floor and rise again in healthy older adults compared with a mean of 20.9 seconds in individuals poststroke.[92] No assistance was allowed in this study and the mean of three trials was used; thus, scores may have been affected by fatigue. The lowering and rising technique was also dictated. The authors found correlation with 5TSTS and the ability of the floor rise test to differentiate between healthy older adults and those with chronic stroke (Sn = 0.92; Sp = 0.72; +LR = 3.29; −LR = 0.28).[92] Bergland and Laake found that difficulty with climbing stairs, walking outdoors, performing IADLs, and self-reported balance were found in those who were unable to rise from the floor. These individuals were also more likely to be living alone and have multiple comorbidities.[93]

Stair Climb Test. The stair climb test (SCT) assesses the ability to ascend and descend a flight of stairs. It is a valid, reliable, and responsive test of the power of the lower extremities.[94] The test has variable elements depending on the number of steps (2 to 12), pace (self-selected or as quickly as feasible), separately timed ascent and descent, outcome of the number of steps in a specified time, or the time of a number of steps.

Directions. It is recommended to perform ascent and descent as a single test on a flight of at least 10 stairs with instructions to go as fast but as safely as possible.[94] If timing ascent and descent separately, instructions are given as to whether the person should stop at the landing. An assistive device and/or the handrail can be used to ensure safety but should be noted. A rate of perceived effort (RPE) may be collected to add to the clinician's interpretation. The number of stairs is divided by the time for stair/s.

Interpretation. A study of 148 Australian adults older than age 60 years found a time of 10.4 s for men and 12.8 s (up and down) for a flight of 11 stairs.[95] A score above or below 15.22 s on 12 stairs (up and down) or 7.51 s (up) was found to best discriminate healthy older adults from stroke survivors (Sn = 1.0; Sp = 0.90; +LR = 10; −LR = 0.11).[96] Nightingale et al. found in their systematic review that SCT time increased with age (mean time of 0.23 s/step in young military personnel compared with 0.49 s/step for 18- to 49-year-olds and 1.38 s ±0.48 s/step for those >65 years), but normative data could not be determined. The review noted descent time was faster than ascent time, reflecting the data from a younger population.[94] The authors hypothesize that descent time slows with aging and may be a more discriminating variable than ascent time.[94] Slower SCT scores are linked with lower self-efficacy for stairs, use of the handrail during descent, and more cautious behavior in women than in men in a group of healthy older adults (>75 years). In fact, four of five men exhibited risky behavior in not using the handrail in spite of clear imbalance.[97]

Timed Up and Go Test. The Timed Up and Go test (TUG) was originally developed as a test of mobility in a frail population and requires balance, sit to stand, walking, and turning.[98] The TUG has many variations including pace (self-selected or fast), distance (2.44 to 3.05 m [8 to 10 ft]), mechanism of turn (walk to line and turn, walk around cone and return, walk to cone and turn), type of chair (with or without arm rests, with or without back rest, chair height [range 40 to 46 cm], and number of trials [range one to four]). The TUG has been tested in many different patient populations including those with stroke, Parkinson disease, dementia, spinal injuries, vestibular disorders, osteoarthritis, brain injury, and more, as well as older adults in various settings.[99] Test–retest reliability is excellent in a variety of populations.[100,101] The TUG is also valid and responsive in geriatric rehabilitation.[98,102]

Although the TUG is not useful in healthy older adults to identify functional decline,[68] it is recommended as a screening tool to determine whether an in-depth mobility assessment and early intervention, such as prescription of a walking aid, home visit, or physical therapy, are necessary.[103] However, the TUG does not provide sufficient information on underlying balance deficits[68] and is not recommended as a tool to identify fall risk in healthy, high-functioning older people.[104–106] The TUG may have more value in less healthy, lower-functioning older people to identify fall risk; however, no cut-point was recommended in one meta-analysis.[106] The TUG is not recommended as an outcome for people with either hip or knee osteoarthritis based on measurement evidence.[107]

Dual-Task Timed Up and Go. The Dual-Task TUG was developed to increase the challenge of the TUG and thus be a better discriminator to identify falls.[108] The Dual-Task TUG is composed of a manual task (carrying a cup of water) or a cognitive task (serial subtraction test) that is combined with the TUG performance. The manual task may stress physical function (balance, gait, transfers), whereas the cognitive task may stress cognitive function. Generally, scores are 1 to 3 s slower than the single-task TUG.[109]

Directions. Directions for the administration of the TUG and Dual-Task TUG are widely available for no cost on the Internet. To decrease test variability, standardized test administration is encouraged. Timing should begin on the command "Go!" (rather than when the individual starts to move), walking pace should be at a self-selected speed,[98] and timing should be stopped when the individual is sitting with the back against the chair. A practice test should precede the actual test. Use of an assistive device is permitted. Scores may reflect the best performance, the average performance of multiple trials, or the worst performance.

Interpretation. Normative scores for the 2.44-m (8-ft) and 3-m tests are listed in Table 7.5 and generally are between 8 and 11 seconds for community-dwelling older adults.[59,78,110,111] A score of 10 s demonstrates functional independence; therefore, that is a minimum threshold.[112,113] Scores ≥9 s predicted risk of disability

TABLE 7.5 Normative Data for Timed Up and Go Test and 8-Foot Up and Go Test

	8-Foot Up and Go[78]		Timed Up and Go[59]	
Age	Men	Women	Men	Women
60–64	4.7	5.2	8 s	8 s
65–69	5.1	5.6		
70–74	5.3	6.0	9 s	9 s
75–79	5.9	6.3		
80–84	6.4	7.2	10 s	11 s
85–90	7.2	7.9		
90–94	8.1	9.4		

(Sn = 0.60; Sp = 0.74; +LR = 2.31; −LR = 0.19).[86] Scores of <20 s indicate independence in basic transfers, basic mobility skills,[98] and a threshold for returning home following rehabilitation.[114] Scores of >30 s indicate dependence in transfers.[98] Mobility disability is identified at ≤12 s.[103] The MDC_{90} of 4.09 s was found for individuals with Alzheimer disease, which increases as dementia severity increases.[101,115] The minimally clinical important difference (MCID) ranges from 0.8 to 1.4 s in individuals with osteoarthritis,[116] 2.9 s in individuals with chronic stroke,[117] and 4.85 in individuals with Parkinson disease.[118] An MDC of 4.0 s was found in older individuals in an adult day center.[119]

In a sample of 120 healthy community-dwelling individuals aged 60 to 87, the mean time to complete the manual Dual-Task TUG was 11.6 s and for the cognitive Dual-Task TUG was 9.8 s.[109]

Distance Walk Tests. Distance walk tests are designed to assess an individual's aerobic capacity/endurance over a specified distance. The most commonly used distance walk test is the 6-minute version, but the 2-minute version is used for those with individuals with poor concentration or endurance and can be useful in busy clinics. The 400-m (0.25-mile) version uses time to cover a set distance rather than distance covered in 6 minutes.

The 6-minute walk test (6MWT) is a submaximal measure of aerobic capacity, useful for measuring functional capacity,[120] and is a valid and reliable indicator of aerobic fitness[121] and lower leg strength.[122] It is responsive with a small meaningful change of 20 m and substantial meaningful change of 50 m.[123]

The 2-minute walk test (2MWT) is a reliable, valid, and responsive test in a variety of populations (including frailty and lower limb amputations) and correlates well with other distance walk tests.[124] It should not be used to measure exercise fitness because of the lack of criterion validity.[124] No MCID has been established for the 2MWT.

The 400-m walk test or long corridor walk is a measure of mobility disability as it represents an equivalent distance of three to four blocks, a standard for community mobility.[7,8] It is considered a test of aerobic capacity[125] and elicits a higher effort than the 6MWT owing to the faster self-selected pace.[125] It is reliable, valid, and responsive.[125–127] The 400-m test has a floor effect in that an individual must be able to complete 400 m to complete the test. In fact, those who are unable to complete the 400 m have a threefold higher risk of death during a 6-year follow-up period compared with those who completed the test, and those who did complete it but took over 7 minutes had an increased mortality risk.[128] Eighty percent of those who walked at a pace of 0.6 m/s or slower could not complete the 400-m test.[129]

Directions. *6MWT:* The 30-m (98 feet) course should be straight (e.g., hallway) and measured in 5-m intervals. Alternatively, an engineer's measuring wheel can be used. Vital signs should be taken prior to and immediately following the test. The RPE should also be recorded. Standing rests are allowed, but as soon as the individual sits down, the test is terminated. Assistive devices may be used. When administering the test, the clinician should not walk with the patient, thus avoiding pacing the individual, but rather the clinician should stand in a central location and share encouragement and amount of time lapsed at 1-minute intervals. Upon completion, the distance completed should be recorded, which is the score.[120]

2MWT: There is not an established protocol for the 2MWT; however, a systematic review proposed a testing protocol as follows[124]: The participant is asked to walk as far as possible in 2 minutes, on a flat, indoor corridor (30-m length preferred), with turnaround points marked by a cone. A starting line should be visible on the floor. The clinician, if needed, should walk half a meter behind the individual so as not to disturb the walking pace. No encouragement should be given to the individual and the individual is not encouraged to talk during the test. Two trials precede the third trial, which is the test. Rest of at least 10 minutes is given between each trial. Distance walked is measured using floor markings or with a measuring wheel. Vital signs are taken before and after the test. The patient may take standing rests, but the test is terminated if the patient needs to sit.

400 meters: A 20-m (65 feet) corridor is used. Each end is marked with a line the individual must cross and turn for each lap until 10 laps are completed. Vital signs are assessed pre- and posttest. An assistive device may be used as preferred. The individual may stop and rest but cannot sit down. If the individual sits down, the test is terminated, and no score is given. The authors of the study recommend assigning a maximum time of 12 minutes (0.56 m/s pace) to nonfinishers.

Interpretation. Normative scores for the 6MWT are listed in Table 7.6. No normative values exist for the 2MWT or 400-m test; however, a distance of 91 to 290 m was the mean distance of the first 2 minutes of the 6MWT (mean distance of 258 to 823 m) in participants aged 3 to 85 years.[130] MDCs for various conditions for both the 6-minute and 2-minute versions are listed in Table 7.7. The MCID of 14 to 30.5 m for the 6MWT was found in one systematic review to be clinically

TABLE 7.6 Normative Values for the 6-Minute Walk Test

	6-Minute Walk Test* (m)	
Age	Men	Women
60–69	560	505
70–79	530	490
80–89	446	382

*Bohannon RW. Six-minute walk test. A meta-analysis of data from apparently healthy elders. *Topics in Geriatric Rehabilitation*. 2007;23(2):155–160.

TABLE 7.7 Minimal Detectable Change for 6- and 2-Minute Walk Tests

Condition	6-Minute Walk Test	2-Minute Walk Test
Osteoarthritis	61.34 m*	
Alzheimer disease	33.47 m[101]	
Geriatrics	58.21 m[123]	12.2 m[§]
Parkinson disease	82 m[100]	
Stroke	60.98 m[123]	13.4 m[214]
Chronic obstructive pulmonary disease	25 m[†]	
Lower extremity amputation		34.4 m[214]
Poliomyelitis		22.9 m[214]

*Kennedy DM, Stratford PW, Wessel J, Gollish JD, Penney D. Assessing stability and change of four performance measures: a longitudinal study evaluating outcome following total hip and knee arthroplasty. BMC Musculoskelet Disord. 2005;6(1):3.

§Connelly DM, Thomas BK, Cliffe SJ, Perry WM, Smith RE. Clinical utility of the 2-minute walk test for older adults living in long-term care. Physiother Can. 2009;61(2):78–87.

†Holland AE, Hill CJ, Rasekaba T, et al. Updating the minimal important distance for six-minute walk distance in patients with chronic obstructive pulmonary disease. YAPMR. 2010;91(2):221–225.

important across multiple patient groups.[131] Distances on 6MWT of <338 m are indicative of increased risk of all-cause mortality.[132] A distance <200 m is predictive of hospitalization or mortality in patients with congestive obstructive pulmonary disease[133,134] and poor postoperative outcome (Sn = 0.82; Sp = 0.84; +LR = 5.13; −LR = 0.02).[134]

In a study of 1300 individuals aged 70 to 79 years with no reported mobility limitations, the median time to complete the 400-m test was approximately 5:09 minutes (range of 4:39 to 5:48) for men and 5:36 minutes (range 5:06 to 6:16) for women.[135] Individuals >60 years of age and unable to walk 400 m (~0.25 miles) in 7 minutes are at risk for significant functional limitations. Those who took longer than 5:30 minutes to walk 400 m may be at risk for impending functional difficulty.[127,136]

Multiactivity Mobility Measures

Short Physical Performance Battery. The Short Physical Performance Battery (SPPB) is used widely in research and increasingly in the clinic as a test of lower extremity function, and global health status and vulnerability in older adults in the hospital and community setting.[137] It consists of three separate tasks: static standing balance, self-selected walking speed, and the 5TSTS. Scores obtained on a 12-point summary scale indicate a gradient of functional decline that has been shown to be predictive of subsequent mobility-related disability, institutionalization, and mortality.[138] The SPPB has a high level of reliability, validity, and responsiveness within an older, community-dwelling population.[139] Power predicts one-third of SPPB performance, underscoring the importance of power in mobility performance.[140] In higher-functioning, healthy older adults, a ceiling effect may occur.[18]

Directions. The SPPB has a specific protocol and scoring sheet that is freely available from the Internet.

The balance component assesses the ability to stand in three positions (feet side by side, semitandem, and tandem) for a maximum of 10 seconds each. The gait portion assesses the time to complete a 3- to 4-m walk in two trials. The lower extremity strength portion measures the time to rise from a standard chair five times. Each task is scored out of 4 points based on criteria, with the three scores summed for a maximum of 12 and a minimum of 0.

Interpretation. Higher scores indicate better lower extremity function. SPPB summary performance of ≤10 indicates mobility disability and is predictive of all-cause mortality.[137,141] Individuals scoring <4 points at discharge had a greater risk for rehospitalization and death than those with scores of 8 or better.[142] A change of 0.5 points is considered a small meaningful change and a change of 1 point is considered a substantial meaningful change.[123]

Physical Performance Test. The Physical Performance Test (PPT) assesses multiple domains of physical function through observed task performance of activities of daily living and mobility.[143] There are two versions, the 9-item that includes stairs and the 7-item. Both are listed in Box 7.4. A maximum score of 28 for the 7-item and of 36 for the 9-item version is possible. A higher totaled score is indicative of better physical performance. Most of the items are timed. The PPT is a reliable, responsive, and valid test demonstrating internal consistency, construct, and criterion validity.[143,144]

Directions. The scoring form and scripted directions are free and available on the Internet. The test takes approximately 10 minutes and requires commonly found equipment of a jacket, a book, a spoon, a coffee can, five dried beans, paper and pen, stairs, and a stopwatch.

Interpretation. Table 7.8 provides means by gender and age for the 7- and 9-item PPT.[145,146] The PPT also predicts ADL functional limitations before ADLs were detected by self-report.[147] The MCID is 2.4 points.[144]

Modified Physical Performance Test. The Modified Physical Performance Test (m-PPT) was modified from the PPT to include components of the SPPB (chair rise and static balance tests) to capture the SPPB's correlations with nursing home placement and loss of independence.[148] The m-PPT is a 9-item test with each item rated

BOX 7.4 Tasks of the 7- and 9-Item Physical Performance and Modified Physical Performance Test Tasks

Physical Performance Test		Modified Physical Performance Test	
9-Item	**7-Item**		
1. Write a sentence	1. Write a sentence	Standing static Balance	Feet together Semitandem Tandem
2. Simulate eating	2. Simulate eating	Chair rise	
3. Lift a book and put it on the shelf	3. Lift a book and put it on the shelf	Book lift	
4. Put on and remove a jacket	4. Put on and remove a jacket	Put on and remove jacket	
5. Pick up a coin from the floor	5. Pick up a coin from the floor	Pick up coin from floor	
6. Turn 360 degrees	6. Turn 360 degrees	Turn 360 degrees	
7. 50-foot walk test	7. 50-foot walk test	50-foot walk test	
8. Climb one flight of stairs		Climb one flight of stairs	
9. Climb up to four flights		Climb four flights of stairs	

TABLE 7.8 Physical Performance Test (PPT) Means and Modified Physical Performance Test Cutoff Score

	7-Item PPT Means (SD) by Age and Gender		9-Item PPT[b] Means (SD) by Age and Gender		Modified PPT Cutoff Scores		
Age	**Male**	**Female**	**Male**	**Female**		**9-Point Scale**	**7-Point Scale**
60–69[146]	24	23	31 (2)	31 (1)	Not frail	32–36	19.4–24.8
70–79[146]	22	22	29 (2)	29 (2)	Mild frailty	25–31	<19.4
80–89[146]	20	20	27 (2)	27 (3)	Moderate frailty	17–24	
90–101[145]	16.1	16.2			Unlikely to be able to function in the community	<17	

on a 0 to 4 scale using descriptive criteria. The maximum score is 36. The test has not been examined for reliability and validity.

Directions. The scoring form and scripted instructions are free and available on the Internet. The test takes approximately 10 minutes and requires commonly found equipment of a jacket, a book, stairs, and a stopwatch. It omits the writing and eating tasks.

Interpretation. The M-PPT was found to be predictive of frailty.[148] Table 7.8 lists cutoff scores for frailty.[148]

BALANCE MEASURES

Static Steady-State Balance Tests

Single Leg Stance Test. The purpose of the single leg stance (SLS) test is to assess static postural and balance control. It is considered the most difficult of three static positions (semitandem and tandem) because of the decreased area of weight bearing and the narrowed base of support.[149] SLS time decreases with age but is not gender dependent.[150] Variations exist for the test performance including shoes on or off, eyes open or closed, how high the nonstance leg is lifted (e.g., 2" or thigh parallel to floor), number of test trials, worst or best performance recorded, and maximum time for test (most common being 30 s). The SLS test has relative reliability[151] and validity with functional measures.[152]

Directions. The test can be performed with or without footwear, as neither leg dominance nor footwear affects test performance.[149] Hands are placed on the hips. The test can be performed with eyes open or eyes closed. When the individual is ready, ask him or her to lift the leg and begin timing. The individual must stand unassisted on one leg, without the lifted leg touching the standing leg. When the leg touches the ground or the standing leg or the hands leave the hips, the test is terminated. The time standing in a steady stance is the score. It is recommended the test be performed to failure, rather than setting a predetermined time as there is considerable ceiling effect.[152]

Interpretation. Normative scores are listed in Table 7.9.[150,152] Men on average held SLS for 5.5 s longer than women.[152] The SLS mean time with eyes closed was 3.7 s (SD = 3.3) for men and 4.1 s (SD = 4.2) for women aged 60 years and over.[95] The MDC_{95} is 24.1 s, exhibiting large measurement error (40.8%) and high minimum change values (113.1%), making it unlikely to be a useful indicator of change in balance performance.[153]

Romberg Test. The Romberg test assesses static standing balance and was originally developed to screen for myelopathies and neuropathies with associated sensory dysfunction. Its reliability and validity have not been established in part because of the integrated systems necessary to maintain this position (nervous system, trunk, and leg muscle tone).[154]

TABLE 7.9 Normative Scores for Single-Leg Stance

Age		Weighted Mean (SD)[152]	Mean (SD)[150]	
Condition		Eyes open	Eyes Closed	
	Time		Men	Women
60–69	30 s	26.4 (1.2)	3.1 (2.7)	2.5 (1.5)
	60 s	31.9 (3.1)		
	≥120 s	63.4 (3.6)		
70–79	30s	17.6 (1.6)	1.9 (0.9)	2.2 (2.1)
	60 s	23.4 (2.9)		
	≥120 s	52.4 (11.3)		
80–89	30 s	10.1 (0.9)	1.3 (0.6)*	1.4 (0.6)*
	60 s	17.3 (3.8)		
	≥120 s	20.5 (3.8)		

*Ages 80–99.

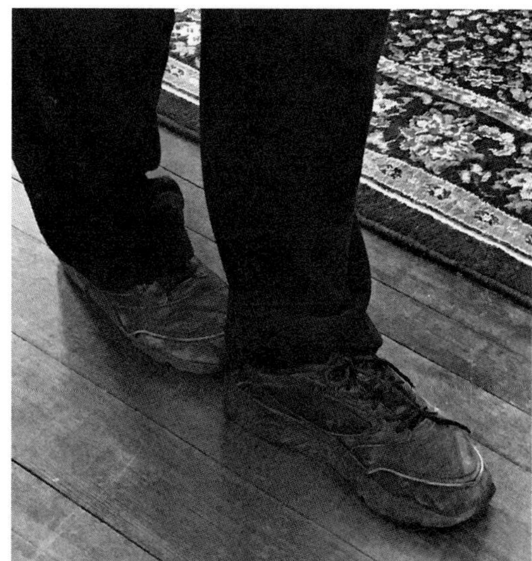

FIG. 7.6 Tandem stance (sharpened Romberg).

Directions. The individual stands on a flat, even surface with feet together. Footwear is optional. Timing commences on "Go." This position is maintained as long possible for 30 seconds. It can be tested with eyes open and with eyes closed, as clinically indicated. Arm position is not standardized but traditionally the individual crosses the arms over the chest.

Interpretation. Decreasing times indicate increased fall risk. A threefold increase in falling was associated with the inability to hold the Romberg position with eyes closed on a foam pad for 20 s.[155]

Tandem (Sharpened Romberg) Test. Along with the SLS, the tandem stance (sharpened Romberg) is the most common measure of balance. The tandem stance requires the individual to stand in a tandem heel-to-toe position. The test commonly includes variations such as footwear (none or preferred), number of trials and which trial is used (e.g., longest vs. shortest trial), maximum length of time of test, assistance used to get into the position, foot forward (dominant vs. nondominant), conditions of test termination (e.g., moving arms from start position, amount of sway allowed), and type of surface (compliant vs. firm). The tandem test has good relative reliability,[151] but validity and responsiveness have not been determined. In a study of young seniors (50 to 70 years old), reliability and validity for the 10-s version was found to be poor.[156]

Directions. The individual is asked to place the heel of one leg in front of and touching the toe of the other leg (often dominant, but both sides can be tested) (Fig. 7.6). If assistance is needed to assume the position, this should be documented. Longer times of 30 seconds are recommended because of ceiling effects.[157] Arm position is not standardized, but it is recommended that the client cross arms across the chest.[30]

Interpretation. Tandem stance balance time predicts future function in healthy older adults.[158,159] Mean scores for eyes open was 49 s (SD = 21 s) and eyes closed was 29 s (SD = 24s) for ages 60 to 80+.[146] Assisting someone who cannot get into the tandem-stance position independently reflects balance deficits and should be a consideration in the decision-making process.[157]

Dynamic Steady-State Balance Tests

Four-Square Step Test. The four-square step test (4SST) is a clinical test of stepping and change of direction to identify multiple falling incidents in older adults. The test requires the individual to step forward, backward, and sideways from right to left while using step clearance. It is a reliable and valid test of dynamic standing balance[160,161] and has been used on a wide variety of conditions such as stroke, osteoarthritis, and vestibular conditions.[162] The time to complete the test is the score.

Directions. Directions are widely available from the Internet. A square is formed with four canes end to end. The canes are used to avoid rolling the cane if the individual were to step on one. Demonstrate the test and then instruct the individual to move from square to square in the sequence shown in Fig. 7.7 as quickly but as safely as possible without touching the canes. If possible, the individual should face forward throughout the sequence. Allow at least one practice trial. Time begins when the first footfall touches square 2 and ends when both feet return to square 4. The time is the score. The individual may use his or her cane as desired, but the test is not appropriate for walker use. The person can start again if he or she does not perform the sequence correctly, touches a cane, or loses balance. Thus, it may take several tries to complete the test. The best of two correctly completed 4SSTs is taken as the score. A score is still provided if the individual is unable to face forward during the entire sequence.

Interpretation. A score of ≥15 seconds (Sn = 0.85; Sp = 0.88 to 1.0; +LR = 7.08; −LR = 0.03) indicates risk for multiple falls.[160,161] A cutoff score of >12 (Sn = 0.80; Sp = 0.92; +LR = 10; −LR = 0.13) identified individuals with vestibular disorders who had one or more risk factors

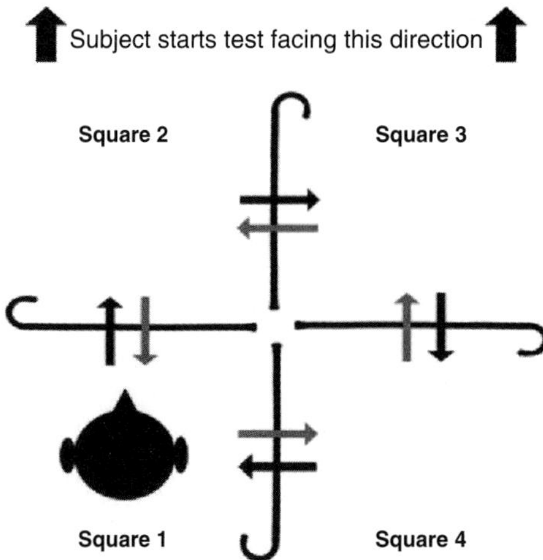

FIG. 7.7 Four-Square Step Test setup and sequence. *(From Cleary KK, Skornyakov E. Predicting falls in older adults using the four square step test. Physiother Theory Pract. 2017;(10):766–771. doi:https://doi.org/10.1080/09593985.2017.1354951. https://www.semanticscholar.org/paper/Predicting-falls-in-older-adults-using-the-four-Cleary-Skornyakov/7916b8c9f3f55d905f3d93c7521d7c4171869e5e.)*

for falls.[163] In individuals with unilateral transtibial amputation, a cutoff score of 24 s (Sn = 0.92; Sp = 0.93; +LR = 13.14; −LR = 0.01) indicated a risk for multiple falls.[164]

Performance Test Batteries

Berg Balance Score. The Berg Balance Score (BBS) is the best-known balance measurement tool, originally designed to measure balance in older individuals. It consists of 14 items scored on an ordinal scale of 0 to 4 for a total of 56 points (a higher score indicates lower fall risk). The items evaluate the ability to maintain static positions of increasing difficulty by decreasing the base of support progressing to dynamic activities of varying difficulty (Box 7.5) The test takes 15 to 20 minutes to administer. The test is reliable, valid, and responsive for a wide range of conditions including dementia.[165,166]

A short version of the BBS was developed to improve the utility of the BBS and remove redundant items (e.g., standing unsupported and transferring).[167] The number of items was reduced from 14 (BBS-14) to 7 (BBS-7) (Box 7.5) with an ordinal scoring system reduced to three levels from the original five. Chou et al. found it to be reliable, valid, and responsive but with a floor effect, thus reducing its utility in people with severe balance deficits.[167]

Directions. Directions for the BBS-14 and scoring form are freely available from the Internet. Equipment needed is a standard chair with armrests, step stool of average height, ruler or yardstick, and slipper or shoe. The BBS-7 requires the same equipment except a stool. The directions allow the individual to choose the preferred leg for the "standing on one foot" item, which may inflate balance scores, especially in stroke or lower limb surgery. Using the impaired limb for scoring may present a more realistic picture.[168]

BOX 7.5 Berg Balance Score 14-Item and 7-Item versions

BBS—Original	Short Version
1. Sitting to standing	1. Reaching forward with outstretched arm
2. Standing unsupported	2. Standing with eyes closed
3. Sitting unsupported	3. Standing with one foot in front
4. Standing to sitting	4. Turning to look behind
5. Transfers	5. Retrieving object from floor
6. Standing with eyes closed	6. Standing on one foot
7. Standing with feet together	7. Sitting to standing
8. Reaching forward with outstretched arm	
9. Retrieving object from floor	
10. Turning to look behind	
11. Turning 360 degrees	
12. Placing alternate foot on stool	
13. Standing with one foot in front	
14. Standing on one foot	

Interpretation. No common interpretation exists. Normative scores are listed in Table 7.10.[59,145,146] Healthy individuals aged approximately 70 years tend to have normal BBS scores (56/56), exhibiting the likelihood of a ceiling effect.[169] In individuals with stroke, scores of 0 to 20 represent balance impairment, of 21 to 40 represent acceptable balance, and of 41 to 56 represent good balance.[170] Lower BBS scores upon admission following stroke predicted a longer length of stay and at 14 and 30 days predicted disability level at 90 days poststroke.[170]

The BBS should not be used alone to determine the risk for falls in older adults as no cutoff score can predict the risk of falls with any certainty.[171] One systematic review identified an MDC of 2.8 to 6.6 points in BBS scores above 20.[166] Table 7.11 lists the MDC for ranges of BBS scores.[172] The MDC increases as independence decreases (e.g., MDC of 3.3 for those who are considered independent with a mean BBS score of 49.2 [SD = 4.4;

TABLE 7.10 Normative Scores for the 14-Item Berg Balance Scale

Age	Group	N	Mean (SD)
60–69	Male	15	55 (1.0)
	Female	22	55 (2)
70–79	Male	14	54 (3)
	Female	22	53 (4)
80–89	Male	4	52 (5)
	Female	14	52 (4)
90–101[145]	Male	2	40 (1.4)
	Female	15	37 (10)

[b]Steffen 2002 and 2005

TABLE 7.11 Berg Balance Score Minimal Detectable Change (MDC) Values

BBS Score Ranges	Mean BBS Score (SD)	MDC_{95}
0–24	20.9 (3.8)	4.6
25–34	30.9 (3.8)	6.3
35–44	39.8 (3.3)	4.9
45–56	49.5 (2.9)	3.3

range 45–56] to an MDC of 5.9 for those requiring standby assistance with a mean BBS score of 30.8 [SD = 7.9; range 25–34]).[172]

Tinetti Performance Oriented Mobility Assessment. The Performance-Oriented Mobility Assessment (POMA) was the first clinical balance assessment tool.[173] It measures an individual's gait and balance abilities using 16 items of balance and gait. Each item is scored on a 3-point ordinal scale (0–2) with 28 possible points. A score of 3 indicates independence on a test item. The balance portion (POMA-B) contains 9 items for a maximum score of 16 and the gait portion (POMA-G) contains 7 items for a maximum score of 12. The test is reliable, valid, and responsive.[174–177] The POMA has excellent test–retest reliability in people with dementia.[178] The gait portion may have a ceiling effect.[176]

Directions. Directions for the administration of the POMA are freely available on the Internet. It takes 10 to 15 minutes to administer.

Interpretation. Mean POMA scores for Korean males and females aged 65 to 79 were found to be 26.21 (SD = 3.4) and 25.16 (SD = 4.3), respectively.[179] The same study found mean scores of 23.39 (SD = 6.02) in males over age 80 years and 17.20 (SD = 8.32) in females over 80 years.[179] The MDC is reported as 4.0 to 4.2.[176] It is a poor discriminator of falls risk.[27,28,180]

Balance Evaluation Systems, Mini-BEST, and Brief-BEST Tests. The Balance Evaluation Systems Test (BESTest) is an extensive 36-item clinical balance tool (Tables 7.12 and 7.13), developed to assess balance

TABLE 7.12 Balance Evaluation System Items for BESTest, Mini-BESTest, and Brief-BESTest

Domain	BESTest 36 items	Mini-BESTest Items 14 Items	Brief-BESTest 8 Items
Biomechanical constraints	1. Base of support		
	2. Center of Mass (CoM) alignment		
	3. Ankle strength and range		
	4. Hip/trunk lateral strength		X
	5. Sit on floor and stand up		
Stability limits	6. Sit verticality and lateral lean		
	7. Functional reach forward		X
	8. Functional reach lateral		
Transitions—anticipatory postural adjustment	9. Sit to stand	X	
	10. Rise to toes	X	
	11. Stand on one leg	X	X (test each leg, counts as two items)
	12. Alternate stair touching		
	13. Standing arm raise		
Reactive postural response	14. In-place response—forward		
	15. In-place response—backward		
	16. Compensatory stepping correction—forward	X	
	17. Compensatory stepping correction—backward	X	
	18. Compensatory stepping correction—lateral	X	X Test both directions (two items)
Sensory orientation	19. Sensory integration for balance (Modified Clinical Test of Sensory Interaction in Balance [CTSIB])	X Eyes open and closed standing on foam surface	X Eyes closed on foam surface
	20. Incline—eyes closed	X	
Stability in gait	21. Gait level surface 20 feet		
	22. Change in gait speed	X	
	23. Walk with head turns—horizontal	X	
	24. Walk with pivot turns	X	
	25. Step over obstacles	X	
	26. Timed "get up and go"		X
	27. Timed "get up and go" with dual task	X	

TABLE 7.13 Normative Scores for the BESTest, Mini BESTest, and Brief BESTest

	60–69	70–79	80–89
Maximum Score			
BESTest %	91.4	85.4	79.4
Mini-BESTest	24.7/28	21.0/28	19.6/28
Brief-BESTest	20.5/24	18.8/24	15.0/24

impairments across six contexts of postural control: mechanical constraints, limits of stability, anticipatory postural adjustments, reactive postural responses, sensory orientation, and gait. The results of the test allow the clinician to tailor interventions to the specific postural control system indicated. The test has a total score of 108 points, calculated to a percentage score. Each context is scored separately on a scale of 0 to 3 (3 = no impairment). The test includes functional reach test, floor rise test, sit to stand, single-leg stance, Romberg (eyes open and closed), items from the Dynamic Gait Index, Timed Up and Go, and Dual-Task Timed Up and Go. It is a reliable and valid test for community-dwelling older adults with and without balance deficits.[181–183] The BESTest takes about 45 minutes to administer. Because of the length of the BESTest, two different versions were developed, the Mini-BESTest and the Brief-BESTest.

The Mini-BESTest is a shortened version of the original BESTest. It has 14 items scored from 0 to 2 with a maximum score of 28.[184] The items chosen had the highest correlation with the overall/complete score of the BESTest using a Rasch analysis.[184] King and Horak[185] clarified an error in the scoring of the Mini-BESTest as proposed by Godi et al. in 2012[186] with clarified testing instructions and scoring form. The Mini version can be administered in 15 to 20 minutes and is as reliable and capable of detecting fall status as the original version.[187] The construct differs from the BESTest as it only considers dynamic balance by omitting items related to mechanical constraints and limits of stability (see Table 7.13).[182] The Mini-BESTest has similar clinimetric properties as the BESTest.[182]

The brief version of the BESTest was developed to improve the clinical utility of the BESTest and to preserve the construct validity of the BESTest. The Brief-BESTest included the most representative item from each of the six domain sections of the original BESTest for a total of 8 items scored 0 to 3 with a maximum score of 24 (see Table 7.13). The Brief-BESTest has similar clinimetric properties as the BESTest and Mini-BESTest.[182]

Directions. Full directions, test forms, and training opportunities can be found at http://bestest.us/ for the original and Mini-BEST versions. Equipment required includes stopwatch, 36" ruler, 4" foam pad (12" × 12"), 10-degree-incline ramp, 6" stair step, two stacked shoe boxes, 5-lb free weight, and chair with arms. The authors emphasize that only the worst performance in items "stand on one leg" and "lateral stepping" are to be scored. Item 14 (Mini-BESTest) is clarified by the authors as "if a person's gait slows >10% between the TUG with and without a dual task, the score should be decreased by a point."[185]

Interpretation. Higher scores indicate better performance. All three versions can detect fallers. With a cutoff score of 59% in the group with fall history and a cutoff score of 95% in the group without fall history, the Brief-BESTest had an Sn and Sp of 1 with an accuracy of 100% to differentiate people with and without a self-reported recent fall history. The cutoff score of 69% on the Mini-BESTest demonstrated an Sn of 0.71 and Sp of 1 (+LR = 71; −LR = 0.28) with an accuracy of 92%. The cutoff score of 77% on the BESTest demonstrated an Sn of 0.86 and Sp of 0.95 (+LR = 17.20; −LR = 0.09) with an accuracy of 92%.[182] Normative data for all three versions is listed in Table 7.14.[188] The BESTest has a calculated MDC of 8.9%.[181]

Fullerton Advanced Balance Scale. The Fullerton Advanced Balance Scale (FAB) assesses static and dynamic balance under varying sensory conditions. It is designed to measure balance in higher-functioning active older adults. The test is made up of 10 performance-based activities scored on an ordinal scale of 0 to 4 (Box 7.6). A total score of 40 points is possible. The test is made of four dimensions: static balance (items 2 and 6), dynamic balance (items 3–5 and 8), sensory reception and integration (items 1, 7, and 9), and reactive postural control (item 10). The FAB takes approximately 10 to 12 minutes to

TABLE 7.14 Comparison of the Dynamic Gait Index (DGI), Functional Gait Assessment, and 4-Item DGI

Dynamic Gait Index Maximum Score = 28	Functional Gait Assessment Maximum Score = 30	4-Item DGI Maximum Score = 12
Gait with level surface (20 feet)	Gait with level surface (20 feet)	Gait with level surface (20 feet)
Change in gait speed	Change in gait speed	Change in gait speed
Gait with horizontal head turns	Gait with horizontal head turns	Gait with horizontal head turns
Gait with vertical head turns	Gait with vertical head turns	Gait with vertical head turns
Gait and pivot turn	Gait and pivot turn	
Step over obstacle	Step over obstacle	
Step around obstacle	Gait with narrow base of support Gait with eyes closed Ambulate backward	
Stairs	Stairs	

BOX 7.6 Fullerton Advanced Balance (FAB) Scale Items

1. Stand with feet together and eyes closed
2. Reach forward to retrieve an object held at shoulder height with outstretched arm
3. Turn 360 degrees in right and left directions
4. Step up onto and over a 6-inch bench
5. Tandem walk
6. Stand on one leg
7. Stand on foam with eyes closed
8. Two-footed jump for distance
9. Walk with head turns
10. Reactive postural control

administer. It is a reliable and valid test to assess balance function in higher-functioning older adults and can discriminate between varying balance abilities.[189,190]

Directions. Instructions for test administration and testing form are freely available from the Internet. Equipment needed includes a stopwatch, 36" ruler, 6" bench, metronome (available as a phone app), two foam Airex pads, and one or more lengths of nonslip material.

Interpretation. Mean scores were 24.7/40 (SD = 7.5) for individuals with a mean age of 76.4 (SD = 7.1).[190] The probability of falling increased by 8% with each 1-point decrease in total FAB scale score.[191]

Community Balance and Mobility Scale. The Community Balance and Mobility Scale (CBM) assesses higher-level balance and mobility skills through performance of tasks that are common to community environments. The purpose of the CBM is to reflect balance and mobility skills necessary for full participation in the community. Thirteen tasks make up the test (Box 7.7) scored from 0 (inability) to 5 for a maximum score of 96. Item arrangement reflects progressive task difficulty. The test takes 20 to 30 minutes to administer. It is reliable, valid, and responsive to change in community-dwelling older adults, those with arthritis, those in cardiac rehabilitation, and those with stroke.[192–195] The CBM does not have the

BOX 7.7 Community Balance and Mobility Scale Tasks

1. Unilateral stance
2. Tandem walking
3. 180-degree tandem pivot
4. Lateral foot scooting
5. Hopping forward
6. Crouch and walk
7. Lateral dodging
8. Walking and looking
9. Running with a controlled stop
10. Forward to backward walking
11. Walk, look, and carry
12. Descending stairs
13. Step-ups × one step

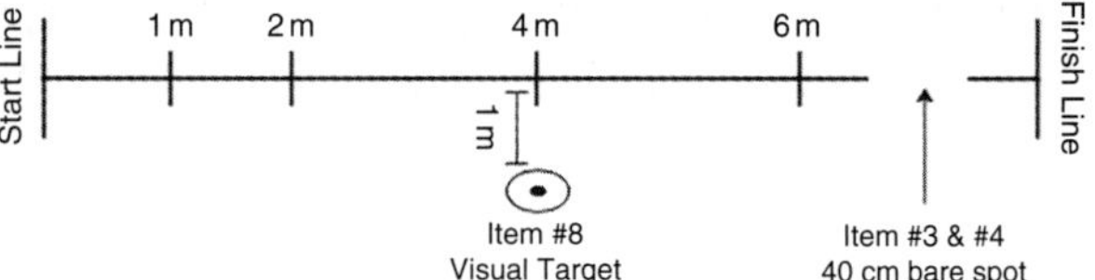

FIG. 7.8 Community balance and mobility scale track setup. *(From Howe J, Inness EL, Wright V. The community balance and mobility scale. The Center for Outcome Measurement in Brain Injury. http://www.tbims.org/combi/cbm. https://www.physio-pedia.com/File:8-meter_measured_track.png.)*

ceiling effects of other measures of balance (e.g., BBS) and correlates with the FAB; therefore, it may be more useful for healthy, higher-functioning, younger community-dwelling older adults.[68,196,197]

Directions. Directions are freely available from the Internet. Equipment needed includes a laundry basket, 2- and 7-lb weights, a bean bag, a visual target, and stairs. Tasks are conducted on an 8-m track that is 2 m wide (Fig. 7.8). The test is to be done without a mobility aid and is tested on both sides.

Interpretation. In a group of older women with low bone mass, a mean score of 42 (SD = 19) was achieved with a range of scores of 0 to 81. In a small sample, normative scores for healthy individuals aged 60 to 69 and 70 to 79 were 65 (SD = 8) and 50 (SD = 7), respectively.[198] An MDC_{90} of 8 points is recommended by the authors.[198] The authors also suggest a score <45 may be a threshold below which community integration could be at risk.[198]

Dynamic Gait Index. The Dynamic Gait Index (DGI) was developed to assess postural stability during gait tasks in the older adult over 60 years of age at risk for falling. It is designed to capture the ability to adapt gait to complex tasks. The test consists of 8 items with varying demands (Table 7.15), scored on a four-level ordinal scale (0–3) with a maximum possible score of 24. The new scoring system, developed in 2013, is reliable and valid.[199]

A 4-item DGI was developed through a Rasch analysis to shorten the test. The 4 items are listed in Table 7.15 and are scored on a scale of 0 to 3 with a maximum score of 12.

Directions. The scoring system for the original 8 item DGI was modified and expanded in 2013.[199] The new scoring system, called the modified DGI, includes time, level of assistance, and gait pattern for each task to attempt to avoid the ceiling effect noted with the original DGI. The test allows the use of an assistive device but results in a loss of points.

Interpretation. A score of 19 or less on the original DGI indicates an increased risk of falling in older adults[200] and in patients with vestibular disorders. It is reliable and valid as well as responsive.[200,201] Fall risk is indicated on the 4-item DGI with a score of <10.[202] An MDC_{95} of 4 points was found for the DGI and it has demonstrated a ceiling effect.[203]

Functional Gait Assessment. The Functional Gait Assessment (FGA) was developed to clarify the ambiguous directions of the DGI and to add more challenging

TABLE 7.15 Recommended Functional Outcome Measures by Setting

Tool	Acute	Subacute/Rehab	Home Health	Outpatient	Wellness
ABC/Falls Efficacy		X	X	X	
Walking Speed	X	X	X	X	X
Sit to Stand		X	X	X	X
Floor Transfer			X	X	X
Stair Climb		X	X	X	
Timed Up and Go	X	X	X		
Distance Walk Tests	2MWT	ALL	2MWT	6MWT 400 meter	400 meter
Short Physical Performance Battery (SPPB)		X	X	X	
Physical Performance Test (PPT)		X	X		
Straight-leg stance (SLS), Romberg, Sharpened Romberg		X	X	X	X
Four-Square Step Test		X	X	X	
Functional Reach Test and Multidirectional Reach Test		X	X	X	
Berg Balance Scale (BBS)		X	X	X	
Performance-Oriented Mobility Assessment (POMA)					
Fullerton				X	X
Community Balance and Mobility Scale				X	X
Balance Evaluation Systems Test (BEST)					
Dynamic Gait Index (DGI)				X	
Functional Gait Assessment				X	
Postural Assessment of Stroke Scale (PASS)	X	X	X		
Stopping Elderly Accidents Deaths and Injuries (STEADI)					

items for people with vestibular disorders. It is composed of 10 items that include 7 of the 8 items from the DGI and 3 new items (Table 7.15). Each item is scored on an ordinal scale of 0 to 3, with 3 indicating better performance. The FGA is reliable and valid, demonstrating consistency with other balance measures with vestibular disorders.[204] The test can have a ceiling effect similar to the DGI.[203]

Directions. Directions and the scoring form are freely available from the Internet.

Interpretation. An FGA cutoff score of 22/30 is effective in classifying fall risk in older adults and predicting unexplained falls in community-dwelling older adults.[205] Reference scores decreased by decade (60 to 69 years = 27.1 [SD = 2.3]; 70 to 79 years = 24.9 [SD = 3.6]; 80 to 89 years = 20.8 [SD = 4.7]).[206] An MDC_{95} of 6 points was found for the FGA.[202]

Postural Assessment Scale for Stroke. The Postural Assessment for Stroke Scale (PASS) is a 12-item performance-based scale used for assessing postural control in people with stroke through a full spectrum of tasks increasing in difficulty from rolling to picking up a pencil from the floor. The test is highly recommended by the American Physical Therapy Association (APTA) Neurology Task Force on Stroke (StrokEDGE). Task activities are listed in Box 7.8 and consist of 5 items of static balance and 7 items considered to represent dynamic tasks. The PASS is reliable and valid in individuals with stroke[207,208] and dementia.[75] The test is responsive in individuals with acute, subacute, and chronic stroke with an MDC of 1 to 3 points.[208,209] Because of the range of tasks, it is unlikely to have a floor effect.

BOX 7.8 Tasks Composing the Postural Assessment of Stroke Scale in Order of Difficulty

STATIC Items

1. Sitting without support (sitting on the edge of exam table with feet touching the floor)
2. Standing with support (feet position free, no other constraints)
3. Standing without support (feet position free, no other constraints)
4. Standing on nonparetic leg (no other constraints)
5. Standing on paretic leg (no other constraints)

DYNAMIC Items

6. Supine to affected side lateral
7. Supine to nonaffected side lateral
8. Supine to sitting up on the edge of the table
9. Sitting on the edge of the table to supine
10. Sitting to standing up
11. Standing up to sitting down
12. Standing, picking up a pencil from the floor

Directions. The directions for the PASS test are freely available on the Internet (https://www.sralab.org/rehabilitation-measures/postural-assessment-scale-stroke#older-adults-and-geriatric-care). Each of the 12 items is assessed on a 4-point scale (0 to 3) with a maximum score of 36.

Interpretation. Cutoff scores of the total PASS indicating patient ambulation at discharge is >12.5 (Sn = 0.79; Sp = 0.84; +LR = 4.94; −LR = 0.06).[210] Static PASS score of >3.5 points were threefold higher than for those scoring <3.5 for walking at discharge (Sn = 0.78; Sp = 0.82).[210] Scores on the dynamic PASS >8.5 had threefold higher odds of walking at discharge compared with those scoring <8.5 (Sn = 0.78; Sp = 0.83; +LR = 4.59; −LR = 0.06).[210]

Stopping Elderly Accidents Deaths and Injuries (STEADI). The Stopping Elderly Accidents Deaths and Injuries (STEADI) tool was designed by the Center for Disease Control and Prevention's Injury Control Center in 2013 to help health care providers in primary care to incorporate best-practice fall prevention assessment into their practices. The STEADI assessment of fall risk uses performance on three tests: TUG, four-stage static balance test, and 30-second sit to stand. With the results of these three tools combined with a falls history and results of a questionnaire, appropriate referral can be made to obtain the appropriate intervention. The questionnaire is composed of 12 questions about risk factors for falls. A score of 4 or more indicates an increased risk of falling and directs the clinician to evaluate gait, strength, and balance through the performance of the TUG, 30-s STS, and four-stage balance test.[211] The toolkit translates the fall risk assessment and treatment process into specific activities through an algorithm that largely follows the American Geriatric Society/British Geriatric Society clinical guideline on falls.[212]

The toolkit includes information for the primary care provider regarding background information about the burden of falls, medications associated with falls, and a table of the most modifiable fall risk factors. It illustrates the use of STEADI in three case studies. The STEADI tool provides customizable referral forms including one for community-based exercise programs, and patient education information including information about preventable risk factors, a home safety checklist, and information about performing the chair rise exercise to address leg strength.

Directions. Training on the implementation and use of the STEADI program can be completed online and all materials are free of cost from the Internet.

Interpretation. Using STEADI criteria, individuals characterized as having moderate fall risk at baseline were 2.6 times as likely to experience a fall in the next 4 years as those with low risk.[213] Those characterized as high risk at baseline were almost five times as likely to experience a fall compared with individuals characterized at baseline as low risk.[213]

SUMMARY

FPMs are a mainstay of the geriatric physical therapy clinician's toolbox. FPMs can provide relevancy to the individual's goals, provide the clinician with actual performance data and likely impairments to inform the treatment plan, and demonstrate progress. The FPMs described in this chapter are commonly used in various settings (see Box 7.3) based on their validity, feasibility, and construct. The accuracy, indicated by the likelihood ratios, may be the least important aspect of the FPM's utility as in most cases, the posttest probability does not change the pretest probability to a meaningful extent. Therefore, it is incumbent on the physical therapist to use evidence-informed clinical reasoning to determine probability of risk, especially related to falls, and to identify the best FPM to inform factors related to the risk.

REFERENCES

1. World Health Organization. *International Classification of Functioning, Disability and Health (ICF).* http://www.who.int/classifications/icf/en/. Published 2018. Accessed July 31, 2018.
2. Reiman MP, Manske RC. The assessment of function: how is it measured? A clinical perspective. *J Man Manip Ther.* 2011;19(2):91–99. https://doi.org/10.1179/106698111X12973307659546.
3. Marko M, Neville CG, Prince MA, Ploutz-Snyder LL. Lower-extremity force decrements identify early mobility decline among community-dwelling older adults. *Phys Ther.* 2012;92(9):1148–1159. https://doi.org/10.2522/ptj.20110239.
4. Tripicchio B, Bykerk K, Wegner C, Wegner J. Increasing patient participation: the effects of training physical and occupational therapists to involve geriatric patients in the concerns-clarification and goal-setting processes. *J Phys Ther Educ.* 2009;23(1):55–63. http://search.ebscohost.com/login.aspx?direct=true&db=rzh&AN=2010324894&site=ehost-live.
5. Rikli RE, Jones CJ. *Senior Fitness Test Manual.* Champaign, IL: Human Kinetics; 2001.
6. Lenze EJ, Host HH, Hildebrand MW, et al. Enhanced medical rehabilitation increases therapy intensity and engagement and improves functional outcomes in postacute rehabilitation of older adults: a randomized-controlled trial. *J Am Med Dir Assoc.* 2012;13(8):708–712. https://doi.org/10.1016/j.jamda.2012.06.014.
7. Andrews AW, Chinworth SA, Bourassa M, Garvin M, Benton D, Tanner S. Update on distance and velocity requirements for community ambulation. *J Geriatr Phys Ther.* 2010;33(3):128–134.
8. Shumway-Cook A, Patla AE, Stewart A, Ferrucci L, Ciol MA, Guralnik JM. Environmental demands associated with community mobility in older adults with and without mobility disabilities. *Phys Ther.* 2002;82(7):670–681. http://www.ncbi.nlm.nih.gov/pubmed/12088464. Accessed January 8, 2019.
9. Cesari M. Role of gait speed in the assessment of older patients. *JAMA.* 2011;305(1):93–94. https://doi.org/10.1001/jama.2010.1970.
10. Puthoff ML, Nielsen DH. Relationships among impairments in lower-extremity strength and power, functional limitations, and disability in older adults. *Phys Ther.* 2007;87:1334–1347.
11. Jan MH, Chai HM, Lin YF, et al. Effects of age and sex on the results of an ankle plantar-flexor manual muscle test. *Phys Ther.* 2005;85(10):1078–1084.
12. Lunsford BR, Perry J. The standing heel-rise test for ankle plantar flexion: criterion for normal. *Phys Ther.* 1995;75(8):694–698. http://www.ncbi.nlm.nih.gov/pubmed/7644573. Accessed January 8, 2019.
13. Zelik KE, Adamczyk PG. A unified perspective on ankle push-off in human walking. *J Exp Biol.* 2016;219(Pt 23):3676–3683. https://doi.org/10.1242/jeb.140376.
14. Corrigan D, Bohannon RW. Relationship between knee extension force and stand-up performance in community-dwelling elderly women. *Arch Phys Med Rehabil.* 2001;82(12):1666–1672.

15. Eriksrud O, Bohannon RW. Relationship of knee extension force to independence in sit-to-stand performance in patients receiving acute rehabilitation. *Phys Ther.* 2003;83 (6):544–551.
16. Keller K, Engelhardt M. Strength and muscle mass loss with aging process. Age and strength loss. *Muscles Ligaments Tendons J.* 2013;3(4):346–350. http://www.ncbi.nlm.nih.gov/pubmed/24596700. Accessed January 8, 2019.
17. Glenn JM, Gray M, Binns A. Relationship of sit-to-stand lower-body power with functional fitness measures among older adults with and without sarcopenia. *J Geriatr Phys Ther.* 2017;40 (1):42–50. https://doi.org/10.1519/JPT.0000000000000072.
18. Brodaty H, Low L, Gibson L, Burns K. What is the best dementia screening instrument for general practitioners to use? *Am J Geriatr Psychiatry.* 2006;14(5):391–400. http://ovidsp.ovid.com.libproxy1.upstate.edu/ovidweb.cgi?T=JS&NEWS=N&PAGE=fulltext&AN=00019442-200605000-00003&D=ovfth.
19. Pescatello LS, Arena R, Riebe D, Thompson PD. *ACSM's Guidelines for Exercise Testing and Prescription.* 9th ed. Baltimore, MD: Wolters Kluwer/Lippincott Williams & Wilkins; 2014.
20. Stratford PW, Kennedy DM. Performance measures were necessary to obtain a complete picture of osteoarthritic patients. *J Clin Epidemiol.* 2006;59(2):160–167. https://doi.org/10.1016/J.JCLINEPI.2005.07.012.
21. Lins L, Carvalho FM. SF-36 total score as a single measure of health-related quality of life: scoping review. *SAGE Open Med.* 2016;4:2050312116671725. https://doi.org/10.1177/2050312116671725.
22. Knäuper B, Carrière K, Chamandy M, Xu Z, Schwarz N, Rosen NO. How aging affects self-reports. *Eur J Ageing.* 2016;13(2):185–193. https://doi.org/10.1007/s10433-016-0369-0.
23. Brach JS, VanSwearingen JM. Physical impairment and disability: relationship to performance of activities of daily living in community-dwelling older men. *Phys Ther.* 2002;82(8):752–761.
24. Kamper SJ, Kamper SJ. Fundamentals of measurement: linking evidence to practice. *J Orthop Phys Ther.* 2019;49 (2):114–115. https://doi.org/10.2519/jospt.2019.0701.
25. Tariq SH, Tumosa N, Chibnall JT, Perry MH, Morley JE. The Saint Louis University Mental Status (SLUMS) | Measurement Instrument Database for the Social Sciences. http://www.midss.org/content/saint-louis-university-mental-status-slums. Published 2019. Accessed March 14, 2019.
26. Portney LG, Watkins MP. *Foundations of Clinical Research.* 3rd ed. Philadelphia: F.A. Davis Company; 2015.
27. Lusardi MM, Fritz S, Middleton A, et al. Determining risk of falls in community dwelling older adults. *J Geriatr Phys Ther.* 2017;40(1):1–36. https://doi.org/10.1519/JPT.0000000000000099.
28. Park S-H. Tools for assessing fall risk in the elderly: a systematic review and meta-analysis. *Aging Clin Exp Res.* 2018;30(1):1–16. https://doi.org/10.1007/s40520-017-0749-0.
29. Leveritt M, Abernethy PJ, Barry BK, Logan PA. Concurrent strength and endurance training. A review. *Sports Med.* 1999;28 (6):413–427. https://doi.org/10.2165/00007256-199928060-00004.
30. AbilityLab Shirley Ryan. Rehabilitation Measures. https://www.sralab.org/rehabilitation-measures. Published 2013. Accessed March 14, 2019.
31. PTNow from APTA. https://www.ptnow.org/Default.aspx. Accessed March 30, 2019.
32. Physiopedia contributors. Category: Older People/Geriatrics. Physiopedia. https://www.physio-pedia.com/Category:Older_People/Geriatrics. Published 2018. Accessed March 25, 2019.
33. Huang T-T, Wang W-S. Comparison of three established measures of fear of falling in community-dwelling older adults: psychometric testing. *Int J Nurs Stud.* 2009;46(10):1313–1319. https://doi.org/10.1016/j.ijnurstu.2009.03.010.
34. Landers MR, Durand C, Powell DS, Dibble LE, Young DL. Development of a scale to assess avoidance behavior due to a fear of falling: the Fear of Falling Avoidance Behavior Questionnaire. *Phys Ther.* 2011;91(8):1253–1265. https://doi.org/10.2522/ptj.20100304.
35. Powell LE, Myers AM. The Activities-specific Balance Confidence (ABC) Scale. *J Gerontol A Biol Sci Med Sci.* 1995;50A(1):M28–M34. http://www.ncbi.nlm.nih.gov/pubmed/7814786. Accessed March 23, 2019.
36. Lajoie Y, Gallagher SP. Predicting falls within the elderly community: comparison of postural sway, reaction time, the Berg balance scale and the Activities-specific Balance Confidence (ABC) scale for comparing fallers and non-fallers. *Arch Gerontol Geriatr.* 2004;38(1):11–26.
37. Portegijs E, Edgren J, Salpakoski A, et al. Balance confidence was associated with mobility and balance performance in older people with fall-related hip fracture: a cross-sectional study. *Arch Phys Med Rehabil.* 2012;93(12):2340–2346. https://doi.org/10.1016/j.apmr.2012.05.022.
38. Wang Y-C, Sindhu B, Lehman L, Li X, Yen S-C, Kapellusch J. Rasch analysis of the activities-specific balance confidence scale in older adults seeking outpatient rehabilitation services. *J Orthop Sport Phys Ther.* 2018;48(7):574–583. https://doi.org/10.2519/jospt.2018.8023.
39. Dewan N, MacDermid JC. Fall Efficacy Scale - International (FES-I). *J Physiother.* 2014;60(1):60. https://doi.org/10.1016/j.jphys.2013.12.014.
40. Yardley L, Beyer N, Hauer K, Kempen G, Piot-Ziegler C, Todd C. Development and initial validation of the Falls Efficacy Scale-International (FES-I). *Age Ageing.* 2005;34 (6):614–619. https://doi.org/10.1093/ageing/afi196.
41. Hauer K, Yardley L, Beyer N, et al. Validation of the Falls Efficacy Scale and Falls Efficacy Scale International in geriatric patients with and without cognitive impairment: results of self-report and interview-based questionnaires. *Gerontology.* 2010;56(2):190–199. https://doi.org/10.1159/000236027.
42. Kempen GIJM, Yardley L, Van Haastregt JCM, et al. The Short FES-I: a shortened version of the Falls Efficacy Scale-International to assess fear of falling. *Age Ageing.* 2007;37 (1):45–50. https://doi.org/10.1093/ageing/afm157.
43. Delbaere K, Crombez G, Vanderstraeten G, Willems T, Cambier D. Fear-related avoidance of activities, falls and physical frailty. A prospective community-based cohort study. *Age Ageing.* 2004;33(4):368–373. https://doi.org/10.1093/ageing/afh106.
44. Cumming RG, Salkeld G, Thomas M, Szonyi G. Prospective study of the impact of fear of falling on activities of daily living, SF-36 scores, and nursing home admission. PubMed - NCBI. *J Gerontol A Biol Sci Med Sci.* 2000;55(5):M299–M305. https://www.ncbi.nlm.nih.gov/pubmed/10819321. Accessed March 26, 2019.
45. Adell E, Wehmhörner S, Rydwik E. The test-retest reliability of 10 meters maximal walking speed in older people living in a residential care unit. *J Geriatr Phys Ther.* 2013;36(2):74–77. https://doi.org/10.1519/JPT.0b013e318264b8ed.
46. Hars M, Herrmann FR, Trombetti A. Reliability and minimal detectable change of gait variables in community-dwelling and hospitalized older fallers. *Gait Posture.* 2013;38(4):1010–1014. https://doi.org/10.1016/j.gaitpost.2013.05.015.
47. Peel NM, Kuys SS, Klein K. Gait speed as a measure in geriatric assessment in clinical settings: a systematic review. *J Gerontol Ser A.* 2013;68(1):39–46. https://doi.org/10.1093/gerona/gls174.

48. Abellan van Kan G, Rolland Y, Andrieu S, et al. Gait speed at usual pace as a predictor of adverse outcomes in community-dwelling older people an International Academy on Nutrition and Aging (IANA) Task Force. *J Nutr Health Aging*. 2009;13(10):881–889.
49. Liu B, Hu X, Zhang Q, et al. Usual walking speed and all-cause mortality risk in older people: a systematic review and meta-analysis. *Gait Posture*. 2016;44:172–177. https://doi.org/10.1016/j.gaitpost.2015.12.008.
50. Kikkert LHJ, Vuillerme N, van Campen JP, Hortobágyi T, Lamoth CJ. Walking ability to predict future cognitive decline in old adults: a scoping review. *Ageing Res Rev*. 2016;27:1–14. https://doi.org/10.1016/j.arr.2016.02.001.
51. Perera S, Patel KV, Rosano C, et al. Gait speed predicts incident disability: a pooled analysis. *J Gerontol Ser A Biol Sci Med Sci*. 2016;71(1):63–71. https://doi.org/10.1093/gerona/glv126.
52. Noce Kirkwood R, de Souza Moreira B, Mingoti SA, Faria BF, Sampaio RF, Alves Resende R. The slowing down phenomenon: what is the age of major gait velocity decline? *Maturitas*. 2018;115:31–36. https://doi.org/10.1016/j.maturitas.2018.06.005.
53. Salbach NM, O'Brien K, Brooks D, et al. Speed and distance requirements for community ambulation: a systematic review. *Arch Phys Med Rehabil*. 2014;95(1):117–128.e11. https://doi.org/10.1016/j.apmr.2013.06.017.
54. Winter DA. Human balance and posture control during standing and walking; *Gait and Posture*. 1995;3(4):193–214.
55. Clark DJ, Manini TM, Fielding RA, Patten C. Neuromuscular determinants of maximum walking speed in well-functioning older adults. *Exp Gerontol*. 2013;48(3):358–363. https://doi.org/10.1016/j.exger.2013.01.010.
56. Middleton A, Fritz SL, Lusardi MM. Walking speed: the functional vital sign. *J Aging Phys Act*. 2015;23(2):314–322. https://doi.org/10.1123/japa.2013-0236.
57. Bohannon RW, Williams Andrews A, Andrews AW. Normal walking speed: a descriptive meta-analysis. *Physiotherapy*. 2011;97(3):182–189. https://doi.org/10.1016/j.physio.2010.12.004.
58. Ng S, Au K, Chan D, et al. Effect of acceleration and deceleration distance on the walking speed of people with chronic stroke. *J Rehabil Med*. 2016;48(8):666–670. https://doi.org/10.2340/16501977.
59. Steffen TM, Hacker TA, Mollinger L. Age- and gender-related test performance in community-dwelling elderly people: six-minute walk test, berg balance scale, timed up & go test, and gait speeds. *Phys Ther*. 2002;82(2):128–137.
60. Artaud F, Singh-Manoux A, Dugravot A, Tzourio C, Elbaz A. Decline in fast gait speed as a predictor of disability in older adults. *J Am Geriatr Soc*. 2015;63(6):1129–1136. https://doi.org/10.1111/jgs.13442.
61. Peel NM, Navanathan S, Hubbard RE. Gait speed as a predictor of outcomes in post-acute transitional care for older people. *Geriatr Gerontol Int*. 2014;14(4):906–910. https://doi.org/10.1111/ggi.12191.
62. McCarthy EK, Horvat MA, Holtsberg PA, Wisenbaker JM. Repeated chair stands as a measure of lower limb strength in sexagenarian women. *J Gerontol A Biol Sci Med Sci*. 2004;59(11):1207–1212. http://www.ncbi.nlm.nih.gov/pubmed/15602077. Accessed January 8, 2019.
63. Goldberg A, Chavis M, Watkins J, Wilson T. The five-times-sit-to-stand test: validity, reliability and detectable change in older females. *Aging Clin Exp Res*. 2012;24(4):339–344.
64. Jones CJ, Rikli RE, Beam WC. A 30-s chair-stand test as a measure of lower body strength in community-residing older adults. *Res Q Exerc Sport*. 1999;70(2):113–119. https://doi.org/10.1080/02701367.1999.10608028.
65. Bohannon RW, Crouch R. 1-Minute sit-to-stand test. *J Cardiopulm Rehabil Prev*. 2018;39(1):1. https://doi.org/10.1097/HCR.0000000000000336.
66. Benton MJ, Alexander JL. Validation of functional fitness tests as surrogates for strength measurement in frail, older adults with chronic obstructive pulmonary disease. *Am J Phys Med Rehabil*. 2009;88(7):579–583. https://doi.org/10.1097/PHM.0b013e3181aa2ff8.
67. Tiihonen M, Hartikainen S, Nykänen I. Chair rise capacity and associated factors in older home-care clients. *Scand J Public Health*. 2018;46(7):699–703. https://doi.org/10.1177/1403494817718072.
68. Bergquist R, Weber M, Schwenk M, et al. Performance-based clinical tests of balance and muscle strength used in young seniors: a systematic literature review. *BMC Geriatr*. 2019;19(1):9. https://doi.org/10.1186/s12877-018-1011-0.
69. Boonstra MC, Schwering PJA, De Waal Malefijt MC, Verdonschot N. Sit-to-stand movement as a performance-based measure for patients with total knee arthroplasty. *Phys Ther*. 2009;90(2):149–156. https://doi.org/10.2522/ptj.20090119.
70. Blennerhassett JM, Jayalath VM. The Four Square Step Test is a feasible and valid clinical test of dynamic standing balance for use in ambulant people poststroke. *Arch Phys Med Rehabil*. 2008;89(11):2156–2161. https://doi.org/10.1016/j.apmr.2008.05.012.
71. French HP, Fitzpatrick M, FitzGerald O. Responsiveness of physical function outcomes following physiotherapy intervention for osteoarthritis of the knee: an outcome comparison study. *Physiotherapy*. 2011;97(4):302–308. https://doi.org/10.1016/j.physio.2010.03.002.
72. Silva PFS, Quintino LF, Franco J, et al. Measurement properties and feasibility of clinical tests to assess sit-to-stand/stand-to-sit tasks in subjects with neurological disease: a systematic review. *Brazilian J Phys Ther*. 2014;18(2):99–110. https://doi.org/10.1590/S1413-35552012005000155.
73. Tiedemann A, Shimada H, Sherrington C, Murray S, Lord S. The comparative ability of eight functional mobility tests for predicting falls in community-dwelling older people. *Age Ageing*. 2008;37(4):430–435. https://doi.org/10.1093/ageing/afn100.
74. Bohannon RW. Test-retest reliability of the five-repetition sit-to-stand test: a systematic review of the literature involving adults. *J Strength Cond Res*. 2011;25(11):3205–3207. https://doi.org/10.1519/JSC.0b013e318234e59f.
75. Blankevoort CG, van Heuvelen MJG, Scherder EJA. Reliability of six physical performance tests in older people with dementia. *Phys Ther*. 2013;93(1):69–78. https://doi.org/10.2522/ptj.20110164.
76. Bohannon RW. Reference values for the five-repetition sit-to-stand test: a descriptive meta-analysis of data from elders. *Percept Mot Skills*. 2006;103(1):215–222. https://www.ncbi.nlm.nih.gov/pubmed/17037663. Accessed March 16, 2019.
77. Jordre B, Schweinle W, Beacom K, Graphenteen V, Ladwig A. The five times sit to stand test in senior athletes. *J Geriatr Phys Ther*. 2013;36(1):47–50. https://doi.org/10.1519/JPT.0b013e31826317b5.
78. Rikli RE, Jones CJ. Functional fitness normative scores for community-residing older adults, ages 60-94. *J Aging Phys Act*. 1999;7:162–181.
79. Schaubert KL, Bohannon RW. Reliability and validity of three strength measures obtained from community-dwelling elderly persons. *J Strength Cond Res*. 2005;19(3):717–720.
80. Rikli RE, Jones CJ. Development and validation of criterion-referenced clinically relevant fitness standards for maintaining physical independence in later years. *Gerontologist*. 2013;53(2):255–267.

81. Jeoung BJ, Lee YC. A Study of relationship between frailty and physical performance in elderly women. *J Exerc Rehabil.* 2015;11(4):215–219. https://doi.org/10.12965/jer.150223.
82. Pinheiro PA, Carneiro JAO, Coqueiro RS, Pereira R, Fernandes MH. "Chair stand test" as simple tool for sarcopenia screening in elderly women. *J Nutr Health Aging.* 2015;20(1):56–59. https://doi.org/10.1007/s12603-015-0621-x.
83. Nishimura T, Arima K, Okabe T, et al. Usefulness of chair stand time as a surrogate of gait speed in diagnosing sarcopenia. *Geriatr Gerontol Int.* 2017;17(4):659–661. https://doi.org/10.1111/ggi.12766.
84. Buatois S, Miljkovic D, Manckoundia P, et al. Five times sit to stand test is a predictor of recurrent falls in healthy community-living subject aged 65 and older. *J Am Geriatr Soc.* 2008;56(8):1575–1577. https://doi.org/10.1111/j.1532-5415.2008.01777.x.
85. Zhang F, Ferrucci L, Culham E, Metter EJ, Guralnik J, Deshpande N. Performance on five times sit-to-stand task as a predictor of subsequent falls and disability in older persons. *J Aging Health.* 2013;25(3):478–492. https://doi.org/10.1177/0898264313475813; 10.1177/0898264313475813.
86. Makizako H, Shimada H, Doi T, et al. Predictive cutoff values of the five-times sit-to-stand test and the timed "up & go" test for disability incidence in older people dwelling in the community. *Phys Ther.* 2017;97(4):417–424.
87. Fleming J, Brayne C, Cambridge City over-75s Cohort (CC75C) Study Collaboration. Inability to get up after falling, subsequent time on floor, and summoning help: prospective cohort study in people over 90. *BMJ.* 2008;337: a2227. https://doi.org/10.1136/bmj.a2227.
88. Ganz DA, Bao Y, Shekelle PG, Rubenstein LZ. Will my patient fall? *JAMA.* 2007;297(1):77–86. https://doi.org/10.1001/jama.297.1.77.
89. Bergland A, Wyller TB. Risk factors for serious fall related injury in elderly women living at home. *Inj Prev.* 2004;10 (5):308–313. http://ip.bmjjournals.com/cgi/content/abstract/10/5/308.
90. Wang C-Y, Olson SL, Protas EJ. Physical-performance tests to evaluate mobility disability in community-dwelling elders. *J Aging Phys Act.* 2005;13(2):184–197. http://www.ncbi.nlm.nih.gov/pubmed/15995264. Accessed March 16, 2019.
91. Ardali G, Brody LT, States RA, Godwin EM. Reliability and validity of the floor transfer test as a measure of readiness for independent living among older adults. *J Geriatr Phys Ther.* 2017;1. https://doi.org/10.1519/JPT.0000000000000142.
92. Ng SSM, Fong SSM, Chan CWL, et al. Floor transfer for assessing people with chronic stroke. *J Rehabil Med.* 2015;47(8):489–494. https://doi.org/10.2340/16501977-1958.
93. Bergland A, Laake K. Concurrent and predictive validity of "getting up from lying on the floor." *Aging Clin Exp Res.* 2005;17(3):181–185.
94. Nightingale EJ, Pourkazemi F, Hiller CE. Systematic review of timed stair tests. *J Rehabil Res Dev.* 2014;51(3):335–350. https://doi.org/10.1682/JRRD.2013.06.0148.
95. Mckay MJ, Baldwin JN, Ferreira P, Simic M, Vanicek N, Burns J. Reference values for developing responsive functional outcome measures across the lifespan. *Neurology.* 2017;88(16):1512–1519.
96. Ng SS, Ng HH, Chan KM, Lai JC, To AK, Yeung CW. Reliability of the 12-step ascend and descend test and its correlation with motor function in people with chronic stroke. *J Rehabil Med.* 2013;45(2):123–129. https://doi.org/10.2340/16501977-1086; 10.2340/16501977-1086.
97. Hamel KA, Cavanagh PR. Stair performance in people aged 75 and older. *J Am Geriatr Soc.* 2004;52(4):563–567. https://doi.org/10.1111/j.1532-5415.2004.52162.x.
98. Podsiadlo D, Richardson S. The timed "Up & Go": a test of basic functional mobility for frail elderly persons. *J Am Geriatr Soc.* 1991;39(2):142–148. http://www.ncbi.nlm.nih.gov/pubmed/1991946. Accessed March 18, 2019.
99. Gallagher R. Timed Up and Go. Shirley Ryan Ability Lab. https://www.sralab.org/rehabilitation-measures/timed-and-go. Published 2013.
100. Steffen T, Seney M. Test-retest reliability and minimal detectable change on balance and ambulation tests, the 36-item short-form health survey, and the unified Parkinson disease rating scale in people with parkinsonism. *Phys Ther.* 2008;88(6):733–746.
101. Ries JD, Echternach JL, Nof L, Gagnon Blodgett M. Test-retest reliability and minimal detectable change scores for the timed "up & go" test, the six-minute walk test, and gait speed in people with Alzheimer disease. *Phys Ther.* 2009;89 (6):569–579. https://doi.org/10.2522/ptj.20080258.
102. Brooks D, Davis AM, Naglie G. Validity of 3 physical performance measures in inpatient geriatric rehabilitation. *Arch Phys Med Rehabil.* 2006;87(1):105–110. http://www.sciencedirect.com/science/article/B6WB6-4J08C1R-R/2/6b6625601de9d75c4bc2c3968804b9b9.
103. Bischoff HA, Stahelin HB, Monsch AU, et al. Identifying a cut-off point for normal mobility: a comparison of the timed "up and go" test in community-dwelling and institutionalised elderly women. *Age Ageing.* 2003;32(3):315–320.
104. Beauchet O, Fantino B, Allali G, et al. Timed Up and Go test and risk of falls in older adults: a systematic review. *J Nutr Health Aging.* 2011;15(10):933–938.
105. Muir SW, Berg K, Chesworth B, Klar N, Speechley M. Quantifying the magnitude of risk for balance impairment on falls in community-dwelling older adults: a systematic review and meta-analysis. *J Clin Epidemiol.* 2010;63(4):389–406. https://doi.org/10.1016/j.jclinepi.2009.06.010.
106. Schoene D, Wu SM, Mikolaizak AS, et al. Discriminative ability and predictive validity of the Timed Up and Go Test in identifying older people who fall: systematic review and meta-analysis. *J Am Geriatr Soc.* 2013;61(2):202–208. https://doi.org/10.1111/jgs.12106; 10.1111/jgs.12106.
107. Dobson F, Hinman RS, Hall M, Terwee CB, Roos EM, Bennell KL. Measurement properties of performance-based measures to assess physical function in hip and knee osteoarthritis: a systematic review. *Osteoarthr Cartil.* 2012;20 (12):1548–1562. https://doi.org/10.1016/j.joca.2012.08.015.
108. Shumway-Cook A. Predicting the probability for falls in community-dwelling older adults using the Timed Up & Go. Test. *Phys Ther.* 2000;80(9):896–903.
109. Hofheinz M, Schusterschitz C. Dual task interference in estimating the risk of falls and measuring change: a comparative, psychometric study of four measurements. *Clin Rehabil.* 2010;24(9):831–842. https://doi.org/10.1177/0269215510367993.
110. Bohannon RW. Reference values for the Timed Up and Go Test: a descriptive meta-analysis. *J Geriatr Phys Ther.* 2006;29(2):64–68.
111. Kear BM, Guck TP, McGaha AL. Timed Up and Go (TUG) Test: normative reference values for ages 20 to 59 years and relationships with physical and mental health risk factors. *J Prim Care Community Health.* 2016;8(1):9–13. https://doi.org/2150131916659282.
112. Hiengkaew V, Jitaree K, Chaiyawat P. Minimal detectable changes of the Berg Balance Scale, Fugl-Meyer Assessment Scale, Timed "Up & Go" Test, gait speeds, and 2-minute walk test in individuals with chronic stroke with different degrees of ankle plantarflexor tone. *Arch Phys Med Rehabil.* 2012;93(7):1201–1208. https://doi.org/10.1016/j.apmr.2012.01.014; 10.1016/j.apmr.2012.01.014.
113. Vereeck L. Clinical assessment of balance: normative data, and gender and age effects. *Int J Audiol.* 2008;47(2):67–76. https://doi.org/10.1080/14992020701689688.

114. Kool J, Oesch P, Bachmann S. Predictors for living at home after geriatric inpatient rehabilitation: a prospective cohort study. *J Rehabil Med.* 2017;49(2):185–190. https://doi.org/10.2340/16501977-2182.
115. McGough EL, Lin S, Belza B, et al. Systematic reviews a scoping review of physical performance outcome measures used in exercise interventions for older adults with Alzheimer disease and related dementias. *J Geriatr Phys Ther.* 2017;1. https://doi.org/10.1519/JPT.0000000000000159.
116. Wright RW, Baumgarten KM. Shoulder outcomes measures. *J Am Acad Orthop Surg.* 2010;18(7):436–444.
117. Lexell J, Flansbjer U-B, Holmbäck AM, Downham D, Patten C. Reliability of gait performance tests in men and women with hemiparesis after stroke. *J Rehabil Med.* 2005;37(2):75–82. https://doi.org/10.1080/16501970410017215.
118. Dal Bello-Haas V, Klassen L, Sheppard MS, Metcalfe A. Psychometric properties of activity, self-efficacy, and quality-of-life measures in individuals with Parkinson disease. *Physiother Can.* 2011;63(1):47–57. https://doi.org/10.3138/ptc.2009-08.
119. Mangione KK, Craik RL, McCormick AA, et al. Detectable changes in physical performance measures in elderly African Americans. *Phys Ther.* 2010;90(6):921–927. http://ptjournal.apta.org/cgi/content/abstract/90/6/921.
120. American Thoracic Society. American Thoracic Society ATS Statement: Guidelines for the Six-minute walk test. *Am J Respir Crit Care Med.* 2002;166:111–117. https://doi.org/10.1164/rccm.166/1/111.
121. Sadaria KS, Bohannon RW. The 6-Minute Walk Test: a brief review of literature. *Clin Exerc Physiol.* 2001;3(3):127–132.
122. Pradon D, Roche N, Enette L, Zory R. Relationship between lower limb muscle strength and 6-minute walk test performance in stroke patients. *J Rehabil Med.* 2013;45(1):105–108. https://doi.org/10.2340/16501977-1059;10.2340/16501977-1059.
123. Perera S, Mody SH, Woodman RC, Studenski SA. Meaningful change and responsiveness in common physical performance measures in older adults. *J Am Geriatr Soc.* 2006;54(5):743–749. https://doi.org/10.1111/j.1532-5415.2006.00701.x.
124. Pin TW. Psychometric properties of 2-minute walk test: a systematic review. *Arch Phys Med Rehabil.* 2014;95(9):1759–1775. https://doi.org/10.1016/j.apmr.2014.03.034.
125. Simonsick EM, Montgomery PS, Newman AB, Bauer DC, Harris T. Measuring fitness in healthy older adults: the Health ABC Long Distance Corridor Walk. *J Am Geriatr Soc.* 2001;49(11):1544–1548.
126. Chalé-Rush A, Guralnik ÃJM, Walkup MP, et al. Relationship between physical functioning and physical activity in the lifestyle interventions and independence for elders pilot. *J Am Geriatr Soc.* 2010;58(10):1918–1924. https://doi.org/10.1111/j.1532-5415.2010.03008.x.
127. Simonsick EM, Fan ÃE, Fleg JL. Estimating cardiorespiratory fitness in well-functioning older adults: treadmill validation of the long distance corridor walk. *J Am Geriatr Soc.* 2006;54(1):127–132. https://doi.org/10.1111/j.1532-5415.2005.00530.x.
128. Vestergaard S, Patel KV, Bandinelli S, Ferrucci L, Guralnik JM. Characteristics of 400-meter walk test performance and subsequent mortality in older adults. *Rejuvenation Res.* 2009;12(3):177. https://doi.org/10.1089/REJ.2009.0853.
129. Rolland YM, Cesari M, Miller ME, Penninx BW, Atkinson HH, Pahor M. Reliability of the 400-M usual-pace walk test as an assessment of mobility limitation in older adults. *J Am Geriatr Soc.* 2004;52(6):972–976. https://doi.org/10.1111/j.1532-5415.2004.52267.x.
130. Bohannon RW, Bubela D, Magasi S, et al. Comparison of walking performance over the first 2 minutes and the full 6 minutes of the Six-Minute Walk Test. *BMC Res Notes.* 2014;7:269. https://doi.org/10.1186/1756-0500-7-269.
131. Bohannon RW, Crouch R. Minimal clinically important difference for change in 6-minute walk test distance of adults with pathology: a systematic review. *J Eval Clin Pract.* 2017;23(2):377–381. https://doi.org/10.1111/jep.12629.
132. Yazdanyar A, Aziz MM, Enright PL, et al. Association between 6-minute walk test and all-cause mortality, coronary heart disease-specific mortality, and incident coronary heart disease. *J Aging Heal.* 2014;26(4):583–599. https://doi.org/10.1177/0898264314525665.
133. Casanova C, Cote CG, Marin JM, et al. The 6-min walking distance: long-term follow up in patients with COPD. *Eur Respir J.* 2007;29(3):535–540. https://doi.org/10.1183/09031936.00071506.
134. Szekely LA, Oelberg DA, Wright C, et al. Preoperative predictors of operative morbidity and mortality in COPD patients undergoing bilateral lung volume reduction surgery. *Chest.* 1997;111(3):550–558. http://www.ncbi.nlm.nih.gov/pubmed/9118686. Accessed March 19, 2019.
135. Simonsick EM, Newman AB, Nevitt MC, et al. Measuring higher level physical function in well-functioning older adults: expanding familiar approaches in the Health ABC study. *J Gerontol A Biol Sci Med Sci.* 2001;56(10):M644–M649. http://www.ncbi.nlm.nih.gov/pubmed/11584038. Accessed March 28, 2019.
136. Lange-Maia BS, Strotmeyer ES, Harris TB, et al. Physical activity and change in long distance corridor walk performance in the health, aging, and body composition study. *J Am Geriatr Soc.* 2015;63(7):1348–1354. https://doi.org/10.1111/jgs.13487.
137. Pavasini R, Guralnik J, Brown JC, et al. Short Physical Performance Battery and all-cause mortality: systematic review and meta-analysis. *BMC Med.* 2016;14(1):215. https://doi.org/10.1186/s12916-016-0763-7.
138. Guralnik JM, Simonsick EM, Ferrucci L, et al. A short physical performance battery assessing lower extremity function: association with self-reported disability and prediction of mortality and nursing home admission. *J Gerontol.* 1994;49(2):M85–M94. http://www.ncbi.nlm.nih.gov/pubmed/8126356.
139. Freiberger E, de Vreede P, Schoene D, et al. Performance-based physical function in older community-dwelling persons: a systematic review of instruments. *Age Ageing.* 2012;41(6):712–721. https://doi.org/10.1093/ageing/afs099.
140. Bean JF, Kiely DK, Herman S, et al. The relationship between leg power and physical performance in mobility-limited older people. *J Am Geriatr Soc.* 2002;50(3):461–467. http://www.ncbi.nlm.nih.gov/pubmed/11943041. Accessed February 17, 2019.
141. Vasunilashorn S, Coppin AK, Patel KV, et al. Use of the Short Physical Performance Battery Score to predict loss of ability to walk 400 meters: analysis from the InCHIANTI Study. *J Gerontol Ser A Biol Sci Med Sci.* 2009;64A(2):223–229. https://doi.org/10.1093/gerona/gln022.
142. Volpato S, Cavalieri M, Sioulis F, et al. Predictive value of the Short Physical Performance Battery following hospitalization in older patients. *J Gerontol A Biol Sci Med Sci.* 2011;66(1):89–96. https://doi.org/10.1093/gerona/glq167.
143. Reuben DB, Siu AL. An objective measure of physical function of elderly outpatients. The Physical Performance Test. *J Am Geriatr Soc.* 1990;38(10):1105–1112.
144. King MB, Judge JO, Whipple R, Wolfson L. Reliability and responsiveness of two physical performance measures examined in the context of a functional training intervention. *Phys Ther.* 2000;80(1):8–16. http://www.ncbi.nlm.nih.gov/pubmed/10623956. Accessed March 21, 2019.

145. Lusardi MM, Pellecchia GL, Schulman M. Functional performance in community living older adults. *J Geriatr Phys Ther.* 2003;26(3). https://journals.lww.com/jgpt/Fulltext/2003/12000/Functional_Performance_in_Community_Living_Older.3.aspx.
146. Steffen TM. Mollinger LA. Age- and gender-related test performance in community-dwelling adults. *J Neurol Phys Ther.* 2005;29(4):181–188.
147. Rozzini R, Frisoni GB, Ferrucci L, Barbisoni P, Bertozzi B, Trabucchi M. The effect of chronic diseases on physical function. Comparison between activities of daily living scales and the Physical Performance Test. *Age Ageing.* 1997;26(4):281–287. http://www.ncbi.nlm.nih.gov/pubmed/9271291. Accessed March 21, 2019.
148. Brown M, Sinacore DR, Binder EF, Kohrt WM. Physical and performance measures for the identification of mild to moderate frailty. *J Gerontol. Med Sci.* 2000;55A(6): M350–M355.
149. Briggs RC, Gossman MR, Birch R, Drews JE, Shaddeau SA. Balance performance among noninstitutionalized elderly women. *Phys Ther.* 1989;69(9):748–756.
150. Springer BA, Marin R, Cyhan T, Roberts H, Gill NW. Normative values for the unipedal stance test with eyes open and closed. *J Geriatr Phys Ther.* 2007;30(1):8–15. http://www.ncbi.nlm.nih.gov/pubmed/19839175. Accessed March 21, 2019.
151. Franchignoni F, Tesio L, Martino MT, Ricupero C. Reliability of four simple, quantitative tests of balance and mobility in healthy elderly females. *Aging (Milano).* 1998;10(1):26–31. http://www.ncbi.nlm.nih.gov/pubmed/9589748. Accessed March 21, 2019.
152. Bohannon RW, Tudini F. Unipedal balance test for older adults: a systematic review and meta-analysis of studies providing normative data. *Physiotherapy.* 2018;104(4):376–382. https://doi.org/10.1016/j.physio.2018.04.001.
153. Goldberg A, Casby A, Wasielewski M. Minimum detectable change for single-leg-stance-time in older adults. *Gait Posture.* 2011;33(4):737–739. https://doi.org/10.1016/j.gaitpost.2011.02.020.
154. Turner MR. Romberg's test no longer stands up. *Pract Neurol.* 2016;16(4):316. https://doi.org/10.1136/practneurol-2016-001365.
155. Agrawa Y, Carey JP, Hoffman HJ, Sklare DA, Schubert MC. The Modified Romberg Balance Test. *Otol Neurotol.* 2011;32(8):1309–1311. https://doi.org/10.1097/MAO.0b013e31822e5bee.
156. Scaglioni-Solano P, Aragón-Vargas LF. Validity and reliability of the Nintendo Wii Balance Board to assess standing balance and sensory integration in highly functional older adults. *Int J Rehabil Res.* 2014;37(2):138–143. https://doi.org/10.1097/MRR.0000000000000046.
157. Hile ES, Brach JS, Perera S, Wert DM, Vanswearingen JM, Studenski SA. Interpreting the need for initial support to perform tandem stance tests of balance. *Phys Ther.* 2012;92(10):1316–1328. https://doi.org/10.2522/ptj.20110283.
158. Guralnik JM, Ferrucci L, Simonsick EM, Salive ME, Wallace RB. Lower-extremity function in persons over the age of 70 years as a predictor of subsequent disability. *N Engl J Med.* 1995;332(9):556–562. https://doi.org/10.1056/NEJM199503023320902.
159. Guralnik JM, Ferrucci L, Pieper CF, et al. Lower extremity function and subsequent disability: consistency across studies, predictive models, and value of gait speed alone compared with the short physical performance battery. *J Gerontol A Biol Sci Med Sci.* 2000;55(4):M221–M231. http://www.ncbi.nlm.nih.gov/pubmed/10811152.
160. Dite W, Temple VA. A clinical test of stepping and change of direction to identify multiple falling older adults. *Arch Phys Med Rehabil.* 2002;83(11):1566–1571. https://doi.org/10.1053/apmr.2002.35469.
161. Cleary K, Skornyakov E. Predicting falls in older adults using the four square step test. *Physiother Theory Pract.* 2017;33(10):766–771. https://doi.org/10.1080/09593985.2017.1354951.
162. Moore M, Barker K. The validity and reliability of the four square step test in different adult populations: a systematic review. *Syst Rev.* 2017;6(1):187. https://doi.org/10.1186/s13643-017-0577-5.
163. Whitney SL, Marchetti GF, Morris LO, Sparto PJ. The reliability and validity of the four square step test for people with balance deficits secondary to a vestibular disorder. *Arch Phys Med Rehabil.* 2007;88(1):99–104. https://doi.org/10.1016/j.apmr.2006.10.027.
164. Dite W, Connor HJ, Curtis HC. Clinical identification of multiple fall risk early after unilateral transtibial amputation. *Arch Phys Med Rehabil.* 2007;88(1):109–114. https://doi.org/10.1016/j.apmr.2006.10.015.
165. Muir-Hunter SW, Graham L, Montero Odasso M. Reliability of the Berg Balance Scale as a clinical measure of balance in community-dwelling older adults with mild to moderate Alzheimer disease: a pilot study. *Physiother Canada.* 2015;67(3):255–262. https://doi.org/10.3138/ptc.2014-32.
166. Downs S, Marquez J, Chiarelli P. The Berg Balance Scale has high intra- and inter-rater reliability but absolute reliability varies across the scale: a systematic review. *J Physiother.* 2013;59(2):93–99. https://doi.org/10.1016/S1836-9553(13)70161-9.
167. Chou CY, Chien CW, Hsueh IP, Sheu CF, Wang CH, Hsieh CL. Developing a short form of the Berg Balance Scale for people with stroke. *Phys Ther.* 2006;86(2):195–204.
168. Straube D, Moore J, Leech K, George Hornby T. Item analysis of the Berg Balance Scale in individuals with subacute and chronic stroke. *Top Stroke Rehabil.* 2013;20(3):241–249. https://doi.org/10.1310/tsr2003-241.
169. Downs S, Marquez J, Chiarelli P. Normative scores on the Berg Balance Scale decline after age 70 years in healthy community-dwelling people: a systematic review. *J Physiother.* 2014;60(2):85–89. https://doi.org/10.1016/j.jphys.2014.01.002.
170. Blum L, Korner-Bitensky N. Usefulness of the Berg Balance Scale in stroke rehabilitation: a systematic review. *Phys Ther.* 2008;88(5):559–566.
171. Lima CA, Ricci NA, Nogueira EC, Perracini MR. The Berg Balance Scale as a clinical screening tool to predict fall risk in older adults: a systematic review. *Physiotherapy.* 2018;104(4):383–394. https://doi.org/10.1016/j.physio.2018.02.002.
172. Donoghue D. Group PR and OP (PROP), Stokes EK. How much change is true change? The minimum detectable change of the Berg Balance Scale in elderly people. *J Rehabil Med.* 2009;41(5):343–346. https://doi.org/10.2340/16501977-0337.
173. Yelnik A, Bonan I. Clinical tools for assessing balance disorders. *Neurophysiol Clin.* 2008;38(6):439–445. https://doi.org/10.1016/j.neucli.2008.09.008.
174. Harada N, Chiu V, Fowler E, Reuben DB. Screening for balance and mobility impairment in elderly individuals living in residential care facilities. *Phys Ther.* 1995;75(6):462–469.
175. Sterke CS, Huisman SL, van Beeck EF, Looman CWN, van der Cammen TJM. Is the Tinetti Performance Oriented Mobility Assessment (POMA) a feasible and valid predictor of short-term fall risk in nursing home residents with dementia? *Int Psychogeriatrics.* 2010;22(02):254. https://doi.org/10.1017/S1041610209991347.
176. Faber MJ, Bosscher RJ, van Wieringen PC. Clinimetric properties of the performance-oriented mobility assessment. *Phys Ther.* 2006;86(7):944–954.

177. Cipriany-Dacko LM, Innerst D, Johannsen J, Rude V. Interrater reliability of the Tinetti Balance Scores in novice and experienced physical therapy clinicians. *Arch Phys Med Rehabil.* 1997;78(10):1160–1164. http://www.ncbi.nlm.nih.gov/pubmed/9339170. Accessed March 23, 2019.
178. Van Iersel MB, Benraad CEM, Olde Rikkert MGM. Validity and reliability of quantitative gait analysis in geriatric patients with and without dementia. *J Am Geriatr Soc.* 2007; 55(4):632–634. https://doi.org/10.1111/j.1532-5415.2007.01130.x.
179. Ko Y-M, Park W-B, Lim J-Y, Kim KW, Paik N-J. Discrepancies between balance confidence and physical performance among community-dwelling Korean elders: a population-based study. *Int Psychogeriatrics.* 2009;21(4):738–747. https://doi.org/10.1017/S1041610209009077.
180. Lin M-R, Hwang H-F, Hu M-H, H-DI Wu, Wang Y-W, Huang F-C. Psychometric comparisons of the timed up and go, one-leg stand, functional reach, and Tinetti balance measures in community-dwelling older people. *J Am Geriatr Soc.* 2004;52(8):1343–1348. https://doi.org/10.1111/j.1532-5415.2004.52366.x.
181. Horak FB, Wrisley DM, Frank J. The Balance Evaluation Systems Test (BESTest) to differentiate balance deficits. *Phys Ther.* 2009;89(5):484–498. https://doi.org/10.2522/ptj.20080071.
182. Padgett PK, Jacobs JV, Kasser SL. Is the BESTest at its best? A suggested brief version based on interrater reliability, validity, internal consistency, and theoretical construct. *Phys Ther.* 2012;92(9):1197–1207. https://doi.org/10.2522/ptj.20120056.
183. O'Hoski S, Sibley KM, Brooks D, et al. Construct validity of the BESTest, mini-BESTest and briefBESTest in adults aged 50 years and older. *Gait Posture.* 2015;42(3):301–305. https://doi.org/10.1016/j.gaitpost.2015.06.006.
184. Franchignoni F, Horak F, Godi M, Nardone A, Giordano A. Using psychometric techniques to improve the Balance Evaluation Systems Test: the mini-BESTest. *J Rehabil Med.* 2010;42(4):323–331. https://doi.org/10.2340/16501977-0537.
185. King L, Horak F. On the Mini-BESTest: scoring and the reporting of total scores. *Phys Ther.* 2013;93(4):571–575. https://doi.org/10.2522/ptj.2013.93.4.571.
186. Godi M, Franchignoni F, Caligari M, Giordano A, Turcato AM, Nardone A. Comparison of reliability, validity, and responsiveness of the Mini-BESTest and Berg Balance Scale in patients with balance disorders. *Phys Ther.* 2013;93(2):158–167. https://doi.org/10.2522/ptj.20120171.
187. Leddy AL, Crowner BE, Earhart GM. Functional gait assessment and balance evaluation system test: reliability, validity, sensitivity, and specificity for identifying individuals with Parkinson disease who fall. *Phys Ther.* 2011;91 (1):102–113.
188. O'Hoski S, Winship B, Herridge L, et al. Increasing the clinical utility of the BESTest, Mini-BESTest, and Brief-BESTest: normative values in Canadian adults who are healthy and aged 50 years or older. *Phys Ther.* 2014;94(3):334–342. https://doi.org/10.2522/ptj.20130104.
189. Rose DJ, Lucchese N, Wiersma LD. Development of a multidimensional balance scale for use with functionally independent older adults. *Arch Phys Med Rehabil.* 2006;8 7(11):1478–1485 https://doi.org/10.1016/j.apmr.2006.07.263.
190. Klein PJ, Fiedler RC, Rose DJ. Rasch analysis of the Fullerton Advanced Balance (FAB) Scale. *Physiother Canada.* 2011;63 (1):115–125. https://doi.org/10.3138/ptc.2009-51.
191. Hernandez D, Rose DJ. Predicting which older adults will or will not fall using the Fullerton Advanced Balance Scale. *Arch Phys Med Rehabil.* 2008;89(12):2309–2315. https://doi.org/10.1016/j.apmr.2008.05.020.
192. Takacs J, Garland SJ, Carpenter MG, Hunt MA. Validity and reliability of the Community Balance and Mobility Scale in individuals with knee osteoarthritis. *Phys Ther.* 2014;94 (6):866–874. https://doi.org/10.2522/ptj.20130385.
193. Knorr S, Brouwer B, Garland SJ. Validity of the Community Balance and Mobility Scale in community-dwelling persons after stroke. *Arch Phys Med Rehabil.* 2010;91(6):890–896. https://doi.org/10.1016/j.apmr.2010.02.010.
194. Martelli L, Saraswat D, Dechman G, Giacomantonio NB, Grandy SA. The Community Balance and Mobility Scale. *J Cardiopulm Rehabil Prev.* 2017;38(2):1. https://doi.org/10.1097/HCR.0000000000000277.
195. Howe JA, Inness EL, Venturini A, Williams JI, Verrier MC. The Community Balance and Mobility Scale-a balance measure for individuals with traumatic brain injury. *Clin Rehabil.* 2006;20(10):885–895. https://doi.org/10.1177/0269215506072183.
196. Balasubramanian CK. The Community Balance and Mobility Scale alleviates the ceiling effects observed in the currently used gait and balance assessments for the community-dwelling older adults. *J Geriatr Phys Ther.* 2015;38(2):78–89. https://doi.org/10.1519/JPT.0000000000000024.
197. Weber M, Van Ancum J, Bergquist R, et al. Concurrent validity and reliability of the Community Balance and Mobility scale in young-older adults. *BMC Geriatr.* 2018; 18(1):156. https://doi.org/10.1186/s12877-018-0845-9.
198. Howe J, Inness EL, Wright V. The Community Balance & Mobility Scale. The Center for Outcome Measurement in Brain Injury. http://www.tbims.org/cbm/cbmfaq.html. Published 2011. Accessed March 29, 2019.
199. Shumway-Cook A, Taylor CS, Matsuda N, Studer MT, Brady K. Expanding the scoring system for the dynamic gait index. *Phys Ther.* 2013;93:1493–1506. https://doi.org/10.2522/ptj.20130035.
200. Shumway-Cook A, Baldwin M, Polissar NL, Gruber W. Predicting the probability for falls in community-dwelling older adults. *Phys Ther.* 1997;77(8):812–819.
201. Whitney SL, Hudak MT, Marchetti GF. The dynamic gait index relates to self-reported fall history in individuals with vestibular dysfunction. *J Vestib Res.* 2000;10(2):99–105. http://www.ncbi.nlm.nih.gov/pubmed/10939685. Accessed March 23, 2019.
202. Marchetti GF, Whitney SL. Construction and validation of the 4-item Dynamic Gait Index. *Phys Ther.* 2006;86 (12):1651–1660. https://doi.org/10.2522/ptj.20050402.
203. Marchetti GF, Lin C-C, Alghadir A, Whitney SL. Responsiveness and minimal detectable change of the Dynamic Gait Index and Functional Gait Index in persons with balance and vestibular disorders. *J Neurol Phys Ther.* 2014;38(2):119–124. https://doi.org/10.1097/NPT.0000000000000015.
204. Wrisley DM, Marchetti GF, Kuharsky DK, Whitney SL. Reliability, internal consistency, and validity of data obtained with the functional gait assessment. *Phys Ther.* 2004;84(10):906–918.
205. Wrisley DM, Kumar NA. Functional gait assessment: concurrent, discriminative, and predictive validity in community-dwelling older adults. *Phys Ther.* 2010;90 (5):761–773. https://doi.org/10.2522/ptj.20090069; 10.2522/ptj.20090069.
206. Walker ML, Austin AG, Banke GM, et al. Reference group data for the functional gait assessment. *Phys Ther.* 2007;87(11):1468–1477.
207. Scrivener K, Sherrington C, Schurr K. A systematic review of the responsiveness of lower limb physical performance measures in inpatient care after stroke. *BMC Neurol.* 2013;13:4. https://doi.org/10.1186/1471-2377-13-4; 10.1186/1471-2377-13-4.

208. Liaw L-J, Hsieh C-L, Lo S-K, Chen H-M, Lee S, Lin J-H. The relative and absolute reliability of two balance performance measures in chronic stroke patients. *Disabil Rehabil.* 2008;30(9):656–661. https://doi.org/10.1080/09638280701400698.
209. Chien CW, Lin JH, Wang CH, Hsueh IP, Sheu CF, Hsieh CL. Developing a short form of the Postural Assessment Scale for people with Stroke. *Neurorehabil Neural Repair.* 2007;21(1):81–90.
210. Huang Y, Wang W, Liou T, Liao C, Lin L, Huang S. Postural Assessment Scale for stroke patients scores as a predictor of stroke patient ambulation at discharge from the rehabilitation ward. *J Rehabil Med.* 2016;48(3):259–264. https://doi.org/10.2340/16501977-2046.
211. Stevens JA. The STEADI Tool Kit: a fall prevention resource for health care providers. *IHS Prim Care Provid.* 2013;39(9):162–166. http://www.ncbi.nlm.nih.gov/pubmed/26766893. Accessed March 24, 2019.
212. Panel on Prevention of Falls in Older Persons AGS and BGS. Summary of the Updated American Geriatrics Society/British Geriatrics Society clinical practice guideline for prevention of falls in older persons. *J Am Geriatr Soc.* 2011;59(1):148–157. https://doi.org/10.1111/j.1532-5415.2010.03234.x; 10.1111/j.1532-5415.2010.03234.x.
213. Lohman MC, Crow RS, DiMilia PR, Nicklett EJ, Bruce ML, Batsis JA. Operationalisation and validation of the Stopping Elderly Accidents, Deaths, and Injuries (STEADI) fall risk algorithm in a nationally representative sample. *J Epidemiol Community Health.* 2017;71(12):1191–1197. https://doi.org/10.1136/jech-2017-209769.
214. Sustakoski A, Perera S, VanSwearingen JM, Studenski SA, Brach JS. The impact of testing protocol on recorded gait speed. *Gait Posture.* 2015;41(1):329–331. https://doi.org/10.1016/j.gaitpost.2014.10.020.

CHAPTER

8

Exercise and Physical Activity for Older Adults

Dale Avers

OUTLINE

INTRODUCTION

Exercise is the single most efficacious intervention for older adults used by physical therapists. Exercise is known to simultaneously impact and mediate chronic disease, many impairments, functional deficits, quality of life, falls, and cognition, and prevent the negative sequelae associated with sedentary lifestyles. Combined with regular physical activity, appropriately prescribed exercise is the mainstay of the geriatric physical therapists' toolbox of interventions. Although many principles of exercise have been known for decades, their application to older adults is relatively recent. A thorough understanding of exercise principles and their benefits should compel the physical therapist to seek creative exercise strategies in application for older adults.

An untapped area of physical therapy is the primary prevention of physical inactivity. In light of the overwhelming and compelling role of physical activity in providing protection from disability and the strong evidence for the effects of exercise, physical therapists have a professional responsibility to apply exercise in the most efficacious manner possible. Understanding the principles of the exercise prescription, and their application to older adults, is a necessary first step. This chapter discusses the role of physical activity and exercise, effects of a sedentary lifestyle, elements of an effective exercise prescription, and the different types of exercise applications for older adults.

PHYSICAL ACTIVITY

The central role of physical activity and exercise is illustrated in the World Health Organization's (WHO) International Classification of Functioning, Disability, and Health (Fig. 8.1). The WHO model not only makes activity central, but also considers the role of environmental and personal factors that may pose barriers to physical activity and exercise. The WHO model is a useful reminder for physical therapists to incorporate physical activity into their plan of care while addressing impairments, activity limitations, and both environmental and personal barriers to participation.[1] Definitions of terms related to physical activity and exercise are included in Box 8.1.[2]

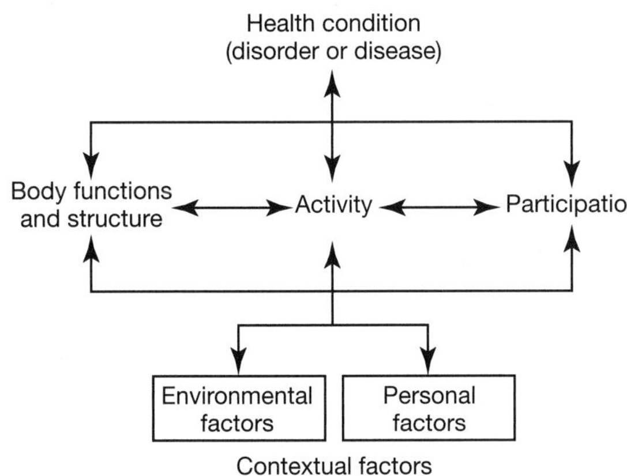

FIG. 8.1 World Health Organization's International Classification of Functioning, Disability, and Health (ICF).

Physical activity declines with age and the incidence of chronic disease increases with age. In 2014, only about 12% of people aged 65 years and over reported participating in leisure-time aerobic and muscle-strengthening activities that met the 2008 federal physical activity guidelines, with lower participation as age increased.[3] In the same year (2014) approximately 60% of older adults reported at least one chronic condition and 12% reported five or more chronic conditions.[4]

The effects of physiologic aging do not occur uniformly across the population. Many aging adults are able to maintain a very high, active lifestyle that includes tennis, skiing, hiking, biking, and running well into late life with little to no disability.[5] Achieving 150 minutes per week of moderate-intense aerobic exercise is associated with at least a 30% lower risk of morbidity, mortality, and functional dependence compared with being inactive.[6,7] Walking 5 to 7 days per week was associated with a 50% to 80% lower risk of mobility impairments,[8] increased longevity by around 4 years, and disability-free life expectancy by around 2 years.[9]

There is strong evidence of an inverse dose–response relationship between the volume of physical activity and risk of disability. Study after study shows the direct correlation between declining levels of physical activity and mobility disability and reduced functional abilities.[10–12] Physical therapists need to recognize the difference between physiological age and physical deconditioning to better implement an effective exercise prescription. A list of the benefits of physical activity supported by evidence is provided in Box 8.2.

Physical inactivity is a significant risk factor for developing many chronic conditions that impact health and functional mobility in older adults, and for increasing the risk of additional disability in someone who already has a chronic condition. Many of these conditions are prevalent in older adults and therefore often seen by physical therapists. For many of these conditions, inactivity has a direct physiological effect on pathology/disease (e.g., the deconditioning of the cardiovascular system). However, for some conditions, the pathology is made worse because of associated impairments that affect function, such as in the accelerated loss of strength that impairs balance and mobility. The loss of mobility rather than the medical condition itself becomes the functional consequence that causes the individual's disability. The good news is that, even in very sedentary individuals, when sedentary activities are broken up by short bouts of just 1 to 10 minutes of physical activity or standing, attenuation of the adverse effects of sedentary behavior can occur.[13,14] For physical therapists, the ultimate goal of activity/exercise is to improve mobility and function and thereby decrease the patient's mobility disability.

Mobility disability is defined as an inability to walk one-quarter of a mile and inability to climb a flight of stairs.[15] Mobility disability can be brought about by an illness-imposed temporary sedentary lifestyle or debilitating illness. For example, the majority of older hospitalized adults experienced a clinically significant decrease in

BOX 8.1 Definition of Terms Related to Physical Activity and Exercise

Term	Definition	Notes
Physical activity	Any self-imposed bodily movement that results in a substantial increase in caloric requirements over resting energy expenditure	Defined by MET level
Exercise	Planned, structured, deliberate physical activity done to improve and/or maintain one or more components of physical fitness	Classified by mode, such as aerobic, resistance, flexibility, and plyometric
Physical fitness	The ability to carry out daily tasks with vigor and alertness, without undue fatigue, and with ample energy to enjoy leisure-time pursuits and respond to emergencies[214]	Cardiovascular fitness, classified by VO_2 max Strength fitness: capacity of the skeletal muscle to move an external load; classified as repetition maximum Balance fitness: ability to control the body's position throughout movement Flexibility fitness: ability to achieve an extended range of motion
Physical inactivity	Physical activity levels less than those required for optimal health and prevention of premature death[214]	

BOX 8.2 Benefits of Physical Activity for Older Adults

Strong Evidence
- ⇒ Lower risk of early death
- ⇒ Lower risk of coronary heart disease
- ⇒ Lower risk of stroke
- ⇒ Lower risk of high blood pressure
- ⇒ Lower risk of adverse blood lipid profile
- ⇒ Lower risk of type 2 diabetes
- ⇒ Lower risk of metabolic syndrome
- ⇒ Lower risk of colon cancer
- ⇒ Lower risk of breast cancer
- ⇒ Weight loss, particularly when combined with reduced calorie intake
- ⇒ Visceral fat loss, even in the absence of overall weight loss
- ⇒ Improved cardiorespiratory and muscular fitness
- ⇒ Improves urinary incontinence through pelvic floor strengthening
- ⇒ Improves balance and agility, thus mediating fall risk and fractures
- ⇒ Decreased pain, especially from osteoarthritis
- ⇒ Reduced depression and improved mental health
- ⇒ Better cognitive function

Moderate to Strong Evidence
- ⇒ Better functional performance in ADLs and IADLs
- ⇒ Reduced abdominal obesity
- ⇒ Prevention of weight gain during menopause and beyond

Moderate Evidence
- ⇒ Lower risk of hip fracture
- ⇒ Lower risk of lung cancer
- ⇒ Lower risk of endometrial cancer
- ⇒ Weight maintenance after weight loss
- ⇒ Increased bone density
- ⇒ Improved sleep quality

ADL, activities of daily living; *IADLs*, instrumental activities of daily living.

community-related mobility in the first month after hospitalization from which 34% had not recovered during the 6 months of follow-up.[16] Physical therapy professionals have a clear and important role to play in preventing and mitigating physical inactivity–related disability at all levels of the health care continuum.

Physical Activity Guidelines

The Centers for Disease Control and Prevention (CDC) has established specific physical activity recommendations for adults and older adults (>65 years of age) to achieve important health benefits and reduce the effects of age-related decline listed in Table 23.2 in the Wellness Chapter 23. Box 8.3 lists the step counts typically associated with sedentary to high activity levels.[17,18] Older adults are encouraged to attain at least 150 minutes of *moderate-intense* physical activity per week, recognizing that more activity (i.e., intensity and volume) has more robust health benefits. However, significant risk reductions for cardiovascular disease and premature mortality begin to be observed at volumes starting at about one-half of the recommended volume.[14] The 2018 update report of the Office of Disease Prevention and Health Promotion[50] emphasizes the robustness of the evidence for the positive impact of physical activity for all older adults, regardless of physical condition. Adapting physical activity for physically challenged older adults is of critical importance and establishes an important role of the physical therapy professional.

BOX 8.3 Physical Activity Step Counts[17,18]

- Sedentary is <5000 steps per day.
- Low active is 5000–7499 steps per day.
- Somewhat active is 7500–9999 steps per day.
- Active is >10,000 steps per day.
- Highly active is >12,500.

Group Exercise

Group exercise, preferred by most older adults (women more than men), is an effective method of achieving recommended doses of physical activity.[19] Group exercise programs have the added benefit of socialization, peer support, supervision, and better long-term adherence even when conducted in long-term care facilities.[20,21] One study of individuals aged 80 and above residing in a nursing home or a residential home found an average 87% adherence to group exercise programs.[21]

Barriers to older adult participation in group programs are many and varied. Environmental factors such as lack of sidewalks, proximity to a park, adverse weather, lack of a convenient exercise facility, or perceived lack of safety can each be a deterrent to exercise,[22] as can lack of transportation, unwillingness to join a group, or aversion to exercise ("I'm not sporty").[23] Factors that increase the likelihood of an older adult engaging in physical activity and exercise include perceived health and proximity to a health facility, self-efficacy, outcome expectations and perceived benefits,[24] proximity to home, exercising outdoors (even in warmer and colder months),[21] programs that were challenging,[25] and those that had functional intent.[23] Older adults who are advised to exercise by their physician are more likely to perform moderate to heavy levels of exercise per week than those who do not receive advice.[26,27] Older adults who participate in group-based programs express a preference for expert guidance because of safety concerns[28] as well as programs that are close to home, offered at little to no cost, and activities that could also be done independently.[29] Ultimately, exercise preferences should be considered on an individual basis as a means to promoting physical activity.

Before beginning a group exercise program, the American College of Sports Medicine (ACSM) recommends completing a preparticipation screening tool.[2] The Canadian Par-Q is freely available and appropriate for community-dwelling elders.[30] The Par-Q+ is appropriate for those who have exercise concerns identified by the Par-Q.[31] Chapter 23 provides more details on preparticipation screening tools.

PHYSICAL STRESS THEORY

The physical stress theory (PST) has been the foundation of exercise prescription for many years. It is alternatively referred to as the specific adaptation of imposed demands (SAID) theory. The PST is defined as the predictable response of tissues, organs, and systems to mechanical and physiological stressors.[32] The PST explains the effect of overload or insufficient load on tissues, organs, or systems, as well as the lack of change in tissues, organs, and systems if a "usual" stress is applied consistently (maintenance). If more than usual stress (overload) is put on a tissue, the tissue responds by increasing its ability to absorb and dissipate that stress. If too much stress is placed on a tissue, the tissue is susceptible to injury (or even death, as in the case of integumentary tissue). Conversely, if too little stress is consistently placed on a tissue, the tissue loses its ability to absorb and dissipate stresses; that is, the tissue atrophies. Every tissue, organ, or system predictably responds to stress or a lack of stress. Applications of the PST to exercise are described in Box 8.4.

The PST is the theory underlying exercise application for the cardiopulmonary and musculoskeletal systems. The effects of too little stress on the cardiopulmonary system are well known to physical therapists, appearing in the form of deconditioning that eventually increases the severity of most, if not all, chronic diseases and conditions. The effects of too little stress on the skeletal system are seen in the condition of osteoporosis and on the muscular system as weakness and mobility disability. Physical therapists use the principles of the PST when they prescribe a specific intensity of aerobic exercise to improve cardiovascular capacity or amount of overload for weight-bearing and resistance exercises to improve bone and muscle strength. Physical activity and exercise that appropriately stress tissues to enhance optimal adaptation to achieve the desired result is the foundation of the exercise prescription.

The ability of tissue to absorb and dissipate forces is dependent on many variables, including the time over which the stressor is applied; the direction, magnitude, and combination of stressors applied; the physiological condition of the tissue, organ, or system; the frequency of the application of a stressor and length of time between the applications; and even the psychological state of the person and the environment or context in which the stressor is applied. In the clinic, physical therapists can modify these variables within an exercise program to achieve a desired outcome. For example, the PST can be used to positively impact the cardiopulmonary, musculoskeletal, and vestibular systems in a frail, sedentary older woman who has increased fall risk and an inability to tolerate walking 1000 feet (community distance) at a reasonable pace. The physical therapist may choose initially to promote safety and reduce the risk of falling by having her use a walker for support and to decrease her unsteadiness, thus adapting the demand of the task to a level that matches the patient's current capabilities. Resistance exercise of an appropriate intensity based on a 10-repetition maximum (RM) can then be prescribed to stress the tissue beyond what is typically experienced and at a level that will promote change in muscle tissue. Balance activities that address a hypoactive vestibular and somatosensory system can be incorporated in a gradually challenging manner to increase response time and accurate reactions. Self-efficacy and motor learning feedback principles can be incorporated to appropriately stress the psychological system. As each system responds, challenges (stressors) are added to that system for continuous adaptation. However, if too little challenge occurs, such as in too little resistance, too short a walking distance, or too slow a pace, little to no change will occur, and in fact, because all systems decline with age, without appropriate stressors, the older person will also decline.[33]

The PST also addresses progression of an activity. Once the tissue, organ, system, and person adapt to being able to absorb and dissipate a certain level of stressor, this level becomes the usual or maintenance level, and increased levels of stress are needed to achieve further gains. Often, hospitalizations and long-term care environments discourage physical activity that supports stress/overload

BOX 8.4 Application of the Physical Stress Theory

Level	Amount	Results	Example
Too much (extreme)	>100% of maximum	Injury or tissue death	Weight bearing on an osteoporotic bone such as ulna, resulting in fracture
Appropriate stress	60%–100% of maximum	Adaptation	Loads of >60% one-repetition maximum (1RM) resulting in strengthening
Usual stress	40%–60% of maximum	Maintenance (no change)	Walking at 5000–7000 steps will maintain current level of fitness
Too little stress	<40% of maximum	Atrophy	Bed rest or sedentary activity
No stress	0% of maximum	Loss of ability to adapt (death)	Prolonged bed rest as in a coma or low responsiveness

outside of supervised sessions. If level of overload achieved in one therapy session is not reinforced outside of therapy, the desired gains may not be realized. This is one of the reasons the Centers for Medicare and Medicaid encourage provision of services in the least restrictive level of care possible.[34]

GENERAL INDICATIONS AND PRECAUTIONS

Although exercise of any type has been shown to be safe and effective with appropriate supervision for nearly all older people[35] (refer to ACSM's list of absolute contraindications[2]), the therapy professional should be aware of extrinsic and intrinsic variables that may adversely affect the desired exercise response in an older adult. For example, when a patient complains of excessive fatigue or muscle pain and does not appear to be gaining strength according to your expectations of the exercise prescription, the state of hydration, electrolyte imbalance, and the use of statins should be considered. Box 8.5 describes the effects of statins on muscle.[36] Chapter 24 lists the electrolyte values and symptoms of electrolyte imbalance of which every therapist should be aware. Because the majority of older adults have chronic diseases and are on multiple medications, individual homeostasis is reduced, and side effects are common. This complexity requires keen observation and awareness of potential causes of unusual or unexpected physiological reactions to exercise. Chapter 18 provides an overview of normal values and typical age-related changes in vital signs, cardiac output, and blood pressure as well as the impact of commonly occurring cardiovascular and pulmonary conditions on exercise capacity. The impact of blood glucose levels and pain are discussed next.

BOX 8.5 Effects of Statins on Muscle

- The most common adverse events of using statins involve muscle pain and weakness (myopathy and rhabdomyolysis). Symptomatically, the urine may appear brown in the presence of rhabdomyolysis.
- Complaints usually occur within a few months of starting a statin or of increasing the dose, but there have been cases occurring after years of stable statin treatment.
- While creatine phosphokinase (CPK) levels are not useful in most cases of myopathy, any complaint of muscle weakness or bilateral proximal muscle pain with no obvious cause such as resistance exercise should be evaluated with a measurement of CPK.
- Stopping statin use reverses these side effects, usually leading to a full recovery within a few weeks.
- Although the risk is low, the risk is elevated with higher doses and interacting drugs.
- Patients with renal involvement, hypothyroidism, serious debility, or frailty, or those who are older than 80 years are more susceptible than others to myopathy.

Blood Glucose

Exercise lowers blood glucose, making individuals prone to hypoglycemia. Persons with diabetes should monitor blood sugars closely during and after physical activity and exercise, recognizing that insulin requirements may decrease with exercise. The risk of incurring exercise-induced hypoglycemia can be mediated by the consumption of an extra 20 to 30 grams of carbohydrates during and after exercise.[37] Also, awareness of an exercise-induced phenomenon in diabetic patients known as delayed-onset hypoglycemia (e.g., low blood glucose concentration 6 to 15 hours after exercise) can help prevent problems through proper education.[2] Eating meals of small portions and at greater frequency can help to avoid delayed-onset low blood glucose response after exercise. If blood glucose falls to or below 100 mg/dL, consuming 15 to 20 grams of carbohydrates is necessary, and then blood sugar should be rechecked, repeating every 15 minutes until blood glucose is at least 100 mg/dL.[38]

Pain

Although pain is a common complaint of an older adult and may present as a barrier to exercise, there is no evidence supporting the decision to curtail exercise in the presence of pain. Certainly, the therapist should be aware of pain caused by acute inflammation or injury, but most pain complaints in older adults may be considered long-standing, or chronic. In fact, a preponderance of studies document the improvement in pain levels with progressive exercise for a variety of conditions that include osteoarthritis, low back pain, and chronic pain.[39] The exercise prescription should be individualized and carefully administered to achieve the pain reduction benefits of exercise. Patient education and patient-centered goal setting are key to working with the patient with chronic pain who will benefit from exercise.

ELEMENTS OF AN EXERCISE PRESCRIPTION

Appropriately designed exercise is a powerful intervention. The basic elements of an exercise program include specificity and progressive overload. Within the elements of specificity are type of contraction, speed of contraction, and variety. Within progressive overload are the individual parameters of intensity, duration, frequency, rest, type of contraction, speed of contraction, reversibility, and variety. To maximize effectiveness, an exercise prescription should reflect an individualized design of the relevant parameters to promote the desired change to the targeted system. When attention is paid to creatively manipulating these parameters of exercise, the outcome of exercise can be more accurately predicted. This section includes a general discussion of parameters that apply to aerobic and resistance modes of exercise. Further detail of specific applications of the parameters occurs later in the chapter.

Specificity

The principle of specificity states that adaptation to the exercise stimulus will be directly related to how the stimulus was generated. Specificity includes the specific exercise, type of muscle contraction, speed of contraction, and consideration of the functional movement inherent in the desired outcome. The closer the training routine is to the conditions of the desired outcome (i.e., specific exercise task or performance criteria), the better will be the outcome.[14] It is commonly accepted that functional improvement occurs when the exercise stimulus closely matches the conditions of the desired outcome. For example, if improved tolerance to exercise is desired, the exercise prescription would call for lower intensity and more time on task such as training for endurance.

Incorporating the same type of muscle contraction (concentric, eccentric, or isometric) that is elicited in a specific movement meets the requirement of specificity in resistance training. Part of a task analysis is to identify the type of muscle contraction needed to complete the activity. For example, trunk muscles are often used as stabilizers during movement and therefore should be trained isometrically in multiple planes and actions.[40]

Specificity is less critical within types of aerobic exercise. One study investigating the effects of exercise mode, training status, and specificity on oxygen uptake (VO_2) found that training level had more effect than the exercise mode.[41] Logically, training on a treadmill will not directly transfer to a swimming task, even in the presence of greater aerobic capacity. Specificity in aerobic exercise may be most critical during maximum effort, such as in competition, but less important in individuals who are not achieving maximal effort.

The specificity concept has led to the contemporary practice of functional training. Functional training is the concept of training a movement rather than a muscle and requires neural activation. Training for speed and power is an application of specificity and overload and a necessary component of functional activities.[42] Functional activities are multiplanar and asymmetrical, incorporate rotation, and are speed and balance dependent. Therefore, exercise aimed at improving function should meet the same criteria. Commercial exercise programs such as CrossFit[43] and Boot Camps for Seniors, which utilize these specificity and functional training concepts, are gaining popularity.[44] Functional training may allow adaptation to a variety of activities more so than strict adherence to the specificity principle. Applications of functional training will be discussed later in this chapter.

Progressive Overload

Applying the theory of physical stress to the exercise prescription to achieve increased strength is called overload. The overload principle states that to achieve adaptation, a stimulus must be greater than what is required to maintain the current state. Parameters that influence overload in resistance training include intensity, sets, repetitions per set, frequency of sessions/week, duration of training (in weeks), rest, and reversibility. These parameters will be discussed in the section on resistance training. Parameters that affect overload in aerobic exercise include intensity, frequency, and duration of training (in weeks). These parameters will be discussed in the section on aerobic exercise.

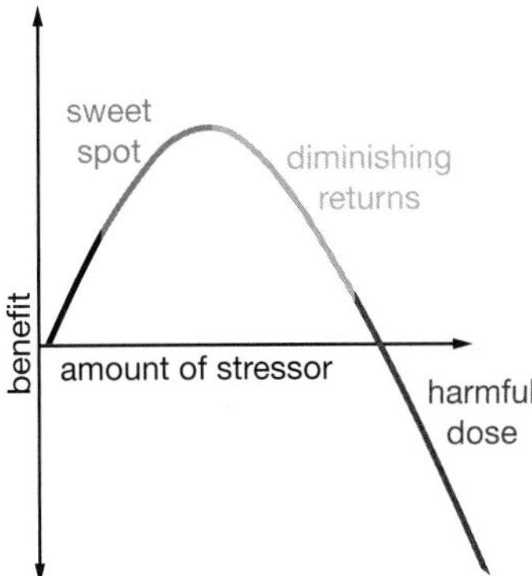

FIG. 8.2 Dose–response curve. *https://www.familyhealthchiropractic.com/3-ways-i-start-my-day-to-boost-productivity/stress-dose-graph/*

The dose or amount of exercise, no matter the mode of exercise, determines the amount of adaptation of the targeted tissue. This dose must be progressively adjusted to promote continued adaptations. The dose–response relationship (curve) illustrates the PST. The dose–response relationship states that with greater doses, greater gains occur, up until the point of diminishing returns (see Fig. 8.2).[45] The dose–response relationship exists between strength increases and training variables such as volume, duration (weeks), and intensity.[46] Training volume in terms of duration appears to be the most important variable of all the elements affecting intensity.[45] Analysis from multiple meta-analyses confirm the training period as the only significant variable to improve muscle strength in the presence of multiple sets, repetitions, and frequency.[45,46] An implication for practice is that the variables of overload can be manipulated to individualize the exercise prescription based on pain, perceived effort, preference, and postexercise soreness *as long as consistency of training is maintained for at least 3 months*, recognizing the principle of reversibility (discussed later) that states that training results diminish upon cessation of the training.

The dose–response relationship appears to hold for resistance exercise for strength gains with an intensity of up to 90% of a one-repetition maximum (1RM),[47] for balance improvements in older adults up to 3 days per week,[48] and for aerobic conditioning up to 80% of the heart rate reserve (HRR).[2] However, health benefits of aerobic exercise eventually reach a point of diminishing returns. Although this point of diminishment is dependent on fitness level, Huang and colleagues found that doses of more than 80% of HRR did not lead to greater enhancement of improvement in VO_2 max but, conversely, resulted in declines.[49] There is some evidence that a dose–response relationship exists between exercise and decreasing the risk of fall-related injury and bone fracture.[50] However, the dose–response relationship does not hold for the relationship between exercise and cognitive function, where shorter sessions of 20 minutes or less showed the largest effects, whereas longer sessions show diminishing results.[51] Performance of functional training such as chair rise and stair climbing does not demonstrate a dose–response relationship, perhaps because of the ceiling effect of the strength necessary to perform specific functional tasks.[47]

The minimum amount of overload to achieve cardiovascular gains is 50% of one's VO_2 maximum (220 – age) or heart rate reserve (maximum heart rate minus resting heart rate).[2] For skeletal muscle strength gains, 60% of the maximum tissue capability should be met, although this level is controversial.[52,53] Traditionally, this 60% threshold applies to untrained individuals, such as most older adults who are not exercising currently. Although strength gains are realized below the 60% threshold, a greater volume of exercise must be undertaken in terms of repetitions, sets, and/or duration. High-intensity and moderate resistance training produce the largest effects on muscle strength in comparison to moderate- or low-intensity training and low-intensity resistance training, respectively.[2,45]

Measuring the amount of aerobic overload is achieved by the cardiac/pulmonary response. For example, the aerobic stimulus that is required to achieve a cardiopulmonary conditioning response is determined by a percentage of a VO_2 max and can be calculated using a variety of methods. The appropriate stimulus for resistance training is classically determined by the 1RM, defined as the resistance that can be moved one time and one time only to muscle failure or when loss of form has occurred.[2] Measuring perceived effort or exertion across exercise types is another low-cost, easy-to-administer method of assessing overload. Rates of perceived exertion (RPE) scales are means of measuring physical intensity levels that originally correlated to heart rate during exercise. RPE is measured using the Borg 6–20 scale,[54] Borg category ratio (CR-10) scale, modality-specific OMNI scales (i.e., walking, cycling, strength training),[55] and the Talk Test.[56] Table 8.1 compares these tools.

Reversibility

Perhaps intuitively, the reversibility principle states that the effects of any exercise form, when stopped, will result in variable declines over time. The level of fitness, age, length of time in training, habitual physical activity, muscle groups involved, and genetic factors add to this variability.[14] Although physiological changes occur as soon as 1 to 2 weeks after cessation of exercise, most well-trained adults will see only modest declines in their fitness and performance over periods of several months.[14] Generally more exercise is required to *improve* cardiopulmonary fitness and cardiometabolic health than is required to *maintain* these improvements.[14] Resistance training–induced improvements in muscle strength and power reverse quickly with complete cessation of exercise, although only one session/week at moderate to hard intensity may be required to maintain muscle and power fitness.[14]

Endurance

Endurance is the ability to sustain an activity for extended periods of time and usually refers to aerobic ability. Local muscle endurance is best described as the ability to resist muscular fatigue and describes how a given type of contraction can be sustained, typically measured in terms of the number of repetitions. Like aerobic endurance, muscular endurance relies on aerobic metabolism. Muscle endurance and muscle strength, both important for everyday life, together constitute muscular fitness. Improving muscular fitness makes everyday activities easier and decreases the risk of injury with activity. Activities that improve cardiovascular endurance also improve muscular endurance. Muscular endurance training programs can produce small, but measurable, gains in muscular strength. As with any fitness program to initiate specific gains, improving muscular endurance requires the application of the overload principle to muscular endurance activities.

Examples of muscular endurance include how many times a full squat, sit-up, or bicep curl with light to moderate weight before breaking form can be performed. Activities that require muscular endurance include sustained walking or running, cycling, resistance training, calisthenics, swimming, circuit training, aerobics, dance, and rope jumping. There are various protocols for muscular endurance training. But, in general, the load applied is relatively low and the number of repetitions is high, as in climbing the stairs.[2] When training for muscular endurance, the number of repetitions and the length of time the muscle or group of muscles contract are more important than the resistance/load or intensity/speed at which the physical activity is performed. However, a minimum training threshold (intensity, frequency, and duration) is required for improvement.

Neuromuscular Training

Neuromuscular activation is the process by which the nervous system produces muscular force through recruitment and rate coding of motor units. Deficits in neuromuscular activation can be seen in reduced muscle power and agonist muscle activation with impairments in acceleration and ability to generate velocity and power. The first and often most rapid improvement in the ability to perform an exercise observed within the first few sessions of training is primarily the result of a learning effect mediated by change in motor skill coordination and level of motivation.[57] In the second phase, lasting up to 3 to

TABLE 8.1 Tools to Measure Perceived Exertion

Borg CR-10 Scale*	Borg 6–20 Scale†	Percentage Effort Scale	OMNI Scale‡	Perceived Workload	Talk Test
0	6		0	No effort	
	7				
1	8	10%–20% effort	1	Very, very easy	Rest
2	9		2	Easy	
	10				
3	11	30% effort	3	Moderate	
	12				
	13				
4	14	40% effort	4	Light/somewhat easy	
5	15	50% effort	5	Difficult/somewhat difficult	Gentle walking or "strolling"
6	16	60% effort	6	Difficult/heavy/hard	Steady pace, not breathless
7	17	70% effort	7		Brisk walking, able to carry on a conversation
8	18	80% effort	8	Very hard/very difficult	Very brisk walking, must take a breath between groups of 4–5 words
9	19	90% effort	9	Extremely difficult	Unable to talk and keep pace
10	20	100% effort	10	Maximal/ exhaustion	

*Borg CR-10 scale correlates with perceived workload indicated for quadriceps muscle (Pincivero DM. Older adults underestimate RPE and knee extensor torque as compared with young adults. *Med Sci Sports Exerc* 2011;43[1]:171–180.)
†Borg 6–20 scale correlates with perceived workload in resistive exercise in sedentary male subjects.
‡OMNI scale is only for use in resistance exercise.
Correlations with percent effort are approximate.
(Adapted from Morishita S, Tsubaki A, Nakamura M, Nashimoto S, Fu JB, Onishi H. Rating of perceived exertion on resistance training in elderly subjects. *Expert Rev Cardiovasc Ther.* 2019;17[2]:135–142.)

4 weeks, strength improvement is attributed to neural adaptation.[58] Neural adaptation elicited by resistance training includes the increased activation of prime mover muscles (through the number of recruited motor units and synchronization of those individual motor units) and better coordination of synergistic and antagonist muscles.[59]

Manini and Clark suggest the loss of muscle strength and power with age (dynapenia) is more related to neural activation impairment and/or reductions in the intrinsic force-generating capacity of skeletal muscle.[60] Neural factors can be facilitated through high-intensity training.[61] Because the majority of motor units are recruited voluntarily in order of increasing size, small motor units (type I) are recruited first, progressing through the fiber types (I < IIA < IIX).[62] Therefore, when low force is required, only type I motor units will be active. Only when force is high will recruitment demand the involvement of the larger motor units, maximizing strength and power gains.

The motor cortex is critical for movement coordination/control and skill acquisition. The role of intracortical inhibition and disorganization with sedentary behavior and disuse is now recognized as a critical determent of muscle strength/weakness.[63,64] Neuromuscular control and integration is necessary to produce controlled movement through coordinated muscle activity. Neuromuscular and sensorimotor dysfunction can be observed in patients with knee osteoarthritis through reduced proprioceptive acuity, instability, and muscle activation deficiency.[65] Neuromuscular exercise is functional exercise involving multiple joints and muscle groups performed in various positions to achieve postural stability. Neuromuscular (functional) exercise incorporates motor skills such as balance, coordination, gait, agility, and proprioceptive training to improve balance, agility, and muscle strength and to reduce the risk of falls.[14]

Numerous neurological and orthopedic conditions are associated with proprioceptive and kinesthetic impairment such as stroke, Parkinson disease, peripheral sensory neuropathies, osteoarthritis, and injuries to ligaments, joint capsules, and muscles.[66] Broadly defined, proprioception refers to the conscious awareness of body and limbs and has several distinct properties: passive motion sense, active motion sense, limb position sense, and a sense of heaviness in the limb.[66] Proprioceptive training is an important aspect of neuromuscular exercise as it induces cortical reorganization.[66] Proprioceptive training through neuromuscular exercise utilizing both passive and active movements with and without visual feedback to achieve meaningful improvements in somatosensory and sensorimotor function is beneficial with large effect sizes of >0.8.[66]

Neuromotor training lasting 6 weeks or longer tended to produce greater benefits than programs of shorter duration.

Enjoyment and Value

A significant challenge of geriatric rehabilitation is engaging older patients to fully participate and adhere to their rehabilitation or physical activity program. Adherence occurs when people are motivated to participate owing to positive experiences that maintain their interest and match their comfort levels.[67] Providing choice and incorporating factors that add personal benefit to older adults who are increasingly self-directed as they mature are important contributors to adherence.

Older adults, as all age groups, need to understand how participation in the physical activity contributes to meeting their personal desires and goals, and then weigh the benefits against potential drawbacks (pain, embarrassment, time and effort, discomfort, etc.). Although many older adults prefer challenging exercise, they must feel confident that the level of challenge is safe.[25] Expert supervision and seeing others model the activity can encourage older adults to move beyond their normal "comfort zone." Miller and colleagues found that participants had developed a preference for the "new" (more challenging) exercises rather than the more traditional (less challenging) exercises previously experienced.[25] Lenze and colleagues demonstrated improved outcomes in frail and deconditioned individuals when they focused on their individually stated goals, were provided with specific kinds of feedback consistent with motor learning, and participated in an exercise prescription that was challenging (high intensity) as compared to standard-of-care rehabilitation.[68] The Enhanced Medical Rehabilitation (EMR) model, illustrated in Fig. 8.3,[68] provides a systematic way of promoting engagement through focus on the patient's goals, linking goals to the rehabilitation activities, and optimizing intensity.

Challenging activities can empower older adults as they succeed at new challenges. Line dancing with other participants in the rehabilitation room using whatever assistive devices that allow them to participate can be immensely enjoyable and empowering. Park and colleagues compared rhythmic dance and walking exercise and found that attendance and physical function improved to a greater extent in the dance group over 12 weeks compared with the walking exercise.[69] Music of the appropriate tempo also adds interest and positive experiences to exercise programs and improves participation, although the authors found that singing distracted the participants and therefore recommend instrumental music.[67]

To increase engagement, therapy, exercise, and physical activity should focus on fun, sociable, and achievable activities in a manner that is individual and relevant to the patient. Variety is also important, to decrease boredom and continue engagement. Exercise circuits of functional activities are easily adapted to all settings while working on speed and performance. Boot camp–style classes or therapy sessions can be easily incorporated by using time on task rather than repetitions, and then immediately progressing to the next activity. Table 8.2 lists some activities for older adults for a circuit or boot camp–style program. The list of potential activities is endless!

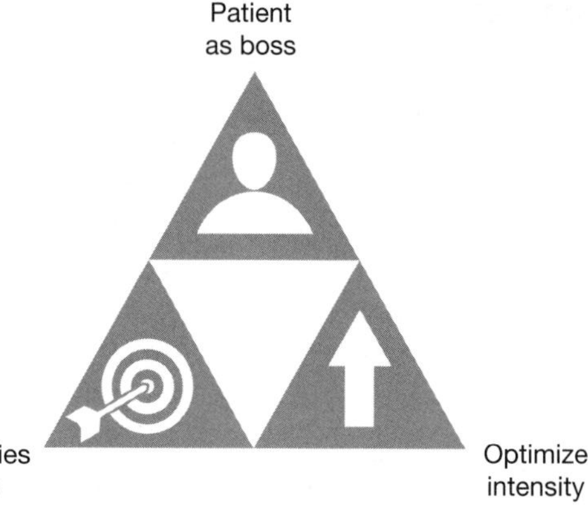

FIG. 8.3 Enhanced Medical Rehabilitation (EMR) model. Three principles make up the EMR model: (1) patient as boss (therapist practices optimal communication, resists taking over the session and lets the patient be in control, and continually looks for opportunities to ask for the patient's input); (2) link activities to personal goals (therapist interviews patient to identify enjoyable, everyday activities that represent aspects of life he or she most wants to restore; emphasizing the why of therapy can enhance participation); (3) optimize intensity (design challenging, intense activities that link to patient's stated goals to elicit maximum effort and physical engagement; the aim is to keep the patient physically engaged in therapy at least 65% of the session). *Copyright Eric Lenze Washington University in St. Louis, School of Medicine. Permission by author.*

TABLE 8.2 Suggested Tasks and Exercises in Exercise Circuits and Boot Camp–Style Sessions Utilizing Time on Task

Possible Formats	Circuit	Boot Camp
30 seconds on task; 10-second rest; multiple sets (3–4); 10 seconds to transition to next exercise	Transferring in and out of bed	Squats
OR	Sit to stands from various surfaces	Dead lifts
40–50 seconds on task; 10 seconds to transition to next station; repeat circuit several times	Floor transfers	Chair pushups
OR	Stair climbing	Step-ups
20 seconds on; 8-second rest emphasizing speed; repeat 6–8 times	Squats	Bosu ball balancing
	Putting jacket on and off	Pushing and pulling plyometric box
	Kneeling and rising	Jump squats
	Farmer's carry	Boxing with therapist
	Folding clothes while standing on a compliant surface	Farmer's carry

Summary

Consideration of the variables of specificity, overload, neuromuscular elements, and enjoyment is key to making an exercise program for any older adults effective. The creative challenge of exercise prescription is how the physical therapist manipulates the variables. With focus on the patient's goals and manipulation of the various exercise prescription elements, engagement is enhanced, and optimal results achieved.

APPLICATION OF PRINCIPLES TO EXERCISE TYPES

Aerobic Exercise

Aerobic exercise increases the body's capacity to absorb, deliver, and utilize oxygen. A training program aimed at enhancing cardiopulmonary performance is indicated for patients who lack the ability to sustain activity for a desired period because of decreased cardiopulmonary and vascular efficiency. Oftentimes, these patients have complaints of fatigue with a given level of exercise, which may be related to disease and/or deconditioning. Either moderate- or vigorous-intensity exercise, or both, can be undertaken to improve aerobic capacity, but it appears that the higher the intensity, the greater the benefits. High-intensity interval training (HIIT) is an example of a feasible form of high-intensity training and is discussed later. Aerobic training at a mean intensity of 66% to 73% HRR with 40 to 50 minutes per session for 3 to 4 days/week for 30 to 40 weeks appears to be effective and optimal for maximum cardiopulmonary benefits in healthy sedentary older adults.[49] A minimum threshold for deriving benefits may exist based on fitness level, with a minimum of 45% oxygen uptake reserve or HRR (<11 metabolic equivalents [METs]) found to provide benefit in untrained older adults.[14,37] The ACSM has suggested that the exercise stimulus of 60% to 80% is necessary to achieve cardiopulmonary adaptation and fitness.[2]

Moderate-intense physical activity may be accumulated in bouts of ≥10 minutes each to attain the daily goal of ≥30 minutes/day; however, it is the volume of activity that will afford health benefits.[14] There is also evidence that sedentary people will benefit from short, regular periods of activity of as little as 1-minute[13] or 10-minute bouts[70] to break up periods of sitting or lying. Although 10-minute bouts of aerobic exercise may be the most feasible for some people, these short bouts must be supplemented with frequency of bouts. Implementing the overload principle with intensity of aerobic exercise will achieve optimal responses of health benefits and cardiorespiratory fitness.

Interval and High-Intensity Interval Training. Interval aerobic training programs are the most efficient to improve cardiopulmonary and endurance performances and general health, even in older adults.[71] Interval training is suitable for healthy adults and those with cardiorespiratory disease, vascular disease, and diabetes.[72,73] The advantages of an interval program over constant-intensity programs are the superior improvements in several cardiovascular outcomes, as well as in fitness and performance,[72,74,75] even in those with cardiopulmonary and vascular disease. Box 8.6 lists the benefits of interval and HIIT training.[76] Interval training may be more effective in untrained individuals than sustained aerobic activity of similar duration in improving cardiopulmonary fitness and blood glucose concentrations but less effective in improving resting heart rate, body composition, and total cholesterol–to–high-density lipoprotein (HDL) ratio.[14]

HITT is a form of interval training exercise in which individuals alternate periods of short, intense, nonoxidative exercise at maximum effort with less intense recovery periods. HIIT allows equal or improved outcomes for markedly less time investment and is associated with greater adherence, with results apparent in as little as 2 weeks.[77] Examples of HITT protocols are listed in Table 8.3. Although few studies have examined HIIT on older adults, the Generation 100 study,[19] using HITT principles, demonstrated 60% adherence to the prescribed intensity (≥15 on the Borg scale) at two times/week over 1 year without strict supervision, although women had a lower adherence rate with high-intensity

BOX 8.6 Benefits of Interval and High-Intensity Interval Training (HIIT) for Older Adults

Healthy Older Adults

- Reduces subcutaneous fat, especially abdominal fat
- Reduces total body mass
- Improves VO_2 max
- Improves insulin sensitivity
- Burns more calories than continuous moderate exercise (CME)
- Increases postexercise fat oxidation and energy expenditure more than CME
- Decreases total cholesterol and low-density lipoprotein cholesterol while increasing high-density lipoprotein cholesterol more than CME
- Improves endothelial function
- Improves blood pressure
- Improves glucose regulation
- Reduces risk of cardiovascular events
- Decreases all-cause mortality

High-Risk Older Adults

- Reduces blood pressure
- Improves endothelial function
- Improves lipid profiles
- Improves VO_2 max
- Improves left ventricular function
- Improves overall myocardial function
- Reverses left ventricular remodeling in heart failure patients

Data from Shiraev T and Barclay G 2012, Australian Family Physician. Vol 41(12) 960–962.

TABLE 8.3 Protocols for High-Intensity Interval Training Shown to Be Effective in Accomplishing the Stated Purpose

Purpose	Second Stage (Once Acclimated to Type of Exercise)
Improve cardiopulmonary function in those participating in cardiac rehabilitation programs[56]	2 × 8-minute interval blocks of 30 seconds at 80%–100% of peak power output interspersed with 30-second active or passive recovery, passive recovery permitted between blocks
Improve aerobic fitness, cardiac function, lipids, and glucose control in patients with cardiometabolic disease[213]	4-minute intervals of high-intensity treadmill walking (usually "uphill") interspersed with periods of moderate-intensity walking
Improve aerobic fitness, cardiac function, and metabolic risk factors in previously sedentary older adults[75]	4 × 4-minute intervals at 90% peak heart rate interspersed by 3 × 3-minute active recovery periods at 70% HR peak for a total of 25 minutes on a non-weight-bearing all-extremity ergometer
Improve vascular function[77]	4 × 4 HIIT at 85%–95% of HR max interspersed with 3 minutes of active recovery at 60%–70% HR max, 3 times/week for 12–16 weeks
Beginners who have been cleared for exercise	2 sessions/week 40%–50% HR max in recovery; 80%–90% HR max in work period 1–4 minutes Recovery is greater than or equal to work period; return HR to 40%–50% HR max through active recovery Progression 1: 60 seconds × 10 Progression 2: 2 minutes × 8 Progression 3: 4 minutes × 4

HR, heart rate; *HIIT*, high-intensity interval training.
All protocols were preceded and followed by a 2- to 10-minute warmup and cooldown.

exercise than did men. HITT is known to be safe for healthy older adults as well as those with diabetes, stable angina, and heart failure, and after myocardial infarct, cardiac stenting, and coronary artery grafting.[73,78]

Measurement. Measuring and interpreting vital signs is the classical way of measuring intensity and response to aerobic exercise. Chapter 18 provides an overview of vital sign measurements for heart rate and blood pressure in healthy older adults and older adults with cardiac or pulmonary dysfunction. As summarized in Table 8.1, various perceived exertion scales are available to help patients gauge their exertion level. The talk test is a valid measure of aerobic intensity based on the premise that exercising at or above the ventilatory (lactate) threshold (50% to 70% VO_2 max) does not allow comfortable, conversational speech and thus serves as a means of estimating the cut point between moderate- and vigorous-intensity exercises.[79] In addition to guiding the intensity of exercise training, the talk test can assist patients in avoiding exertional ischemia[80] and those with atrial fibrillation.[79] The talk test may not be as practical for monitoring exercise intensity in HIIT because of the shorter duration of exercise bouts at higher intensity.[79] Protocols include reciting a standard paragraph of 10 to 15 seconds out loud or counting out loud. The individual is asked at rest and before exercising to count as high as possible before having to take a second breath. This establishes a baseline target during exercise and corresponds to moderate- to vigorous-intensity exercise (46% to 100% VO_2 max).[81]

OMNI scales for walking and resistance exercise are illustrated in Fig. 8.4. The OMNI perceived aerobic exercise scale is a valid measure of aerobic capacity that visually reflects effort in response to aerobic exercise (cycle and walking) with more accuracy at higher loads of exertion for older adults.[82–84]

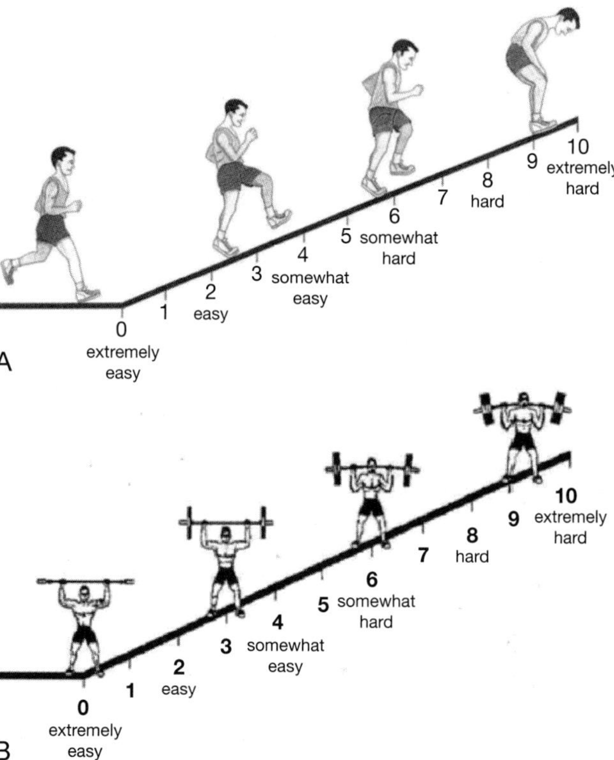

FIG. 8.4 A, OMNI Scale for walking and resistance exercise. **B,** OMNI scale for aerobic exercise. *(From Shinya Yamauchi SM, Yamauchi S, Fujisawa C, Domen K. Rating of perceived exertion for quantification of the intensity of resistance exercise. Int J Phys Med Rehab. 2013;1[9]:1–4.)*

Functional Measures of Aerobic Capacity. Tests that assess exercise response to common functional activities such as walking and climbing stairs are commonly used. These tests are described in Chapter 7. The 6-minute walk test (6MWT) is a measure of how far a person can walk in 6 minutes and is a valid and reliable indicator of aerobic fitness.[85] The 400-m walk test (long corridor walk) is useful for measuring aerobic capacity and thus identifying cardiovascular disease[86] but can also identify the risk of developing mobility disability.[87,88] The 2-minute step test has established norms, and is commonly used in fitness circles. This author has perceived it to be a more strenuous test by older individuals than the distance walk tests.

Mode. The modality of aerobic exercise should be rhythmic and repetitive in nature and involve large muscle groups. Common modes include walking, stair climbing, hiking, jogging, running, social dancing, cycling, swimming, cross-country skiing, skating, rowing, and playing tennis, racquet sports, basketball, soccer, volleyball, and others. A host of equipment can be used indoors for aerobic conditioning of the older individual, including a treadmill, elliptical trainer, stair stepper, rower, stationary bike, and recumbent-type bike. Outdoor activities include walking or hiking, cross-country skiing, skating, jogging, and cycling. Each activity has advantages and disadvantages. The individual's preference should be the basis for recommending a specific type of aerobic exercise. In addition, the physical requirements for each activity should be considered, matching the requirements with the person's abilities. The best activity is the one that the individual will do consistently. Once an aerobic exercise program is established, there is typically little need for physical therapist supervision other than to periodically adjust the intensity of the program as the patient progresses.

Aerobic exercise may be one aspect of a complete exercise program for an older adult. Considerations of physical impairments, functional deficits, and patient goals need to be considered and the exercise mode individualized. Strengthening exercises may need to be done prior to participation in aerobic conditioning to enable aerobic conditioning to occur, especially if the person complains of pain or fatigue.

Aquatic Exercise

Aquatic exercise allows the application of the physical stress theory for individuals who cannot tolerate the stresses of land-based exercises. The buoyancy of the water allows a deconditioned individual or an individual with significant joint pathology to exercise by lessening the impact on the joints, thus serving as a viable environment for individuals who have pain. The buoyancy of water decreases compressive forces within joints by 36% to 55% while offering hydrostatic support to the upright position.[89] Older adults may have lower body density and a higher level of buoyancy owing to body composition.

Aquatic exercise can be used to improve cardiorespiratory fitness, strength, power, bone density,[90] flexibility, and agility.[91] Aquatic exercise may have moderate-sized effects on physical functioning in healthy older adults when compared with no training, and may be at least as effective as land-based exercise.[91] In a meta-analysis of the effect of aquatic exercise in older adults, the authors found that younger participants (<68 years of age) may benefit more, which may result from the higher intensity used. This review found no difference between two and three sessions/week. When compared with control interventions of usual care, education, telephone calls, social attention, and no intervention, aquatic exercise has small short-term (immediately after treatment) improvement in pain, disability, and quality of life in people with knee and hip osteoarthritis or both. These effects on pain and disability were considered clinically relevant.[92,93]

The effects of water turbulence offer periods of instability that must be overcome and can result in positive changes in balance and postural stability compared with the more static nature of land-based exercise. Additionally, most pools are heated, which may have a therapeutic effect on painful joints.[93] Patients who have osteoarthritis, are overweight, or have recently undergone surgery may initially benefit from aquatic exercise. Also, those patients who have significant balance disorders or a fear of falling may derive some initial benefits from the water before progressing to land-based exercises.

When designing the exercise prescription for the individual undergoing aquatic exercises, the goal and desired outcome should drive the prescription. For example, if improving physical activity and/or aerobic capacity is the goal, achieving all or part of the recommended 150 minutes in variable session length and intensity is appropriate. If the goal is improved lower extremity strengthening, then intensity would be key, employing aquatic equipment such as floats and paddles to increase or decrease resistance.

Regardless of the goal, monitoring exercise tolerance through an RPE or heart rate that is adjusted for the aquatic environment is critical. The heart rate reduction model was determined by Luiz Fernando Martins Kruel and is sometimes referred to as the Kruel protocol.[94] An aquatic heart rate reduction is determined by subtracting a 1-minute in-pool heart rate from a 1-minute land-based heart rate (Table 8.4). The difference is referred to as the aquatic reduction. Because heart rate decreases in response to water immersion, vital signs can overestimate the response.[95] RPE correlates well with the percentage of VO_2 peak in aquatic exercise in younger women.[96] RPE intensities of 12 to 13 corresponded to 46% to 63% VO_2 max (moderate) and those of 14 to 17 corresponded to 64% to 90% VO_2 max (vigorous).[96]

The use of aquatic exercise allows a patient, who may otherwise be unable to exercise because of pain or instability, the ability to be more physically active and to gain initial levels of strength to permit land-based exercise.

TABLE 8.4 Calculating Target Heart Rate for a 70-Year-Old Woman with a Resting Heart Rate of 75 bpm

Variable	Traditional (ACSM) Method	Karvonen Method	Aquatic Reduction
Maximum heart rate given the example of a **70-year-old woman**	220−age = **150 bpm**	206−88% of age = **144.4 bpm**	220−age−5 bpm aquatic adjustment = **145 bpm**
Heart rate reserve (maximum heart rate − resting heart rate); given the example of a resting **heart rate of 75 bpm**	150−75 = **75 bpm**	144.4−75= **69.4 bpm**	145−75 = **70 bpm**
Target heart rate = 80% of maximum heart rate, given example	150 × 80% = **120 bpm**	144.4 × 80% = **116 bpm**	145 × 80% = **116 bpm**

Resistance Training

Functional capacity shows a progressive decline with aging, as does the increased incidence of mobility disability. This is not surprising, because older adults lose as much as 40% of their strength between 60 and 90 years.[97] Compounding this decline is the amount of strength lost with bed rest, of an order of 1% to 3% per day.[98] The relationship between strength and functional ability places enormous responsibility on physical therapists to create and deliver effective progressive resistance exercise (PRE) programs. PRE is the most effective intervention to elicit improvements in muscle strength and functional performance and to develop muscle hypertrophy.[99] PRE can also add reserve to provide a protective effect in the event the person has a period of reduced activity or bed rest secondary to injury or illness. Much recent research has determined that strength training is a first-line intervention for many of the symptoms and consequences of chronic diseases such as chronic obstructive pulmonary disease, osteoporosis, and falls.[100]

Specificity and progressive overload are critical parameters of PRE. The elements of intensity, duration, sets, repetitions, and frequency can be manipulated within the exercise program design to individualize the program to match each person's baseline abilities, desires, and limitations.

Intensity. Strength training intensity explains improvements in maximal strength.[45,47,53,101] A recent meta-analysis of studies of older adults found that resistance training improved muscle strength by 13% to 90% (25 studies) and, to a smaller extent, improved muscle morphology (by 1% to 21%; 9 studies).[45] The ACSM and others have suggested that an intensity of 80% of an 1RM is a preferred workload to obtain optimal results.[2,100]

The intensity of resistance training to achieve muscle strengthening is influenced by the amount of overload (a load greater than what is required to maintain current status), amount of time the muscle is under tension, and volume of exercise (repetitions and sets). Although higher loads have superior strength outcomes compared with lower loads (<50% 1RM) for both untrained individuals[45,102] and people with frailty,[103] both high- and low-load exercise can increase muscle strength, functional ability, and hypertrophy given sufficient volume of exercise. Despite superior strength gains with high-intensity/low-repetition exercise, beginning at an intensity of 20% to 30% and progressing to 80% of an 1RM may be better tolerated by frail and untrained individuals and allow for gradual accommodation and neural adaptation while decreasing the negative effects of delayed-onset muscle soreness and high perceived effort. Training to failure (the inability to continue to perform the exercise through full range and in good form), rather than to a predetermined number of repetitions, may require less volume and therefore less time but is prone to creating muscle soreness and creating a stressful cardiovascular response secondary to effort. Training at a submaximal level may require more volume (sets and repetitions) and thus more time but creates a less stressful cardiovascular response.[101,102] However, it is clear that both strategies achieve the intensity required to increase muscle strength.

Time under tension is also a strategy to increase intensity because total time under tension has a strong effect on strength gains.[45] Time under tension is important for mechanobiological adaptations, motor unit recruitment, and motor unit firing rates. The longer a contraction is maintained, the more motor units are recruited until maximum contraction occurs. Time under tension differs for different types of contractions. Borde and colleagues, in their review of a study of healthy older adults, found that isometric contractions required constant tension of 2.0 seconds, concentric contractions required 2.5 seconds, and eccentric contractions required 3.0 seconds for maximum effect.[45] Six seconds total appeared to be the most effective length of time under tension in this review, thus providing opportunity to vary the contraction speed.

Training eccentrically is another strategy for achieving overload and time under tension. When performing an eccentric contraction, slowing the speed of the movement overloads the activity, as in having a patient sit down in a controlled manner. Eccentric contractions have an additional advantage in that they have been found to produce larger gains in muscle strength and size compared with concentric muscle actions.[45,105]

Sets. Improved strength occurs in two to four sets of resistance exercise per muscle group in most individuals.

However, in untrained and frail individuals, a single set may also significantly improve strength and size. A recent meta-analysis of studies of healthy older adults revealed little or no effect of number of sets per exercise and number of repetitions per set on strength gains.[45] The analysis found the largest effects were from two to three sets; however, in the short term (6 weeks), no difference existed between single versus multiple sets.[106] The number of sets performed to failure does not appear to impact neural adaptations as measured by electromyography activation of the quadriceps muscles in groups of older women (60 to 74 years) who trained using single or multiple sets.[106]

Repetitions. A systematic analysis found that the largest effects in strength gains occurred when older adults used seven to nine repetitions per set to failure (high intensity).[45] However, this finding is impacted by the number of repetitions performed to failure. Training to muscular failure explains how benefits of strength training occur with different magnitudes of overload (20% to 90% 1RM). It is the effort of achieving failure that is critical to strength gains, rather than the number of repetitions at a certain load.[100]

Other Principles. Other specific parameters known to affect maximum results of strength training include a rest of 60 seconds between sets, a training frequency of two sessions per week, and performance of two to three sets per exercise with seven to nine repetitions per set and 4 seconds between repetitions. Any of these training variables are known to optimize the effects of resistance training in improving maximal voluntary strength in healthy older adults.[2,14,45,47]

Application to Inpatient environment. Although adapting recommended frequencies can be done easily in an outpatient or group training program, an inpatient environment presents unique challenges to designing the optimal exercise prescription where daily or twice-daily sessions are delivered, 5 to 7 days/week. Adaptions in the rehabilitation environment can be made by adjusting intensity and limiting resistance training to limited muscle groups in a given session. Table 8.5 provides examples of how to apply the frequency principle to an inpatient environment.

Strength Measurement. The 1RM method is the gold standard to measure strength across a variety of individuals, including athletes.[2] The 1RM test is a maximum exertion test that is safe for older adults but may result in muscle soreness and blood pressure spikes.[107] A multiple RM can also be obtained, which is the number of repetitions an individual achieves before muscle failure. For example, when an individual can leg press 200 pounds for six repetitions before losing form or being unable to complete another repetition, the individual has achieved a 6RM. There are numerous online tables that convert a multiple RM to a 1RM or a 10RM for the purpose of assessing an individual over time and for determining the weight that will equate to a percentage maximum for training purposes. An example of a conversion is listed in Table 8.6.

TABLE 8.5 Example of Applying Frequency Recommendations in an Inpatient Environment

	Monday	Tuesday	Wednesday	Thursday	Friday
Strengthening High intensity	Ankle and knee Quadriceps Dorsiflexors Gastrocnemius	Core strength Abdominals Gluteus maximus Gluteus medius Erector spinae	Ankle and knee Quadriceps Dorsiflexors Gastrocnemius	Core strength Abdominals Gluteus maximus Gluteus medius Erector spinae	Ankle and knee Quadriceps Dorsiflexors Gastrocnemius
Functional training for gait	Short bouts of fast gait speed and directional changes	Ambulation distance	Work on gait speed	Ambulation distance	Short bouts of fast gait speed
Balance and agility	Static balance (reaching, head turning, eyes closed) Dynamic balance Stability ball	Dynamic gait (head turning, obstacle course, ramps, curbs, uneven and compliant surfaces)	Static balance Dynamic balance (squats, lunges, reaching with foot, ARROM with elastic while balancing on other foot)	Dynamic gait (head turning with forward, backward, and sideways stepping), obstacle course, uneven and compliant surfaces)	Static balance (reaching, head turning, eyes closed) Dynamic balance Stability ball
Functional training for specific tasks	Task specific (ADLs, transfers, bed mobility, wheelchair mobility) timed or weighted	Task specific (reaching, squatting, bending, lifting, rotation, etc.) timed or weighted	Task specific (ADLs, transfers, bed mobility, wheelchair mobility) timed or weighted	Task specific (reaching, squatting, bending, lifting, rotation, etc.) timed or weighted	Task specific (ADLs, transfers, bed mobility, wheelchair mobility) timed or weighted

ADLs, activities of daily living; *ARROM*, active resistive range of motion
This sample exercise program could be utilized with a patient requiring BID physical therapy treatments 5 days per week consistent with any functional profile.

TABLE 8.6 Maximum Weight That Can Be Lifted Decreases with the Number of Repetitions

Given:	1RM	2RM	3RM	4RM	5RM	6RM	7RM	8RM	9RM	10RM
The load (in pounds)	100	95	93	90	87	85	83	80	77	75
Number of repetitions	1	2	3	4	5	6	7	8	9	10

Avers D, Brown M. Daniel and Worthingham's Muscle Testing. 10th ed. St Louis: Elseiver; 2019.

Measuring an RM for a functional movement such as a chair rise requires some creativity. For example, if an older individual is not able to rise from a standard chair without using his or her arms, the therapist must create a situation where the person can be successful, such as raising the surface to allow the individual to complete the task independently. The number of times the person can rise from the raised surface becomes that person's repetition maximum and the appropriate training stimulus can be determined. For example, if the surface height is 21 inches and the person can stand 10 times without using his or her arms, the person has achieved a 10RM from a 21-inch-high surface, representing an 80% training stimulus (10RM = 75% to 80% 1RM). The height of the surface can be increased or decreased to achieve the desired training stimulus. With some creativity and an eye for objectivity, this method can be used for any movement such as bridges, lunges, wall squats, and step-ups and step-downs.

Similar to aerobic exercise, perceived exertion scales, summarized in Table 8.1, can be used to measure intensity and to target a desired amount of intensity during resistance training. Increases in strength are well documented at perceived levels of exertion over 4 (Borg CR-10 and OMNI scales) and 12 (Borg 6–20 scale) and are validated against the repetition maximum method.[55,108,109] Perceived exertion, reported similarly by men and women,[109] is affected by the number of sets performed and muscle group activated,[108] perhaps related to differing patterns of muscle recruitment. Some reports indicate that older adults overestimate their perceived exertion when using upper extremity muscles.[110,111] The OMNI resistance scale (Fig. 8.4) has been robustly investigated on older adults participating in resistance training.[55,112–115] The OMNI scale may be easier to use because it is a visual scale. In older adults, perceived effort is an important indicator of training intensity.[116] Therefore, it is recommended that the RPE be used with the 1RM method to regulate training intensity.[45,62]

Manual muscle testing (MMT) has been used in the clinic to quantify strength, but its application is somewhat limited. Although MMT is a valid way to determine strength below or at a grade of 3/5, it is not valid above the grade of 3, especially when considering the strength required for functional, mobility-type movements involving lower extremities. Bohannon has determined that the minimum amount of force necessary to rise from a chair unassisted and without the use of the individual's arms is 45% of a person's body weight, equating to a bilateral MMT of the quadriceps of 5/5 on one side and 4+/5 on the other.[117] Clearly, an MMT has a ceiling effect, especially for functional movements involving lower extremities.

Handheld muscle dynamometry is easy to use and valid but is influenced by the tester's strength, the subject's position, the ability to stabilize the limb, and the technique used.[118] Handheld muscle dynamometers, because of their quantitative nature, have published norms that can be useful for therapists.[119–122]

Specificity

The importance of specificity in strength training is well documented. By not matching the exercise to the outcome, the principle of specificity is too frequently violated in research and the clinic. A common example of this violation is the frequent yet inappropriate use of open-chain leg extension exercises for patients who need to perform functional movements such as sit-to-stand transfers from the chair and/or bed or stair climbing. The specificity principle applied to this example would be to strengthen the quadriceps through a slowed (3-second) eccentric squatting movement. Because eccentric contractions produce a greater strength response, assisted concentric movements to standing can be used, with the slowed eccentric movement used for the going-down movement. Even adapting the chair height to allow independent standing would be more effective than open-chain, full-arc extension, even with overload using ankle weights. Likewise, there would be little basis for the use of straight-leg raises or open-chain knee extension to achieve a functional movement such as walking or stair climbing.

Additionally, awareness of the specific actions of the muscles involved in a movement (task analysis) is critical for application of the specificity concept. For example, hip abduction controls the position of the knee in weight bearing.[129] Because many older people demonstrate weakness of the hip abductors and thus exhibit valgus when getting up from a chair (often associated with knee pain), strengthening the hip abductors to better perform the sit-to-stand movement would be in order. Specificity in this example is accomplished through motor learning of visual cueing (watching and controlling the position of the knee in a mirror) and verbal cueing (pushing the feet apart), using an elastic band loop encircling the thighs to provide sensory feedback, and performing an eccentric contraction while squatting.

Core Stability. Core stability, defined as proximal stability for distal mobility, provides a solid base for movement and forces generated by the limbs. Prior to limb movement or contraction, contraction of core muscles of up to 30% (maximum voluntary contraction [MVC]) has been recorded, supporting the need for core strength/activation and stability in day-to-day activity and prevention of injury.[130,131] Training core muscles to stabilize limb movement effectively can be done on stable and unstable surfaces and with the unilateral movement of one limb or both. For example, raising one arm requires the opposing obliques to contract. The clinician should be aware that standing on unstable surfaces to elicit core muscle activation is not the same as challenging balance. Here, as always, specificity is important.

Core strength may not be as important as core activation, depending on the task for which stabilization is needed. Relatively low levels of activation are required for most activities of daily living (ADLs); therefore, an awareness of core activation *while performing other activities* is an appropriate method of training for stability. Additionally, a variety of activities in which to train core activation is important in keeping with the different patterns of activation that occur in response to movement.[40] Figs. 8.5 and 8.6 demonstrate two of the author's favorite core exercises for older adults.

Equipment. A variety of equipment can be utilized to provide overload and specificity. Weight machines, body weight elastic bands, cuff and hand weights, dumbbells, kettlebells, handheld blades, and so forth can offer overload to a specific task while adding variety and progression to any program. There does not seem to be a difference in effectiveness among types of external resistance with proper supervision, and each may have its advantages and disadvantages. The key is to individualize the program, honor the principle of specificity, be creative in how to provide the optimal training stimulus for any given individual, and keep the program fun and interesting. Variety often helps clients maintain their enthusiasm for the strengthening exercise program. Mixing and matching the equipment to the prescribed exercise can achieve variety. This variety can promote functional strengthening by training a given muscle to react in many different ways. Some authors have referred to this phenomenon of changing the exercise stimulus to prevent "staleness" as muscle confusion. Ultimately the decision of what type of resistance to use becomes personal preference and is based on the clinician's clinical judgment.

Protein Supplementation. The muscle adaptations induced by resistance-type exercise training can be augmented by dietary protein ingestion as skeletal muscle is nutritionally responsive to amino acid availability, particularly in older adults.[123] Older adults display anabolic resistance to amino acid intake with less sensitivity to smaller doses of ingested protein (<20 g),[124,125] necessitating protein supplementation for optimal results of a resistance exercise program.[126] Thus, the dose of protein needed to achieve a robust stimulation of protein synthesis during recovery of resistance exercise is twice as high in older adults as younger adults.[125] However, the volume of resistance exercise also stimulates protein synthesis, with one study showing increased muscle protein synthesis rates occurring with an increased exercise intensity from three sets to six sets, regardless of load, unlike with younger adults. Exercise intensity may provide another strategy for increasing protein synthesis.[127] Generally, there is agreement that an older adult should strive to achieve the number of grams of protein equal to half his or her body weight (160 pounds = 80 g of protein) with approximately 40 g of protein at breakfast and lunch.[125] Protein supplementation has not been shown to retard the loss of lean muscle mass in nonexercising older adults.[128]

Summary. Resistance exercise at sufficient intensity to achieve a strength training effect is the hallmark of any skilled physical therapy intervention for older adults because of its substantive functional impact. Much research has been done on the most effective exercise prescription for resistance exercise in older adults, yet much controversy exists, in part because of method (e.g., to muscular fatigue or not). Regardless, it is clear there is a dose–response relationship of resistance exercise to strength that can be achieved through sets, repetitions, and intensity. The variety of strength-training exercises is endless and only requires creativity and knowledge of functional movements and specificity. It is the opinion of this author that many older adults are uninterested in their exercise program because of insufficient challenge, lack of progress, or the appearance of irrelevancy of the exercise program to their personal goals. This is unfortunate because of the preponderance of evidence that describes the effectiveness of well-designed strengthening exercise programs to achieve improved function, decrease the impact of chronic disease, and improve balance, coordination, speed of movement, and overall mobility. Physical therapists who treat older adults would do well to become exercise experts in applying the evidence to resistance exercise programs for older adults in all practice settings and across all functional levels of their patients.

Speed, Power, and Plyometrics

Speed and Power. Power is defined as the force exerted multiplied by the velocity of movement. Muscular power is a function of strength, neuromuscular activation, and speed of movement. Power rather than strength is a better predictor of functional abilities such as stair climbing, gait speed, and chair rise.[104,132,133] Power is observed in the ability to move quickly and powerfully, with stability. The loss of muscle power is associated with slowness, an increased risk of falling, impaired functional performance, and frailty.[134,135] Slowness occurs in part because of a preferential loss of type II or fast-twitch muscle fibers, which happens at twice the rate as strength loss and in part because of disuse.[136]

Power Training. High-velocity power training is feasible, is well tolerated, and can effectively improve lower

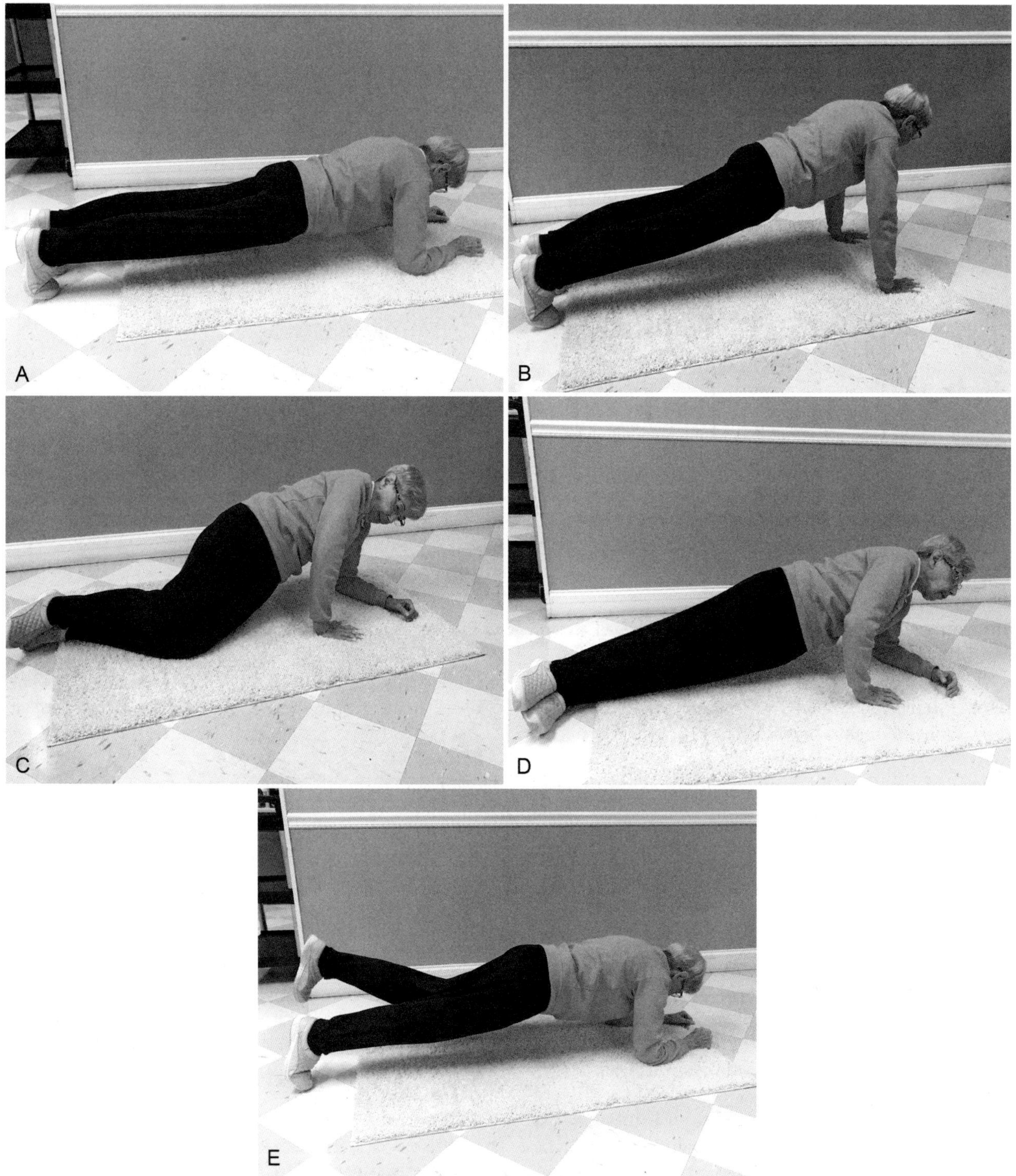

FIG. 8.5 Plank progression. **A,** Prone on elbows. **B,** Prone on hands. **C,** Side plank with increased leg support. **D,** Side plank. **E,** Prone plank with one leg extended.

extremity muscle power and function in healthy older men and women, older women with self-reported disability, older adults with mobility limitations, and frail women over 80 years of age.[104,133,137] Because many movements intrinsic to balance require a response in milliseconds, the risk of accidental falls and injury indicates the need for a power component in an older adult's exercise program.

Power training is distinguished from resistance training by the intention to move with maximal velocity.[137] Moving a load "as fast as possible" has a moderate advantage over resistance training at any load in improving physical function, and is an equal or better predictor of functional performance than maximal force.[137] Although power improves with any resistance (20% to 80% 1RM), there appears to be a dose–response relationship to resistance

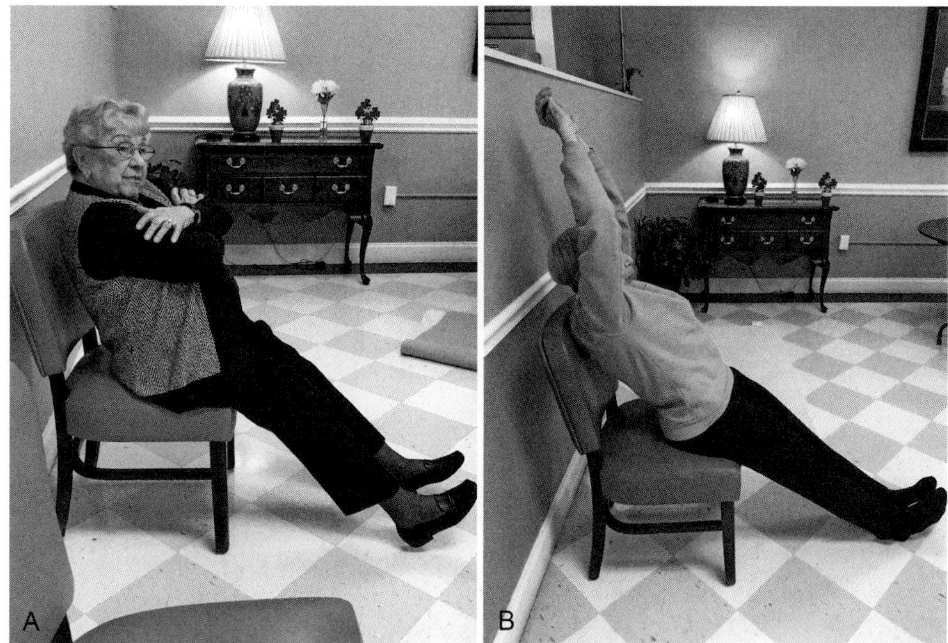

FIG. 8.6 Sit-backs. **A,** Easier version with arms crossed, leaning back without touching the back of the chair. **B,** Harder version of sit-backs (with arms elevated).

training and velocity, with the largest gains achieved with the highest loading intensity (80% 1RM).[133,137] However, lower loads allow for greater emphasis on speed and power and possibly postural control.[137] Additionally, Reid et al. observed that lower loads with power training created a lower rate of perceived exertion with similar improvements in muscle power and physical performance, which may be an advantage for more frail or debilitated older adults.[138]

Significant improvements in muscle power and physical function can be gained through simple resisted functional task exercises performed with maximum intended movement velocity.[137] De Vreede et al. reported that a 12-week intervention using functional tasks performed as quickly as possible with progressive resistance through weighted vests resulted in significant improvements in functional task performance.[139]

For a group of older women residing in a nursing home, utilizing body weight with traditional lower extremity exercises such as hip abduction, hip extension, heel rises, hamstring curls, and squats, and progressing to elastic bands and gradually adding a speed component demonstrated improvements in the timed up and go (improvement of 6.3 s), chair stand (increased by four repetitions), and gait speed (decreased by 4 seconds) over 10 weeks.[140]

Once an older adult achieves two sets of a resistive exercise or movement with good form and no pain, it is appropriate to add power challenges to the exercise program. The goal is to move as quickly as possible through the concentric phase of the exercise, followed by a slow and controlled lowering of the load through the eccentric phase back to starting position.[141] When training for power, care should be taken to not overload the movement so that it alters the desired movement pattern. In other words, quality of movement prevails over speed. Finally, better training results are reported for frail older adults in programs where speed and power training are supervised.[104,142]

Assessment of Speed and Power. Speed and power are typically measured through timed tests such as gait speed over a set distance (e.g., 4 meters or 10 meters), timed chair stands (e.g., 30 seconds or the amount of time it takes to stand five times), and the amount of time it takes to climb a flight of stairs. However, any task can be timed to measure speed and power. For example, the time it takes to complete a bed transfer, rise from the floor, or get dressed could all be useful measures of power depending on the patient's goal and desired outcome. Other speed- and power-based tests include the short physical performance test (SPPB), timed up-and-go test, four-square step test, and fast gait speed.

Plyometric Training. Plyometric exercise, a form of power-based exercise, usually consists of an eccentric contraction followed by a concentric contraction of the same muscles. Plyometric exercise attempts to use the stretch reflex of the muscle spindle and the elastic energy that is stored in a stretched muscle to enhance an immediate reciprocal contraction in that muscle. For example, a patient would rapidly squat and then immediately jump through a ballistic contraction. In this example, energy is stored in the gastrocnemius as the ankle dorsiflexes and in the quadriceps as the knee flexes. As the person begins to jump, a strong and rapid contraction of the gastrocnemius and quadriceps propels the patient into a jumping motion.

Plyometrics may aid in bone formation, according to Wolff's law, by increasing the compressive forces that the bone is required to absorb.[143,144] Other authors have suggested that using plyometrics for increasing upper extremity power, such as in a boxing-type movement, aids in decreasing hip and head injuries associated with falling by allowing the person to get his or her arms out to absorb some of the force from the fall.[145] Jumping has been shown to have a positive effect on decreasing fall risk in long-term care residents when combined with strengthening, stretching, and aerobic conditioning.[146] Jump training in older adults (>50 years) was found to be safe and effective in increasing muscle power in a recent meta-analysis.[147] Jump landings train balance and promote joint stability through proprioceptive control and eccentric activation.[147] Low-impact jumps such as bunny hops and quick heel raises can be used initially. Double-leg jumps (e.g., long jumps) and landings can afford greater stability than single-leg variations and may be a better place to start. Jumps onto a box can reduce impact forces compared with landing on the ground. Figs. 8.7 through 8.9 illustrate some plyometric exercises.

A conservative approach to plyometrics should be taken because beginning exercisers may not have the soft tissue and muscle integrity that is required. Therefore, as older adults progress in their exercise program, speed of contraction should be used first, before plyometrics is added. Quick unilateral movements performed functionally, as in a skipping-type exercise, is one way to achieve increased speed of muscle contraction with a load. Then bilateral movements, such as jumping in place, can be added. Refer to Table 8.7 for ideas of how to progress a jumping program.

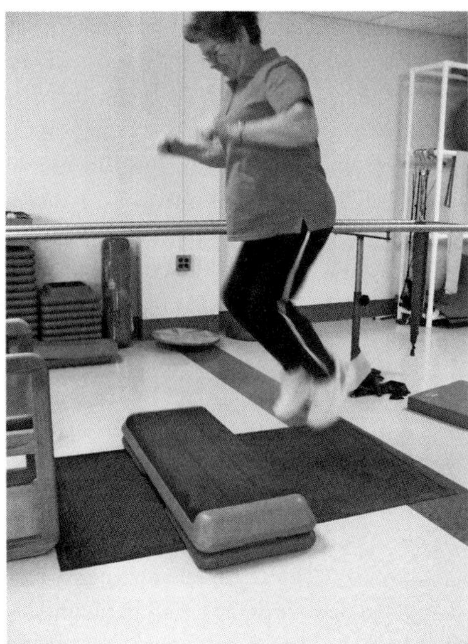

FIG. 8.7 Plyometric exercise jumping onto and off of a step.

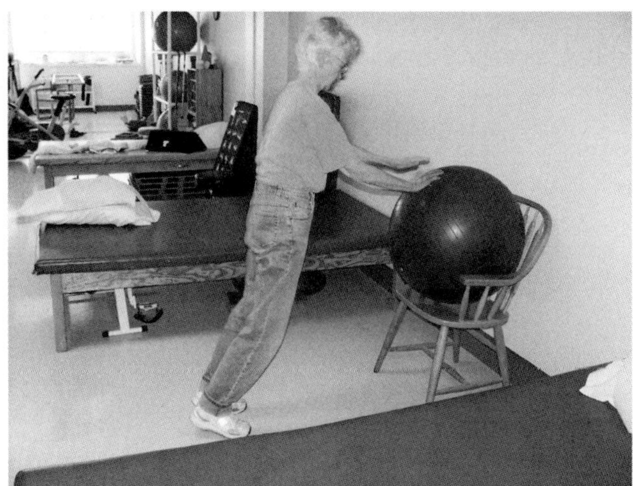

FIG. 8.8 Plyometrics, falling forward onto gym ball to increase upper extremity power.

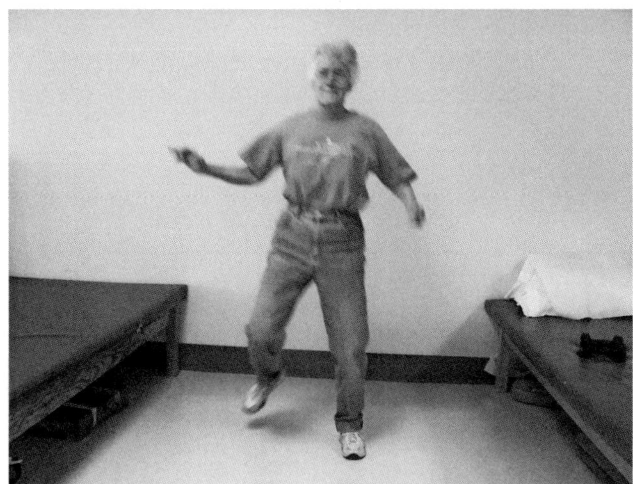

FIG. 8.9 Plyometrics, jumping from foot to foot.

While plyometrics—specifically jump training—is safe, adequate supervision to monitor and coach form is critical.[147] A baseline strength of >80% in both limbs and 90% to 95% pain-free range of motion in the weightbearing limbs are required before power and plyometric activities are added,[148] which is indicated by correct technique without adaptations. Core and proximal strength are necessary for adequate postural control and stability. Adequate proprioception indicated by adequate joint stability is also necessary. In addition to creating a challenge to produce a quick contraction, plyometrics may also impose an overload to the cardiopulmonary system that may need to be monitored. Plyometrics should not be used in the presence of significant pain, inflammation, or joint stability.[148]

Coaching techniques such as demonstrating proper joint positioning and encouraging correct landing techniques (e.g., listening to the sound of the landing) can be effective ways of teaching force absorption skills. Twenty-five jumps per session seems to be the lower limit for effectiveness, which can be divided between exercises.

TABLE 8.7 Progression of Jumps and Plyometrics

Beginner	Intermediate	Advanced
Balls of feet in contact with floor, hinge at hips, emphasize quickness of movement, agility, reciprocal movements of arms and legs, postural control	Emphasize lightness in landing with "soft knee" rather than velocity or distance, reciprocal movements, postural control	Emphasize lightness with power to achieve velocity and distance
Quick calf raises, single and double	Small jump, double stance	High jumps with arms outstretched
Bunny hops	Long jumps	Lateral jumps (up and over) on Bosu
Pivot and turn on floor	Donkey kicks	Box jumps
Weight shifting from foot to foot in multiple directions	Jump rope	Line hops
Jumping jacks without leaving the floor	Jumping jacks	Squat jumps
Scissors (rapidly criss-crossing feet in standing)	Skipping Forward bounding	Diagonal and side jumps
Upper body: emphasize shoulder stability, postural stability		
Wall pushups	Wall bounces or catches	Stability ball body bounces
Bosu modified full plank (on hands)	Bosu rocks in full plank (flat side up)	Bosu ball plank shifts with arms (one arm on ball, one arm off, then switch)
Simulated boxing, emphasizing quickness of arms, varied stances	Combine boxing moves emphasizing foot work and quickness (upper cuts, jabs, hooks, etc.)	Combination boxing moves emphasizing power and foot work (e.g., jab–jab–cross; jab–right hand; jab–right hand–left hook)
Bouncing ball in double stance	Squats while bouncing ball, staggered stance	Squats while throwing ball Sit-ups combined with throwing ball

Building up to 25 repetitions is recommended, focusing on alignment and landing technique and form.[147]

An innovative application of overload and plyometrics, described as the LIFTMOR trial, utilized high-resistance exercise with plyometrics to investigate the effect on bone mineral density and physical functioning in postmenopausal women with osteopenia and osteoporosis.[144] The 8-month, twice-weekly intervention consisted of four exercises during a 30-minute supervised program. The program gradually increased load over 1 month to achieve correct form performing deadlift, overhead press, and back-squat exercises. Program volume was high at five sets of five repetitions maintaining an intensity of 80% to 85% 1RM. Impact loading via jumping chin-ups with drop landings was performed with close supervision for five sets of five repetitions each. Eight-month results indicated increases in body height versus a loss in height for the control group (non-impact, low-load balance and mobility program of similar length), improved bone mineral density in most participants compared with a loss of bone in 73% of the control participants, and improved functional performance. Additionally, compliance was slightly higher than the control group (both were >80%). Importantly, there were no injuries other than one mild low back strain and no evidence of vertebral fractures in the intervention group.[149] This novel intervention demonstrates the safety of high-intensity resistance exercise and plyometrics even in high-risk groups such as those with osteoporosis, promoting confidence to therapists in utilizing evidence-based principles in the design of exercise interventions.

Functional Training and Multicomponent Programs

Functional training is particularly effective in improving performance in ADLs of older adults.[47] Improvements in functional abilities are likely a result of strength and power training but are more likely to occur if the functional task is also practiced. Simply walking on level surfaces at the same speed is not likely to transfer to more complex gait activities such as changes in speed or direction unless those parameters are specifically practiced. Because muscle power shows a higher correlation to functional performance than muscle strength, training for speed with body weight improves chair rising and stair climbing ability more so than with traditional strength training.[150] Interventions incorporating multiple training components (e.g., training resistance, balance, endurance, coordination, and power using multicomponent exercises) demonstrate better functional outcomes than single-focus exercise.[104] Exercise types such as tai ji (tai chi), qigong, and yoga involve varying combinations of neuromotor exercise, resistance exercise, and flexibility exercise and may offer functional carryover.

Functional training can incorporate tasks while challenging balance through the progression from parallel stance to staggered stance to tandem stance and finally to unilateral stance. At the same time, the patient can be challenged to perform activities further and further away from his or her base of support and through multiple planes of movement, eyes closed or gaze off the feet, moving head side to side, and progressing to a compliant surface. Squats and lunges can be incorporated into functional training using the same base of support and principles of progression. Examples of techniques to overload the patient's gait training session include increasing walking speed or directional movements or adding dual tasking (e.g., carrying a full glass of water), uneven surfaces and obstacles, head turns while walking, or carrying a large object such as a laundry basket that blocks direct vision of the feet. Mall walking requires a person to move with and around other people and navigate environmental challenges.[151] Table 8.8 and Figs. 8.10 through 8.19 provide examples of functional training exercises specific to common functional tasks.

The optimal intensity of functional training has not been determined. However, improvements in functional performance from frequencies of ≥2 to 3 days/week with exercise sessions of ≥20 to 30 minutes in duration for a total of ≥60 minutes of neuromuscular exercise per week were found in one review.[14] There does not seem to be an intensity effect on functional training as measured by walking speed and timed up-and-go tests. However, high-intensity training favored improvements in stair climbing.[47]

Integrating functional exercises into daily life is an alternative to structured exercise programs, especially for the very old and frail. Integrated functional exercise programs aim to turn daily routines into opportunities for exercising rather than performing separate exercises, such as purposeful walking (to store, church), tandem walking on the way to the kitchen, stair climbing, obstacle crossing, or rising from a chair. The Lifestyle-integrated Functional Exercise (LiFE) program is a physical therapist–led, evidence-based program focusing on embedding functional activities into daily life, thereby enhancing overall level of physical activity. The program is taught by professional trainers during five to seven home visits and two follow-up phone calls over a 6-month period.[152,153] LiFE activities are linked to daily tasks by using situational and environmental cues (e.g., tooth brushing) as prompts to action. The idea of LiFE is to perform the activities intentionally and consciously until they become a habit. Outcomes of the program included improved balance, reduced falls (31%), lower extremity strength, functional performance, and improved physical activity.[23]

Circuit Training. Circuit training (CT) is a shorter form of resistance training that can be less physically challenging but still improves muscular strength, aerobic fitness, and body composition.[154] CT is composed of a group of exercises, each activating a different muscle group for a specified number of repetitions (e.g., 10 to 12) or time period (e.g., 10 to 120 seconds). The participant moves quickly (transitions) to each exercise "station" with little (e.g., 8 to 30 seconds) or no rest. One to three cycles can be performed per session at modest (~40% to 60% of 1RM) exercise intensity. CT has several advantages. The number of stations, composition of stations, time at each station, and rest periods can be varied to fit the specific environment and needs of the participant. CT can be

TABLE 8.8 Functional Tasks and Suggested Functional Training

Task	Functional Training
Bed mobility	Bridge progression (Fig. 8.15) Sit-backs (Fig. 8.6) Plank (modified and full) (Fig. 8.5) Side plank (regular and modified) (Fig. 8.5) Rolling
Transfers and squats	Sit to stand from various heights and types of surfaces (compliant and firm) with arms extended (Fig. 8.13) Squats with knees abducted and hips externally rotated Leg press, wall slides
Reaching overhead	Overhead press Jump squats
Walking and stair climbing	Plank (modified and full) (Fig. 8.5) Lunges (partial and full) Step-ups (varied heights) Eccentric step-downs (Fig. 8.16) Box steps or agility ladder for directional steps Heel raises (single and double) Toe tapping with and without resistance and speed Concentric followed by eccentric dorsiflexion Pushing large object Speed work Farmer's carry (Fig. 8.17)
Floor transfers	Kneeling with trunk rotations, extension, upper extremity movements Quadruped trunk rotations and hip extensions Lunges (Fig. 8.18) Kneeling to half kneeling Mountain climbers (Fig. 8.19)
Bending over to pick up something from floor	Hip hinge to dead lifts; lifting from varying heights (Fig. 8.12)
Carrying	Farmer's carry
Mobility training	Standing weighted ball tosses Kettle bell swings Carrying laundry basket

Includes information from Senior Rehab Project podcast 8/27/18 by Alyssa Kuhn. http://seniorrehab.libsyn.com/high-intensity-functional-exercise

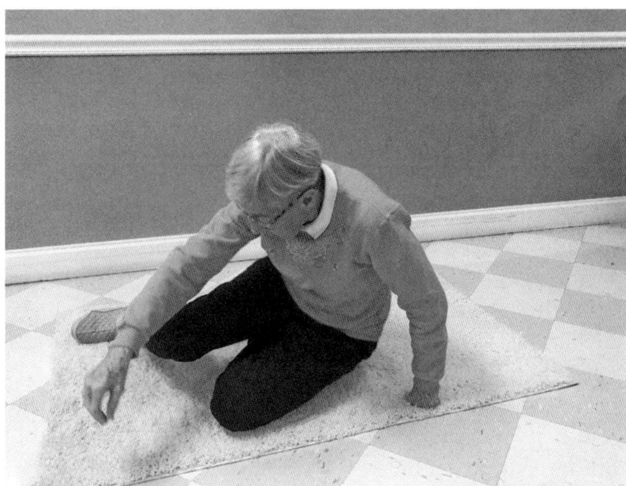
FIG. 8.10 Floor rise.

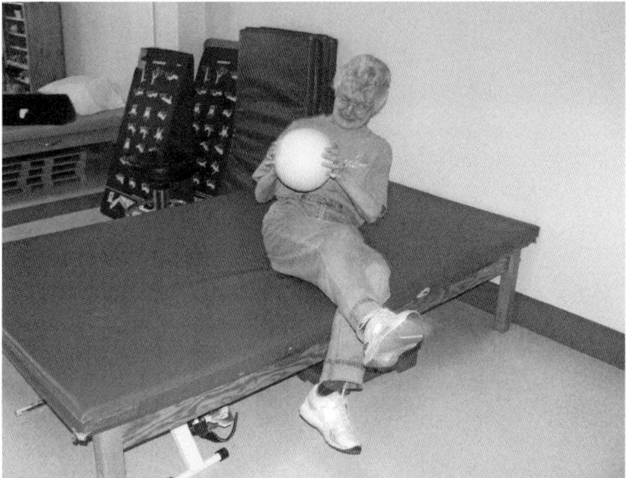
FIG. 8.11 Overload principle applied to supine-to-sit transfer.

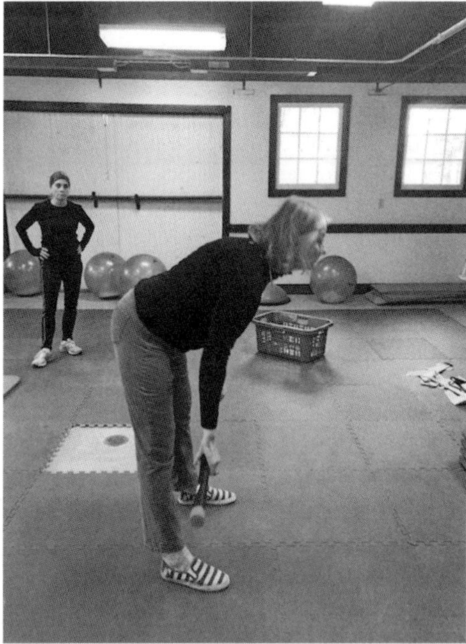
FIG. 8.12 Dead lift.

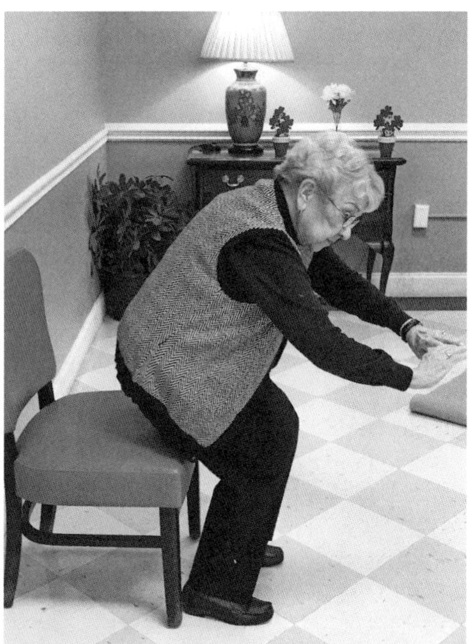
FIG. 8.13 Sit-to-stand or -squat progression.

adapted for a home or clinic environment as well as a group or exercise class situation. CT can be designed for specificity of a patient's needs, addressing specific ADLs and functional tasks, and can utilize common household items or exercise equipment. Stations can also include recreational activities such as kicking a ball at a target, throwing darts, shooting a basketball, or swinging a golf club. It can also be designed to include strengthening, balance, and functional training exercises. Table 8.9 lists examples of circuit stations suitable for a wide range of older adults' abilities. The possibilities for stations are endless.

A recent systematic review and meta-analysis on CT in older adults found that CT could be safely applied and enhanced both lower and upper body muscle strength in a diverse population of older adults including those with stroke, post–myocardial infarction, coronary bypass, hypertension, and obesity.[154] The intensity of the muscle strengthening did not seem to affect the results, indicating that even at lower intensities, CT improved strength and may have a positive effect on adherence rates.

Flexibility and Joint Mobility

Flexibility is the ability to voluntarily move a joint through its full range of motion. Older adults have less flexibility than younger adults, in part because of connective tissue, hydration, and other soft tissue changes. But movement patterns or the absence of movement also affects flexibility. This decline occurs with an average of a 10% decrease every 10 years.[155] Fixed postures and joint stiffness can result in pain syndromes, abnormal movement patterns, and difficulty in or loss of function.

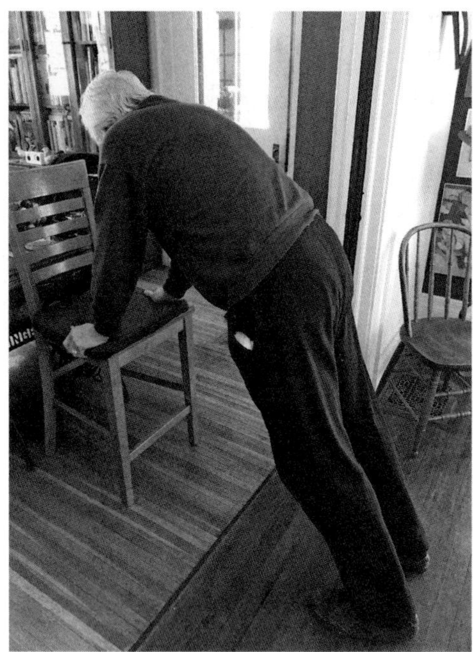

FIG. 8.14 Squat thrust from chair.

Consideration of the potential for future painful conditions and loss of function may indicate a need for stretching intervention even when a loss of motion has not yet led to pain or disability. Stretching may be indicated to promote adaptation of shortened muscles to a more lengthened position to achieve better posture and movement patterns.

Flexibility can be improved in older adults,[14] although the mechanism is unclear. In one review, the authors found that improvement in range of motion was achieved independently from stretching technique.[155] All stretching techniques showed increases in range of motion after a period of at least 4 weeks, although in one study, relatively greater gains occurred with static stretching compared with ballistic stretching or proprioceptive neuromuscular facilitation stretching.[14] Figs. 8.20 through 8.22 illustrate examples of stretching exercises used for common movement restrictions in older adults.

A systematic review found that 5 days was the minimum weekly recommended frequency to achieve significant improvements and 5 minutes per week per muscle appeared to elicit a greater response.[14,155] Hold times

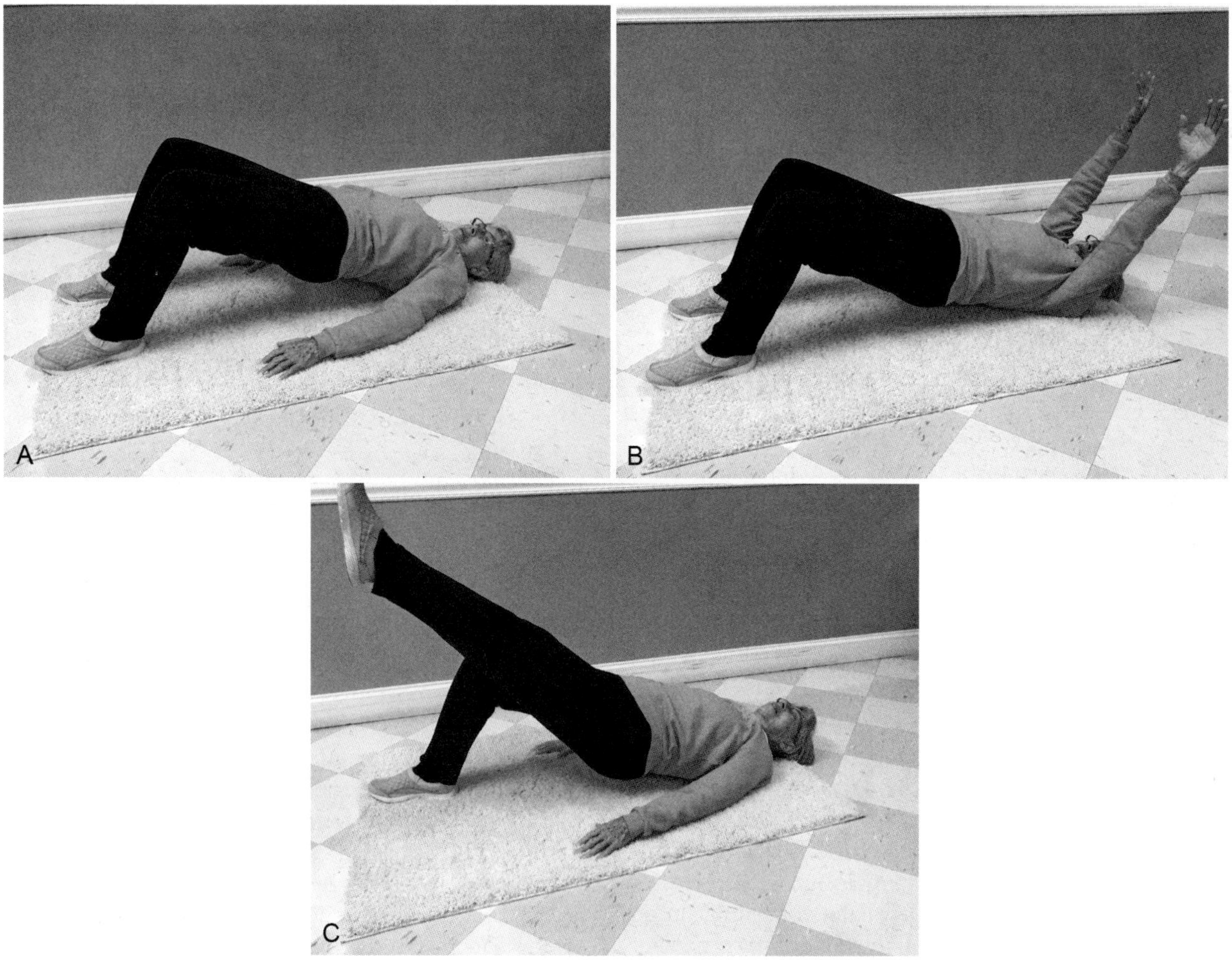

FIG. 8.15 Bridge progression. **A,** Bridge with arms to side. **B,** Bridge with arms elevated. **C,** Single-leg bridge.

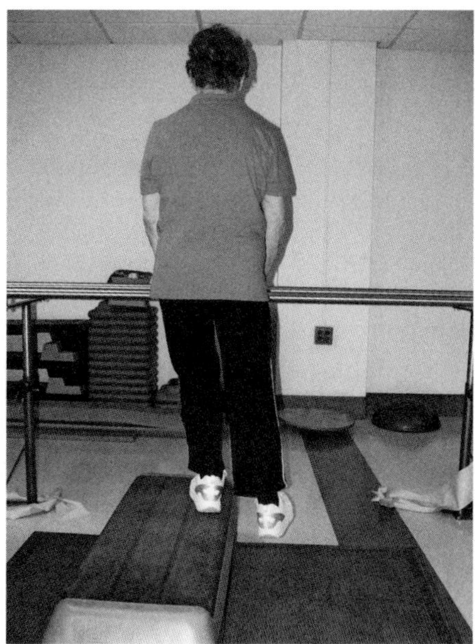

FIG. 8.16 Eccentric step-down.

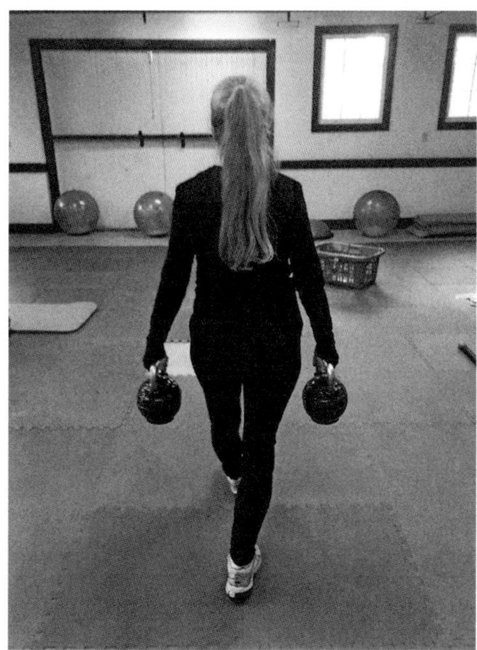

FIG. 8.17 Farmer's carry.

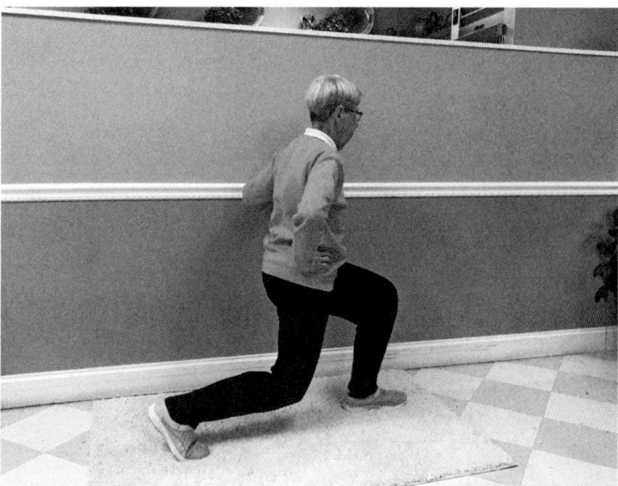

FIG. 8.18 Lunges.

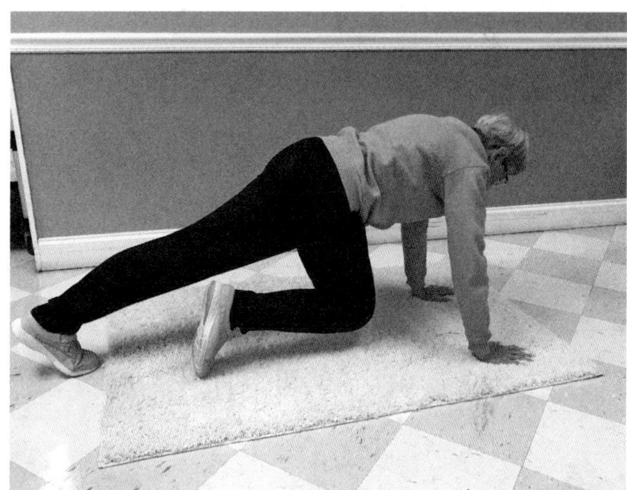

FIG. 8.19 Mountain climbers.

varied with no differences noted between durations. Although Feland et al. found that a 60-second hold time was necessary for adults aged 65 years and older compared with a 30-second hold time in younger adults, these results have not been replicated.[156] Dynamic movements are recommended prior to engaging in exercise, whereas static stretching should be performed after exercising when the muscle is warm. In addition to the muscle, soft tissue, including the joint capsule or ligaments, fascia, and connective tissue, may also be involved. Joint mobilization techniques are recommended to stretch the joint capsule, and slow static stretching is recommended for stretching collagen tissue that is the substance of these structures. The author has found hip capsule mobilization beneficial in some lumbar, hip, and knee pain and stiffness presentations.

Yoga. Yoga is a general term used for the practice of Hatha Yoga, a centuries-old health and well-being system from India that involves a combination of physical postures or poses (asana), breathing exercises (pranayama), integrated breath movement sequences, relaxation, and concentration/meditation. Many styles of Hatha Yoga have developed with subtle differences. All Hatha Yoga classes require participants to hold and move between various stationary positions with the goal of developing strength, balance, and flexibility. Typically, depending on ability level, a mixture of standing, seated, kneeling, supine, and prone stationary positions are used, with transitions incorporating forward bends, back bends, side bends, twists, inversions, and balances.

TABLE 8.9 Examples of Circuit Stations for Older Adults of Various Abilities

Stepping onto a stair or bench or stair climbing
Chair stands or squats (add speed)
Pushups
Various forms of sit-ups
Planks (various forms)
Transfers in and out of bed, off table
Heel lifts
Hip exercise in standing (various planes)
Shoulder exercises (various planes)
Sprint walking
Leg press
Obstacle course
Floor transfer
Shelf reaches
Standing, folding laundry (modified to sitting if necessary)
Vacuuming and sweeping
Tossing a basketball into a hoop
Throwing darts
Balancing on Bosu ball or other compliant surface such as a sofa cushion
Putting dishes away (bending and reaching)
Triceps pushups

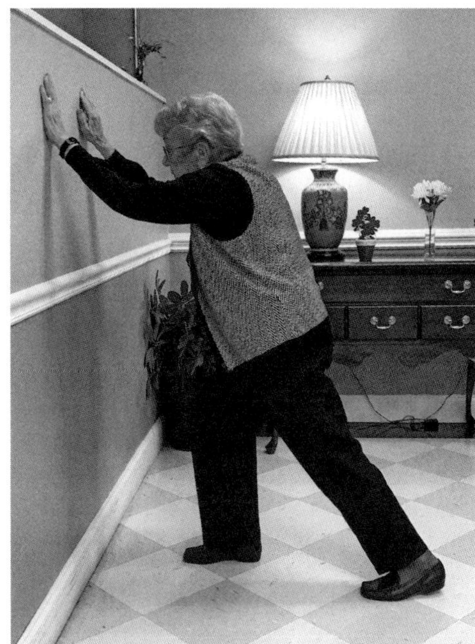

FIG. 8.21 Gastrocnemius soleus stretch.

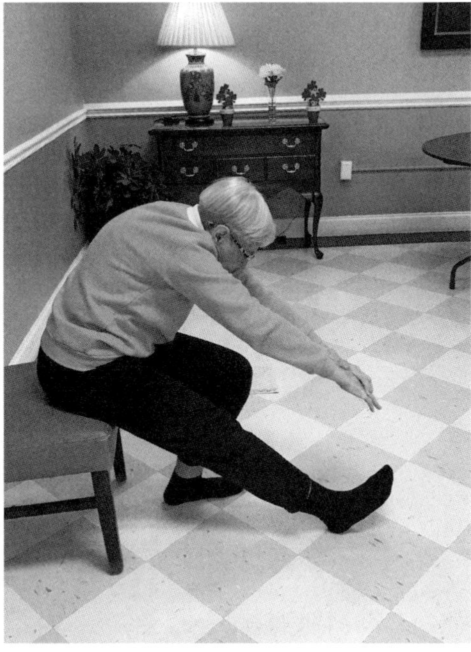

FIG. 8.22 Sit and reach hamstring and low back stretch.

The British Wheel of Yoga Gentle Years Yoga[157] is a 12-week, one-class-per-week program of 75 minutes of group-based classes for physically inactive older adults with various comorbidities. The classes adapted Hatha Yoga poses for the seated and standing positions, reduced hold time in a single pose, and slowed class pace to allow greater time for breath control and recovery. In a study of older adults with a mean age of 74 years, results indicated an improvement in lower body flexibility with reported enjoyment by participants compared with the control group.[158]

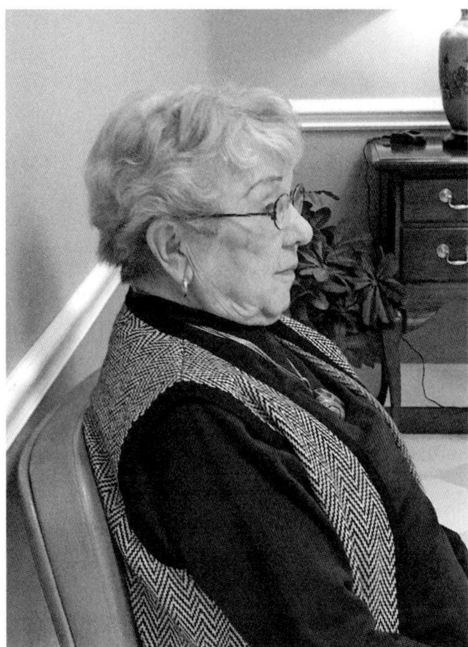

FIG. 8.20 Chin tuck.

Proprioceptive Neuromuscular Facilitation. Proprioceptive neuromuscular facilitation (PNF) has been used effectively to elongate the musculotendinous unit and, as a result, increase the range of motion of a specific joint.

A static (isometric) contraction (traditionally maximal) of a stretched target muscle and/or a shortening (concentric) contraction of an opposing muscle to lengthen the target muscle, together with a slow and controlled approach to the stretch, is generally what differentiates PNF stretching from static and dynamic alternatives,[159] although others have disputed this.[155] Autogenic and reciprocal inhibition are traditionally the accepted neurophysiological explanations for the superior range-of-motion gains. Increasing tolerance may be a likely explanation.[159] Although stretching is effective at enhancing joint range of motion, PNF stretching is reported to yield greater gains and at a faster rate than static stretching and a no-stretching control, and to improve both passive and active flexibility.[159,160]

The review of PNF by Sharman et al. resulted in several applicable recommendations.[159] A PNF technique of combining a shortening contraction of the opposing muscle and a static contraction of the target muscle is most effective. One repetition of PNF is sufficient to increase range of motion from anywhere between 3 and 9 degrees, with subsequent repetitions resulting in minor gains. Twice-a-week sessions, even with one repetition, effectively increase range of motion. Variable durations of 1 day to 12 weeks produces changes in range of motion, with most of the change occurring in the first half of the duration. Because improvements decrease within a week of PNF, it is recommended to conduct PNF once or twice weekly to maintain range-of-motion gains. Sharman and colleagues recommend holding the static contraction for 3 seconds with a low intensity (20% of a maximum voluntary contraction). The stretch component of the procedure should be maintained until the sensation of stretch abates.[159,161] Of note, the review did not specifically address the application of PNF to older adults.

Summary. Muscle shortening often occurs from the lack of movement through its full range, a common effect of a sedentary lifestyle. Often, physical activity, especially when accompanied by strengthening exercises, will improve flexibility.[162] Therefore, emphasis may be better placed on functional training rather than on specific stretching. When specific stretching is indicated, 5 minutes per muscle, per week appears to have benefit. The type of stretch seems to be less important.

Balance Training and Fall Prevention

Balance is a complex interaction of physiological and cognitive variables that combine to keep a person upright during stance and movement-based activities in a variety of environments. The most effective balance programs address as many components of balance as possible including vestibular, vision, reaction time, cognition, weight shifting, strength, power, range of motion, and behavior to name a few.[163] Fortunately, exercise can improve balance, decrease falls, and decrease injuries from falls in community-dwelling older adults.[164–166] Appropriately designed exercise interventions that target balance, gait, muscle strength, coordination, and function are demonstrated to decrease falls in community-dwelling older adults over 65 years of age by 23%.[163,164] Additionally, when balance programs are supervised by a health professional such as a physical therapist, larger effects of exercise on balance and falls reduction were seen.[164] Recommendations for specific elements of a balance program to increase the effectiveness of the exercise intervention are listed in Box 8.7.[163,167]

BOX 8.7 Evidence-Based Recommendations for Exercise to Improve Balance and Reduce Falls

- Exercise must provide a moderate to high challenge to balance
  - Standing with little to no upper extremity support
  - Reducing base of support
  - Altering the center of gravity
- Exercise must be progressed and ongoing
- Two to 3 hours per week for a minimum of 12 weeks
- Can be group based or home based
- Multidimensional stepping more effective than walking (e.g., walking backward, tandem walking, reaching, stooping, turning)
- Walking training may be included, but high-risk individuals should not be prescribed brisk walking programs
- Strength training may be included but must be of sufficient overload
- Obstacle training
- Functional exercises

Because balance is a complex function, no single-mode intervention is sufficient to effectively improve balance skills. In fact, a single-mode exercise program such as walking in isolation is not an exercise that prevents falls, and can even increase falls in at-risk populations if delivered in an unstructured manner, such as instructions to "walk daily."[168,169] And the need to integrate multiple approaches to balance may be why no clear fall-preventative effect could be shown for resistance training alone.[170]

The ability to rapidly generate force decreases to a greater extent and more rapidly with age than declines in strength. The ability to generate force in a fall-threatening situation is more relevant for preventing a fall than the capacity to produce maximal strength. In an actual fall risk situation, the time taken to produce maximal strength is too long to recover successfully from the balance threat. Power-based ballistic (rapid)-type contractions are needed and should be incorporated into resistance training for older adults.[170,171] Many studies have demonstrated the effectiveness of multidirectional stepping such as teaching the crossover step strategy to recover balance (requiring a strong gluteus medius),[172] backward walking,[173] and stepping interventions that were associated with a falls reduction rate of 50%.[174] Based on these studies, balance training should include several exercise stimuli such as tandem foot standing, multidirectional weight lifts, heel–toe walking, line walking, stepping practice, standing on one leg, weight transfers (from one leg to the other), and even modified tai chi exercises and dance. Box 8.8 lists exercises appropriate for different levels of balance.

Dancing. Dance can promote enhanced balance, balance confidence, postural control through its cognitive demands, multidirectional stepping patterns, and demands of the dance itself.[69,175–177] Salsa,[175,178] jazz,[179] ballroom,[180] and other types of dance[181] have shown benefits in socialization, sense of well-being, improved balance confidence, and in some cases balance control. Importantly, improved balance through dance was seen in those with cognitive difficulty.[182,183]

Other Balance Training. To improve postural control, core exercises are effective such as performance of planks, bird-dogs, and bridges.[184–186] Perturbation training may be a way to enhance reaction times and improve stepping strategies. Various strategies that invoke sudden and unexpected perturbations include sudden stops and starts on a treadmill or with manual cues and lean and release to promote the recovery the balance.[187,188] The use of a cable harness may provide a sense of confidence and safety.[25] Box 8.8 lists some examples of core and perturbation training.

Foot pain is a known risk factor for balance impairment and can contribute to falls.[189] Foot exercise that addresses foot pain was shown to positively affect balance,[190] as was foot and ankle strengthening.[191,192] Box 8.8 lists some examples of ankle exercises from these studies.

To address visual contributions to balance, Park and colleagues developed a unique program of eyeball exercises that challenge visual perturbations while standing, thus combining postural control with visual challenge.[193] Adding multidirectional stepping as discussed previously is a natural progression to visual exercises. Box 8.8 lists some visual exercises.

Training under single-task conditions does not transfer to dual-task conditions. Therefore, dual-task training should be integrated into an effective balance program.[194–196] Dual tasking can incorporate motor tasks and cognitive tasks, both of which should be included for maximum effectiveness. Specific strategies are listed in Box 8.9. Power training performed at a low intensity (20% of 1RM) was associated with the greatest improvement in balance performance compared to training performing at 50% and 80% of the 1RM.[197] Typically, skill and balance activities are practiced 20 to 30 minutes per session. Motor learning theory suggests that several thousand repetitions or several hours of practice are needed on a daily basis to learn a new movement pattern.[198] Motor learning also suggests that reaching motor fatigue is a necessary factor for skill development, implying that fatigue, and not time, should be used as a target.[199]

The *Otago Exercise Program* is a home-based program developed by and for physiotherapists that shows a fall reduction of 35% over 1 year and substantially reduces

BOX 8.8 Challenging Balance Exercises and Progressions Suitable for Older Adults

Exercise and/or Target	Progression
Reaching outside base of support	Narrower foot placement Reaching further and in different directions Reaching for heavier objects Pulling (such as a refrigerator door) Reaching down to a stool or the floor employing deadlift movement Standing on a compliant surface Stepping while reaching
Stepping in multiple directions	Longer or faster steps Step over obstacles Pivot on nonstepping foot Clock exercise Clock yourself game*
Walking practice	Tandem walk Increase step length and speed Walking in different directions Walking on different surfaces Walking around and over obstacles Heel and toe walking
Foot and ankle	Heel raises Decrease hand support Hold raise for longer One leg at a time Add weight (vest or hand weights) Toe curls Rhythmical and speed-based toe taps Elastic band resistance at ankle and foot Walking barefoot on different surfaces Standing on unstable surface such as Bosu ball or wobble board, progressing to stepping on and off to speed stepping Multidirectional stepping
Step-ups, forward and lateral	Decrease hand support Increase step height Add weight vest
Squats	Variations of sit to stands (adjust height and compliance of surface) Hold squat at various levels Add weight Use staggered stance
Core exercises	Bird dogs (single-limb raise to alternate double-limb raise) Planks (saws, one leg, dropping knees, side planks, side planks with rotation) Bridges (double, single leg, on platform, arms up) (Fig. 8.15) Sit-backs (Fig. 8.6)
Perturbations	Starting and stopping treadmill Boxing (hitting bag) Lean and release Manual perturbations
Visual	Focusing on single objective while performing balance task Moving head while maintaining gaze on object Following object with eyes Low vision stepping in multiple directions Closed eyes while stepping in multiple directions and turning
Dual tasking	Carrying objects while performing gait activities Cognitive exercises (counting backward, etc.)

*Lowry M, Wallace D. Clock Yourself. http://clockyourself.com.au/. Published 2018. Retrieved March 9, 2019.

BOX 8.9 Dual-Task Activities to Improve Balance

Motor	Cognitive
Walking	
Forward	Listening to music
Backward	Listening to talk-radio
Obstacles	Verbal fluency
	Answering autobiographical questions
Balancing	
Sensory organization training (SOT) (e.g., eyes closed)	Serial-3 subtraction
Dynamic weight shifting	Information processing tasks
External perturbations	Counting backward
External Cueing	
Speed	Auditory choice reaction time task
Stride length	Visuospatial task of pattern matching
Timing/metronome	

Courtesy of Nora Fritz, PhD, PT, DPT, NCS

injurious falls.[200] The program includes five to six physiotherapist visits delivered over 8 weeks in home or outpatient settings.[201] The program utilizes standard balance and strength exercises (from 17 total) performed at home 30 minutes/week three times per week. The patient performs and progresses exercises independently. The program includes walking up to 30 minutes three times per week and follow-up visits and phone calls for up to a year. The Otago program is now freely available from the North Carolina Area Health Education Center[202] and has been modified for community-group delivery.

Tai chi originated as a form of martial art but now has multiple forms and styles that have been adapted from the original form. The largest body of research about tai chi focuses on fall risk benefits. Tai chi involves learning multiple poses that are linked together with slow movements that emphasize control and balance. These routines or "forms" can range from the classic 109 postures to as few as 42. The focus required to complete the movements and postures and recalling the sequence of postures has been credited with both the mental calm and the cognitive benefits associated with tai chi. Improvement in balance and decreased fall risk are attributed to the slow repetitive work and the emphasis on control and coordination especially at the ankle.

Tai chi has long been used to improve balance and reduce falls. However, there is conflicting evidence of the effects of tai chi on balance and falls. Although earlier evidence demonstrated the tai chi decreases the number of falls, lowers the risk of falling, and improves balance and physical functioning in older inactive adults,[203] newer evidence is more equivocal.[164,204–207] Tai Chi Quan: Moving for Better Balance is one form of tai chi identified by the National Council on Aging[208] and the Administration on Community Living as an effective and evidence-based community-based falls prevention program.[209]

Slow body movements superimposed on the ankle musculature that must react rapidly to maintain the position provides an overload stimulus for ankle power and proprioception that likely contribute to its beneficial effect. Most patients enjoy the practice of tai chi and are compliant with its practice.

SAFETY

The ACSM, the Centers for Disease Control and Prevention, and others state that exercise is generally safe for older people to perform without the need to consult with a health care practitioner.[2,210] However, there are relative and absolute contraindications for aerobic exercise (see Box 18.1) of which the clinician should be aware. For patients with unstable cardiac conditions or risk signs for cardiac disease, the monitoring of blood pressure and heart rates should be routinely performed. Individuals can be instructed in how to self-monitor their status and to take their own heart rate and blood pressure. Patients should be instructed to report untoward effects of lightheadedness, dizziness, profuse sweating, or nausea. Physical therapists should be knowledgeable about an individual's medications, particularly those that have a potential effect on an individual's ability to exercise or that affect the response to exercise. β-Blockers decrease both the force of contraction of heart muscle and heart rate, keeping the heart rate artificially low during exercise. An RPE is an acceptable alternate to taking a pulse in the presence of β-blockers. Exercise also changes the need for insulin in patients with diabetes; therefore, close monitoring of the patient with insulin-dependent diabetes is required. Education regarding precautionary measures such as adequate hydration, cushioned shoes (especially if reduced sensation is identified), and close monitoring of blood glucose is part of the exercise prescription.

It stands to reason that exercise, and balance exercises in particular, may increase the risk of falls, particularly in higher-risk individuals. The risk may be increased if an exercise participant becomes fatigued during exercise or is not encouraged to use support when needed.[211] Very few problems have been reported with strength training or balance training despite the fact that fairly high levels of systolic and diastolic pressures have been reported.[212] Even with high-intensity training, no long-term injuries have been reported. In fact, in many studies where control groups are used to measure the effects of strength training in older adults, the more sedentary control group had more injuries and falls than the exercising group.[8] Of studies that report adverse events following exercise training, the most severe injury is musculoskeletal in nature, generally of soreness, stiffness, or muscle strain. It cannot be stressed enough that older adults seen in the rehabilitation setting require one-on-one supervision during the entirety of the exercise training to ensure appropriate form, intensity, and response. An older adult may need encouragement to maintain proper form, to breathe properly, and to attend to his or her level of joint or muscle discomfort.

SUMMARY

Exercise is *the* most powerful intervention for maintaining well-being, the remediation of impairment, and the promotion of function in all age groups. For older adults, exercise is a robust application for the prevention and treatment of chronic diseases and mobility disability and maintaining quality of life. Because of the robust evidence for the effectiveness of exercise on most if not all the conditions affecting older adults, geriatric physical therapists are compelled to be exercise experts across all practice settings by applying our knowledge of the relationships between physical activity, pathology, impairment, functional abilities, and disability.

REFERENCES

1. World Health Organization. International Classification of Functioning, Disability and Health (ICF). http://www.who.int/classifications/icf/en/. Published 2018. Accessed July 31, 2018.
2. Pescatello LS, Arena R, Riebe D, Thompson PD. *ACSM's Guidelines for Exercise Testing and Prescription*. 9th ed. Baltimore, MD: Wolters Kluwer/Lippincott, Williams & Wilkins; 2014.
3. Edwards JJ, Khanna M, Jordan KP, et al. Older Americans 2016: Key Indicators of Well-Being. *Federal Interagency Forum on Aging-Related Statistics*. https://doi.org/10.1136/annrheumdis-2013-203913. https://acl.gov/agng-and-disability-in-america/data-and-research/key-indicators-well-being. Published March 29, 2018. Accessed July 6, 2019.
4. Buttorff C, Ruder T, Bauman M. Multiple chronic conditions in the United States. Santa Monica: Rand Corporation; 2017. https://www.rand.org/content/dam/rand/pubs/tools/TL200/TL221/RAND_TL221.pdf.
5. Chakravarty EF, Hubert HB, Lingala VB, Fries JF. Reduced disability and mortality among aging runners: a 21-year longitudinal study. *Arch Intern Med*. 2008;168(15):1638–1646. https://doi.org/10.1001/archinte.168.15.1638.
6. Chou W-T, Tomata Y, Watanabe T, Sugawara Y, Kakizaki M, Tsuji I. Relationships between changes in time spent walking since middle age and incident functional disability. *Prev Med (Baltim)*. 2014;59:68–72. https://doi.org/10.1016/j.ypmed.2013.11.019.
7. Paterson DH, Warburton DE. Physical activity and functional limitations in older adults: a systematic review related to Canada's Physical Activity Guidelines. *Int J Behav Nutr Phys Act*. 2010;7(1):38. https://doi.org/10.1186/1479-5868-7-38.
8. McPhee JS, French DP, Jackson D, Nazroo J, Pendleton N, Degens H. Physical activity in older age: perspective for healthy ageing and frailty. *Biogerontology*. 2016;17:567–580. https://doi.org/10.1007/s10522-016-9641-0.
9. Ferrucci L, Guralnik ÃJM, Studenski S, Fried LP, Jr BC, Walston JD. Delaying functional decline and disability in frail, older persons. *JAGS*. 2004;52:625–634.
10. Hackstaff L. Factors associated with frailty in chronically ill older adults. *Soc Work Health Care*. 2009;48(8):798–811. https://doi.org/10.1080/00981380903327897.
11. Ryan A, Murphy C, Boland F, Galvin R, Smith SM. What is the impact of physical activity and physical function on the development of multimorbidity in older adults over time? A population-based cohort study. *Journals Gerontol Ser A*. 2018;73(11):1538–1544. https://doi.org/10.1093/gerona/glx251.
12. Olaya B, Moneta MV, Doménech-Abella J, et al. Mobility difficulties, physical activity, and all-cause mortality risk in a nationally representative sample of older adults. *J Gerontol Ser A*. 2018;73(9):1272–1279. https://doi.org/10.1093/gerona/glx121.
13. Healy G, Dunstan D, Salmon J, et al. Breaks in sedentary time: beneficial associations with metabolic risk. *Diabetes Care*. 2008;31:661–666.
14. Garber CE, Blissmer B, Deschenes MR, et al. American College of Sports Medicine position stand. Quantity and quality of exercise for developing and maintaining cardiorespiratory, musculoskeletal, and neuromotor fitness in apparently healthy adults: guidance for prescribing exercise. *Med Sci Sports Exerc*. 2011;43(7):1334–1359. https://doi.org/10.1249/MSS.0b013e318213fefb.
15. Gill TM, Allore HG, Hardy SE, Guo Z. The dynamic nature of mobility disability in older persons. *J Am Geriatr Soc*. 2006;54(2):248–254. http://www.blackwell-synergy.com/doi/abs/10.1111/j.1532-5415.2005.00586.x.
16. Loyd C, Beasley TM, Miltner RS, Clark D, King B, Brown CJ. Trajectories of community mobility recovery after hospitalization in older adults. *J Am Geriatr Soc*. 2018;66(7):1399–1403. https://doi.org/10.1111/jgs.15397.
17. Tudor-Locke C, Bassett DR. How many steps/day are enough? *Sport Med*. 2004;34(1):1–8. https://doi.org/10.2165/00007256-200434010-00001.
18. Tudor-Locke C, Craig CL, Aoyagi Y, et al. How many steps/day are enough? For older adults and special populations. *Int J Behav Nutr Phys Act*. 2011;8:80. https://doi.org/10.1186/1479-5868-8-80.
19. Reitlo LS, Sandbakk SB, Viken H, et al. Exercise patterns in older adults instructed to follow moderate- or high-intensity exercise protocol - the generation 100 study. *BMC Geriatr*. 2018;18(1):208. https://doi.org/10.1186/s12877-018-0900-6.
20. Farrance C, Tsofliou F, Clark C. Adherence to community based group exercise interventions for older people: a mixed-methods systematic review. *Prev Med (Baltim)*. 2016;87:155–166. https://doi.org/10.1016/j.ypmed.2016.02.037.
21. van der Bij AK, Laurant MGH, Wensing M. Effectiveness of physical activity interventions for older adults: a review. *Am J Prev Med*. 2002;22(2):120–133. http://www.ncbi.nlm.nih.gov/pubmed/11818183. Accessed February 23, 2019.
22. Schutzer KA, Graves BS. Barriers and motivations to exercise in older adults. *Prev Med (Baltim)*. 2004;39(5):1056–1061. https://doi.org/10.1016/j.ypmed.2004.04.003.
23. Weber M, Belala N, Clemson L, et al. Feasibility and effectiveness of intervention programmes integrating functional exercise into daily life of older adults: a systematic review. *Gerontology*. 2018;64(2):172–187. https://doi.org/10.1159/000479965.
24. van Stralen MM, De Vries H, Mudde AN, Bolman C, Lechner L. Determinants of initiation and maintenance of physical activity among older adults: a literature review. *Health Psychol Rev*. 2009;3(2):147–207. https://doi.org/10.1080/17437190903229462.
25. Miller CT, Teychenne M, Maple J-L. The perceived feasibility and acceptability of a conceptually challenging exercise training program in older adults. *Clin Interv Aging*. 2018;13:451–461. https://doi.org/10.2147/CIA.S154664.
26. Taylor D. Physical activity is medicine for older adults. *Postgr Med J*. 2014;90:26–32.
27. Balde A, Figueras J, Hawking DA, Miller JR. Physician advice to the elderly about physical activity. *PsycNET J Aging Phys Act*. 2003;11(1):90–97. https://psycnet.apa.org/record/2003-04330-006. Accessed 23 February 2019.

28. Mehra S, Dadema T, Kröse BJA, et al. Attitudes of older adults in a group-based exercise program toward a blended intervention; a focus-group study. *Front Psychol.* 2016;7:1827. https://doi.org/10.3389/fpsyg.2016.01827.
29. van Uffelen JGZ, Khan A, Burton NW. Gender differences in physical activity motivators and context preferences: a population-based study in people in their sixties. *BMC Public Health.* 2017;17(1):624. https://doi.org/10.1186/s12889-017-4540-0.
30. Canadian Exercise Physiology Society. Par-Q & you. http://www.paguide.com. Published 2018. Accessed March 7, 2019.
31. 2018 PAR-Q+ The Physical Activity Readiness Questionnaire for Everyone. www.who.int/dietphysicalactivity/en/. Accessed 7 March 2019.
32. Mueller MJ, Maluf KS. Tissue adaptation to physical stress: a proposed "physical stress theory" to guide physical therapist practice, education, and research. *Phys Ther.* 2002;82 (4):383–403.
33. Bortz WM. A conceptual framework of frailty: a review. *J Gerontol.* 2002;57A(5):M283–M288.
34. Bishop CE, Stone R. Implications for policy: the nursing home as least restrictive setting. *Gerontologist.* 2014;54(Suppl 1): S98–S103. https://doi.org/10.1093/geront/gnt164.
35. Taylor NF, Dodd KJ, Shields N, Bruder A. Therapeutic exercise in physiotherapy practice is beneficial: a summary of systematic reviews 2002–2005. *Aust J Physiother.* 2007;53(1):7–16. https://doi.org/10.1016/S0004-9514(07)70057-0.
36. Armitage J. The safety of statins in clinical practice *Lancet.* 2007;6736(07):1–10. https://doi.org/10.1016/S0140-6736 (07)60716-8.
37. Liang M, Lin S. Aerobic exercise prescription for the older population: a short review. *Nov Physiother.* 2014;4(2): 1000201.
38. American Diabetes Association. Blood glucose and exercise. American Diabetes Association. http://www.diabetes.org/food-and-fitness/fitness/get-started-safely/blood-glucose-control-and-exercise.html. Published 2017. Accessed February 23, 2019.
39. Geneen LJ, Moore RA, Clarke C, Martin D, Colvin LA, Smith BH. Physical activity and exercise for chronic pain in adults: an overview of Cochrane Reviews. *Cochrane Database Syst Rev.* 2017;4(4):CD011279. https://doi.org/10.1002/14651858.CD011279.pub3.
40. Lederman E. The myth of core stability. *J Bodyw Mov Ther.* 2010;14(1):84–98. https://doi.org/10.1016/j.jbmt.2009.08.001.
41. Caputo F, Denadai BS. Effects of aerobic endurance training status and specificity on oxygen uptake kinetics during maximal exercise. *Eur J Appl Physiol.* 2004;93(1–2):87–95. https://doi.org/10.1007/s00421-004-1169-3.
42. Behm DG, Sale DG. Velocity specificity of resistance training. *Sports Med.* 1993;15(6):374–388.
43. Mallia S. CrossFit: forging elite fitness. *The Journal.* https://journal.crossfit.com/article/lift-to-live-well-2. Published 2016. Accessed February 23, 2019.
44. Are Boot Camp Workouts for Seniors? BOOTCAMPSF blog. http://www.bootcampsf.com/blog/?p=1256. Published 2017. Accessed February 23, 2019.
45. Borde R, Hortobagyi T, Granacher U. Dose-response relationships of resistance training in healthy old adults: a systematic review and meta-analysis. *Sports Med.* 2015;45(12): 1693–1720. https://doi.org/10.1007/s40279-015-0385-9.
46. Silva NL, Oliveira RB, Fleck SJ, Leon AC, Farinatti P. Influence of strength training variables on strength gains in adults over 55 years-old: a meta-analysis of dose-response relationships. *J Sci Med Sport.* 2014;17(3):337–344. https://doi.org/10.1016/j.jsams.2013.05.009.
47. Steib S, Schoene D, Pfeifer K. Dose–response relationship of resistance training in older adults: a meta-analysis. *Med Sci Sports Exerc.* 2010;42(5):902–914. https://doi.org/10.1249/MSS.0b013e3181c34465.
48. Lesinski M, Hortobagyi T, Muehlbauer T, Gollhofer A, Granacher U. Effects of balance training on balance performance in healthy older adults: a systematic review and meta-analysis. *Sports Med.* 2015;45(12):1721–1738. https://doi.org/10.1007/s40279-015-0375-y.
49. Huang G, Wang R, Chen P, Huang SC, Donnelly JE, Mehlferber JP. Dose–response relationship of cardiorespiratory fitness adaptation to controlled endurance training in sedentary older adults. *Eur J Prev Cardiol.* 2016;23(5):518–529. https://doi.org/10.1177/2047487315582322.
50. Office of Disease Prevention and Health Promotion. 2018 Physical Activity Guidelines Advisory Committee Scientific Report. 2018. https://health.gov/paguidelines/second-edition/report/pdf/PAG_Advisory_Committee_Report.pdf. Accessed July 24, 2018.
51. Sanders LMJ, Hortobágyi T, la Bastide-van Gemert S, van der Zee EA, van Heuvelen MJG. Dose-response relationship between exercise and cognitive function in older adults with and without cognitive impairment: a systematic review and meta-analysis. In: Regnaux J-P, ed. *PLoS One*; 2019: e021003614(1)2019. https://doi.org/10.1371/journal.pone.0210036.
52. Rhea MR, Alvar BA, Burkett LN, Ball SD. A meta-analysis to determine the dose response for strength development. *Med Sci Sports Exerc.* 2003;35(3):456–464. https://doi.org/10.1249/01.MSS.0000053727.63505.D4.
53. Peterson MD, Rhea MR, Sen A, Gordon PM. Resistance exercise for muscular strength in older adults: a meta-analysis. *Ageing Res Rev.* 2010;9:226–237. https://doi.org/10.1016/j.arr.2010.03.004.
54. Borg G. *Borg's Perceived Exertion and Pain Scales.* Champaign, IL: Human Kinetics; 1998.
55. Morishita S, Tsubaki A, Nakamura M, Nashimoto S, Fu JB, Onishi H. Rating of perceived exertion on resistance training in elderly subjects. *Expert Rev Cardiovasc Ther.* 2019;17(2):135–142. https://doi.org/10.1080/14779072.2019.1561278.
56. Reed JL, Pipe AL. The talk test: a useful tool for prescribing and monitoring exercise intensity. *Curr Opin Cardiol.* 2014;29:475–480.
57. Donatelli RA, Dimond D. Strength training concepts in the athlete. In: Donateli R, ed. *Sports-Specific Rehabilitation.* St Louis: Churchill Livingstone; 2007.
58. Moritani T, de Vries HA. Neural factors versus hypertrophy in the time course of muscle strength gain. *Am J Phys Med.* 1979;58(3):115–130. http://www.ncbi.nlm.nih.gov/pubmed/453338. Accessed February 26, 2019.
59. Sale DG. Neural adaptation to resistance training. *Med Sci Sports Exerc.* 1988;20(5 Suppl):S135–S145. http://www.ncbi.nlm.nih.gov/pubmed/3057313. Accessed February 23, 2019.
60. Manini TM, Clark BC. Dynapenia and aging: an update. *J Gerontol Ser A.* 2012;67A(1):28–40. https://doi.org/10.1093/gerona/glr010.
61. Gabriel DA, Kamen G, Frost G. Neural adaptations to resistive exercise. *Sport Med.* 2006;36(2):133–149. https://doi.org/10.2165/00007256-200636020-00004.
62. Toigo M, Boutellier U. New fundamental resistance exercise determinants of molecular and cellular muscle adaptations. *Eur J Appl Physiol.* 2006;97(6):643–663. https://doi.org/10.1007/s00421-006-0238-1.
63. Clark BC, Mahato NK, Nakazawa M, et al. The power of the mind: the cortex as a critical determinant of muscle strength/

weakness. *J Neurophysiol*. 2014;112:3219–3226. https://doi.org/10.1152/jn.00386.2014.

64. Taub E, Uswatte G, Mark VW, Morris DM. The learned nonuse phenomenon: implications for rehabilitation. *Eura Medicophys*. 2006;42(3):241–256.
65. Ageberg E, Roos EM. Neuromuscular exercise as treatment of degenerative knee disease. *Exerc Sport Sci Rev*. 43(1):2015, 14–22.
66. Aman JE, Elangovan N, Konczak J. The effectiveness of proprioceptive training for improving motor function: a systematic review. *Hum Neurosci*. 2014;8:1075.
67. Johnson G, Otto D, Clair AA. The effect of instrumental and vocal music on adherence to a physical rehabilitation exercise program with persons who are elderly. *J Music Ther*. 2001;38 (2):82–96. http://www.ncbi.nlm.nih.gov/pubmed/11469917. Accessed February 24, 2019.
68. Lenze EJ, Host HH, Hildebrand MW, et al. Enhanced medical rehabilitation increases therapy intensity and engagement and improves functional outcomes in postacute rehabilitation of older adults: a randomized-controlled trial. *J Am Med Dir Assoc*. 2012;13(8):708–712. https://doi.org/10.1016/j.jamda.2012.06.014.
69. Park YS, Koh K, Yang JS, Shim JK. Efficacy of rhythmic exercise and walking exercise in older adults' exercise participation rates and physical function outcomes. *Geriatr Gerontol Int*. 2017;17(12):2311–2318. https://doi.org/10.1111/ggi.13046.
70. Powell K, Pauluch A, Blair S. Physical activity for health: what kind? How much? How intense? On top of what? *Annu Rev Public Health*. 2011;32:349–365.
71. Bouaziz W, Vogel T, Schmitt E, Kaltenbach G, Geny B, Olivier P. Health benefits of aerobic training programs in adults aged 70 and over: a systematic review. *Arch Gerontol Geriatr*. 69:2017, 110–127.
72. MacDonald MJ, Currie KD. Interval exercise is a path to good health, but how much, how often and for whom? *Clin Sci*. 2009;116(4):315–316. https://doi.org/10.1042/CS20080632.
73. Wormgoor SG, Dalleck LC, Zinn C, Harris NK. Effects of high-intensity interval training on people living with type 2 diabetes: a narrative review. *Can J Diabetes*. 2017;41 (5):536–547. https://doi.org/10.1016/j.jcjd.2016.12.004.
74. Molmen HE, Wisloff U, Aamot IL, Stoylen A, Ingul CB. Aerobic interval training compensates age related decline in cardiac function. *Scand Cardiovasc J*. 2012;46(3):163–171. https://doi.org/10.3109/14017431.2012.660192.
75. Hwang C-L, Yoo J-K, Kim H-K, et al. Novel all-extremity high-intensity interval training improves aerobic fitness, cardiac function and insulin resistance in healthy older adults. *Exp Gerontol*. 2016;82:112–119. https://doi.org/10.1016/j.exger.2016.06.009.
76. Guiraud T, Nigam A, Gremeaux V, Meyer P, Juneau M, Bosquet L. High-intensity interval training in cardiac rehabilitation. *Sport Med*. 2012;42(7):587–605. https://doi.org/10.2165/11631910-000000000-00000.
77. Ramos JS, Dalleck LC, Tjonna AE, Beetham KS, Coombes JS. The impact of high-intensity interval training versus moderate-intensity continuous training on vascular function: a systematic review and meta-analysis. *Sport Med*. 2015;45 (5):679–692. https://doi.org/10.1007/s40279-015-0321-z.
78. Shiraev T, Barclay G. Evidence based exercise - clinical benefits of high intensity interval training. *Aust Fam Physician*. 2012;41(12):960–962. http://www.ncbi.nlm.nih.gov/pubmed/23210120. Accessed 3 March 2019.
79. Reed JL, Pipe AL. The talk test. *Curr Opin Cardiol*. 2014;29 (5):475–480. https://doi.org/10.1097/HCO.00000000000-00097.
80. Cannon C, Foster C, Porcari JP, Skemp KM, Fater DCW, Backes R. The talk test as a measure of exertional ischemia. *Am J Med Sci*. 2004;1:52–56.
81. Loose BD, Christiansen AM, Smolczyk JE, et al. Consistency of the counting talk test for exercise prescription. *J Strength Cond Res*. 2012;26(6):1701–1707. https://doi.org/10.1519/JSC.0b013e318234e84c.
82. Kilpatrick MW, Robertson RJ, Powers JM, Mears JL, Ferrer NF. Comparisons of RPE before, during, and after self-regulated aerobic exercise. *Med Sci Sport Exerc*. 2009;41(3):682–687. https://doi.org/10.1249/MSS.0b013e31818a0f09.
83. Utter AC, Robertson RJ, Green JM, Suminski RR, McAnulty SR, Nieman DC. Validation of the Adult OMNI Scale of perceived exertion for walking/running exercise. *Med Sci Sports Exerc*. 2004;36(10):1776–1780. http://www.ncbi.nlm.nih.gov/pubmed/15595300. Accessed 7 March 2019.
84. Guidetti L, Sgadari A, Buzzachera CF, et al. Validation of the OMNI-cycle scale of perceived exertion in the elderly. *J Aging Phys Act*. 2011;19(3):214–224. http://www.ncbi.nlm.nih.gov/pubmed/21727302. Accessed 20 February 2019.
85. Sadaria KS, Bohannon RW. The 6-Minute Walk Test: a brief review of literature. *Clin Exerc Physiol*. 2001;3(3):127–132.
86. Newman AB, Simonsick EM, Naydeck BL. Association of long-distance corridor walk performance with mortality, cardiovascular disease, mobility limitation, and disability. *JAMA*. 2006;295(17):2018–2026. https://doi.org/10.1001/jama.295.17.2018.
87. Simonsick EM, Montgomery PS, Newman AB, Bauer DC, Harris T. Measuring fitness in healthy older adults: the Health ABC Long Distance Corridor Walk. *J Am Geriatr Soc*. 2001;49(11):1544–1548.
88. Fletcher GF, Ades PA, Kligfield P, et al. Exercise standards for testing and training: a scientific statement from the American Heart Association. *Circulation*. 2013;128(8):873–934. https://doi.org/10.1161/CIR.0b013e31829b5b44.
89. Kutzner I, Richter A, Gordt K, et al. Does aquatic exercise reduce hip and knee joint loading? In vivo load measurements with instrumented implants. *PLoS One*. 2017;12(3):e0171972. https://doi.org/10.1371/journal.pone.0171972.
90. Rotstein A, Harush M, Vaisman N. The effect of a water exercise program on bone density of postmenopausal women. *J Sports Med Phys Fitness*. 2008;48(3):352–359. http://www.ncbi.nlm.nih.gov/pubmed/18974722. Accessed 2 March 2019.
91. Waller B, Ogonowska-Słodownik A, Vitor M, et al. The effect of aquatic exercise on physical functioning in the older adult: a systematic review with meta-analysis. *Age Ageing*. 2016;45 (5):594–602. https://doi.org/10.1093/ageing/afw102.
92. Franco MR, Morelhão PK, de Carvalho A, Pinto RZ. Aquatic exercise for the treatment of hip and knee osteoarthritis. *Phys Ther*. 2017;97(7):693–697. https://doi.org/10.1093/ptj/pzx043.
93. Bartels EM, Lund H, Hagen KB, Dagfinrud H, Christensen R, Danneskiold-Samsoe B. Aquatic exercise for the treatment of knee and hip osteoarthritis. *Cochrane Database Syst Rev*. 2007;4:CD005523.
94. Kruel LFM, Peyre-Tartaruga LA, Alberton CL, Muller FG, Petkowizc R. Effects of hydrostatic weight on heart rate during water immersion. *Int J Aquat Res Educ*. 2009;3:178–185.
95. Pinto SS, Alberton CL, Zaffari P, et al. Rating of perceived exertion and physiological responses in water-based exercise. *J Hum Kinet*. 2015;49:99–108. https://doi.org/10.1515/hukin-2015-0112.
96. Alberton CL, Pinto SS, Gorski T, et al. Rating of perceived exertion in maximal incremental tests during head-out water-based aerobic exercises. *J Sports Sci*. 2016;34 (18):1691–1698. https://doi.org/10.1080/02640414.2015.1134804.
97. Rikli RE, Jones CJ. Development and validation of criterion-referenced clinically relevant fitness standards for

maintaining physical independence in later years. 2013;53: 255–267. https://doi.org/10.1093/geront/gns071.
98. Tieland M, Trouwborst I, Clark BC. Skeletal muscle performance and ageing. *J Cachexia Sarcopenia Muscle.* 2018;9(1):3–19. https://doi.org/10.1002/jcsm.12238.
99. Liu CJ, Latham NK. Progressive resistance strength training for improving physical function in older adults. *Cochrane Database Syst Rev.* 2009;(3):CD002759. https://doi.org/10.1002/14651858.CD002759.pub2.
100. Fisher J, Steele J, Bruce-Low S, Smith D. Evidence-based resistance training recommendations. *Med Sport.* 2011;15 (3):147–162. https://doi.org/10.2478/v10036-011-0025-x.
101. da Silva LN, Teodoro JL, Menger E, et al. Repetitions to failure versus not to failure during concurrent training in healthy elderly men: a randomized clinical trial. *Exp Gerontol.* 2018;108:18–27. S0531-5565(18)30142-6.
102. Rooney KJ, Herbert RD, Balnave RJ. Fatigue contributes to the strength training stimulus. *Med Sci Sports Exerc.* 1994; 26(9):1160–1164. http://www.ncbi.nlm.nih.gov/pubmed/7808251. Accessed 4 March 2019.
103. Schoenfeld BJ, Wilson JM, Lowery RP, Krieger JW. Muscular adaptations in low- versus high-load resistance training: a meta-analysis. *Eur J Sport Sci.* 2016;1:1–10. https://doi.org/10.1080/17461391.2014.989922.
104. Izquierdo M, Cadore EL. Brief review: muscle power training in the institutionalized frail: a new approach to counteracting functional declines and very late-life disability. 2014;908175: 1–6. https://doi.org/10.1185/03007995.2014.908175.
105. Roig M, O'Brien K, Kirk G, et al. The effects of eccentric versus concentric resistance training on muscle strength and mass in healthy adults: a systematic review with meta-analysis. *Br J Sports Med.* 2009;43(8):556–568. https://doi.org/10.1136/bjsm.2008.051417.
106. Radaelli R, Wilhelm EN, Botton CE, et al. Effects of single vs. multiple-set short-term strength training in elderly women. *Age (Omaha).* 2014;36(6):9720. https://doi.org/10.1007/s11357-014-9720-6.
107. Lovell DI, Cuneo R, Gass GC. The blood pressure response of older men to maximum and sub-maximum strength testing. *J Sci Med Sport.* 2011;14(3):254–258. https://doi.org/10.1016/j.jsams.2010.12.005.
108. Pincivero DM. Older adults underestimate RPE and knee extensor torque as compared with young adults. *Med Sci Sport Exerc.* 2011;43(1):171–180. https://doi.org/10.1249/MSS.0b013e3181e91e0d.
109. Morishita S, Yamauchi S, Fujisawa C, Domen K. Rating of perceived exertion for quantification of the intensity of resistance exercise. *Int J Phys Med Rehabil.* 2013;1(9):1–4. https://doi.org/10.4172/2329-9096.1000172.
110. Allman BL, Rice CL. Perceived exertion is elevated in old age during an isometric fatigue task. *Eur J Appl Physiol.* 2003;89 (2):191–197. https://doi.org/10.1007/s00421-002-0780-4.
111. John EB, Liu W, Gregory RW. Biomechanics of muscular effort. *Med Sci Sport Exerc.* 2009;41(2):418–425. https://doi.org/10.1249/MSS.0b013e3181884480.
112. Gearhart RF, Riechman SE, Lagally KM, Andrews RD, Robertson RJ. RPE at relative intensities after 12 weeks of resistance-exercise training by older adults. *Percept Mot Skills.* 2008;106(3):893–903. https://doi.org/10.2466/pms.106.3.893-903.
113. Lagally KM, Robertson RJ. Construct validity of the OMNI resistance exercise scale. *J Strength Cond Res.* 2006;20 (2):252. https://doi.org/10.1519/R-17224.1.
114. Naclerio F, Rodríguez-Romo G, Barriopedro-Moro MI, Jiménez A, Alvar BA, Triplett NT. Control of resistance training intensity by the Omni perceived exertion scale. *J Strength Cond Res.* 2011;25(7):1879–1888. https://doi.org/10.1519/JSC.0b013e3181e501e9.
115. Gearhart RF, Riechman SE, Lagally KM, Andrews RD, Robertson RJ. Safety of using the adult OMNI resistance exercise scale to determine 1-Rm in older men and women. *Percept Mot Skills.* 2011;113(2):671–676. https://doi.org/10.2466/10.15.PMS.113.5.671-676.
116. Robertson RJ, Goss FL, Rutkowski J, et al. Concurrent validation of the OMNI perceived exertion scale for resistance exercise. *Med Sci Sport Exerc.* 2003;35(2):333–341. https://doi.org/10.1249/01.MSS.0000048831.15016.2A.
117. Bohannon RW. Knee extension strength and body weight determine sit-to-stand independence after stroke. *Physiother Theory Pr.* 2007;23(5):291–297.
118. Avers D, Brown M. *Daniel and Worthingham's Muscle Testing.* 10th ed. St. Louis: Elseiver; 2019.
119. McKay MJ, Baldwin JN, Ferreira P, Simic M, Vanicek N, Burns J. Normative reference values for strength and flexibility of 1,000 children and adults. *Neurology.* 2017;88:36–43.
120. Andrews AW, Thomas MW, Bohannon RW. Normative values for isometric muscle force measurements obtained with hand-held dynamometers. *Phys Ther.* 1996;76(3): 248–259.
121. Bohannon RW. Reference values for extremity muscle strength obtained by hand-held dynamometry from adults aged 20 to 79 years [Comment]. *Arch Phys Med Rehabil.* 1997;78(1): 26–32.
122. Phillips BA, Lo SK, Mastaglia FL. Muscle force measured using "break" testing with a hand-held myometer in normal subjects aged 20 to 69 years. *Arch Phys Med Rehab.* 2000;81:653–661. https://doi.org/10.1053/mr.2000.4413.
123. Hruby A, Sahni S, Bolster D, Jacques PF. Protein intake and functional integrity in aging: the Framingham Heart Study offspring. *J Gerontol Ser A.* 2018. [e-pub ahead of print] https://doi.org/10.1093/gerona/gly201.
124. Yang Y, Breen L, Burd NA, et al. Resistance exercise enhances myofibrillar protein synthesis with graded intakes of whey protein in older men. *Br J Nutr.* 2012;108(10):1780–1788. https://doi.org/10.1017/S0007114511007422.
125. Churchward-Venne TA, Holwerda AM, Phillips SM, van Loon LJ. What is the optimal amount of protein to support post-exercise skeletal muscle reconditioning in the older adult? *Sports Med.* 2016;46(9):1205–1212. https://doi.org/10.1007/s40279-016-0504-2.
126. Robinson MJ, Burd NA, Breen L, et al. Dose-dependent responses of myofibrillar protein synthesis with beef ingestion are enhanced with resistance exercise in middle-aged men. *Appl Physiol Nutr Metab.* 2013;38(2):120–125. https://doi.org/10.1139/apnm-2012-0092.
127. Kumar V, Atherton PJ, Selby A, et al. Muscle protein synthetic responses to exercise: effects of age, volume, and intensity. *J Gerontol A Biol Sci Med Sci.* 2012;67(11):1170–1177. https://doi.org/10.1093/gerona/gls141.
128. Oikawa SY, McGlory C, D'Souza LK, et al. A randomized controlled trial of the impact of protein supplementation on leg lean mass and integrated muscle protein synthesis during inactivity and energy restriction in older persons. *Am J Clin Nutr.* 2018;108(5):1060–1068. https://doi.org/10.1093/ajcn/nqy193.
129. Hollman JH, Ginos BE, Kozuchowski J, Vaughn AS, Krause DA, Youdas JW. Relationships between knee valgus, hip-muscle strength, and hip-muscle recruitment during a single-limb. *Journal of Sport Rehab.* 2009;18:104–117. Figure 1.
130. Tarnanen SP, Ylinen JJ, Siekkinen KM, Malkia EA, Kautiainen HJ, Hakkinen AH. Effect of isometric upper-extremity exercises on the activation of core stabilizing muscles. *Arch Phys Med Rehabil.* 2008;89:513–521.
131. Lee J-H, Choi J-D. The effects of upper extremity task training with symmetric abdominal muscle contraction on

trunk stability and balance in chronic stroke patients. *J Phys Ther Sci.* 2017;29(3):495–497. https://doi.org/10.1589/jpts.29.495.

132. Bean JF, Kiely DK, LaRose S, Goldstein R, Frontera WR, Leveille SG. Are changes in leg power responsible for clinically meaningful improvements in mobility in older adults? *J Am Geriatr Soc.* 2010;58(12):2363–2368. https://doi.org/10.1111/j.1532-5415.2010.03155.x.
133. Reid KF, Fielding RA. Skeletal muscle power: a critical determinant of physical functioning in older adults. *Exerc Sport Sci Rev.* 2012;40(1):4–12. https://doi.org/10.1097/JES.0b013e31823b5f13.
134. Millor N, Lecumberri P, Gómez M, et al. Gait velocity and chair sit-stand-sit performance improves current frailty-status identification. *IEEE Trans Neural Syst Rehabil Eng.* 2017;25(11):2018–2025. https://doi.org/10.1109/TNSRE.2017.2699124.
135. Bean JF, Kiely DK, Herman S, et al. The relationship between leg power and physical performance in mobility-limited older people. *J Am Geriatr Soc.* 2002;50(3):461–467. http://www.ncbi.nlm.nih.gov/pubmed/11943041. Accessed 17 February 2019.
136. Keller K, Engelhardt M. Strength and muscle mass loss with aging process. Age and strength loss. *Muscles Ligaments Tendons J.* 2013;3(4):346–350. http://www.ncbi.nlm.nih.gov/pubmed/24596700. Accessed 8 January 2019.
137. Byrne C, Faure C, Keene DJ, Lamb SE. Ageing, muscle power and physical function: a systematic review and implications for pragmatic training interventions. *Sports Med.* 2016;46(9):1311–1332. https://doi.org/10.1007/s40279-016-0489-x.
138. Reid KF, Martin KI, Doros G, et al. Comparative effects of light or heavy resistance power training for improving lower extremity power and physical performance in mobility-limited older adults. *J Gerontol A Biol Sci Med Sci.* 2015;70(3):374–380. https://doi.org/10.1093/gerona/glu156.
139. de Vreede PL, Samson MM, van Meeteren NLU, Duursma SA, Verhaar HJJ. Functional-task exercise versus resistance strength exercise to improve daily function in older women: a feasibility study. *Arch Phys Med Rehabil.* 2004;85(12):1952–1961. https://doi.org/10.1016/j.apmr.2004.05.006.
140. Hruda KV, Hicks AL, McCartney N. Training for muscle power in older adults: effects on functional abilities. *Can J Appl Physiol.* 2003;28(2):178–189.
141. Avers D, Brown M. White paper: strength training for the older adult. *J Geriatr Phys Ther.* 2009;32(4):148–153. https://doi.org/10.1519/00139143-200932040-00002.
142. Ramirez-Campillo R, Martinez C, de La Fuente CI, et al. High-speed resistance training in older women: the role of supervision. *J Aging Phys Act.* 2017;25(1):1–9. https://doi.org/10.1123/japa.2015-0122.
143. Kemmler W, Lauber D, Weineck J, Hensen J, Kalender W, Engelke K. Benefits of 2 years of intense exercise on bone density, physical fitness, and blood lipids in early postmenopausal osteopenic women: results of the Erlangen Fitness Osteoporosis Prevention Study (EFOPS). *Arch Intern Med.* 2004;164(10):1084–1091. https://doi.org/10.1001/archinte.164.10.1084.
144. Watson SL, Weeks BK, Weis LJ, Harding AT, Horan SA, Beck BR. High-intensity resistance and impact training improves bone mineral density and physical function osteoporosis: the LIFTMOR randomized controlled. *J Bone Miner Res.* 2018;33(2):211–220. https://doi.org/10.1002/jbmr.3284.
145. Sran MM, Stotz PJ, Normandin SC, Robinovitch SN. Age differences in energy absorption in the upper extremity during a descent movement: implications for arresting a fall. *J Gerontol A Biol Sci Med Sci.* 2010;65(3):312–317. https://doi.org/10.1093/gerona/glp153.
146. Cakar E, Dincer U, Kiralp MZ, et al. Jumping combined exercise programs reduce fall risk and improve balance and life quality of elderly people who live in a long-term care facility. *Eur J Phys Rehabil Med.* 2010;46(1):59–67.
147. Moran J, Ramirez-Campillo R, Granacher U. Effects of jumping exercise on muscular power in older adults: a meta-analysis. *Sport Med.* 2018;48(12):2843–2857. https://doi.org/10.1007/s40279-018-1002-5.
148. Kisner C, Colby LA, Borstad J. *Therapeutic exercise: foundations and techniques.* 7th ed. Philadelphia: F. A. Davis Company; 2018.
149. Watson SL, Weeks BK, Weis LJ, Harding AT, Horan SA, Beck BR. High-intensity exercise did not cause vertebral fractures and improves thoracic kyphosis in postmenopausal women with low to very low bone mass: the LIFTMOR trial. *Osteoporos Int.* 2019;30:957–964f. https://doi.org/10.1007/s00198-018-04829-z.
150. Zech A, Steib S, Sportwiss D, Freiberger E, Pfeifer K. Functional muscle power testing in young, middle-aged, and community-dwelling nonfrail and prefrail older adults. *Arch Phys Med Rehabil.* 2011;92:967–971. https://doi.org/10.1016/j.apmr.2010.12.031.
151. Rose DJ. *Fall proof! A comprehensive balance and mobility training program.* Champaign, IL: Human Kinetics; 2010.
152. Clemson L, Fiatarone Singh MA, Bundy A, et al. Integration of balance and strength training into daily life activity to reduce rate of falls in older people (the LiFE study): randomised parallel trial. *BMJ.* 2012;345. https://doi.org/10.1136/bmj.e4547. e4547.
153. Clemson L, Fiatarone MA. Integration of balance and strength training into daily life activity to reduce rate of falls in older people (the LiFE study): randomised parallel trial. *BMJ.* 2012;345:1–15. https://doi.org/10.1136/bmj.e4547. e4547.
154. Buch A, Kis O, Carmeli E, et al. Circuit resistance training is an effective means to enhance muscle strength in older and middle aged adults. *Ageing Res Rev.* 2017;37:16–27. https://doi.org/10.1016/j.arr.2017.04.003.
155. Thomas E, Bianco A, Paoli A, Palma A. The relation between stretching typology and stretching duration: the effects on range of motion. *Int J Sports Med.* 2018;39(4):243–254. https://doi.org/10.1055/s-0044-101146.
156. Feland JB, Myrer JW, Schulthies SS, Fellingham GW, Measom GW, Words K. The effect of duration of stretching of the hamstring muscle group for increasing range of motion in people age 65 years or older. *Phys Ther.* 2001; 81(5): 1100–1117. http://www.ncbi.nlm.nih.gov/pubmed/11319936. Accessed March 2, 2019.
157. About the British Wheel of Yoga. https://www.bwy.org.uk/about/. Published 2019. Accessed March 10, 2019.
158. Tew GA, Howsam J, Hardy M, Bissell L. Adapted yoga to improve physical function and health-related quality of life in physically-inactive older adults: a randomised controlled pilot trial. *BMC Geriatr.* 2017;17(1):131. https://doi.org/10.1186/s12877-017-0520-6.
159. Sharman MJ, Cresswell AG, Riek S. Proprioceptive neuromuscular facilitation stretching. *Sport Med.* 2006;36(11):929–939. https://doi.org/10.2165/00007256-200636110-00002.
160. Cayco CS, Labro AV, Gorgon EJR. Hold-relax and contract-relax stretching for hamstrings flexibility: a systematic review with meta-analysis. *Phys Ther Sport.* 2019;35:42–55. https://doi.org/10.1016/j.ptsp.2018.11.001.
161. Rees SS, Murphy AJ, Watsford ML, McLachlan KA, Coutts AJ. Effects of proprioceptive neuromuscular facilitation stretching on stiffness and force-producing characteristics of the ankle in active women. *J Strength Cond Res.* 2007;21(2):572. https://doi.org/10.1519/R-20175.1.

162. Barbosa AR, Santarem JM, Filho WJ, Marucci MF. Effects of resistance training on the sit-and-reach test in elderly women. *J Strength Cond Res*. 2002;16(1):14–18.
163. Sherrington C, Tiedemann A. Physiotherapy in the prevention of falls in older people. *J Physiother*. 2015;61(2):54–60. https://doi.org/10.1016/j.jphys.2015.02.011.
164. Sherrington C, Fairhall NJ, Wallbank GK, et al. Exercise for preventing falls in older people living in the community. *Cochrane Database Syst Rev*. 2019;1:CD012424. https://doi.org/10.1002/14651858.CD012424.pub2.
165. Sherrington C, Tiedemann A, Fairhall N, Close JC, Lord SR. Exercise to prevent falls in older adults: an updated meta-analysis and best practice recommendations. *N S W Public Health Bull*. 2011;22(3–4):78–83. https://doi.org/10.1071/NB10056.
166. Karinkanta S, Kannus P, Uusi-Rasi K, Heinonen A, Sievänen H. Combined resistance and balance-jumping exercise reduces older women's injurious falls and fractures: 5-year follow-up study. *Age Ageing*. 2015;44(5):784–789. https://doi.org/10.1093/ageing/afv064.
167. Sherrington C, Fairhall NJ, Wallbank GK, et al. Exercise for preventing falls in older people living in the community. *Cochrane Database Syst Rev*. 2019;1. https://doi.org/10.1002/14651858.CD012424.pub2 CD012424.
168. Sherrington C, Tiedemann A, Cameron I. Physical exercise after hip fracture: an evidence overview. *Eur J Phys Rehabil Med*. 2011;47(2):297–307.
169. Cadore EL, Rodriguez-Manas L, Sinclair A, Izquierdo M, Rodrı L. Effects of different exercise interventions on risk of falls, gait ability, and balance in physically frail older adults: a systematic review. *Rejuvenation Res*. 2013;16(2):105–114. https://doi.org/10.1089/rej.2012.1397.
170. Granacher U, Muehlbauer T, Zahner L, Gollhofer A, Kressig RW. Comparison of traditional and recent approaches in the promotion of balance and strength in older adults. *Sports Med*. 2011;41(5):377–400. https://doi.org/10.2165/11539920-000000000-00000.
171. Cadore EL, Izquierdo M. New strategies for the concurrent strength-, power-, and endurance-training prescription in elderly individuals. *J Am Med Dir Assoc*. 2013;14(8):623–624. https://doi.org/10.1016/j.jamda.2013.04.008.
172. Addison O, Inacio M, Bair W, Beamer BA, Ryan AS, Rogers MW. Role of hip abductor muscle composition and torque in protective stepping for lateral balance recovery in older adults. *Arch Phys Med Rehabil*. 2016;98:1223–1228. https://doi.org/10.1016/j.apmr.2016.10.009.
173. Fritz NE, Worstell AM, Kloos AD, Siles AB, White SE, Kegelmeyer DA. Backward walking measures are sensitive to age-related changes in mobility and balance. *Gait Posture*. 2013;37(4):593–597. https://doi.org/10.1016/j.gaitpost.2012.09.022.
174. Okubo Y, Osuka Y, Jung S, et al. Walking can be more effective than balance training in fall prevention among community-dwelling older adults. *Geriatr Gerontol Int*. 2016;16:118–125. https://doi.org/10.1111/ggi.12444.
175. Granacher U, Muehlbauer T, Bridenbaugh SA, et al. Effects of a salsa dance training on balance and strength performance in older adults. *Gerontology*. 2012;58(4):305–312. https://doi.org/10.1159/000334814.
176. Howe TE, Rochester L, Neil F, Skelton DA, Ballinger C. Exercise for improving balance in older people. *Cochrane Database Syst Rev*. 2011;11:CD004963. https://doi.org/10.1002/14651858.CD004963.pub3.
177. Keogh JW, Kilding A, Pidgeon P, Ashley L, Gillis D. Physical benefits of dancing for healthy older adults: a review. *J Aging Phys Act*. 2009;17(4):479–500.
178. Marquez DX, Wilbur J, Hughes S, et al. B.A.I.L.A. - a Latin dance randomized controlled trial for older Spanish-speaking Latinos: rationale, design, and methods. *Contemp Clin Trials*. 2014;38:397–408. S1551-7144(14)00094-9.
179. Wallmann HW, Gillis CB, Alpert PT, Miller SK. The effect of a senior jazz dance class on static balance in healthy women over 50 years of age: a pilot study. *Biol Res Nurs*. 2009; 10(3):257–266. https://doi.org/10.1177/1099800408322600.
180. Noreau L, Martineau H, Roy L, Belzile M. Effects of a modified dance-based exercise on cardiorespiratory fitness, psychological state and health status of persons with rheumatoid arthritis. *Am J Phys Med Rehabil*. 1995;74(1):19–27.
181. Murrock CJ, Higgins PA, Killion C. Dance and peer support to improve diabetes outcomes in African American women. *Diabetes Educ*. 2009;35(6):995–1003. https://doi.org/10.1177/0145721709343322.
182. Palo-Bengtsson L, Winblad B, Ekman SL. Social dancing: a way to support intellectual, emotional and motor functions in persons with dementia. *J Psychiatr Ment Health Nurs*. 1998;5(6):545–554.
183. Hokkanen L, Rantala L, Remes AM, Harkonen B, Viramo P, Winblad I. Dance and movement therapeutic methods in management of dementia: a randomized, controlled study. *J Am Geriatr Soc*. 2008;51(4):771–772. https://doi.org/10.1111/j.1532-5415.2008.01611.x.
184. Granacher U, Gollhofer A, Hortobagyi T, et al. The importance of trunk muscle strength for balance, functional performance, and fall prevention in seniors: a systematic review. *Sports Med*. 2013;43(7):627–641. https://doi.org/10.1007/s40279-013-0041-1.
185. Akuthota V, Ferreiro A, Moore T, Fredericson M. Core stability exercise principles. *Curr Sports Med Rep*. 2008;7(1):39–44. https://doi.org/10.1097/01.CSMR.0000308663.13278.69.
186. Kahle N, Tevald MA. Core muscle strengthening's improvement of balance performance in community-dwelling older adults: a pilot study. *J Aging Phys Act*. 2014;22(1):65–73. https://doi.org/10.1123/JAPA.2012-0132.
187. Mansfield A, Aqui A, Danells CJ, et al. Does perturbation-based balance training prevent falls among individuals with chronic stroke? A randomised controlled trial. *BMJ Open*. 2018;8(8):e021510. https://doi.org/10.1136/bmjopen-2018-021510.
188. Gerards MHG, McCrum C, Mansfield A, Meijer K. Perturbation-based balance training for falls reduction among older adults: current evidence and implications for clinical practice. *Geriatr Gerontol Int*. 2017;17(12):2294–2303. https://doi.org/10.1111/ggi.13082.
189. Menz HB, Auhl M, Spink MJ. Foot problems as a risk factor for falls in community-dwelling older people: a systematic review and meta-analysis. *Maturitas*. 2018;118:7–14. https://doi.org/10.1016/j.maturitas.2018.10.001.
190. Spink MJ, Fotoohabadi MR, Wee E, Hill KD, Lord SR, Menz HB. Foot and ankle strength, range of motion, posture, and deformity are associated with balance and functional ability in older adults. *Arch Phys Med Rehabil*. 2011;92(1):68–75. https://doi.org/10.1016/j.apmr.2010.09.024.
191. Fujimoto M, Hsu WL, Woollacott MH, Chou LS. Ankle dorsiflexor strength relates to the ability to restore balance during a backward support surface translation. *Gait Posture*. 2013;38(4):812–817. https://doi.org/10.1016/j.gaitpost.2013.03.026.
192. Maritz CA, Silbernagel KG. A prospective cohort study on the effect of a balance training program, including calf muscle strengthening, in community-dwelling older adults. *J Geriatr Phys Ther*. 2016;39:125–131. https://doi.org/10.1519/JPT.0000000000000059.
193. Park JH. The effects of eyeball exercise on balance ability and falls efficacy of the elderly who have experienced a fall: a single-blind, randomized controlled trial. *Arch Gerontol Geriatr*. 2017;68:181–185. S0167-4943(16)30186-8.

194. Muir-Hunter SW, Wittwer JE. Dual-task testing to predict falls in community-dwelling older adults: a systematic review. *Physiotherapy*. 2016;102(1):29–40. https://doi.org/10.1016/j.physio.2015.04.011.
195. Agmon M, Belza B, Nguyen HQ, Logsdon R, Kelly VE. A systematic review of interventions conducted in clinical or community settings to improve dual-task postural control in older adults. *Clin Interv Aging*. 2014;9:477. https://doi.org/10.2147/CIA.S54978.
196. Menant JC, Schoene D, Sarofim M, Lord SR. Single and dual task tests of gait speed are equivalent in the prediction of falls in older people: a systematic review and meta-analysis. *Ageing Res Rev*. 2014;16:83–104. https://doi.org/10.1016/j.arr.2014.06.001.
197. Orr R, de Vos NJ, Singh NA, Ross DA, Stavrinos TM, Fiatarone-Singh MA. Power training improves balance in healthy older adults. *J Gerontol A Biol Sci Med Sci*. 2006;61(1):78–85. http://www.ncbi.nlm.nih.gov/pubmed/16456197. Accessed March 3, 2019.
198. Lang CE, Macdonald JR, Gnip C. Counting repetitions: an observational study of outpatient therapy for people with hemiparesis post-stroke. *J Neurol Phys Ther*. 2007;31(1):3–10. https://doi.org/10.1097/01.NPT.0000260568.31746.34.
199. Voelcker-Rehage C. Motor-skill learning in older adults — a review of studies on age-related differences. *Eur Rev Aging Phys Act*. 2008;5:5–16. https://doi.org/10.1007/s11556-008-0030-9.
200. Thomas S, Mackintosh S, Halbert J. Does the "Otago exercise programme" reduce mortality and falls in older adults? A systematic review and meta-analysis. *Age Ageing*. 2010;39(6):681–687. https://doi.org/10.1093/ageing/afq102.
201. Robertson MC, Campbell AJ, Gardner MM, Devlin N. Preventing injuries in older people by preventing falls: a meta-analysis of individual-level data. *J Am Geriatr Soc*. 2002;50(5):905–911. http://www.ncbi.nlm.nih.gov/pubmed/12028179. Accessed March 5, 2019.
202. Falls & Otago Resources | Carolina Geriatric Education Center (CGEC). 2019. https://www.med.unc.edu/aging/cgec/exercise-program/. Accessed March 9, 2019.
203. Li F, Harmer P, Fisher KJ, et al. Tai Chi and fall reductions in older adults: a randomized controlled trial. *J Gerontol A, Biol Sci Med Sci*. 2005;60(2):187–194.
204. Leung DP, Chan CK, Tsang HW, Tsang WW, Jones AY. Tai chi as an intervention to improve balance and reduce falls in older adults: a systematic and meta-analytical review. *Altern Ther Health Med*. 2011;17(1):40–48.
205. Logghe IH, Verhagen AP, Rademaker AC, et al. The effects of Tai Chi on fall prevention, fear of falling and balance in older people: a meta-analysis. *Prev Med (Baltim)*. 2010;51(3–4):222–227. https://doi.org/10.1016/j.ypmed.2010.06.003.
206. Rand D, Miller WC, Yiu J, Eng JJ. Interventions for addressing low balance confidence in older adults: a systematic review and meta-analysis. *Age Ageing*. 2011;40(3):297–306. https://doi.org/10.1093/ageing/afr037.
207. Cameron ID, Gillespie LD, Robertson MC, et al. Interventions for preventing falls in older people in care facilities and hospitals. *Cochrane Database Syst Rev*. 2012;12:CD005465. https://doi.org/10.1002/14651858.CD005465.pub3.
208. National Council on Aging. Program Summary: Tai Ji Quan: Moving for Better Balance. https://www.ncoa.org/resources/program-summary-tai-ji-quan-moving-for-better-balance/. Accessed March 17, 2019.
209. Leung J. Implementing Tai Ji Quan: moving for better balance in real world settings: succeses and challenges. *J Sport Heal Sci*. 2014;3:34–35.
210. Centers for Disease Control and Prevention. Physical Activity Basics | Physical Activity. https://www.cdc.gov/physicalactivity/basics/index.htm. Published 2019. Accessed March 7, 2019.
211. Skelton DA, Beyer N. Exercise and injury prevention in older people. *Scand J Med Sci Sports*. 2003;13:77–85.
212. de Vos NJ, Singh NA, Ross DA, et al. Continuous hemodynamic response to maximal dynamic strength testing in older adults. *Arch Phys Med Rehabil*. 2008;89(2):343–350. https://doi.org/10.1016/j.apmr.2007.08.130.
213. Tjønna AE, Lee SJ, Rognmo Ø, et al. Aerobic interval training versus continuous moderate exercise as a treatment for the metabolic syndrome: a pilot study. *Circulation*. 2008;118(4):346–354.
214. Booth FW, Roberts CK, Laye MJ. Lack of exercise is a major cause of chronic diseases. *Compr Physiol*. 2012;2(2):1143–1211. https://doi.org/10.1002/cphy.c110025.

CHAPTER

9

Age-Related Changes in Gait and Mobility

Julie D. Ries

OUTLINE

INTRODUCTION

Physical therapists play a unique and important role when examining the older adult with gait dysfunction. Although "gait training" may sound like a simple and straightforward task, this is rarely the case with older adult clients. Bipedal locomotion is a uniquely human skill that requires multiple systems (neurologic, musculoskeletal, cardiopulmonary, cognition) to work in a congruent and sophisticated manner. Normal age-related decline across these systems, even in healthy individuals, has a predictable impact on gait in the older adult.

Often, health care professionals look to physical therapists to "clear" an older adult for safe discharge from the inpatient environment, or a patient or primary care physician requests a consultation from a physical therapist to assess mobility concerns. A high level of clinical skill is required to adequately analyze and identify specific problems in the complex task of functional ambulation, particularly in older adults who have multiple potential contributing factors to impaired mobility. Safe ambulation requires the ability to appropriately and sometimes quickly accelerate and decelerate, engage proactive and reactive balance control mechanisms, and address myriad different environmental and specific task demands. Before clearing a patient for discharge, a professional judgment that implies the individual is safe and independent in ambulation in various environments, or making suggestions that would restrict independent community mobility, a skilled assessment of ambulation capabilities and safety must be conducted.

To perform a comprehensive and accurate examination of ambulation capabilities and effective interventions for identified dysfunctions, a physical therapist should have (1) extensive knowledge of normal gait and changes that occur with aging, (2) a clear understanding of the functional requirements of ambulation with and without assistive devices, (3) a repertoire of tests and measures appropriate for gait assessment, and (4) an ability to evaluate examination findings and create an appropriate and effective evidence-based plan of care.

This chapter begins with a discussion of locomotor functions, primary tasks of locomotion, and phases of the normal gait cycle. The chapter then describes anticipated gait changes that occur with normal aging and provides an analysis of the complex functional gait requirements of community ambulation related to speed, distance, and navigation of various terrains. The chapter then continues with a discussion of planning and justifying a comprehensive, yet efficient, examination of gait for a given older individual using appropriate tests and measures and ends with an analysis of evidence for various treatment interventions used in gait-training the older adult.

NORMAL GAIT

A solid understanding of the biomechanics of normal gait is a prerequisite of the highest-quality care. Generally speaking, humans all walk similarly, striving to move forward and keep the center of gravity over the base of support in the most energy-efficient manner possible. Perry and Burnfield's[1] traditional framework for describing the gait cycle, organized from a biomechanical perspective around the sagittal plane, highlights the basic components of normal gait. This chapter assumes the reader is familiar with the basic principles of kinetics, kinematics, and muscle activity that are relevant to human walking. Only a brief review of the major tasks and phases of the gait cycle is provided. An understanding of normal gait is a necessary foundation for identifying and problem solving gait abnormalities.

The four locomotor functions of gait[1] include shock absorption, stance stability, propulsion, and energy conservation. Shock absorption is the result of muscle activity when loading the stance extremity. Eccentric dorsiflexor activity, eccentric knee extensor activity (both in the sagittal plane), and eccentric hip abductor activity (in the frontal plane) all work to absorb shock as the limb is loaded. Stance stability is determined by ground reaction force vectors (GRFVs), ligament and joint support, and muscle activity. Using GRFVs to determine the flexion or extension moment at each joint of the lower extremity, one can determine the static (joint and ligamentous structures) and dynamic (muscle activity) components required to control movement of the lower extremity segment during stance. It is acknowledged and accepted that GRFVs are an imperfect and simplistic way of conceptualizing the physics of gait; however, GRFVs serve as a useful framework for examining basic principles of muscle activity within the phases of gait.

Forward propulsion in gait is the result of the body's forward fall, rocker mechanisms (i.e., heel, ankle, forefoot, and toe rockers) that allow smooth translation of weight over the distal lower extremity, momentum created by the swing of the contralateral lower extremity, and active push-off of the stance lower extremity.

Energy conservation is thought to be maximized by selective muscle recruitment and the determinants of gait. Selective muscle recruitment is the efficiency achieved by using muscles strategically so as not to require excess or redundant muscle activity (e.g., short head of biceps femoris can flex the knee without unwanted extension of the hip early in swing phase; biarticular hamstrings can eccentrically slow both hip flexion and knee extension during late swing). The determinants of gait are biomechanical adjustments that are purported to decrease the excursion of the body's center of mass in all planes, thereby decreasing the energy required to maintain stability over the base of support throughout the gait cycle. It should be noted, however, that the assumptions underlying this long-standing and well-accepted biomechanical theory have undergone very little empirical testing.

The gait cycle is conceptualized as eight phases within three major tasks: (1) weight acceptance, (2) single limb support, and (3) limb advancement.[1] In normal gait, weight acceptance includes the phases of *initial contact* and *loading response,* during which the heel is the first to contact the support surface (during initial contact) and the limb absorbs shock as the weight of the individual is translated onto the stance lower extremity (loading response). Single limb support includes the phases *midstance* and *terminal stance.* During *midstance,* the opposite limb advances as the body begins posterior to the weight-bearing foot but moves anterior by the end of the phase, controlled primarily by eccentric soleus and gastrocnemius activity. In *terminal stance,* body weight moves anterior to the forefoot and the heel rises from the support surface. Perry and Burnfield identify this as "roll off," suggesting that "push off" occurs later in the preswing phase of gait, but others consider that terminal stance offers a propulsive "push off" with concentric plantar flexor activity, which aids in the forward momentum of the body during gait.[2] Limb advancement is successfully carried out by the combination of *preswing* (final unloading of the lower extremity), *initial swing* (preparing the swinging leg for foot clearance), *midswing* (ensuring continued clearance), and *terminal swing* (slowing of the leg in preparation for initial contact).

Table 9.1 provides a general summary of the normal gait cycle, including the primary tasks of gait, the phases of gait, and some of the key events that occur within each of the phases. An appreciation for the range of motion (ROM), muscle activity, and motor control requirements of the various phases of gait makes for efficient clinical problem solving related to gait deviations.

Gait Characteristics: Typical Changes with Aging

Aging is accompanied by multiple changes in sensory, motor, and central nervous system (CNS) functioning that interact to bring about predictable changes in gait performance. Common sensory (affector system) changes include decreased abilities of visual and auditory systems and diminished input from somatosensory, proprioceptive, and vestibular systems. These changes can lead to inaccurate appraisal of environmental demands or erroneous self-assessment of positioning and/or movement. Common motor (effector system) changes include decreased motor neuron conduction velocity, decrease in numbers of motor fibers, and periarticular connective tissue stiffness. Combined effects may result in limitations in ROM and muscle strength. CNS functioning and integrative changes might include loss of neuronal connectivity and altered level of neurotransmitter production, resulting in slowed reaction time and decreased facility of movement presenting as motor control deficits.

Armed with an understanding of the specific requirements of normal gait, a physical therapist can anticipate

TABLE 9.1 Summary of the Normal Gait Cycle: Three Primary Tasks and Eight Gait Phases

	Three Primary Tasks of Gait							
	Weight Acceptance		Single-Limb Support		Limb Advancement			
Eight Phases of Gait	**Initial Contact**	**Loading Response**	**Midstance**	**Terminal Stance**	**Preswing**	**Initial Swing**	**Midswing**	**Terminal Swing**
Temporal location of each phase along the gait cycle	~0%–2%	~3%–10%	~10%–30%	~31%–50%	~50%–60%	~61%–75%	~75%–85%	~86%–100%
Objectives/critical events within each phase	Heel strike Stable, upright trunk is key to *all* phases	Shock absorption Weight-bearing stability Preservation of progression	Progression over stationary foot (controlled tibial advancement) Limb and trunk stability	Push-off; heel rise Progression of body beyond supporting foot (free forward fall)	Transfer of body weight unloads limb Knee flexion in preparation for foot clearance	Foot clears floor (knee flexion essential) Limb advances from its trailing position	Ankle dorsiflexion to neutral key for foot clearance Continued limb advancement	Hip and knee deceleration, complete limb advancement Limb prepares for stance with knee extension and ankle neutral
Rocker mechanism	Heel rocker	Heel rocker	Ankle rocker	Forefoot rocker	Toes rocker			
Selected muscle activity	Firing of lower extremity extensors in preparation for weight bearing Isometric dorsiflexor activity keeps ankle in neutral for heel contact	Period of maximal muscle activity Hip extensors help progress body Eccentric knee extensors, hip abductors, and ankle dorsiflexors aid in shock absorption	Hip abductors stabilize pelvis Eccentric plantar-flexors allow controlled forward progression of tibia over fixed foot to dorsiflexion 10 degrees	Ankle plantar-flexor activity provides "push-off"	Hip flexors and adductors assist in actively initiating hip flexion (passive hip and knee flexion are the result of the tibia rolling forward)	Momentum carries limb to great extent Some hip and knee flexion activity Pretibials fire to begin to bring foot back into dorsiflexion	Primarily momentum carrying limb Pretibials bring ankle to neutral	Eccentric hamstring activity to slow the swinging limb at both hip and knee Isometric pretibials keep ankle in neutral

how specific changes in ROM, strength, and motor control can lead to predictable gait changes. Take, for example, a subtle decrease in hip extension ROM in an older adult. Hip extension ROM is required late in the stance phase. If the trailing limb is not extended at the hip during terminal stance, this will affect the efficiency of swing for that leg: The stretch to hip flexors in preparation for swing will not be effectively applied, and the leg loses some of its swing preparation time, making foot clearance during swing more difficult. A loss of terminal knee extension ROM will affect the gait cycle during loading response, making shock absorption at the knee difficult or ineffective because it eliminates the excursion of the range where the eccentric activity of the quadriceps works to load the limb in a controlled manner.

Alignment and arthrokinematic changes can *result from* or be *caused by* changes in strength and flexibility with aging. It is difficult to know which came first—the gait deviation or the ROM limitation—but they are clearly interrelated. Consider the previous example. A loss of hip extension ROM necessitates shorter step length on the contralateral limb, and shorter step length requires less hip extension ROM. One of the more common habitual postures of the older adult is that of succumbing to gravity (kyphotic trunk, often with flexion at the hips and knees). This flexed posture changes the influence of GRFVs at each joint and alters the excursion of movement and the demand on muscle activity during the gait cycle. Anticipating the incompatibilities between a habitual posture and the requirements of normal gait prepare the physical therapist to conduct an efficient evaluation of gait.

Although patients are unique in their clinical presentation and impairments, there are generalizations that can be made about gait changes associated with aging. There is a dearth of data related to middle-aged adult gait,[3] but in comparing healthy younger versus healthy older adults, the most predictable gait changes repeatedly demonstrated in the literature and represented in recent systematic reviews[3–5] are presented in Box 9.1. Older adults who are physically active experience benefits to all bodily systems. Although there is general agreement that gait changes are seen with the typical or usual aging process, physically active older adults can mitigate some of these changes.[6]

Decrease in self-selected gait speed (SSGS) (also called "preferred" or "comfortable" gait speed) is a consistent finding with aging; however, as evidenced in Box 9.1, older adult gait is not simply a slower version of young adult gait. It is important to note that the kinematic and kinetic changes associated with aging are not simply a function of slower gait. When comparing younger and older adults at matched velocities, these changes persist.[4] Older adults display a more conservative gait pattern and a decreasing step and stride length; they spend a progressively longer time and percentage of the gait cycle in double-limb support and display an increasing step width[7–9] in an effort to be safer and more stable in upright. Electromyography suggests greater coactivation of muscles around the ankle and knee in older as compared to young adults.[10] Additionally, where young adults rely on distal propulsive forces (power generation from the plantar flexors) during terminal stance and into preswing, older adults demonstrate a decrease in this distal mechanism and may shift the demand for power proximally to the hip, especially in efforts to walk with increased speed.[4] Lower extremity ROM excursions during the gait cycle are less in older than young adults, and the extremes of all joint ranges in the sagittal plane are decreased with the exception of hip flexion. Older adults display greater hip flexion in terminal swing and initial contact than young adults and diminished terminal knee extension in these phases. Combined with reduced hip extension late in the stance phase, the result is a less upright posture throughout the gait cycle.[4]

Increased gait variability (with a variety of different operational definitions) has consistently been associated with an increased risk of falls.[11] Many identified gait changes in older adults represent an effort to increase stability and safety in gait (e.g., decreased speed, decreased step and stride length, increased step width, increased double-limb support time). Variability of gait does not appear to be under such deliberate control, as variability of many gait parameters increases with age.[4,5] In healthy older adults, variability is magnified at higher speeds, under the influence of postural threat, or under dual-task demands.[12] Variability within a movement pattern is not inherently detrimental. In fact, variability is typically associated with adaptability and flexibility of movement performance, which is critical to an adaptive control system. However, in the older adult, increasing gait variability seems to translate to increasing instability. Older adults adopt a more conservative gait pattern in an effort to increase stability and reduce the likelihood of falls, yet they demonstrate an increased variability, which paradoxically increases falls risk.

BOX 9.1 Typical Gait Changes in Older Adults

- Decreased self-selected gait speed
- Decreased step and stride length
- Increased stance time and double-limb support time
- Increased step width (not a universal finding across studies)
- Increased variability of gait (operationally defined as variability in step or stride time, length, or width)
- Decreased excursion of movement at lower extremity joints
- Decreased reliance on ankle kinetics and power
- Less upright posture

PATHOLOGIC GAIT CHANGES

Although normal aging brings about predictable gait changes, clinicians need to be able to distinguish between normal age-related changes and those resulting from pathology. Verghese et al.[13] studied the epidemiology of gait disorders in community-residing older adults ($n = 468$).

Classifying subjects as "normal" and "abnormal," and further identifying "neurologic" and "nonneurologic" gait patterns, the authors demonstrated that the prevalence of abnormal gait was 35% in their study population. Nonneurologic abnormal gait characteristics were more common than neurologic, and mild abnormalities were more common than severe. The incidence of abnormal gait increased with advanced age and was associated with progressive risk of institutionalization and death. If these findings can be generalized to all older adults, clinicians might expect up to one-third of their older adult community-residing clients to display gait changes beyond those demonstrated with typical aging.

Slowed gait beyond the typical expectations of aging is a defining feature of frailty,[14,15] and decreases in SSGS are predictive of activities of daily living (ADL) and mobility disability,[15,16] cognitive decline,[17] and mortality.[18] Physical therapists should be especially astute in identifying individuals who are transitioning to frailty (i.e., classified as prefrail). These individuals may not have a discrete diagnosis, but may demonstrate a pronounced decline in temporal and spatial parameters of gait as compared to healthy older adults, specifically decreased step length and increased variability of step width.[14] Deterioration of performance within a transitionally frail group is not necessarily associated with age, suggesting that other factors (e.g., muscle weakness, depression, fear of falling) may be more related to gait performance within this group than age alone.[14,19] Gill et al.[20] suggest that mobility disability is an extremely dynamic process involving transitions from no disability to intermittent disability to continuous disability, and back again. They concede that transitions from disability back to no disability are less common than trends in the direction of disability, but certainly improvement is possible for some individuals. They state a case for physical therapists to focus not only on prevention of mobility impairments but also on restoration of mobility in those who become disabled, especially frail older women, as they are most susceptible to mobility disability. Age-related changes in gait also appear to be magnified when looking at older individuals prone to falls.[11] Older adults who have fallen are slower than their age-matched peers without a fall history and they demonstrate shorter step and stride length, and increased gait variability.

An exhaustive listing and description of common gait deviations observed with different diagnostic groups is beyond the scope of this chapter; however, some generalizations can be made about gait characteristics associated with specific pathologies, all of which will demonstrate slowed SSGS, and a hallmark of neurologic disorders is an increase in gait variability.[21] Older adults with hemiplegia due to stroke present with significant asymmetries in gait that are often motivated by avoidance of weight bearing through the involved lower extremity, affecting both the hemiplegic and uninvolved side.[22] Given various compensatory strategies and the intricacies related to abnormal tone in these individuals, evaluating and treating hemiplegic gait is a unique challenge. Parkinson disease is associated with decreased speed, decreased step length, and increased variability of gait[23] and often presents with the classic shuffling or festinating gait. Difficulty with initiation and freezing episodes provide an added dimension to the management of parkinsonian gait. Individuals with dementias generally display amplified findings of the typical aging changes, although there is some evidence of subtle differences between different types of dementias.[24,25] Evaluating and working with individuals with cognitive impairment brings with it a whole new set of challenges. Regardless of diagnosis, each client will require careful examination of the unique clinical presentation of gait. The underlying diagnosis may cue the therapist to look for certain gait characteristics, but there is variability within each diagnostic group.

INTERRELATEDNESS OF GAIT AND COGNITION

The act of walking was once considered to be an automatic function with very little need for cognitive oversight. In fact, much of the excitement over locomotor treadmill training with partial body weight support as an intervention for restoring gait was predicated on the theory that central pattern generators in the spinal cord could potentially drive walking with little or no supraspinal input. There is now, however, clear evidence of the interrelatedness of gait and cognition, including proposed shared mechanisms in the brain driving clinical changes that affect both gait and cognition with aging and pathology (e.g., neurodegenerative, vascular, and inflammatory processes).[26,27] Poor gait performance, most often defined by slow speed, has been demonstrated to precede cognitive decline and clinical diagnosis of dementia.[17,24] In fact, gait slowing over time is a more sensitive predictor of dementia than cognitive decline, and individuals showing downward trajectories in gait and cognition have a higher risk of developing dementia than those showing decline in one area or the other.[28] Motoric cognitive risk syndrome (MCRS), a relatively new area of study, describes the condition of slowed gait ($\geq$1 standard deviation below age- and sex-matched gait speed norms) combined with subjective cognitive or memory complaint in the absence of dementia or mobility/ADL disability. Evidence is mounting to show that individuals with MCRS are two to three times more likely to develop dementia than those without MCRS, with some studies suggesting these numbers are much higher.[29,30] While the predictive capabilities of gait speed as related to cognitive decline are important, so is the concept of shared pathology. Neural plasticity in response to activity-based interventions is well supported and perhaps, with the appropriate level of challenge and training, both physical and cognitive, older adults can delay, slow, or avoid declining function. Systematic reviews of combined physical and cognitive exercises for older adults with varying levels of cognitive impairment demonstrate improved gait and balance performance.[31,32] Physical therapists are movement experts, but given the intertwined relationship between gait and cognition, clinicians must be equipped to strategically integrate cognitive demands within mobility and gait training.

FUNCTIONAL AMBULATION REQUIREMENTS

If functional mobility in the real world were confined to the demands of walking on a level, cleared, well-lit pathway, then individuals walking a lap around the physical therapy clinic or a length of the facility hallway would easily demonstrate their readiness for safe discharge from physical therapy. Clearly, this is not the case. The International Classification of Functioning, Disability, and Health (ICF) model demonstrates the significant impact that environment and personal factors have on activity and participation of our older adult clients. Functional mobility in the real world depends on what the individual brings to the encounter, as well as what the task and the environment demand (e.g., variations in speed, distance, and terrain; obstacle clearance/avoidance; dual- or multitasking while walking). Individual, task, and environmental constraints determine the ultimate movement strategies used within specific gait challenges.

Individual Constraints

At the level of the individual, potential constraints (disabling factors) to walking ability at home and in the community may be physiological and/or psychological. Physiological factors may include impairments in range of motion, strength, motor control, somatosensation, vestibular function, or cardiopulmonary endurance. The experience of pain is another frequent culprit impacting walking characteristics and ability. There is no direct formula to predict the correlation between impairments and gait performance. Familiarity with the requirements for normal gait and understanding common individual constraints to ambulation in older adults enhance the physical therapist's ability to organize and prioritize the examination to quickly uncover impairments that will affect gait.

Often overlooked is the enabling or disabling influence of an individual's psychological status on gait performance. Perceptions about aging, personal abilities, and self-efficacy related to gait and balance may be useful indicators for gait performance. A positive perception of self-rated health is protective against decline in gait speed and other performance measures.[33,34] Depressive symptoms negatively influence gait speed, even in the absence of a major depressive episode.[35] Anxiety or fear related to falls is common in older adults and is highly correlated with measures of gait and balance and indicative of whether individuals will venture into the community.[36,37] Tools to assess individuals' perceptions about their gait and balance (e.g., Activities-specific Balance Confidence [ABC] Scale, Balance Self-Efficacy Scale) are useful in this context. Older adults with excessive concerns about falling may display maladaptive behaviors to enhance stability when they feel posturally threatened, and these behaviors (i.e., decreased speed, decreased step length, increased double-limb support time) may paradoxically increase fall risk.[38] Although patients should not have a false confidence about their abilities in the community, unwarranted fears that limit community mobility or increase the risk of falls are undesirable. In conjunction with exercise interventions to improve fall risk and fear of falling,[39] therapists can work with older adults to build confidence for community mobility. Talkowski et al.[40] demonstrated that individuals who perceived their own health and balance to be good walked more than those who did not, and Hausdorff et al.[41] showed that exposing older adults to positive stereotyping about aging increased their gait speed, suggesting that therapists might be able to exploit the relationship between self-perception and function. Building confidence and alleviating fears about community mobility is an underutilized and potentially powerful tool.

A comprehensive patient interview will reveal patients' perceived risks for community ambulation, which are as important as patients' real risks. Individuals may have less than obvious perceived risks associated with community mobility that might include concerns about self-image related to appearance while walking, inability to access public necessities easily (e.g., restrooms), and fear of physical harm at the hand of individuals in the environment. Perceived neighborhood safety has been found to correlate with physical activity and walking in older adults.[42,43] Individuals are unlikely to venture walking into their communities if they feel threatened by the people or the environment, and this is sometimes the case in socioeconomically deprived neighborhoods. In addition to safety, other important environment themes in supporting older adults in being physically active in their communities and walking to community destinations include pedestrian infrastructure (e.g., sidewalk status, protection from traffic), access to destinations/facilities (e.g., pragmatic locations [stores, senior center, public transit], parks, benches, restrooms), aesthetics, and environmental/weather conditions.[43] Dog ownership is a positive influence on neighborhood walking. Older adult dog owners participate in significantly more community walking than their non-dog-walking peers.[44] Therapists support individual clients to enhance their community mobility on a daily basis. It is important to remember that the vision of the American Physical Therapy Association (APTA) is "transforming society by optimizing movement to improve the human experience" and the APTA strategic plan identifies reducing, among other things, community barriers to movement.[45] To facilitate the ability to age in place and encourage active living into older adulthood, therapists are well situated to advocate on a large scale by consulting and advising on neighborhood planning and policy that supports ease of community mobility.

A final consideration in interviewing older adults about community ambulation is that individuals may report that they are independent in the community, but upon further investigation, the therapist might discover that the individual has significantly modified his or her community outings, and adjusted his or her community lifestyles, to meet his or her decreased mobility level. This could be an appropriate and realistic adjustment, or it could be a premature withdrawal from community activities that has a negative impact on quality of life (e.g., an individual may order grocery delivery to avoid outings to the grocery store, but also might forfeit enjoyable outings to the community center for weekly social events). A comprehensive assessment of individual capabilities and a realistic understanding of the demands of the community will help the therapist identify the optimal goals related to community mobility. Therapists can survey their patients to determine what challenges they have encountered and which ones they have avoided in their recent outings. Sometimes, the reality is that independent community ambulation is no longer safe for an older adult and helping to problem-solve ways in which individuals can continue community activities that are important to them in a safe manner becomes the focus of the physical therapist's attention. But sometimes, individuals may pull out of community activities prematurely, and physical therapy can positively affect quality of life by preparing patients for and reintroducing them to community ambulation. Accompanied ambulation in the community may be a useful intervention to facilitate patients' community mobility. When an individual successfully performs community ambulation under the watchful eye of a health care professional, this achievement can be an excellent confidence builder.

Speed and Distance Requirements for Functional Ambulation

Physical therapists generally consider mobility on a continuum: nonfunctional ambulation, household ambulation, limited community ambulation, independent community ambulation; however, universally accepted operational definitions of these terms are lacking. Oftentimes in the clinic environment, guidelines are arbitrarily identified—the distance to lap a section of the hospital floor or the perimeter around the physical therapy gym becomes the distance to which physical therapists aspire to have their patients walk.

Preserving community mobility in older adults has been the subject of much study, as has the effort to understand the relationship between environmental demands and community ambulation.[46–53] Mobility decline in older adults not only is a physical event but also has significant social and psychological consequences,[54] which is important for therapists to acknowledge and understand.

How does one define *mobility disability*? What does it mean to state that an individual is an "independent community ambulator"? The answer depends on who is asked. Box 9.2 presents several different operational definitions for mobility disability and community ambulation from the published literature. Many physical therapy clinics use 150 feet (45.72 m) as the criterion for community ambulation. This may originate from the widely used Functional Independence Measure (FIM), which defines the highest level of locomotion (FIM score 7) as the ability to walk 150 feet safely and without assistance in a reasonable time period.[55] When third-party payers see documentation that a patient is ambulating 150 feet, they may question the need for continued physical therapy, and they certainly will challenge the need for home health care. The reality, however, is that successful community mobility requires ambulation of distances well over 150 feet. In addition, although short-distance gait speed tests are valid and reliable for self-comparison, they may not generalize well to community distances. For instance, gait speed during a 4-meter walk test may not accurately project how an older adult will fare when crossing a large intersection that spans more than 20 meters.

A systematic review by Salbach et al.[56] synthesized data from studies of community ambulation speed and distance requirements. When considering similar methods of measurement and reporting in U.S.-based studies, data suggests that a trip to the grocery store requires a mean walking distance of between 294 and 381 meters. These measures can be considered conservative because the measurement protocols involved parking in the closest handicap-accessible space and walking one-half of the

BOX 9.2 Variations Among Commonly Used Operational Definitions of Terms Related to Mobility

Mobility Disability

"The impaired ability to move independently from one location to another and reach the desired destination."[53]

"The inability to walk one-quarter mile or climb a flight of stairs without assistance."[20]

"The inability to walk one-half mile or climb a flight of stairs without assistance."[113]

Community Ambulation

"Walking in the community to pursue recreational, social, or employment goals, and to destinations significant for participation in activities that fulfill quality of life."[48]

"The ability to walk with or without a gait aid to destinations important for participation in community life."[49]

"Independent mobility outside the home which includes the ability to confidently negotiate uneven terrain, private venues, shopping centers and other public venues."[51]

The ability "to ambulate a distance sufficient to conduct business in a variety of locations, . . . ascend and descend curbs, and cross a street within the time provided by a crossing signal."[114]

aisles of the store and returning to the parking space. One study[57] represented values for superstores (e.g., Target, Walmart) and club warehouses (e.g., Costco, Sam's Club) requiring mean walking distances of 607 and 677 meters, respectively, but these are also quite conservative as the walking path included the perimeter and central aisles only. Mean gait speeds required to cross streets within the allotted time of the crosswalk signal in the United States were impacted by city size and ranged from 0.49 to 1.32 m/s and mean crosswalk distances ranged from 10 to 27 meters. It is apparent that being independently ambulatory in a highly populated city will require walking faster and further than in a more rural, less populated town. The authors make a case for understanding the community environment each individual will be returning to after discharge and using this information in goal setting.[56]

Task and Environment Demands

True independence in the community requires so much more than specific distance or speed requirements. Box 9.3 identifies some of the many environmental demands that characterize community mobility. A conceptual framework introduced some time ago by Patla and Shumway-Cook[53] provides a comprehensive way to analyze environmental factors or "dimensions" that can operationally define the complexity of a specific mobility task. They identify eight environmental dimensions that can be classified or measured to characterize the external demands an individual may face in an effort to be independently mobile within a specified community. The dimensions are minimum walking distance, time constraints, ambient conditions (light, weather), terrain characteristics, external physical load, attentional demands, postural transitions, and traffic level. What is unique and intriguing about this model is that it informs mobility training such that it can meet the needs of a particular client. The interactions among the dimensions have not been elucidated and only some aspects of this framework have been systematically evaluated.[46,52] Regardless, the paradigm underscores the multifaceted nature of community mobility.

BOX 9.3 Environmental Demands Commonly Encountered During Community Ambulation

- Starts and stops
- Acceleration and deceleration
- Sideways stepping
- Backward stepping
- Changing directions and turning around
- Obstacle clearance/avoidance
- Picking up/carrying/putting down objects
- Pushing/pulling doors
- Managing displacement forces
- Terrain changes
- Lighting changes
- Weather changes
- Stepping up and down curbs/stairs/ramps of different heights and grades
- Concurrent execution of other tasks (cognitive and physical)

Ambulation with Assistive Devices

The use of assistive devices can have a significant impact on the mobility of older adults, providing much-needed support and confidence that may enhance household and community locomotion. Bertrand et al., in a systematic review, demonstrate that mobility devices improve the activity and participation of mobility-impaired adults.[58] They do acknowledge that there are obstacles that must be overcome with assistive device use, including environmental barriers and social stigma, and that the role of the therapist includes supporting individuals to overcome obstacles and integrate assistive device use into their daily lives. There are clear trends of increased assistive device use with aging and increased use in more recent years.[59,60] This is attributable, in part, to the increasing number of older adults, but also to increased prescription and availability of assistive devices. Recent survey studies of nationally representative samples report prevalence of assistive device use in community dwelling older adults to be 16.6% to 24%.[59,61] The most commonly used assistive devices are canes, although it is notable that Gell et al. found that one-third of assistive device users reported use of more than one type of device.[59]

Physical therapists are responsible for optimal assistive device prescription. Finding the best possible solution for each patient on the stability–mobility continuum is an ongoing challenge. The goal is to prescribe the least restrictive assistive device that provides the degree of stability and support required by the client. Proper adjustment and maintenance of assistive devices is a key factor to safe mobility. Clear instruction as to the optimal use of an assistive device and assessment of patient understanding of assistive device use is an important component of a comprehensive physical therapy program. Although assistive devices are useful in aiding patients' stability, clinicians need to remember that these devices also require considerable attention for proper use, creating a superimposed cognitive as well as physical task (manipulation of assistive device) on the primary motor task of walking. This may require a good deal of practice and instruction. Another consideration is that energy consumption is greater for ambulation with an assistive device than without, although this is confounded by the underlying cause of assistive device use.[62] Individuals using assistive devices ambulate more slowly than those without[63]; however, it is not known whether they are slower in an effort to preserve energy or to enhance stability. Also of note, for all walking and mobility activities, the importance of appropriate footwear for optimal safety and function should always be taken into account.

Some older adults take great pride in their ability to ambulate without a cane or walker and are resistant to the notion and the appearance of needing external support. In fact, the decision to use an assistive device can be monumental for some clients. Negative ageist stereotypes may drive an individual's resistance to assistive device use.[54] Although the physical therapist will actively listen to and acknowledge a person's concerns related to use of assistive devices, safety should be the driving force in device prescription, followed closely by function. There is some indication of improved satisfaction and use of assistive devices that are personalized for "fun, function, and fashion"[64] or are more mainstream or athletic in appearance (think trekking pole vs. cane). Convincing an older adult that an assistive device will afford the safest and most functional independent access to the home and/or community can be a difficult but necessary discussion. Framing the conversation to demonstrate what is *gained* by assistive device use (improved safety, mobility, stability, independence, and peace of mind) versus what is lost is a recommended strategy.

Stair Negotiation

Successful stair negotiation requires greater ROM (hip and knee flexion, ankle dorsiflexion) and muscle strength (extensors of the lower extremity working concentrically in ascent and eccentrically in descent) than level ground walking. Individuals may identify difficulty with ascent or descent or both. Speed for stair negotiation in older adults correlates with walking speed and lower extremity strength,[65–67] and a study by Hinman et al. demonstrated that SSGS and single-limb stance time are the two best indicators of stair climbing speed and explain 63% of the variance in performance.[67] Self-efficacy on stairs relates to speed and safety precautions undertaken (e.g., use of rails).[66] Because stairs are one of the most common environmental obstacles that are encountered both at home and in the community, it is important to consider the prerequisite actions and tasks needed for this activity and prioritize stair training within the plan of care.

EXAMINATION AND EVALUATION OF GAIT

A comprehensive examination of gait will include gathering a patient history, reviewing all pertinent systems, and carrying out appropriate tests and measures related to ambulation. A thorough gait assessment has significant redundancy with balance assessment, and the reader is directed to the Chapter 10 for complementary content.

A survey or interview of a patient's perception of difficulty with walking is a reasonable component of the physical therapy examination; however, patients frequently underreport gait difficulties. Goals related to gait activities are pivotal in planning an intervention, as the intervention strategies will need to demonstrate specificity to goals. Prior level of function, and the duration of that level, is a key factor to appropriate intervention selection in a rehabilitation program. If an older adult was nonambulatory prior to admission to an inpatient setting, it is important to quantify the duration of this status (i.e., days, weeks, months, or years) as this information will significantly affect the goal setting for the rehabilitation program. An individual who has only recently stopped walking owing to acuity of illness or a progressive condition that is now being medically managed might return to prior level of functioning very quickly. A careful evaluation of patient potential and an individualized plan of care might even lead to an individual exceeding his or her previous level of function. Individuals whose ambulation disability is long-standing (e.g., months or even years) are also deserving of careful evaluation even if the preexisting nonambulatory status might not be completely reversible.

Careful review of comorbidities and medications is another important component of the patient history. Some musculoskeletal and neurologic diagnoses affect gait in fairly predictable ways as previously noted. Many medications have systemic side effects that can affect a patient's tolerance for therapy or alter movement strategies. The reader is directed to Chapter 6 for more in-depth discussion related to the impact of medications on mobility in older adults.

Choice of physical therapy tests and measures for an older adult with mobility issues will be driven by screening body systems and may include specific assessment of ROM, strength, joint pain, motor control, and coordination; somatosensation, proprioception, and vestibular function; and functional mobility (bed mobility and transfers). Observational gait analysis (OGA) is a reasonable place to initiate a gait assessment but cannot be considered the sole "test" of gait within an examination as there is lack of standardization and an absence of support for psychometric properties of OGA. Nevertheless, OGA may be a useful starting point to make some general observations about an individual's gait. It can be done without interrupting the flow of other parts of the examination, such as when the patient walks from the door back to the living room after letting the home care therapist into the house, or from the bed to the bathroom in the inpatient environment, or when the patient enters the outpatient clinic and walks to a treatment table. The therapist can make general observations about speed, symmetry, stability, and efficiency of gait. Observations made during OGA, including any specific gait deviations, will help direct the appropriate selection of more objective outcome measures. There are many gait-specific outcome measures from which to choose, and the clinician should have a reasonable rationale for selecting and combining specific measures. Gait speed will be the only outcome measure reviewed in detail here; for an extensive list and description of other relevant tools, reference values, and psychometric properties, see Chapter 7 on outcome measures.

Gait Speed

Using a timed walk of a specific distance is an easy, reliable, and efficient way to measure gait performance. The strong psychometric properties of walking speed, the clinical usefulness, and the flexibility of this measure have led to its identification as a "functional vital sign" in older adults.[68] A commonly used SSGS threshold that delineates older adult community ambulators from those who are more limited is 1 m/s. This is a useful reference value to keep in mind when relating SSGS to functional mobility. Table 9.2 represents descriptive and predictive capabilities of older adult gait speeds as represented in review studies.[68,69]

Gait speed is an outcome measure physical therapists should use with all ambulatory older adults. SSGS tends to be the most individually efficient gait speed. It is often useful to collect both self-selected and fast gait speed capabilities, as there are environmental challenges that sometimes demand increased gait speeds (e.g., crossing streets). The difference between an older adult's fast gait speed and SSGS gives insight into the gait speed "reserve." A large reserve might suggest that therapeutic goals toward increasing SSGS are realistic, whereas a small reserve indicates that the individual is functioning close to his or her threshold, which may be dictated by confidence/safety, cardiopulmonary status, or neuromuscular issues.

Comfortable gait speed in older adults, both community dwelling and in residential settings, is highly valid and reliable.[70,71] Gait speed can be assessed with sophisticated equipment (e.g., portable computerized walkways, two- or three-dimensional motion analysis systems, triaxial accelerometry) but can just as reliably be assessed with a measured course and a stopwatch/timer phone app. A classic method of data collection is the use of a 20-m pathway, where the central 10 m is marked for timed testing allowing for acceleration (5 m) and deceleration (5 m) outside of the timed walking course, such that the measured distance represents a steady state of speed. Given that a straight 20-m walkway may not be available in all settings, a frequent variation is to use a 10-m pathway where the central 6 m are marked for timed testing with 2 m for acceleration and deceleration.[68] Four-meter or 5-m paths of steady-state walking are also viable alternatives.[5,68] A portable gait speed "tool kit" consisting of a timer and a length of rope (sold by the foot at hardware stores) measured and marked with bright tape to indicate the central timed walkway distance(s) provides an efficient and consistent ability to create a temporary test walkway. For SSGS allow ≥2 m for acceleration, and for fast gait speed allow ≥3 m. Timing begins when the individual breaks the vertical plane of the mark to begin the timed/steady-state component of the walk and ends upon breaking the plane to exit the timed component. Published protocol distances for gait speed calculation are extremely variable, and environmental constraints may dictate which distance is used, but the critical feature is that the same protocol is used to assess for changes over time, as concurrent validity between speeds calculated at different distances does not allow for direct comparison.[68,72] Distances of as little as 8 feet with a static start (i.e., acceleration within the timed test) have been used to assess gait speed, demonstrating that even in the home care environment, assessing SSGS is feasible.[73,74]

TABLE 9.2 Gait Speed Descriptors and Predictive Capabilities from Review Studies[68,69]

Cut Point	Interpretation
>1.3 m/s	Extremely fit; can cross street safely
>1.0 m/s	Healthy older population with lower risk of hospitalization or adverse health events; independent in ADLs
<1.0 m/s (vs. ≥1.0)	Increased risk for cognitive decline within 5 years; increased risk for death and hospitalization within 1 year
<0.8 m/s	Increased risk of mortality and mobility/ADL disability at 2 years; limited community ambulator
<0.7 m/s	Increased risk of death, hospitalization, institutionalization, and falls
<0.4 m/s	Functional dependence; severe walking disability
<0.2 m/s	Extremely frail; highly dependent

ADLs, activities of daily living.

Data from systematic reviews and meta-analyses provide reference values for gait speed in older adults, often separated by sex, although size is arguably a confounding variable in these findings. Gait speed is a product of step length and cadence, and there is some evidence that in adulthood, men take longer step lengths and women have higher cadence.[75] Bohannon and William Andrews published a meta-analysis based on descriptive data for >23,000 subjects across studies to establish SSGS reference values by decade and sex.[76] It is worth mentioning that the authors offered no quality assessment of included studies. Salbach et al. included 18 studies in a systematic review of timed walks of measured distances to establish reference values for healthy adults.[77] Reference values from these studies are presented in Table 9.3. An individual's SSGS may be expressed as a percentage of the reference value to portray level of deficit related to healthy older adults; this may help to express the impact of the clinical condition on walking in a way that is easily understood by patients, families, and the health care team. There is limited published data relating norms for SSGS with assistive device use,[5] but slower SSGS and slower "fast gait speeds" as compared to those without assistive devices are to be expected.[63] Systematic reviews of studies in geriatric clinical settings are also helpful for comparative clinical values. For instance, Peel et al. identified that

TABLE 9.3 Older Adult Gait Speed Reference Values from Review Studies

	Age in Years	Male	Female
Bohannon and Andrews[76] MEAN gait speed from 41 studies with varied distance (3.7–30 m) and assessment protocols (e.g., stopwatch, gait mat, camera system) Reported here with 95% confidence interval Originally reported as cm/s	60–69	1.34 m/s (1.03–1.59 m/s)	1.24 m/s (0.97–1.45 m/s)
	70–79	1.26 m/s (0.96–1.42 m/s)	1.13 m/s (0.83–1.50 m/s)
	80–99	0.97 m/s (0.60–1.22 m/s)	0.94 m/s (0.56–1.17 m/s)
Salbach et al.[56] MEDIAN gait speed from 18 studies with varied distance (3–40 m) and assessment protocols (e.g., stopwatch, GaitRite, lab system)	60–70	1.27 m/s	1.24 m/s
	70–79	1.18 m/s	1.13 m/s

mean SSGSs in clinical settings of individuals ≥70 years in acute care, subacute/rehab, and outpatient settings are 0.46 m/s, 0.53 m/s, and 0.75 m/s, respectively.[78] Kuys et al. determined that the mean SSGS for ambulatory long-term care residents was 0.48 m/s.[79] While these values for healthy community dwelling or geriatric clinical settings are useful for reference, the most important comparison is an individual's repeated performance over time to his or her initially assessed SSGS.

Table 9.4 represents SSGS norms of community-dwelling older adults by decade as presented in four different studies. The differences in values in Table 9.4 may be

TABLE 9.4 Comfortable Gait Speed Reference Values for Community-Dwelling Older Adults as Reported in Four Different Studies

Author (year) and mechanism of gait speed measurement		Subset of National Health & Nutrition Examination Survey 2001–2002[73] Stopwatch timed 6 m from static start Mean (SD) in m/s*	Lusardi et al. (2003)[63] GaitRite walkway Mean (SD) in m/s	Steffen et al. (2002)[80] Stopwatch timed central 6 m of 10-m walkway Mean (SD) in m/s	Beauchet et al. (2017)[5] GaitRite walkway (data extracted from databases of ongoing studies) Mean (SD) in m/s†
Subject population		Assistive device users excluded (n = 1331 ≥60 years)	Included subjects with and without assistive devices (n = 76)	Subjects able to walk 6 minutes without complaints or assistive device (n = 96)	"Very healthy" older adults (no cognitive decline, fall history, or polypharmacy) (n = 954)
Female	60–69	1.01 (0.23)	1.24 (0.12)	1.44 (0.25)	—
	65–74	—	—	—	1.26 (0.22)
	70–79	0.93 (0.23)	1.25 (0.18)	1.33 (0.22)	—
	75–84	—	—	—	1.10 (0.24)
	≥80	0.78 (0.22)	—	—	—
	80–89	—	0.80 (0.20)	1.15 (0.21)	—
	≥85	—	—	—	0.88 (0.19)
	90–101	—	0.71 (0.23)	—	—
Male	60–69	1.03 (0.21)	1.26 (n = 1)	1.59 (0.24)	—
	65–74	—	—	—	1.25 (0.22)
	70–79	0.96 (0.23)	1.25 (0.23)	1.38 (0.23)	—
	75–84	—	—	—	1.18 (0.25)
	≥80	0.83 (0.22)	—	—	—
	80–89	—	0.88 (0.23)	1.21 (0.18)	—
	≥85	—	—	—	0.90 (0.15)
	90–101	—	0.72 (0.14)	—	—

— Not reported.
*Originally reported in ft/sec.
†Originally reported in cm/sec.

explained by methodological differences in the studies. Steffen et al.[80] and Beauchet et al.[5] reported the fastest self-selected gait speeds and had the most stringent inclusion criteria (e.g., no assistive devices, "very healthy"). Lusardi et al.[63] included individuals with assistive devices, as they felt that this inclusion was representative of the population of study. Bohannon[73] presented times for walks that were initiated from a static standing position, including acceleration within the recorded time, accounting for why these values are slower than the others. Understanding the differences among studies provides the clinician with a choice of reference values for particular clients in specific settings.

Responsiveness is the ability of a measure to detect meaningful change (progress or decline in performance) over time. Minimally clinically important difference (MCID) values represent the amount of change required to be considered clinically relevant (i.e., important to the patient and/or clinician). Studies across a variety of older adults (community dwelling, sedentary, mobility impaired) have suggested a change in gait speed of >0.05 m/s represents a small but clinically meaningful change,[81,82] and a change >0.10 m/s represents a substantially meaningful change in gait performance (i.e., MCID).[81,83]

Gait speed is considered the most critical of the gait parameters, but there are ways in which other parameters of interest can be assessed in the clinic. The GaitRite walkway is a valid and reliable quantitative gait analysis system that uses imbedded sensors in a portable mat that are triggered when mechanical pressures (footfalls) are applied. The software program provides a diagrammatic representation and extensive profile of the subject's temporal and spatial gait parameters. This type of equipment is not often found in a typical clinic because of its expense. An inexpensive alternative for measuring step length, stride length, step width, and cadence is to have the individual perform a timed walk down a measured paper walkway (brown roll paper works well) with water footprints, measure the relevant distances between footfalls (therapist can outline wet footprints with a marker to be measured later), and calculate mean values for the walk.

Other outcome measures commonly combined with gait speed are the timed up and go (TUG, time required for individuals to stand from a standard-height arm chair, walk forward 3 m to a target mark, and walk back to the chair and sit) and the 6-minute walk test (6MWT, distance traversed over 6-minute period), which was initially introduced as a measure of endurance in patients with cardiac and pulmonary problems but has come to be considered a broader measure of mobility and function. Tests that add more environmental and task challenges to walking include the dynamic gait index (DGI) and functional gait assessment (FGA), and of course, combining balance assessment tools, like the modified Clinical Test of Sensory Interaction on Balance (CTSIB), Berg Balance Scale, or Mini-BESTest, can augment the clinician's understanding of a patient's challenges. These assessment tools are described more fully in Chapter 7. Choosing from the available tools may seem overwhelming, but careful history taking and keen observational gait analysis of the patient on walking into the clinic can help the physical therapist to focus the gait examination and make appropriate decisions about which tool(s) to use. An SSGS measure is always a good starting point, and fast gait speed is an easy measure to add. The TUG gives the physical therapist an opportunity to assess more functional components of mobility: transitioning sit–stand and turning, which may be very important if the history or the observation of the individual reveals that these components of mobility are challenging. When a person presents with a history that implicates diminished endurance for walking activities (e.g., "I feel less steady after I have been walking for a while"), then the 6MWT is an excellent tool for both an objective measure of distance covered and perhaps a more subjective observation of changes in gait quality from start to finish. For individuals with a high level of function but complaints of gait difficulty within challenging environments, the DGI and FGA may be useful tools, as they provide higher-level challenges to the individual. With so many tests and measures to choose from, the physical therapist needs to consciously decide what data would be most useful for a given individual and focus the gait examination accordingly.

PLAN OF CARE AND INTERVENTIONS

Through thoughtful evaluation of examination findings, the physical therapist considers the older adult's participation restrictions, activity limitations, and impairments. Most relevant to older adults are life's roles that they cannot fully realize (participation restrictions), so the clinician must team with patients to determine and prioritize the plan of care for highest impact. Interventions might include addressing impairments as well as activity limitations, but the ultimate goal is to enhance participation. Clinicians who do not have extensive experience in geriatrics may have a tendency to underchallenge older adults during treatment sessions, limiting activities by a preset determination of repetitions of exercises or tasks, or offering frequent (but unnecessary) rest breaks. This is a disservice that will undermine the effectiveness of the intervention. Therapists should rely on their expertise to provide a sufficient level of challenge and intensity while observing the older adult for decompensation of movement strategies or physiological indications of need for rest breaks.

Treatment at the Impairment Level

Intuitively, it makes sense that specific impairments would have a significant effect on gait performance. Yet there is a dearth of evidence to draw the direct relationships between impairments at the body systems level and activity limitations at the functional level. Nevertheless, training to address impairments identified upon initial examination is an appropriate component of the plan of care.

Flexibility Training. Normal gait requires a considerable arc of motion at each of the lower extremity joints. According to Perry and Burnfield's[1] model:

- The hip moves from 30 degrees of flexion early in stance to 10 degrees of extension late in stance.
- The knee is nearly fully extended at initial contact and again in midstance and reaches its peak of 60 degrees of flexion by the end of initial swing.
- The ankle displays its maximal amount of dorsiflexion (10 degrees) when the tibia rolls over the foot at the end of midstance and its maximal amount of plantar flexion (20 degrees) during the transition from preswing to initial swing.

It is prudent to strive toward increasing ROM in older adults who have flexibility limitations. As previously mentioned, decreased excursion of movement of the lower extremity joints during gait may be the cause or the result of diminished ROM. Flexibility training may have the potential to improve gait parameters, but improvements in flexibility alone will not translate into functional gains. Flexibility gains must be consciously integrated into gait and other functional tasks for gains to be appreciable and maintained. Flexibility training is one component of a comprehensive program, and it is often an element that the patient can independently work on as part of a home exercise program.

Strength, Power, and Agility Training. Lower extremity muscle weakness has been associated with decreased speed of gait and decreased performance on functional measures, and there is substantial evidence to suggest that improved lower extremity strength and power correlate with improved gait speed, TUG time, and function in older individuals ranging from frail to healthy.[84–88] Strength training has an undisputed place as a component of a gait intervention program. There is some evidence that lower extremity progressive resistance training will not only strengthen but also improve muscle power,[89] but purposefully integrating power training provides a value-add. Loss of muscle power in aging may be more functionally relevant than loss of strength and has been associated with decreased mobility and increased falls.[90] Exercises that emphasize rapid bursts of muscle activity are likely the best way to train reactive balance control mechanisms, which require fast force production. Additionally, the previously mentioned predictable shift in muscle demands in older adult gait from distal to proximal suggests that ankle strength and power training may be a high-impact intervention for gait.

Speed and agility training are not well defined or well studied in the older adult, although many comprehensive balance training protocols have representative components of agility training. To date, systematic reviews tend to categorize agility training with other interventions as "coordination" or "rhythmic" training exercises and suggest discernable benefit to gait outcomes.[86,87] A framework by Donath et al. suggests that components of agility training for older adults should include explosive and reactive strength training, static and dynamic balance activities, acceleration and deceleration practice, and directional changes including cuts and rotations.[91] These components are all instrumental in managing the challenges of community mobility. In the context of exercise sessions, brisk walking, lower extremity target identification, timed drills involving varied directional movements, and dance or video game interventions with stepping and weight-shifting components or that challenge reaction time while upright are all examples of activities that might enhance agility. Like power training, agility training is underutilized in rehabilitation of the older adult.

Cardiovascular Training. Certainly, cardiovascular training in the form of walking or another aerobic exercise program will enhance endurance for walking activities. Aerobic training in isolation does not appear to impact SSGS in older adults, with the exception of sedentary overweight or obese individuals, in which case both aerobic and resistance training have been shown to improve SSGS.[92] As part of a comprehensive exercise program, aerobic training represents a component of successful interventions to improve gait speed in older adults.[86,93–95] Striving for general health and fitness in the older adult is a consistent emphasis of the physical therapist, and a walking program is an excellent mode of delivery for cardiovascular exercise, providing it is of appropriate intensity.

Multimodal Training. Multimodal interventions, combinations of the aforementioned types of training with balance training, have demonstrated beneficial impact on gait speed in community-dwelling and mobility-impaired older adults.[86,87,95] The omission of the description of balance training in this section is purposeful, as Chapter 10 provides detail related to balance interventions. This should not be interpreted as an effort to minimize the importance of balance interventions in a well-rounded program to address gait in older adults. In fact, balance and strength training represent the top priorities in a multimodal program for older adults with reduced physical capacity.[95]

Specific Interventions for Gait Training

Gait Training Versus Assisted Ambulation. All individuals needing assistance with ambulation may not be appropriate for physical therapy. Sometimes physical therapists are consulted for individuals who may not benefit from skilled services for various reasons. If an individual requires the assistance of another for ambulation activities, this does not necessarily equate to the need for gait training. Educating physicians and other health care professionals about the roles and responsibilities of a physical therapist can be beneficial. If an older adult's long-standing ambulation status has required assistance of another for safety, or he or she has no personal goals to increase or improve ambulation abilities, "assisted ambulation" is appropriate and can be carried out by any caregiver after appropriate training. "Gait training" is a skilled intervention using the education, experience, and expertise of a physical therapist. It implies that an analysis of gait and an evaluation of what specific interventions might enhance gait performance precede the training.

Specificity of Training: Community Mobility. Motor learning theory indicates that optimal learning occurs when the learner receives task-specific training, appropriate in level of challenge and intensity, with abundant practice opportunity. Learning is facilitated when learners repeatedly solve their own motor problems. If preservation or recovery of community walking function is a therapy goal, then community walking should be part of the treatment plan. Simonsick et al. made a case for having older adults "just get out the door!" in a study that demonstrated that functionally limited older women who walked as little as eight blocks per week maintained their functional abilities better than women who walked less or not at all.[50] Encouraging individuals to push the limits of their ambulation mobility, under supervision for safety if necessary, is an integral part of rehabilitation. Gradually increasing ambulation challenges while always respecting the importance of "safety first" is an effective training tool. Individuals limited to their households may venture to the mailbox with guidance. Individuals who avoid community mobility may agree to a supervised outing. The first step out the door is often the hardest.

It may be useful to monitor distance covered or time spent in outings in individuals who are working toward increasing their community mobility. Commercial-grade activity trackers (e.g., Fitbit, Jawbone) are a reasonable mechanism of monitoring activity and community mobility over time, and it can be motivating for individuals to have objective data and goals relative to walking, but these devices do have some limitations. A recent systematic review of commercial activity tracker use in older adults (seven studies, $n = 290$) revealed that devices tend to overestimate step count and, to a lesser extent, physical activity,[96] but this need not be an impediment to monitoring change over time with consistent use and placement of a single device. Some devices showed greater percentage error in data collection with slowed walking speed and/or lower activity levels, and this is an important consideration for use with this population.

Training Speed. For most older adults, working toward improvements in gait speed is a critical goal substantiated by the evidence associating slow gait speed with decreased activity and function, frailty, disability, and mortality.[15,16,18,97] Although SSGS is known to decline with age, older adults may be capable of faster gait speeds but reluctant to use them. Despite patient perception, faster gait speed in the healthy older adult does not inherently translate to less stability,[98] but does require more energy consumption. As mentioned in previous sections, improvement in gait speed has been demonstrated in a variety of review studies of older adults (healthy, frail, and mobility impaired) as a result of strengthening and multimodal exercise programs, providing the interventions are appropriately intense.[84–88,95,99] The protected therapeutic environment is a perfect place for specificity of training of fast walking. If training on a treadmill, clinicians should be advised that an older adult's SSGS on the treadmill will likely be significantly slower than his or her over-ground SSGS.[100] Spontaneous increases in speed are more the result of increasing cadence over increasing step length in healthy older adults,[98] which is relevant to training speed and can be exploited with the use of music or a metronome for superimposed timing. Incremental improvement in SSGS of as little as 0.1 m/s is predictive of a significant risk reduction in disability and mortality.[101] This alone should warrant consideration of training speed as a component of interventions to improve gait.

Progression of Tasks: Modification of Task or Environment. Frank and Patla suggested a framework for structuring rehabilitation programs for older adults for enhancing adaptive locomotion.[47] They discuss the importance of reactive control (recovery from extrinsic destabilizing forces), predictive control (minimizing intrinsically derived destabilizing forces), and anticipatory control (adjusting walking pattern to avoid obstacles). They identify vision as the most critical sensory modality to community mobility and suggest that training include tasks that challenge the visual system. Training activities might include (1) step-by-step modifications to hitting targets and avoiding obstacles of varying heights, (2) ambulating while carrying an object that obscures view of legs, (3) training under challenging lighting conditions, and (4) scanning the environment prior to and during locomotion.[47] Use of obstacle courses, directional training, and dual-task paradigms can provide deliberately selected challenges to gait training the older adult.

Obstacle Courses and Stair Training. When faced with altered terrain, obstacle negotiation, or stairs, healthy older adults adopt a slower and more conservative movement strategy than younger adults.[102–104] When there are time constraints during obstacle negotiation, older adults are more likely to come into contact with the object they are trying to avoid.[103,105] A recent systematic review shows some limited evidence for effectiveness of exercise interventions on obstacle negotiation, but the exercise programs were extremely variable, with few studies training to the obstacle negotiation task.[106] Obstacle course training is an excellent intervention aimed at improving mobility and safety, and can address altered terrain, obstacle avoidance, and possibly even steps or ramps, all within one therapeutic activity. A course may include stepping up and over a step or stool, walking on different surfaces (e.g., foam, floor mat, ropes on floor) including rugged terrain (e.g., can put small items and/or towels haphazardly under a series of yoga mats), toe walking, heel walking, walking around cones, picking up items, kicking balls, and carrying objects. Adding a time constraint during training is an important component, as strategies for clearance may be altered under stress and this could be a contributing factor to trips and falls.[105] Stair and ramp training can be part of an obstacle or walking course or can be practiced in isolation. Practicing strategies that encourage enhanced independence on stairs (e.g., working without the handrail, progressing step over step vs. step to step) might be appropriate for some individuals. Stair descent appears to be more hazardous than ascent and responsible for more falls,[107] and therefore should be the focus of discrete training.

Directional Training. Lateral stepping; turning 90, 180, or 360 degrees; and backward walking have functional implications for mobility in small spaces or for high-level mobility activities and are all appropriate components of a gait training program. Functionally, backward stepping is used in anticipatory (e.g., opening refrigerator door) and reactive contexts (e.g., in response to posterior displacement force), yet it is often overlooked as a training activity. Backward walking in older adults, as compared to middle-aged and young adults, is characterized by decreased speed, shorter stride length, increased double-limb support phase, decreased swing time, and increased variability,[108,109] and these changes are generally magnified in fallers versus nonfallers. In fact, Fritz et al. identified that older adults who walk backward slower than 4.0 m/s have a 3.2 times greater likelihood of falling than those who walked faster.[108] Lateral stepping strategies do not seem to be inherently associated with age, but older adults who use a more protracted weight-shifting strategy for lateral stepping are more susceptible to falls, and step initiation latency may be responsive to training.[110]

Dual Tasking. Given the inarguable association between gait and cognition, deliberate use of dual-tasking assessment and treatment activities is a must. A systematic review and meta-analysis by Smith et al. demonstrates the impact of superimposing a cognitive task on gait performance in healthy older adults (i.e., those whose SSGS is ≥1.0 m/s).[12] Gait speed slows significantly, primarily through cadence reduction, and gait variability increases. Complex cognitive tasks (e.g., serial seven subtraction) resulted in mean slowing of >20% SSGS, but even simple cognitive tasks (e.g., backward counting) had a significant impact, resulting in mean slowing of ≥12% SSGS. Changes in gait parameters with dual tasking may be a more sensitive predictor of falls in older adults than single-task gait assessment, but the literature in this area is not yet robust enough to direct clinicians as to the optimal assessment strategies and interpretations.[111] Beauchet et al. suggest that a "full dataset" regarding gait of older adults should include steady-state gait speed for (1) comfortable pace, (2) fast pace, (3) superimposed task of counting backward by 1 from 50, and (4) superimposed task of naming animals.[5] These baseline values provide the clinician with points of comparison for posttreatment. Dual-task interference (degradation of task performance with competing demands for attentional resources) may be the result of the attentional demand exceeding capacity, difficulty allocating attention appropriately, or both. Gait-related dual-task interference is responsive to training,[112] and Table 9.5 represents some dual-task training challenges. There is no evidence to support the transfer

TABLE 9.5 Tasks to Be Superimposed on Gait, Posture, or Mobility Activities

Superimposed Cognitive Tasks	Recite alternate letters of the alphabet Name words starting with a particular letter or in a discrete category Spell words backward Recall of word list Count backward by 1, 3, or 7 (progressively harder) from arbitrary start Calculations Visual target searches Selective attention to visual or auditory cues (e.g., visual cue [arrow, pointing] says "right" but verbal instruction says "left" and client is cued up front to prioritize one over the other)
Superimposed Motor Tasks	Carry, manipulate object with upper extremities (e.g., bounce ball, self-catch, toss ball or balloon with partner while mobile) Carry, manipulate object with lower extremities (e.g., soccer dribbling, kick ball to target or with partner) Choreographed dance or scripted/instructed movements to music
Classic Cognitive Tests Modified for Motor Performance	Trail Making Test: Floor targets with letters and numbers placed around the room and the client moves from target to target in order (1–A–2–B–3–C...) Stroop Test: Floor targets with names of colors printed in color other than the named color (e.g., "green" is printed in "pink" ink) and the client states the color of ink (vs. word) as he or she moves from target to target, or is directed to targets by ink color (vs. word)
Task Prioritization	No overt instruction leaves the client to prioritize performance Prioritize motor task ("The most important thing is to keep up your walking speed") Prioritize cognitive task ("The most important thing is that you don't make any math errors")

of dual-task training to novel dual-task conditions; thus, training should be progressed and purposefully planned to meet dual-task demands anticipated for individual clients.

SUMMARY

An understanding of the normal gait cycle allows the therapist to easily identify deviations from typical gait in older adults and make an informed hypothesis as to why an individual may present with a particular gait deviation. Older adults walk slower and with greater variability of gait parameters than young adults. Psychological and physiological factors may contribute to mobility disability in older adults and limit their community ambulation (a term that is not clearly defined). Physical therapists should train their patients to ambulate the distances required for patient-specific functional community ambulation. Mobility in the community requires great flexibility in gait skills to meet the varied distance, speed, and terrain demands as well as allow for management of ambient conditions and multitasking as the environment demands. An examination of an older adult with gait dysfunction may include the assessment of ROM, strength, and motor control as well as the use of a variety of different gait tests and measures that complement one another in terms of information gleaned. Physical therapists will be deliberate and creative in putting together the optimal intervention techniques for a given individual's deficits. There is some evidence to support a variety of different therapeutic interventions to enhance gait and mobility in the older adult. Treatment sessions should be engaging and challenging, with specific functional goals driving the intervention. The consistent observation that functional ambulation in the community requires walking distances of well over 300 m has been specifically emphasized so that training of such distances is warranted if community ambulation is a goal. Repeated use of consistent outcome measures, especially gait speed, over the course of treatment and comparison to established norms will aid the physical therapist in goal setting and reevaluation of client performance. The ability to ambulate is key to an individual's sense of independence, self-reliance, general health and fitness, and overall function. Physical therapists play an important part in restoring or enhancing this ability in many older adult clients, thereby significantly influencing quality of life.

REFERENCES

1. Perry J, Burnfield J. *Gait Analysis: Normal and Pathological Function.* 2nd ed. Thorofare, NJ: Slack Incorporated; 2010.
2. Rose J, Gamble JG. *Human Walking.* 3rd ed. Philadelphia, PA: Lippincott Williams & Wilkins; 2006.
3. Herssens N, Verbecque E, Hallemans A, Vereeck L, Van Rompaey V, Saeys W. Do spatiotemporal parameters and gait variability differ across the lifespan of healthy adults? A systematic review. *Gait Posture* 2018;64:181–190.
4. Boyer KA, Johnson RT, Banks JJ, Jewell C, Hafer JF. Systematic review and meta-analysis of gait mechanics in young and older adults. *Exp Gerontol* 2017;95:63–70.
5. Beauchet O, Allali G, Sekhon H, et al. Guidelines for assessment of gait and reference values for spatiotemporal gait parameters in older adults: the Biomathics and Canadian Gait Consortiums Initiative. *Front Hum Neurosci* 2017;11:article 353.
6. Boyer KA, Andriacchi TP, Beaupre GS. The role of physical activity in changes in walking mechanics with age. *Gait Posture* 2012;36(1):149–153.
7. Hollman JH, McDade EM, Petersen RC. Normative spatiotemporal gait parameters in older adults. *Gait Posture* 2011;34(1):111–118.
8. Verlinden VJA, van der Geest JN, Hoogendam YY, Hofman A, Breteler MMB, Ikram MA. Gait patterns in a community-dwelling population aged 50 years and older. *Gait Posture* 2013;37(4):500–505.
9. Aboutorabi A, Arazpour M, Bahramizadeh M, Hutchins SW, Fadayevatan R. The effect of aging on gait parameters in able-bodied older subjects: a literature review. *Aging Clin Exp Res* 2016;28(3):393–405.
10. Schmitz A, Silder A, Heiderscheit B, Mahoney J, Thelen DG. Differences in lower-extremity muscular activation during walking between healthy older and young adults. *J Electromyogr Kinesiol* 2009;19(6):1085–1091.
11. Mortaza N, Abu Osman NA, Mehdikhani N. Are the spatio-temporal parameters of gait capable of distinguishing a faller from a non-faller elderly? *Eur J Phys Rehabil Med* 2014;50(6):677–691.
12. Smith E, Cusack T, Cunningham C, Blake C. The influence of a cognitive dual task on the gait parameters of healthy older adults: a systematic review and meta-analysis. *J Aging Phys Act* 2017;25(4):671–686.
13. Verghese J, LeValley A, Hall CB, Katz MJ, Ambrose AF, Lipton RB. Epidemiology of gait disorders in community-residing older adults. *J Am Geriatr Soc* 2006;54(2):255–261.
14. Schwenk M, Howe C, Saleh A, et al. Frailty and technology: a systematic review of gait analysis in those with frailty. *Gerontology* 2014;60(1):79–89.
15. Apóstolo J, Cooke R, Bobrowicz-Campos E, et al. Predicting risk and outcomes for frail older adults: an umbrella review of frailty screening tools. *JBI Database Syst Rev Implement Rep* 2017;15(4):1154–1208.
16. Perera S, Patel KV, Rosano C, et al. Gait speed predicts incident disability: a pooled analysis. *J Gerontol A Biol Sci Med Sci* 2016;71(1):63–71.
17. Kikkert LHJ, Vuillerme N, van Campen JP, Hortobágyi T, Lamoth CJ. Walking ability to predict future cognitive decline in old adults: a scoping review. *Ageing Res Rev* 2016;27:1–14.
18. Studenski S, Perera S, Patel K, et al. Gait speed and survival in older adults. *JAMA J Am Med Assoc* 2011;305(1):50–58.
19. Kressig RW, Gregor RJ, Oliver A, et al. Temporal and spatial features of gait in older adults transitioning to frailty. *Gait Posture* 2004;20(1):30–35.
20. Gill TM, Allore HG, Hardy SE, Guo Z. The dynamic nature of mobility disability in older persons. *J Am Geriatr Soc* 2006;54(2):248–254.
21. Moon Y, Sung J, An R, Hernandez ME, Sosnoff JJ. Gait variability in people with neurological disorders: a systematic review and meta-analysis. *Hum Mov Sci* 2016;47:197–208.
22. Balaban B, Tok F. Gait disturbances in patients with stroke. *PM R* 2014;6(7):635–642.

23. Debû B, De Oliveira Godeiro C, Lino JC, Moro E. Managing gait, balance, and posture in Parkinson's disease. *Curr Neurol Neurosci Rep* 2018;18(5):23.
24. Beauchet O, Annweiler C, Callisaya ML, et al. Poor gait performance and prediction of dementia: results from a meta-analysis. *J Am Med Dir Assoc* 2016;17(6):482–490.
25. Valkanova V, Ebmeier KP. What can gait tell us about dementia? Review of epidemiological and neuropsychological evidence. *Gait Posture* 2017;53(Suppl C):215–223.
26. Parihar R, Mahoney JR, Verghese J. Relationship of gait and cognition in the elderly. *Curr Transl Geriatr Exp Gerontol Rep* 2013;2(3):1–11.
27. Cohen JA, Verghese J, Zwerling JL. Cognition and gait in older people. *Maturitas* 2016;93:73–77.
28. Montero-Odasso M, Speechley M, Muir-Hunter SW, et al. Motor and cognitive trajectories before dementia: results from gait and brain study. *J Am Geriatr Soc* 2018;66(9):1676–1683.
29. Verghese J, Wang C, Lipton RB, Holtzer R. Motoric cognitive risk syndrome and the risk of dementia. *J Gerontol A Biol Sci Med Sci* 2013;68(4):412–418.
30. Chhetri JK, Chan P, Vellas B, Cesari M. Motoric cognitive risk syndrome: predictor of dementia and age-related negative outcomes. *Front Med* 2017;4:article 166.
31. Booth V, Hood V, Kearney F. Interventions incorporating physical and cognitive elements to reduce falls risk in cognitively impaired older adults: a systematic review. *JBI Database Syst Rev Implement Rep* 2016;14(5):110–135.
32. Lipardo DS, Aseron AMC, Kwan MM, Tsang WW. Effect of exercise and cognitive training on falls and fall-related factors in older adults with mild cognitive impairment: a systematic review. *Arch Phys Med Rehabil* 2017;98(10):2079–2096.
33. Martinez DJ, Kasl SV, Gill TM, Barry LC. Longitudinal association between self-rated health and timed gait among older persons. *J Gerontol B Psychol Sci Soc Sci* 2010;65 (6):715–719.
34. Brenowitz WD, Hubbard RA, Crane PK, Gray SL, Zaslavsky O, Larson EB. Longitudinal associations between self-rated health and performance-based physical function in a population-based cohort of older adults. *PloS One* 2014;9 (11). e111761.
35. Brandler TC, Wang C, Oh-Park M, Holtzer R, Verghese J. Depressive symptoms and gait dysfunction in the elderly. *Am J Geriatr Psychiatry Off J Am Assoc Geriatr Psychiatry* 2012;20(5):425–432.
36. Delbaere K, Crombez G, van Haastregt JCM, Vlaeyen JWS. Falls and catastrophic thoughts about falls predict mobility restriction in community-dwelling older people: a structural equation modelling approach. *Aging Ment Health* 2009;13 (4):587–592.
37. Lord SE, Weatherall M, Rochester L. Community ambulation in older adults: which internal characteristics are important? *Arch Phys Med Rehabil* 2010;91(3):378–383.
38. Delbaere K, Sturnieks DL, Crombez G, Lord SR. Concern about falls elicits changes in gait parameters in conditions of postural threat in older people. *J Gerontol A Biol Sci Med Sci* 2009;64A(2):237–242.
39. Kumar A, Delbaere K, Zijlstra GA, et al. Exercise for reducing fear of falling in older people living in the community: Cochrane systematic review and meta-analysis. *Age Ageing* 2016;45(3):345–352.
40. Talkowski JB, Brach JS, Studenski S, Newman AB. Impact of health perception, balance perception, fall history, balance performance, and gait speed on walking activity in older adults. *Phys Ther* 2008;88(12):1474–1481.
41. Hausdorff JM, Levy BR, Wei JY. The power of ageism on physical function of older persons: reversibility of age-related gait changes. *J Am Geriatr Soc* 1999;47(11):1346–1349.
42. Won J, Lee C, Forjuoh SN, Ory MG. Neighborhood safety factors associated with older adults' health-related outcomes: a systematic literature review. *Soc Sci Med* 2016;165:177–186.
43. Moran M, Van Cauwenberg J, Hercky-Linnewiel R, Cerin E, Deforche B, Plaut P. Understanding the relationships between the physical environment and physical activity in older adults: a systematic review of qualitative studies. *Int J Behav Nutr Phys Act* 2014;11:79.
44. Gretebeck KA, Radius K, Black DR, Gretebeck RJ, Ziemba R, Glickman LT. Dog ownership, functional ability, and walking in community-dwelling older adults. *J Phys Act Health* 2013;10(5):646–655.
45. APTA. Vision Statement for the Physical Therapy Profession and Guiding Principles to Achieve the Vision. http://www.apta.org/Vision/. Published 2013.
46. Shumway-Cook A, Patla AE, Stewart A, Ferrucci L, Ciol MA, Guralnik JM. Environmental demands associated with community mobility in older adults with and without mobility disabilities. *Phys Ther* 2002;82(7):670–681.
47. Frank JS, Patla AE. Balance and mobility challenges in older adults: implications for preserving community mobility. *Am J Prev Med* 2003;25(3 Suppl 2):157–163.
48. Corrigan R, McBurney H. Community ambulation: influences on therapists and clients reasoning and decision making. *Disabil Rehabil* 2008;30(15):1079–1087.
49. Corrigan R, McBurney H. Community ambulation: environmental impacts and assessment inadequacies. *Disabil Rehabil* 2008;30(19):1411–1419.
50. Simonsick EM, Guralnik JM, Volpato S, Balfour J, Fried LP. Just get out the door! Importance of walking outside the home for maintaining mobility: findings from the women's health and aging study. *J Am Geriatr Soc* 2005;53 (2):198–203.
51. Lord SE, McPherson K, McNaughton HK, Rochester L, Weatherall M. Community ambulation after stroke: how important and obtainable is it and what measures appear predictive? *Arch Phys Med Rehabil* 2004;85(2):234–239.
52. Shumway-Cook A, Patla A, Stewart A, Ferrucci L, Ciol MA, Guralnik JM. Environmental components of mobility disability in community-living older persons. *J Am Geriatr Soc* 2003;51(3):393–398.
53. Patla AE, Shumway-Cook A. Dimensions of mobility: defining the complexity and difficulty associated with community mobility. *J Aging Phys Act* 1999;7:7–19.
54. Goins RT, Jones J, Schure M, et al. Older adults' perceptions of mobility: a metasynthesis of qualitative studies. *Gerontologist* 2015;55(6):929–942.
55. Guide for the Uniform Data Set for Medical Rehabilitation. In: *The Functional Independence Measure (FIM);* Published 1996. https://www.udsmr.org/WebModules/FIM/Fim_About.aspx.
56. Salbach NM, O'Brien K, Brooks D, et al. Speed and distance requirements for community ambulation: a systematic review. *Arch Phys Med Rehabil* 2014;95(1):117–128.e11.
57. Andrews AW, Chinworth SA, Bourassa M, Garvin M, Benton D, Tanner S. Update on distance and velocity requirements for community ambulation. *J Geriatr Phys Ther* 2010;33(3):128–134.
58. Bertrand K, Raymond M-H, Miller WC, Martin Ginis KA, Demers L. Walking aids for enabling activity and participation: a systematic review. *Am J Phys Med Rehabil* 2017;96(12):894–903.
59. Gell NM, Wallace RB, LaCroix AZ, Mroz TM, Patel KV. Mobility device use in older adults and incidence of falls and worry about falling: findings from the 2011-2012 national health and aging trends study. *J Am Geriatr Soc* 2015;63 (5):853–859.

60. Spillman BC. *Assistive Device Use Among the Elderly: Trends, Characteristics of Users, and Implications for Modeling*. The Urban Institute. Prepared for the Office of Disability, Aging and Long-Term Care Policy Office of the Assistant Secretary for Planning and Evaluation, U.S. Department of Health and Human Services. Contract #HHS-100-97-0010. https://aspe.hhs.gov/system/files/pdf/73181/astdev.pdf. 2005.
61. West BA, Bhat G, Stevens J, Bergen G. Assistive device use and mobility-related factors among adults aged ≥65years. *J Safety Res* 2015;55:147–150.
62. Bateni H, Maki BE. Assistive devices for balance and mobility: benefits, demands, and adverse consequences. *Arch Phys Med Rehabil* 2005;86(1):134–145.
63. Lusardi MM, Pellecchia GL, Schulman M. Functional performance in community living older adults. *J Geriatr Phys Ther* 2003;26(3):14–22.
64. Gardner P. MAPx (Mobility Aid Personalization): examining why older adults "pimp their ride" and the impact of doing so. *Disabil Rehabil Assist Technol* 2017;12(5):512–518.
65. Verghese J, Wang C, Xue X, Holtzer R. Self-reported difficulty in climbing up or down stairs in nondisabled elderly. *Arch Phys Med Rehabil* 2008;89(1):100–104.
66. Tiedemann AC, Sherrington C, Lord SR. Physical and psychological factors associated with stair negotiation performance in older people. *J Gerontol A Biol Sci Med Sci* 2007;62(11):1259–1265.
67. Hinman MR, O'Connell JK, Dorr M, Hardin R, Tumlinson AB, Varner B. Functional predictors of stair-climbing speed in older adults. *J Geriatr Phys Ther* 2014;37(1):1–6.
68. Middleton A, Fritz SL, Lusardi M. Walking speed: the functional vital sign. *J Aging Phys Act* 2015;23(2):314–322.
69. Abellan van Kan G, Rolland Y, Andrieu S, et al. Gait speed at usual pace as a predictor of adverse outcomes in community-dwelling older people an International Academy on Nutrition and Aging (IANA) Task Force. *J Nutr Health Aging* 2009;13 (10):881–889.
70. Rydwik E, Bergland A, Forsén L, Frändin K. Investigation into the reliability and validity of the measurement of elderly people's clinical walking speed: a systematic review. *Physiother Theory Pract* 2012;28(3):238–256.
71. Mijnarends DM, Meijers JMM, Halfens RJG, et al. Validity and reliability of tools to measure muscle mass, strength, and physical performance in community-dwelling older people: a systematic review. *J Am Med Dir Assoc* 2013;14(3):170–178.
72. Peters DM, Fritz SL, Krotish DE. Assessing the reliability and validity of a shorter walk test compared with the 10-Meter Walk Test for measurements of gait speed in healthy, older adults. *J Geriatr Phys Ther* 2013;36(1):24–30.
73. Bohannon RW. Population representative gait speed and its determinants. *J Geriatr Phys Ther* 2008;31(2):49–52.
74. Bohannon RW. Measurement of gait speed of older adults is feasible and informative in a home-care setting. *J Geriatr Phys Ther* 2009;32(1):22–23.
75. Frimenko R, Goodyear C, Bruening D. Interactions of sex and aging on spatiotemporal metrics in non-pathological gait: a descriptive meta-analysis. *Physiotherapy* 2015;101(3):266–272.
76. Bohannon RW, Williams Andrews A. Normal walking speed: a descriptive meta-analysis. *Physiotherapy* 2011;97 (3):182–189.
77. Salbach NM, O'Brien KK, Brooks D, et al. Reference values for standardized tests of walking speed and distance: a systematic review. *Gait Posture* 2015;41(2):341–360.
78. Peel NM, Kuys SS, Klein K. Gait speed as a measure in geriatric assessment in clinical settings: a systematic review. *J Gerontol A Biol Sci Med Sci* 2013;68(1):39–46.
79. Kuys SS, Peel NM, Klein K, Slater A, Hubbard RE. Gait speed in ambulant older people in long term care: a systematic review and meta-analysis. *J Am Med Dir Assoc* 2014;15(3):194–200.
80. Steffen TM, Hacker TA, Mollinger L. Age- and gender-related test performance in community-dwelling elderly people: Six-Minute Walk Test, Berg Balance Scale, Timed Up & Go Test, and gait speeds. *Phys Ther* 2002;82(2):128–137.
81. Perera S, Mody SH, Woodman RC, Studenski SA. Meaningful change and responsiveness in common physical performance measures in older adults. *J Am Geriatr Soc* 2006;54(5):743–749.
82. Perera S, Studenski S, Newman A, et al. Are estimates of meaningful decline in mobility performance consistent among clinically important subgroups? (Health ABC study). *J Gerontol A Biol Sci Med Sci* 2014;69(10):1260–1268.
83. Bohannon RW, Glenney SS. Minimal clinically important difference for change in comfortable gait speed of adults with pathology: a systematic review. *J Eval Clin Pract* 2014;20(4):295–300.
84. Beijersbergen CMI, Granacher U, Vandervoort AA, DeVita P, Hortobágyi T. The biomechanical mechanism of how strength and power training improves walking speed in old adults remains unknown. *Ageing Res Rev* 2013;12(2):618–627.
85. Papa EV, Dong X, Hassan M. Resistance training for activity limitations in older adults with skeletal muscle function deficits: a systematic review. *Clin Interv Aging* 2017;12:955–961.
86. Hortobágyi T, Lesinski M, Gäbler M, VanSwearingen JM, Malatesta D, Granacher U. Effects of three types of exercise interventions on healthy old adults' gait speed: a systematic review and meta-analysis. *Sports Med Auckl NZ* 2015;45 (12):1627–1643.
87. Van Abbema R, De Greef M, Crajé C, Krijnen W, Hobbelen H, Van Der Schans C. What type, or combination of exercise can improve preferred gait speed in older adults? A meta-analysis. *BMC Geriatr* 2015;15:72.
88. Jadczak AD, Makwana N, Luscombe-Marsh N, Visvanathan R, Schultz TJ. Effectiveness of exercise interventions on physical function in community-dwelling frail older people: an umbrella review of systematic reviews. *JBI Database Syst Rev Implement Rep* 2018;16(3):752–775.
89. Straight CR, Lindheimer JB, Brady AO, Dishman RK, Evans EM. Effects of resistance training on lower-extremity muscle power in middle-aged and older adults: a systematic review and meta-analysis of randomized controlled trials. *Sports Med Auckl NZ* 2016;46(3):353–364.
90. McKinnon NB, Connelly DM, Rice CL, Hunter SW, Doherty TJ. Neuromuscular contributions to the age-related reduction in muscle power: mechanisms and potential role of high velocity power training. *Ageing Res Rev* 2017;35:147–154.
91. Donath L, van Dieën J, Faude O. Exercise-based fall prevention in the elderly: what about agility. *Sports Med Auckl NZ* 2016;46(2):143–149.
92. Henderson RM, Leng XI, Chmelo EA, et al. Gait speed response to aerobic versus resistance exercise training in older adults. *Aging Clin Exp Res* 2017;29(5):969–976.
93. Timmons JF, Minnock D, Hone M, Cogan KE, Murphy JC, Egan B. Comparison of time-matched aerobic, resistance or concurrent exercise training in older adults. *Scand J Med Sci Sports* 2018;28(11):2272–2283. https://doi.org/10.1111/sms.13254.
94. Chase J-AD, Phillips LJ, Brown M. Physical activity intervention effects on physical function among community-dwelling older adults: a systematic review and meta-analysis. *J Aging Phys Act* 2017;25(1):149–170.
95. Liu C-J, Chang W-P, Araujo de Carvalho I, Savage KEL, Radford LW, Amuthavalli Thiyagarajan J. Effects of physical exercise in older adults with reduced physical capacity: meta-analysis of resistance exercise and multimodal exercise. *Int J Rehabil Res Int* 2017;40 (4):303–314.

96. Straiton N, Alharbi M, Bauman A, et al. The validity and reliability of consumer-grade activity trackers in older, community-dwelling adults: a systematic review. *Maturitas* 2018;112:85–93.
97. Middleton A, Fulk GD, Beets MW, Herter TM, Fritz SL. Self-selected walking speed is predictive of daily ambulatory activity in older adults. *J Aging Phys Act* 2016;24(2):214–222.
98. Fan Y, Li Z, Han S, Lv C, Zhang B. The influence of gait speed on the stability of walking among the elderly. *Gait Posture* 2016;47:31–36.
99. Lopopolo RB, Greco M, Sullivan D, Craik RL, Mangione KK. Effect of therapeutic exercise on gait speed in community-dwelling elderly people: a meta-analysis. *Phys Ther* 2006;86 (4):520–540.
100. Malatesta D, Canepa M, Menendez Fernandez A. The effect of treadmill and overground walking on preferred walking speed and gait kinematics in healthy, physically active older adults. *Eur J Appl Physiol* 2017;117(9):1833–1843.
101. Hardy SE, Perera S, Roumani YF, Chandler JM, Studenski SA. Improvement in usual gait speed predicts better survival in older adults. *J Am Geriatr Soc* 2007;55(11):1727–1734.
102. Marigold DS, Patla AE. Age-related changes in gait for multi-surface terrain. *Gait Posture* 2008;27(4):689–696.
103. Galna B, Peters A, Murphy AT, Morris ME. Obstacle crossing deficits in older adults: a systematic review. *Gait Posture* 2009;30(3):270–275.
104. Benedetti MG, Berti L, Maselli S, Mariani G, Giannini S. How do the elderly negotiate a step? A biomechanical assessment. *Clin Biomech* 2007;22(5):567–573.
105. Maidan I, Eyal S, Kurz I, et al. Age-associated changes in obstacle negotiation strategies: does size and timing matter? *Gait Posture* 2018;59:242–247.
106. Guadagnin EC, da Rocha ES, Duysens J, Carpes FP. Does physical exercise improve obstacle negotiation in the elderly? A systematic review. *Arch Gerontol Geriatr* 2016;64:138–145.
107. Startzell JK, Owens DA, Mulfinger LM, Cavanagh PR. Stair negotiation in older people: a review. *J Am Geriatr Soc* 2000;48(5):567–580.
108. Fritz NE, Worstell AM, Kloos AD, Siles AB, White SE, Kegelmeyer DA. Backward walking measures are sensitive to age-related changes in mobility and balance. *Gait Posture* 2013;37(4):593–597.
109. Laufer Y. Effect of age on characteristics of forward and backward gait at preferred and accelerated walking speed. *J Gerontol A Biol Sci Med Sci* 2005;60(5):627–632.
110. Sparto PJ, Jennings JR, Furman JM, Redfern MS. Lateral step initiation behavior in older adults. *Gait Posture* 2014;39 (2):799–803.
111. Muir-Hunter SW, Wittwer JE. Dual-task testing to predict falls in community-dwelling older adults: a systematic review. *Physiotherapy* 2016;102(1):29–40.
112. Plummer P, Zukowski LA, Giuliani C, Hall AM, Zurakowski D. Effects of physical exercise interventions on gait-related dual-task interference in older adults: a systematic review and meta-analysis. *Gerontology* 2015;62(1):94–117.
113. Strawbridge WJ, Kaplan GA, Camacho T, Cohen RD. The dynamics of disability and functional change in an elderly cohort: results from the Alameda County Study. *J Am Geriatr Soc* 1992;40(8):799–806.
114. Lerner-Frankiel M, Vargas S, Brown M, Krusell L, Schoneberger W. Functional community ambulation: what are your criteria? *Clin Manag Phys Ther* 1986;6(2):12–15.

CHAPTER 10

Balance and Falls in Older Adults

Alia A. Alghwiri, Susan L. Whitney

OUTLINE

INTRODUCTION

Falls are common throughout the life span. Young children fall frequently but rarely suffer more than minor bumps and bruises. However, falls are the leading cause of death from injury as well as injury-related hospitalization in older adults.[1] The 2014 Behavioral Risk Factor Surveillance System (BRFSS) survey of Medicare recipients reported that nearly 29% of individuals over the age of 65 self-reported a fall during 2014, and this increased to 36.5% of individuals over the age of 84.[2] Having fallen once, particularly having fallen and been injured, is a significant risk factor for future injurious falls.[1] Of older adults who fell, 37.5% sustained an injury serious enough to require medical attention or activity self-restriction for at least 1 day.[2] According to the U.S. Centers for Disease Control and Prevention, in 2015, medical treatment for falls among people older than age 65 years cost the United States more than $50 billion in health care costs.

In addition to the medical costs, there are also enormous societal and personal costs. Falls are associated with pain, loss of confidence, functional decline, and institutionalization. Falls affect quality of life for the older adult, typically decreasing participation in instrumental activities of daily living (IADLs) and/or social activities. Falling will producc a fear of falling in 20% to 30% of people who fall, which can lead to a further decrease in activity.[3] Falls can seriously threaten the functional activities, participation, and well-being of older adults.

DEFINITION AND CLASSIFICATION OF FALLS

A fall is defined as "an unintentional loss of balance that leads to failure of postural stability" or "a sudden and unexpected change in position which usually results in landing on the floor.[4]" Recurrent fallers are those who have fallen two or more times in either 6 or 12 months.[4] A fall without injury is still a fall. A challenge in examining studies focused on falls is the wide variety of operational definitions used to categorize someone as having "fallen" or, more commonly, the lack of any operational definition of a fall. Hauer et al., in a systematic review of falls, reported that falls were not defined in 44 of 90 studies reviewed.[5] Falls can be classified as accidental versus nonaccidental, syncopal versus nonsyncopal, intrinsically versus extrinsically driven, falls with injury versus falls without injury, and a single fall incident versus recurrent falling. Schwenk et al. recommend a standardized definition of injurious falls with four severity levels from no injury to severe injury.[6]

FALL RISK FACTORS

Identifying specific risk factors for falls in older adults and using these risk factors to predict who will fall is complex. Although the underlying "causes" of a fall are typically divided into extrinsic (environmental) and intrinsic (e.g., postural control mechanisms, age, race, gender, chronic physical or psychological diseases),[7] falls often represent a complex interaction of environmental challenges (tripping, slipping) and compromises across multiple components of the postural control systems (somatosensory inputs, central processing, musculoskeletal effectors) in responding to a postural challenge.[8,9] When utilizing fast walking as a predictor of falls, both the frail older adult using short shuffling steps and the healthy older adult with more risk factors were found at high risk of falls.[10] Intrinsic factors that place one at risk of falling could stem from an accumulation of multiple age-related changes in postural control structures, particularly in those older than age 80 or 85 years, or, more commonly, a combination of health/medical conditions that compromise the postural control system superimposed on age-related changes. Deteriorating cognitive skills such as executive function, working memory, and attention result in increased gait instability and decreased gait speed, both contributing to increased risk of falls for those with cognitive impairments such as dementia.[11]

Identifying those at risk for falling and the factors placing them at risk can guide an intervention program to ameliorate or accommodate risk. To provide a more precise assessment of fall risk, most studies choose a relatively narrow category of older adult, chosen either by their current health status (community dwelling, nursing home, acutely ill, frail, or active) or because they have a specific disease or chronic condition likely to affect one or more specific components of the postural control system. Specific risk factors can vary widely across these groups. Similar themes do emerge, however. These include common age-related changes that, when combined with health-related conditions across several body systems, serve as intrinsic factors contributing to falls. Fig. 10.1 provides a summary of the many intrinsic factors that are commonly associated with falls in older adults.

The American Academy of Neurology (2008) fall guidelines[12] suggested that people with the diagnoses of stroke, dementia, walking and balance problems, or a history of recent falls, plus people who use walking aids such as a cane or a walker, are at the highest risk of falling. This group also identifies Parkinson disease, peripheral neuropathy, lower extremity weakness or sensory loss, and substantial loss of vision as probable predictors of fall risk. For patients undergoing treatment for cancer, the use of neurotoxic chemotherapy can result in chemotherapy-induced peripheral neuropathy (CIPN). Patients experiencing CIPN symptoms are three times more likely to experience a fall or near fall.[13] In those who are experiencing cognitive impairment, the reduced speed of processing and impairment in executive functions have shown to be a predictor of falls as well.[14]

Polypharmacy, and issues of drug interactions and drug adverse effects, can add substantially to impaired balance and risk of falls. A fall rate of 43% was reported for patients with heart failure, most frequently attributed to medications such as benzodiazepines and digoxin as well as loop diuretics.[15] Antidepressants, antianxiety drugs, sedatives, tranquilizers, diuretics, and sleep medications are all related to increasing the risk of falling in older adults.[14] Thus, a review of medications for potential contributions to fall risk, with referral for medical management as indicated, should be part of every fall risk screening.

Vitamin D and calcium are helpful when prescribed to the older adult in long-term care in an attempt to help prevent fractures from falls.[14] The International Osteoporosis Foundation also recommends reaching and maintaining a vitamin D level of 75 nmol/L (30 ng/mL) by supplementing 800 to 1000 IU/day, with adjustments being made for those who are obese, those with osteoporosis, and those with limited sun exposure.[16] The U.S. Preventative Service Taskforce, in a 2018 update, no longer recommends vitamin D supplementation to prevent falls unless the person has osteoporosis or is vitamin D deficient.[17] Medications used to manage some health conditions can have an unintended consequence of increasing fall risk. For example, receiving femoral peripheral nerve blocks following knee and hip arthroplasty is associated with an increased risk of falls during the early postoperative period.[18]

Environmental hazards, discussed in more detail in Chapter 5, such as a slippery walking surface, loose rug, poor lighting, and obstacles in the walking path, can increase risk of falling, particularly in individuals with already compromised balance. Overall, as the number of risk factors increases, the chance of falling increases. Decreasing the number of risk factors can decrease the person's risk of falling, although it does not always reduce anxiety and continued fear of falling.[19]

One-third of older adults who experience a fall develop a fear of falling.[20] Fear of falling may lead to a more sedentary lifestyle with subsequent deconditioning that creates an ongoing downward spiral leading to frailty and increased risk of future falls.[19,21] Caregiver fear that an older adult might fall can result in the caregiver limiting an older adult's participation in activities.[19] Fear of falling has been associated with the use of a walking device, balance impairment, depression, trait anxiety, female gender, and a previous history of a fall or falls.[22]

POSTURAL CONTROL AND AGING

Postural control is achieved by continually positioning the body's center of gravity (COG) over the base of support

INTRINSIC FALL RISK FACTORS

	AGE-RELATED CHANGES	HEALTH CONDITION RELATED*
Somatosensory	• Decreased light touch • Decreased proprioception • Decreased two-point discrimination • Decreased vibration sense • Decreased muscle spindle activity	• Diabetic/idiopathic neuropathy • Spinal stenosis • Stroke • Multiple sclerosis
Visual	• Decreased visual acuity • Decreased contrast sensitivity • Decreased depth perception	• Cataracts • Macular degeneration • Glaucoma • Diabetic retinopathy • Stroke • Use of progressive, bifocal, or trifocal corrective lenses
Vestibular	• Decreased vestibular hair cells • Decreased vestibular nerve fibers • Changes in VOR[a]	• Benign paroxysmal positional vertigo • Unilateral vestibular hypofunction • Meniere disease • Bilateral vestibular hypofunction
CNS	• Decreased coordination	• Parkinson disease • Stroke • Cerebellar atrophy
Neuromuscular	• Slowing of muscle timing/sequencing • Decreased ROM/flexibility • Decreased muscle endurance • Decreased lower extremity muscle strength, torque, and power • Delayed distal muscle latency • Increased cocontraction • Impaired postural alignment (such as kyphosis)	• Impaired postural alignment • Osteoporosis with vertebral fracture and kyphosis • Diabetes with distal motor neuropathy • Lower limb joint diseases (such as arthritis) • Spinal stenosis
Cardiovascular		• Conditions associated with syncope or lightheadedness (arrhythmia, orthostatic hypotension, etc.)
Psychosocial	• Fear of falling • Cognitive impairment	• Depression
Other		• Incontinence • Alcohol abuse

*Selected health conditions commonly associated with fall risk in older adults and responses to medications used to manage the condition
[a]Vestibular ocular reflex

FIG. 10.1 Commonly identified factors associated with increased fall risk, organized by postural control–related body systems. *ROM*, range of motion; *VOR*, vestibular ocular reflex.

(BOS) during both static and dynamic situations. Physiologically, postural control depends on the integration and coordination of three body systems: sensory, central nervous (CNS), and neuromuscular. The sensory system gathers essential information about the position and orientation of body segments in space. The CNS integrates, coordinates, and interprets the sensory inputs and then directs the execution of movements. The neuromuscular system responds to the orders provided by the CNS. All postural control components undergo changes with aging. Deficits within any single component are not typically sufficient to cause postural instability, because compensatory mechanisms from other components prevent that from happening. However, accumulation of deficits across multiple components may lead to instability and eventually falls.

Sensory System

Sensory information plays a significant role in updating the CNS about the body's position and motion in space. Sensory inputs are gathered through the somatosensory, visual, and vestibular systems. Advancing age is accompanied by diverse structural and functional changes in most of the sensory components of postural control.

Somatosensory Input. Somatosensory information, gathered from receptors located in joints, muscles, and tendons, provides the CNS with crucial information regarding body segment position and movement in space relative to each other, as well as the amount of force generated for the movement. There are age-related declines in two-point discrimination, muscle spindle activity, proprioception, and cutaneous receptors in the lower extremities, plus changes in vibration sense. Normal thresholds for vibration sensory perception decrease with age,[23] with substantial losses in those over 75 years of age.[24] Kristinsdottir et al.[25] compared postural control of younger adults (mean age of 37.5 years) and older adults (mean age of 74.6 years), some with intact and others with impaired vibration perception in their lower extremities. Vibration perception in the lower extremities was found to be the main determinant for postural control in these older individuals. Postural control in older adults with intact vibration perception was comparable to that of the younger adults, whereas older individuals with impaired vibration perception had increased high-frequency sway. Proprioceptive and cutaneous inputs have been identified as the primary sensory information used to maintain balance.[26] The frequently referenced study of Judge et al.[27] compared the contribution of proprioception and vision on balance in older adults by using the EquiTest sensory organization test (SOT), discussed later in this chapter, of the computerized dynamic posturography (CDP). Reduction in vision with reduced proprioceptive inputs increased the odds ratio of a fall during testing by 5.7-fold.[27] Therefore, somatosensory sensation including vibration, proprioception, and cutaneous inputs is important to consider in the evaluation and intervention processes in older adults who have or who are at risk for postural instability.

Visual Input. Visual input provides the CNS with upright postural control information important in maintaining the body in a vertical position with the surrounding environment. Visual acuity, contrast sensitivity, depth perception, and peripheral vision are all essential visual components that provide the CNS with the required information about objects in the surrounding environment. Visual acuity, contrast sensitivity, and depth perception diminish with advanced age[28] and have been associated with a higher number of falls in older adults. Addressing visual problems can substantially decrease this risk factor. For example, glasses with prisms can compensate for peripheral-field deficits, tinted glasses can increase contrast sensitivity, and different glasses for near and far vision can reduce problems associated with bifocals. Lord et al. suggest that multifocal lenses impair both edge-contrast sensitivity and depth perception.[29] Significant visual restrictions from cataracts may require cataract surgery to improve vision and decrease fall risk. Maximizing vision in both eyes appears to be critical. For macular degeneration in older adults, medication and careful observation by an ophthalmologist can slow its progression. Health professionals working with older adults with balance complaints should always inquire about eye health and whether the individual has had an eye examination within the last year and encourage regular eye exams to ensure undetected eye impairments are not contributing to balance deficits.

Vestibular. The vestibular system provides the CNS with information about angular acceleration of the head via the semicircular canals and linear acceleration via the otoliths. This information is considered key sensory data for postural control. The vestibular system regulates the head and neck position and movement through two outputs: the vestibular ocular reflex (VOR) and vestibular spinal reflex (VSR). The VOR is important for stabilizing visual images on the retina during head movements. The VSR allows for reflex control of the neck and lower extremity postural muscles so that the position of the head and trunk can be maintained accurately and correlated with eye movements. Information from sensory receptors in the vestibular apparatus interacts with visual and somatosensory information to produce proper body alignment and postural control.

Anatomic and physiological changes occur in the vestibular system of older adults. Anatomically, progressive loss of peripheral hair cells[30] and vestibular nerve fibers[31] has been reported in people older than 55 years of age. Physiologically, changes in the VOR and the VSR were attributed to the anatomic changes in the vestibular system. However, these changes do not cause vestibular disorders unless another insult happens to older individuals. For people with unilateral vestibular hypofunction, Norré et al.[32] found that their central adaptive mechanisms become less effective with advancing age. Thus, the VSR becomes "dysregulated" and, as a result, postural sway disturbances and imbalance take place with any balance perturbation.[32]

Central Processing

Central processing is an important physiological component of the postural control system. The CNS receives sensory inputs, interprets and integrates these inputs, then coordinates and executes the orders for the neuromuscular system to provide corrective motor output. The cortex, thalamus, basal ganglia, vestibular nucleus, and cerebellum are all involved in postural control processes.

In real-life circumstances, postural responses are elicited in both feedback and feed-forward situations. However, researchers have primarily examined the automatic postural responses in feedback paradigms. Four main conditions have been studied to examine postural control: standing without any perturbations, standing with sudden perturbation using movable platforms, postural control during execution of voluntary movement, and sudden perturbation during voluntary movement execution.

Movable platforms have been used to create perturbations in forward, backward, and rotational directions. Muscle responses then have been recorded using electromyography to determine muscle sequencing and timing. The latency and the sequence of muscle responses have been identified to define strategies of postural control in such perturbations.

Response Strategies to Postural Perturbations. Five basic strategies, depicted in Fig. 10.2, have been identified as responses to unexpected postural perturbations. The strategy elicited depends on the amount of force created and the size of the BOS during the perturbation:

- An *ankle strategy* is the activation of muscles around the ankle joint after a small disturbance of BOS when standing on a "normal" support surface. The latency is approximately 73 to 110 ms with a distal-to-proximal muscle sequence.[33] One might use an ankle strategy to maintain balance with a slight perturbation of the trunk or center of mass such as reaching for objects in front of you without taking a step. Horak and Nashner have suggested that one may be able to "train" people to execute an ankle or hip strategy based on training paradigms.[33] Ankle strength and mobility is a requisite for successful execution of an ankle strategy. Significant improvements in lower limb muscle strength and ankle force generation have been reported in adults over the age of 65 after a 10-week strength training program.[34]
- A *hip strategy* is the activation of muscles around the hip joint as a result of a sudden and forceful disturbance of BOS while standing with a narrow support surface. The latency is the same as in the ankle strategy; however, the muscle sequence follows a proximal-to-distal pattern.[33]

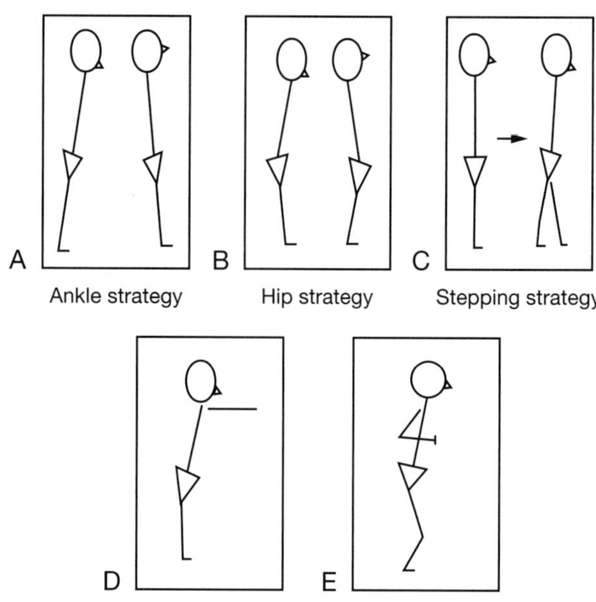

FIG. 10.2 Five basic postural strategies used in response to postural perturbations. **A,** Ankle strategy: activation of muscles around the ankle joint after a small disturbance of base of support (BOS) when standing on a "normal" support surface. **B,** Hip strategy: activation of muscles around the hip joint as a result of a sudden and forceful disturbance of BOS while standing in a narrow support surface. **C,** Stepping strategy: taking a forward or backward step rapidly to regain equilibrium when the center of gravity is displaced beyond the limits of the BOS. **D,** Reaching strategy: moving the arm to grasp or touch an object for support. **E,** Suspensory strategy: bending the knees during standing or ambulation to enhance stability.

A combination of both ankle and hip strategies was reported while standing in an intermediate support surface.[33] In both ankle and hip strategies, muscle activity is generated to keep the COG within the BOS. However, if the disturbances are more forceful, other movements must occur that change the BOS to prevent falling.

- The *stepping strategy* has been defined as taking a forward or backward step rapidly to regain equilibrium when the COG is displaced beyond the limits of the BOS. This can be observed clinically by resisting the patient enough at the hips to cause a significant loss of balance requiring one or more steps to maintain postural control.[35]
- The *reaching strategy* includes moving the arm to grasp or touch an object for support.[36] Arm movements play a significant role in maintaining stability by altering the COG or protecting against injury. Stepping and reaching strategies are the only compensatory reactions to large perturbations; thus, they have a significant role in preventing falls.[36] In unexpected disturbances of balance, older adults tend to take multiple steps to recover, with the later steps usually directed toward recovering lateral stability.[36]
- The *suspensory strategy* includes bending knees during standing or ambulation for the purpose of maintaining a stable position during a perturbation. Bending of the

knees usually lowers the COG to be closer to the BOS, thereby enhancing postural stability.

The sequencing and timing of muscle contraction appears to undergo changes with advanced age including delay in distal muscle latency and increases in the incidence of co-contraction in antagonist muscle groups.[37] Older adults with a history of falls demonstrate greater delay in muscle latency when compared to age-matched nonfallers.[38] In a study, healthy older adults showed slower reaction times to change the direction of the whole body in response to an auditory stimulus compared to healthy young individuals, and moved in more rigid patterns indicating altered postural coordination.[39] These changes make it harder for older adults to respond quickly enough to "catch" themselves when challenged with a large unexpected perturbation.

Neuromuscular System

The neuromuscular system represents the biomechanical apparatus through which the CNS executes postural actions. Muscle strength, endurance, latency, torque and power, flexibility, range of motion (ROM), and postural alignment all affect the ability of a person to respond to balance perturbations effectively. Most of those factors change with advanced age in a way that decreases the capacity of the older adult to respond effectively to balance disturbances.

Muscle strength, especially for lower extremity muscles, plays a significant role in maintaining a balanced posture. There is an average reduction of muscle strength of 30% to 40% over a lifetime. Marked reduction in muscle strength of the lower extremities has been noted among older adult fallers.[38] Muscle endurance is maintained with aging much more effectively than muscle strength.[40] Prolonged latency in lower extremity muscles, especially those around the ankle joint, was found to be related to frequent falling among older adults.[39] Studenski et al. determined that older adult fallers produce significantly less distal lower extremity torque than healthy older adults.[38] Similarly, Whipple et al. found that nursing home residents with a history of recurrent falls demonstrated diminished torque production of both the ankle and knee.[41]

Reduction of joint flexibility and ROM are the main consequences of joint diseases that affect postural stability and may contribute to falls. Stooped posture or kyphosis is one of the impaired postural alignment problems in older adults that interfere with balance and stability.

EXAMINATION AND EVALUATION OF BALANCE AND RISK OF FALLS

Fig. 10.3 provides an evidence-based, expert panel–approved conceptual framework for best-practice steps to reduce falls in vulnerable older adults. The framework is built around 12 quality indicators for fall risk reduction listed in Box 10.1. The conceptual framework is grounded

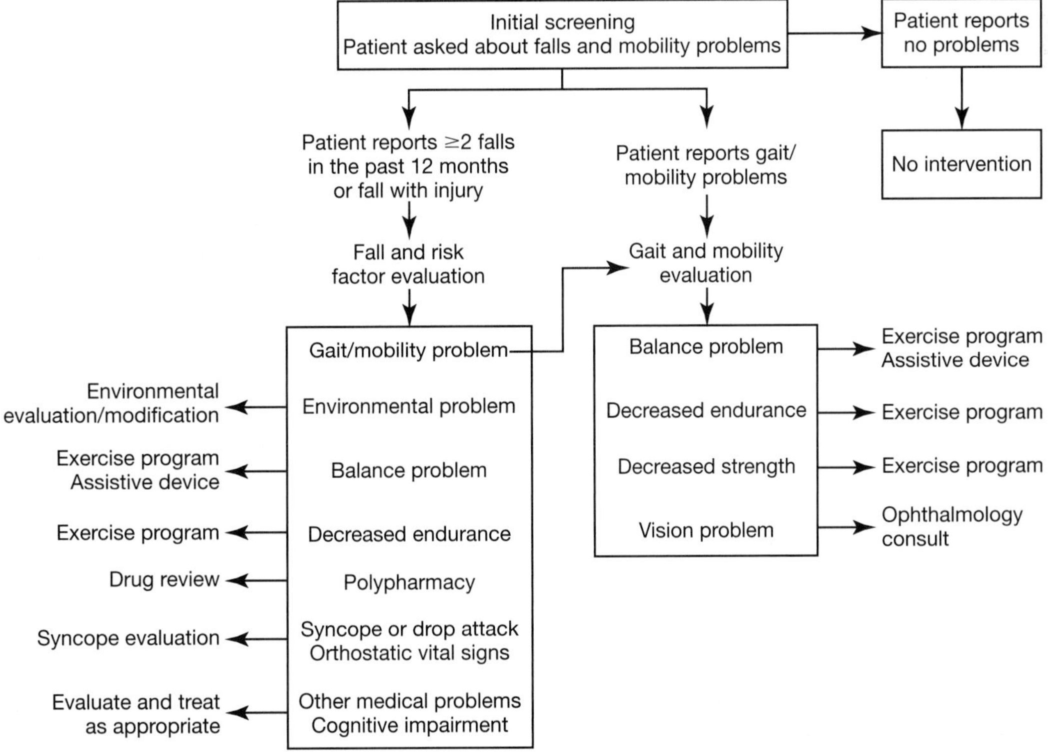

FIG. 10.3 Conceptual framework for "best practice" steps to reducing falls in vulnerable older adults. *(Reprinted, with permission, from Chang JT, Ganz DA. Quality indicators for falls and mobility problems in vulnerable elders. J Am Geriatr Soc. 2007; 55:S327–S334.)*

BOX 10.1 12 Evidence-Based Quality Indicators for Best Practice in Managing Older Adults at Risk for Falling[48]

For all vulnerable older adults regardless of history of falls there should be documentation of the following:

1. Inquiry about falls within the past 12 months
2. Basic gait, balance, and muscle strength assessment for anyone expressing new or worsening gait difficulties
3. Assessment for possible assistive device prescription IF demonstrating poor balance, impairments of proprioception, or excessive postural sway
4. Participation in a structured or supervised exercise program IF found to have a problem with gait, balance, strength, or endurance

In addition to the above, for all older adults who have fallen two times or more in the past year, or who have fallen once with an injury, there should be documentation that:

1. A basic fall history has been obtained
2. An assessment for orthostatic hypotension has been done
3. Visual acuity has been examined
4. Basic gait, balance, and muscle strength have been assessed
5. Home hazard assessment has been completed
6. Medication side effects have been assessed with special note if the person is taking a benzodiazepine
7. The appropriateness of the device has been assessed
8. Cognitive status has been assessed

(Adapted from Chang JT, Ganz DA. Quality indicators for falls and mobility problems in vulnerable elders. *J Am Geriatr Soc.* 2007;55[Suppl 2]: S327–S334.)

in the work of Rubenstein et al.[42] with a more recent update by Chang and Ganz.[43] The Centers for Disease Control and Prevention (CDC) embeds this general framework approach into the STEADI toolkit algorithm for falls risk screening, assessment, and intervention,[44] discussed later in this section.

Determining the underlying cause of balance deficits and related fall risk is a complex undertaking. Most typically, balance dysfunctions emerge gradually from the accumulation of multiple impairments and limitations across many components of postural control, some associated with normal age-related changes and others with acute and chronic health conditions. The redundancies built into the postural control system often allow one system to compensate for deficiencies in another, thus masking developing deficits. Once the deficits reach a critical point or an acute illness incident exceeds the "deficit" threshold, the patient can no longer consistently manage challenges to balance and begins to fall.

Ideally, the physical therapist would intervene at an early point in the process to remediate, compensate, or accommodate the impairment. Frequently, however, the physical therapist is only called upon after one or multiple falls have occurred, for individuals at risk of frailty. A hypothetical functional progression along the "slippery slope" of aging, including critical thresholds for functional ability, is graphically depicted in Chapter 1. This slippery slope is partially modifiable: The physically fit and healthy older adult has less downward slope in the curve; the unfit or unhealthy individual has a sharper downward slope. Interventions to improve physiological factors contributing to functional ability can move the entire curve upward (and perhaps above key critical thresholds); illness and deconditioning can move the entire curve downward. Although the trajectory can be modified at all levels of the curve, it is much easier to modify the curve upward when the person is starting from the "fun" or "functional" levels than when he or she has reached the frailty level.

Although it is important to assess all physiological and anatomic factors likely to contribute to a given patient's fall risk, the physical therapist must develop strategies to narrow down the factors considered so as not to overwhelm the patient with tests and measures. A simple movement screen is indicated to determine which body areas require additional investigation. Each test and measure should have a reasonable likelihood of revealing significant contributors underlying the balance dysfunction and to be of assistance in guiding a balance intervention program. The data gathered from a preliminary medical history and review of systems helps guide the choice of specific tests and measures deemed important to understanding the postural control and functional performance issues of the patient, as well as the impact of environmental factors and current health conditions on psychosocial status and participation.

There is no "one" best way to structure examination activities. For extremely frail individuals or individuals with marked balance deficits, the examiner may start with the least challenging static postural tasks and move to more dynamic tasks as deemed appropriate. For the person walking independently with less obvious signs of balance deficits, starting by completing one or two functional movement tests (Timed Up and Go, Berg Balance Scale, or Dynamic Gait Index) allows for the observation of movement under various postural challenge conditions while identifying a norm-based estimate for fall risk. The quality of the individual's performance of specific items within these functional tests can provide invaluable clues about possible impairments to guide subsequent examination activities.

Tools assessing functional balance typically aim to examine balance challenges across many conditions and situations. Functional balance tests can also examine activity across each of the multiple systems contributing to postural control. Assessing factors contributing to the risk of falls requires a substantial "toolbox" with careful consideration of the floor and ceiling effects of functional assessment tools as well as amount of new information to be gleaned and the ability of the test findings to contribute to the decision about plan of care.

The physical therapist is uniquely qualified to assess the components of gait, mobility, and balance that contribute to fall risk and then, in conjunction with information about environmental and personal factors, guide an intervention program to improve or accommodate many of these risk factors. The physical therapist will also screen for balance and fall risk conditions that may be outside the scope of physical therapy and refer to, or consult with, the appropriate practitioner (e.g., vision consult when significant undiagnosed visual issues are uncovered; medical consult when orthostatic hypotension is identified).

History and Screening

During the initial interview the physical therapist gathers medical history data and listens carefully to the patient's self-report of any gait and balance deficits or fall incidents. Interview data can provide critical information about the etiology and likely problems contributing to falling incidents and to risk for future falls. A thorough exploration of both intrinsic and extrinsic factors surrounding the circumstances of previous falls or near-falling episodes helps guide and inform the patient examination, evaluation, and diagnosis.

This exploration should start with open-ended questions that become progressively narrowed (Box 10.2). It is important to ask about the onset of falls, activities at the time of falls, symptoms at or prior to falls, direction of falls, medications, and environmental conditions at the time of the fall. A history of a recent fall (within 3 months to 2 years) is an important indicator for future falls, and recurrent fallers are at particularly high risk for additional fall events.[12] Determining an individual's activities at the time of a fall and symptoms prior to a fall event provide valuable clues. Falling to the side is much more likely to result in a hip fracture than a fall forward or backward.[45]

The risk of falling increases when taking multiple medications and with use of specific medications such as antidepressants, tranquilizers, and benzodiazepines (see Chapter 6, Pharmacology). Although lower systolic or diastolic blood pressure while standing has been associated with higher risk of falling in some studies, recent regression analyses of large sample sizes suggest that fall risk is more strongly associated with accompanying frailty[46,47] and number and type of medications[47] than blood pressure levels. Thus, the past and current medication history should be noted for possible contribution to unsteadiness. Orthostatic hypotension, with its sudden drop in blood pressure, is associated with an increased risk of a falling, especially if the orthostatic hypotension occurs two or more times.[48]

Cognitive changes complicate the taking of a fall history, as the patient may not be a reliable source of information about fall history or the conditions surrounding a falling incident. Family members are a valuable resource while taking a history of a person with significant cognitive impairment. Careful examination of the skin can help identify recent or new injuries from falls. Particular attention should be paid to the knees, elbows, back of the head, and hands.

By understanding the risk factors for falls, health care providers can help to minimize the risk of a first or subsequent falls. Screening tools are useful in assessing balance and gait in the older adult, indicating areas that need to be improved to prevent falls. Common tests used by health care providers that can serve as screening tools (as well as outcome measures) to assess balance and gait include the Timed Up and Go test, Tinetti Balance and Gait test, and Berg Balance Scale, among many others.

BOX 10.2 Key Questions to Ask Someone About Falling

1. Have you fallen?
   - If yes, in the past month how many times have you fallen?
   - How many times have you fallen in the past 6 months?
2. Can you tell me what happened to cause you to fall?
   - If they cannot tell you why they fell, this clearly deserves more questions and is a "red flag" to question them more thoroughly. (Consider cardiovascular or neurologic causes carefully if they are cognitively intact and cannot tell you why they fell.)
3. Did someone see you fall? If yes, did you have a loss of consciousness (LOC)?
   - If they had an LOC, make sure that their primary care physician is aware of this finding.
   - Often with a hit to the head with an LOC, persons may develop benign paroxysmal positional vertigo (BPPV).
   - The Dix-Hallpike test is indicated to rule out benign paroxysmal positional vertigo after an LOC with a hit to the head.
4. Did you go to the doctor as a result of your fall or did you have to go to the emergency room?
5. Did you get hurt?
   - No injury
   - Bruises
   - Stitches
   - Fracture
   - Head injury
6. Which direction did you fall?
   - To the side
   - Backward
   - Forward
7. Did you recently change any of your medicines?
   - If yes, what was changed?

Stopping Elderly Accidents, Deaths, and Injuries

The CDC Injury Center's program STEADI (Stopping Elderly Accidents, Deaths and Injuries) was developed in 2013[49] as a toolkit for health care providers to screen older adults for risk of falling. It includes tools and resources for providers to assess and educate their patients on the risks of falls and risk reduction. The main aim of the toolkit is to provide a quick and simple way to incorporate this screening into the everyday practice of health care practitioners. Training on the implementation and use of the STEADI program can be completed online and all materials are available free of charge online as well.[50] The toolkit begins with an algorithm adapted from the Clinical Practice Guidelines of the British and American Geriatric Societies to assess the patient's risk of falls. Once the patient's fall risk has been assessed, the toolkit then provides guidance and educational materials for the health care provider, as well as the patient, and assists in creating an individualized plan for fall interventions.

Several studies have been undertaken to assess the feasibility and validity of the STEADI. In 2017, Lohman et al. adapted the STEADI for use with the National Health and Aging Trends study (NHATS). The STEADI screening tool was adapted to be usable with survey cohort data and sought to determine any predictive abilities of the STEADI. The adapted screening tool was valid in predicting future fall risk. Participants classified as having a moderate fall risk had a 2.62 times greater probability of falling at follow-up than those at low risk, and those classified as high fall risk had a 4.76 times greater probability of falling than those at low risk.[44] The results of the STEADI assessment correlated with the results of the Feet Side-by-Side (FSS), Instep-Touching-Toe (ITT), and Standing-on-One-Foot (SOF) portions of the 4-Stage Balance Test.[51]

Utilizing the STEADI algorithm and toolkit provided an effective way to assist health care providers (specifically advanced practice nurses for this study) in assessing and preventing falls in older adults.[52] Eckstrom et al. also noted that the integration of the STEADI program in clinical practice resulted in 64% of patients being screened and 22% of those screened being categorized as high falls risk. Interventions offered included further assessment of and intervention on gait, orthostatic hypotension, vision, adequate vitamin D, foot issues, and, at a lower percentage, medication examination. For their study, they also created a three-question short form of the Stay Independent questionnaire to test alongside the original 12-item questionnaire and found that the short version was more efficient, as well as more effective, in identifying older patients at risk for falls.[53] The three questions on the short form are as follows: (1) Have you fallen in the past year? (2) Do you feel unsteady when standing or walking? (3) Do you worry about falling?

Greenberg et al. found that patients seen in an emergency room setting who were provided with written materials from the CDC STEADI program as well as written treatment options/ideas for practice at home were more likely to be able to relate activities that would decrease their risk of falling.[54]

EXAMINATION OF IMPAIRMENTS IN POSTURAL CONTROL

Based on the International Classification of Functioning, Disability and Health (ICF) model of functioning and disability, postural instability in older adults is multifactorial and results from an interaction between impairments in structures and functions contributing to postural control with the environmental and personal characteristics, which all lead to activity limitations and participation restrictions. Therefore, the next step after history taking is to examine the components of postural control to determine the etiology of the imbalance problem. Systems review should always include an assessment of vital signs. Blood pressure should be assessed for signs of orthostatic hypotension with positional changes in older adults who have fallen, particularly those who complained of lightheadedness at the time of the fall or who are taking medication to control their blood pressure.

Sensory

Sensory changes may play an integral role in determining the etiology of falls. Abnormal or insufficient sensory input due to injury or disease in one of the sensory systems (vision, vestibular, or somatosensory) may predispose a person to falling. Therefore, it is important to examine each of these sensory components contributing to postural control.[55] Chapter 5, which discusses accommodating sensory changes in environmental design, provides additional insights into physiological changes in sensory structure with aging and environmental adaption to accommodate these changes.

Vision. Vision is an important sensory component of intrinsic postural control as well as an important mechanism for avoiding balance challenges from environmental hazards. Significantly impaired visual acuity and impaired contrast sensitivity and depth perception have been associated with falls, as well as health conditions resulting in central or peripheral visual field cuts.[56]

Visual Acuity. Visual acuity can be estimated clinically by having the patient read a Snellen chart with both eyes and then, as deemed appropriate, with each eye separately, both with and without any eyeglasses the patient typically wears while walking. An extreme loss of visual acuity is associated with gait instability in older adults.[28] Bifocals, trifocals, and progressive lenses often used by older adults can increase the likelihood of a fall event, especially on steps.[57] Several prevention programs found that the use of single-lens glasses[58] or intermediate ones[59] reduces the risk of falls in older adults.

Contrast Sensitivity. Contrast sensitivity is the ability to detect subtle differences in shading and patterns. Contrast sensitivity is important in detecting objects without clear outlines and discriminating objects or details from their background, such as the ability to discriminate steps covered with a patterned carpet. Contrast sensitivity declines with increased age and with health conditions such as cataracts and diabetic retinopathy. Brannan et al.[60] found that falls decreased from 37% prior to cataract surgery to 19% by 6 months following cataract surgery. Contrast sensitivity can be measured clinically by using a contrast sensitivity chart such as the Hamilton-Veale contrast test chart depicted in Fig. 10.4. Persons are asked to read the letters they can see on the special visual chart.

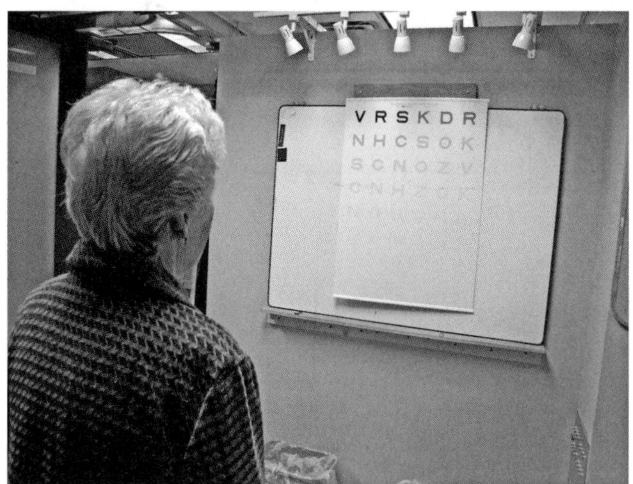

FIG. 10.4 An older adult reading letters from a contrast sensitivity chart.

The letters at the top of the chart are dark with a greater number of pixels and then gradually become lighter until they are almost impossible to visualize. The chart has eight lines of letters. Each line of letters has corresponding line numbers associated with the person's performance. Scoring is based on the ability to see the letters. Persons fail when they have guessed incorrectly two of the three letters out of a combination of three letters. The score is based on when the person has last guessed two of three correctly. Poor performance has been associated with persons requiring a low vision assessment and disease such as macular degeneration or glaucoma.

Depth Perception. Depth perception is the ability to distinguish distances between objects. One simple clinical depth perception screening test, depicted in Fig. 10.5, is to hold your index fingers pointing upward in front of the patient at eye level, one finger closer to the patient than the other. Gradually move the index fingers toward each other (one forward, one back) until the patient identifies when the fingers are parallel or lined up. If the patient's perception of parallel is off by 3 inches or more, depth perception may be a problem and referral to an ophthalmologist for additional investigation is warranted.

Visual Field Restrictions. Peripheral vision is the ability to see from the side while looking straight ahead. To test peripheral vision, the examiner brings his or her fingers from behind the patient's head at eye level while the patient looks straight ahead. The patient identifies when he or she first notices the examiner's finger in his or her side view. A significant field cut unilaterally or bilaterally would be important to notice. Loss of central vision, most typically seen with macular degeneration, has also been related to falling.

Vestibular. Persons with impaired vestibular function may be more likely to fall. In one cross-sectional survey of over 5000 adults over the age of 40 years, those who reported vestibular symptoms had a 12-fold increase in the odds of falling.[61] Vestibular evaluation may be necessary if the patient is complaining of dizziness or significant postural instability. Vestibular assessment ranges from simple tests and measures to highly sophisticated examination tools. Visual impairments may reflect vestibular dysfunction because of the complex central connections between the vestibular system and eye movements. A more detailed discussion of vestibular system examination tools can be found in Whitney et al.[62]

Three clinical tests to assess VOR function, which controls gaze stability, are briefly described here. VOR can be tested clinically by asking the patient to focus on a fixed target and move the head to the right and left (horizontally) and then up and down (vertically) with various speeds. Normally, a person should be able to maintain gaze without blurring of the target. Inability to maintain gaze fixation on the target indicates abnormal VOR function as a result of peripheral or central vestibular lesion.[62] VOR function can also be tested clinically by assessing the patient's response to rapid head thrusts, with the patient seated.[63] Ask the patient to relax and allow you to move

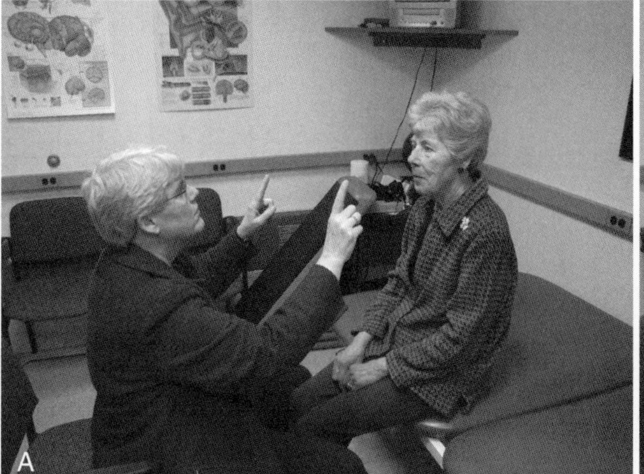

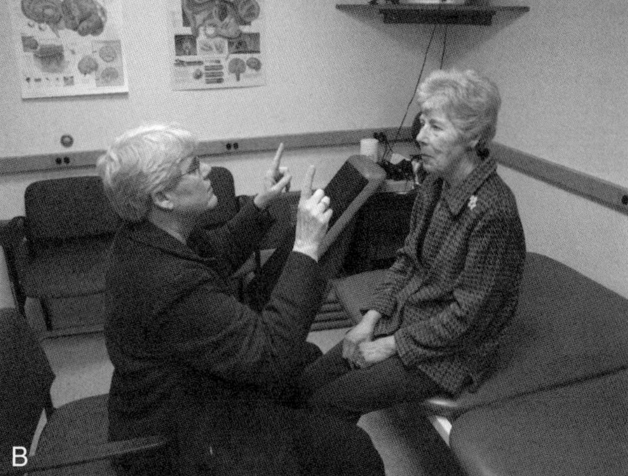

FIG. 10.5 Assessing depth perception. **A,** The right hand is closer and is slowly moved away from the patient until the fingers align an equal distance from the patient's face. **B,** The patient reports that the fingers are of equal distance from the face.

his or her head and check his or her cervical ROM. Then ask the patient to focus on a fixed target directly in front of him or her (usually your nose) while you move the patient's head rapidly over a small amplitude. Observe the patient's ability to sustain visual fixation on the target and look for corrective saccades plus note the head thrust direction if a saccade occurs. A positive head thrust test indicates an impaired VOR due to a peripheral lesion.

A third clinical test of VOR function is the assessment of static/dynamic visual acuity. This test is performed by asking the patient to read a visual acuity chart to the lowest possible line (until he or she cannot identify all the letters on a line) with the head held stationary. Then, the patient reads the chart again while the examiner moves the patient's head side to side at 2 Hz. A drop in visual acuity of three or more lines indicates an impaired VOR as a result of either peripheral or central lesion.[64]

Patients with an acute peripheral vestibular disorder will have positive test results with the head thrust test, have abnormalities with the VOR, and have impairments of static and dynamic visual acuity. With a central vestibular disorder, one would expect to see impairments of saccades or smooth pursuit. Therefore, if the therapist is expecting a peripheral vestibular disorder, then testing the head thrust, the VOR, and the static and dynamic visual acuity will be a priority to perform. While inspecting abnormalities with saccadic eye movement or smooth pursuit, the therapist's attention should be directed to a central vestibular disorder. The assessment of the VSR requires examination of gait, locomotion, and balance, including walking with head rotation.

Somatosensory

A somatosensory examination includes proprioception, vibration, and cutaneous sensation. Proprioception (sense of position and sense of movement) can be tested clinically by a joint position matching test beginning distally with a "toe up/down" test with eyes closed, and moving more proximally to the ankle and knee if impairments are noted in the toes. A patient with normal proprioception should be able to detect very subtle movements of the big toe. Vibratory sense can be tested by placing a tuning fork at the first metatarsal head. Proprioception testing, vibration testing, cutaneous pressure sensation, and two-point discrimination were together found to have reliable results in assessing sensory changes that affect balance.[65]

Sensory Integration Testing

The interaction between all sensory modalities (vision, vestibular, somatosensory) can be tested in different ways. The Clinical Test of Sensory Interaction and Balance (CTSIB) is a commonly used measure to examine the interaction between the vision, vestibular, and somatosensory systems.[66] Traditionally, the CTSIB has been performed by assessing a person's balance under six different standing conditions. The person stands on a solid surface with eyes open, with eyes closed, and with altered visual feedback by wearing a visual conflict dome and then repeats each visual condition while standing on a foam surface. The magnitude of the sway (minimal, mild, or moderate) and fall occurrence are then reported or the performance can be timed with a stopwatch. The CTSIB was able to classify 63% of people at risk for falling.[67] More recently, based on studies finding little difference between the eyes closed and the visual conflict dome conditions, the visual conflict dome condition has been omitted in many tests.[68]

The sensory organization test (SOT) of computerized dynamic posturography, depicted in Fig. 10.6, is a quantitative test that objectively identifies abnormalities in the sensory components that contribute to postural control during standing balance. The subject stands on a movable force plate with a movable surrounding wall. Visual and somatosensory elements are manipulated in various combinations to provide six different sensory conditions, described in Box 10.3. Functional responses of subjects and occurrence of falls are reported.

Patients who fall under conditions 5 and 6 are often assumed to have vestibular dysfunction. However, many older adults will fall under conditions 5 and 6 without any vestibular loss because they are difficult balance tests. Patients who fall under conditions 4, 5, and 6 are surface dependent. The SOT is a very helpful tool in guiding interventional approach. SOT scores are less effective in older adults compared to younger individuals.[69] The composite SOT score can improve over time in older adults who have undergone rehabilitation.[70]

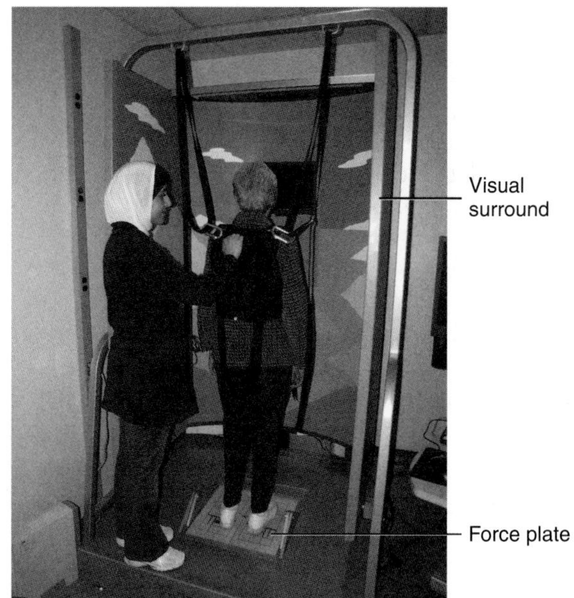

FIG. 10.6 The sensory organization test (SOT) of computerized dynamic posturography. The physical therapist is guarding the patient but *not* touching her during the testing.

BOX 10.3 Six Testing Conditions of Sensory Organization Testing Using Posturography

Condition 1	Person stands on the force plate with eyes open, feet together. There is no movement of the force plate or the visual surround.
Condition 2	Person stands on the force plate with eyes closed, feet together. There is no movement of the force plate or the visual surround.
Condition 3	Person stands on the force plate with eyes open and the platform surface is sway referenced to visual surround (the floor moves commensurate with the person's sway).
Condition 4	Person stands on the force plate with eyes open while the force plate is sway referenced, and fixed visual surround.
Condition 5	Person stands on the force plate with eyes closed while the force plate is sway referenced.
Condition 6	Person stands on the force plate with eyes open while both the force plate and the visual surround are sway referenced.

Neuromuscular Testing

Muscle strength, range of motion, and endurance should be assessed in all older adults. The ability of the neuromuscular system to react quickly to postural perturbations declines with aging and thus can become an important risk factor for falling. A loss of muscle mass, strength, and endurance especially in the lower extremities has been found to increase the risk of falling by four to five times.[71] Small changes within multiple systems may reduce physiological reserve, resulting in challenges in the postural control system.

Strength. Testing strength in older adults provides essential information regarding the ability to generate sufficient muscle force to recover from balance disturbances. Manual muscle testing (MMT), a traditional mechanism for examining isolated muscle strength at slow speeds, may not provide the most useful information regarding balance control. It does not assess the ability to produce muscle force quickly or functionally, essential components of effective postural response.

The five times sit-to-stand test (FTSST)[72] and the 30-second chair rise time[73] are both functional performance tests that assess multiple components of neuromuscular effectors of balance, with both requiring good lower extremity muscle strength to complete at age-appropriate norms. See Chapter 7, Functional Outcome and Assessments, for descriptions of these functional tests and key interpretation of findings. Poor performance in rising from a chair is a strong predictor of fall risk in community-dwelling older adults when combined with other fall risk factors such as medications, comorbid disease, or at least one other fall risk factor.[74]

ROM and Flexibility. Assessing the ROM of the ankle, knee, hip, trunk, and cervical spine is particularly important in uncovering ROM impairments that can negatively affect balance. Assessment of ROM can be accomplished by using standard goniometric methods. Reduced ROM of the ankle or hip joints may affect the ability to use ankle or hip strategies, respectively, in recovering from external perturbations.

Aerobic Endurance

Endurance is another important factor to be carefully assessed. General endurance estimates an individual's ability to generate adequate force during tasks that require continued effort, such as walking for a long distance. The 6-minute walk test, described in Chapter 7, is a commonly used quantitative test to assess endurance and may be particularly useful in assessing endurance in frail older adults.

Environmental Assessment

Environmental factors can either facilitate or hinder the ability to function within one's surroundings. A home safety checklist appraises the home environment and highlights extrinsic fall hazards for incorporation into patient education interventions. An "in-home" safety check should be a routine part of home-care physical therapy and part of discharge activities of a patient from rehabilitation. A safety check examines things like home lighting, types of flooring, grab bars in the tub or shower, and handrails for stairways. The physical therapist may need to watch the patient's performance during routine activities within his or her home. The therapist may observe the patient getting in and out of bed and in and out of the shower or bathtub. In addition, it is important to assess the patient's access to light switches. Obstacles, cords, and clutter become particularly relevant to the patient with serious visual deficits or gait abnormality but need to be addressed only to the extent that they pose a threat to the patient's safe function. Chapter 5 provides a detailed discussion of environmental fall risk factors and home modification strategies.

Psychosocial Assessment

Social support and behavioral/cognitive function should be addressed in the comprehensive evaluation of patients experiencing recurrent falls. Memory deficits, dementia, and depression are health conditions seen with greater prevalence in older adults and that have been associated with increased fall risk. Impaired cognition, especially executive functions, have a strong relationship with risk of falls[75] as the cognitively impaired person may not recognize a fall-risk situation or make prudent choices to prevent a fall. Strong social support can help minimize fall risk by providing a safe and supportive environment that allows the cognitively impaired person to function maximally within his or her environment.

Fear of Falling

The Activities-specific Balance Confidence (ABC) Scale attempts to quantify fear of falling in older adults. The test items, with varying degrees of difficulty, were generated by clinicians and older adults. The Falls Efficacy Scale (FES) is a 10-item test rated on a 10-point scale from not confident at all to completely confident.[76] It is correlated with difficulty getting up from a fall and level of anxiety. The Falls Efficacy Scale International (FES-I), which is gaining increasing popularity, consists of either 7[77] or 16[78] items that are very similar to the 16-item ABC Scale.[21] See Chapter 7 for more details on fear-of-falling assessment tools.

INTERVENTION

The main goal of physical therapy management of falls is to maximize mobility and functional independence and to prevent further falls. Physical therapists are the health professionals most uniquely prepared to analyze and address balance and gait limitations and physical functional impairments contributing to movement dysfunctions associated with falling. Table 10.1 provides a listing of common fall risk factors and strategies available to physical therapists to decrease or eliminate these risk factors. When the physical therapist identifies a risk factor outside the scope of physical therapy, referral to or collaboration with other health professionals, as applicable, should occur.

Overall prevention and intervention management of risk factors can be restorative, compensatory, or accommodating to medical conditions, rehabilitative approaches, or environmental strategies. For example, therapeutic exercise is a primary restorative approach; footwear that provides increased sensory cues in the presence of decreased position sense serves as a compensatory approach; and wearing hip protectors or using an assistive device serves an accommodating role. Muscle strengthening, gait training, balance training, and flexibility or range-of-motion exercises are all key ingredients for a successful physical therapy program to address balance deficits.

Individuals who are frail and thus at high risk for falling can often benefit greatly from a comprehensive fall risk assessment and subsequent targeted interventions that include physical therapy. Frail individuals have low physiological reserve and impairments across multiple physiological systems, thus making them particularly vulnerable to stressors. Fig. 10.7 provides examples of the many therapeutic interventions that should be considered for “frail” and “very frail” older adults.

Fear of falling needs to be considered when developing and implementing the plan of care. The exercise environment and exercise activities should be structured to minimize fear while ensuring adequate challenge to lead to improvements. Particular attention should be paid to home exercise programs. Exercises perceived as too challenging are less likely to be carried out because of fear of falling. For all except the extremely frail, it is essential that balance exercises be performed in upright stance to adequately challenge balance responses. Seated balance exercises do little to affect standing balance responses. It is also important to move the older adult beyond low-level elastic resistance exercise in order to use overload principles to increase muscle strength.[79] Often frail older adults will need more supervision to perform their exercise program. Those older adults who are very frail in outpatient settings may initially need to be seen more frequently so that they can be closely supervised during their exercise program.

Balance Training

One aspect of balance training is improving the speed and accuracy of response to unexpected perturbations by improving ankle, hip, stepping, or reaching strategies. Ankle strategy response can be progressively enhanced through exercises such as simple weight shifts and rocking forward and backward to the edge of BOS followed by rocking forward and backward against resistance at the shoulders and then “letting go” (done carefully to protect the patient from falling). An option to train hip strategy response is to ask the patient to practice leaning forward at the hips while maintaining foot position (touch the nose to the mat table) or pulling the patient off balance at the hip enough that he or she must lean at the trunk to control balance.

Standing, standing with fast and slow weight shifts in all directions, standing and reaching, or standing with small pushes and then reaching for an object with a slight push each progresses the patient’s standing balance. During any weight shift, it is important to teach the patient to be more aware of lower extremity sensation and better recognize where the weight is under his or her feet. Activating distal sensation has been reported to be one of the possible reasons that tai chi may be successful in reducing falls in older persons.[80]

Tai Chi. Tai chi (TC) is considered a balance training program because it contains slow movements that stress postural control. Tai chi can be performed in groups or independently and requires the person to move body parts gently and slowly while breathing deeply. Tai chi has a positive effect on balance in older adults[81] and has been demonstrated to reduce fear of falling, risk of falls, and lower blood pressure.[82] Richerson and Rosendale found that both older adults with diabetes and healthy older persons who participated in TC demonstrated improvements in their distal sensation.[80]

Vestibular Training. Dizziness is never normal in older adults. Persons with vestibular deficits (dizziness, lightheadedness, or vertigo complaints) benefit from exercise and balance programs. Often older adults do not complain of spinning but may only report lightheadedness during movement. Other conditions that cause dizziness must be ruled out to ensure that you are treating a vestibular condition. Not all persons with vestibular disorders have both dizziness and balance problems. The exercise

TABLE 10.1 Fall Risk Factors and Strategies a Physical Therapist Should Consider to Ameliorate the Risk Factor and Improve Patient Function

Fall Risk Factor	Strategies to Ameliorate the Fall Risk Factor
Weakness	• Individualized muscle strengthening program followed by • Community exercise program for continued participation in strength training
Loss of flexibility and range of motion	• Stretching program • Modifications if range of motion cannot be achieved
Low/high body mass index	• Refer patient for consultation with a physician • Refer patient for consultation with a nutritionist • Assess for depression
Impaired vision	• Determine when the patient received his or her most recent glasses • Refer patient for consultation with an ophthalmologist if any undiagnosed or changing visual impairments • Patient education on environmental strategies to minimize risk in the presence of impaired vision • (Be sure physical therapist's environment adequately accommodates low vision needs)
Impaired recreation	• Careful listening to the patient's interests and desires for specific recreational activities, and strategizing options to achieve participation (in typical or adaptive form) • Building a rehabilitative program to address the specific skills required to participate in the activities • Recommendations for local programs that provide recreational opportunities consistent with the individual's capabilities

Impaired sensation	• Exercises to maintain or improve distal muscle strength
	• Tai chi demonstrated to be successful at enhancing distal sensation
	• Patient education in skin checks to prevent injury to feet:
	  • Daily checking of skin on feet
	  • Wearing cotton socks
	  • Checking shoe wear and condition frequently
	• Patient education in use of alternative balance systems (visual and vestibular) to maximize balance function
	• Future direction could be subthreshold vibration in the shoe

Cognitive impairment	• Review of medication, with particular emphasis on medications with a sedative effect • Attempt to keep the environment consistent • Evaluate the environment for safety hazards • Family education on safety and monitoring in the home setting • Participation in exercise and physical activity programs appropriate to individuals with cognitive impairment • Referral to primary physician if cognitive impairment is new or has demonstrated substantial change recently
Incontinence	• Patient and caretaker education in establishing a regular toileting program • Patient and caretaker education about effects of caffeine and particular risks of excessive fluids late in the day requiring trips to the bathroom at night • Consultation with physician, as indicated, for medication management

Environmental hazards	• Provide an environmental assessment:
	  • Stability of furniture likely to be used to assist with ambulation in the home
	  • Need for grab bar, tub floor mat installation in the bathroom
	  • Recommend handrails on steps
	  • Adequacy of lighting and accessibility of light switches
	• Assess clothing and footwear

Postural hypotension	• Consult with the physician about a medication review or need for a cardiovascular referral
	• Patient assessment for, and education in, physiological maneuvers beneficial in decreasing an orthostatic event:
	  • Active movements of the lower extremities prior to moving from sit to stand
	  • Use of elastic pressure stockings or an abdominal binder
	  • Slowly move from supine to sit
	  • Ankle pumps or upper extremity movement prior to changing position

Osteoporosis	• Standing exercises/weight-bearing exercise • Consider hip pads • Patient education in the benefits of medications and vitamin D supplementation
Polypharmacy	• Review of medications: Consult with physician if signs that an adverse medication response may be affecting balance, particularly those causing postural hypotension or confusion • Attempt, with the help of the team, to determine if benzodiazepines are necessary
Impaired gait	• Determine factors contributing to the gait disturbance • Balance exercises • Establish a walking program • Assistive device use or modification
Impaired balance	• Exercises performed in standing • Attempts to increase the person's limits of stability in all directions
Joint pain	• Strengthening program • Physical agents as an adjunct

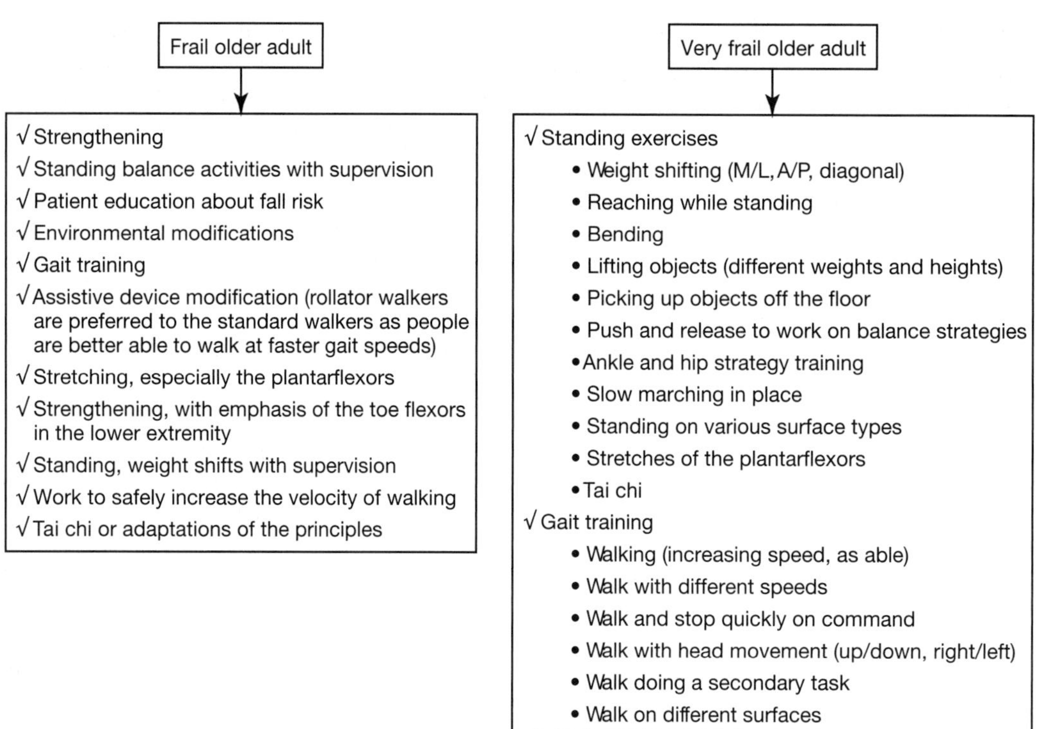

FIG. 10.7 Illustrative ideas for physical therapy intervention based on the degree of frailty. *A/P*, anteroposterior; *M/L*, mediolateral.

program should specifically address the impairments and functional deficits noted.

The most common intervention for older adults is the use of the canalith repositioning maneuver (modified Epley maneuver) for benign paroxysmal positional vertigo (BPPV).[83] BPPV is extremely common in older persons and reports of dizziness in people older than age 40 years are related to reported falls.[61] The canalith repositioning maneuver is highly effective in resolving dizziness that is associated with a change of head position relative to gravity,[84] and with the resolution of BPPV, older adults fall less.[85]

Eye/head movements are often used with visual fixation to attempt to normalize the gain of the VOR in persons with vestibular dysfunction.[86] Patients are often asked to stare at a fixed target and then move their head either up/down, right/left, or ear to their shoulder while keeping the image on the fovea (keeping the target in focus). As they improve, the patient is asked to increase the speed of the head movement and also to try to perform the exercise with various backgrounds and during standing and gait.[87] It is thought that retinal slip drives the adaptation of the VOR.[86]

Progressive standing balance and gait exercises for individuals with vestibular disorders include several key concepts[87]: (1) starting in more static and advancing toward more dynamic movements; (2) considering subject learning style and key motor learning concepts such as knowledge of results and performance; (3) increasing the difficulty of the environment (closed to open skills, quiet vs. busy environment); (4) varying from no head movement to complex head movement during standing and gait; (5) adding secondary tasks to the balance or gait task (talking, holding/carrying, calculating); and (6) manipulation of the support surface from flat/stable surface to a dynamic surface (foam pad, gravel, grass, etc.).[87]

Exercise Interventions: Strength, ROM, and Endurance

To the extent that muscle strength, ROM, and aerobic endurance contribute to a patient's instability, each needs to be addressed in the intervention program. Research indicates that lower extremity weakness is significantly associated with recurrent falls in older adults,[88,89] and that improved lower extremity strength is associated with improvements in static and dynamic balance.[90] A multidimensional training program that included stretching, flexibility, balance, coordination, and mild strengthening exercise has demonstrated improvements in physical functioning and oxygen uptake in community-dwelling older adults.[91] Similarly, a strength and balance training program improved muscle strength, functional performance, and balance in older adults with a history of recurrent or injurious falls.[92] Although it is clear that exercise is important to balance training, the optimal type, duration, and frequency of exercise programs are still unclear.[93] In general, exercise programs should address static and dynamic balance, coordination, strength, endurance, and ROM. Most exercise/balance programs that have demonstrated effectiveness lasted for >10 weeks. See Chapter 8 for a more detailed discussion of general exercise principles for the older adult.

Assistive and Accommodative Devices

Ambulation devices, such as different types of canes and walkers, may provide older fallers with greater stability and reduce risk of falling. These devices increase the BOS in standing and walking by increasing the ground contact. Ambulation devices may also help in reducing fear of falling by providing physical support and by adding tactile cues to enhance somatosensory contributions to postural control and sense of where the person is in space. The proper ambulatory device can be prescribed according to older adults' needs based on a comprehensive balance assessment.

Hip pads are most commonly used with patients in nursing homes who are at very high risk for injury from a fall. Hip pads reduce the fracture rate marginally in older adults.[94] Compliance is a concern as the hip pads are somewhat cumbersome and unattractive worn under clothing. However, for some older adults who are fearful of falling, wearing hip protectors has a psychological benefit.

Properly fitting footwear with a low heel and high sole/surface contact area decreases the risk of falling. Because decline in distal somatosensory function with advanced age can lead to instability and increased risk of falling, special insoles have been designed to enhance somatosensory input. A facilitatory insole, as depicted in Fig. 10.8, improved lateral stability during gait and decreased the risk of falling in older adults.[95] Vibrating insoles have also been used to enhance sensory and motor function in older adults.[96] The use of vibrating insoles has been associated with a large reduction in older adults' sway during standing trials, reduced Timed Up and Go scores, and improved gait speed.[97] Therefore, vibrating shoe insoles might contribute to enhanced stability of older adults during dynamic balance activities.[98,99] Gait variability in the laboratory was reduced for older adults plus older fallers while wearing the subthreshold vibratory device during gait.[100]

The Use of Technology for Balance and Gait

Technology is utilized for both interventions and monitoring fall risk in older adults. Wearable technology can monitor activity levels and alert families/caregivers of a change in normal activity levels. Common devices such as a Fitbit can monitor steps as an activity tracker, heart rate, and even sleep via a mobile app. There are apps for smartphones that can detect unanticipated movements of the phone that might be a fall event and notify key contacts of a potential fall occurrence (Fallception). Wearable technology has become much more affordable and should continue to become more affordable and effective over time.

Vibrotactile feedback applied to the trunk continues to be developed around the world with the goal of reducing falls.[101] A cell phone balance trainer that delivers vibrotactile feedback has been implemented in community-living healthy older adults with success via telehealth. Data from the cell phone, electronically sent to a physical therapist, allowed the physical therapist to adjust a program based on this feedback. Balance improved and all participants were able to utilize the cell phone technology. Older adults at mild fall risk who used exoskeleton devices to provide external support to maintain stance experienced fewer falls and had less pain at 6 and 12 months than a comparison group of exercise only.[102]

An exercise program targeted to older adults delivered via tablet technology[103] was successful at motivating older adults via game and interactive features that allowed participants to compare their scores to others, work as a group to win a game based on points, and write messages of encouragement to perform the exercise program. Making exercise fun and including a group experience produced a low dropout rate.

Gaming technology with force plates and/or sensors (Nintendo Wii, Microsoft Kinect, Dance Dance Revolution, and PlayStation EyeToy) are being utilized by seniors to improve postural control. A recent meta-analysis using Preferred Reporting Items for Systematic Reviews and Meta-analyses (PRISMA) guidelines suggests that virtual reality exercise is better than no exercise but is slightly less effective than a supervised exercise program in persons over 60 years of age.[104] Innovative technology-assisted approaches supporting interventions that decrease risk of falling during standing and gait will be a direction of the future. Although not all of the technological devices are readily acceptable to seniors at this time,[105] subsequent generations of older adults who are currently regular users of technology will expect availability of user-friendly and affordable assistive technologies when they move into older age.

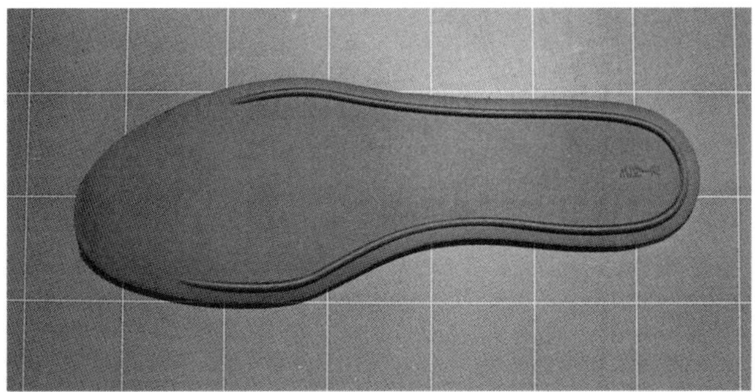

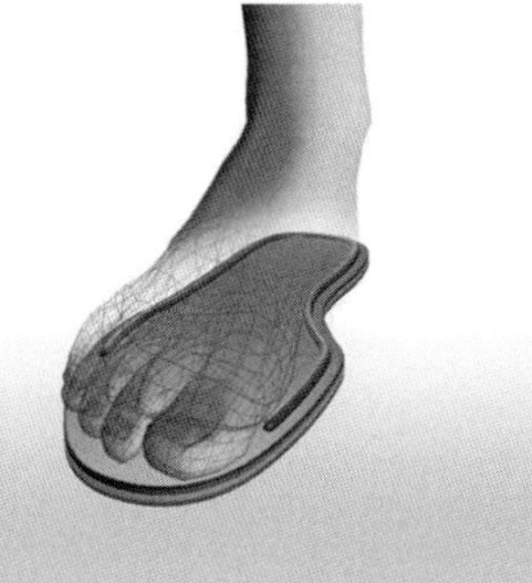

FIG. 10.8 An insole that provides increased lateral cues to older adults when they move close to their limits of medial/lateral stability. *(From Perry S, Radtke A, McIlroy W, et al. Efficacy and effectiveness of a balance-enhancing insole. J Gerontol. 2008;63A:595–602.)*

Environmental Modifications

Environmental modifications may prevent falls and reduce the risk of falling significantly. Chapter 5 provides an in-depth discussion of environmental modifications. Slippery floor surfaces, trip risk factors (scatter rugs, electrical cords, clutter, etc.), lack of hand railings on stairs, and absence of grab bars in the tub/shower have all been identified as significant risk factors for falls in the home.[106] Motion detection lighting and lamps that are turned on via touch or voice command are two of the more affordable methods that can be utilized to enhance safety in the home.

Pre- or Postrehabilitation Community-Based Programs for Falls Prevention

In recent years, there has been increased recognition of the importance of community-based disease prevention and health promotion programs delivered affordably and on a large scale. There is substantial evidence that these programs can reduce the need for costly medical interventions and enhance quality of life. Physical therapists are often asked by their patients for recommendations about community exercise or educational programs to join following discharge to minimize likelihood of future falls. Physical therapists should be knowledgeable about the various programs available in their community to recommend programs that best fit an individual patient following discharge from physical therapy.

In 2017, the Administration on Community Living (ACL) recognized 12 community-delivered falls prevention programs as "evidence based," determined by quality standards established by an ACL advisory committee.[107] Both exercise programs and risk factor self-management programs are included, with target audiences ranging from the reasonably fit to the more frail older adult. A review committee assesses new programs and new evidence annually. The quality standards a program must meet to be designated evidence based by the ACL are summarized in Box 10.4. A list of these programs can be found on the National Council on Aging (NCOA) website.[107] Having this designation allows senior-serving community centers to utilize Title III-D funding of the Older Americans Act to support these evidence-based health promotion programs. Various insurance entities and employers have also provided some support to community organizations offering these approved programs. Most of these programs function primarily with lay leaders often with some level of health professional collaboration. Physical therapists could (and should) have a role in screening participants, training lay leaders, and consulting with program leaders on exercise program components, progression, or modification.

Most of the programs include some combination of exercise, participant education, and self-efficacy training for fall risk management. Target audiences vary from low to high risk of falling older adults. Programs like A Matter of Balance (AMOB) focus on decreasing fear of falling, participant education, and increasing self-efficacy. Stay Active and Independent for Life (SAIL) is a group exercise program for community-dwelling older adults that emphasizes strength training, flexibility, balance, and overall fitness with tips on reducing falls as part of each exercise class. The Otago Exercise Program (OEP) is an individually tailored exercise program found most effective for near-frail or frail older adults who have fallen in the past year and have moderate to severe decreases in strength and balance. The traditional OEP program combines periodic physical therapist visits with independent or caregiver-supervised ongoing exercise, often delivered to home-bound individuals. Reviewing the full list of ACL-approved programs can help match an individual patient's need for ongoing exercise with available programs in your region.

BOX 10.4 ACL Definition of an Evidence-based Disease Prevention and Health Promotion Program

1. Has been demonstrated through evaluation to be effective for improving the health and well-being or reducing disease, disability, and/or injury among older adults; *and*
2. Has been proven effective with older adult population, using experimental or quasi-experimental design*; *and*
3. Has research results published in a peer-review journal; *and*
4. Has been fully translated** in one or more community site(s); *and*
5. Includes developed dissemination products that are available to the public.

*Experimental designs use random assignment and a control group. Quasi-experimental designs do not use random assignment.
**For purposes of the Title III-D definitions, being "fully translated in one or more community sites" means that the evidence-based program in question has been carried out at the community level (with fidelity to the published research) at least once before. Sites should only consider programs that have been shown to be effective within a real-world community setting.
(From https://acl.gov/programs/health-wellness/disease-prevention)

SUMMARY

Falls in older adults are a major concern and are a major cause of morbidity and mortality. Falls are multifaceted and a heterogeneous problem. A comprehensive evaluation of pathophysiological, functional, and environmental factors of falls is important for effective management. The goal of intervention should always be to maximize functional independence in a manner that moves the person up higher on the "slippery slope," away from the line that indicates frailty and closer to the line that indicates "fun," and to do this safely so that older persons can participate in their community.

REFERENCES

1. Pohl P, Nordin E, Lundquist A, Bergstrom U, Lundin-Olsson L. Community-dwelling older people with an injurious fall are likely to sustain new injurious falls within 5 years—a prospective long-term follow-up study. *BMC Geriatr*. 2014;14:120.

2. Bergen G, Stevens MR, Burns ER. Falls and fall injuries among adults aged >/=65 years - United States, 2014. *MMWR Morb Mortal Wkly Rep*. 2016;65(37):993–998.
3. Scheffer AC, Schuurmans MJ, van Dijk N, van der Hooft T, de Rooij SE. Fear of falling: measurement strategy, prevalence, risk factors and consequences among older persons. *Age Ageing*. 2008;37(1):19–24.
4. Gregg EW, Pereira MA, Caspersen CJ. Physical activity, falls, and fractures among older adults: a review of the epidemiologic evidence. *J Am Geriatr Soc*. 2000;48 (8):883–893.
5. Hauer K, Lamb SE, Jorstad EC, Todd C, Becker C. Systematic review of definitions and methods of measuring falls in randomised controlled fall prevention trials. *Age Ageing*. 2006;35(1):5–10.
6. Schwenk M, Lauenroth A, Stock C, et al. Definitions and methods of measuring and reporting on injurious falls in randomised controlled fall prevention trials: a systematic review. *BMC Med Res Methodol*. 2012;12:50.
7. Ambrose AF, Paul G, Hausdorff JM. Risk factors for falls among older adults: a review of the literature. *Maturitas*. 2013;75(1):51–61.
8. Fabre JM, Ellis R, Kosma M, Wood RH. Falls risk factors and a compendium of falls risk screening instruments. *J Geriatr Phys Ther*. 2010;33(4):184–197.
9. Park JH, Mancini M, Carlson-Kuhta P, Nutt JG, Horak FB. Quantifying effects of age on balance and gait with inertial sensors in community-dwelling healthy adults. *Exp Gerontol*. 2016;85:48–58.
10. Callisaya ML, Blizzard L, McGinley JL, Srikanth VK. Risk of falls in older people during fast-walking—the TASCOG study. *Gait Posture*. 2012;36(3):510–515.
11. Montero-Odasso M, Annweiler C, Hachinski V, Islam A, Yang N, Vasudev A. Vascular burden predicts gait, mood, and executive function disturbances in older adults with mild cognitive impairment: results from the gait and brain study. *J Am Geriatr Soc*. 2012;60(10):1988–1990.
12. Thurman DJ, Stevens JA, Rao JK. Practice parameter: assessing patients in a neurology practice for risk of falls (an evidence-based review): report of the Quality Standards Subcommittee of the American Academy of Neurology. *Neurology*. 2008;70(6):473–479.
13. Kolb NA, Smith AG, Singleton JR, et al. The association of chemotherapy-induced peripheral neuropathy symptoms and the risk of falling. *JAMA Neurol*. 2016;73(7):860–866.
14. Beegan L, Messinger-Rapport BJ. Stand by me! Reducing the risk of injurious falls in older adults. *Cleve Clin J Med*. 2015;82(5):301–307.
15. Lee K, Pressler SJ, Titler M. Falls in patients with heart failure: a systematic review. *J Cardiovasc Nurs*. 2016;31(6):555–561.
16. Dawson-Hughes B, Mithal A, Bonjour J, et al. IOF position statement: vitamin D recommendations for older adults. *Osteoporos Int*. 2010;21:1151–1154.
17. Grossman DC, Curry SJ, Owens DK, et al. Vitamin D, calcium, or combined supplementation for the primary prevention of fractures in community-dwelling adults: US Preventive Services Task Force Recommendation Statement. *JAMA*. 2018;319(15):1592–1599.
18. Crumley Aybar BL, Gillespie MJ, Gipson SF, Mullaney CE, Tommasino-Storz M. Peripheral nerve blocks causing increased risk for fall and difficulty in ambulation for the hip and knee joint replacement patient. *J Perianesth Nurs*. 2016;31(6):504–519.
19. Honaker JA, Kretschmer LW. Impact of fear of falling for patients and caregivers: perceptions before and after participation in vestibular and balance rehabilitation therapy. *Am J Audiol*. 2014;23(1):20–33.
20. Fletcher PC, Berg K, Dalby DM, Hirdes JP. Risk factors for falling among community-based seniors. *J Patient Saf*. 2009;5(2):61–66.
21. Delbaere K, Crombez G, Vanderstraeten G, Willems T, Cambier D. Fear-related avoidance of activities, falls and physical frailty. A prospective community-based cohort study. *Age Ageing*. 2004;33(4):368–373.
22. Sharaf AY, Ibrahim HS. Physical and psychosocial correlates of fear of falling: among older adults in assisted living facilities. *J Gerontol Nurs*. 2008;34(12):27–35.
23. Lin YH, Hsieh SC, Chao CC, Chang YC, Hsieh ST. Influence of aging on thermal and vibratory thresholds of quantitative sensory testing. *J Peripher Nerv Syst*. 2005;10(3):269–281.
24. Brocklehurst JC, Robertson D, James-Groom P. Clinical correlates of sway in old age—sensory modalities. *Age Ageing*. 1982;11(1):1–10.
25. Kristinsdottir EK, Fransson PA, Magnusson M. Changes in postural control in healthy elderly subjects are related to vibration sensation, vision and vestibular asymmetry. *Acta Otolaryngol*. 2001;121(6):700–706.
26. Bacsi AM, Colebatch JG. Evidence for reflex and perceptual vestibular contributions to postural control. *Exp Brain Res*. 2005;160(1):22–28.
27. Judge JO, King MB, Whipple R, Clive J, Wolfson LI. Dynamic balance in older persons: effects of reduced visual and proprioceptive input. *J Gerontol A Biol Sci Med Sci*. 1995;50(5):M263–M270.
28. Lord SR, Dayhew J. Visual risk factors for falls in older people. *J Am Geriatr Soc*. 2001;49(5):508–515.
29. Lord SR, Dayhew J, Howland A. Multifocal glasses impair edge-contrast sensitivity and depth perception and increase the risk of falls in older people. *J Am Geriatr Soc*. 2002;50 (11):1760–1766.
30. Rosenhall U. Degenerative patterns in the aging human vestibular neuro-epithelia. *Acta Otolaryngol*. 1973;76 (2):208–220.
31. Iwasaki S, Yamasoba T. Dizziness and imbalance in the elderly: age-related decline in the vestibular system. *Aging Dis*. 2015;6(1):38–47.
32. Norre ME, Forrez G, Beckers A. Vestibular dysfunction causing instability in aged patients. *Acta Otolaryngol*. 1987;104(1–2):50–55.
33. Horak FB, Nashner LM. Central programming of postural movements: adaptation to altered support-surface configurations. *J Neurophysiol*. 1986;55(6):1369–1381.
34. Hess JA, Woollacott M, Shivitz N. Ankle force and rate of force production increase following high intensity strength training in frail older adults. *Aging Clin Exp Res*. 2006;18(2):107–115.
35. Horak FB, Wrisley DM, Frank J. The Balance Evaluation Systems Test (BESTest) to differentiate balance deficits. *Phys Ther*. 2009;89(5):484–498.
36. Maki BE, McIlroy WE. Control of rapid limb movements for balance recovery: age-related changes and implications for fall prevention. *Age Ageing*. 2006;35(Suppl 2):ii12–ii18.
37. Woollacott MH, Shumway-Cook A, Nashner LM. Aging and posture control: changes in sensory organization and muscular coordination. *Int J Aging Hum Dev*. 1986;23(2):97–114.
38. Studenski S, Duncan PW, Chandler J. Postural responses and effector factors in persons with unexplained falls: results and methodologic issues. *J Am Geriatr Soc*. 1991;39(3):229–234.
39. Tucker MG, Kavanagh JJ, Barrett RS, Morrison S. Age-related differences in postural reaction time and coordination during voluntary sway movements. *Hum Mov Sci*. 2008;27 (5):728–737.
40. Laforest S, St-Pierre DM, Cyr J, Gayton D. Effects of age and regular exercise on muscle strength and endurance. *Eur J Appl Physiol Occup Physiol*. 1990;60(2):104–111.

41. Whipple RH, Wolfson LI, Amerman PM. The relationship of knee and ankle weakness to falls in nursing home residents: an isokinetic study. *J Am Geriatr Soc.* 1987;35(1):13–20.
42. Rubenstein LZ, Powers CM, MacLean CH. Quality indicators for the management and prevention of falls and mobility problems in vulnerable elders. *Ann Intern Med.* 2001;135 (8 Pt 2):686–693.
43. Chang JT, Ganz DA. Quality indicators for falls and mobility problems in vulnerable elders. *J Am Geriatr Soc.* 2007;55 (Suppl 2):S327–S334.
44. Lohman MC, Crow RS, DiMilia PR, Nicklett EJ, Bruce ML, Batsis JA. Operationalisation and validation of the Stopping Elderly Accidents, Deaths, and Injuries (STEADI) fall risk algorithm in a nationally representative sample. *J Epidemiol Community Health.* 2017;71(12):1191–1197.
45. Smeesters C, Hayes WC, McMahon TA. Disturbance type and gait speed affect fall direction and impact location. *J Biomech.* 2001;34(3):309–317.
46. Bromfield SG, Ngameni CA, Colantonio LD, et al. Blood pressure, antihypertensive polypharmacy, frailty, and risk for serious fall injuries among older treated adults with hypertension. *Hypertension.* 2017;70(2):259–266.
47. Sagawa N, Marcum Z, Boudreau R, et al. Low blood pressure levels for fall injuries in older adults: the Health, Aging and Body Composition Study. *Eur J Ageing.* 2018;15(3):321–330.
48. Ooi WL, Hossain M, Lipsitz LA. The association between orthostatic hypotension and recurrent falls in nursing home residents. *Am J Med.* 2000;108(2):106–111.
49. Stevens JA, Phelan EA. Development of STEADI: a fall prevention resource for health care providers. *Health Promot Pract.* 2013;14(5):706–714.
50. Sarmiento K, Lee R. STEADI: CDC's approach to make older adult fall prevention part of every primary care practice. *J Safety Res.* 2017;63:105–109.
51. Miciano AS, Bissen B, Cross CL. Poster 8 the STEADI measure from the Center for Disease Control & Prevention (CDC) and its correlation with clinical observation assessments. *PM R.* 2016;8(9S):S163.
52. Mark JA, Loomis J. The STEADI toolkit: incorporating a fall prevention guideline into the primary care setting. *Nurse Pract.* 2017;42(12):50–55.
53. Eckstrom E, Parker EM, Lambert GH, Winkler G, Dowler D, Casey CM. Implementing STEADI in academic primary care to address older adult fall risk. *Innov Aging.* 2017;1(2):igx028.
54. Greenberg MR, Nguyen MC, Stello B, et al. Mechanical falls: are patients willing to discuss their risk with a health care provider? *J Emerg Med.* 2015;48(1):108–114. e102.
55. Menz HB, Morris ME, Lord SR. Foot and ankle risk factors for falls in older people: a prospective study. *J Gerontol A Biol Sci Med Sci.* 2006;61(8):866–870.
56. Freeman EE, Munoz B, Rubin G, West SK. Visual field loss increases the risk of falls in older adults: the Salisbury eye evaluation. *Invest Ophthalmol Vis Sci.* 2007;48 (10):4445–4450.
57. Johnson L, Buckley JG, Scally AJ, Elliott DB. Multifocal spectacles increase variability in toe clearance and risk of tripping in the elderly. *Invest Ophthalmol Vis Sci.* 2007;48 (4):1466–1471.
58. Haran MJ, Cameron ID, Ivers RQ, et al. Effect on falls of providing single lens distance vision glasses to multifocal glasses wearers: VISIBLE randomised controlled trial. *BMJ.* 2010;340:c2265.
59. Elliott DB, Hotchkiss J, Scally AJ, Foster R, Buckley JG. Intermediate addition multifocals provide safe stair ambulation with adequate "short-term" reading. *Ophthalmic Physiol Opt.* 2016;36(1):60–68.
60. Brannan S, Dewar C, Sen J, Clarke D, Marshall T, Murray PI. A prospective study of the rate of falls before and after cataract surgery. *Br J Ophthalmol.* 2003;87(5):560–562.
61. Agrawal Y, Carey JP, Della Santina CC, Schubert MC, Minor LB. Disorders of balance and vestibular function in US adults: data from the National Health and Nutrition Examination Survey, 2001-2004. *Arch Intern Med.* 2009;169(10):938–944.
62. Whitney S, Alghwiri A, Alghadir A. An overview of vestibular rehabilitation. In: JFAT Lempert, ed. *Handbook of Clinical Neurology.* Elsevier; 2016:137.
63. Halmagyi GM, Curthoys IS, Cremer PD, et al. The human horizontal vestibulo-ocular reflex in response to high-acceleration stimulation before and after unilateral vestibular neurectomy. *Exp Brain Res.* 1990;81(3):479–490.
64. Longridge NS, Mallinson AI. The dynamic illegible E (DIE) test: a simple technique for assessing the ability of the vestibulo-ocular reflex to overcome vestibular pathology. *J Otolaryngol.* 1987;16(2):97–103.
65. Shaffer SW, Harrison AL. Aging of the somatosensory system: a translational perspective. *Phys Ther.* 2007;87(2):193–207.
66. Shumway-Cook A, Horak FB. Assessing the influence of sensory interaction of balance. Suggestion from the field. *Phys Ther.* 1986;66(10):1548–1550.
67. Di Fabio R, Seay R. Use of the "fast evaluation of mobility, balance, and fear" in elderly community dwellers: validity and reliability. *Phys Ther.* 1997;9:904–917.
68. Whitney SL, Wrisley DM. The influence of footwear on timed balance scores of the modified clinical test of sensory interaction and balance. *Arch Phys Med Rehabil.* 2004;85(3):439–443.
69. Cohen H, Heaton LG, Congdon SL, Jenkins HA. Changes in sensory organization test scores with age. *Age Ageing.* 1996;25 (1):39–44.
70. Tsang WW, Hui-Chan CW. Effect of 4- and 8-wk intensive tai chi training on balance control in the elderly. *Med Sci Sports Exerc.* 2004;36(4):648–657.
71. Guideline for the prevention of falls in older persons. American Geriatrics Society, British Geriatrics Society, and American Academy of Orthopaedic Surgeons Panel on Falls Prevention. *J Am Geriatr Soc.* 2001;49(5):664–672.
72. Lord SR, Murray SM, Chapman K, Munro B, Tiedemann A. Sit-to-stand performance depends on sensation, speed, balance, and psychological status in addition to strength in older people. *J Gerontol A Biol Sci Med Sci.* 2002;57(8): M539–M543.
73. Rikli R, Jones C. *Senior Fitness Test Manual.* Champaign, IL: Human Kinetics; 2001.
74. Nandy S, Parsons S, Cryer C, et al. Development and preliminary examination of the predictive validity of the Falls Risk Assessment Tool (FRAT) for use in primary care. *J Public Health (Oxf).* 2004;26(2):138–143.
75. Muir SW, Gopaul K, Montero Odasso MM. The role of cognitive impairment in fall risk among older adults: a systematic review and meta-analysis. *Age Ageing.* 2012;41 (3):299–308.
76. Tinetti ME, Richman D, Powell L. Falls efficacy as a measure of fear of falling. *J Gerontol.* 1990;45(6):P239–P243.
77. Kempen GI, Yardley L, van Haastregt JC, et al. The Short FES-I: a shortened version of the falls efficacy scale-international to assess fear of falling. *Age Ageing.* 2008;37(1):45–50.
78. Yardley L, Beyer N, Hauer K, Kempen G, Piot-Ziegler C, Todd C. Development and initial validation of the Falls Efficacy Scale-International (FES-I). *Age Ageing.* 2005;34 (6):614–619.
79. Liu CJ, Latham NK. Progressive resistance strength training for improving physical function in older adults. *Cochrane Database Syst Rev.* 2009;3:CD002759.

80. Richerson S, Rosendale K. Does tai chi improve plantar sensory ability? A pilot study. *Diabetes Technol Ther.* 2007;9(3):276–286.
81. Hakim R, DiCicco J, Burke J, Hoy T, Roberts E. Differences in balance related measures among older adults participating in tai chi, structured exercise, or no exercise. *J Geriatr Phys Ther.* 2004;27:13–17.
82. Wolf SL, Barnhart HX, Kutner NG, McNeely E, Coogler C, Xu T. Reducing frailty and falls in older persons: an investigation of tai chi and computerized balance training. Atlanta FICSIT Group. Frailty and Injuries: Cooperative Studies of Intervention Techniques. *J Am Geriatr Soc.* 1996;44(5):489–497.
83. Epley JM. The canalith repositioning procedure: for treatment of benign paroxysmal positional vertigo. *Otolaryngol Head Neck Surg.* 1992;107(3):399–404.
84. Bhattacharyya N, Baugh RF, Orvidas L, et al. Clinical practice guideline: benign paroxysmal positional vertigo. *Otolaryngol Head Neck Surg.* 2008;139(5 Suppl 4):S47–S81.
85. Jumani K, Powell J. Benign paroxysmal positional vertigo: management and its impact on falls. *Ann Otol Rhinol Laryngol.* 2017;126(8):602–605.
86. Shelhamer M, Tiliket C, Roberts D, Kramer PD, Zee DS. Short-term vestibulo-ocular reflex adaptation in humans. II. Error signals. *Exp Brain Res.* 1994;100(2):328–336.
87. Klatt BN, Carender WJ, Lin CC, et al. A conceptual framework for the progression of balance exercises in persons with balance and vestibular disorders. *Phys Med Rehabil Int.* 2015;2(4):1044.
88. Moreland JD, Richardson JA, Goldsmith CH, Clase CM. Muscle weakness and falls in older adults: a systematic review and meta-analysis. *J Am Geriatr Soc.* 2004;52(7):1121–1129.
89. Ding L, Yang F. Muscle weakness is related to slip-initiated falls among community-dwelling older adults. *J Biomech.* 2016;49(2):238–243.
90. Reeves ND, Narici MV, Maganaris CN. Myotendinous plasticity to ageing and resistance exercise in humans. *Exp Physiol.* 2006;91(3):483–498.
91. Hughes KJ, Salmon N, Galvin R, Casey B, Clifford AM. Interventions to improve adherence to exercise therapy for falls prevention in community-dwelling older adults: systematic review and meta-analysis. *Age Ageing.* 2018;39(8):709–713.
92. Hauer K, Rost B, Rutschle K, et al. Exercise training for rehabilitation and secondary prevention of falls in geriatric patients with a history of injurious falls. *J Am Geriatr Soc.* 2001;49(1):10–20.
93. Farlie MK, Robins L, Haas R, Keating JL, Molloy E, Haines TP. Programme frequency, type, time and duration do not explain the effects of balance exercise in older adults: a systematic review with a meta-regression analysis. *Br J Sports Med.* 2018. [epub ahead of print] https://doi.org/10.1136/bjsports-2016-096874.
94. Santesso N, Carrasco-Labra A, Brignardello-Petersen R. Hip protectors for preventing hip fractures in older people. *Cochrane Database Syst Rev.* 2014;3:CD001255.
95. Perry SD, Radtke A, McIlroy WE, Fernie GR, Maki BE. Efficacy and effectiveness of a balance-enhancing insole. *J Gerontol A Biol Sci Med Sci.* 2008;63(6):595–602.
96. Hijmans JM, Geertzen JH, Zijlstra W, Hof AL, Postema K. Effects of vibrating insoles on standing balance in diabetic neuropathy. *J Rehabil Res Dev.* 2008;45(9):1441–1449.
97. Aboutorabi A, Arazpour M, Bahramizadeh M, Farahmand F, Fadayevatan R. Effect of vibration on postural control and gait of elderly subjects: a systematic review. *Aging Clin Exp Res.* 2018;30(7):713–726.
98. Aboutorabi A, Arazpour M, Farahmand F, Bahramizadeh M, Fadayevatan R, Abdollahi E. Design and evaluation of vibratory shoe on balance control for elderly subjects: technical note. *Disabil Rehabil Assist Technol.* 2018;13(2):173–177.
99. Lipsitz LA, Lough M, Niemi J, Travison T, Howlett H, Manor B. A shoe insole delivering subsensory vibratory noise improves balance and gait in healthy elderly people. *Arch Phys Med Rehabil.* 2015;96(3):432–439.
100. Galica AM, Kang HG, Priplata AA, et al. Subsensory vibrations to the feet reduce gait variability in elderly fallers. *Gait Posture.* 2009;30(3):383–387.
101. Lin C, Whitney S, Loughlin P, et al. The use of vibrotactile feedback during dual-task standing balance conditions in people with unilateral vestibular hypofunction. *Otol Neurotol.* 2018;39(5):e349–e356.
102. Verrusio W, Gianturco V, Cacciafesta M, Marigliano V, Troisi G, Ripani M. Fall prevention in the young old using an exoskeleton human body posturizer: a randomized controlled trial. *Aging Clin Exp Res.* 2017;29(2):207–214.
103. Silveira P, van de Langenberg R, van Het Reve E, Daniel F, Casati F, de Bruin ED. Tablet-based strength-balance training to motivate and improve adherence to exercise in independently living older people: a phase II preclinical exploratory trial. *J Med Internet Res.* 2013;15(8). e159.
104. Donath L, Rossler R, Faude O. Effects of virtual reality training (exergaming) compared to alternative exercise training and passive control on standing balance and functional mobility in healthy community-dwelling seniors: a meta-analytical review. *Sports Med.* 2016;46(9):1293–1309.
105. Cohen C, Kampel T, Verloo H. Acceptability of an intelligent wireless sensor system for the rapid detection of health issues: findings among home-dwelling older adults and their informal caregivers. *Patient Prefer Adherence.* 2016;10:1687–1695.
106. Gill TM, Williams CS, Robison JT, Tinetti ME. A population-based study of environmental hazards in the homes of older persons. *Am J Public Health.* 1999;89(4):553–556.
107. National Council on Aging. Falls prevention programs: evidence-based falls prevention program review council. https://www.ncoa.org/center-for-healthy-aging/basics-of-evidence-based-programs/apply-ebp/falls-prevention-programs/. Published 2017.

CHAPTER

11

Patient Education: Implications for Physical Therapist Practice

Elizabeth Ruckert, Katherine Beissner

OUTLINE

INTRODUCTION

Educating patients is perhaps the most important and impactful role of the physical therapist. Long after a patient completes an exercise regimen prescribed in the therapy plan of care, what he or she learned about movement and health ideally remains as knowledge gain and/or behavior change. Indeed, patient learning is certainly an underlying goal of physical therapy. Although this goal may not be achieved for every client or patient, there are best practices the physical therapist should consider when designing educational interventions.

In 1985, a Delphi study was performed to develop a consensus definition of patient education: "a planned learning experience using a combination of methods such as teaching, counseling, and behavior modification techniques which influence patient knowledge and health behavior."[1] This definition provides an important foundation for conceptualizing patient education—it is a planned (but can also be spontaneous!) encounter in the clinical environment; it involves not only teaching but also coaching and mentoring to encourage behavior modification; and it impacts the individual patient's unique knowledge and behavioral needs. Fig. 11.1 demonstrates the interplay between the learner, teacher, and environment in patient education delivery. Each of these areas must be considered in the context of a unique learning session to provide effective education. We will dig deeper into each of these areas throughout the chapter.

PATIENT EDUCATION IN PHYSICAL THERAPY

Patient education is not just a goal for our patients; it is considered an essential competency of health professionals, regardless of specialty area. The U.S. Institute of Medicine published *Health Professions Education: A Bridge to Quality,* which outlined core competencies needed for health care professionals in the 21st century.[2] The first professional competency, "provide patient-centered care," specifically denotes the need for health providers to "listen to, clearly inform, communicate with, and educate patients." The report emphasizes that knowledge and information sharing between practitioner and patient are essential to promote health and outcomes. In fact, patient education has been linked to improved self-efficacy, self-care, pain control, and function for patients with many chronic conditions, including chronic obstructive pulmonary disease,[3] osteoporosis,[4] breast cancer,[5] and others.[6] These chronic conditions, although potentially impacting individuals in all age ranges, especially affect older adults and support the demand for quality patient education.

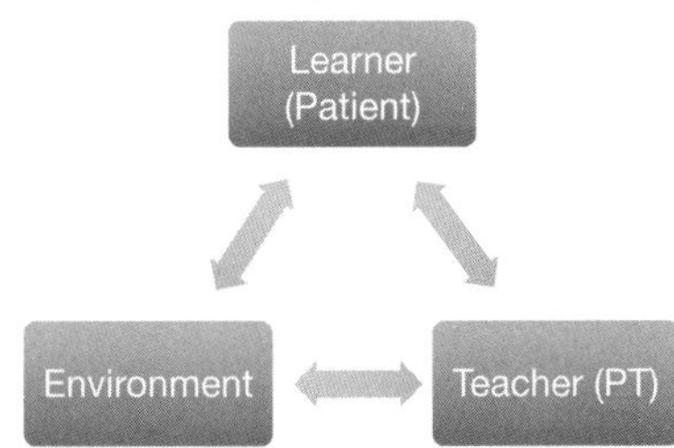

FIG. 11.1 Delivery of patient education considers the learner, the teacher, and the environment. *PT*, physical therapist.

The *Guide to Physical Therapist Practice* describes "patient/client instruction" (or patient education) as an integral component of the physical therapist's patient/client management model. The guide states that patient education should be an intervention "used with *every* patient and client" throughout the plan of care. This includes examination, evaluation, diagnosis, prognosis, interventions, and outcomes. Table 11.1 describes the role of patient education in each part of the patient management process as it relates to a patient poststroke.

What does patient education "throughout the plan of care" really mean? Some studies have suggested that patient education is delivered most frequently in the initial visits of a plan of care and then tapers off,[7] whereas others suggest it occurs in a distributed manner across the plan of care.[8] Physical therapists should avoid providing education only at evaluation and discharge sessions. Instead, consider sharing information in smaller amounts (known in teaching literature as "micro-learning") revisited across many sessions in the plan of care.[9] Planning to provide education in a distributed manner over many sessions in the plan of care is most consistent with the neuroscience of learning[10] and also helps memory.[8] This also means that the therapist should avoid the commonly performed discharge patient education overload, or "last-minute information dumping." Research highlights the importance of quality discharge education and planning to prevent hospital readmissions and adverse events following hospitalization in older adults,[11] including those with heart failure[12] and total joint replacement.[13] There are excellent resources available for patients to take a more active role in ensuring quality discharge instruction. Medicare's "Discharge Planning Checklist Worksheet"[14] highlights many aspects related to physical therapy (PT) including medical equipment information, assistance with daily activities, and what care is planned for the patient after discharge. The Family Caregiver Alliance's "Hospital Discharge Planning:

TABLE 11.1 Patient Education Across the Patient Management Model

Element	Sample Patient EducationTopic Areas	Sample PT Education
Examination	• Rationale for tests/measures selected • Test procedures, including verbal instructions and demonstration	"I am going to use a test called the Berg Balance Scale to assess your risk for falls and see what body system changes (sensory, motor, others) may be contributing to that fall risk."
Evaluation	• Interpretation of test/measure results	"You are having trouble feeling where your left leg is in space. We call that impaired proprioception. As a result, you may have difficulty moving safely in dark environments (like at night)."
Diagnosis	• Primary limitations amenable to PT • Referral to other interdisciplinary team members	"There are many aspects of your mobility that a PT program can help you to address, including your safety around your house and in the community. It also sounds like you are looking to be more connected to the community. I think a referral to a social worker would be helpful to find community resources to increase your social engagement and network in your local neighborhood."
Prognosis	• Focus of PT plan of care (recovery vs. compensation) • Relevant prognostic factors influencing care • Factors important for prevention of long-term disability	"We are going to focus your therapy plan on getting you to walk without the cane. This seems possible given the rate of your recovery since leaving the hospital, your improving awareness of the left side of your body, and your balance reactions."
Intervention	• Specific training interventions: aerobic, muscle activation, sensory retraining, range of motion, others • Home exercise program	"Do you know why aerobic training is so important for us to include in your exercise program? This is a very prevalent problem after stroke and contributes to inactivity, decreased quality of life, and increased risk for future cardiac events."
Outcomes	• Changes on outcome measure performance (positive or negative) • Progress toward therapy goals • Establishing new therapy goals • Referral to other interdisciplinary team members • Community support resources	"You have achieved three of your four therapy goals to date. These related to improving your balance, increasing your walking speed, and getting down and back up from the floor with supervision. Great job!"

PT, physical therapy.

TABLE 11.2 Resources for Commonly Avoided Patient Education Topics for Older Adults

General Health Resources	Stress Management Resources
• **Exercise:** Go4Life Program, http://www.nia.nih.gov/Go4Life (National Institute on Aging) • **Physical activity:** Healthy Aging in Parks Program, http://www.nrpa.org/health-aging-in-parks (National Recreation and Park Association) • **Sleep:** "Aging and Sleep," http://www.sleep.org (National Sleep Foundation) • **Diet:** "Choosing Healthy Meals as You Get Older," http://www.ChooseMyPlate.gov/olderadults (U.S. Department of Agriculture) • **Cognitive Health:** "Talking About Brain Health & Aging: The Basics," http://www.acl.gov (Administration for Community Living) • **Engagement:** Arts & Aging Toolkit, http://www.creativeaging.org/resources/toolkits (National Center for Creative Aging)	• http://www.healthfinder.gov (Office of Disease Prevention and Health Promotion) • http://www.Healthtools.aarp.org (AARP) • "Coping with Stress and Anxiety" (American Psychological Association)

A Guide for Families and Caregivers"[15] empowers caregivers to advocate for information, resources, and assistance for a loved one being discharged home or to other medical facilities. These are just two examples of web-based or print resources that a physical therapist can provide an older patient and his or her family to improve discharge planning and education.

Sluijs and colleagues defined five common areas of physical therapy education: (1) illness related, (2) home exercise, (3) advice/information, (4) general health information, and (5) stress-related problems.[16] Information related to the health condition and home exercises is the most frequently provided by physical therapists, whereas education on general health and stress management is the least frequently provided.[7] This may be surprising—isn't promotion of health and wellness an essential part of the physical therapist's role? These results are a helpful reminder for physical therapists to provide education in these areas, especially when treating the older adult. A plethora of resources exist to help promote a healthy lifestyle of physical activity, diet, sleep, cognitive health, and stress management in older clients. Refer to Table 11.2 for easy-to-access resources designed specifically for the older adult. Physical therapists should consider the importance of education for prevention and wellness with all older adults, in addition to specific injury or health condition information and home exercise instruction.

Although many physical therapists did not enter the profession with the primary goal of teaching, physical therapists report teaching as a necessary skill in clinical practice.[17] Resnik and Jensen's theory of expert physical therapist practice highlights an "emphasis on education" as a hallmark of the expert physical therapist's clinical practice style.[18] In a qualitative study of physical therapists providing care to outpatients with low back pain, a central theme included education as the most important part of physical therapy intervention.[8] Patients expect to be educated as well. Current literature investigating patient preferences for the patient–physician relationship highlights patient desire for education and information as top priorities.[19] In terms of patient expectations for their relationship with physical therapists, a study by Grannis investigated what older adults considered the "ideal physical therapist."[20] The sample population, all born before 1920, reported that three of the seven most important qualities of a physical therapist were related to teaching and communication: (1) "presents instructions to the patient in a clear and concise manner"; (2) "instructs the patient clearly in the purpose of a procedure"; and (3) "effectively demonstrates while instructing." Other items were related to thoroughness, empathy, humor, and patient comfort during the session.[20] Of note, the study subjects were "Traditionalists," or part of the "Silent Generation" (born before 1942). These preferences toward teaching are consistent with viewing the teacher (or therapist) as an expert and expecting clear instructions for activities.[21] This paternalistic preference for health care by some older adults comes in direct challenge to current views on how patients should participate. The current era of health care, characterized by an emphasis on patient choice, autonomy, and shared decision making,[2] may be more reflective of preferences of aging baby boomers. Thus, physical therapists may find themselves educating some older clients on *why* the physical therapist offers choice and opportunity for decision making within treatment sessions and how important an understanding of the older patient's learning preferences and perceptions are to creating a successful plan of care.

We have now established the need and desire for teaching as a part of physical therapist practice. There are challenges, however, to delivering patient education effectively. Table 11.3 considers barriers to patient education across three areas: patient factors, therapist factors, and environmental factors. Understanding these barriers and designing patient education in anticipation of these barriers will help to make patient learning outcomes positive and effective. We will now discuss the "education basics" behind patient education, starting with learning theory.

TABLE 11.3 Barriers to Patient Education Among Health Care Providers

	Perceived Barriers to Patient Education	Strategy to Overcome
Patient Factors	• Literacy/health literacy[4]	Assess patient literacy level
	• Attitudes about illness or disability[17]	Ask questions to understand patient's view of illness/disability to frame education
	• Preference for passive role in therapy[17]	Describe why active patient role is desired in therapy; once goals are established, minimize choices offered if passive role is preferred
	• Unrealistic expectations for therapy outcomes[17]	Break down unrealistic expectations into smaller, meaningful, and attainable outcomes
	• Impaired cognitive status[17]	Empower patient as able; target education to caregiver (incorporating both patient's needs and caregiver's needs)
	• Emotional lability[17]	Seek resources or support from psychology or mental health providers to assist in education delivery
	• Lack of family/caregiver participation[17]	Consider role of other health care advocate or LTC ombudsman (http://www.eldercare.acl.gov)
Therapist Factors	• Priority for hands-on clinical care[94]	Reprioritize patient sessions to include both physical interventions *and* education. Education should be viewed as equal priority
	• Limited time[17]	Consider "bare minimum" education that should be provided in each therapy session to minimize time constraints; spread out education across multiple sessions in small amounts
	• Lack of knowledge[79,94]	Assess personal strengths and weaknesses in education topics and seek out colleagues and other professional resources to help fill knowledge gaps; the WHO has created profiles of patient education competencies for some chronic diseases like diabetes and asthma[79]
	• Lack of confidence or comfort with diagnosis[94]	Seek out colleagues and professional resources to help fill knowledge gaps; observe a colleague or supervisor provide education to patients with this diagnosis; set up mentoring opportunities
	• Poor communication skills[95]	Seek mentoring from peers or supervisors to improve communication approach with patients
	• Limited reimbursement[94]	Create therapeutic culture where education is valued regardless of reimbursement; provide education while performing other billable activities
Environmental Factors	• Space layout and equipment setup[17]	Establish areas in clinic or care areas where education is more conducive; reserve quiet treatment room if available
	• Distractions[17]	Provide education when distractions are minimal (e.g., during middle of treatment vs. beginning/end; when engaged in 1:1 activities vs. large gym equipment)
	• Organizational culture does not value education[95]	Raise concerns regarding priority for patient education at staff meetings or during staff feedback opportunities for the health care system
	• Fractionated education across health care team members[95]	Encourage communication and sharing of education resources across team members for consistent approach and message
	• Limited available resources or poor quality (print, media, etc.)[76]	Seek out opportunities for quality improvement projects (or student projects) to improve educational material availability/quality; encourage patients to provide feedback on strengths and areas for improvement in education resources

LTC, long-term care; *WHO*, World Health Organization.

LEARNING THEORY: UNDERSTANDING HOW WE LEARN

Adult Learning Theory

Helping older adults comprehend, retain, and apply what is taught in therapy requires an understanding of how one learns. Older adults are, by nature, adult learners. Malcolm Knowles developed the theory of andragogy, which emphasizes six key characteristics of adult learners[22]:

1. Adults bring prior experience to the learning environment.
2. Adults learn best when there is a need for immediate application.
3. Adults learn most when the topic is related to their life context and roles.
4. Adults want some control and responsibility over what they learn.
5. Adults possess internal motivation to learn.
6. Adults need to know *why* they should learn.

A physical therapist should take these principles of adult learning into account when educating older adults. Some aspects of adult learning theory may come more naturally in the physical therapist's educational design, whereas others require more effort. For example, using patient goals to help frame education toward a patient's immediate needs (tenet 2) or linking education to family, work, and leisure roles (tenet 3) may inherently come from information collected during the patient's subjective intake. More deliberate structuring of the patient education may be required to provide the patient with a feeling of control over his or her learning. In addition, the physical therapist should inquire about and build upon prior learning experiences the patient brings to the PT session. This includes not only learning in prior physical therapy (as applicable) but also experiences about learning in other facets of life, including work, hobbies, and leisure time. Table 11.4 provides examples of how adult learning principles relate to patient education in PT.

TABLE 11.4 Applying Adult Learning Theory to Patient Education

Principles of Adult Learning	Sample Questions to Ask Older Patient to Tailor Patient Education
1. Adults bring prior experience to the learning environment	• What do you already know about this health condition? • How did you learn best in prior episodes of PT? • What have been positive learning experiences you have had related to your health? Negative ones? • Can you tell me about any new work-related tasks or hobbies that you have learned recently? What strategies helped your learning?
2. Adults learn most when there is a need for immediate application	• What are your goals for PT? • What is the most important thing for you to leave PT knowing about today? • How do you hope to apply what you learn in PT?
3. Adults learn most when the topic is related to their life context and roles	• Tell me more about your work. • What other roles are important to you? • What is your home setup?
4. Adults want some control and responsibility over learning	• Do you have ideas on how you would like to learn more about this? • Would you prefer to talk about exercises related to your walking or exercises related to your strength today? • Would you like to learn about how to prevent a similar issue in the future today or save that for another session?
5. Adults possess internal motivation to learn	• Why do you want to know more about this? • What motivates you to come to PT today?
6. Adults need to know *why* they should learn	• Do you know why this topic is important for reaching your PT goals? • Do you see how this information relates to your current movement problems? • Do you know how this will impact the progression of your disease?

PT, physical therapy.

Experiential Learning Cycle

The role of experience in learning is not only highlighted in adult learning theory but also central to Kolb's Experiential Learning Cycle (ELC). David Kolb describes learning as a cyclical process that centers around one's experience and reflection.[23] According to Kolb, learning stems from experiences that require the individual to interpret, process, and make meaning. The process of reflecting on and interpreting experiences creates new learning that is applied to other experiences and continues the learning cycle. Kolb further describes learning styles or preferences that individuals have with initiating learning in certain parts of this experiential cycle. We will discuss this more later in this chapter.

The ELC provides a helpful framework for patient education. The physical therapist may have a role at any part of the learning cycle: creating meaningful patient learning experiences, helping the patient reflect on experiences, and/or providing context for conceptualizing experiences. To optimize learning it is important to create a clinical environment that encourages patients to share their life experiences, allowing the physical therapist to relate new learning to those patient experiences. Creating an open atmosphere for sharing on the part of the patient requires the therapist to build a trusting relationship with the patient. This is another important component of expert physical therapist practice: the patient–therapist relationship.[18] Refer to Fig. 11.2 for ideas on how to use the experiential learning cycle to create patient education and learning opportunities in physical therapy sessions.

To create meaningful learning out of patient experiences, the physical therapist must listen carefully when a patient shares updates in therapy. Consider these scenarios:

- An older patient shares an experience related to his or her injury or health but has inaccurately drawn conclusions that require the physical therapist to

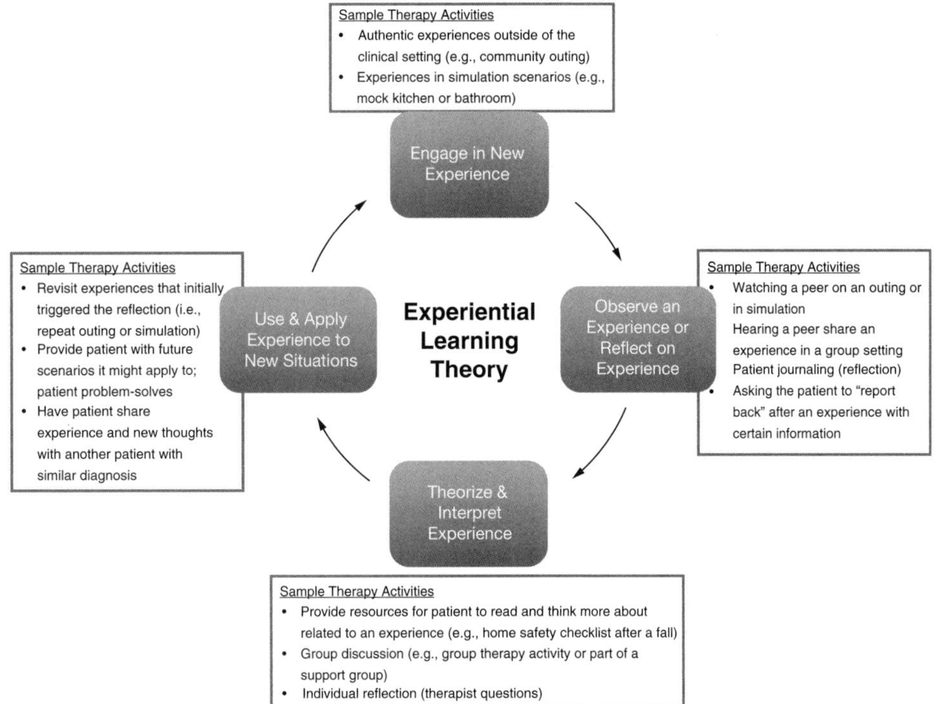

FIG. 11.2 Applying Kolb's experiential learning theory to patient education.

recalibrate—for example, a patient who experienced muscle soreness that then went away within 24 hours of a PT session, but the patient discontinued the exercise because he or she thought it was an adverse reaction.

- An older patient shares an experience with the physical therapist but the patient fails to see the learning moment—for example, the older adult who reports a near fall at home but dismisses the link to his or her health condition. Therapist questioning can help the patient to draw links between the patient's lower extremity sensory impairment from diabetes and tripping over a floor rug. The patient would gain new insight for how this can be prevented in the future.
- An older patient shares a frustration with an aspect of his or her health condition that other patients have also identified as a frustration—for example, a patient with diabetes feels frustrated about the fluctuations in glycemic control with diet and exercise. The physical therapist can identify another patient with a history of diabetes who may be willing to share his or her experiences and strategies for addressing this frustration of the disease.

Social Cognitive Theory

Derived from social learning theory, social cognitive theory (SCT) provides the framework for educational interventions in a variety of contexts and has demonstrated effectiveness in interventions geared toward increasing physical activity in older populations.[24,25] SCT describes learning in a social context, affected by personal, environmental, and behavioral factors. We will first focus on the personal factors and consider behavioral and environmental factors later in the chapter.

Two personal factors that older adults bring to the therapy learning environment are beliefs about one's own ability to adopt a new behavior (self-efficacy) and beliefs about the potential of the new behavior to produce desired results (outcome expectancies). Another fundamental premise of SCT is the concept of vicarious experience as fundamental to instruction—individuals learn by observing the behaviors and the behavioral consequences of others. Thus, credible role models are used to learn and reinforce desired behavior change.

The role of personal factors should not be underestimated when trying to promote learning and behavior change with patients, and the therapist should inquire about these areas when initiating patient education: *What areas of PT do you feel confident with? Where do you feel less confident? What outcomes are you expecting?*

There are four main ways that self-efficacy can be bolstered to maximize learning[26,27]:

1. Performance accomplishments: Successful accomplishment of a given activity or task will help to improve self-efficacy for learning. Physical therapists should create goals with small, measurable, achievable components for older adults to experience success.
2. Vicarious experience: Seeing or hearing about other individuals with similar characteristics (e.g., age, health condition, disability, life roles) learning about or accomplishing a given task helps to improve self-efficacy of learning. Physical therapists can utilize peer educators to help older adults have role models for learning in therapy.

3. Verbal encouragement: Positive feedback and verbal support are important in boosting self-efficacy for learning. Praise and encouragement from physical therapists and health care providers are especially effective for older adults.
4. Personal perceptions: Accurate interpretation of a person's response (physiologically or affectively) to a given task is important for self-efficacy for learning. Physical therapists can provide realistic interpretations for how well a skill is learned or how an activity is performed to help an older adult measure success.

Interestingly, for behavior change and learning to occur, outcome expectancy for physical activity appears to be more important for older adults than younger individuals.[28] Careful attention to the patient's beliefs about the perceived benefit of a course of therapy or a desired behavior change is especially important. The following are suggestions for improving outcome expectations:

1. Create opportunities for patients to experience positive outcomes of desired behavior (e.g., reduced pain or improved pain after a brief bout of physical activity). Cue the patient to reflect on these outcomes.
2. Discuss research outcomes in a user-friendly manner, perhaps by using infographics.
3. Provide therapy near credible peer role models who have had successful outcomes, or show pictures/videos demonstrating positive behavior outcomes using credible peer models.
4. Address concerns with the physical environment that might interfere with the desired behavior.

Bolstering self-efficacy and outcome expectations for your older patient can be easy: "With time and effort, patients I have worked with like you do really well with learning and understanding these concepts."[29,30] Yes, the therapist simply verbalizing to the patient that he or she expects positive outcomes from the patient based on past experience has been shown to improve learning!

Peer education can be helpful in enhancing self-efficacy through the sharing of experiences that are relatable for a patient with a given health condition or disability, and standardized programs for self-management of chronic conditions are available in many communities. Peer education has been shown to facilitate learning and behavior change for older adults in a variety of areas, including fall prevention,[31] osteoporosis management,[32] and end-of-life care planning.[33] A Cochrane review of self-management programs for chronic conditions found that layperson education had short-term improvements in self-efficacy, self-rated health, cognitive symptom management, and frequency of aerobic exercise.[34] The benefits of peer education go beyond just the patient, or receiver of information. Literature investigating the benefits of these models for the peer teacher suggest the experience improved his or her own learning and knowledge on the topic, as well as skills for facilitating groups.[35] The benefits of peer education are highlighted in Fig. 11.3.

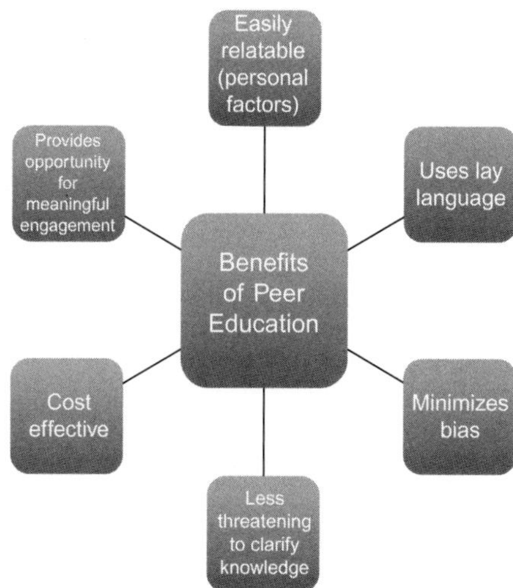

FIG. 11.3 Benefits of peer education for older adults. *(Data from Peel NM, Warburton J. Using senior volunteers as peer educators: what is the evidence of effectiveness in falls prevention? Australas J Ageing. 2009;28[1]:7–11.)*

There are, however, some drawbacks for the physical therapist to consider when referring patients to peer education programs. Notably, peer educators require training and support,[36] and the quality of instruction may therefore vary, even with the use of standardized instructional materials. Even with considerable training peer educators do not replace medical professionals in terms of knowledge or ability to provide medical advice.[37]

Reflection

Reflection is a component of several learning theories (e.g., Kolb's ELC, transformative learning theory[38]), but here we will discuss it as an educational strategy. Reflection is the process of thinking deeply about an experience to make meaning, arrive at new insights, or change perspective.[21] Reflection requires a variety of skills on the part of the learner to create learning: self-awareness, description, critical analysis, synthesis, and evaluation.[39] These are high-level learning skills based on Bloom's taxonomy and may not come easily for many learners.[40] Therefore, using reflection as a learning tool may not be appropriate for all patients and when used will require mentoring and patience on the part of the therapist and increased effort on the part of the patient. In their systematic review of reflection and reflective practice in health care, Mann and colleagues emphasized that reflection requires "purposeful critical analysis of knowledge and experience."[41] This skill—purposeful critical analysis or "critical thinking"—is an important one for patients to possess for independence in life roles at home and in the community.

Reflection is a three-staged process.[42] The first stage involves a "trigger event" that creates discomfort or uneasiness. Next, the learner must analyze the feelings and make sense of those feelings. Lastly, a new perspective is learned and adopted.[39] Questions are the main tool that physical therapists use to drive the reflective process with patients.

Purposeful and systematic questioning is necessary. Plack and Greenberg describe two helpful frameworks for engaging a learner in reflection: time dependent and content dependent.[42] Time-dependent reflective questions are based on the work of Schon[43] and Killion and Todnem.[44] They engage the learner in thinking critically "in-action," or during the experience; "on-action," or after the experience; and "for action," or for a future experience. Content-dependent questions stem from the work of Mezirow,[38] who proposed that reflection can occur based on the *content* of an experience, the *process* of an experience, or the *premise* of an experience.

Let's put Mezirow's reflective framework in a patient context. A patient experienced difficulty maneuvering his wheelchair in public places, including accessing a public bus on a community outing. Content reflection by the patient would focus on what the background of the problem was: *What did the patient know about the adapted capacity of the bus? What was the procedure for requesting the bus to stop? What position should he have been in while waiting on the curb?* Process reflection would focus on how the patient tried to solve the problem: *How did he solve the problem for getting onto the bus? What was an alternate strategy for getting onto the bus?* Premise reflection focuses on the values, biases, and assumptions the patient brought to the experience, and consideration of alternate perspectives: *Why did he get angry about the way he had to get on the bus? What did he assume the bus driver would assist him with? How did the situation make the bus driver feel?* As you can see, reflective questioning requires the therapist to dig much deeper than simply asking "How did that go?" or "What would you do differently next time?" Helping a patient reflect for learning involves the therapist deliberately prompting the patient with questions that help him or her become more self-aware, descriptive, analytic, and evaluative of a given situation.[42]

So far, this section has described the reflective process as driven by the therapist. But another important aim of patient education should be for the patient to develop this reflective process within himself or herself. Reflection is what will help the patient become a critical thinker and problem solver in future situations outside of PT. The physical therapist should fade his or her reflective questions over the course of the plan of care to enable the patient to develop the skills for critical analysis and self-reflection. The therapist might consider explicitly sharing aspects of the Plack and Greenberg frameworks[42] for the patient to think about and report back on. For example, "Did you only think about how it felt in the moment? Did you consider how the experience might impact your future approach to that situation?" or "Did you think about your process along with the assumptions or biases you brought to the situation?" Refer to Table 11.5 for examples of applying these frameworks to a patient case.

TABLE 11.5 Applying Principles of Reflection to Facilitate Patient Learning

Case example: Mr. O'Day is a 75-year-old male s/p knee replacement in an inpatient rehabilitation facility. Today's task: ascending/descending a curb. Mr. O'Day has been limited in rehabilitation by pain, ROM limitations, and weakness in the right LE. During ascent, Mr. O'Day starts with placing his right leg on the step first. He attempts to push up but is limited by pain and decreased ability to generate force. The physical therapist asks, "Is this going how you expected? How might you change what you're doing to be more effective?" Mr. O'Day changes legs, initiates the step with his left LE, and completes the task with moderate assistance. He requests a rest break. The physical therapist facilitates additional reflection on his performance.

Time-Dependent Reflective Questions	Content-Dependent Reflective Questions

• Reflection-in-Action
  • Is this going how you expected?
  • How might you change your approach to be more effective?
  • What did you want to happen now?
• Reflection-on-Action
  • What happened?
  • Were you successful? Why or why not?
  • Do you feel good about the outcome?
  • Is this what you had hoped would occur?
• Reflection-for-Action
  • How will you approach this task next time? Similarly or differently?
  • How will you plan for dealing with a curb next time?
  • What do you think would help you achieve a better outcome?
	• Content (think "What" questions)
	  • What did you know about approaching a curb or stair?
	  • What additional information would you like to know?
	  • What do you know about the resources or capabilities you bring to the task?
	• Process (think "How" questions)
	  • How did you learn from this process?
	  • How did you solve the problem?
	  • What strategies did you use to be successful?
	  • How did you approach the task? How could you approach it differently next time?
	  • How effective were you in completing the task? How could you be more effective next time?
	• Premise (think "Why" questions)
	  • Why did you react like that to the challenge of the task?
	  • Why did you assume the task would be easy or hard?
	  • Did you bring any biases to the situation?

LE, lower extremity; *ROM*, range of motion; *s/p*, status post.
(Adapted from Plack & Greenberg.[42])

Keep in mind that reflective questioning will be important for the physical therapist to utilize when facilitating caregiver learning as well. A caregiver can also be trained by the therapist to ask the patient reflective, problem-solving questions as part of a home education program to develop patient insight, independence, and autonomy.

In this section, we reviewed educational theory that relates to patient education. Consideration of adult learning, experiential learning, social learning, and reflective theories will help the physical therapist to design patient education more effectively. Next we will think about the contributions that the older adult learner, the physical therapist (as teacher), and the environment bring to the learning situation.

THE OLDER LEARNER

Without consideration of the unique characteristics of the patient and the environment, a physical therapist runs the risk of providing generic education that does not meet the learner's needs or the therapist's goal.[45] Fig. 11.4 highlights those influences that should be considered and assessed by the therapist *before* initiating patient education. Keep in mind that patient education applies to many learners outside of just the patient! Although the focus of this chapter is on the older patient, don't forget that family members, caregivers, and other health care providers all require PT education to maximize the older patient's response to PT. As you read, consider how the information may apply to these other learners in health care.

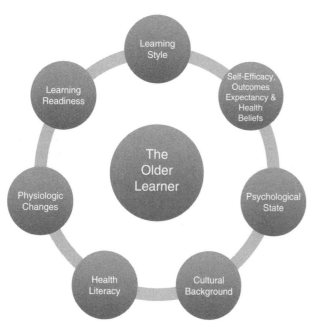

FIG. 11.4 Factors influencing the older adult's learning capacity.

Learning Style

Most people have a preferred way to take in and learn new information. Some prefer to see new information presented visually, some prefer to hear new information presented orally, and some prefer to touch and feel new information kinesthetically. Table 11.6 describes these preferences and educational methods a therapist might use to appeal to each of these styles. Although people can learn through any of these modalities, usually one is a favored method. This does not mean that all information throughout therapy needs to be presented in one manner, but it can be helpful to use the patient's preferred modality to engage and motivate him or her to learn. Teaching best practices encourages health care providers to assess patient learning styles prior to providing education.[45] The therapist can get an idea of a patient's preferred learning methods by asking simple questions: "There is a lot of information to understand about your diagnosis and therapy care. What is the best way to help you learn? We can use tools that involve reading materials, listening, watching videos, or getting hands-on practice."[46] Or, "When you learn new things, how do you like to first be exposed to the information? Seeing it? Hearing it? Feeling it?" Asking these questions during a patient's

TABLE 11.6 Learning Styles and Patient Education Methods[17,45]

	Description	Clinical Teaching Strategies
Visual	Learner prefers to *see* information presented visually—in pictures, diagrams, graphs, charts	• Use printed handouts • Use videos • Use gestures and demonstrations to supplement information
Auditory	Learner prefers to *hear* information presented through speaking, discussion, and talking things out	• Use verbal explanations • Patient or therapist read printed materials out loud • Use auditory recordings (podcasts) or videos • Verbal explanations over simulation/ demonstration
Kinesthetic	Learner prefers to *feel, touch, and experience* information presented kinesthetically	• Use physical activities and simulations • Use models and equipment for patients to touch • Use demonstrations that patient actively participates in

evaluation or therapy session will help to tailor the learning to the patient's ideal strategy.

Visual, auditory, and kinesthetic learning styles help to describe how a learner prefers to perceive information, or take information in. Another aspect of learning styles that is important to consider is how a learner prefers to *process* information.[21] This brings us back to David Kolb and his experiential learning cycle. Kolb suggested that four learning styles emerge depending on how learners prefer to take in information and how learners process information.[23] Think about these styles as fluctuating between preferring to *think* about information (i.e., compare experiences to theories) versus *experience* learning hands on (i.e., actively participate in specific examples of concepts), and then fluctuating between processing information through *observation* versus *experimentation*. Here is how Kolb described each of the learning styles that emerges from these preferences and how they might apply in clinic with an older patient with osteoporosis who needs education about the role of exercise in maintaining bone health and preventing future fractures.

- **Assimilators** prefer to learn through analyzing and comparing theory with experience. They like to spend time thinking about and understanding the premise of a concept first. These learners process information by observing experiences and gathering more information. Background information is very important for this learning style. An older patient who is an assimilator would likely benefit from having a resource to review before having the therapist explain more about a topic. For example, an older patient who is learning about his or her risk for future fractures with osteoporosis might benefit from first reading about osteoporosis and the benefits of exercise in print materials or on the web. Assimilators are less apt to want to actively "dig in" when learning through application, but instead to think and reflect.
- **Convergers** like to learn through understanding theory (like assimilators) but then prefer applying information actively. They spend some time using theory and background information to provide understanding, but then like to solve problems and use information for "real world" application. Older patients who are convergers would likely benefit from reviewing background information and then thinking about how it directly applies to them. They solve problems practically and are realistic. For example, an older patient who is learning about his or her risk for future fractures with osteoporosis might benefit from reading about strategies to reduce fracture risk immediately followed by considering how to apply the recommendations to his or her own life with concrete diet and exercise strategies.
- **Accommodators** like to learn information through experience and active involvement. These learners are less concerned with theory and do not spend much time reflecting. These are active problem solvers who like to dive into practicing, thinking about solutions, and trying out different approaches. This type of learner wants to actively "do" and does not want to read and think when learning. For example, an older patient who is learning about his or her risk for future fractures with osteoporosis would benefit from jumping right into problem-solving ways to decrease fracture risk. Immediately practicing exercises or creating ideas for lifestyle modifications will be more beneficial for this patient's learning than an informational brochure.
- **Divergers** prefer to learn through experience and reflection. Divergers are very interested in how information or problems apply to them by thinking about lots of possibilities. This person is a social learner and prefers to talk and think out loud. For example, an older patient who is learning about his or her risk for future fractures would be interested in thinking about all of the different risk factors that contribute to fractures and brainstorming ways to address each one. The patient's brainstorming will be directly applicable to his or her own life and experience.

It might be a little harder in clinic to figure out a patient's learning style based on Kolb's theory compared to the sensory learning–style preferences. Often, patients will have preferences related to more than one of these learning styles. Knowing how to frame education around these learning styles can be determined by asking your patient a few simple questions: "Is background information and theory important to your learning or are you more concerned in how the information directly applies to you?" "Are you more interested in learning by 'doing' your home exercise program, or would you prefer to learn about why each exercise is being proposed and have time to think about the exercises before performing them?" "When learning about your health, are you motivated by facts and resources or are you motivated by thinking through your personal needs and problems?" The answers to these questions can help you determine the best frame for your education: theory versus practice, thinking versus doing, brainstorming and creativity versus practicality. Another helpful hint to determining your patient's learning style is to listen to the types of questions or comments the patient brings to the learning environment. Consider these patient-generated questions posed about a prescribed exercise program: "Why do I have to do this exercise?" (the assimilator), or "Why give me all these options when I like this exercise best?" (the converger), or "What if I did this type of exercise or tried that type of exercise?" (the diverger), or "Why don't you give me more information while I'm trying the exercise?" (the accommodator). Fig. 11.5 helps to pull all of this information together and utilize different teaching/education methods depending on the learning style of your patient.

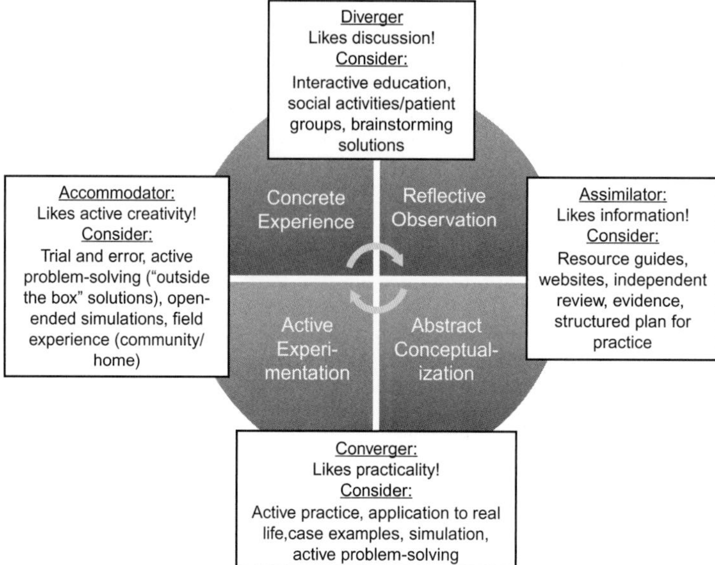

FIG. 11.5 Kolb's learning styles applied to patient education activities. *(Data from Kolb D. Experiential Learning: Experience as the Source of Learning and Development. Englewood Cliffs, NJ: Prentice-Hall; 1984.)*

Self-Efficacy, Outcomes Expectations, and Health Beliefs

Health beliefs are another important consideration for the therapist in crafting education for patients. The health beliefs model (HBM) incorporates concepts from social cognitive theory[47] and describes factors associated with older adults' adoption of desirable health behaviors. As shown in Fig. 11.6, this model defines five factors that contribute to adherence to recommended health behavior:

1. Perceived severity: the individual's perception of the seriousness of the health condition or the seriousness of not treating the health condition
2. Perceived susceptibility: the individual's perception of his or her likelihood of acquiring a condition or obtaining a poor outcome. Combined, perceived susceptibility and perceived severity define a level of "perceived threat." Higher perceived threat increases the likelihood of action.
3. Outcome expectations: the perceived effectiveness of the intervention, similar to SCT. The HBM balances the perceived benefits of action with the barriers.
4. Perceived barriers: obstacles to initiating or sustaining treatment, for example, inconvenience, cost, pain.
5. Cues to action: stimuli to encourage behavior change, including therapist or family member encouragement.

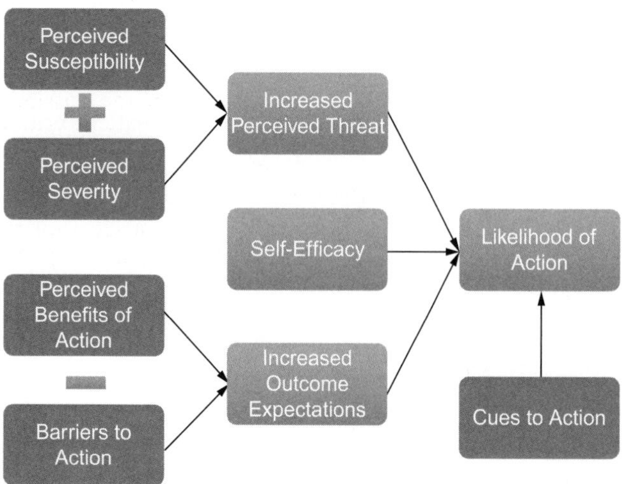

FIG. 11.6 Health beliefs model.

Although not explicitly designed as a model for tailored patient education, the HBM can be used by the physical therapist to guide careful questioning of patients in order to identify education areas that may enhance behavior change. Helping patients understand the "threat" of their condition and potential for positive intervention outcomes, along with enhanced self-efficacy, should increase the likelihood of behavior change. Research shows that perceived benefits, perceived barriers, and perceived susceptibility to dementia are associated with older adults' intent to be screened for cognitive decline,[48] and perceived benefits and barriers and stronger cues to action were associated with participation in community-based cardiac rehabilitation programming.[49]

Psychological State

Understanding your patient's frame of mind in therapy is an important prerequisite for learning. A patient who is approaching physical therapy with anxiety, depression, or fear will likely have difficulty learning. Literature shows that depression in older adults is related to cognitive deficits, including decreased memory, processing speed, attention, and executive functioning.[50,51] In fact, depression has been linked to medial temporal lobe atrophy and increased risk for cognitive impairment, including Alzheimer disease and dementia.[51] Anxiety, on the other hand, has more mixed effects on cognition. Some studies suggest a "U-shaped" interference of anxiety on cognition: Moderate levels of anxiety improve attention and memory, but low or high levels of anxiety are detrimental to cognition.[50] Pietrzak and colleagues found that healthy older adults with "mild worry symptoms" had difficulty learning a new task, and this also predicted cognitive decline at 2-year follow-up.[52]

Does this mean that patient education does not apply to older adults with an impaired psychological state? Certainly not. Education, however, must be tailored to the unique patient's needs. First, the therapist needs to establish trust and understanding with the patient. Provide time for the patient to share how he or she is feeling. Acknowledgment of the patient's emotional state and its impact on learning and performance in therapy should be discussed. Providing personal anecdotes of a therapist's own struggles with health or physical activity may help to create a common ground with a patient and establish rapport.[53] The therapist should try to alleviate any sources of stress within the therapy session. Therapists should avoid quizzing, which may be anxiety producing for the patient. Instead, posing open-ended questions and providing extra time for the patient to process and respond is helpful.[53] Fear of falling, pain, and additional injury are commonly experienced by older adults and should be validated and addressed by the therapist in education interventions. The therapist should find positives in the patient's presentation and learning, as praise and positive reinforcement can help learning.[54] Therapists can consider asking a patient if he or she is in a good mindset for education that day. The patient may be experiencing information overload and may want to focus on performing familiar tasks rather than confronting new material. In some cases, postponing education to another session may be more beneficial if the patient is having an especially challenging day. Similarly, education should be approached throughout the PT plan of care and not provided in large amounts in one session. Given the working memory and processing challenges that anxiety and depression can create, providing multiple exposures to education on a given topic may be necessary. Older adults with anxiety or depression may need breaks during patient education to facilitate learning; consider a walk or other exercise activity as a "motor break" between education interventions. Lastly, patients with emotional or cognitive challenges may appreciate attending group education but should not be put on the spot to actively participate. Observing others may be a helpful learning strategy.[53]

Another helpful psychological state to consider with the older learner is determining the presence of a fixed or growth mindset. Older patients bring with them a lot of past experiences related to learning—at home, as a student, at work, in hobbies and other situations. The mindset with which they approached prior learning can impact learning in PT. Carol Dweck, a psychologist from Stanford University, has studied the effect of mindset on learning for individuals across many age groups and situations (school, business, interpersonal relationships, etc.).[55] A person with a fixed mindset thinks that he or she is born with an innate set of abilities that can't be changed or grown. An older adult who approaches PT with a fixed mindset might think, "I have always been a terrible student, so learning this health information is going to be impossible for me" or "I've never been good at exercise—it's not something I can learn or do well." In contrast, a person with a growth mindset is one who believes that effort and challenges create new learning. With persistence and effort, one's learning and abilities can improve and change. An older adult who approaches PT with a growth mindset will think, "Understanding new things about my health and body is hard, but I am up for the effort" or "Learning and remembering these exercises is a fun challenge!"

The good news is that mindsets can change! People with a fixed mindset can change to a growth mindset perspective with education and coaching. Here are four quick questions[55] that can be used to assess growth versus fixed mindset in patients: "Tell me how much you agree or disagree with the following statements":

- "Your intelligence is something very basic about you that you can't change very much" (agree = fixed mindset; disagree = growth mindset).
- "You can learn new things, but you can't really change how intelligent you are" (agree = fixed mindset; disagree = growth mindset).
- "No matter how much intelligence you have, you can always change it quite a bit" (agree = growth mindset; disagree = fixed mindset).
- "You can always substantially change how intelligent you are" (agree = growth mindset; disagree = fixed mindset).

If a patient is presenting with a fixed mindset, consider providing education on their ability to learn new things. Providing the patient with information about the plasticity and potential for the older brain to learn may be an important prerequisite to other health-related education. Neuroplasticity can serve as a powerful educational tool for helping an older patient see the potential and possibility within themselves (growth mindset!).[56] The National Institute on Aging has many resources for cognitive health for older adults.[57] Clearly, consideration of mindset and strategies to enhance an older patient's mindset prior to education should be a structured component of PT education.

Cultural Background

Culture is defined as "the customary beliefs, social forms, and material traits of a racial, religious, or social group; the characteristic features of everyday existence shared by people in a place or time."[58] These definitions support the view that culture is much more than just language. The need to consider cultural background and beliefs may be more apparent when working with a patient whose primary language is not English, but this is a potential shortfall for clinicians! Acknowledging and appreciating the role of culture, especially cultural views of health, health care, and communication, are significant when approaching patient education with an older adult.

As stated in the definition, culture impacts all features of "everyday existence" for a person. The health care professional may need to ask questions to attain a full understanding of how culture may influence a patient's learning. Communication preferences may be the best place to start. Ask the patient and family members or caregivers how they prefer to be addressed. Determining cultural communication norms, including interpersonal space distances, volume, tone, use of touch, gestures, and eye contact, is important.[59] Paying close attention through observation but also asking direct questions regarding communication norms is appropriate. It is also important to ascertain information about the patient's cultural views of health, health care, and traditional (non-Western) medicinal practices that may be relevant to his or her current therapy care.[59] Even the expression of pain, an impairment often addressed in PT with older clients, is influenced by culture. Past experiences in health care, both positive and negative, may provide the physical therapist with a context for how to maximize adherence to education provided. Social organization within the culture can also impact patient education. Knowing about family structure, social/community organization, and gender roles will enable the physical therapist to involve and educate the most important people to the patient for positive health outcomes.[59]

Finally, consideration of language proficiency is important. For patients who speak English as a second language, the therapist should anticipate that some aspects of medical language may be hard to understand. In addition, stress can influence how well a person understands and speaks a second language. Consider offering an interpreter to maximize learning during a health crisis, even to patients who speak English as a second language well.[59] Demonstration and illustration of concepts should supplement any verbal instructions provided. Return demonstration on the part of the patient, after education has occurred, will be of primary importance to ensure that the patient truly understands and can perform the instructed skills. Involving a professional medical interpreter is beneficial to ensure patients and family members are on the same page. Best practice for translation services involves use of a professional medical interpreter, instead of using family members, to avoid misunderstanding of medical information.

Cultural competence and cultural humility are essential skills for physical therapists. The therapist should fully consider the impact of culture on all aspects of therapeutic intervention, including patient education. Literature shows that patients working with culturally competent health care providers experience greater satisfaction, are more open and trusting, and have improved adherence to medical recommendations.[60] Many resources exist for health care providers to improve culturally appropriate and effective interactions. The Office of Minority Health of the Department of Health and Human Services has a "Think Cultural Health" curriculum designed for health care professionals who seek to improve cultural competency.[61] Above all, the best resource for cultural competence is the patient. Demonstrating cultural humility by asking appropriate questions and demonstrating a desire to learn from them will go a long way!

Literacy and Health Literacy

The formal assessment of an older adult's health literacy is necessary to determine the level of communication (written and verbal) that should be utilized in therapy. Assuming that an older patient is capable of understanding and applying health education is dangerous for health care providers. Health literacy encompasses a wide variety of skills related to a person's ability to obtain, process, and make sense of health information and services. This includes being able to verbalize health needs, find and navigate health services, collaborate with health care providers, and understand and act on health-related advice.[62] Even basic health literacy skills are lacking for most older adults. The 2003 National Assessment of Adult Literacy found that adults over age 65 had the highest proportion of individuals with literacy below the basic literacy level as compared to any other adult age group.[63] Adults over 65 also made up the lowest number of individuals rated as "proficient" in health literacy. A staggering 3% of older adults in the survey attained this level; 97% of those surveyed fell in the intermediate (38%), basic (30%), or below basic (29%) health literacy levels[63] (Fig. 11.7). This data supports the need for physical therapists to assess health literacy among older adults.

Assuming literacy level based on the patient's level of education attained or completed is problematic. In fact, the health literacy level can be up to five grade levels *below* the level of education completed by the individual.[64] However, older adults may not be forthcoming about low literacy. Red flags that suggest a patient should be screened for literacy level include patients avoiding completion of forms, suggesting they "forgot their glasses," wanting to wait until a caregiver arrives to discuss information, providing an incomplete description of information that is focused on pictures/visuals, and reporting physical impairments such as headache or stomachache when asked to complete forms.[65]

A number of assessments of literacy are available to assess a patient's reading skills and literacy level. The Rapid Estimate [changed based on Table 11.7 title] of Adult Literacy in Medicine (REALM) is among the most utilized.[66] The REALM is a well-established tool to assess

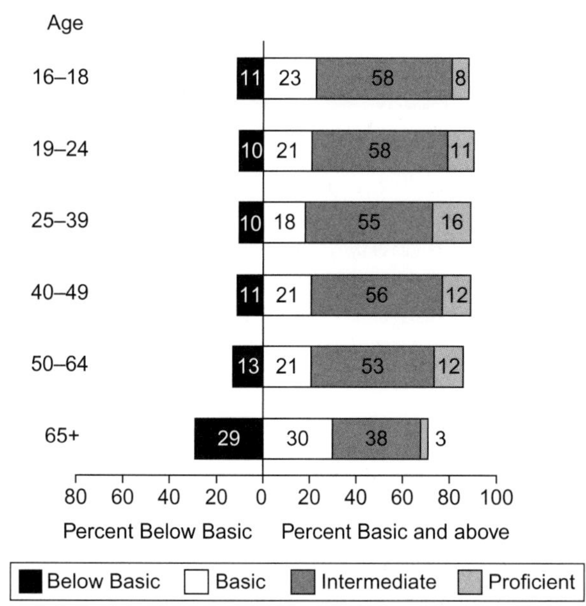
Percentage of adults in each health literacy level, by age: 2003
Age
16–18 11 23 58 8
19–24 10 21 58 11
25–39 10 18 55 16
40–49 11 21 56 12
50–64 13 21 53 12
65+ 29 30 38 3
80 60 40 20 0 20 40 60 80 100
Percent Below Basic
Percent Basic and above
Below Basic
Basic
Intermediate
Proficient
NOTE: Detail may not sum to totals because of rounding. Adults are defined as people 16 years of age and older living in households or prisons. Adults who could not be interviewed because of language spoken, or cognitive or mental disabilities (3 percent in 2003), are excluded from this figure. SOURCE: U.S. Department of Education, Institute of Education Sciences, National Center for Education Statistics, 2003 National Assessment of Adult Literacy.

FIG. 11.7 Health literacy rates for adults in the United States by age. *(From Kutner M, Greenberg E, Jin Y, Paulsen C. The Health Literacy of America's Adults: Results from the 2003 National Assessment of Adult Literacy. Washington, DC: U.S. Department of Education, National Center for Education Statistics; 2006.)*

literacy based on a patient reading and pronouncing a list of words of increasing complexity (number of syllables) (Table 11.7). The patient is instructed to read each word or say "blank" if unable to read the word. The practitioner counts the number of correct words, as well as the number of words with errors in pronunciation or skipped words. The patient is then scored out of a total of 66. Based on this score, the patient's literacy level is ranked by reading grade level (third grade and below, fourth to sixth grade, seventh to eighth grade, high school). The REALM can be completed in a few minutes.

Another more recent tool, the Newest Vital Sign (NVS), is helpful for assessing patient health literacy.[67] Here the patient reads a nutrition label and answers six questions based on the information on the label (Fig. 11.8). A benefit of this assessment is that it requires the patient to not only read information but also interpret and make decisions based on what is read.[66] For example: Is it safe to eat this food based on a given allergy? Some of the questions involve mathematical calculation as well. The total score classifies the patient as high likelihood of limited literacy, possible limited literacy, and adequate literacy. Literature suggests this tool takes more than 10 minutes to complete with a patient, which may be impractical in some clinical settings.[66] However, the benefits of knowing a patient's health literacy and being able to adequately structure therapeutic interventions and education around that literacy level may outweigh the challenges of time.

If it is determined that an older adult has low literacy levels, how should the physical therapist modify education and instructions? Because of low literacy levels, listening will likely be a preferred modality for learning. Therefore, personalized, face-to-face communication is encouraged.[68] Use the patient's personal context to apply the information so that it is meaningful. Avoid medical jargon and use simple words and phrases when possible, without talking down to the patient.[65] Limit the amount of education and information provided to patients to only the "need to know." Ask yourself, "Is this information absolutely necessary for the patient to understand or is it more 'nice to know' information?" Focusing on only the most important information reduces the overall quantity of information for the patient to process. Provide the most important education and information at the beginning or end of the education—information delivered at these times tends to be remembered best.[65] As discussed in earlier sections of this chapter, distributing patient education across multiple sessions, and even repeating information across multiple sessions, will help boost learning. Providing extra time for processing information will also be helpful—so don't rush!

In addition to those verbal education strategies, consider the following tips for written education and instructions. Printed handouts should be at no higher than a sixth-grade reading level.[64] Grade level can easily be calculated by using web-based "readability calculators."[69] After entering sample text, the calculator will provide the user with a reading grade level or level of difficulty information according to a variety of rating scales including Simple Measure of Gobbledygook (SMOG) and Flesch-Kinkaid Index. Using a large font size (>12) and easily readable font style is also good practice (e.g., "Arial" front type) on handouts.[64] Pictures and graphs supplement narrative information to boost understanding. The time spent ensuring that design of health-related patient education materials is geared to lower literacy levels will help to support the overall learning environment in therapy.

Physiologic Changes

As noted in Chapter 3, aging is associated with many normal changes in body systems, including those related to learning and memory. Assessing for and accommodating these age-related changes can help to improve the older adult's ability to obtain and process patient education. The sensory systems are, perhaps, most important to accommodate when framing education for an older adult. First, the visual system: Does the patient have adequate visual acuity for reading therapy handouts? Perhaps the font needs to be larger or have more contrast. Does the

TABLE 11.7 Rapid Estimate of Adult Literacy in Medicine Assessment (REALM)

TABLE C-l REALM

Patient Name/ Subject # ____________ Date of Birth ____________ Reading Level ____________

Date ____________ Clinic ____________ Examiner ____________ Grade Completed____________

List 1	List 2	List 3
Fat	Fatigue	Allergic
Flu	Pelvic	Menstrual
Pill	Jaundice	Testicle
Dose	Infection	Colitis
Eye	Exercise	Emergency
Stress	Behavior	Medication
Smear	Prescription	Occupation
Nerves	Notify	Sexually
Germs	Gallbladder	Alcoholism
Meals	Calories	Irritation
Disease	Depression	Constipation
Cancer	Miscarriage	Gonorrhea
Caffeine	Pregnancy	Inflammatory
Attack	Arthritis	Diabetes
Kidney	Nutrition	Hepatitis
Hormones	Menopause	Antibiotics
Herpes	Appendix	Diagnosis
Seizure	Abnormal	Potassium
Bowel	Syphilis	Anemia
Asthma	Hemorrhoids	Obesity
Rectal	Nausea	Osteoporosis
Incest	Directed	Impetigo
		SCORE
		List 1 ____________
		List 2 ____________
		List 3 ____________
		Raw Score ____________

Directions:

1. Give the patient a laminated copy of the REALM and score answers on an unlaminated copy that is attached to a clipboard. Hold the clipboard at an angle so that the patient is not distracted by your scoring procedure. Say:
   "I want to hear you read as many words as you can from this list. Begin with the first word on List 1 and read aloud. When you come to a word you cannot read, do the best you can or say "blank" and go on to the next word."
2. If the patient takes more than 5 seconds on a word, say "blank" and point to the next word, if necessary, to move the patient along. If the patient begins to miss every word, have him or her pronounce only known words.
3. Count as an error any word not attempted or mispronounced. Score by marking a plus (+) after each correct word, a check (✓) after each mispronounced word, and a minus (–) after words not attempted. Count as correct any self-corrected word.
4. Count the number of correct words for each list and record the numbers in the "SCORE" box, total the numbers, and match the total score with its grade equivalent in the table below (Table C-2).

TABLE C-2 Scores and Grade Equivalents for the REALM

GRADE EQUIVALENT

Raw Score	Grade Range
0–18	Third grade and below * Will not be able to read most low-literacy materials; will need repeated oral instructions, materials composed primarily of illustrations, or audio or videotapes
19–44	Fourth to sixth grade * Will need low-literary materials; may not be able to read prescription labels
45–60	Seventh to eighth grade * Will struggle with most patient education materials; will not be offended by low-literacy materials
61–66	High school * Will be able to read most patient education materials

(Excerpts taken from Davis TC, Long SW, Jackson RH, et al. Rapid estimate of adult literacy in medicine: a shortened screening instrument. *Fam Med.* 1993;25(6):391–385.)

REALM-SF Score Sheet

Select for PDF Version [- 179 KB]

Patient ID #: ____________ Date: ____________ Examiner Initials: __________

Behavior ____
Exercise ____
Menopause ____
Rectal ____
Antibiotics ____
Anemia ____
Jaundice ____

TOTAL SCORE ____

Administering the REALM-SF:

Suggested Introduction:

"Providers often use words that patients don't understand. We are looking at words providers often use with their patients in order to improve communication between health care providers and patients. Here is a list of medical words.

Starting at the top of the list, please read each word aloud to me. If you don't recognize a word, you can say 'pass' and move on to the next word."

Interviewer: Give the participant the word list. If the participant takes more than 5 seconds on a words, say "pass" and point to the next word. Hold this scoring sheet so that it is not visible to the participant.

Scores and Grade Equivalents for the REALM-SF

Score	Grade range
0	Third grade and below; will not be able to read most low-literacy materials; will need repeated oral instructions, materials composed primarily of illustrations, or audio or video tapes.
1-3	Fourth to sixth grade; will need low-literacy materials, may not be able to read prescription labels.
4-6	Seventh to eighth grade; will struggle with most patient education materials; will not be offended by low-literacy materials.
7	High school; will be able to read most patient education materials.

FIG. 11.8 REALM-SF score sheet. *(From U.S. Department of Health & Human Services. https://www.ahrq.gov/professionals/quality-patient-safety/quality-resources/tools/literacy/index.html#rapid.)*

patient have sensitivity to glare? If yes, adjusting lighting or treating in a room with more lighting control may help. Next, consider hearing. Presbycusis is a common age-related sensorineural hearing loss that especially impacts the ability to hear high-tone sounds. The therapist should be sure to speak in a low tone, and speak in a quiet space with minimal background noise to help accommodate for this change. Gestures, demonstrations, and facial expression will also boost patient understanding in the presence of hearing impairment.[70] Avoid overenunciating words and gum chewing, which may interfere with an older patient's ability to read lips.

Another important system to consider for educating the older population is the aging neurologic system. Cognition, including memory, changes with age. Short-term memory is most impacted with aging, so this affects the ability to learn and recall new information.[71] Repeating important aspects of patient education and spreading education out across sessions is important. Providing visual aids and reminders that a patient can place around his or her house can also assist memory and recall of information. Another strategy to accommodate memory changes with age is the "Power of 3" education tool.[72] Power of 3 utilizes alliteration in a simple three-word combination to help patients remember key aspects of care—for example, "wash, weigh, and walk" after open heart surgery or "monitor, medicine, and mobility" to prevent deep vein thrombosis after joint replacement. This strategy of focusing on three words is likely helpful for older adults owing to age-related decline in word recall (average 5 words; 2.5 words for those with low health literacy).[72] Keeping the patient as an active participant in the learning, and avoiding passive "dumping" of information while providing education, will also help learning. Learning is facilitated by hearing, seeing, feeling, touching, and teaching. Can you have the patient apply his or her education by teaching caregivers or other patients the information? Consider providing "active" education using practical situations and applications and in real or simulated environments to help the patient remember.

Learning Readiness and Expectations

If your patient is not ready to learn, your education will be ineffective. Even the best-planned educational methods are worthless if a learner is not motivated or engaged to take in the information. The PEEK framework is a helpful way to pull together much of the information we have discussed in this section of characteristics of the older learner.[73] PEEK encourages the therapist to consider physical, emotional, environmental, and knowledge-related readiness in the learner. As you approach education with your older patient, ask yourself the following questions:

- P (Physical) readiness: Is the patient awake, alert, and comfortable? Have physiologic changes been accommodated for (i.e., hearing or visual impairments)? Is your patient positioned in an ideal way to receive information (i.e., sitting up or head of bed elevated)?
- E (Emotional) readiness: Is the patient emotionally present and stable? Have you considered psychological effects that may limit learning (i.e., anxiety, depression, self-efficacy)? Have you provided the opportunity for open communication to acknowledge any emotional concerns prior to initiating education?
- E (Environmental) readiness: Is the physical environment amenable to education delivery? Is the light adequate? Are distractions limited? Is the environment quiet? (We will talk more about environmental factors influencing learning later in this chapter.)
- K (Knowledge) readiness: What is the patient's preferred learning style for taking in new information? How does the patient process information? What literacy level should be used? What cultural knowledge or understanding does the patient have that may influence acquiring new knowledge?

Once you have established your learner's readiness for learning, you can start to teach your patient.

THE THERAPIST AS TEACHER

Learning is not just about the learner! The physical therapist, as teacher, has an equal role in the learning process through preparation, content selection, and delivery of information. For physical therapists to be effective in patient education, they must *value* their role as educators and take steps to design their patient education with intent and purpose.[8] See Fig. 11.9 for a summary of the competencies discussed here.

Therapist Patient Education Competencies

Effective patient education delivery requires specific therapist competencies. In 2018, Forbes and colleagues published a Delphi study to establish patient education competencies for physical therapists.[74] The competencies extend across therapist knowledge, skills, and attitudes and were agreed upon by physiotherapist experts in Australia. Table 11.8 includes the 22 competencies across these three domains and poses questions in the form of a self-assessment for therapists to consider their own strengths and knowledge gaps in each area. Therapists can take steps to improve competency in those areas they marked as "neutral," "disagree," or "strongly disagree."

Preparation and Timing

Although patient education can happen spontaneously in a patient's plan of care, we advocate that planned education should occur regularly. First, the therapist should consider how older adults learn best. Refer back to earlier in this chapter for a review of relevant learning theories for the older patient (e.g., adult learning theory, experiential learning theory, social learning theory, and reflective practice). When a therapist initially designs the patient's plan of care according to the physical therapist management model, goals should be set regarding specific educational competencies the patient should attain. SMART

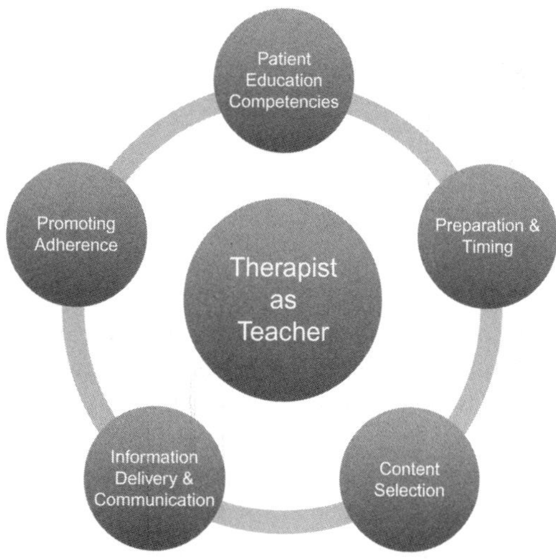

FIG. 11.9 Therapist teaching competencies.

TABLE 11.8 Therapist Patient Education Competency Self-Assessment

To what extent do you agree or disagree with the following statements?
(Strongly Disagree Disagree Neutral Agree Strongly Agree)

Knowledge	1. I know the role of patient education in PT practice. 2. I understand the principles of adult learning. 3. I provide education within limits of practice, seeking advice or referring to another professional where appropriate.
Attitudes	4. I consider the impact of social, cultural, and behavioral variables on patient learning. 5. I ask patients about their perceptions and concerns. 6. I use shared decision making in therapy. 7. I provide content that is in the best interests of the patient.
Skills	8. I integrate evidence-based practice into patient education. 9. I ask questions to understand the patient's learning needs. 10. I utilize reflective questioning in patient education. 11. I utilize a range of learning content tailored to the patient. 12. I utilize communication styles, language, and materials that are tailored to the patient. 13. I effectively explain the patient's condition. 14. I provide self-management education and reinforce the patient's ability to manage. 15. I provide family or caregivers with information where present. 16. I control attention and engagement throughout the educational intervention. 17. I effectively summarize information. 18. I consistently and regularly review progress of patient learning. 19. I use the "teach back" method to evaluate understanding. 20. I identify where educational needs have been met. 21. I recognize and manage barriers to effective education. 22. I continue to develop patient education skills.

PT, physical therapy.
(Adapted from Forbes et al.[74])

goals that are Specific, Measurable, Achievable, Recorded, and Time based are necessary.[75] Breaking SMART goals down into smaller pieces will help the therapist to plan learning distribution across the episode of care. Within a given therapy session, the therapist should factor in the patient's response to therapeutic interventions when deciding the time to implement therapy. When is the patient's attention most focused during the session? How can cognitive fatigue be avoided? Timing of education is important to consider, as well as keeping education short (<15 minutes).[76]

Patient education should start with a "hook" to grab the attention of the learner.[21] There are endless options for a hook! For example, you can relate the education topic to an interesting fact, a joke, an experience the patient told you about in the last session, or maybe an observation you had about the patient's movement or lifestyle. The key is that the hook is something to get your patient engaged and interested in hearing more about the topic.

Content Selection

Content selection may be one of the hardest parts of patient education because there are so many health education resources available today. Encouraging patients to share what they already know about the topic provides the therapist with a targeted starting point.[77] Marjorie Whitman is a nurse educator who encourages health care providers to ask the patient, "What worries you most?" and use this as a jumping-off point for education.[78] We discussed earlier the importance of sharing "need to know" information with patients at basic and low levels of health literacy, but this is a helpful principle for all teaching. Start teaching with more basic information and then move into more complex information. In general, try to focus education on specific behaviors and skills and less on background knowledge and content information.[76] Being able to select and target information to the patient's needs helps to prevent overload and promote retention of information over time.

How does the therapist ensure the most necessary information is being discussed with the patient? The physical therapist has a responsibility to be current in his or her field. For example, recent changes in neuroscience of chronic pain have created new approaches to patient education in this area.[8] Colleagues are another great resource to share experiences with key "learning pearls" for patients. Lastly, professional resources may be available. For example, the World Health Organization, in its publication regarding "Therapeutic Patient Education," established key competencies for patients related to two common chronic diseases, diabetes and asthma, which include physical activity competencies that are physical therapist related.[79]

Delivery of Information and Communication

Even with adequate preparation and content selection, a therapist's patient education can be rendered ineffective with poor delivery of the information. Using different modes of information delivery (visual, verbal, media, others) will help the brain learn.[8] Delivery should incorporate strategies that appeal to adult learners, incorporate authentic experiences, involve social participation, and encourage reflection on the part of the patient. In addition, we have discussed the benefit of education that is provided over multiple time points (not all at once).

Ideally, the therapist should consider making learning active.[76] Therapists should avoid making patients be passive receivers of information and instead encourage the patient to engage and ask questions, apply the information to his or her life, and consider potential challenges and roadblocks to learning and behavior change.

Another essential consideration for patient education is communication: How is the therapist going to share relevant information with the patient? Communication is essential in creating a therapist–patient relationship and establishing trust between parties. This is especially important for older adults who feel undervalued and disrespected in the medical system.[80] Research has shown that health care providers interacting with older adults spend less time with them, are more controlling, and provide less information compared to other age populations.[70] Table 11.9 includes a number of "dos and don'ts" for communicating patient education with older adults. Perhaps the biggest takeaway for the therapist to consider in education delivery with older adults is the importance of rapport building. Allocating adequate time with the patient, using verbal and nonverbal communication that exudes empathy, and providing opportunities for the patient to share their knowledge and concerns are critical communication strategies for the physical therapist to utilize.

Promoting Adherence and Behavior Change

Most often in practice the intent of patient education time is to get patients to do something specific, such as adopting self-management strategies for a chronic condition, performing a home exercise program, or becoming more physically active. However, there is ample evidence that adherence to health care providers' recommendations is poor. For example, following a physical therapy program for fall prevention, 37% of the older adult participants indicated that they no longer performed their individualized home exercise program, and only 13% continued to do the complete program.[81] Reasons for nonadherence to therapist recommendations vary by the individual, and behavior change models can be helpful in identifying patient-specific barriers to uptake of the new behavior. Using models can guide therapists toward patient education approaches that address the patient's most pertinent concerns. Social cognitive theory and the health beliefs model were discussed earlier. A third model, the transtheoretical model (TTM), is among the most commonly known behavior change models, developed in the early 1980s to describe how people adopt new health behaviors.[82] According to the TTM, individuals adopt new behaviors in a series of stages. The patient's receptivity to education to support the desired behaviors varies by stage. There is substantial evidence that the amount of change in physical activity is associated with the stage of change in general populations,[83] and a large community-based TTM-based intervention for older adults was shown to be effective in progressing the stage of change related to adoption of physical activity.[84] The key feature of TTM is the stage approach in that different strategies and interventions are used for individuals at different stages of readiness to change or adopt new behaviors. Table 11.10 describes the stages and the appropriate types of educational intervention for each stage.

Technology is another consideration for patient education and behavioral change. Use of technology, such as activity monitors, has the potential to increase adherence to a variety of positive health behavior changes.[85] Short-term studies on the effect of technology-based interventions (e.g., gaming system exercise programs) for older adults suggest a higher adherence rate than with traditional exercise programs, but little research has investigated tailoring such interventions to older adults or to the individual.[86] An ongoing study is investigating the impact of mobile technology to motivate and guide exercise in older adults with the ability to tailor interventions to the individual.[87] Tailored interventions with

TABLE 11.9 Dos and Don'ts of Communication During Education

Dos	Don'ts
• Encourage the patient to take an active role in education by giving him or her time to speak and ask questions.[77] • Pay attention to patient nonverbals and body language. • Lean in.[96] • Use facial expressions (smiling, frowning, others).[96] • Encourage sharing of information, including what the patient already knows about health condition.[70] • Ask open-ended questions[75] and encourage the patient to share information.[77] • Accommodate aging sensory changes (visual and hearing impairment especially).[70] • Be empathetic by addressing concerns and fears.[77] • Be patient and open when listening.[70] • Use verbal strategies such as providing rationale, paraphrasing, and summarizing.[75]	• Avoid grouping all older adults together as the "same" type of patient requiring the same education. Each patient is unique. • Avoid "elderspeak" or talking to older adults like a child.[70] • Avoid patient taking only a passive listening role.[77] • Avoid stereotyping older adults. Common stereotypes include that older adults are challenging and exhausting to work with.[80] • Avoid medical jargon.[77] • Avoid distancing behaviors[96] like standing over the patient or talking to the patient from across the room. • Avoid taking control over the encounter in a "doctor knows best" approach.[70,80]

TABLE 11.10 Transtheoretical Model of Behavior Change

Stage	Learner Characteristics	Educational Intervention
Precontemplation—no acknowledgment of a problem or intent to take action	Resistant to change, if thinking about change at all May fear failure May lack information	Consciousness raising, including personalized information about benefits of targeted activity and risks of current behavior
Contemplation—acknowledges a problem with behavior but not ready to change	May be open to information about benefits of new behavior May be curious about results that could be obtained from changing Ambivalence is common	Work with the individual to identify and reduce barriers to targeted behavior Use role models to reinforce benefits of the targeted behavior Continue to provide education about personal risks and benefits
Preparation—a commitment to behavior change but uncertainty on how to approach	May take small steps toward change	Assist in developing specific plans Identify alternatives to targeted behavior that will accomplish same goal Encourage the individual to make a public commitment to action Involve peers or caregivers in the plan
Action—behavioral change is initiated	Requires commitment and energy to make it work May be looking for reinforcement and encouragement	Provide frequent positive reinforcement Log of activity Provide support networks
Maintenance—behavioral change is ongoing	Challenge is to sustain behavior and overcome barriers	Encourage setting long-term goals Encourage use of support groups and networks

individualized feedback are superior to generic feedback,[85] and as technology develops there may be more easily customizable products to guide and measure adherence.

There may be barriers to the adoption of mobile or other digital technologies in the older population. A recent study showed widespread use of the internet to access information or communicate with others among non-Hispanic adults aged 65 to 79, but substantially less use among black, Latino, Filipino, or Chinese elders. This pattern is paralleled in older adults' interest in using online programs to view live or recorded online webinars or to receive information, respond to questions, and get feedback online (except Chinese). Further, across all racial/ethnic groups there is little interest in using health-related apps. Thus, while there may be potential for use of mobile or digital technology to influence health behaviors, the technology is less likely to reach those racial/ethnic groups with a higher prevalence of chronic conditions and more barriers to health care access.[88] This may change with the baby boomer cohort.

ENVIRONMENTAL INFLUENCES

The environment has an important role in learning. The SCT, discussed earlier, specifically considers the role of environmental factors in influencing behavior change. Environmental factors must be anticipated (in the best-case scenario) or assessed (in the less ideal scenario) and be addressed. These include both physical aspects of the environment and social aspects of the environment.

First consider the space. A quiet area with limited distractions helps the learner to attend to the information being delivered. Lighting will be an important consideration depending on the learning style/preference of the patient, the visual abilities the patient has, and the teaching modality the therapist has planned. In most cases, avoiding glare will be helpful in accommodating for aging visual changes. Temperature is a factor that should be considered in learning, although it may be hard for the therapist to control. Acknowledging that excessive heat or cold might influence the patient's attention and learning could help the therapist to set appropriate expectations. Perhaps the education should be delayed until the next session, or maybe the patient should plan to bring a jacket or wear lighter clothing so that the conditions are more ideal for learning next time. Position of the therapist and patient within the environment should also be considered. Is the therapist situated in front of the patient to facilitate eye contact, lip reading (if necessary), and ability to see demonstrations or handouts utilized? Also consider patient position. A patient who is seated in a chair or in bed with the head elevated will likely have more focused attention on education provided than a patient who is lying flat in bed. Weather, transportation, and building accessibility should be considered when assessing physical environment factors impacting physical activity participation and adherence.[89]

Lastly, the social aspects of the environment can impact learning. We discussed social cognitive theory and the use of peer educators and role models earlier in this chapter. Peers or other patients and health care providers can provide helpful motivation for learning.[27] Shared experiences, relatedness, and real-world application are incentives to learning with peers. Other social facilitators and barriers to behavior change include family support, peer support, interdisciplinary team support, and socioeconomic factors. Specifically, physician encouragement for patients to participate in physical activity and home exercises, in addition to therapist-led education, has been shown to improve adherence for older adults with osteoarthritis.[89] Be sure to analyze these factors when considering a social environment for learning.

The contributions of the learner (older patient), teacher (therapist), and environment have been analyzed in their contribution to patient education (see Fig. 11.1). Next we will discuss the "nuts and bolts" of putting it all together in a patient education process that creates learning and behavior change.

PATIENT EDUCATION: PUTTING IT ALL TOGETHER

In this chapter, we have described how patient education must interlace an understanding of learning and behavior change theory with characteristics of the adult learner, competencies of the therapist as teacher, and the environment. This takes careful planning and deliberate intention on the part of the therapist. The foundation of the learning should be rooted in educational theory and behavior change theory. The process should be driven primarily by the patient with the therapist as guide. Fig. 11.10 shows the whole process put together.

The entire patient education process is started based on patient needs. Completing a formal needs assessment cannot be emphasized enough: What are the patient's learning goals? What is the patient's motivation to learn? What is the patient's readiness to learn?[90] For example, a patient who has just found out she has osteoporosis may not be ready to take in information about diet and exercise. Take time to understand these factors with open-ended questions for the patient. A needs assessment is not only about content knowledge! Part of the therapist's questioning should include factors discussed in the previous section from this chapter about the older learner (i.e., cultural background, health literacy level, physiologic changes with age, etc.), especially the PEEK framework for learner readiness.

The needs assessment helps the therapist to provide context for patient education. This helps to show the patient how the information applies to the "big picture" of PT care. Research supports patient education that is not generalized, but tailored to the individual.[91] To tailor education, the therapist needs to know what the patient already knows and what gaps in knowledge exist. Beth Fahlberg is a nurse who advocates for the "no education about me without me" mantra for patient education by nurses, and the same applies for physical therapists. Helping patients to approach education as a shared effort is helpful for understanding and retention. Fahlberg asserts, "A top-down, prepackaged approach to education, based on a standardized teaching plan, doesn't acknowledge the patient's expertise about her body, health, resources, beliefs and values."[92]

The educational intervention design will take time and planning on the part of the therapist. The therapist should assess his or her own educational competencies and seek feedback from patients, peers, and supervisors for improved efficacy. The therapist must consider strategies to support behavior change and adherence. The transtheoretical model, social cognitive theory, and health belief models were discussed in this chapter as important theories to support and guide the educational design, along with educational learning theories.

Providing education requires attention to timing, as well as environmental factors (both social and physical). The therapist should consider multiple modalities for information delivery, including oral, visual, kinesthetic, and virtual tools to support learning.

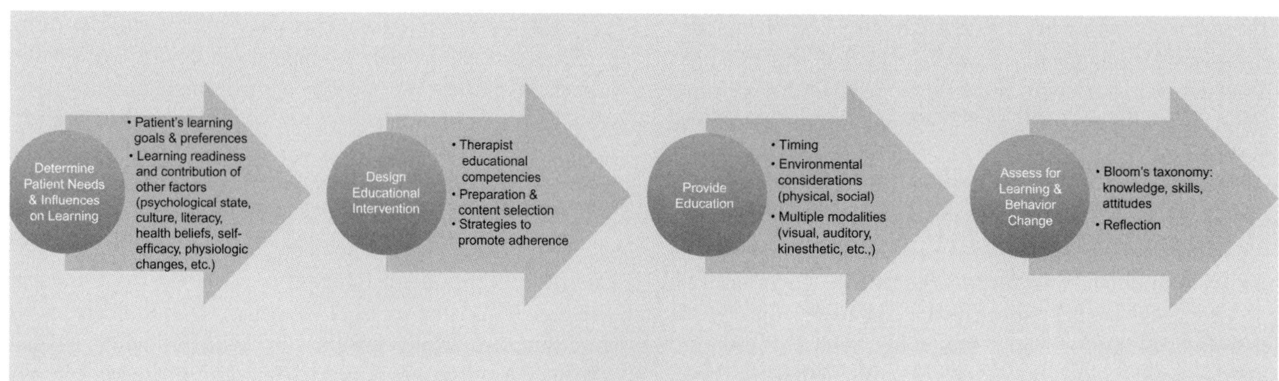

FIG. 11.10 Pulling it all together: the patient education process.

LEARNING ASSESSMENT

Even with thoughtful consideration of the learner and the environment, as well as therapist competency in delivering education, one might ask: *How does the physical therapist ensure that a patient actually learns what is taught in therapy?* Regular assessment of learning confirms that the individual understands what has been taught, can perform the desired physical skills, and values any intervention taught enough to adhere to it. These three areas of assessment reflect the three domains of learning often described as part of Bloom's taxonomy: cognitive, psychomotor, and affective.[40] The techniques used to assess learning vary by domain.

The cognitive domain involves what a person knows and how he or she can use that knowledge. Exams or quizzes are usually used in traditional educational settings, but these have limited use in clinical settings. The "teach back" method, in which the individual explains the content of interest in his or her own words, is a more effective approach. Alternatively, through careful questioning therapists can identify areas that need further instruction. Well-structured open-ended questions can help assess the patient's understanding and recall, and give cues to the effectiveness of the instruction.[93]

The psychomotor domain of learning involves the learning and execution of physical skills. Assessment in the psychomotor domain is part of everyday PT practice, most commonly done through observation of exercises, functional activities, or desirable postures or positions. Oftentimes this type of evaluation is referred to as "return demonstration." With all patients it is preferable to request return demonstrations in multiple settings, for example, ambulating with walkers on smooth surfaces, over carpet, and on uneven surfaces, or doing exercises on a mat in the clinic as well as a softer surface like a mattress, such as would be used at home. It is important to evaluate psychomotor performance under conditions relevant to the individual patient, particularly with older adults who may have environmental challenges in the home setting. Return demonstration is also an important strategy for patients at low health literacy levels or who are not primary English speakers.

The affective domain involves individuals' values and beliefs. It is often said that the way we use our time is the best indicator of our values, and that if something is important enough we take the time to do it. Take the example of teaching older patients about the importance of an active lifestyle. The physical therapist can teach the facts about the dangers of sedentary behaviors and activity guidelines, but if the individual does not value the lifestyle, he or she is unlikely to adopt it. Therefore, instruction in the affective domain should be geared toward helping the patient value an intervention enough to adhere to it. Often this is done by linking the desired behaviors (e.g., becoming more active) to salient and meaningful things that the patient already values through patient-specific goal setting. As discussed in the section on reflection, careful questioning can help the patient reconsider prior biases and adopt new beliefs and values that foster adherence to education. Questioning, therefore, is a helpful assessment tool to determine changes in the affective domain.

Activity logs and other self-report methods are the most common ways to assess adherence, though increasingly activity monitors are used for this purpose. It is important to not interpret adherence as merely a measure of affective learning, as sometimes the individual may not understand the instructions, or there might be environmental challenges or social demands that interfere. As discussed in the section on behavior change, if an individual is not adhering to instructions, it is imperative that the therapist carefully question the patient to determine the reason for nonadherence.

Assessment does not just happen in a summative manner at the end of education. Assessment should occur throughout the PT management process in a formative, ongoing manner.[21] Think back to the earlier discussion on the role of reflection in learning. Reflection is a great assessment tool for the therapist! The therapist should ask questions to the patient throughout the learning process ("in-action," "on-action," and "for-action") to grasp a patient's understanding of content across domains of learning.

Consideration for all of these variables within patient education interventions will optimize the success of the patient's learning. The therapist should remember that patient education is a process, not a one-time event, and using the best practices recommended in this chapter will help to support learning and behavior change goals for the patient.

REFERENCES

1. Bartlett BE. At last, a definition. *Patient Educ Couns*. 1985;7:323.
2. Institute of Medicine. *Health Professions Education: A Bridge to Quality*. (Greiner AC, Knebel E, eds.). Washington, DC: National Academies Press; 2003. https://www.ncbi.nlm.nih.gov/books/NBK221519/.
3. Tan JY, Chen JX, Liu XL, et al. A meta-analysis on the impact of disease-specific education programs on health outcomes for patients with chronic obstructive pulmonary disease. *Geriatr Nurs (Minneap)*. 2013;22(4):280–296.
4. Gold DT, McClung B. Approaches to patient education: emphasizing the long-term value of compliance and persistence. *Am J Med*. 2006;119(4 Suppl 1):S32–S37. https://doi.org/S0002-9343(05)01201-5.
5. Shahsavari H, Matory P, Zare Z, Taleghani F, Kaji MA. Effect of self-care education on the quality of life in patients with breast cancer. *J Educ Health Promot*. 2015;4:70. https://doi.org/10.4103/2277-9531.171782.
6. Fernsler JI, Cannon CA. The whys of patient education. *Semin Oncol Nurs*. 1991;7(2):79–86. https://doi.org/0749-2081(91)90085-4.
7. Gahimer JE, Domholdt E. Amount of patient education in physical therapy practice and perceived effects. *Phys Ther*. 1996;76(10):1089–1096.
8. Harman K, Bassett R, Fenety A, Hoens AM. Client education: communicative interaction between physiotherapists and clients

with subacute low back pain in private practice. *Physiother Canada.* 2011;63(2):212–223. https://doi.org/10.3138/ptc.2009-52P.

9. Brown PC, Roediger 3rd, HL, McDaniel MA. *Make It Stick: The Science of Successful Learning.* Cambridge, MA: Belknap Press of Harvard University Press; 2014.
10. Weinstein Y, Madan CR, Sumeracki MA. Teaching the science of learning. *Cogn Res Princ Implic.* 2018;3(1):2. https://doi.org/10.1186/s41235-017-0087-y.
11. Polster D. Preventing readmissions with discharge education. *Nurs Manage.* 2015;46(10):30–38. https://doi.org/10.1097/01.NUMA.0000471590.62056.77.
12. Paul S. Hospital discharge education for patients with heart failure: what really works and what is the evidence? *Crit Care Nurse.* 2008;28(2):66–82. https://doi.org/28/2/66.
13. Choi J. Effect of pictograph-based discharge instructions on older adults' comprehension and recall: a pilot study. *Res Gerontol Nurs.* 2016;9(2):66–71. https://doi.org/10.3928/19404921-20150513-05.
14. Centers for Medicare and Medicaid Services. Your Discharge Planning Checklist: For Patients and their Caregivers. https://www.medicare.gov/sites/default/files/2018-07/11376-discharge-planning-checklist.pdf. Accessed August 6, 2018.
15. Family Caregiver Alliance. Hospital Discharge Planning: A Guide for Families and Caregivers. https://www.caregiver.org/hospital-discharge-planning-guide-families-and-caregivers. Published 2018. Accessed August 6, 2018.
16. Sluijs EM. Patient education in physiotherapy: towards a planned approach. *Physiotherapy.* 1991;77:503–508.
17. Chase L, Elkins JA, Readinger J, Shepard KF. Perceptions of physical therapists toward patient education. *Phys Ther.* 1993;73:787–796.
18. Resnik L, Jensen GM. Using clinical outcomes to explore the theory of expert practice in physical therapy. *Phys Ther.* 2003;83(12):1090–1106.
19. Dormohammadi G, Asghari F, Rashidian A. What do patients expect from their physicians? *Iran J Publ Heal.* 2010;39(1):70–77.
20. Grannis CJ. The ideal physical therapist as perceived by the elderly patient. *Phys Ther.* 1981;61(4):479–486.
21. Plack M, Driscoll MA. *Teaching and Learning in Physical Therapy: From Classroom to Clinic.* Thorofare, NJ: SLACK Incorporated; 2011.
22. Taylor DC, Hamdy H. Adult learning theories: implications for learning and teaching in medical education: AMEE Guide No. 83. *Med Teach.* 2013;35(11):e1561–e1572. https://doi.org/10.3109/0142159X.2013.828153.
23. Kolb D. *Experiential Learning: Experience as the Source of Learning and Development.* Englewood Cliffs, NJ: Prentice-Hall; 1984.
24. Speelman AD, van Nimwegen M, Bloem BR, Munneke M. Evaluation of implementation of the ParkFit program: a multifaceted intervention aimed to promote physical activity in patients with Parkinson's disease. *Physiotherapy.* 2014;100(2):134–141. https://doi.org/10.1016/j.physio.2013.05.003.
25. Stacey FG, James EL, Chapman K, Courneya KS, Lubans DR. A systematic review and meta-analysis of social cognitive theory-based physical activity and/or nutrition behavior change interventions for cancer survivors. *J Cancer Surviv.* 2015;9(2):305–338. https://doi.org/10.1007/s11764-014-0413-z.
26. Bandura A, Adams NE, Beyer J. Cognitive processes mediating behavioral change. *J Pers Soc Psychol.* 1977;35(3):125–139.
27. Lee LL, Arthur A, Avis M. Using self-efficacy theory to develop interventions that help older people overcome psychological barriers to physical activity: a discussion paper. *Int J Nurs Stud.* 2008;45(11):1690–1699. https://doi.org/10.1016/j.ijnurstu.2008.02.012.
28. Williams DM, Anderson ES, Winett RA. A review of the outcome expectancy construct in physical activity research. *Ann Behav Med.* 2005;29(1):70–79. https://doi.org/10.1207/s15324796abm2901_10.
29. Wulf G, Lewthwaite R. Optimizing performance through intrinsic motivation and attention for learning: the OPTIMAL theory of motor learning. *Psychon Bull Rev.* 2016;23(5):1382–1414. https://doi.org/10.3758/s13423-015-0999-9.
30. Winstein C, Lewthwaite R, Blanton SR, Wolf LB, Wishart L. Infusing motor learning research into neurorehabilitation practice: a historical perspective with case exemplar from the accelerated skill acquisition program. *J Neurol Phys Ther.* 2014;38(3):190–200. https://doi.org/10.1097/NPT.0000000000000046.
31. Khong L, Farringdon F, Hill KD, Hill AM. "We are all one together": peer educators' views about falls prevention education for community-dwelling older adults—a qualitative study. *BMC Geriatr.* 2015;15:23–28. https://doi.org/10.1186/s12877-015-0030-3.
32. Kloseck M, Fitzsimmons DA, Speechley M, Savundranayagam MY, Crilly RG. Improving the diagnosis and treatment of osteoporosis using a senior-friendly peer-led community education and mentoring model: a randomized controlled trial. *Clin Interv Aging.* 2017;12:823–833. https://doi.org/10.2147/CIA.S130573.
33. Abba K, Byrne P, Horton S, Lloyd-Williams M. Interventions to encourage discussion of end-of-life preferences between members of the general population and the people closest to them - a systematic literature review. *BMC Palliat Care.* 2013;12(1):40. https://doi.org/10.1186/1472-684X-12-40.
34. Foster G, Taylor SJ, Eldridge SE, Ramsay J, Griffiths CJ. Self-management education programmes by lay leaders for people with chronic conditions. *Cochrane Database Syst Rev.* 2007;(4);CD005108. https://doi.org/10.1002/14651858.CD005108.pub2 .
35. Seymour JE, Almack K, Kennedy S, Froggatt K. Peer education for advance care planning: volunteers' perspectives on training and community engagement activities. *Health Expect.* 2013;16(1):43–55. https://doi.org/10.1111/j.1369-7625.2011.00688.x.
36. Sanders C, Seymour J, Clarke A, Gott M, Welton M. Development of a peer education programme for advance end-of-life care planning. *Int J Palliat Nurs.* 2006;12(5):214, 216–223.
37. Peel NM, Warburton J. Using senior volunteers as peer educators: what is the evidence of effectiveness in falls prevention? *Australas J Ageing.* 2009;28(1):7–11. https://doi.org/10.1111/j.1741-6612.2008.00320.x.
38. Mezirow J. Transformative learning theory: theory to practice. *New Dir Adult Cont Ed.* 1997;1997(74):5–12.
39. Atkins S, Murphy K. Reflection: a review of the literature. *J Adv Nurs.* 1993;18(8):1188–1192.
40. Bloom B, Englehart M, Furst E, Hill W, Krathwohl D. *Taxonomy of Educational Objectives: The Classification of Educational Goals. Handbook I: Cognitive Domain.* New York, Toronto: Longmans, Green; 1956.
41. Mann K, Gordon J, MacLeod A. Reflection and reflective practice in health professions education: a systematic review. *Adv Health Sci Educ Theory Pract.* 2009;14(4):595–621. https://doi.org/10.1007/s10459-007-9090-2.
42. Plack MM, Greenberg L. The reflective practitioner: reaching for excellence in practice. *Pediatrics.* 2005;116:1546–1552.
43. Schon DA. *The Reflective Practitioner: How Professionals Think in Action.* New York: Basic Books; 1983. https://doi.org/0-465-06874-X.
44. Killion J, Todnem G. A process for personal theory building. *Educ Leadersh.* 1991;48(6):171–175.

45. Inott T, Kennedy BB. Assessing learning styles: practical tips for patient education. *Nurs Clin North Am*. 2011;46(3):313–320. vi. https://doi.org/10.1016/j.cnur.2011.05.006.
46. Chase TM. Learning styles and teaching strategies: enhancing the patient education experience. *SCI Nurs*. 2001;18 (3):138–141.
47. Rosenstock IM, Strecher VJ, Becker MH. Social learning theory and the health belief model. *Health Educ Behav*. 1988;15 (2):175–183. https://doi.org/10.1177/109019818801500203.
48. Harada K, Lee S, Shimada H, et al. Psychological predictors of participation in screening for cognitive impairment among community-dwelling older adults. *Geriatr Gerontol Int*. 2017;17(8):1197–1204. https://doi.org/10.1111/ggi.12841.
49. Horwood H, Williams MJ, Mandic S. Examining motivations and barriers for attending maintenance community-based cardiac rehabilitation using the health-belief model. *Heart Lung Circ*. 2015;24(10):980–987. https://doi.org/10.1016/j.hlc.2015.03.023.
50. Dotson VM, Szymkowicz SM, Kirton JW, McLaren ME, Green ML, Rohani JY. Unique and interactive effect of anxiety and depressive symptoms on cognitive and brain function in young and older adults. *J Depress Anxiety*. 2014; Suppl 1:22565.
51. Shimada H, Park H, Makizako H, Doi T, Lee S, Suzuki T. Depressive symptoms and cognitive performance in older adults. *J Psychiatr Res*. 2014;57:149–156. https://doi.org/10.1016/j.jpsychires.2014.06.004.
52. Pietrzak RH, Maruff P, Woodward M, et al. Mild worry symptoms predict decline in learning and memory in healthy older adults: a 2-year prospective cohort study. *Am J Geriatr Psychiatry*. 2012;20(3):266–275. https://doi.org/10.1097/JGP.0b013e3182107e24.
53. Student First Project. School and Classroom Strategies: Depression. http://studentsfirstproject.org/wp-content/uploads/School-and-Classroom-Depression-Strategies.pdf. Accessed August 29, 2018.
54. Mental Health America. Tips for Teachers: Ways to Help Students Who Struggle with Emotions or Behavior. http://www.mentalhealthamerica.net/conditions/tips-teachers-ways-help-students-who-struggle-emotions-or-behavior. Accessed September 4, 2018.
55. Dweck CS. *Mindset: The New Psychology of Success*. New York: Ballantine Books; 2006.
56. Park DC, Bischof GN. The aging mind: neuroplasticity in response to cognitive training. *Dialogues Clin Neurosci*. 2013;15(1):109–119.
57. National Institute on Aging. Cognitive Health and Older Adults. https://www.nia.nih.gov/health/cognitive-health-and-older-adults. Accessed August 26, 2018.
58. Merriam-Webster. Culture. https://www.merriam-webster.com/dictionary/culture. Published 2018. Accessed September 5, 2018.
59. Chang M, Kelly AE. Patient education: addressing cultural diversity and health literacy issues. *Urol Nurs*. 2007;27 (5):411–417. quiz 418.
60. Brunett M, Shingles RR. Does having a culturally competent health care provider affect the patients' experience or satisfaction? A critically appraised topic. *J Sport Rehabil*. 2018;27(3):284–288. https://doi.org/10.1123/jsr.2016-0123.
61. U.S. Department of Health & Human Services. Guide to Providing Effective Communication and Language Assistance Services. https://hclsig.thinkculturalhealth.hhs.gov/. Accessed August 28, 2018.
62. Levasseur M, Carrier A. Do rehabilitation professionals need to consider their clients' health literacy for effective practice? *Clin Rehabil*. 2010;24(8):756–765. https://doi.org/10.1177/0269215509360752.
63. Kutner M, Greenberg E, Jin Y, Paulsen C. *The Health Literacy of America's Adults: Results from the 2003 National Assessment of Adult Literacy*. Washington, DC: U.S. Department of Education, National Center for Education Statistics; 2006.
64. Davidhizar RE, Brownson K. Literacy, cultural diversity, and client education. *Health Care Manag (Frederick)*. 1999;18 (1):39–47.
65. Murphy PW, Davis TC. When low literacy blocks compliance. *RN*. 1997;60(10):58–63. quiz 64.
66. Chesser AK, Keene Woods N, Smothers K, Rogers N. Health literacy and older adults: a systematic review. *Gerontol Geriatr Med*. 2016;2:1–13. https://doi.org/10.1177/2333721416630492 2333721416630492-Dec.
67. Weiss BD, Mays MZ, Martz W, et al. Quick assessment of literacy in primary care: the newest vital sign. *Ann Fam Med*. 2005;3(6):514–522. doi:3/6/514.
68. Centers for Disease Control and Prevention. Improving Health Literacy for Older Adults: Expert Panel Report. Atlanta, GA: U.S. Department of Health and Human Services; *2009*: 2009.
69. Readability Formulas Automatic Readability Checker. http://www.readabilityformulas.com/free-readability-formula-tests.php.
70. The Gerontological Society of America. *Communicating with Older Adults: An Evidence-Based Review of What Really Works*. Washington, DC: Gerontological Society of America; 2012.
71. Dellasega C, Clark D, McCreary D, Helmuth A, Schan P. Nursing process: teaching elderly clients. *J Gerontol Nurs*. 1994;20(1):31–38.
72. Sanchez LM, Cooknell LE. The Power of 3: using adult learning principles to facilitate patient education. *Nursing (Lond)*. 2017;47(2):17–19. https://doi.org/10.1097/01.NURSE.0000511819.18774.85.
73. Bastable SB, Gramet P, Jacobs K, Sopczyk DL. *Health Professional as Educator*. Sudbury, MA: Jones & Bartlett Learning; 2011.
74. Forbes R, Mandrusiak A, Smith M, Russell T. Identification of competencies for patient education in physiotherapy using a Delphi approach. *Physiotherapy*. 2018;104(2): 232–238.
75. Lonsdale C, Hall AM, Murray A, et al. Communication skills training for practitioners to increase patient adherence to home-based rehabilitation for chronic low back pain: results of a cluster randomized controlled trial. *Arch Phys Med Rehabil*. 2017;98(9):1732–1743. e7.
76. Wingard R. Patient education and the nursing process: meeting the patient's needs. *Nephrol Nurs J*. 2005;32(2):211–214. quiz 215.
77. Marcus C. Strategies for improving the quality of verbal patient and family education: a review of the literature and creation of the EDUCATE model. *Heal Psychol Behav Med*. 2014;2 (1):482–495. https://doi.org/10.1080/21642850.2014.900450.
78. Whitman M. Patient education: what worries the patient most? *Nursing (Lond)*. 2015;45(1):52–54. https://doi.org/10.1097/01.NURSE.0000453722.00617.69.
79. Europe WHORO for Europe Compenhagen. *Therapeutic Patient Education: Continuing Education Programmes for Health Care Providers in the Field of Prevention of Chronic Diseases: A Report of a WHO Working Group*. http://www.who.int/iris/handle/10665/108151.
80. Roberts L, Cornell C, Bostrom M, et al. Communication skills training for surgical residents: learning to relate to the needs of older adults. *J Surg Educ*. 2018;75(5):1180–1187.
81. Forkan R, Pumper B, Smyth N, Wirkkala H, Ciol MA, Shumway-Cook A. Exercise adherence following physical

therapy intervention in older adults with impaired balance. *Phys Ther*. 2006;86(3):401–410.

82. Prochaska JO, DiClemente CC. Stages and processes of self-change of smoking: toward an integrative model of change. *J Consult Clin Psychol*. 1983;51(3):390–395.
83. Marshall SJ, Biddle SJ. The transtheoretical model of behavior change: a meta-analysis of applications to physical activity and exercise. *Ann Behav Med*. 2001;23(4):229–246. https://doi.org/10.1207/S15324796ABM2304_2.
84. Greaney ML, Riebe D, Ewing Garber C, et al. Long-term effects of a stage-based intervention for changing exercise intentions and behavior in older adults. *Gerontologist*. 2008;48(3):358–367.
85. Krebs P, Prochaska JO, Rossi JS. Defining what works in tailoring: a meta-analysis of computer tailored interventions for health behavior change. *Prev Med*. 2010;51(3–4):214–221. https://doi.org/10.1016/j.ypmed.2010.06.004. DEFINING.
86. Valenzuela T, Okubo Y, Woodbury A, Lord SR, Delbaere K. Adherence to technology-based exercise programs in older adults: a systematic review. *J Geriatr Phys Ther*. 2018;41(1):49–61. https://doi.org/10.1519/JPT.0000000000000095.
87. Mehra S, Visser B, Dadema T, et al. Translating behavior change principles into a blended exercise intervention for older adults: design study. *JMIR Res Protoc*. 2018;7(5):e117. https://doi.org/10.2196/resprot.9244.
88. Gordon NP, Hornbrook MC. Older adults' readiness to engage with eHealth patient education and self-care resources: a cross-sectional survey. *BMC Health Serv Res*. 2018;18(1):220. https://doi.org/10.1186/s12913-018-2986-0.
89. Petursdottir U, Arnadottir SA, Halldorsdottir S. Facilitators and barriers to exercising among people with osteoarthritis: a phenomenological study. *Phys Ther*. 2010;90(7):1014–1025. https://doi.org/10.2522/ptj.20090217.
90. Phillips LD. Patient education. Understanding the process to maximize time and outcomes. *J Intraven Nurs*. 1999;22(1):19–35.
91. Kuhlenschmidt ML, Reeber C, Wallace C, Chen Y, Barnholtz-Sloan J, Mazanec SR. Tailoring education to perceived fall risk in hospitalized patients with cancer: a randomized, controlled trial. *Clin J Oncol Nurs*. 2016;20(1):84–89. https://doi.org/10.1188/16.CJON.84-89.
92. Fahlberg B. "No education about me without me": a shared decision-making approach to patient education. *Nursing (Lond)*. 2015;45(2):15–16. https://doi.org/10.1097/01.NURSE.0000459549.75744.3a.
93. Rigdon AS. Development of patient education for older adults receiving chemotherapy. *Clin J Oncol Nurs*. 2010;14(4):433–441. https://doi.org/10.1188/10.CJON.433-441.
94. Lelorian S, Bachelet A, Bertin N, Bourgoin M. French healthcare professionals' perceived barriers to and motivation for therapeutic patient education: a qualitative study. *Nurs Health Sci*. 2017;19:331–339.
95. Farahani MA, Mohammadi E, Ahmadi F, Mohammadi N. Factors influencing patient education: a qualitative research. *Iran J Nurs Midwifery Res*. 2013;18(2):133–139.
96. Ambady N, Koo J, Rosenthal R, Winograd CH. Physical therapists' nonverbal communication predicts geriatric patients' health outcomes. *Psychology Aging*. 2002;17(3):443–452.

CHAPTER
12

Caregiving of the Older Adult

Elizabeth J. Bergman, Brian W. Pulling

OUTLINE

INTRODUCTION

As we age, many of us will need assistance with tasks such as personal care (e.g., bathing, dressing), transportation, meal preparation, and health maintenance, and often this assistance will be needed over a sustained period of time. These long-term services and supports (LTSSs), also called long-term care, will be provided by caregivers, either professional (e.g., physicians, physical therapists, home health aides) or unpaid (e.g., spouses, adult children, friends). LTSSs may be provided in nursing homes or other residential settings but are most often provided in the home by unpaid family caregivers, who serve as the backbone of the LTSS system in the United States and in many nations across the world.[1]

Health care professionals are caregivers, of course, but so too are parents, grandparents, children, friends, neighbors, and volunteers. Caregivers are not always professionally trained, but care is always contextually delivered and experientially informed. That is, all caregivers provide care based on their assessment of need, and the ways in which they provide care are informed by their own experience. This chapter will demonstrate the relevance of caregiving in a variety of contexts (e.g., dementia caregiving, grandparents raising grandchildren) as well as from the perspectives of clinicians, family caregivers, and patients. Caregivers perform a seemingly endless array of duties and roles, and are essential to the health and wellness of all people. Caregiving is not nearly so linear as described in the institutional setting; it is often a circular process, and we aim to present it as such.

This chapter will focus primarily on the experience of providing unpaid care to older adults. Given the realities of family life today, we use the term *family caregiver* to refer not just to those with a familial or legal relationship with the care recipient (e.g., spouses, adult children, and other relatives), but also to other nonprofessional sources of care (e.g., neighbors, partners, friends) who help older adults manage the trajectory of disease and/or disability. All uses of the terms *caregiving* and *caregiver* will refer to unpaid family caregivers, unless explicitly stated. This review of the caregiving literature will examine the types of care provided, the nature and flow of exchanges within families, specific roles family members may take, and the impacts of family caregiving. This literature is important to physical therapists in treating patients who may be caregivers themselves and in treating patients who receive care from a family caregiver.

We will also examine the experience of physical therapists as professional caregivers. Through the exploration of the caregiving literature provided here, we aim to provoke geriatric physical therapists to remain cognizant of the pivotal role of caregivers *and* to remember to see themselves as caregivers. It is useful to remember that being a caregiver is often a very prominent and salient role and is a significant part of lived experience when serving in the role of caregiver, whether informal or formal, unpaid or paid. "However one looks at caregiving and the mechanisms that drive it over time, one finds that its demands and activities are dynamic and change. The caregivers are likely to confront a shifting assortment of conditions requiring a rather constant structuring and restructuring of their lives."[2]

CAREGIVING CONTEXT AND STATISTICS

The demographics of the U.S. population are covered elsewhere in this text. It is important to note here that even by their most conservative projections, the U.S. Census Bureau estimates that by the year 2050 one in five (20%) Americans will be aged 65 or older, up from 13% in 2010.[3] The vast majority of Americans prefer to live in the least restrictive environment as they age and opt for institutionalization only as it becomes a necessity. Many families accommodate this preference through a commitment to caring for their aging loved ones. The need for caregivers will therefore inevitably increase.[4]

A recent, nationally representative study of family caregiving in the United States[5] found that an estimated 34.2 million adults had served as an unpaid caregiver to another adult age 50 or older in the last 12 months.[5] This represents 14.3% of American adults, or one in seven. Approximately 60% of caregivers are female. The age of caregivers in the United States spans the life course. This study found that 21% of caregivers were aged 18 to 34, 24% were aged 35 to 49, 35% were aged 50 to 64, 12% were aged 65 to 74, and 8% were aged 75 or older. Average age varies by race/ethnicity, with the highest average age among white caregivers (53.4) and the lowest age among Hispanic caregivers (44.2). Approximately one-third of caregivers provide more than 21 hours of care each week. Older caregivers are more likely to provide more intense care in terms of hours per week.[5]

Estimates of the type of relationship between caregiver and care recipient vary. Spillman and colleagues[6] found that approximately 20% of caregivers are spouses and approximately 50% are adult children. The same nationally representative study referenced in the previous paragraph[5] estimated that a minority of caregivers (14%) were caring for a nonrelative (e.g., friend, neighbor, other).[5] A majority (86%) were caring for a relative—most frequently a parent (47%) or parent-in-law (8%). Eleven percent of caregivers were caring for a spouse or partner. The remaining 20% were caring for other relatives (e.g., grandparent, aunt/uncle, sibling).

A *primary caregiver* is one who is either the sole caregiver or one who provides the majority of care. A *secondary caregiver* is a family caregiver who supports a primary caregiver. Approximately one-half of primary caregivers say that their loved one receives support from another family caregiver and one-third say that their loved one receives support from a paid, formal caregiver (e.g., aide, housekeeper). One-third of primary caregivers report that they are the sole source of support, formal or informal, to their loved one. These sole family caregivers are more likely than other family caregivers to be older, higher-hour caregivers (57%) who care for a spouse or partner (78%).[7]

Family caregivers have been described as the "invisible workforce." The estimated economic value of the unpaid care provided by U.S. caregivers in 2013 was approximately $470 billion. This is roughly equivalent to the economic value of Walmart, the world's largest corporation based on revenue.[8] Without family caregivers, health care and LTSS costs would escalate dramatically.[9] Instead, many of these costs are transferred to caregivers and families. These costs are financial, but also social, emotional, and physical, as will be explored later in this chapter.

Members of this invisible workforce often struggle to balance caregiving commitments with workforce participation. Approximately one-third of caregivers work full time and one-quarter work part time.[5] Caregivers make sacrifices to provide care to their loved one(s) in the form of curtailed workforce participation, loss of wages and job benefits such as health insurance, and loss of retirement savings and Social Security benefits. One study estimated the average lifetime losses in income and benefits to a caregiver who leaves the workforce to be $303,880.[10]

Reciprocity and Exchange

Despite the language of "caregiver" and "care recipient," it is important to remember that the exchanges that occur within families are not unidirectional. Older adults who are the recipients of care very often contribute to the family system as well. Depending on the family's circumstances, these contributions may be financial, emotional, instrumental (e.g., childcare), or otherwise. The caregiving experience is more reciprocal and nonlinear than in the professional health care setting. This affects both the caregiver and care recipient in unique ways, which stand apart from other medical care.

Implications for Geriatric Physical Therapy

Within the context of family caregiving, the nature of care exchanges, the types of care performed, and caregiving outcomes are diverse and vary widely. Understanding the broader demographic and social changes occurring within their patient population while also seeking to better understand the unique individual aspects of their patient's experience will allow professional and unpaid caregivers to work dynamically together. Family caregiving relationships are complicated and based on the experience of those providing and receiving care. Geriatric physical therapists can maximize the effect of their interventions by working dynamically with other caregivers, respecting their role while facilitating best practice care through their professional training and expertise.

DOMAINS OF CAREGIVER ACTIVITIES

Every situation involving the exchange of elder care within families is unique. Most, however, involve some combination of the activities summarized in Table 12.1, which organizes the many tasks and activities of family caregivers into domains. These include household tasks; self-care, supervision, and mobility; emotional and social support; health and medical care; advocacy and care coordination; and surrogacy.[1]

The first two domains, *household tasks* and *self-care, supervision, and mobility*, are those most often associated with family caregiving. Household tasks include the day-to-day activities associated with living and maintaining a home, such as preparing meals, doing laundry, and paying

TABLE 12.1 What Family Caregivers Do for Older Adults

Domain	Caregiver Activities and Tasks
Household tasks	• Help with bills, deal with insurancessss claims, and manage money • Home maintenance (e.g., install grab bars, ramps, and other safety modifications; repairs, yard work) • Laundry and other housework • Prepare meals • Shopping • Transportation
Self-care, supervision, and mobility	• Bathing and grooming • Dressing • Feeding • Supervision • Management of behavioral symptoms • Toileting (e.g., getting to and from the toilet, maintaining continence, dealing with incontinence) • Transferring (e.g., getting in and out of bed and chairs, moving from bed to wheelchair) • Help getting around inside or outside
Emotional and social support	• Provide companionship • Discuss ongoing life challenges with care recipient • Facilitate and participate in leisure activities • Help care recipient manage emotional responses • Manage family conflict • Troubleshoot problems
Health and medical care	• Encourage healthy lifestyle • Encourage self-care • Encourage treatment adherence • Manage and give medications, pills, or injections • Operate medical equipment • Prepare food for special diets • Respond to acute needs and emergencies • Provide wound care
Advocacy and care coordination	• Seek information • Facilitate person and family understanding • Communicate with doctors, nurses, social workers, pharmacists, and other health care and long-term service and support (LTSS) providers • Facilitate provider understanding • Locate, arrange, and supervise nurses, social workers, home care aides, home-delivered meals, and other LTSSs (e.g., adult day services) • Make appointments • Negotiate with other family member(s) regarding respective roles • Order prescription medicines • Deal with insurance issues
Surrogacy	• Handle financial and legal matters • Manage personal property • Participate in advanced planning • Participate in treatment decisions

(From Schulz R, Eden J, eds. *Families Caring for an Aging America*. Washington, DC: National Academies Press; 2016. https://doi.org/10.17226/23606; Spillman BC, Wolff J, Freedman VA, Kasper JD. *Informal Caregiving for Older Americans: An Analysis of the 2011 National Study of Caregiving.* Washington, DC: Office of the Assistant Secretary for Planning and Evaluation; 2014. http://aspe.hhs.gov/report/informal-caregiving-older-americansanalysis-2011-national-health-and-aging-trends-study; Wolff J, Dy SE, Frick K, Kasper JD. End-of-life care: Findings from a National Survey of Informal Caregivers. *Arch Int Med.* 2007;167(1):40–46.

bills. This domain also includes one-time activities (e.g., installing grab bars or ramps) as well as longer-term duties (e.g., dealing with insurance claims). The domain of self-care, supervision, and mobility includes assistance with activities of daily living (ADLs) and instrumental activities of daily living (IADLs).

The *emotional and social support* domain includes a broad range of activities, from making it possible for the care recipient to engage in leisure activities to providing companionship to listening to the care recipient and helping resolve life challenges or family conflict, if possible. This domain of activity is likely to take on greater importance as the care recipient's disease or disability progresses, and the care recipient may become increasingly isolated and susceptible to loneliness.

The domain of *health and medical care* varies in intensity based on the care recipient's diagnosis, stage of progression, and ability. Early on, a caregiver's role within this domain may be to provide encouragement regarding lifestyle, self-care, and treatment adherence. As the intensity of the caregiver role increases, the caregiver may be increasingly responsible for more complex care, such as operating medical equipment, giving injections, and providing wound care.

Advocacy and care coordination include activities related to seeking and facilitating an understanding of health and other care-related information as well as activities related to communication across specialists and other professionals involved in the care recipient's care. It also involves coordinating care, including negotiating the roles of other family members involved in providing care, managing prescription orders, and managing the delivery of services provided by professional LTSS providers.

Surrogacy involves communicating for, and sometimes acting on behalf of, care recipients when they are unable to do so for themselves. This most frequently occurs in the context of financial and legal matters and in health care decision making. Surrogacy often goes hand in hand with advocacy and care coordination and is most likely to increase in intensity as the care recipient's disease or condition progresses into the later stages. Caregivers may be called upon to serve as the agent of a health care proxy, a legal document in which the care recipient appoints a surrogate health care decision maker.

Despite the fact that they are often overlooked or minimized in analyses of health care policy and practice, family caregivers are a crucial and indispensable part of the health care delivery system, especially for older adults.[11,12] Historically, research and policy have defined the role of family caregiver based on the provision of assistance with ADLs and IADLs.[13,14] It is increasingly the case, however, that caregivers assist with much more. In a recent, nationally representative survey of caregivers in the United States,[7] 57% reported assisting with complex medical and nursing activities. Another recent study[15] found that nearly half (46%) of all family caregivers reported similar responsibilities. Caregivers reported the following complex medical and nursing activities to be most challenging, in order of frequency: managing incontinence and the use of incontinence equipment and treatments (67%); wound and ostomy care (66%); managing medications (including IVs and injections; 61%); adhering to special diets (53%); and operating medical equipment (e.g., mechanical ventilators, oxygen, home dialysis equipment; 49%).

Owing to medical specialization and fragmentation of the health care system, family caregivers increasingly find themselves responsible for managing the care recipient's interactions with and across the health care system. They must effectively articulate the experiences and needs of the care recipient to multiple specialists in an attempt to provide continuity between health care providers and see that medical orders are made to address the care recipient's needs. Within this fragmented health care system, the caregiver is often the only person to have experienced the full trajectory of his or her loved one's illness and related health care experience.[12] Unfortunately, however, caregivers are often left out of the care recipient's medical record and are not adequately included in important treatment-planning decisions, even though they are often expected to carry out these treatment plans without adequate training and knowledge. Only 14% of family caregivers report receiving preparation or training to provide medical and nursing assistance.[5] As the care recipient's disability or disease progresses, these tasks take on greater importance and the lack of preparation and instruction can be a significant source of caregiver stress.

Caregiver activities vary based on a number of factors, including caregiver characteristics, the care recipient's diagnosis and abilities, and proximity to the care recipient. In addition to the fact that women are more likely to be in the role of family caregiver, they are also more likely to provide basic care, such as assistance with dressing, feeding, and bathing. Male caregivers, on the other hand, are more likely to provide financial assistance.[10]

Caregiver activities also vary based on the care recipient's diagnosis or disability. Kim and Schulz[16] compared the experiences of four groups of caregivers: those caring for loved ones with cancer, dementia, diabetes, and frailty. They found that caregivers of people with cancer or dementia were providing the most assistance with ADLs and IADLs and were more likely to be coordinating outside services provision than were caregivers of people with diabetes or frailty. Although caregivers for people with dementia were more likely to assist with the management of incontinence, people with cancer were more likely to need assistance feeding and transferring.

Proximity to the care recipient is yet another factor that impacts caregiver tasks and activities. Long-distance caregivers (who live more than an hour away) are more likely to provide emotional and social support and advocacy and care coordination, for example, whereas more proximal caregivers are more likely to provide assistance with self-care, supervision, and mobility and with household tasks. It is not uncommon for multiple family caregivers of varying distances to collaborate in the care of an older relative.[1]

Implications for Geriatric Physical Therapy

Caregivers at all levels of the professional and informal spectrum are driven to provide what care they are able in response to the needs of the care recipient. This is best demonstrated by observing the dynamic nature of an interdisciplinary care team in an institutional care environment. Health professionals here communicate and plan as a unit to provide customized and multimodal care with the intention to maximize the patient's function. However, consider that the vast majority of caregivers for older adults are informally trained and have different support structures than those of professionals. As such, an individual caregiver provides a much wider array of tasks and roles for the care recipient.

Many of these domains include duties that require, or at least benefit significantly from, formal training (e.g., transfers, wound care, etc.). In the absence of such training, a caregiver makes do. There are frequent opportunities for physical therapists to significantly improve the care provided to their older adult patients by offering expertise on the safety and efficacy of a task. Consider both that a family caregiver may benefit from the expertise of a health care provider and that the care recipient may benefit from the expert adapting to his or her informal caregiver. Caregiving occurs in the context of the family system, so accommodate care planning and interventions to this context. Gauge the knowledge and comfort level of the caregiver before prescribing that he or she assist with specific tasks, and ensure that prescribed recommendations are feasible within the family system. This is also an opportunity to include the caregiver in problem solving and to provide the caregiver with specific knowledge on how to perform skills like guarding or cueing exercise form. It can also be an opportunity for the health professional to learn from the caregiver, because the caregiver is likely to have performed the task on the family member many times more than the health professional.

THE CAREGIVER ROLE TRAJECTORY

People with serious illness or disability are likely to make frequent transitions between health care settings. Such settings include but are not limited to the emergency department, hospital, skilled nursing facility subacute unit, assisted living, and home (with or without skilled home care services). Eventually they may transition to long-term care in a nursing facility. Death may occur here or in the hospital, perhaps involving the transition to palliative care and/or hospice.[12] Together with these frequent transfers in setting, the health care system has shifted more responsibility onto family caregivers to provide complex medical care, which they are not usually trained to do.

Within this context, family caregiving has been described as a "career" and involves an ever-changing set of circumstances and multiple transitions as the needs of the care recipient change (Table 12.2).[4,17] Viewing caregiving from a career perspective allows for the examination of both the stress processes and rewards that cut across all stages and the particular characteristics and experiences of each stage of the caregiving career. Among the first to describe caregiving as a career, Aneshensel and colleagues[4] divided caregiving into three phases: role acquisition, role enactment, and role disengagement. Others[1,18] have expanded on this early work to map onto the caregiving trajectory the kinds of tasks and activities typical of each phase. It is important to note that the trajectory of the caregiving career is not always linear. As noted in the introduction of this chapter, caregivers are constantly adjusting their activities, priorities, and approaches based on the ever-changing needs and experiences of their care recipient. Care recipients' conditions may improve or decline rapidly, they may need hospitalization or short-term or long-term skilled nursing facility care, they may die suddenly, or other changes may occur that affect the trajectory of the caregiving career.

Role Acquisition

During the role acquisition phase, caregivers may not even yet think of themselves as such. This is the phase during which the awareness of the need for care emerges, loved ones communicate with one another and negotiate roles relative to the care of their older family member, and caregiving roles are accepted. Role acquisition may happen quickly, as in the case of a stroke, or it may happen more gradually, as in the case of a progressive dementia.[1]

The pathway to becoming a caregiver is paved with sometimes competing social norms of reciprocity and obligation. It is also influenced by the history and quality of relationships within families, cultural norms and expectations, gender roles, geographic proximity, and other factors.[19] Potential caregivers often willingly accept the caregiving role, yet the work remains largely invisible and is often done in social isolation.[4]

Role Enactment

During the role enactment phase, caregiving tasks and activities often expand from monitoring and IADL assistance to more complex medical and nursing care, assistance with ADLs, care coordination, and hiring and managing outside care providers. This phase may also be characterized by one or more hospitalizations, admission to a long-term care facility, the provision of palliative care, and/or the transition to hospice care.[1] Some caregivers will experience this phase in a pattern described by Aneshensel and colleagues[4] as *sustained caregiving,* or the continued provision of in-home care until the death of the care recipient. *Comprehensive caregiving* refers to the pattern in which the care recipient moves to a long-term care facility of some kind and the caregiver maintains the provision of substantial care. In contrast, in the *withdrawal from*

TABLE 12.2 Common Experiences, Tasks, and Experiences by Phase of the Caregiver Career

Phase	Role Acquisition	Role Enactment	Role Disengagement
Common experiences	• Emerging awareness of loved one's need for care • Illness/disability onset • Onset of care	• Increasing care demands • In-home care • Possible admission to LTC facility • Hospitalizations • End-of-life care	• Care recipient death • Bereavement • Social reengagement
Common tasks and activities	• Communicate with health care providers • Accompany CR to appointments • Errands/shopping and other IADL support • Encourage treatment adherence • Monitor and check in	• Manage finances • Hire and manage care providers • IADL and ADL support • Supervision • Companionship, listening, and other emotional and social support • Medication and medical equipment management • Wound care and other complex medical/ nursing care • Care coordination and advocacy with health care providers and LTC staff • Communicate with and negotiate roles with other caregivers • Oversee admission and transition to hospice • Advance care planning • Surrogacy	• Financial and legal matters • Resolve insurance issues • Dispenses of CR's personal property • Grief support • Reconnect with and establish new social supports and leisure pursuits

ADL, activities of daily living; *CR*, care recipient; *IADL*, instrumental activities of daily living; *LTC*, long-term care.
(Adapted from Aneshensel CS, Pearlin LI, Mullan JT, Zarit SH, Whitlatch CJ. *Profiles in Caregiving*: The *Unexpected Career*. San Diego, CA:Academic Press; 1995; Schulz R, Tompkins CA. Informal caregivers in the United States: prevalence, caregiver characteristics, and ability to provide care. In: National Research Council. In: *The Role of Human Factors in Home Health Care: Workshop Summary.* Washington, DC: National Academies Press; 2010. Retrieved from, https://www.ncbi.nlm.nih.gov/books/NBK210056/pdf/Bookshelf_NBK210056.pdf; Schulz R, Eden J, eds. *Families Caring for an Aging America*. Washington, DC: National Academies Press; 2016. https://doi.org/10.17226/23606.)

caregiving pattern, caregivers step out of their role as caregiver upon the care recipient's admission to a facility. Finally, in the *foreshortened caregiving* pattern, the care recipient dies very shortly after admission to a facility.

Role Disengagement

The last phase of the caregiving career is role disengagement, which most often begins with the death of the care recipient but may also result when the caregiver dies or shifts caregiving responsibilities to another caregiver owing to illness or inability to sustain the role.[2] During this phase, the caregiver may need to resolve any lingering financial or legal matters and oversee the dispensation of the care recipient's personal property. Caregivers may also experience grief and utilize one or more services designed to support them in their grief. This is also a phase during which many bereaved caregivers begin to resume previous leisure and social pursuits, reinvest in social relationships, and establish new interests and social connections.[4]

Implications for Geriatric Physical Therapy

Caregivers are expected to integrate care across medical settings, often involving frequent changes in providers. It should come as no surprise that family caregivers often feel stressed and overwhelmed within this context of fragmented and complicated care. At the same time, given that they are likely to have experienced the entire trajectory of their loved one's illness and/or disability, they are an extremely important resource to health care providers, including physical therapists, who can provide a context that may otherwise be unavailable, and which may very well drive treatment goals and care decisions.

Although this trajectory has been presented as a linear series of transitions, keep in mind that the caregiver role is dynamic and may not occur in predictable steps. This trajectory is dependent on many factors, which include the influence of professionals on directing and facilitating care. Anticipating key components of the caregiver experience allows the professional to support family caregivers by providing insight and expertise.

THE STRESS PROCESS

The stress process framework has been an important and prominent theoretical perspective guiding caregiving research since its articulation by Pearlin and colleagues.[20] According to the stress process framework, as applied to family caregiving, factors affecting the caregiving experience can be divided into four primary domains. These include the (1) background characteristics of the caregiver/caregiving context, (2) stressors, (3) mediators, and (4) the outcomes or manifestations of stress.[21]

The background and caregiving context include the set of factors with the potential to impact, directly or indirectly, the other domains within the caregiving stress process framework. Examples of factors in this domain include caregiver age, socioeconomic and employment status, gender, race/ethnicity, educational attainment, relationship to the care recipient (e.g., adult child, spouse), and the nature of the relationship between caregiver and care recipient, both in the present and in the past (e.g., closeness, level of conflict).[21]

According to this framework, stressors can be either primary or secondary. *Primary stressors* are those that are directly related to the experience of caregiving. They may be objective (e.g., care recipient's functional or cognitive status, severity of disease/disability) or subjective (e.g., caregiver's perception or appraisal of the situation as stressful; role captivity). *Secondary stressors* are related to or caused by primary stressors but fall outside of the caregiving experience (e.g., family conflicts, financial strains, loss of social or leisure activities, or employment challenges related to the caregiver role).[22] *Proliferation* occurs when stressors in one domain or role overflow into or affect other domains or roles. This may occur, for example, when changes in one's financial situation impact the caregiving role or vice versa.[2,21]

Mediators include those factors that serve as coping resources (e.g., mindfulness practice, maintaining hobbies and other interests, maintaining sense of humor)[23] or social supports (e.g., assistance from family, friends, and church or other community organization; use of formal caregiver supports). Coping is defined by Pearlin and Schooler[24] as behavior that protects individuals from the negative psychological effects of stress, either by changing the conditions causing the stress or by altering the emotional response to stress, thereby eliminating or reducing its potential to cause distress. Lazarus and Folkman[25] refer to efforts to change the conditions causing the stress as *problem-focused coping*, examples of which include identifying the problem, determining potential approaches to altering the situation, weighing the advantages and disadvantages of potential solutions, and taking action to bring about the necessary alterations to the situation. An example of problem-focused coping as it applies to family caregiving involves the hiring of outside help, such as a home health aide, to alleviate some of the workload and allow a caregiver to focus on other essential familial and occupational roles. *Emotion-focused coping*, on the other hand, is described by Lazarus and Folkman[25] as involving efforts to change the meaning of an event or situation. For example, an individual may attempt to minimize the negative outcomes of caregiving by engaging in efforts to reframe the situation as more positive, selectively focusing on the enjoyable aspects of caregiving, or distancing themselves from the caregiving role.

Additionally, a caregiver's perception, or appraisals, of his or her coping resources and supports as adequate to meet the demands of the caregiving context serve to mediate the effects of stressors, whereas caregiving stressors that are appraised or perceived as potentially overwhelming, threatening, or harmful may lead to more negative caregiving outcomes. These mediating factors help to explain the fact that different caregivers experience, respond to, and are affected by the same stressors differently.[21]

Caregiving has outcomes related to physical health (e.g., diminished objective and subjective health, injury, heightened risk of mortality)[26,27] and mental health (e.g., depression, anxiety).[20,26,28] Within the stress process framework, these outcomes are seen as having the potential to affect caregiver well-being and the ability to sustain the caregiver role.[21]

Caregiver Outcomes

The caregiving experience is highly individual and the potential effects extremely varied. Caregiving for older adults is often rigorous and time consuming, and may include costs across a spectrum of physical, psychological, social, and financial conditions.[5] It is often unclear how long a person will require care, and further unclear how long a person will be able to provide it. Burnout is commonly observed institutionally, and this phenomenon is complicated at the informal level because caregivers cannot usually "clock out." There are measurable costs to caregiving, but there are also significant rewards reported by caregivers and recipients alike.[26] In fact, even high levels of distress related to the caregiver role and the derivation of benefits and rewards may occur simultaneously.[6]

Physical Health

The most direct effects of caregiving on caregivers' physical health include the strains and injuries that may result from the lifting, transferring, bathing, dressing, and repetitive actions associated with the role. This is true both for home care and both other professional caregivers[1] and family caregivers.[29] Geriatric physical therapists should make every effort to assess the home environment, the physical demands imposed by caregiving, and the abilities of the caregiver, and factor this information into their treatment plans and assignments that require the assistance of a caregiver.

In comparison to noncaregivers, caregivers self-report poorer health.[26] Caregiver status is independently predictive of risk for cardiovascular disease,[30] coronary heart disease, stroke,[31] frailty,[32] and mortality.[27,33,35] Caregivers may also neglect their own health, engaging in fewer health-promoting self-care behaviors (e.g., rest, preventive health care, exercise) and in more health risk behaviors (e.g., substance abuse, poor diet, smoking).[1]

Psychological Health and Quality of Life

It is well documented that caregiving impacts psychological health and quality of life. In an analysis of National

Study of Caregiving data, Spillman and colleagues[6] found that nearly half of all caregivers reported some degree of emotional difficulty and more than one-quarter reported substantial emotional difficulty. Level of emotional difficulty and negative aspects of caregiving were associated with care recipient health and intensity of care. Many studies have established a relationship between caregiving and lower subjective well-being, depression,[26,34,36,37] and anxiety.[38] This emotional distress persists for caregivers across settings, including after the care recipient transitions to a long-term care facility.[39,40]

Social Well-Being

The social effects of caregiving include changes and potential conflict in family relationships and restrictions on access to one's wider network of social support.[1] In one survey, 55% of caregivers reported feeling overwhelmed by the caregiving role.[41] Caregivers report exhaustion, having too much to do, and not having time for themselves. This results in a lack of time to engage in social and leisure pursuits, including visiting with family and friends, attending religious services, engaging in volunteer work, or going out for enjoyment.[6]

Caregiving also holds the potential for familial conflict, a situation that may be exacerbated by a caregiver's diminished ability to effectively communicate or engage in conflict resolution owing to physical or emotional distress. Studies have documented caregiving-related family discord linked to boundary setting, the nature of the care recipient's condition, perceived inadequacy of support from others, the quality of care, financial matters, and perceived underappreciation of the demands of the caregiver role.[1]

Economic Well-Being

There are a range of potential financial costs of caregiving, including the provision of direct financial assistance to the care recipient, reduced personal savings or ability to meet personal expenses, taking on of debt, and the consequences of employment changes, such as lost income, benefits, or reduced private pension and Social Security benefits.[9] Caregiving has been found to be associated with reduced labor force participation as well as reduced net worth for caregivers.[42] Furthermore, 20% of caregivers reported that the out-of-pocket medical costs of their care recipient accounted for their highest expense.[6] Nearly 40% report that caregiving results in a moderate to high degree of financial strain.[5]

Rewards of Caregiving

Family caregivers very often report experiencing positive aspects of caregiving simultaneously with caregiver strain. Examples of the commonly experienced positive aspects of caregiving include satisfaction in reciprocating care, feeling appreciated, passing on a tradition of care within the family by modeling caring behavior, closer familial relationships, increased meaning and purpose, enhanced confidence and personal growth, increased self-esteem, mastery, satisfaction in keeping the care recipient(s) safe and healthy, and pride in maintaining family well-being and identity.[1,36,43] It is also possible that caregivers' perception of other stressful situations in their lives will be mediated by the successes and rewards they experience as a caregiver.

Costs and Rewards to the Care Recipient

Being the recipient of care also has costs and rewards, as examined by Reinhard et al.[15] Costs of receiving care included constantly being reminded of their illness or disability (24%); pain, discomfort, and embarrassment (16%); and limited activity (11%). Most frequently reported rewards included avoiding nursing home placement (51%); more independence (43%); lessened pain and symptoms (40%); and permitting more family involvement and outside activities (31%).

Implications for Geriatric Physical Therapy

Experiences surrounding stress and coping will be familiar to any health care professional, and training and resources are commonly available to them in dealing with the complex challenges they face. In this way, geriatric physical therapists can better empathize with family caregivers in the shared coping experience. There is, however, an added layer to the experience in that family caregivers are caring for loved ones, and their relationship to the care recipient is not exclusively centered around the giving of care. This additional context may be a mediator of the stress experience as described earlier but more generally will have profound effects on the entire experience of caregiving in more emotional ways than are typical to a professional caregiving relationship. Geriatric physical therapists are particularly suited to provide resources to caregivers to help them cope with the stressors they face. These may be offered by the physical therapist directly, such as with expert opinion or experience in dealing with a complex medical situation at home, or in identifying and accessing resources in the community.

SPECIFIC CAREGIVING RELATIONSHIPS

As stated throughout this chapter, the caregiving experience is dynamic, nonlinear, and highly individualized. However, it is useful to have an understanding of some of the most common caregiving relationships, their unique challenges and rewards, and their clinical implications. Our exploration of the first three caregiving relationships—spousal caregiving, parental caregiving, and dementia caregiving—focuses on older adults as the recipients of care. With respect to the final two caregiving relationships—caring for adults with developmental/intellectual disability and kinship caregiving—we focus on older adults as the providers of care.

Spousal/Partner Caregiving

The spouse/partner, if there is one, is often the most likely caregiver. This is often by choice—indeed, many spouses say that honoring their marriage vow of "in sickness and in health" is a particular reward of caregiving. Sometimes, however, the spouse/partner as primary caregiver is more a reflection of societal and familial pressures.[2] Nearly one in five (18%) of all caregivers to older adults are spouses or partners,[44] and they provide nearly a third of the total hours of care provided to older adults.[6]

Covinsky and colleagues[45] conducted a large-scale cross-sectional study of patients with dementia and their caregivers, which revealed that 32% of participating caregivers presented with depressive symptomatology and that female spousal caregivers were at particular risk. Pinquart and Sörensen[26] also found that spousal caregivers, regardless of gender, reported more stress, lower levels of feelings of self-efficacy, and poorer physical health than nonspousal caregivers, potentially owing to the compounding effects of age-related losses.

Parental Caregiving

In the absence of a spouse/partner, adult children are the next most likely caregivers (Table 12.3). Nearly half (42%) of all caregivers are children[44] and they provide nearly half of the total hours of care.[6] In some cases, more than one adult child is available and willing to serve in the role. In other cases, the role of caregiver falls to a particular adult child. This could be because he or she is an only child, the most geographically proximate, unpartnered or without dependent children, or female in a family that divides responsibilities according to traditional gender norms.[2] Regardless of how an adult child acquires the role, he or she often cites the ability to reciprocate for the love and care the parent showed him or her as a particular reward of caregiving. In other cases, parental care occurs in the context of a historically conflictual or even abusive relationship. It can be difficult for some adult children to accept the role reversal that occurs in the context of parental caregiving. This can be particularly salient when the care recipient and caregiver are of the opposite sex and the parent requires assistance with, for example, bathing or personal hygiene.

A majority of parental caregivers are employed (57%), according to a 2011 analysis of parental caregivers aged 50+ by the MetLife Mature Market Institute. Many of these parental caregivers also have children living at home and are members of the "sandwich generation" of caregivers with responsibilities to more than one generation at a time.

Dementia Caregiving

Dementia involves cognitive decline related to learning and memory, language, executive function, complex attention, perceptual–motor function, and/or social cognition.[46] Dementia is not a disease, but rather a term that refers to a set of symptoms related to these areas of cognitive function and severe enough to interfere with everyday activities. Alzheimer disease is the most common form of dementia, accounting for 60% to 80% of cases, but dementias can also be vascular (occurring after a stroke) or related to a number of other conditions (e.g., Lewy body dementia, Parkinson disease). The average length of survival after an Alzheimer diagnosis among individuals aged 65 and older is 4 to 8 years, having significant implications for the caregiver. Some conditions that cause symptoms of dementia are reversible in nature, such as thyroid problems and vitamin deficiencies.[48]

Dementia caregiving has been characterized in the literature as particularly stressful and uniquely demanding. In addition to memory loss, people with dementia may have communication impairments or exhibit behavior changes, such as emotional outbursts or dramatic changes in sleeping or eating patterns, that may be stressful for caregivers. It can be a particularly emotionally taxing experience to see a loved one "lose themselves" and the often long duration of the caregiving role has other implications for

TABLE 12.3 A Comparison of Spousal/Partner and Parental Caregiving

Relationship	Caregiver	Care Recipient	Needs and Intensity
Spouse/partner	68-year-old white unemployed female currently providing care for 44.4 hours a week for an average of 5.6 years without other unpaid help	71-year-old male spouse who had surgery/wounds or heart disease	Helps with more ADLs (2.2) and IADLs (5.3), and more likely to help with medical/nursing tasks (83%) and have a high burden of care (73%)
Parent (or in-law)	48-year-old employed daughter, currently providing care for 23.9 hours per week for an average of 4.0 years with other unpaid help	77-year-old mother or mother-in-law who has "old age" issues, Alzheimer disease, or mobility problems	More likely to help with arranging services (37%); helps with 4.3 IADLs; more likely wanting information about financial help

ADLs, activities of daily living; *IADLs*, instrumental activities of daily living.
(Data from National Alliance for Caregiving & AARP Public Policy Institute. Caregivers of Older Adults: A focused Look at Those Caring for Someone Age 50+. Washington DC. https://www.aarp.org/content/dam/aarp/ppi/2015/caregivers-of-older-adults-focused-look.pdf Published 2015.)

emotional, social, and physical health.[47] It can be challenging to sustain motivation, coping resources, and physical stamina over the long duration of caregiving while the intensity of care progressively increases. It is also not uncommon for people with dementia to transition between different health care settings and levels of care. Although these transitions can sometimes bring caregivers some relief, they can also be accompanied by a heightened need for advocacy, care coordination, and/or surrogacy.

Unfortunately, a dementia diagnosis can have implications for the quality of the health care made available to people. Although the presence of dementia may factor into health care decision making, it does not in and of itself mean that a person is any less worthy of care, and the goals of rehabilitation should still be the restoration of function and the maintenance of activity and mobility. Physical therapists and other health care providers should strive to avoid "professional nihilism," or the attitude that because a patient has dementia their efforts as health care providers are not worthwhile.[47] Instead, identify and partner with caregivers to understand patients' needs and values, and provide the caregivers with the information and training they need to support the goals of rehabilitation.

Caring for an Adult Child with Intellectual/Developmental Disability

People with intellectual and developmental disabilities (I/DDs) are living longer than ever before and their care is primarily provided by family members, often a parent.[49] As they age, individuals with I/DDs are at risk for undetected and/or poorly managed health conditions and accelerated aging associated with their condition.[50] At the same time, approximately one in four family caregivers of people with I/DDs are over age 60 and may themselves experience changes in their health and need the assistance of family or paid caregivers.[49]

Many parents caring for an adult child with an I/DD have done so for the entire life of the child, and as such the caregiving role has become a routinized part of life. However, planning is necessary for the likely possibility that alternate caregivers will be needed after the parents pass away. The process of developing a plan for the continued care of an adult child with an I/DD is often stressful in and of itself. If there are siblings, they may find themselves in the role of family caregiver to both their parents and sibling with an I/DD.[51]

Yamaki et al.[52] found that female caregivers of adults with I/DDs were more likely to have arthritis, high blood pressure, obesity, and activity limitations compared with females in the general U.S. population. These or other conditions may result in a need for physical therapy for caregivers, which alternately can present a challenge to caregivers in finding time to participate in therapy, as well as potentially offering them a respite from their duties.

Kinship Care/Grandparents as Caregivers

Kinship care refers to grandparents and other relatives caring for young children. In 2012, 6% of all children in the United States lived in grandparent-maintained households and 2.7 million grandparents had primary responsibility for their minor grandchildren who lived with them. Many of these grandparents (39%) had been caring for their grandchildren for more than 5 years.[53]

Grandparents who care for their grandchildren are not representative of all grandparents in the United States. They are younger, less educated, and more likely to be divorced or widowed, living in poverty, black or Hispanic, and unable to work owing to disability or illness.[53] Very often, grandparents find themselves raising their grandchildren owing to potentially difficult or stressful circumstances, such as the death, extended illness, or incarceration of the parent, or owing to parental substance abuse or military deployment.[54] In these cases, both the grandparent(s) and grandchildren may need significant external support. Grandparents may also have needs related to housing their grandchildren, meeting their educational needs, or obtaining legal custody and financial supports.

Grandparents who are raising their grandchildren present to physical therapy with very specific needs, and usually very specific goals as well. The motivation for improving mobility and increasing activity level is often external, having to do with their desire to "keep up" with their grandchild(ren). These patients have significant responsibilities outside of their rehabilitation, and geriatric physical therapists should consider this when planning treatment.

For example, John is a 67-year-old man who has been referred to outpatient physical therapy after a right total knee arthroplasty. He and his wife have recently started caring for their 8-year-old granddaughter, whose parents very recently passed away in an accident. It is August, and the granddaughter is supposed to go back to school in a few weeks. John's only priority is to take care of his granddaughter, comfort and support her, make her feel at home in a new city, and get her back to school. In other words, rehabilitation is not a priority, but helping out with his granddaughter's soccer practice is, and so rehabilitation becomes a means to a very specific end. The most meaningful rehabilitative goals for grandparents caring for grandchildren are those in the context of that relationship.

Implications for Geriatric Physical Therapy

There are two primary considerations for geriatric physical therapy in the context of caregiver roles, both of which present unique challenges for physical therapists in the way they design and adapt their treatments to best suit the needs of their patient. First, a physical therapist may be providing care for someone who also has a family caregiver. In this case, it is mainly important that care be designed and implemented in a way that is supplemented by or supplementary to the other care being provided. Second, caregivers themselves may require physical therapy while also providing care for someone else. In this case, it is crucial that treatment at the very least not hinder the caregiver's work, and potentially support it. And last, physical therapists are caregivers too, and by better understanding the experience of other caregivers, they can provide better care themselves.

MULTICULTURAL ISSUES IN CAREGIVING

"The older adult population" is not one homologous demographic, and beyond the differences in their health care needs, it is absolutely necessary to consider that the way in which people provide (and indeed receive) care is a function of their culture. We have intentionally chosen not to elaborate on the specific details of any one group, culture, or identity to avoid the potential for oversimplification and/or marginalization. Instead, we have created several vignettes (Table 12.4) that integrate the concepts outlined here, with specific implications for physical therapy practice.

It is through the lens of our culture that we learn to understand the world and our place in it. Our culture and our cultural values dictate our behaviors and influence our perception of health. For example, culture influences our decision-making processes (e.g., collective vs. individual), our perception of and response to pain,[55] our health services utilization, and the ways in which we define a health problem, report symptoms, and respond to treatment guidance.[56] Geriatric physical therapists must, therefore, remain keenly attuned to the role of culture in each individual patient's experience and in each patient's care exchange network.

Cultural Competence

The American Physical Therapy Association defines cultural competence as "a set of congruent behaviors, attitudes, and policies that come together in a system, agency, or among professionals and enable that system, agency, or those professionals to work effectively in cross-cultural situations."[57] Cultural competence is a long-term developmental process, not an end point, and it requires ongoing self-assessment and a commitment to inclusion.[58] Essentially, building cultural competence is to expand on one's knowledge of culture and the implications it may have on all aspects of life, but in this case more directly on physical therapy treatment outcomes. It is clear that culture affects caregiving experiences, and that both individuals and groups have explicit rules for how caregiving develops.[58] It may not always be clear why or how specific cultural differences manifest for caregivers or care recipients,[59] but recognizing the complexity and diversity of the older adult population is a necessity for all caregivers.

Cultural Humility

Cultural humility allows the health care practitioner to take a step further toward a more comprehensive awareness and integration of culture and individuality.[60] Cultural humility expands on cultural competence by adding that while there are many specific and consistent factors related to culture that may impact the health care experience, these factors equally may impact that experience in previously unexpected ways, or even not at all.[61] Health care practitioners should always question and analyze their own biases and preconceptions with reflection and humility.

Studying culture to better understand others is a very positive component of clinical practice, but categorizing and compartmentalizing any person is a great disservice both to one's clinical practice and, moreover, to the dignity of the patient. It is impractical to expect to study and learn all the potential implications of culture on health care. Rather, ask questions, reflect, and, most of all, listen with the intention of learning, rather than judging. There is value in seeking to understand an individual, with respect and appreciation for his or her culture, values, and experiences. Attune specifically to such things as body language and potential expressions of anxiety or discomfort. Remain nonjudgmental in verbal and nonverbal communications and ask open-ended questions in your attempt to understand your patient's cultural values relative to such things as eye contact, volume of voice, perceptions of control over and cause of illness, response to pain, and use of names.[56]

Intersectionality

Intersectionality helps us understand the ways in which people are shaped by the interaction of multiple social locations (e.g., age, race, ethnicity, ability, religion, gender, class) and to examine the context of interconnected systems of power (e.g., governments, laws, religious institutions, media) within which these interactions occur and through which privilege and oppression are created.[62]

The intersection of multiple aspects of identity shape and inform the caregiving experience. It is not sufficient to say that because someone falls into one group (e.g., transgender, African American, etc.) he or she will experience or enact caregiving in a particular way. It is necessary to examine the intersections of multiple aspects of identity, including caregiver status.[63] To understand the impact of caregiving within the health care system, or indeed from any perspective, you need to consider how all of these variables may interact and influence one another. Moreover, you must have the humility to respect the fact that variables may not interact in the way you expect.

For example, it is important to be aware of the lasting effects of historical oppression and discrimination and continued structural racism that result in delayed treatment and poorer prognosis for many African American patients. However, social class, level of education,

TABLE 12.4 Culture and Geriatric Physical Therapy Practice Vignettes

Vignette 1

Profile

David is a 77-year-old male, presenting to physical therapy with an idiopathic onset of neck pain beginning 6 months ago. He has radiating symptoms down the right arm and intermittent numbness and tingling on the back of his neck. He is a retired banker who has lived in New York City his entire adult life. David is gay, lives alone, is currently unpartnered, and has no children. Owing to his sexual orientation, he has experienced significant discrimination and was estranged from his family as a young adult, though he now has a good relationship with his older sister in California.

Possible Intersections

David is relatively affluent and has good health insurance, but his experiences with the health care system have discouraged him from seeking treatment, to the point where he is now in significant pain. He says that he has always feared revealing a full picture of his lifestyle to his health care providers, a fear that was reinforced by his now-deceased partner's experiences during his diagnosis and treatment of HIV/AIDS. David's privilege afforded by his gender, race, and socioeconomic status intersects with his experience of discrimination and isolation based on his sexual orientation.

Clinical Considerations

David lives alone and avoids interactions with the health care system. He is very concerned that there is nothing anyone can do for his pain and is skeptical that physical therapy or any medical intervention can help him. He doesn't have anyone to help him with his home exercise program.

Vignette 2

Profile

Carlos is a 70-year-old man presenting to physical therapy with deconditioning secondary to chronic obstructive pulmonary disorder (COPD). His left leg was amputated above the knee after being wounded while serving as an infantryman in the Vietnam War, and he reports occasional phantom limb pain distal to his residual limb. Carlos is Puerto Rican and lives in Florida with his wife. He has three children, with one daughter who lives nearby.

Possible Intersections

Carlos was wounded in action and was awarded the Purple Heart. After his leg was amputated he received significant physical therapy at the Veteran's Administration (VA) hospital and was fitted with a prosthetic leg. He has become less and less active over the years and has not sought any counseling or care for posttraumatic stress disorder (PTSD), which has affected him since the war. Carlos has a very supportive family, his wife is his primary caregiver, and his youngest daughter comes over twice a week to help him walk around the neighborhood (though lately he has preferred to stay inside and play with his grandson). Carlos is tremendously proud of his three children and five grandchildren, though he wishes he could see them more often. He doesn't want to be a burden to his wife, but she insists on coming to all his physical therapy sessions and helping him with his home exercise program so that "he will get strong and take me dancing again."

Clinical Considerations

Carlos has many unresolved issues with the VA system and from his experience in Vietnam. He is, however, extremely motivated to continue to be able to play with his grandson and to dance with his wife. He is disinterested in discussing or confronting the roots of his illness: Agent Orange exposure leading to COPD, and PTSD worsening his phantom limb pain. He does reliably complete his home exercise program though, and has expressed interest in trying aquatics therapy.

Vignette 3

Profile

Anna is a 62-year-old woman who lives with her husband in the Southwest as members of the Navajo Nation. She presents to physical therapy in preparation for knee replacement surgery in 2 months, to plan subsequent rehabilitation.

Possible Intersections

Many Navajo people do not implicitly trust doctors, particularly those who are not themselves Navajo people, or from the reservation. Furthermore, discussions about illness and future care planning are in conflict with traditional values. Anna was referred by her physician and may be initially averse to discussing any long-term care plan. She may prefer that close or highly revered family members of her care exchange network, such as her husband, sister, or parents, are informed about her health care first or concurrently. She also may prefer that her health care providers speak about medical interventions in the third person, rather than describing them in direct relation to her personally* (Carrese & Rhodes, 2000).

Clinical Considerations

There is research on specific intersections between Navajo culture and the U.S. health care system. However, keep in mind the importance of cultural humility when interpreting the research on these intersections with an individual patient. Aim to provide compassionate care, offering support while prioritizing the patient's values, dignity, and well-being.

*From: Carrese JA, Rhodes LA. Bridging cultural differences in medical practice. The case of discussing negative information with Navajo patients. *J Gen Intern Med.* 2000;15(2):92–96. PubMed PMID: 10672111; PubMed Central PMCID: PMC1495335.

TABLE 12.5	Cultural Competence, Cultural Humility, and Intersectionality Resources
Harvard Project Implicit, *Implicit Association Test:* https://implicit.harvard.edu/implicit/takeatest.html	
National Center for Elder Abuse, *Fact Sheets for Cultural Issues:* https://ncea.acl.gov/resources/publications.html	
American Physical Therapy Association, *Cultural Competence in Physical Therapy:* http://www.apta.org/CulturalCompetence/	
National Seed Project, Unpacking the Invisible Knapsack by Peggy McIntosh: https://nationalseedproject.org/images/documents/Knapsack_plus_Notes-Peggy_McIntosh.pdf	
The Cross Cultural Health Care Program, *Cultural Competence Resources Guides:* http://xculture.org/resources/general-resource-guides/cultural-competence-resources/	

religion, or other aspects of identity may intersect with race and result in different health behaviors, health services utilization, and outcomes than would be the case based on race alone.

Implications for Geriatric Physical Therapy

Understanding that the absence of cultural competence and humility, both individually and systemically, is directly related to the existence of health disparities[55] and identifying the intersectionality of identity with both cultural humility and competence are foundations of good clinical practice, and essential to caregiving. There are no shortcuts here, but self-awareness is a primary tool in developing these practices. There are specific concerns for the physical therapist that directly affect patient care, beyond building rapport and protecting patient dignity. The previous availability of formal medical resources may impact the stage of disability or disease at which a patient presents to physical therapy. A history of discrimination, limited availability of resources on reservations, and residence in very rural or very urban areas all may impact care. Physical therapists may not see their patients until later stages of disease progression or may see them in more restrictive settings, limiting the availability of treatment options.

These ideas will be further explored in the vignettes in Table 12.5, intended as case studies of the ways in which culture and identity may intersect, and how those intersections could impact physical therapy practice.

ELDER ABUSE

A potential result of caregiver stress, elder abuse is defined by the Centers for Disease Control and Prevention (CDC) as "an intentional act or failure to act by a caregiver or another person in a relationship involving an expectation of trust that causes or creates a risk of harm to an older adult."[64]

Types of Elder Abuse

There are many different categories of elder abuse (Table 12.6). *Physical abuse* includes the deliberate use of force that results in illness, injury, pain, impairment, or death. Examples include hitting, choking, pushing, shaking, and force-feeding. The inappropriate use of medications and restraints is also considered physical abuse. *Emotional/psychological abuse* includes both verbal and nonverbal behaviors that inflict mental pain,

TABLE 12.6	Signs of Elder Abuse
Geriatric physical therapists should use clinical reasoning to recognize these and other potential signs of elder abuse, recognizing that some of these signs can be innocuous or unrelated, but that in context they may be indicative of something far more serious than the diagnostic presentation might suggest.	
Physical or Sexual Abuse	
• Bruising or welts on the skin, especially those appearing on the face, or lateral and anterior region of the arms • Broken glasses • Fingerprints or handprints visible on the face, neck, arms, or wrists • Burns from scalding, from cigarettes, or in shapes of objects such as an iron • Cuts, lacerations, or puncture wounds • Sprains, fractures, or dislocations • Internal injuries or vomiting • Unexplained sexually transmitted diseases	
Neglect	
• Weight loss with no apparent explanation • Appearing disheveled, in soiled/torn clothing, or inappropriately attired for climate • Appearing hungry, malnourished, disoriented, or confused • Lack of medical aids (e.g., hearing aid, medications, glasses, walker) • Bed sores or other preventable conditions • Report of drug overdose or not taking medications/not refilling medications	
Psychological Abuse	
• Caregiver refusing to let you see patient alone • Disappearing from contact with neighbors, friends, or family • Uncharacteristic changes in behavior (e.g., withdrawal from normal activities, changes in alertness)	
Financial Abuse or Exploitation	
• Lack of amenities elder could afford • Elder has signed property transfers • Elder "voluntarily" gives uncharacteristically excessive financial reimbursement or gifts for needed care or companionship • Caregiver has control of the elder's money but is failing to provide for his or her needs	

(Adapted from National Center on Elder Abuse, https://ncea.acl.gov/resources/publications.html; National Institute on Aging, https://www.nia.nih.gov/health/elder-abuse#types; National Adult Protective Services Association, http://www.napsa-now.org/get-informed/what-is-abuse/.)

distress, or fear. This category of abuse is further categorized into four domains: humiliation/disrespect, threats, harassment, and isolation/coercive control. *Sexual abuse* includes any unwanted and/or forced sexual interaction. This includes acts that involve touching, such as attempted or completed penetration, as well as non-touching acts, such as sexual harassment and forced viewing of pornography. *Financial abuse/exploitation* involves the improper, unauthorized, or illegal use of an elder's financial resources or property, or preventing an elder's access to information or use of personal resources. Cash may be stolen, checks written and erroneously signed, and credit cards misused. In other cases, legal documents are changed for financial gain (such as rewriting a will) or insurance policies changed without permission of the older adult.[64] *Neglect* is when a caregiver ignores or refuses to respond to a person's physical, social, or emotional needs, which results in risk of compromised health or safety. This can include withholding food, water, clothing, medications, or assistance.[1]

Prevalence and Risk Factors for Elder Abuse

In a 2010 study, Acierno and colleagues[65] reported that approximately 1 in 10 adults over the age of 60 experienced some form of elder abuse. The same study revealed that most of this abuse went unreported. The New York State Elder Abuse Prevalence Study[66] found that for every case of financial abuse that was reported, 44 went unreported, and that for every case of abuse that programs and agencies were aware of, they were unaware of 23.5 others. Risk factors for elder abuse include dementia diagnosis, reliance on others for ADL assistance, female gender, frailty, and social isolation.[1,67] Substance abuse and mental health issues for either or both the elder and the caregiver are also risk factors.[68]

Responding to Elder Abuse

All states have legal statutes addressing elder abuse that identify specific persons as mandatory reporters and define the conditions under which they must make a report. In general, mandatory reporters are required to make a report if they have reasonable cause to suspect or believe that a vulnerable older person has been abused or is living in hazardous conditions. Physical therapists are often identified specifically in state statutes as mandatory reporters, though in some states the law simply identifies all persons as mandatory reporters.[69] If you suspect elder abuse, neglect, or mistreatment of any kind, report your concerns. If the suspected abuse relates to an older adult living in the community, contact your local adult protective services agency. If the suspected abuse relates to an older adult living in a long-term care facility, contact your local long-term care ombudsman (Table 12.7).

TABLE 12.7 Elder Abuse Resources

National Eldercare Locator Hotline: 1-800-677-1116
National Eldercare Locator Online: https://eldercare.acl.gov/Public/Index.aspx
National Center on Elder Abuse: https://ncea.acl.gov/
National Domestic Violence Hotline: http://www.thehotline.org/
National Adult Protective Services Association: http://www.napsa-now.org/get-help/help-in-your-area/
National Institute on Aging: http://www.nia.nih.gov
National Long-Term Care Ombudsman Resource Center: http://theconsumervoice.org/get_help
Stetson Law Center for Excellence in Elder Law, state-by-state breakdown of mandatory reporting statutes for elder abuse: http://www.stetson.edu/law/academics/elder/ecpp/media/Mandatory%20Reporting%20Statutes%20for%20Elder%20Abuse%202016.pdf

Supporting Caregivers

A range of interventions to support family caregivers have been developed (Table 12.8). Most caregiver intervention programs are multidimensional,[70] and these interventions should be categorized as professional support, psychoeducational, behavior management/skills training, counseling/psychotherapy, self-care/relaxation techniques, and environmental redesign. Although their exploration is beyond the scope of this chapter, examples of evidence-based interventions that have been shown to improve caregiver outcomes include Resources for Enhancing Alzheimer's Caregiver Health II (REACH II),[71] $Skills_2Care$,[72] the New York University Caregiver Intervention (NYUCI),[73] the Savvy Caregiver Program,[74] and Powerful Tools for Caregivers.[75] As an illustration of the common features of caregiver intervention programs, the NYUCI program had three components: tailored individual and family counseling, caregiver support groups, and

TABLE 12.8 Caregiver Resources and Supports

National Association of Area Agencies on Aging: https://www.n4a.org/
National Alliance for Caregiving: http://www.caregiving.org/
Family Caregiver Alliance: https://www.caregiver.org/
Family Caregiver Alliance State-by-State Family Care Navigator: https://www.caregiver.org/family-care-navigator
U.S. Department of Health & Human Services, *Eldercare Locator:* https://eldercare.acl.gov/Public/Index.aspx
U.S. Administration for Community Living, *National Family Caregiver Support Program:* https://www.acl.gov/programs/support-caregivers/national-family-caregiver-support-program
AARP Resources for Caregivers: https://www.aarp.org/caregiving/
National Institute on Aging Caregiver Resources: https://www.nia.nih.gov/health/caregiving
The Alzheimer's Association: http://www.alz.org
24/7 Helpline: 1-800-272-3900
Next Step in Care, *Family Caregivers and Health Care Professionals Working Together:* https://www.nextstepincare.org/

"ad hoc" counseling available to caregivers by telephone or in-person at any time during their participation in the program. The improved caregiver outcomes achieved by the NYUCI have also been demonstrated to persist into the caregiver's adjustment to bereavement.[76]

Federal and state policies have been enacted to support family caregivers in a variety of ways. Enacted in 2000, the U.S. National Family Caregiver Support Program provides grants to states and territories to support caregivers with information about available services, assistance gaining access to services, counseling/support groups/caregiver training, respite, and supplemental services.[77] Many family caregivers are overwhelmed by the number of different organizations and requirements they encounter when they seek LTSSs, something they often do not do until they are in a time of crisis. Unfortunately, this sometimes means that decisions are made and LTSSs purchased or used that are not sufficiently aligned with the specific needs of the caregiver and his or her family. In recognition of these challenges, the federal government has implemented a system to support states in the establishment of Aging and Disability Resource Centers that operate as a "No Wrong Door" single-point-of-entry system designed to provide caregivers with information, one-on-one counseling, and simplified access to LTSSs.[78]

In an effort to support family caregivers and care recipients during particularly vulnerable times of transition to or from the hospital, the AARP has led an effort to ensure passage of the Caregiver Advise, Record, Enable (CARE) Act. This legislation, now enacted in a majority of states, requires hospitals to identify family caregivers in medical records, inform them of the care recipient's discharge, and provide them with education and training pertaining to the medical tasks they will be required to perform and the needs of the care recipient as he or she transitions home.[79]

SUMMARY

In this chapter, we have presented and discussed caregiving as an integrated and person-centered practice. We have explored relevant statistics, the reciprocity and exchanges that occur in families, types of caregiving tasks and activities, caregiving relationships, and the caregiver role trajectory. We have situated family caregiving within a system of health care that is currently in a state of transition. Using the stress process framework to guide our discussion of caregiving, we have explored the factors that shape the experience of caregiving and mediate its outcomes. We explored these potential outcomes in detail—physical, emotional, social, and economic—and we have described the rewards of caregiving. Furthermore, we have reminded readers not to make assumptions and to consider the ways in which various aspects of identity and culture intersect with one another to shape the experiences, values, and goals of their patients and their families. We suggest that practitioners constantly strive to further expand their cultural competence and to develop an approach to practice characterized by cultural humility. Finally, we presented information on elder abuse, which can happen when caregivers are under extreme stress, and about supporting caregivers in their important work.

We hope to have left readers with an appreciation for the ways in which geriatric physical therapists can integrate themselves into the larger context of care exchanges often occurring for their patients. In addition, we encourage geriatric physical therapists to utilize the full scope of resources that caregivers can offer to the broader mission of improving the health and well-being of their patients. We hope to have left readers with the conceptualization of physical therapy as a caregiving profession. Physical therapists are caregivers too, and as such they stand to learn a great deal from the dynamic, holistic, and multimodal approach of informal family caregivers, a great deal of which can be implemented in their formal practice of physical therapy. Finally, we stress that it is important for geriatric physical therapists to consider the vast array of factors that shape their patients' lived experience. These factors may not, on first consideration, directly relate to a patient's functional outcomes. However, to the extent that these factors shape and inform a patient's and his or her family's perceptions of health and health care, health behaviors, and treatment adherence, they do in fact directly relate to that patient's functional outcomes.

REFERENCES

1. Schulz R, Eden J, eds. *Families Caring for an Aging America*. Washington, DC: National Academies Press; 2016. https://doi.org/10.17226/23606.
2. Pearlin LI, Aneshensel CS. Caregiving: the unexpected career. *Social Justice Res*. 1994;7:373–390. https://doi.org/10.1007/BF02334863.
3. Ortman JM, Velkoff VA, Hogan H. *An Aging Nation: The Older Population in the United States. Current Population Reports*. Washington, DC: U.S. Census Bureau; 2014. https://www.census.gov/prod/2014pubs/p25-1140.pdf.
4. Aneshensel CS, Pearlin LI, Mullan JT, Zarit SH, Whitlatch CJ. *Profiles in Caregiving: The Unexpected Career*. San Diego, CA: Academic Press; 1995.
5. National Alliance for Caregiving & AARP Public Policy Institute. Caregivers of Older Adults: A Focused Look at Those Caring for Someone Age 50+. Washington, DC. https://www.aarp.org/content/dam/aarp/ppi/2015/caregivers-of-older-adults-focused-look.pdf. Published 2015.
6. Spillman BC, Wolff J, Freedman VA, Kasper JD. *Informal Caregiving for Older Americans: An Analysis of the 2011 National Study of Caregiving*. Washington, DC: Office of the Assistant Secretary for Planning and Evaluation; 2014. http://aspe.hhs.gov/report/informal-caregiving-older-americans-analysis-2011-national-health-and-aging-trends-study.
7. National Alliance for Caregiving & AARP Public Policy Institute. Caregiving in the U.S. 2015. Washington, DC. http://ww1.prweb.com/prfiles/2015/06/03/12765231/2015_CaregivingintheUS_Final%20Report_WEB.pdf. Published 2015.
8. Fortune. *Fortune Global*. 2018;500. http://fortune.com/global500/. Published 2018.

9. Reinhard SC, Feinberg LF, Choula R, Houser A. *Valuing the Invaluable: 2015 Update, Undeniable Progress, but Big Gaps Remain*. Washington, DC: AARP Public Policy Institute; 2015. http://www.aarp.org/content/dam/aarp/ppi/2015/valuing-the-invaluable-2015-update-new.pdf.
10. MetLife Mature Market Institute. The MetLife study of caregiving costs to working caregivers: double jeopardy for Baby Boomers caring for their parents. Westport, CT. Retrieved from http://www.caregiving.org/wp-content/uploads/2011/06/mmi-caregiving-costs-working-caregivers.pdf. Published 2011.
11. Gitlin LN, Wolff J. Family involvement in care transitions of older adults: what do we know and where do we go from here? *Ann Rev Gerontol Geriatr*. 2011;31(1):31–64. https://doi.org/10.1891/0198-8794.31.31.
12. Levine C, Halper D, Peist A, Gould DA. Bridging troubled waters: family caregivers, transitions, and long-term care. *Health Aff*. 2010;29(1):116–124. https://doi.org/10.1377/hlthaff.2009.0520.
13. Giovannetti ER, Wolff JL. Cross-survey differences in national estimates of numbers of caregivers of disabled older adults. *Milbank Q*. 2010;88:310–349. https://doi:10.1111/j.1468-0009.2010.00602.x.
14. LaPlante MP, Harrington C, Kang T. Estimating paid and unpaid hours of personal assistance services in activities of daily living provided to adults living at home. *Health Serv Res*. 2002;37(2):397–415.
15. Reinhard S, Levine C, Samis S. *Home Alone: Family Caregivers Providing Complex Chronic Care*. Washington, DC: AARP and United Hospital Fund; 2012. Retrieved from, https://www.aarp.org/content/dam/aarp/research/public_policy_institute/health/home-alone-family-caregivers-providing-complex-chronic-care-rev-AARP-ppi-health.pdf.
16. Kim Y, Schulz R. Family caregivers' strains: comparative analysis of cancer caregiving with dementia, diabetes, and frail elderly caregiving. *J Aging Health*. 2008;20(5):483–503. https://doi.org/10.1177/0898264308317533.
17. Brody EM. Parent care as a normative family stress. *Gerontologist*. 1985;25(1):19–29. https://doi.org/10.1093/geront/25.1.19.
18. Schulz R, Tompkins CA. Informal caregivers in the United States: prevalence, caregiver characteristics, and ability to provide care. In: National Research Council. In: *The Role of Human Factors in Home Health Care: Workshop Summary*. Washington, DC: National Academies Press; 2010. Retrieved from, https://www.ncbi.nlm.nih.gov/books/NBK210056/pdf/Bookshelf_NBK210056.pdf.
19. Cavaye JE. From dawn to dusk: a temporal model of caregiving: adult carers of frail parents. Paper presented at CRFR conference, Edinburgh, UK, October 2008. Retrieved from http://oro.open.ac.uk/27974/1/CRFR%20Conf%20Paper%20October%2008%20Final.pdf.
20. Pearlin LI, Mullan JT, Semple SJ, Skaff MM. Caregiving and the stress process: an overview of concepts and their measures. *Gerontologist*. 1990;30(5):583–594. http://psycnet.apa.org/doi/10.1093/geront/30.5.583.
21. Montgomery RJV, Kwak J, Kosloski KD. Theories guiding support services for family caregivers. In: Bengtson VL, Settersten RA, eds. *Handbook of Theories of Aging*. New York, NY: Springer; 2016:443–462.
22. Skaff MM, Pearlin LI, Mullan JT. Transitions in the caregiving career: effects on sense of mastery. *Psychology Aging*. 1996;11(2):247–257. https://doi.org/10.1037/0882-7974.11.2.247.
23. Ekwall AK, Sivberg B, Hallberg IR. Older caregivers' coping strategies and sense of coherence in relation to quality of life. *J Adv Nurs*. 2007;57(6):584–596. https://doi:10.1111/j.1365-2648.2006.03994.x.
24. Pearlin LI, Schooler C. The structure of coping. *J Health Social Behav*. 1978;19(1):2–21. https://doi.org/10.2307/2136319.
25. Lazarus RS, Folkman S. *Stress, Appraisal, and Coping*. New York: Springer; 1984.
26. Pinquart M, Sörensen S. Differences between caregivers and noncaregivers in psychological health and physical health: a meta-analysis. *Psychology Aging*. 2003;18(2):250–267. http://psycnet.apa.org/doi/10.1037/0882-7974.18.2.250.
27. Schultz R, Beach SR. Caregiving as a risk factor for mortality: the Caregiver Health Effects Study. *JAMA*. 1999;282(23):2215–2219. http://psycnet.apa.org/doi/10.1001/jama.282.23.2215.
28. Haley WE, Levine EG, Brown SL, Bartolucci AA. Stress, appraisal, coping, and social support as predictors of adaptational outcome among dementia caregivers. *Psychology Aging*. 1987;27:323–330.
29. Brown AR, Mulley GP. Injuries sustained by caregivers of disabled elderly people. *Age Ageing*. 1997;26(1):21–23.
30. Capistrant BD, Moon JR, Berkman LF, Glymour MM. Current and long-term caregiving and onset of cardiovascular disease. *J Epidemiol Community Health*. 2012;66(10):951–956. https://dx.doi.org/10.1136%2Fjech-2011-200040.
31. Ji J, Zöller B, Sundquist K, Sundquist J. Increased risks of coronary heart disease and stroke among spousal caregivers of cancer patients. *Circulation*. 2012;125(14):1742–7. doi: 10.1161/CIRCULATIONAHA.111.057018. Epub 2012 Mar 13. PubMed PMID: 22415143.
32. Dassel KB, Carr DC. Does dementia caregiving accelerate frailty? Findings from the Health and Retirement Study. *Gerontologist*. 2016;56(3):444–450. https://doi.org/10.1093/geront/gnu078.
33. Perkins M, Howard VJ, Wadley VG, et al. Caregiving strain and all-cause mortality: evidence from the REGARDS Study. *J Gerontol B Psychol Sci Social Sci*. 2013;68(4):504–512. https://dx.doi.org/10.1093%2Fgeronb%2Fgbs084.
34. Cuijpers P. Depressive disorders in caregivers of dementia patients: a systematic review. *Aging Mental Health*. 2005;9(4):325–330. https://doi.org/10.1080/13607860500090078.
35. Nielsen M, Hansen J, Ritz B, et al. Cause-specific mortality among spouses of Parkinson disease patients. *Epidemiology*. 2014;25(2):225–232. https://doi.org/10.1097/EDE.0000000000000042.
36. Haley WE, Allen JY, Grant JS, Clay OJ, Perkins M, Roth DL. Problems and benefits reported by stroke family caregivers: results from a prospective epidemiological study. *Stroke*. 2009;40(6):2129–2133. https://doi.org/10.1161/STROKEAHA.108.545269.
37. Kim Y, Shaffer KM, Carver CS, Cannady RS. Prevalence and predictors of depressive symptoms among cancer caregivers 5 years after the relative's cancer diagnosis. *J Consult Clin Psychology*. 2014;82(1):1–8. http://psycnet.apa.org/doi/10.1037/a0035116.
38. Cannuscio CC, Jones C, Kawachi I, Colditz GA, Berkman L, Rimm E. Reverberations of family illness: a longitudinal assessment of informal caregiving and mental health status in the Nurses' Health Study. *Am J Public Health*. 2002;92(8):1305–1311.
39. Gaugler JE. Family involvement in residential and long-term care: a synthesis and critical review. *Aging Mental Health*. 2005;9(2):105–118. http://psycnet.apa.org/doi/10.1080/13607860412331310245.
40. Schulz R, Belle SH, Czaja SJ, McGinnis KA, Stevens A, Zhang S. Long-term care placement of dementia patients and caregiver health and well-being. *JAMA*. 2004;292(8):961–967. https://doi.org/10.1001/jama.292.8.961.
41. American Psychological Association. *Stress in America: Our Health at Risk*. Washington, DC: American Psychological Association; 2012. https://www.apa.org/news/press/releases/stress/2011/final-2011.pdf.

42. Butrica B, Karamcheva N. *The Impact of Informal Caregiving on Older Adults' Labor Supply & Economic Resources*. Washington, DC: U.S. Department of Labor; 2014. https://www.dol.gov/sites/default/files/ebsa/researchers/analysis/retirement/impactofinformalcaregivingonolderadults.pdf.
43. Coon DW. Resilience and family caregiving. *Ann Rev Gerontol Geriatr*. 2012;32(1):231–250. https://doi.org/10.1891/0198-8794.32.231.
44. Freedman VA, Spillman BC. Disability and care needs of older Americans: an analysis of the 2011 National Health and Aging Trends Study. In: *Report to the U.S. Department of Health and Human Services Assistant Secretary for Planning and Evaluation Office of Disability, Aging and Long-Term Care Policy*; 2014. http://aspe.hhs.gov/daltcp/reports/2014/NHATS-DCN.cfm.
45. Covinsky KE, Newcomer R, Fox P, et al. Patient and caregiver characteristics associated with depression in caregivers of patients with dementia. *J Gen Intern Med*. 2003;18(12):1006–1014. https://dx.doi.org/10.1111%2Fj.1525-1497.2003.30103.x.
46. American Psychiatric Association. In: *Diagnostic and Statistical Manual of Mental Disorders*. 5th ed. Arlington, VA: American Psychiatric Publishing; 2013.
47. Cohen D, Eisdorfer C. *The Loss of Self: A Family Resource for the Care of Alzheimer's Disease and Related Disorders*. New York: W.W. Norton & Company; 2001.
48. Alzheimer's Association. 2018 Alzheimer's disease facts and figures. *Alzheimer's Dementia*. 2018;14(3):367–429. https://doi.org/10.1016/j.jalz.2018.02.001.
49. Factor A, Heller T, Janicki M. *Bridging the Aging and Developmental Disabilities Service Networks: Challenges and Best Practices*. Chicago: Institute on Disability and Human Development, University of Illinois at Chicago; 2012. http://www.acf.hhs.gov/sites/default/files/aidd/bridgingreport_3_15_2012.pdf.
50. Perkins EA, Moran JA. Aging adults with intellectual disabilities. *JAMA*. 2010;304(1):91–92. http://psycnet.apa.org/doi/10.1001/jama.2010.906.
51. Heller T, Caldwell J, Factor A. Aging family caregivers: policies and practices. *Dev Res Rev*. 2007;13(2):136–142. https://doi.org/10.1002/mrdd.20138.
52. Yamaki K, Hsieh K, Heller T. Health profile of aging family caregivers supporting adults with intellectual and developmental disabilities at home. *Intellect Dev Disabil*. 2009;47(6):425–435. https://doi.org/10.1352/1934-9556-47.6.425.
53. Ellis RR, Simmons T. Coresident grandparents and their grandchildren: 2012. In: *Current Population Reports, P20-576*. Washington, DC: U.S. Census Bureau; 2014. https://www.census.gov/content/dam/Census/library/publications/2014/demo/p20-576.pdf.
54. Rubin D, Springer SH, Zlotnik S, Kang-Yi CD. Needs of kinship care families and pediatric practice. *Pediatrics*. 2017;139(4):e20170099. https://doi.org/10.1542/peds.2017-0099.
55. Coolen PR. Cultural relevance in end-of-life care. *Ethnomed*. https://ethnomed.org/clinical/end-of-life/cultural-relevance-in-end-of-life-care. Published 2012.
56. Wright EM. Cultural competence: a vital piece in the puzzle of health literacy. Paper presented at the Finger Lakes Geriatric Education Center Healthy Aging in Rural New York Conference, Watkins Glen, NY, April 18, 2018.
57. American Physical Therapy Association. *Cultural competence in physical therapy*. http://www.apta.org/CulturalCompetence.
58. Dilworth-Anderson P, Williams IC, Gibson BE. Issues of race, ethnicity, and culture in caregiving research: a twenty year review (1980-2000). *Gerontologist*. 2002;42(2):237–272.
59. Pinquart M, Sörensen S. Ethnic differences in stressors, resources, and psychological outcomes of family caregiving: a meta-analysis. *Gerontologist*. 2005;45(1):90–106. https://doi.org/10.1093/geront/45.1.90.
60. Hook JN, Davis DE, Owen J, Worthington EL, Utsey SO. Cultural humility: measuring openness to culturally diverse clients. *J Couns Psychol*. 2013;60(3):353–366. https://doi.org/10.1037/a0032595.
61. Tervalon M, Murray-Garcia J. Cultural humility versus cultural competence: a critical distinction in defining physician training outcomes in multicultural education. *J Health Care Poor Underserved*. 1998;9(2):117–125. https://doi.org/10.1353/hpu.2010.0233.
62. Hankivsky O. Intersectionality 101. In: *Institute for Intersectionality Research & Policy, Simon Fraser University*; 2014. https://alumni.northeastern.edu/wp-content/uploads/2017/02/Intersectionality-101-Week-1.pdf.
63. Crenshaw K. Demarginalizing the intersection of race and sex: a black feminist critique of antidiscrimination doctrine, feminist theory and antiracist politics. *University of Chicago Legal Forum*. 1989;1989(1). http://chicagounbound.uchicago.edu/uclf/vol1989/iss1/8.
64. Hall JE, Karch DL, Crosby AE. Elder abuse surveillance: uniform definitions and recommended core data elements for use in elder abuse surveillance, Version 1.0. Atlanta, GA: National Center for Injury Prevention and Control. Centers for Disease Control and Prevention. 2016. Retrieved from https://www.cdc.gov/violenceprevention/pdf/EA_Book_Revised_2016.pdf.
65. Acierno R, Hernandez MA, Amstadter AB, et al. Prevalence and correlates of emotional, physical, sexual, and financial abuse and potential neglect in the United States: the National Elder Mistreatment Study. *Am J Public Health*. 2010;100(2):292–297. https://dx.doi.org/10.2105%2FAJPH.2009.163089.
66. Lifespan of Greater Rochester, Cornell University, and New York City Department for the Aging. Under the Radar: New York State Elder Abuse Prevalence Study. https://ocfs.ny.gov/main/reports/Under%20the%20Radar%2005%2012%2011%20final%20report.pdf. Published 2011.
67. Beach SR, Schulz R, Williamson GM, Miller LS, Weiner MF, Lance CE. Risk factors for potentially harmful informal caregiver behavior. *J Am Geriatr Soc*. 2005;53(2):255–261. https://doi.org/10.1111/j.1532-5415.2005.53111.x.
68. National Center on Elder Abuse. *Red Flags of Elder Abuse*. Washington, DC: National Center on Elder Abuse; 2015. https://ncea.acl.gov/resources/docs/Red-Flags-Elder-Abuse-NCEA-2015.pdf.
69. Stetson University Law School. Mandatory reporting statutes for elder abuse. http://www.stetson.edu/law/academics/elder/ecpp/media/Mandatory%20Reporting%20Statutes%20for%20Elder%20Abuse%202016.pdf. Published 2016.
70. Gitlin LN, Marx K, Stanley IH, Hodgson N. Translating evidence-based dementia caregiving interventions into practice: state-of-the-science and next steps. *Gerontologist*. 2015;55(2):210–226. https://doi.org/10.1093/geront/gnu123.
71. Belle SH, Burgio L, Burns R, et al. Enhancing the quality of life of dementia caregivers from different ethnic or racial groups: a randomized, controlled trial. *Ann Intern Med*. 2006;145(10):727–738. https://doi.org/10.7326/0003-4819-145-10-200611210-00005.
72. Gitlin LN, Winter L, Corcoran M, Dennis MP, Schinfeld S, Hauck WW. Effects of the Home Environmental Skill-Building Program on the caregiver–care recipient dyad: 6-month outcomes from the Philadelphia REACH Initiative. *Gerontologist*. 2003;43(4):532–546. https://doi.org/10.1093/geront/43.4.532.
73. Mittelman MS, Roth DL, Coon DW, Haley WE. Sustained benefit of supportive intervention for depressive symptoms in Alzheimer's caregivers. *Am J Psychiatry*. 2004;161:850–856. https://doi.org/10.1176/appi.ajp.161.5.850.

74. Hepburn KW, Lewis M, Sherman CW, Tornatore J. The Savvy Caregiver Program: developing and testing a transportable dementia family caregiver training program. *Gerontologist.* 2003;43(6):908–915. https://doi.org/10.1093/geront/43.6.908.
75. Boise L, Congleton L, Shannon K. Empowering family caregivers: the Powerful Tools for Caregiving Program. *Educ Gerontol.* 2005;31(7):573–586. https://doi.org/10.1080/03601270590962523.
76. Haley WE, Bergman EJ, Roth DL, McVie T, Gaugler JE, Mittelman MS. Long-term effects of bereavement and caregiver intervention on dementia caregiver depressive symptoms. *Gerontologist.* 2008;48(6):732–740. https://doi.org/10.1093/geront/48.6.732.
77. U.S. Administration for Community Living. National Family Caregiver Support Program. https://www.acl.gov/programs/support-caregivers/national-family-caregiver-support-program
78. U. S. Administration on Aging. FY 2015 Report to Congress: Older Americans Act. https://www.acl.gov/about-acl/reports-congress-and-president. Published 2015.
79. Coleman EA. Family caregivers as partners in care transitions: the Caregiver Advise, Record, and Enable Act. *J Hosp Med.* 2016;11(12):883–885. https://doi.org/10.1002/jhm.2637.

CHAPTER 13

The Older Adult Who Is Frail

Dale Avers

OUTLINE

INTRODUCTION

Frailty is a concept that most clinicians recognize when they see it, yet it often defies a clear definition. The condition of frailty strongly influences what the clinical presentation of a given disease may look like. For example, a person with kidney disease who also has frailty may present with acute delirium and exhaustion and take an unexpectedly long time to recover from an acute episode of fluid imbalance. Having frailty also adversely influences outcomes of surgery and rehabilitation discussed later in this chapter. Because having frailty has a broad clinical impact on the older adult, recognizing and understanding frailty is key to understanding age- related disease. This chapter will explore the models, background, measurement, intervention, and prevention of frailty.

The aging process, a slow but insidious decline in the functioning of each biological system, typically occurs at a rate of 8% to 10% per decade after age 30. Bortz saw nearly 20 years ago that all organ systems have built-in redundancy and function.[1] For example, the oxygen, digestive, and metabolic systems interact and work together to deliver needed fuel to the right structures at the right time. A decline or dysfunction in one system can lead to an increased contribution of another system, thus maintaining adequate fuel delivery. This built-in redundancy permits most organ systems to function adequately until a 30% minimum functional threshold is crossed. Commonly recognized biological structures and functions known to benefit from this redundancy are listed in Box 13.1. When losses exceed this approximate 30% threshold, diminished function and illness occur. Although frailty is not created when one organ system reaches this minimal functional threshold, when several systems reach this level, the biological stress becomes greater than the organism's capacity to maintain homeostasis.

A key hallmark of frailty, agreed upon by most, is decreased physiological reserve across multiple organ systems leading to identifiable alterations in physical functioning beyond what is expected for normal aging.[2] A cycle of declining energetics and decreasing physiological reserve diminishes one's ability to tolerate day-to-day or acute stressors, leading to a loss in homeostasis and thus increasing vulnerability to adverse health events (Fig. 13.1).[3] Interestingly, Bortz notes that it is when the musculoskeletal system declines to this minimal functional level that frailty becomes apparent.[1] Indeed, weakness is the most common initial manifestation of frailty.[4] Individuals who regularly exercise and stay physically active experience this physiological loss at a much slower rate, remaining free of frailty into their 90s. No matter how frequently observed, frailty should not be considered inevitable until extreme old age. Fig. 13.2 illustrates this generalized decline. Further description of this graphic is found elsewhere in this text.

There is no universally agreed-upon definition of frailty. However, frailty is most often characterized as a biologic syndrome of decreased reserve and resistance to stressors, resulting from cumulative declines across multiple physiologic systems, and causing vulnerability to adverse outcomes.[3] This definition has produced two major models for recognizing frailty. The first model is operationalized by five clinical attributes of weakness, slowness, shrinking, low energy, and inactivity

BOX 13.1 Commonly Recognized Biological Structures and Functions That Benefit from Cross-System Redundancy, Providing an Approximate 70% Safety Margin Before Frank Dysfunction Appears[1]

Oxygen transport
Myocardial oxygen consumption
Arterial cross-sectional area
Hemoglobin–oxygen dissociation
Maximum breathing capacity
Forced expiratory volume
Hematologic values
Hepatic and renal function
Blood sugar
Sensory capacity (vision and hearing)
Cognitive skills
Brain dopamine content
Musculoskeletal (sarcopenia and osteoporosis)

Note: Nerve conduction velocity and red blood cell mass have less redundancy than those listed.[1]

known as the phenotype of frailty. The second model is operationalized by the cumulative effect of age-related disorders, functional conditions, and psychosocial issues, known as the Frailty Index. Both descriptions of frailty are anchored by the impact of loss of physiological reserve, vulnerability to physiological stress, and dysregulation across multiple organ systems.

PREVALENCE

The prevalence of frailty depends on which model is used to evaluate frailty and ranges from 4.0% to 59.1% in community-dwelling older adults.[5] However, when only the frailty phenotype model was used, the prevalence ranged from 4.0% to 17%.[5] Similarly, a 2011 study using the same frailty phenotype model found the prevalence of frailty to be 15.3% of a nationally representative sample of over 7000 community-dwelling, Medicare enrollees ≥65 years of age. This same study found that 45.5% of these older adults were prefrail (having one or two of the five attributes).[6] Frailty increases with age. For example, the proportion of individuals identified as frail rose from only 8.9% of individuals in the 65- to 69-year age bracket to 37.9% of individuals in the age bracket of 90+ years.[6] Although the number of individuals classified as prefrail also increases with age, the increase was less steep, with 39.5% of individuals in the 65- to 69-year age bracket classified as prefrail compared to 48.7% of individuals in the age bracket of 90+ years.[6] Frailty prevalence occurs at higher rates among older women, racial/ethnic minorities, and those with lower incomes.[6] Frailty prevalence is 65% to 85% higher for blacks and Hispanics than whites.[6] Frailty occurs at the highest rate in nursing homes, with some estimates as high as 76% depending on the frailty measurement used, with the remainder considered prefrail.[7,8]

MODELS OF FRAILTY

The phenotype of frailty, developed by Linda Fried and others, consists of five clinical attributes: (1) unintentional weight loss, (2) self-reported exhaustion, (3) muscle weakness, (4) slow walking speed, and (5) low physical activity.[3] The phenotype has been used to classify individuals as not frail (zero characteristics), prefrail (one to two

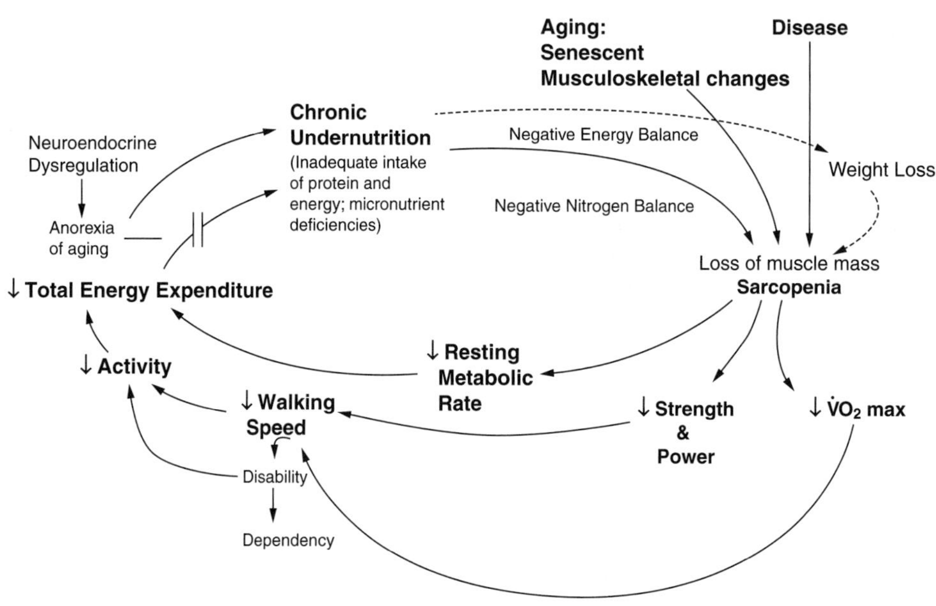

FIG. 13.1 Operational model of frailty. *(From Fried LP, Walston J. Frailty and failure to thrive. In: Hazzard WR, Blass JP, Ettinger WH Jr, Halter JB, Ouslander J, eds. Principles of Geriatric Medicine and Gerontology. 4th ed. New York: McGraw Hill; 1998:1387–1402.)*

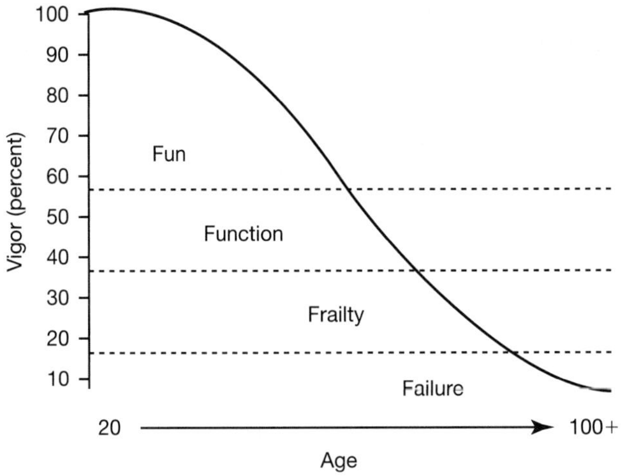

FIG. 13.2 Slippery slope of aging. *(Adapted from Schwartz RS. Sarcopenia and physical performance in old age: introduction. Muscle Nerve. 1997;Suppl 5:S10–S12.)*

characteristics), or frail (three or more characteristics) in studies examining frailty outcomes, transitions through the various stages of frailty, and interventions to reverse or decrease frailty. The frailty phenotype model is the most commonly used method of recognizing frailty.[5] The phenotype is particularly useful to physical therapists as each of the five attributes can be addressed through specific interventions within the physical therapist's scope of care. Table 13.1 provides details of the phenotype's operational definition.

In contrast to the phenotype of frailty, the Frailty Index characterizes the extent of a person's frailty by creating a frailty risk index. The actual number of health deficits an individual has accumulated over time is divided by the total number of wide-ranging potential health deficits considered. The resultant index represents a continuous scale ranging from 0 to 1.[9] The risk index is derived from a survey of 70 clinical indicators in the original form (30- or 40-item indicators in more recent short forms) that includes items of physical and cognitive impairments, diseases and syndromes, disability, and psychosocial risk factors.[9,10] Box 13.2 displays the 70-item list of the original Frailty Index.[11] Lending credibility to the cumulative deficit model is the finding that an individual with four or more comorbid indicators is 40 times more likely to be frail than nonfrail.[6] The Frailty Index may better predict the stages of moderate and severe frailty.[12] An important take-home is that when a patient presents with a long list of comorbidities and functional deficits, the clinician should consider the context of frailty. The most obvious difference between the two models is that Rockwood and colleagues[11] considered any clinical indicator associated with an adverse health outcome as a clinical deficit, whereas the frailty phenotype focuses on five specific physical attributes as key indicators of frailty.

DOMAINS OF FRAILTY

Although the study of frailty has focused almost exclusively on the physical aspect of frailty, there is some contention that a more conceptual perspective of frailty should be considered, one that recognizes that there are other pathways or domains to frailty in addition to physical.[13] The factors most closely associated with the physical domain of frailty, and the attributes of the frailty phenotype, include nutrition, mobility, physical activity, strength, endurance, and balance. However, some researchers advocate for the consideration of the cognitive, psychological (mood, emotions, control), and social domains of frailty. Cognition, psychological, and social domains of frailty will be briefly described next as they are relevant to the physical therapist. These domains have unique features and may overlap with each other.

Cognitive Frailty

There is growing recognition that older adults with physical frailty may exhibit poorer cognitive performance and steeper cognitive decline than those without physical frailty.[14] In a large sample of over 6000 individuals, cognitive impairment (defined as the lowest quartile of two cognitive tests) was observed in approximately 20% (92 of 421) of frail individuals living in the community.[15] Cognitive frailty is linked to a reduction in cognitive reserve, where reserve is defined as the capacity of an individual to resist cognitive impairment or decline.[16,17] Cognitive frailty may be the intermediary between "normal aging" and brain disease[18] and may be reversible with management of underlying causes.[19]

The frequency of the apolipoprotein E ε4 allele (a strong genetic risk factor for Alzheimer disease) does not differ between those who are frail and those who are not,[15] thus supporting the contention that cognitive frailty is independent of Alzheimer disease. Cognitive frailty is strongly associated with both physical frailty and cognitive impairment excluding a clinical diagnosis of Alzheimer disease or another dementia.[16] Thus, recognizing physical frailty as a possible risk factor for cognitive frailty may aid in identifying appropriate interventions to prevent or reverse cognitive decline. Gait speed and grip strength, the physical components of frailty most strongly associated with cognitive function,[18] can be key to identifying beneficial interventions.

Multiple risk factors that influence cognitive impairment are also associated with the development and worsening of physical frailty.[19] Fig. 13.3 illustrates the relationship between specific risk factors for frailty and cognitive impairment. These factors include cardiovascular events (e.g., diabetes, dyslipidemia, hypertension), nutritional deficiencies (e.g., malnutrition, vitamin D deficiency), hormonal imbalance (e.g., reduced testosterone, insulin resistance), inflammation, accumulation of neurotoxic β-amyloid in the brain, nigral neuronal loss,

TABLE 13.1 Phenotype of Frailty

Criteria	Description	Measurement
Weight loss	Unintentional weight loss of 10 pounds or more in past year or more than 5% in past year	Scale or self-report
Fatigue	Complaint of exhaustion with normal activity	Meets criteria for frailty if answer is positive for the question: • Felt that everything I did was an effort in last week or could not get going in last week Meets criteria for frailty if a self-report of "moderate or most of the time" is given for either statement: • I felt that everything I did was an effort in the last week. • I could not get going in the last week. Mobility Tiredness Scale[148] A point is given for an affirmative response to the question: • Do you feel tired when Climbing stairs? Walking outside? Walking indoors? Getting outside? Bathing lower body? Dressing lower body? Items are ranked by hierarchy of most strenuous to least strenuous. Scoring is dichotomous on scale of 0 to 6 with higher scores indicating fatigue.[148]
Low physical activity	History of sedentary behavior <383 kcal/week men <270 kcal/week women	Goal is to capture sedentary activity. Ask: • Do you get any physical exercise for the sake of exercising? • How often do you leave your house? IF help is needed to leave home, OR if less than three times per week, assume frailty. Activity scale with subset of six activities: Walking Chores Gardening General exercise Mowing Golfing
Slowness	Usual gait speed over 4.57 meters (15 feet)	Women: ≥7 s for height ≤159 cm (0.65 m/s) Women: ≥6 s for height >159 cm (0.76 m/s) Men: ≥7 s for height ≤173 cm (0.65 m/s) Men: ≥6 s for height >173 cm (0.76 m/s)
Weakness	Grip strength	Lowest 20% of handgrip strength for BMI indicated Men BMI — Grip strength (kg) ≤24 — ≤29 kg 24.1–26 — ≤30 kg 26.1–28 — ≤30 kg >28 — ≤32 kg Women BMI — Grip strength (kg) <23 — ≤17 kg 23.1–26 — ≤17.3 kg 26.1–29 — ≤18 kg >29 — ≤21 kg Gold standard for strength <30 kg for men and <20 kg for women in EWGSOP or <8 sit to stands in 30 s

BMI, body mass index; *EWGSOP*, European Working Group on Sarcopenia in Older People.

BOX 13.2 70 Criteria of the Cumulative Deficit Model or Frailty Index

Changes in everyday activities
Head and neck problems
Poor muscle tone in neck
Bradykinesia, facial
Problems getting dressed
Problems with bathing
Problems carrying out personal grooming
Urinary incontinence
Toileting problems
Bulk difficulties
Rectal problems
Gastrointestinal problems
Problems cooking
Sucking problems
Problems going out alone
Impaired mobility
Musculoskeletal problems
Bradykinesia of the limbs
Poor muscle tone in limbs
Poor limb coordination
Poor coordination, trunk
Poor standing posture
Irregular gait pattern
Falls
Mood problems
Feeling sad, blue, depressed
History of depressed mood
Tiredness all the time
Depression (clinical impression)
Sleep changes
Restlessness
Memory changes
Short-term memory impairment
Long-term memory impairment
Changes in general mental functioning
Onset of cognitive symptoms
Clouding or delirium
Paranoid features
History relevant to cognitive impairment or loss
Family history relevant to cognitive impairment or loss
Impaired vibration
Tremor at rest
Postural tremor
Intention tremor
History of Parkinson disease
Family history of degenerative disease
Seizures, partial complex
Seizures, generalized
Syncope or blackouts
Headache
Cerebrovascular problems
History of stroke
History of diabetes mellitus
Arterial hypertension
Peripheral pulses
Cardiac problems
Myocardial infarction
Arrhythmia
Congestive heart failure
Lung problems
Respiratory problems
History of thyroid disease
Thyroid problems
Skin problems
Malignant disease
Breast problems
Abdominal problems
Presence of snout reflex
Presence of palmomental reflex
Other medical history

Variables constructed from the Canadian Study of Health and Aging Rockwood.
(From Rockwood K, Andrew M, Mitnitski A. A comparison of two approaches to measuring frailty in elderly people. *J Gerontol A Biol Sci Med Sci*. 2007;62[7]:738–743.)

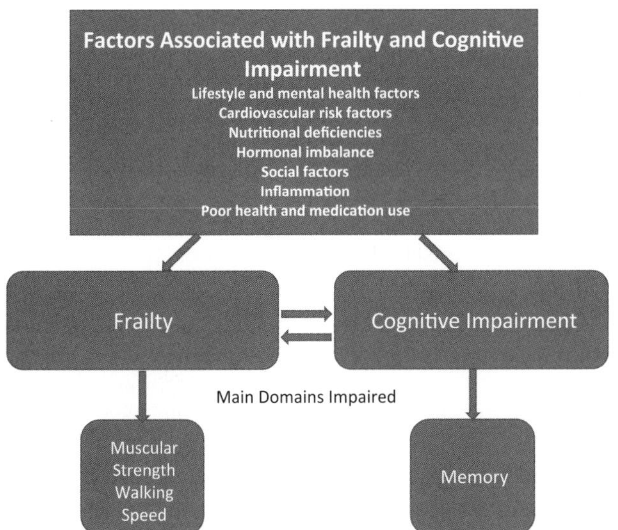

FIG. 13.3 Relationship between frailty and cognitive impairment. The factors associated with frailty and cognitive impairment are similar. The risk of cognitive impairment increases as the degree of frailty increases. *(Brigola AG, Rossetti ES, Neri AL. Relationship between cognition and frailty in elderly: a systematic review. Dementia & Neuropsychologia. 2015:9;110–119 available from http://www.scielo.br/scielo.php?script=sci_arttext&pid=S1980-57642015000200110.)*

lifestyle (social network, cognitive leisure activity, physical activity), and depression.[19] New insights about changes in the brain and cognition and how compensatory mechanisms work are being revealed by neural imaging. For example, older adults recruit more prefrontal circuits with greater cognitive demand than younger adults. This greater demand results in eventual decompensation when challenge overrides ability.[20] In another study, women who developed frailty had impaired executive functioning (Trail Making Test, part B).[14] Executive functioning often precedes declines in memory.[21] The implication of these sorts of findings is that a biological marker for cognitive frailty might be an inability to exhibit a minimal level of compensation for a cognitive task that most healthy older persons could perform.[18] Inability to adapt to increased stress and cognitive load, such as when an older adult has a sudden change in his or her environment (e.g., hospitalization or emergency department), may be the essential determinant of cognitive frailty.[17]

Psychological Frailty

Psychological frailty encompasses mood (fear, anxiety, anger, etc.), resilience, depression, self-efficacy, and control. These attributes are difficult to tease out from the physical presentation of frailty, and research is not clear on their relationships to frailty. However, depressive symptoms are common in people who are frail, with prevalence between 20.7% and 53.8% depending on how frailty was measured.[22] Perhaps the prevalence is strong because of the shared attribute of exhaustion found in many models.[22] Several moderators of the depression and frailty relationship have been studied including anemia,[23] sarcopenia/osteopenia,[24] and antidepressant use.[25]

Little is known about the ability of psychological factors to modify frailty outcomes. For example, the characteristics of high anxiety levels, low levels of well-being and sense of control, the need for caregiver assistance, having few social activities, and having low home/neighborhood satisfaction were associated with frailty and an increased likelihood of adverse outcomes such as being admitted to the emergency department within 1 month of hospital discharge.[26] Alternatively, higher levels of wellness, self-mastery (sense of control), and self-efficacy were associated with decreased odds of functional decline and can protect older individuals from transitioning from a state of lower physical performance into further disability and nursing home placement.[5] Those men and women with higher levels of psychological well-being were less likely to become frail over a 4-year follow-up period.[27] It may be that psychological resources can serve as a safeguard against adverse outcomes such as functional decline and mortality in older adults who are frail.[28]

Resilience is an example of a psychological resource that seems to protect against frailty. Resilience is the capacity to adapt to changing environmental challenges, whereas frailty is described as a loss of resilience. Resilience is significantly associated with frailty. High levels of resilience were found in those people less likely to be frail, especially men.[29] Conversely, low resilience and depressive symptoms can predict frailty.[29] Interestingly, in a group of nuns, fast gait speed was positively associated with resilience.[30] For men and women, active engagement in social activities can reduce depressive symptoms. Social support is a protective factor for women. Traumatic life events can be a contributing factor for frailty and are associated with resilience. Traumatic life events are associated with long-term effects on health and with early mortality in late life.[31] Trauma severity and trauma count were positively associated with frailty in men only.[29] Reminiscence approaches to cope with traumatic experiences may help to build resilience.[29]

Social Frailty

Social supports are important determinants of well-being throughout life and may promote well-being and protect against a variety of other life stresses, including the stress related to aging. Financial well-being (adequacy of income) is associated with frailty in separate studies of English and Chinese older adults.[32,33] Less is known about the association of wealth and frailty in the United States; however, poorer economic status is associated with functional limitations, worse cognitive function, and greater disease burden.[34] Wealth disparities negatively impact frailty, with those older adults who are poorer having a greater risk to become frail as compared with wealthier older adults.[35]

Social frailty is defined using criteria such as having few contacts, little involvement in social activities, and living alone; loneliness is defined as a subjective feeling of dissatisfaction with one's social relationships.[36] Frailty is indirectly associated with loneliness and social isolation.[27] For example, in those who were frail at baseline, loneliness increased over 3 years studied.[28] Steptoe et al. found that social factors and loneliness are linked with increased mortality, incident heart disease, and functional decline.[37] Woo et al. found an association between a lack of social support network and increasing frailty.[32] For example, prefrail and frail adults had a smaller network size and higher levels of loneliness compared with nonfrail peers; however, it may be that people with smaller social networks have a higher chance of becoming physically frail in later life.[36] In a study of nearly 2500 Chinese participants in Singapore, the authors found that social frailty was closely related to physical frailty, sharing many risk factors in common with physical frailty, even to being able to independently predict instrumental activities of daily living (IADL) difficulty and severe disability.[38]

Loneliness may increase the likelihood of sarcopenia.[39] Loneliness and social isolation are associated with a decline in both typical and fast gait speed[40] as well as less resilience.[30] Poor physical functioning may promote physical isolation; however, it is controversial whether social engagement has a positive impact on physical functioning, although those who have lower physical function may benefit more from increased social engagement.[41] Because low physical activity is a cause of sarcopenia, physical activity may be a mechanism underlying loneliness and the progression of physical frailty. Lonely people are more likely to be inactive, and such inactivity increases the risk of physical frailty.[42]

Although there are many tools to measure psychological/cognitive and social frailty, the Tilburg Frailty Indicator (TFI) is a comprehensive, multidimensional questionnaire that addresses physical, psychological/cognitive, and social components of frailty. It consists of two parts. Part A consists of 10 questions on frailty determinants (e.g., age, gender, marital status, education level, and way of life), and Part B consists of 15 frailty elements arranged according to three different subdomains. The physical aspect consists of items related to physical health, similar to the phenotype attributes. The psychological aspect includes components related to cognition, depression, anxiety, and coping. The social aspect consists of elements associated with living alone, social relationships, and social support.[13] Much research needs to be done before a more conceptual view of frailty is fully understood, incorporating the nonmedical attributes of cognition, mood, depression, and social factors.

FRAILTY TRANSITIONS

The state of frailty is dynamic, rather than static, having particular implications for physical therapists. Table 13.2 summarizes the findings of a 4.5-year longitudinal study examining the natural progression of frailty among 754 community-dwelling older adults over the age of 70 years using a modified version of the frailty

TABLE 13.2 Transitions Across Categories of Frailty Among Community-Dwelling Older Adults over an 18-Month Period[43]

Transition from nonfrail to:		Direction of Change
Nonfrail	51.5%	No change
Prefrail	40.1%	Declined
Frail	4.2%	Substantial decline
Transition from prefrail to:		
Nonfrail	11.9%	Improved
Prefrail	58.3%	No change
Frail	24.9%	Declined
Transition from frail to:		
Frail	63.9%	No change
Prefrail	23%	Improved
Nonfrail	0%	Substantial improvement

phenotype. Over the first 18-month time period, the majority of people did not change from their initial category. However, of those who transitioned, most transitioned to a greater state of frailty, and once frail, no one transitioned back to a nonfrail status.[43] These downward transitions highlight the need to identify a vulnerability to prefrailty and frailty so as to determine appropriate interventions. Although moving into greater degrees of frailty is more common, transitions into lesser degrees are also possible, but they are more likely when moving from prefrail to not frail.[44] The most frequent transition is to move from nonfrail to prefrail and from frail to death.

The fluidity of degrees of frailty is seen in response to a stressor such as illness (e.g., pneumonia). The independent but vulnerable patient who is admitted for a short stay in the hospital but who is unable to return home in a short time period because of increased mobility disability is an illustration of this exaggerated reaction to a stressor.[45] As Fig. 13.4 indicates, a person who is not frail and managing well is likely to withstand an external stressor with only a minor and short-lasting decline in functioning. However, with increasing degrees of frailty, that same stressor causes a more pronounced decline in function and requires more time to return to the prior level of functioning, if return to prior function occurs at all. Thus, degrees of frailty should be identified with the view of improving outcomes and avoiding all unnecessary external stressors such as those that might occur with nonessential medical interventions or surgeries. Because the potential for adverse outcomes increases with increasing severity of frailty, identifying highly vulnerable individuals and adjusting interventions accordingly may improve outcomes. The markers of various stages described in Table 13.3 may assist the clinician.

Vigorous physical activity carried out at least once weekly appears to be the most effective means to reduce the progression of frailty in older adults. However, even moderate physical activity at least once weekly was associated with the decreased extent and progression of frailty in individuals over 65 as well as those 50 to 54 years of age. A pilot study of home exercise found that prefrail and nonfrail adults had similar interventional effects from 4 months of exercise. In this small study, none of the prefrail subjects transitioned to frailty and 4 of 17 originally prefrail subjects became nonfrail.[46] But in nonfrail adults over age 50, mild physical activity does not appear to be a sufficient stimulus to prevent a downward transition from nonfrail to frail compared with being sedentary. Of note, the substantial influence of physical activity on the transitions of frailty may be because of the frailty measurement used, because attributes of frailty (physical strength, energy, and mobility) contribute the most in explaining differences in frailty status and are most amenable to change via physical activity.[47]

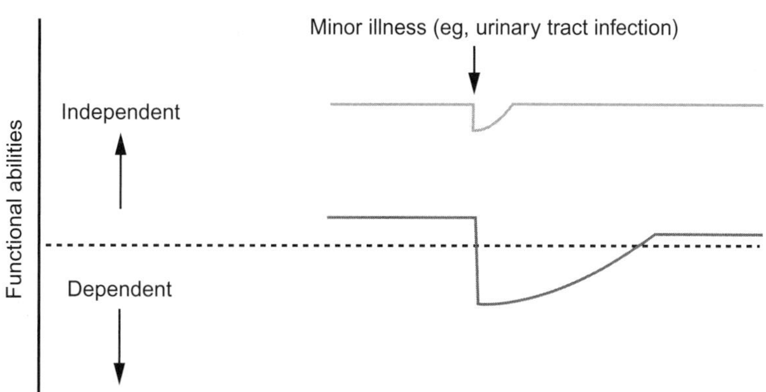

FIG. 13.4 Response to a stressor. Managing well: a fit older adult who, following a minor stressor, experiences a minor deterioration in function and then returns to homeostasis. Frailty: a frail older adult who, following a similar stressor, experiences more significant deterioration and does not return to baseline homeostasis. With more severe frailty, this may lead to functional dependency or death. *(From Clegg A: Frailty in elderly people. https://www.ncbi.nlm.nih.gov/pubmed/23395245 Lancet. 2013 Mar 2;381(9868):752–62. © Elsevier.)*

TABLE 13.3 Degrees of Frailty

Degree of Frailty	Description	Functional Characteristics
1. Fit (not frail)	Few long-term conditions and those are well controlled. Physically active, no functional limitations.	Gait speed of >1.2 m/s TUG <10 s 6MWT > 548 meters 30s chair rise ≥15 Can get up from floor easily
2. Mild frailty (prefrail)	Slowing, may need help with IADLs, making adaptations to functional mobility. Beginning to restrict life space mobility. Vulnerable and often makes a poor recovery from illness or injury.	Gait speed = 0.8–1.2 m/s TUG 10–15 s 6MWT = 400–548 m 30s chair rise 8–15 May modify getting up from floor Frailty Index of ~0.25[11]
3. Moderate frailty	Demonstrates difficulty with outdoor mobility and may need some help with ADLs. Life space is increasingly restricted and loss of independence is apparent.	Gait speed = 0.5–0.8 m/s TUG 15–20 s 6MWT > 400 m 30s chair rise <8 Difficult or unable to get up from floor unassisted
4. Severe frailty (end stage)	Dependent in ADLs, actively or inactively dying. Life expectancy 6 to 12 months.	Gait speed <0.5 m/s TUG >20 s 6MWT = unable 30s chair rise = unable Floor rise = unable

Ranges are approximate and should inform clinical reasoning rather than be used as definitions of each category.
6MWT, 6-minute walk test; *ADLs*, activities of daily living; *IADLs*, instrumental activities of daily living; *TUG*, Timed Up and Go Test.

IMPLICATIONS OF FRAILTY

In addition to increased vulnerability to stressors leading to adverse health events, frailty is linked to, but not synonymous with, a decrease in mobility, dependence in IADLs and activities of daily living (ADLs), higher rates of hospitalization, 6-month mortality,[48] institutionalization,[49] and poor surgical outcomes. As displayed in Table 13.4, the prevalence of self-reported difficulty in common mobility activities is much higher in frail individuals as compared to nonfrail.[50] Although it is tempting to see mobility disability and frailty as similar, even synonymous, constructs, they are different, but they may coexist.[51] Mobility disability may be more related to sarcopenia than to frailty because of the characteristic of weakness but can be seen in both conditions.[12] In fact, it is not unreasonable to view mobility disability, sarcopenia, and frailty as a continuum. Frailty should be viewed as a decline in an individual's homeostatic function, strength, and physiologic reserves leading to increased vulnerability, whereas sarcopenia describes a loss of muscle mass and function with age. Sarcopenia is twice as common in the general population as frailty,[52] and with weakness the most common attribute in frailty, the two conditions are closely related.

Many geriatric syndromes, including falls, mobility disability, delirium, incontinence, osteoporosis, sarcopenia, and susceptibility to adverse drug reactions (ADRs), are each associated with frailty and are often associated with the adverse events outlined in Box 13.3.[6] Although each of these conditions is discussed elsewhere in this text, recognizing these syndromes within the context of frailty will aid in the comprehensive management of the patient. For example, preventing osteoporosis and sarcopenia may help reduce the risk of frailty.[53]

TABLE 13.4 Prevalence of Mobility Disability in Frail and Nonfrail Older Adults

Self-Report Difficulty In:	Frail	Not Frail
Mobility	93.2%	58.1%
Walking 100 m	48.4%	5.68%
Getting out of chair	55.3%	21.8%
Climbing several flights of stairs	79.1%	32.6%
Climbing one flight	53.4%	8.45%

BOX 13.3 Prevalence of Adverse Events in Frail Compared with Nonfrail Older Adults

Adverse Event	Nonfrail	Frail
Falling in previous year	18.1%	54.9%
Worried about falling in past month	12.4%	56.9%
Multiple falls in past year	5%	35.2%
Hospital stay in past year	11.1%	42.4%
Need for help with self-care	2%	45%
Need for help with mobility	1%	50%

(Modified from Bandeen-Roche K, Seplaki CL, Huang J, et al. Frailty in older adults: a nationally representative profile in the United States. *J Gerontol Ser A Biol Sci Med Sci*. 2015;70[11]:1427–1434.)

Finally, frailty's cost to society cannot be overestimated. In the United States, adverse health effects associated with increased vulnerability are related to considerably higher costs to the Medicare program, particularly related to inpatient hospitalization stays, as complications are more frequent and recovery is longer.[54,55] Frail older adults account for 32% of all Medicare spending, even though only 15% of the Medicare population is considered frail.[56] The prevalence of a hospital stay in the past year is fourfold higher in frail compared to nonfrail individuals.[6]

In a large, prospective, longitudinal epidemiological study in Germany that used the frailty phenotype classification, health care costs of nonfrail and prefrail older adults did not differ from each other. In contrast, health care costs of frail individuals displaying three of five frailty phenotype attributes were 55% higher than nonfrail older adults. Health care costs were 101% higher for frail individuals displaying four or five of the frailty phenotype attributes than for nonfrail individuals.[55] The health care costs of Australian individuals classified as "moderate frail" using a frailty index were 22% higher than those classified "low frail"; individuals classified "high frail" were 43% higher than individuals classified as "low frail."[57]

Surgical Implications

The increase in health care costs related to surgery is particularly concerning as over 20% of all operations performed in the United States are on those individuals over 65 years of age.[58] Frailty is found to be a better predictor of mortality than chronological age in studies on the association between surgical outcomes and frailty.[59,60] The prevalence of frailty in the surgical population varies by procedure, with frailty occurring in 52% of those undergoing vascular procedures.[61] Adverse surgical outcomes in individuals with frailty include an increased rate of complications and length of stay, increased institutional rate, and delirium.[2] Those individuals over 80 years of age undergoing arterial surgery had twice the risk of adverse outcomes than those between ages 60 and 69.[62] The risk in mortality increases dramatically when a complication occurs (3.7% risk without complications compared to 26.1% when one or more complications occur). Surgical costs are higher too. One study found that the cost of elective surgical procedures for those with frailty was three times the cost of those without frailty ($76,363 ± $48,495 compared to $27,731 ± $15,693).[63]

Frailty can occur in degrees. The degree of frailty may serve as a prognostic indicator of rehabilitation potential.[64] Recognizing the degree of frailty allows management to be directed at the appropriate level. With increased levels of frailty, there is a longer and incomplete time to recovery of mobility skills and some level of independence, a significant issue for physical therapists.[64] Furthermore, recognizing the degree of frailty and intervening appropriately may delay the transition to a lower state of frailty, thus allowing the individual to live in the environment he or she prefers for a satisfying quality of life. Fried's original work on the phenotype model, confirmed in more recent studies, supports the concept of frailty as a unique physiological syndrome, related to but separate from disability and comorbidity. Table 13.3 provides descriptions of four different degrees of frailty with objective markers for each degree that can be used to help direct management and contribute to prognosis.

PATHOPHYSIOLOGY OF FRAILTY

The state of frailty is associated with multisystem dysregulations, leading to a loss of energetics, homeostasis, and physiological reserve.[65] Although the two major models of frailty have done much to describe characteristics and attributes of frailty, neither the phenotype model nor the cumulative deficit model explains how multisystem dysregulation occurs. Perhaps the most pervasive homeostatic dysregulation feature of aging is the acquisition of a proinflammatory state, demonstrated by chronically elevated levels of cytokines (cytokine interleukin [IL]-6 and C-reactive protein) as well as white blood cell and monocyte counts.[66] Thus, frailty is associated with a blunted immune response to vaccination and/or to infection, which leads to a predisposition to infections.[66] Kidney function in frailty is often substantially impaired beyond what is expected by aging. Anemia and malnutrition are also common features of aging and frailty contributing to reduced energetics. The three main portions of the nervous system (central, peripheral, and autonomic) likely have some degree of involvement and play an important role in the physical and cognitive manifestations of frailty.[66] Motor neuron loss and fragmentation of the neuromuscular junction probably contribute to sarcopenia and poor mobility. Impaired orthostatic hemodynamics and heart rate control and reduced intestinal peristalsis are signs of autonomic dysfunction. And finally, the endocrine system is implicated through sex steroid effects on skeletal muscle.[66] Although many studies have considered relationships of frailty with single physiologic and pathologic features, the consistent involvement of multiple physiologic systems in frailty suggests that most of them are driven by some unifying cause, but this is still unknown and hidden.

In more recent years, researchers' attention has focused on identifying etiological factors that contribute to the frail state. These include genetic factors, metabolic factors, environmental and lifestyle stressors, and acute and chronic diseases.[66] Fig. 13.5 illustrates the relationship between the molecular, physiologic, and clinical manifestations of frailty.[65] The physiologic markers or biomarkers are hypothesized and may provide some information on possible mechanisms of the clinical manifestations. Research on frailty consistently supports the

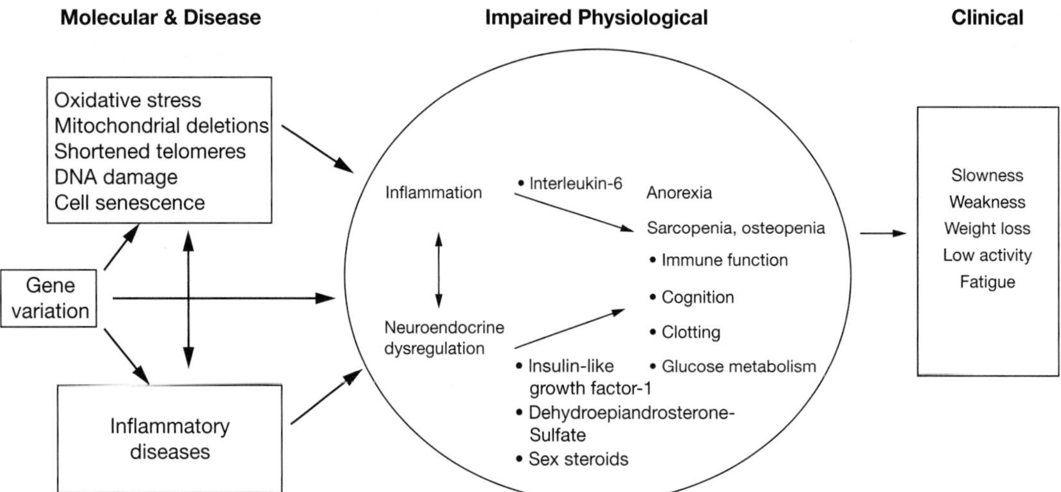

FIG. 13.5 Molecular, physiological, and clinical manifestations of frailty. *(From Walston JD, Hadley EC, Ferrucci L, et al. Research agenda for frailty in older adults: toward a better understanding of physiology and etiology: summary from the American Geriatrics Society/National Institute on Aging Research Conference on Frailty in Older Adults. JAGS. 2006;54:6.)*

presence of multisystem impairments across multiple physiologic systems and organs. For example, the musculoskeletal system experiences reduced muscle mass and strength with increased fat mass and bone fragility over and beyond what is expected from the pure effect of aging. This decline is exacerbated in the individual with a sedentary lifestyle. Low fitness is accompanied by altered resting metabolic rate and reduced energetic efficiency, which likely contributes to fatigue and reduced mobility. Some homeostatic mechanisms are impaired as evidenced by low reserves, reduced ability to respond to perturbation, and reduced ability to recover a stable level of equilibrium.

Aging is thought to be a proinflammatory state. Aging and frailty may share the same features of chronic inflammation, with frailty exhibiting an advanced state, which is thus sometimes referred to as "accelerated aging." This is consistent with the idea that aging negatively affects physical resilience and increases susceptibility to stressful events, which disrupts homeostatic equilibrium, thus lowering the potential for regaining the lost equilibrium. The accumulation of damage due to loss of physical resilience across different physiologic systems leads to multimorbidity, the development of frailty, and decline in many functions that ultimately impact physical and cognitive performance, triggering events that eventually lead to death. If frailty and aging are made of the same fabric, then understanding the biological mechanisms of frailty may inform our understanding of aging.

FRAILTY AND SARCOPENIA

Sarcopenia is a prime component of the frailty syndrome, and both sarcopenia and frailty are associated with increased disability, falls, hospitalization, nursing home placement, and mortality.[67] Sarcopenia is widely defined as the age-related loss of skeletal muscle. It is a condition characterized by progressive and generalized loss of skeletal muscle mass and strength with a risk of adverse outcomes such as physical disability, poor quality of life, and death.[68] Many disabling conditions are associated with an accelerated loss of lean muscle mass, including cachexia, cancer, diabetes, kidney disease, and certain neurological diseases. Sarcopenia is thought to be a precursor of the physical manifestations of frailty, even a main driver of frailty, but is distinct from frailty, with sarcopenia being twice as common as frailty.[52] Although weakness is often the first manifestation of the prefrail person,[4,69] weakness in and of itself does not imply sarcopenia. Other factors shared by frailty and sarcopenia are mobility difficulties and a decrease in physical function. The most common criteria of frailty are weakness (54%) and slow gait speed (43%), which share attributes with the functional definition of sarcopenia.[4] The decrease in physical function, especially gait speed, may reflect the need to conserve energy for essential metabolic functions.[70,71] The relationship between frailty and sarcopenia continues to evolve, especially regarding a shared physiologic pathway thought to be increased systemic inflammation.[12] Importantly, both are thought to be amenable to interventions and thus reversible.[72] Sarcopenia is discussed in more detail elsewhere in this text.

ASSESSMENT OF FRAILTY

There is no gold standard for the assessment of frailty, in part because there is a lack of consensus on the components of frailty. However, there are several options that suit the continuum of screening to evaluation as listed in Table 13.5.

Comprehensive Geriatric Assessment (CGA). The most comprehensive method of assessing frailty is the Comprehensive Geriatric Assessment (CGA). The CGA is a multidimensional and usually interdisciplinary diagnostic process to determine the medical conditions, mental health, functional capacity, and social circumstances of the person with frailty.[73] The older individual is central to the evaluation process. If the person's capacity to

TABLE 13.5 Frailty Assessment Tools

Tool	Purpose	Description
Comprehensive Geriatric Assessment (CGA)	Documents a plan to optimize and maintain health and function, an escalation plan advising when the patient/carer might need to seek further advice, an urgent care plan, and, when appropriate, an end-of-life care plan	Includes domains of: Medical (including urinary or fecal incontinence) Function (including vision and hearing) Psychological Social Environmental Advance care planning Spirituality Sexuality and intimacy
PRISMA-7	Screening tool to identify those in need of a more comprehensive evaluation	7 self-report items; 3 or more items present indicate potential disabilities or frailty[74]: 1. Are you older than 85 years? 2. Male? 3. In general do you have any health problems that require you to limit your activities? 4. Do you need someone to help you on a regular basis? 5. In general do you have any health problems that require you to stay at home? 6. In case of need, can you count on someone close to you? 7. Do you regularly use a stick, walker, or wheelchair to get about?
Clinical Frailty Scale	Assess the severity of frailty	9 items (Fig. 13.7) and score is assigned based on clinical judgment.
Phenotype of Frailty (Fried)	Identification of frailty based on the Cardiovascular Health Model (CHS)	Uses 5-point scale of objective criteria. Score of 1 to 2 indicates prefrailty, and score of 3 or more indicates frailty.
FRAIL[149,150]	Frailty screening in African American males and older women, modeled on the CHS	Total score = 5 No frailty = 0 Prefrail = 1 or 2 deficits Frailty = 3 more deficits Five criteria include: F: Are you *F*atigued? R: *R*esistance: Can you walk up a flight of stairs? A: *A*mbulation: Can you walk a block? I: Do you have more than five *I*llnesses L: Have you *L*ost 5% of weight in the past 6 months?
Gait speed	To assess frailty	Distance walked over 4 m or more. Frailty is indicated with gait speeds of 0.8 m/s or less.
Edmonton Frail Scale	Identifies aspects of frailty amenable to preoperative optimization	Multidimensional scale used frequently for surgery patients to assess risk of postoperative complications. Total score = 17. 0–5 = Not frail 6–7 = Vulnerable 8–9 = Mild frailty 10–11 = Moderate frailty 12–17 = Severe frailty
Life space assessment	Identify risk of frailty and loss of social role	UAB Life Space Assessment OR two questions: In the previous 4 weeks during a typical week: Did you leave your neighborhood? Weather permitting, did you go outside your house? If yes, follow up with frequency. If help is needed to leave home OR if less than three times per week, assume frailty.
Physical Performance Test[151] (PPT) and Modified Physical Performance Test (M-PPT)[152]	Assess frailty (7- to 9-item version)	Measures time to complete ADL and mobility skills; 9-item version includes stairs. M-PPT, which includes balance tests rather than the writing and eating task, determined out of a score 36: 32–36 = Not frail 25–32 = Mild frailty 17–24 = Moderate frailty <17 = Unlikely to function in community

ADLs, activities of daily living; UAB, University of Alabama at Birmingham.

Level of the ICF	Pattern of frailty	Common causes	Other causes
Health condition	Unstable health conditions	Infections, injuries, cardiorespiratory disease	Frequent transition between primary care and acute care Sub-optimal management
	Undernutrition[a]	Inability to prepare meals	Inability to purchase food Exhaustion
Impairment of the body's structure/function	Psychological factors[a]	Depression, grief	Negative outlook
	Impaired cognition	Dementia	Lack of compensatory strategies
	Impaired vision / hearing	Macular degeneration, cataracts / presbycusis	Lack of appropriate equipment /aids / eye surgery
Activity limitation[b]	Decreased mobility[a] / decreased self care	Impaired balance/co-ordination and /or strength Environmental barriers Recent traumatic event	Decreased cardiovascular endurance Fear of falling
Participation restriction[c]	Lack of participation in life roles	Social barriers Limited family contact Environmental barriers	Decreased self-efficacy
Environmental contextual factors	Problems with services or support systems	Services not readily available Lack of service coordination	Carer stress Interaction with support network Low income Physical or social isolation

Figure 1 Important factors to assess in the frail patient and the interactions between them. [a]Captured in the Frailty Phenotype; [b]Defined as difficulty experienced by an individual when executing activities (International Classification of Functioning (ICF)[26]); [c]Defined as problems experienced by an individual in their involvement in life situations (ICF).

FIG. 13.6 Relationship of frailty factors to International Classification of Functioning, Disability, and Disease (ICF) model. *(From Fairhall N, Langron C, Sherrington C, et al. Treating frailty – a practical guide. BMC Med. 2011;9:83.)*

participate voluntarily is lacking, a system to address his or her needs in an ethical fashion is developed. Circumstances that drive the CGA include an acute illness associated with a significant change in functional ability, transfers of care for rehabilitation or continuing care, consideration of surgery, and experiencing two or more "geriatric syndromes" of falls, delirium, incontinence, or immobility. Other reasons to refer for a CGA may be age, medical comorbidities such as heart failure or cancer, psychosocial disorders such as depression or isolation, previous or predicted high health care utilization, consideration of change in living situation, and specific acute care situations of fractures, failure to thrive, recurrent pneumonia, and pressure sores in addition to the geriatric syndromes mentioned earlier.[73] Fig. 13.6 illustrates the relationship of the factors to assess in frailty and their relationship to the International Classification of Functioning, Disability, Disease and Health (ICF) perspective.

The CGA is performed by an interdisciplinary team headed by the geriatrician, nurse practitioner, or physician's assistant. Traditionally a nurse, social worker, pharmacist, and physical and/or occupational therapist also are on the team. Different members may complete unique parts of the CGA. For example, the physical therapist might complete the functional abilities and fall history aspects, whereas a social worker might assess sources of social support and advance care preferences.

PRISMA-7. The PRISMA-7 is a brief 7-item screening tool recommended by the British Geriatric Society to detect frailty.[74] It was designed to identify considerably disabled older adults in order to prevent or delay functional decline. With a score of 3 or greater, it has a sensitivity of 78.3% and specificity of 74.7% for detecting significant disabilities.[75] With a score of 3 or greater, the PRISMA-7 can provide a quick screen for frailty with a sensitivity and specificity of 0.83 but with considerable uncertainty secondary to its wide confidence limits.[45] Using the frailty phenotype and expert clinical judgment as the reference, the PRISMA-7 performed better than any of the other 10 tools used to identify frailty.

Frailty Index. The Frailty Index (FI) was originally developed from the Canadian Study of Health and Aging.[76] The FI, also referred to as the deficit accumulation index, theorizes that the more deficits one has, the more that disease and frailty burden exists. The number of deficits that accumulate as one ages is considered a more accurate estimate of biologic age and associated morbidity and death than chronological age.[77] The original FI consisted of 70 items representing deficits in a wide range of domains including presence of diseases, abilities in ADLs, physical signs from clinical exams, and social issues. A person with seven deficits was determined to have an index score of 0.1 by dividing the number of deficits by the total number of items. An FI score of > 0.45 (31.5 deficits out of 70) was associated with a 100% mortality within 7 years. An FI score of approximately 0.25 is the cut point between nonfrailty and prefrailty, and an FI score of 0.3 to 0.4 indicates moderate frailty.[11] In the general population, more than 99% of people have an FI value of <0.7. Of those who had an FI value of >0.5 (based on a CGA), 100% were dead about 20 months later.[59] The 40-item version is the more common version of the FI, but its psychometrics have not been determined. A list of the 70 deficits is found in Box 13.2. It follows that the therapist should be aware of the prognostic implications of the number of diagnoses, clinical deficits, and social contributions of an individual.

Clinical Frailty Scale. The Clinical Frailty Scale (CFS), illustrated in Fig. 13.7, was developed by the same group that developed the FI as a more user-friendly tool with wide applicability. The CFS is used to measure the severity of frailty on a 9-point scale; however, it predicts death better than it predicts frailty.[76,78] It has not been validated for responsiveness or accuracy but does have a strong correlation with the FI ($r = 0.80$). Many physicians find the tool easy to use because of its descriptions, thus explaining its growing use; however, the British Geriatric Society recommends its use only after a CGA is performed.

Phenotype of Frailty. The phenotype of frailty, developed by Fried and others, arguably provides the most widespread criteria for frailty and is used frequently in research. It is particularly relevant to physical therapists because of its focus on physical attributes with an emphasis on strength and gait speed. It is also valuable because it can predict prefrailty, which may be the most optimum time to intervene. However, it may only be appropriate for nondisabled persons and may not be feasible for acute care where mobility is limited. Each of the five criteria has a sensitivity and specificity of more than 80%, with the exception of weight loss (8.3% and 97.4%, respectively).[79] One study found that the positive predictive value for frailty was 87.5% when gait speed and grip strength are combined.[79]

The frailty phenotype uses handgrip strength to measure strength as a criterion for frailty; however, handgrip strength may not be an appropriate measure to evaluate changes in muscle strength during an exercise intervention in older people with frailty.[80] The 30-second sit-to-stand test may be better suited for the construct of frailty than the handgrip measure and is responsive to change.[81] The 30-second sit-to-stand test can assess the fatigue effect caused by the number of sit-to-stand repetitions.[82] Additionally, the 30-second sit to stand can reflect power demands that are reduced in individuals with frailty. A score of fewer than eight chair rises can be used to reflect frailty.[82] Millor et al. also found that the way an individual performed the sit-to-stand maneuver is indicative of frailty. For example, the presence of additional backward and forward lean was seen in frail individuals.[82]

Timed Up and Go and Gait Speed. Two single-item assessments have been proposed in best-practice guidelines in Great Britain for rapid identification of frailty and are well known to physical therapists.[74] The first is the Timed Up and Go Test (TUG). A cutoff of 10 seconds is proposed for detecting frailty. With 10 seconds as a cutoff, the tool performs well as a screening measure (0.93 sensitivity) but will overestimate the incidence of frailty

Clinical Frailty Scale*

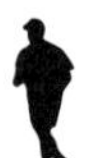

1 **Very Fit** – People who are robust, active, energetic, and motivated. These people commonly exercise regularly. They are among the fittest for their age.

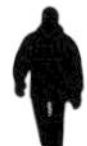

2 **Well** – Pepole who have **no active disease symptoms** but are less fit than category I. Often, they exercise or are very **active occasionally**, e.g. seasonally.

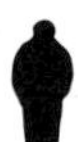

3 **Managing Well** – People whose **medical problems are well controlled,** but are **not regularly active** beyond routine walking.

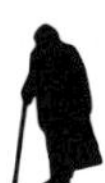

4 **Vulnerable** – While **not dependent** on others for daily help, often **symptoms limit activities.** A common complaint is being "slowed up",and/or being tired during the day

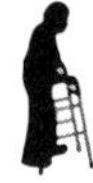

5 **Mildly Frail** – These people often have **more evident slowing,** and need help in **high order IADLs** (finances, transportation, heavy housework, medications). Typically, mild frailty progressively impairs shopping and walking outside alone, meal preparation, and housework.

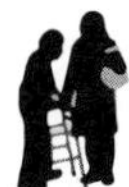

6 **Moderately Frail** – People need help with **all outside activities** and with **keeping house.** Inside, they often have problems wirh stairs and need **help with bathing** and might need minimal assistance (cuing, standby) with dressing.

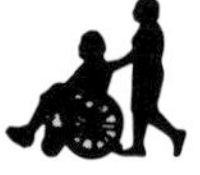

7 **Severely Frail** – **Completely dependent for personal care,** from whatever cause (physical or cognitive). Even so, they seem stable and not at high risk of dying (within ~ 6 months).

8 **Very Severely Frail** – Completely dependent, approaching the end of life. Typically, they could not recover even from a minor illness.

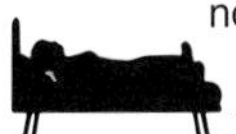

9 **.Terminally Ill** – Approaching the end of life. This category applies to people with **a life expectancy <6 months**, who are **not otherwise evidently frail.**

Scoring frailty in people with demantia

The degree of frailty corresponds to the degree of dementia. Common **symptoms in mild dementia** include forgetting the details of a recent event, though still remembering the event itself, repeating the same question/story, and social withdrawal.

In **moderate dementia**, recent memory is very impaired, even though they seemingly can remember their past life events well. They can do personal care with prompting.

In **severe dementia,** they cannot do personal care without help.

* 1. Canadian Study on Health & Aging, Revised 2008.
2. K. Rockwood et. al. A global clinical measure of fitness and frailty in elderly people. CMAJ 2005;173:489-495.

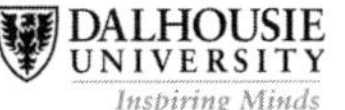

FIG. 13.7 Clinical Frailty Scale. *(From Dalhousie University, Geriatric Medicine Research, © 2007–2009, Halifax Canada.)*

(0.63 specificity). The TUG is discussed in detail elsewhere in this text. Gait speed has also been used to assess frailty.[10,83,84] Ninety percent of frail individuals have walking speeds of <0.8 m/s.[50] A cutoff score of <0.8 m/s has high sensitivity (0.99) and moderate specificity (0.64) for identifying frailty, with narrow confidence limits.[45] A cutoff value of <0.7 m/s has lower sensitivity (0.93) but higher specificity (0.77).[45]

Life Space. Constricted life space is a behavioral adaptation to meet environmental challenges made in response to declining physiologic reserve and capacity.[69] Measuring how much a person moves about the environment may be illuminating regarding mobility and participation in social activities. Assessing life space may reflect actual mobility performance not otherwise captured in self-reports or physical performance tests. It may identify changes in community mobility that often precede ADL and IADL difficulty. Life space constriction may indicate a decline in a person's social participation with associated decrease in quality of life.[85] The University of Alabama (UAB) Life Space Questionnaire measures movement to specific life space levels ranging from within one's own dwelling to beyond one's own town in the preceding 4 weeks.[86] The questionnaire captures frequency of movement and use of assistance (from equipment or another person). It is scored out of 120 points, with >60 points indicating the ability to move freely and independently beyond walking distance of the home. Individuals with scores of <60 were at 4.4 times higher risk of nursing home placement during the subsequent 6 years than individuals with scores ≥60.[85] Greater levels of life space constriction are correlated with higher levels of frailty.[87] Other instruments are described in Table 13.5.

MANAGEMENT OF FRAILTY

Management of the frail older adult is challenging on multiple levels. The lack of clear consensus on how to assess or diagnose frailty in the clinical setting, the complex interaction of multiple morbidities, vulnerability to deterioration, and increased social needs all make the management of the patient with frailty a complex undertaking. This complexity is compounded by our fragmented health care delivery system that does not effectively support consistent ongoing management. General consensus is that frailty should be identified through a validated tool and a multidisciplinary approach to address comorbidities, nutrition, sarcopenia (weakness), and physical inactivity. The most popular intervention methods include exercise and physical activity, nutritional management, and hormone replacement.

Although physical activity and resistance exercise continue to be hallmarks for the intervention of frailty and sarcopenia, it is important to thoroughly evaluate comorbidities for contributions to the frail state and to the loss of muscle mass. Awareness of the consequences of muscle loss and management of many medical conditions compounding frailty and sarcopenia, such as osteoporosis, osteopenia, obesity, type 2 diabetes, and breast cancer, may improve physical function and quality of life. Importantly, no drugs are registered for the treatment of sarcopenia; however, two drugs, myostatin antibody (REGN-1033) and activin receptor inhibitor (BMY-338), are in phase 2 and 3 trials, although their effectiveness is in doubt.[88]

Physical Activity and Exercise

The ESCEO Experts Group[89] recommends physical activity and progressive resistive exercise (PRE), vitamin D supplementation, adequate protein intake, and education as the front-line management of frailty. Simple recommendations to improve physical activity include reducing sedentary time, encouraging walking in 10-minute bouts or more, and performing functional exercises that mimic daily activities. However, practitioners should be aware that adherence to physical activity programs among older adults is poor for a variety of reasons. These reasons, such as fear of falling, low self-efficacy and coping strategies, poor attitude toward physical activity, and adverse social and environmental influences, require individual interventions, perhaps best done by a physical therapist. To support this recommendation, it is known that older adults are more likely to adhere to a physical activity program if the program is supervised, is individually tailored, and contains self-efficacy training, and if the referring practitioner encourages participation.[90]

Each category of frailty will require different goals. For individuals found to be prefrail, the goal will be to prevent the transition to frailty. For individuals who are frail, the goal may be to maintain the current level of function and prevent further decline. Aerobic exercise may be the exercise of choice for individuals who are frail, especially if they cannot perform resistance exercise.[91] Likewise, different stages of frailty may require different approaches. The concept of building reserve is an important consideration for nonfrail and prefrail adults. Because reserve diminishes with age, building reserve through aerobic and strengthening activities may provide the individual with a cushion of reserve if an injury or illness occurs. Individuals with greater reserve often have an easier time recuperating. Individuals with little to no reserve may use their entire bank of energy stores just to perform ADLs. Although no universal exercise prescription exists for older adults with frailty, Bray et al. recommend an exercise prescription that includes PRE, aerobic training, and balance and flexibility exercises in specific doses depending on the level of frailty, with the goal of accumulating 60 minutes per session for prefrail adults and 45 minutes per session for frail adults (Fig. 13.8).[91]

As discussed elsewhere in this text, PRE has profound effects on the untrained older adult, including those with frailty. PREs can decrease biological age by changing the

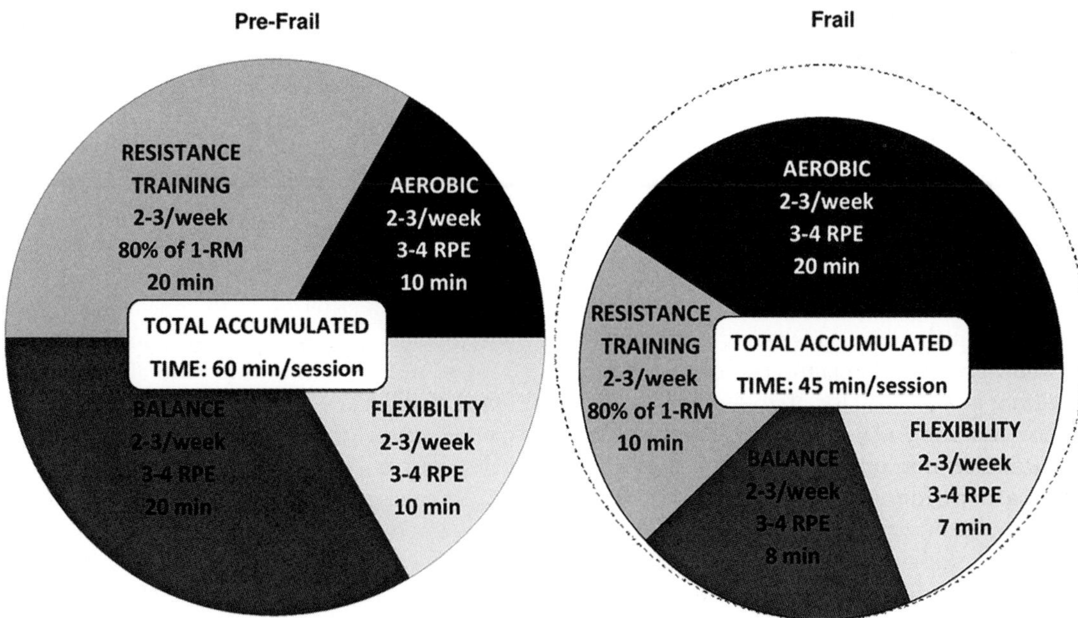

FIG. 13.8 Exercise prescription for frailty. The outer circle on the frail figure identifies the prefrail total exercise duration relative to the frail.[91] The inner circle and quadrants on the frail figure represent the exercise time accumulated, which differs for each component of exercise, as well as reduction in total accumulated exercise time. *RPE,* rating of perceived exertion; *1-RM,* 1-repetition maximum; *min,* minutes.

mitochondrial characteristics to reflect a younger age. For example, after 6 months of resistance exercise, participants who were an average age of 68 showed mitochondrial characteristics similar to persons with a mean age of 24 years.[92] PREs remain the key intervention for the treatment of frailty.[93,94] Concurrently, an emphasis on increasing physical activity should be a focus of any home program and prevention program, working toward the goal of accumulating 150 minutes per week of exercise, consistent with the Centers for Disease Control and Prevention recommendations.[95] Within these 150 minutes is the recommendation for resistance exercise. Because sarcopenia is a significant component of age-related weakness and frailty, resistance training is the ideal and preferred option for improving function and reducing the likelihood of falls. It may take as many as 3 months for resistance training effects to become evident.[96] Therefore, it is critical to use strategies to promote behavior change in concert with the exercise prescription.

High-intensity effort is the key to strength gains (50% to 90% 1-Repetition Maximum [1-RM]) even when a minimal dose approach to resistance training may be necessary in some individuals with frailty.[97] Supervision may be highly important for adherence and optimal outcomes as it produces higher work intensity.[97] Low-dose exercise of 20 to 25 minutes for 3 days per week has resulted in strength effects in frail individuals. Interestingly, these individuals did not show a consistent benefit beyond one set of low-dose resistance exercise.[98] One minimal dose prescription consists of the use of 3 to 10 weight stack machines performed for a single set. Essential exercises include chest press, leg press, and seated row. Supplementary exercises include the overhead press, latissimus pull-down, lumbar extension, abdominal flexion, and neck extension. In this prescription, the dose was low to moderate at <60 minutes per session for 2 days per week and was supervised to promote adherence.[97]

To examine the feasibility of a physical therapist–led high-intensity walking training (HIWT) on prefrail and frail older adults, five assisted living residents with an average age of 87 years (four frail, one prefrail) underwent a supervised 12-session intervention. The intervention consisted of 30 minutes of HIWT at 70% to 80% of heart rate reserve or ratings of 15 to 17 (hard to very hard) on the Borg Rating of Perceived Exertion Scale while wearing ankle cuff weights to increase limb loading. Training included walking at fast speeds, in multiple directions, upstairs, and on outdoor surfaces with and without an assistive device and obstacle negotiation. Training significantly reduced frailty, as evidenced by improved fast gait speed (0.7 to 0.9 m/s), improved 6-minute walk test distance (217 ± 150 to 401 ± 202 m), and enhanced Berg Balance Scale scores (32.2 ± 9.23 to 37.8 ± 9). Two participants were able to transition from walking with a walker to no device or walking with a walker to a straight cane. There were no adverse events and all participants reached target training intensity in all 12 sessions. Usual gait speed and step count did not statistically improve, perhaps because of the study being underpowered. Participants viewed the walking intervention as highly satisfactory and 100% recommended that the assisted living facility should offer HIWT as part of routine programming.[99] HIWT may be a feasible option to increase reserve in frail older adults.

Although exercise and its prescription are discussed elsewhere in this text, a few specifics deserve mentioning here. Progressive resistance training should be 40% to 80% one-repetition maximum (1RM) with a volume increasing from one set of eight repetitions to three sets of eight repetitions three times a week for 60 minutes for a duration of at least 10 weeks.[100] Detraining will occur without adequate stimulus. This prescription for strengthening results in improved functional and ADL performance in institutionalized older people who are frail.[100] The prescription should include the principle of specificity through functional training of activities done commonly throughout the day, which may be sufficient overload to promote strengthening in very weakened individuals. Functional gait training for 30 to 45 minutes two times per week in frail nursing home residents for 4 weeks led to substantial gains in gait speed and balance.[101] Agility should be incorporated to promote balance reactions. Power should be a part of any exercise prescription for the continuum of frailty as power declines at a faster rate than resistance and with sufficient power, individuals will be more able to stand from a chair with less effort and walk at a more efficient speed. Balance exercises should be progressively challenged with a frequency of three times per week for 60 minutes per session for at least 3 months.[100] Endurance is improved through a progressive resistance training of an intensity of 80% 1RM, with volume, frequency, and duration similar to the strengthening recommendations stated earlier.[100] When people who are frail cannot exercise at the volumes and intensity recommended by the research cited previously, the therapist should adjust the program to allow the person to exercise as intensely as feasible, knowing the more intense and more volume program will create optimal results. Because undertreating is a concern for physical therapists, every effort should be made to be creative in an exercise prescription to promote sufficient intensity and volume.[102] Finally, to improve quality of life, a progressive functional training program of similar volume, frequency, and duration that includes walking, stepping, gamelike exercises, and sportlike exercises are recommended for a duration of 6 months.[100]

Lower extremity exercises should take priority over upper extremity exercises to maintain and improve mobility. Core strength provides proximal stability for distal mobility and aids in anticipatory postural adjustments at the trunk to provide more efficient gait and enhance balance.[103] Therefore, the core musculature should be addressed to combat the stooped posture, posterior pelvic tilt, and need to bear weight on the arms that occurs from prolonged sitting and weakened core musculature. Orthostatic hypotension is prevalent in those with frailty and may even be a clinical marker of frailty.[104] Because orthostatic hypotension is linked with an increased risk of falls, the physical therapist would do well to monitor blood pressure during and before activity. Finally, individuals should be taught to get up from the floor, in case of a fall. There are myriad strategies and the best strategy should be identified and practiced so the individual can achieve confidence in being able to recover if a fall should occur. Several clever floor-rise strategies are available on the Internet.[105] Some suggested exercises showing adaptations for progressive frailty are listed in Table 13.6.

Nutrition

Proper nutrition provides energy and essential nutrients while helping to maintain homeostasis. Unintentional weight loss, a criterion of the phenotype model of frailty, is associated with morbidity and mortality, and occurs in 15% to 20% of older adults and 50% to 60% of nursing home residents.[106] Involuntary weight loss can lead to muscle wasting, decreased immunocompetence, depression, and an increased rate of disease complications. Cachexia, loss of muscle mass with or without loss of fat, is associated with increased infections, pressure ulcers, and failure to respond to medical treatments.[106] Because weight loss is a key feature of frailty, it should be addressed. Physical therapists can use the Mini Nutritional Assessment (MNA) to screen for weight loss.[107] The MNA is a simple and sensitive tool for nutritional screening and assessment and is available in many languages. It can identify adults who are frail.[10]

The pathophysiology of unintentional weight loss is not well understood. It is unclear whether the presence of elevated biomarkers such as inflammatory cytokines is a direct cause or a marker for an underlying condition.[108] Reversible causes of weight loss include illness and cancer, dementia, medications, and swallowing difficulty.[109] Social isolation and having difficulty leaving the home can also affect appetite and thus be a factor in weight loss. The Meals on Wheels mnemonic[110] shown in Box 13.4 is one tool to increase awareness of the myriad potential causes of unintended weight loss.

Treatment for unintended weight loss should focus on the underlying cause. This may involve members of the interdisciplinary team such as dietitians; dentists; speech, occupational, and/or physical therapists; and social service workers. Common strategies to address unintentional weight loss include dietary changes, environmental modifications, nutritional supplements, flavor enhancers, and appetite stimulants.

Adequate amounts of protein may help preserve muscle mass and strength, but strong evidence is lacking.[111] Although no robust studies definitively show that increasing protein intake alone increases muscle strength, increased protein intake while engaging in resistance exercise is considered an effective strategy for the prevention and treatment of sarcopenia and frailty.[112] One study of 1172 participants investigated the effects of oral nutrition supplementation plus physical exercise on the physical function and quality of life of frail institutionalized older adults aged 70 years and older.[113] A supplement of 20 g of protein, prebiotic fiber, and 500 IU vitamin D was given two times a day for 2 weeks. Concurrently, physical exercise supervised by a physical therapist was delivered 5 days

TABLE 13.6 Suggested Exercises for Individuals on the Continuum of Frailty

Region	Nonfrail at Risk for Frailty	Prefrail	Frail
Core	Side planks on extended legs	Side planks on bent knees	Side-lying transfers on compliant surfaces (e.g., bed transfers) progressing to reduced arm support
	Prone planks on extended legs	Planks on bent knees	Prone press-ups
	Sit-backs with arms overhead or sit ups against gravity	Sit-backs with arms folded across chest	Sitting unsupported with arms extended (e.g., reaching activities) at various positions
	Single leg bridges with arms at sides or crossed	Bridges (both legs) with arms overhead	Bridges with arms at sides or crossed
	Pushups on knees	Pushups on raised surface such as table	Pushups against wall
Lower extremity	Side-lying hip abduction (if hip flexors are sufficient length)	Side stepping with/without elastic band with minimal to no support	Standing hip abduction with minimal support
	Squats with weight on heels to appropriate height surface (to produce overload) to rising on heels to progress to power squats	Sit to stands with arms crossed or arms elevated and trunk extended	Sit to stands on raised surface with no arm support
	Lunges	Partial lunges	Forward stepping with knee bend
	Heel raises on unstable platforms (wobble boards, compliant surfaces)	Heel raises, walking on toes	Ankle plantar flexion against STRONG elastic resistance
Gait activities	Agility course or ladder	Agility course with appropriate obstacles in low light	Corridor walking negotiating busy hallway or obstacles
	Speed walking with rapid changes in speed and direction	Speed walking with focus on recovering balance	Corridor walking with focus on length of step and reduced upper extremity support

BOX 13.4 "Meals on Wheels": A Mnemonic for Common Treatable Causes of Unintentional Weight Loss in the Elderly

M Medication effects
E Emotional problems, especially depression
A Anorexia nervosa, alcoholism
L Late-life paranoia
S Swallowing disorders
O Oral factors (e.g., poorly fitting dentures, caries)
N No money
W Wandering and other dementia-related behaviors
H Hyperthyroidism, hypothyroidism, hyperparathyroidism, hypoadrenalism
E Enteric problems
E Eating problems (e.g., inability to feed self)
L Low-salt, low-cholesterol diet
S Stones, social problems (e.g., isolation, inability to obtain preferred foods)

(From Morley JE, Silver AJ. Nutritional issues in nursing home care. *Ann Intern Med.* 1995;123[11]:850.)

per week for 2 weeks. Physical exercise consisted of standing leg exercises, sitting exercises using a 1-pound weight, chair rises using arms, and flexibility exercises. In spite of the low dose of exercise, 53% of participants improved at least 1 point on the Short Physical Performance Battery at week 6, and 48.4% improved at least 1 point at week 12. There was no significant improvement in function at 12 weeks, but nutritional status was improved. Nutritional status improvement was greater in those with more frailty criteria, lower functional level, lower vitamin D levels, and poor nutritional status.

The recommended daily protein intake for sarcopenic older adults is 1.2 g/kg of body weight with the exception of those with severe kidney dysfunction.[114] Although most nutritional investigations involve protein supplementation, other nutritional supplements have been researched. Supplementation with essential amino acids (EAAs) has been suggested for older people with frailty. EAAs are proteins the body cannot manufacture itself and are therefore essential to obtain from dietary intake. These EAAs include valine, leucine, isoleucine, lysine, threonine, tryptophan, methionine, phenylalanine, and histidine. Several studies have found that older adults improve in their physical function when supplemented with 2.5 g of leucine-enriched EAAs. For instance, Deutz et al.[114] reported that leucine-enriched whey protein increased muscle mass and leg function in older adults with sarcopenia. Leucine is metabolized to β-hydroxy-β-methylbutyrate (HMB) in cells, and it appears that an HMB-enriched protein mixture enhances muscle mass and function.[115] HMB, creatine, and some milk-based proteins may have beneficial effects on protein balance in skeletal muscle.[115] Correction of vitamin D deficiency is also needed for proper muscle function.[115]

Adherence to a Mediterranean diet was associated with significantly lower risk of frailty in a systematic review of nearly 6000 people followed for 4 years.[116] The diet consisted of abundant plant foods (fruits, vegetables, cereals, potatoes, beans, nuts, and seeds), olive oil as the principle source of fat, dairy products, fish and poultry in low to moderate amounts, zero to four eggs per week, red meat consumed in low amounts, and wine in low to moderate amounts, normally taken with meals. Those women who consumed the most components of the Mediterranean Diet had significantly higher fat-free mass and leg muscle power than those who consumed the least. The improved leg muscle power and fat-free mass may be related to increased physical activity and walking speed reported in those participants who adhered to the diet.[117,118] Interestingly, a meta-analysis found that a Mediterranean diet is protective of frailty and functional disability, but not of sarcopenia.[119] In a cross-sectional study of 923 older Taiwanese adults, a similar diet with the exception of wine and olive oil was protective against frailty.[120] The mechanism of these diets is thought to lower oxidative stress and inflammation.[121]

Pharmaceuticals

Individuals with frailty have multiple comorbidities and thus are susceptible to polypharmacy. General consensus guidelines recommend the regular review of medications to identify potential inappropriate prescriptions, to reconcile medications with diagnoses, and to deprescribe medications whose risk–benefit ratio is not advantageous to the individual.[74] Some drugs to consider for deprescribing include statins, glucocorticoids, anticholinergics, and benzodiazepines. Addressing unwanted side effects, such as an increase in fall risk that comes with benzodiazepines, is a benefit of regular review of a patient's medications.[122]

Hormonal Management

Testosterone levels decline in men at a rate of 1% per year from age 30, paralleling declines in muscle mass and strength.[67] The clinical presentation of androgen deficiency in men shares common features with frailty, creating interest in treating the weakness, fatigue, reduced muscle mass, osteoporosis, sexual dysfunction, depression, and memory impairment associated with aging in men with hormone deficiency. One study discovered that higher androgen levels may protect older men from worsening frailty; however, the authors urged further investigation.[123] Although the administration of testosterone, whether by transdermal patches, gels, subcutaneous pellets, injectables, or transbuccal delivery systems, increases muscle strength, high doses are necessary and have been reported to be associated with increased cardiovascular disease.[67] Similar findings are reported for women.[67]

Selective androgen receptor molecules (SARMs) produce the positive effects of testosterone without the negative effects. Nandrolone, an injectable SARM, has produced a variety of positive effects on muscle in older persons.[88] Enobosarm (ostarine) is a SARM associated with increased muscle mass and stair-climbing power.[124] However, hormone replacement, either with dehydroepiandrosterone (DHEA) and atamestane or transdermal testosterone, did not improve frailty.[125] However, many authors and pharmaceutical companies believe testosterone and SARMs show promise in treating sarcopenia and frailty but require larger, more definitive trials. Additionally, it is not known if the effects are seen only in men with hypogonadism.

Vitamin D (25-hydroxy) levels decline over the life span. Low vitamin D levels are common in older persons, and many studies have linked low levels of vitamin D to muscle weakness and frailty. However, the results of research on outcomes of strength, function, and falls is mixed. It appears that the benefit of vitamin D may be limited to those with low levels (<20 ng/mL) of vitamin D. The effects may be on the neuromuscular function rather than directly on muscle.[67]

Self-Management Programs Aimed at Preventing or Managing Frailty

Self-management programs to improve self-efficacy, empower individuals, and promote targeted behaviors such as physical activity or improved nutrition may have promise in addressing individuals at risk for or with frailty. The Stanford Chronic Disease Self-Management Program (CDSMP) was among the first widely adopted community-based self-management support interventions. The CDSMP is anchored in a philosophy that, regardless of a participant's specific chronic health conditions, all individuals living with one or multiple chronic health condition(s) can benefit from education for effective self-management. The CDSMP is designed to increase participants' confidence in their ability to self-manage their chronic health conditions. Topics include managing symptoms (pain, fatigue, depression, etc.), appropriate use of medications, appropriate exercise, talking with family members about their condition, talking with health care providers, nutrition, decision making, and evaluating new treatments.

The CDSMP program is based on Bandura's social cognitive theory of self-efficacy. In the CDSMP model, participants with chronic diseases meet weekly for 6 weeks in a small group workshop with the goals of becoming more confident and skillful in their ability to manage their symptoms. The CDSMP program is now widely utilized in the United States and around the world, generally includes high representation of older adult participants, and is particularly applicable to individuals who are prefrail to prevent or delay movement into frailty.

Two recent and large-scale systematic reviews have evaluated the effectiveness of the CDSMP.[126,127] The most notable health outcomes were in psychological health. Specific indicators included improved self-efficacy and decreased cognitive symptoms, depression, and health distress.[126] A significant but small improvement in physical health behaviors such as exercise was also noted. The overall picture is an intervention that has a modest effect on cognitive symptoms and confidence in self-control of chronic conditions, with smaller improvements in physical functioning. Although the effect on physical functioning such as participation in stretching/strengthening or aerobic exercise was small, it should be recognized that effects can be cumulative and any positive change is notable.

Later modifications of the CDSMP, still structured around the basic tenets of the original CDSMP, provide self-management programs targeted toward specific chronic conditions (diabetes, falls prevention, arthritis, etc.) in an expectation that a more tailored program may improve the physical functioning outcomes. Condition-specific CDSMPs have similar outcomes as the CDSMP for a general population with chronic diseases, with the added benefit of more targeted patient education in managing the medical conditions associated with the chronic condition. Additionally, the original, small group, in-person, structured format is now offered in a range of delivery modes using emerging electronic technologies. Physical therapists should be aware of the various programs available in their community to provide an evidence-informed option to help their patients decide on the most appropriate program for their needs.

Self-management programs that focus on individuals with multiple chronic diseases may be specifically appropriate for individuals with prefrailty or frailty.[135] These individuals may benefit more from a self-management intervention aimed at preventing age-related decline. Multiple cognitive and behavioral strategies for dealing with the different kinds of age-related problems so common to the condition of frailty may be particularly valuable. One such program, a bibliography program called "Grip on Life," found that self-management abilities and subjective well-being improved, although improvements in subjective well-being were not sustained at 6 months.[135]

It is especially challenging to improve engagement and self-management in individuals with frailty who reside in long-term care facilities secondary to cognitive challenges and a passive approach to life.[136] However, a systematic review of 10 educational interventions to empower residents found self-efficacy and self-care were significantly improved by interventions that included interactive group education and individually tailored counseling as well as positive feedback.[136] The authors suggest that goal setting, pacing information and time to perform ADL tasks, and providing relevant information that is individual to the resident are effective strategies to empower residents.[136] For example, though not primarily aimed at frailty, the successful Stepping On program, a multifaceted, community-based program, utilizes various strategies in the home environment to improve self-efficacy in fall-risk situations, explore barriers and options for reducing risk for falls, and offer adult learning principles to self-manage risk.[137,138]

Finally, confounding factors common to frailty such as poor health and lower education make self-management programs challenging but potentially more valuable for this vulnerable group. Cramm and colleagues found that those who reported poor health tended to be frail and have lower self-management abilities that were also associated with lower education.[128] The authors recommended that self-management strategies be aimed at the physical health aspects of aging as well as social and psychological aspects of life for these vulnerable elders. One CDSMP program found the benefit of the CDSMP program to benefit those with lower education more so than those with higher education.[129] Another study evaluating a 12-month self-management intervention that stratified participants by robust, frail, and complex care status found health, well-being, and self-management abilities decreased in all three groups as compared with a usual care group.[130] The authors suggest that the length of the program may not have been sufficient and that the usual care group may not have been sufficiently different from the intervention group. Regardless, this study and others[131–134] demonstrate both the potential and difficulty in employing self-management interventions in individuals who are already frail and who have complex health needs. Table 13.7 describes several self-management programs.

Others

Screening for reversible causes of fatigue, combined with targeted interventions, can improve the outcomes of adults with frailty. Treatable causes of fatigue include sleep apnea, depression, anemia, hypotension, hypothyroidism, and B_{12} deficiency.[25] Importantly, selective serotonin reuptake inhibitors (SSRIs) used to treat depression may actually worsen frailty.[25] Further, addressing psychological issues such as depression, social isolation, impaired vision and hearing, and impaired cognition may yield small to large gains in quality of life and promote a greater sense of well-being that may positively impact the person with frailty.[83]

Palliative Care

Frailty predicts functional decline and progression of dependency at the end of life. Severe frailty (four to five

TABLE 13.7 Self-Management Programs Targeting Individuals with Frailty

Program	Target	Population	Description	Results
Stepping On*	Falls prevention program	Community-dwelling elders with fall risk	2 hours/7 weeks; cognitive-behavioral learning in a small group environment with Otago Exercise Program	31% to 50% reduction in falls 6 months after the program
Enhanced Medical Rehabilitation†	Promote and enhance patient engagement through personal goal setting, therapeutic connection, and patient autonomy	Residents of a skilled nursing facility receiving physical (PT) and occupational therapy (OT)	PT and OT training to promote interactive patient direction and frequent feedback as well as high-intensity therapy. Five training sessions of 30 to 60 minutes each; individual and group coaching sessions	More active time in therapy (47 ± 13.5 min for high intensity condition vs. 16.7 ± 10.1 min for standard intensity condition) and longer duration (76.2 ± 12 min vs. 34.2 ± 14.7 min) in standard-intensity session**; more improved gait speed, 6-minute walk, and more engaged with therapy[134]
Grip on Life: A Bibliotherapy‡	Increase self-management abilities so that sustainable positive well-being is achieved	Slightly to moderately frail individuals	Self-managed, interactive course consisting of five books of 11 to 19 pages each that address developing a positive frame of mind, being self-efficacious, taking initiative, investing in resources, and taking care of a multifunctionality of resources	Intervention group increased self-management abilities, whereas control group decreased. Subjective well-being improved more in the intervention group but was not sustained at 6 months
Embraced§	Support older adults to age in place through a self-management support and prevention program focused on staying healthy and independent for as long as possible	Older adults aged 75 and over stratified by level of frailty and complexity of care needs	Group meetings for education about self-management abilities including health maintenance, physical and social activities, and dietary recommendations. Frail people received additional individual support from a case manager with input from the individual	No differences in health, well-being, or self-management
Chronic Disease Self-Management Program (CDSMP)¶	Improve coping resources and well-being of people with frailty and multiple chronic diseases	Older adults (mean age 81 years) from an elderly daycare facility with several locations	6 weekly sessions using CDSMP protocol	Sense of mastery improved only in lower-educated group and a stabilizing effect on valuation of life. No differences in cognitive function or depression were noted

*Clemson L, Cumming RG, Kendig H, Swann M, Heard R, Taylor K. The effectiveness of a community-based program for reducing the incidence of falls in the elderly: a randomized trial. *J Am Geriatr Soc*. 2004;52(9):1487–1494. http://www.blackwell-synergy.com/links/doi/10.1111/j.1532-5415.2004.52411.x/abs.
†Bland MD, Birkenmeier RL, Barco P, Lenard E, Lang CE, Lenze EJ. Enhanced medical rehabilitation: effectiveness of a clinical training model (Danzl M, Etter N, eds.). *NeuroRehabilitation*. 2016;39(4):481–498. https://doi.org/10.3233/NRE-161380.
‡Frieswijk N, Steverink N, Buunk BP, Slaets JPJ. The effectiveness of a bibliotherapy in increasing the self-management ability of slightly to moderately frail older people. *Patient Educ Couns*. 2006;61(2):219–227. https://doi.org/10.1016/J.PEC.2005.03.011.
§Spoorenberg SLW, Wynia K, Uittenbroek RJ, Kremer HPH, Reijneveld SA. Effects of a population-based, person-centered and integrated care service on health, wellbeing and self-management of community-living older adults: a randomised controlled trial on Embrace (Evans CJ, ed.). *PLoS One*. 2018;13(1):e0190751. https://doi.org/10.1371/journal.pone.0190751.
¶Jonker AAGC, Comijs HC, Knipscheer KCPM, Deeg DJH. Benefits for elders with vulnerable health from the Chronic Disease Self-Management Program (CDSMP) at short and longer term. *BMC Geriatr*. 2015;15:101. https://doi.org/10.1186/s12877-015-0090-4.
**Host HH, Lang CE, Hildebrand MW, et al. Patient Active Time During Therapy Sessions in Postacute Rehabilitation: Development and Validation of a New Measure. *Phys Occup Ther Geriatr.* 2014;32(2):169–178. https://doi.org/10.3109/02703181.2014.915282.

attributes of the frailty phenotype model) and metabolic abnormalities of low cholesterol and albumin predict particularly high short-term mortality rates in frail older adults.[139] These characteristics can mark a predeath phase of severe frailty. Poor responses to treatment are recognized with end-stage frailty, and the adoption of palliative care approaches may be appropriate.

However, one could argue that advanced biological aging, such as extreme frailty, signals that the end of life is approaching. Palliative care focuses on improving life and providing comfort to people of all ages with serious, chronic, and life-threatening illnesses. Frailty could be considered a chronic and serious condition that has the potential of being life-threatening. Patient-centered and holistic care, the hallmark of palliative care, focuses on the patient's priorities and what is important to the person. The role of the physical therapist in palliative care, also discussed elsewhere in this text, is multifaceted and applicable to the individual with frailty. Establishing patient-centered goals and the interventions to best address these goals, patient and family education, and the prevention of hospitalization are the primary roles of a physical therapist in the palliative care setting. Optimizing independence and function through an appropriate exercise and physical activity program may be key while minimizing risk of adverse events such as falls. Key to a palliative approach to frailty is to identify and treat reversible causes of decline as has been discussed previously.

Reducing the mobility disability that often results from inpatient stays is an important role of the physical therapist. Strategies can include the encouragement of wearing comfortable shoes and clothing while an inpatient, standing orders for activity, patient and family education regarding physical activity, and involving the family in mobility. Empowering the patient to do as much as possible—that is, function-focused care—can improve the sense of well-being. And finally, using trained individuals to serve as walking aides may address the pervasive physical inactivity that occurs in the inpatient environment.

PREVENTION

Frail older adults are heavy users of health and social care. Reducing the costs associated with frailty should be a priority for any health care system. Addressing frailty through prevention may be the most effective intervention. Recognizing frailty as a long-term condition that needs to be diagnosed and treated *before* a health crisis arises rather than when a person is in the midst of a crisis is a major goal for the coordinated management of frailty.[140] Healthy behaviors throughout the life span, cognitive stimulation, and maintaining a purpose in life are keys to aging as optimally as possible and thus avoiding or delaying frailty. Additionally, having a positive attitude toward aging and general participation in life has a powerful effect on health and engagement.

It is concerning that several studies have found that more recently born cohorts of older adults are more frail than earlier born cohorts.[35,141] Regular engagement in moderate to vigorous physical activity is protective behavior against frailty in older adults and is best to develop a lifestyle that is physically active, an increasing challenge in this technology-driven world.[142]

The culture of sedentary activity and an acceptance of the attitude that frailty is part of aging and therefore inevitable and unavoidable lead to frailty. Sedentary behavior should be avoided. The amount of sitting time that predicted frailty was greater than 495 minutes (8.25 hours) per day in men and over 536 minutes (8.9 hours) per day in women.[143] Reducing sedentary time by even 1-minute bouts of activity lowered the incidence of frailty.[144] Another study found that moderate to vigorous activity is required to reduce the trajectory of frailty progression.[142]

Restricting the factors that contribute to frailty (inactivity, muscle weakness, and negative attitudes about physical activity) while increasing protective factors can reduce the frailty condition.[145] However, frail adults, especially those who are quite old, may be unable to self-manage their health and health care as is expected with many other chronic conditions.[146] Although poor health negatively impacts being physically active, it is uncertain whether poor health is implicated by a lack of physical activity. Therefore, the recommendation is to increase physical activity even in the presence of poor health to avoid frailty.[145]

Prevention and treatment require multifactorial interventions at inter- and intrapersonal levels as well as environmental and policy levels. Primary preventative intervention for cognitive frailty includes the promotion of physical activities, cognitive stimulation, exercise and a healthy diet such as the Mediterranean diet, cessation of smoking, promoting emotional recovery, engaging in an active and socially integrated lifestyle, an ideal amount of daily sleep, maintenance of proper body weight, and metabolic control (including control of dyslipidemia, diabetes, and blood pressure).[112] Secondary prevention, for those with prefrailty, utilizes a CGA to determine the key underlying deficits that can guide an individualized multimodal intervention. This multimodal intervention could include drug treatment for chronic diseases, fall prevention interventions, and exercise and nutritional support as well as social and psychological support.

In summary, physical activity interventions (of all types and combinations) are the most effective means of preventing or reducing the level of frailty.[147] Clearly physical therapists have an important role to play in reducing the incidence and severity of frailty.

REFERENCES

1. Bortz WM. A conceptual framework of frailty: a review. *J Gerontol.* 2002;57A(5):M283–M288.
2. Mosquera C, Spaniolas K, Fitzgerald TL. Impact of frailty on surgical outcomes: the right patient for the right procedure. *Surgery.* 2016;160(2):272–280. https://doi.org/10.1016/j.surg.2016.04.030.
3. Fried LP, Tangen CM, Walston J, et al. Frailty in older adults: evidence for a phenotype. *J Gerontol Med Sci.* 2001;56A(3):M146–M156. https://doi.org/10.1093/gerona/56.3.M146.
4. Rothman MD, Leo-Summers L, Gill TM. Prognostic significance of potential frailty criteria. *J Am Geriatr Soc.* 2008;56(12):2116–2211. https://doi.org/10.1111/j.1532-5415.2008.02008.x.
5. Collard RM, Boter H, Schoevers RA, Oude Voshaar RC. Prevalence of frailty in community-dwelling older persons: a systematic review. *J Am Geriatr Soc.* 2012;60(8):1487–1492. https://doi.org/10.1111/j.1532-5415.2012.04054.x.
6. Bandeen-Roche K, Seplaki CL, Huang J, et al. Frailty in older adults: a nationally representative profile in the United States. *Journals Gerontol Ser A Biol Sci Med Sci.* 2015;70(11):1427–1434. https://doi.org/10.1093/gerona/glv133.
7. Buckinx F, Reginster J-Y, Gillain S, Petermans J, Brunois T, Bruyère O. Prevalence of frailty in nursing home residents according to various diagnostic tools. *J Frailty Aging.* 2017;6(3):122–128. https://doi.org/10.14283/jfa.2017.20.
8. Kojima G. Prevalence of frailty in nursing homes: a systematic review and meta-analysis. *J Am Med Dir Assoc.* 2015;16(11):940–945. https://doi.org/10.1016/j.jamda.2015.06.025.
9. Rockwood K, Hogan DB, MacKnight C. Conceptualisation and measurement of frailty in elderly people. *Drugs Aging.* 2000;17(4):295–302.
10. Abellan van Kan G, Rolland Y, Bergman H, Morley JE, Kritchevsky SB, Vellas B. The I.A.N.A Task Force on frailty assessment of older people in clinical practice. *J Nutr Health Aging.* 2008;12(1):29–37.
11. Rockwood K, Andrew M, Mitnitski A. A comparison of two approaches to measuring frailty in elderly people. *Journals Gerontol Ser A Biol Sci Med Sci.* 2007;62(7):738–743. https://doi.org/10.1093/gerona/62.7.738.
12. Wilson D, Jackson T, Sapey E, Lord JM. Frailty and sarcopenia: the potential role of an aged immune system. *Ageing Res Rev.* 2017;36:1–10. https://doi.org/10.1016/J.ARR.2017.01.006.
13. Gobbens RJJ, Luijkx KG, Wijnen-Sponselee MT, Schols JMGA. Towards an integral conceptual model of frailty. *J Nutr Health Aging.* 2010;14(3):175–181. http://www.ncbi.nlm.nih.gov/pubmed/20191249. Accessed July 27, 2018.
14. Gross AL, Xue Q-L, Bandeen-Roche K, et al. Declines and impairment in executive function predict onset of physical frailty. *Journals Gerontol Ser A Biol Sci Med Sci.* 2016;71(12):1624–1630. https://doi.org/10.1093/gerona/glw067.
15. Avila-Funes JA, Amieva HH, Barberger-Gateau P, et al. Cognitive impairment improves the predictive validity of the phenotype of frailty for adverse health outcomes: the three-city study. *J Am Geriatr Soc.* 2009;57(3):453–461. https://doi.org/10.1111/j.1532-5415.2008.02136.x.
16. Kelaiditi E, Cesari M, Canevelli M, et al. Cognitive frailty: rational and definition from an (I.A.N.A./I.A.G.G.) International Consensus Group. *J Nutr Health Aging.* 2013;17(9):726–734. https://doi.org/10.1007/s12603-013-0367-2.
17. Woods AJ, Cohen RA, Pahor M. Cognitive frailty: frontiers and challenges. *J Nutr Health Aging.* 2013;17(9):741–743. https://doi.org/10.1007/s12603-013-0398-8.
18. Fitten LJ. Psychological frailty in the aging patient. *Nestle Nutr Inst Workshop Ser.* 2015;83:45–54. https://doi.org/10.1159/000382060.
19. Fougère B, Delrieu J, del Campo N, Soriano G, Sourdet S, Vellas B. Cognitive frailty. *Clin Geriatr Med.* 2017;33(3):339–355. https://doi.org/10.1016/j.cger.2017.03.001.
20. Cappell KA, Gmeindl L, Reuter-Lorenz PA. Age differences in prefrontal recruitment during verbal working memory maintenance depend on memory load. *Cortex.* 2010;46(4):462–473. https://doi.org/10.1016/j.cortex.2009.11.009.
21. Carlson MC, Xue Q-L, Zhou J, Fried LP. Executive decline and dysfunction precedes declines in memory: the Women's Health and Aging Study II. *J Gerontol Ser A Biol Sci Med Sci.* 2009;64A(1):110–117. https://doi.org/10.1093/gerona/gln008.
22. Vaughan L, Corbin AL, Goveas JS. Depression and frailty in later life: a systematic review. *Clin Interv Aging.* 2015;10:1947–1958. https://doi.org/10.2147/CIA.S69632.
23. Chang SS, Weiss CO, Xue Q-L, Fried LP. Patterns of comorbid inflammatory diseases in frail older women: the Women's Health and Aging Studies I and II. *J Gerontol Ser A Biol Sci Med Sci.* 2010;65A(4):407–413. https://doi.org/10.1093/gerona/glp181.
24. Rolland Y, Abellan van Kan G, Bénétos A, et al. Frailty, osteoporosis and hip fracture: causes, consequences and therapeutic perspectives. *J Nutr Health Aging.* 2008;12(5):335–346. http://www.ncbi.nlm.nih.gov/pubmed/18443717. Accessed July 27, 2018.
25. Lakey SL, LaCroix AZ, Gray SL, et al. Antidepressant use, depressive symptoms, and incident frailty in women aged 65 and older from the Women's Health Initiative Observational Study. *J Am Geriatr Soc.* 2012;60(5):854–861. https://doi.org/10.1111/j.1532-5415.2012.03940.x.
26. Dent E, Hoogendijk EO. Psychosocial factors modify the association of frailty with adverse outcomes: a prospective study of hospitalised older people. *BMC Geriatr.* 2014;14(1):108. https://doi.org/10.1186/1471-2318-14-108.
27. Gale CR, Cooper C, Deary IJ, Aihie Sayer A. Psychological well-being and incident frailty in men and women: the English Longitudinal Study of Ageing. *Psychol Med.* 2014;44(4):697–706. https://doi.org/10.1017/S0033291713001384.
28. Hoogendijk EO, van Hout HPJ, van der Horst HE, et al. Do psychosocial resources modify the effects of frailty on functional decline and mortality? *J Psychosom Res.* 2014;77(6):547–551. https://doi.org/10.1016/j.jpsychores.2014.09.017.
29. Freitag S, Schmidt S. Psychosocial correlates of frailty in older adults. *Geriatrics.* 2016;1(4):26. https://doi.org/10.3390/geriatrics1040026.
30. Wells M, Avers D, Brooks G. Resilience, physical performance measures, and self-perceived physical and mental health in older Catholic nuns. *J Geriatr Phys Ther.* 2012;35(3):126–131. https://doi.org/10.1519/JPT.0b013e318237103f.
31. Ogle CM, Rubin DC, Siegler IC. The impact of the developmental timing of trauma exposure on PTSD symptoms and psychosocial functioning among older adults. *Dev Psychol.* 2013;49(11):2191–2200. https://doi.org/10.1037/a0031985.
32. Woo J, Goggins W, Sham A, Ho SCC. Social determinants of frailty. *Gerontology.* 2005;51(6):402–408. https://doi.org/10.1159/000088705.
33. Lang IA, Hubbard RE, Andrew MK, Llewellyn DJ, Melzer D, Rockwood K. Neighborhood deprivation, individual socioeconomic status, and frailty in older adults. *J Am Geriatr Soc.* 2009;57(10):1776–1780. https://doi.org/10.1111/j.1532-5415.2009.02480.x.
34. Louie GH, Ward MM. Socioeconomic and ethnic differences in disease burden and disparities in physical function in older adults. *Am J Public Health.* 2011;101(7):1322–1329. https://doi.org/10.2105/AJPH.2010.199455.
35. Marshall A, Nazroo J, Tampubolon G, Vanhoutte B. Cohort differences in the levels and trajectories of frailty among older people in England. *J Epidemiol Community Health.* 2015;69(4):316–321. https://doi.org/10.1136/jech-2014-204655.

36. Hoogendijk EO, Heymans MW, Deeg DJH, Huisman M. Socioeconomic inequalities in frailty among older adults: results from a 10-year longitudinal study in the Netherlands. *Gerontology*. 2018;64(2):157–164. https://doi.org/10.1159/000481943.
37. Steptoe A, Shankar A, Demakakos P, Wardle J. Social isolation, loneliness, and all-cause mortality in older men and women. *Proc Natl Acad Sci*. 2013;110(15):5797–5801. https://doi.org/10.1073/pnas.1219686110.
38. Teo N, Gao Q, Nyunt MSZ, Wee SL, Ng T-P. Social frailty and functional disability: findings from the Singapore Longitudinal Ageing Studies. *J Am Med Dir Assoc*. 2017;18(7):637.e13–637.e19. https://doi.org/10.1016/j.jamda.2017.04.015.
39. Gale CR, Mõttus R, Deary IJ, Cooper C, Sayer AA. Personality and risk of frailty: the English Longitudinal Study of Ageing. *Ann Behav Med*. 2017;51(1):128–136. https://doi.org/10.1007/s12160-016-9833-5.
40. Shankar A, McMunn A, Demakakos P, Hamer M, Steptoe A. Social isolation and loneliness: prospective associations with functional status in older adults. *Health Psychol*. 2017;36(2):179–187. https://doi.org/10.1037/hea0000437.
41. Cherry KE, Walker EJ, Brown JS, et al. Social engagement and health in younger, older, and oldest-old adults in the Louisiana Healthy Aging Study. *J Appl Gerontol*. 2013;32(1):51–75. https://doi.org/10.1177/0733464811409034.
42. Peterson MJ, Giuliani C, Morey MC, et al. Physical activity as a preventative factor for frailty: the health, aging, and body composition study. *J Gerontol A Biol Sci Med Sci*. 2009;64(1):61–68. https://doi.org/10.1093/gerona/gln001.
43. Gill TM, Gahbauer EA, Allore HG, Han L. Transitions between frailty states among community-living older persons. *Arch Intern Med*. 2006;166(4):418–423. https://doi.org/10.1001/.418.
44. Xue QL. The frailty syndrome: definition and natural history. *Clin Geriatr Med*. 2011;27(1):1–15. https://doi.org/10.1016/j.cger.2010.08.009.
45. Clegg A, Rogers L, Young J. Diagnostic test accuracy of simple instruments for identifying frailty in community-dwelling older people: a systematic review. *Age Ageing*. 2015;44(1):148–152. https://doi.org/10.1093/ageing/afu157.
46. Takano E, Teranishi T, Watanabe T, et al. Differences in the effect of exercise interventions between prefrail older adults and older adults without frailty: a pilot study. *Geriatr Gerontol Int*. 2017;17(9):1265–1269. https://doi.org/10.1111/ggi.12853.
47. Sourial N, Bergman H, Karunananthan S, et al. Contribution of frailty markers in explaining differences among individuals in five samples of older persons. *J Gerontol Ser A*. 2012;67(11):1197–1204. https://doi.org/10.1093/gerona/gls084.
48. Joosten E, Demuynck M, Detroyer E, Milisen K. Prevalence of frailty and its ability to predict in hospital delirium, falls, and 6-month mortality in hospitalized older patients. *BMC Geriatr*. 2014;14(1):1. https://doi.org/10.1186/1471-2318-14-1.
49. Kojima G, Iliffe S, Walters K. Frailty index as a predictor of mortality: a systematic review and meta-analysis. *Age Ageing*. 2018;47(2):193–200. https://doi.org/10.1093/ageing/afx162.
50. Gale CR, Cooper C, Aihie Sayer A. Prevalence of frailty and disability: findings from the English Longitudinal Study of Ageing. *Age Ageing*. 2015;44(1):162–165. https://doi.org/10.1093/ageing/afu148.
51. Theou O, Rockwood MR, Mitnitski A, Rockwood K. Disability and co-morbidity in relation to frailty: how much do they overlap? *Arch Gerontol Geriatr*. 2012;55(2):e1–e8. https://doi.org/10.1016/j.archger.2012.03.001.
52. von Haehling S, Morley JE, Anker SD. An overview of sarcopenia: facts and numbers on prevalence and clinical impact. *J Cachexia Sarcopenia Muscle*. 2010;1(2):129–133. https://doi.org/10.1007/s13539-010-0014-2.
53. Yoshimura N, Muraki S, Oka H, et al. Do sarcopenia and/or osteoporosis increase the risk of frailty? A 4-year observation of the second and third ROAD study surveys. *Osteoporos Int*. 2018;29(10):2181–2190. https://doi.org/10.1007/s00198-018-4596-4.
54. Boyd CM, Ricks M, Fried LP, et al. Functional decline and recovery of activities of daily living in hospitalized, disabled older women: the Women's Health and Aging Study I. *J Am Geriatr Soc*. 2009;57(10):1757–1766. https://doi.org/10.1111/j.1532-5415.2009.02455.x.
55. Hajek A, Bock J-O, Saum K-U, et al. Frailty and healthcare costs—longitudinal results of a prospective cohort study. *Age Ageing*. 2018;47(2):233–241. https://doi.org/10.1093/ageing/afx157.
56. Gleckman H. *Frail Seniors Are Most At-Risk and Costliest to Treat*. https://www.forbes.com/sites/howardgleckman/2012/07/06/frail-seniors-are-most-at-risk-and-costliest-to-treat/#6e44d473540d. Published 2012. Accessed July 10, 2018.
57. Comans TA, Peel NM, Hubbard RE, Mulligan AD, Gray LC, Scuffham PA. The increase in healthcare costs associated with frailty in older people discharged to a post-acute transition care program. *Age Ageing*. 2016;45(2):317–320. https://doi.org/10.1093/ageing/afv196.
58. Elderkind. *The Most Common Surgeries Needed by Older Patients*. http://elderkind.com/common-surgeries-needed-older-patients/. Published 2018. Accessed July 30, 2018.
59. Song X, Mitnitski A, Rockwood K. Prevalence and 10-year outcomes of frailty in older adults in relation to deficit accumulation. *J Am Geriatr Soc*. 2010;58(4):681–687. https://doi.org/10.1111/j.1532-5415.2010.02764.x.
60. Rockwood K, Howlett SE, MacKnight C, et al. Prevalence, attributes, and outcomes of fitness and frailty in community-dwelling older adults: report from the Canadian Study of Health and Aging. *J Gerontol A Biol Sci Med Sci*. 2004;59(12):1310–1317. http://biomed.gerontologyjournals.org/cgi/content/abstract/59/12/1310.
61. Partridge JSL, Fuller M, Harari D, Taylor PR, Martin FC, Dhesi JK. Frailty and poor functional status are common in arterial vascular surgical patients and affect postoperative outcomes. *Int J Surg*. 2015;18:57–63. https://doi.org/10.1016/j.ijsu.2015.04.037.
62. Chung J-Y, Chang W-Y, Lin T-W, et al. An analysis of surgical outcomes in patients aged 80 years and older. *Acta Anaesthesiol Taiwanica*. 2014;52(4):153–158. https://doi.org/10.1016/j.aat.2014.09.003.
63. Sheetz KH, Waits SA, Terjimanian MN, et al. Cost of major surgery in the sarcopenic patient. *J Am Coll Surg*. 2013;217(5):813–818. https://doi.org/10.1016/j.jamcollsurg.2013.04.042.
64. Hatheway OL, Mitnitski A, Rockwood K. Frailty affects the initial treatment response and time to recovery of mobility in acutely ill older adults admitted to hospital. *Age Ageing*. 2017;46(6):920–925. https://doi.org/10.1093/ageing/afw257.
65. Clegg A, Young J, Iliffe S, Rikkert MO, Rockwood K. Frailty in older people. *Lancet*. 2013;381(9868):752–762. https://doi.org/10.1016/S0140-6736(12)62167-9.
66. Chen X, Mao G, Leng SX. Frailty syndrome: an overview. *Clin Interv Aging*. 2014;9:433–441. https://doi.org/10.2147/CIA.S45300.
67. Morley JE, Malmstrom TK. Frailty, sarcopenia, and hormones. *Endocrinol Metab Clin N Am*. 2013;42:391–405. https://doi.org/10.1016/j.ecl.2013.02.006.
68. Liguori I, Russo G, Aran L, et al. Sarcopenia: assessment of disease burden and strategies to improve outcomes. *Clin Interv Aging*. 2018;13:913–927. https://doi.org/10.2147/CIA.S149232.
69. Xue QL, Fried LP, Glass TA, Laffan A, Chaves PH. Life-space constriction, development of frailty, and the competing risk of mortality: the Women's Health and Aging Study I. *Am J Epidemiol*. 2008;167(2):240–248. https://doi.org/10.1093/aje/kwm270.

70. Schrack JA, Zipunnikov V, Simonsick EM, Studenski S, Ferrucci L. Rising energetic cost of walking predicts gait speed decline with aging. *J Gerontol Ser A Biol Sci Med Sci.* 2016;71(7):947–953. https://doi.org/10.1093/gerona/glw002.
71. Schrack JA, Simonsick EM, Chaves PHM, Ferrucci L. The role of energetic cost in the age-related slowing of gait speed. *J Am Geriatr Soc.* 2012;60(10):1811–1816. https://doi.org/10.1111/j.1532-5415.2012.04153.x.
72. Gill TM, Allore HG, Hardy SE, Guo Z. The dynamic nature of mobility disability in older persons. *J Am Geriatr Soc.* 2006; 54(2):248–254. http://www.blackwell-synergy.com/doi/abs/10.1111/j.1532-5415.2005.00586.x.
73. Parker SG, McCue P, Phelps K, et al. What is Comprehensive Geriatric Assessment (CGA)? An umbrella review. *Age Ageing.* 2018;47(1):149–155. https://doi.org/10.1093/ageing/afx166.
74. Turner G, Clegg A, British Geriatrics Society, et al. Best practice guidelines for the management of frailty: a British Geriatrics Society, Age UK and Royal College of General Practitioners report. *Age Ageing.* 2014;43(6):744–747. https://doi.org/10.1093/ageing/afu138.
75. Raiche M, Hebert R, Dubois M-F. PRISMA-7: a case-finding tool to identify older adults with moderate to severe disabilities. *Arch Gerontol Geriatr.* 2008;47(1):9–18.
76. Rockwood K, Song X, MacKnight C, et al. A global clinical measure of fitness and frailty in elderly people. *CMAJ.* 2005;173(5):489–495 173/5/489.
77. Kulminski AM, Ukraintseva SV, Kulminskaya IV, Arbeev KG, Land K, Yashin AI. Cumulative deficits better characterize susceptibility to death in elderly people than phenotypic frailty: lessons from the Cardiovascular Health Study. *J Am Geriatr Soc.* 2008;56(5):898–903. 10.1111/j.1532-5415.2008.01656.x.
78. Theou O, Walston J, Rockwood K. Operationalizing frailty using the frailty phenotype and deficit accumulation approaches. *Interdiscip Top Gerontol Geriatr.* 2015;41:66–73. https://doi.org/10.1159/000381164.
79. Lee L, Patel T, Costa A, et al. Screening for frailty in primary care: accuracy of gait speed and hand-grip strength. *Can Fam Physician.* 2017;63(1):e51–e57. http://www.ncbi.nlm.nih.gov/pubmed/28115460. Accessed June 19, 2018.
80. Tieland M, Verdijk LB, de Groot LCPGM, van Loon LJC. Handgrip strength does not represent an appropriate measure to evaluate changes in muscle strength during an exercise intervention program in frail older people. *Int J Sport Nutr Exerc Metab.* 2015;25(1):27–36. https://doi.org/10.1123/ijsnem.2013-0123.
81. Millor N, Lecumberri P, Gomez M, et al. Gait velocity and chair sit-stand-sit performance improves current frailty-status identification. *IEEE Trans Neural Syst Rehabil Eng.* 2017;25(11):2018–2025. https://doi.org/10.1109/TNSRE.2017.2699124.
82. Millor N, Lecumberri P, Gómez M, Martínez-Ramírez A, Izquierdo M. An evaluation of the 30-s chair stand test in older adults: frailty detection based on kinematic parameters from a single inertial unit. *J Neuroeng Rehabil.* 2013;10:86. https://doi.org/10.1186/1743-0003-10-86.
83. Fairhall N, Langron C, Sherrington C, et al. Treating frailty—a practical guide. *BMC Med.* 2011;9:83. https://doi.org/10.1186/1741-7015-9-83.
84. Abellan van Kan G, Rolland Y, Andrieu S, et al. Gait speed at usual pace as a predictor of adverse outcomes in community-dwelling older people an International Academy on Nutrition and Aging (IANA) Task Force. *J Nutr Health Aging.* 2009;13(10):881–889.
85. Sheppard KD, Sawyer P, Ritchie CS, Allman RM, Brown CJ. Life-space mobility predicts nursing home admission over 6 years. *J Aging Health.* 2013;25(6):907–920. https://doi.org/10.1177/0898264313497507.
86. Baker PS, Bodner EV, Allman RM. Measuring life-space mobility in community-dwelling older adults. *J Am Geriatr Soc.* 2003;51(11):1610–1614.
87. Portegijs E, Rantakokko M, Viljanen A, Sipilä S, Rantanen T. Is frailty associated with life-space mobility and perceived autonomy in participation outdoors? A longitudinal study. *Age Ageing.* 2016;45(4):550–553. https://doi.org/10.1093/ageing/afw072.
88. Morley JE. Pharmacologic options for the treatment of sarcopenia. *Calcif Tissue Int.* 2016;98(4):319–333. https://doi.org/10.1007/s00223-015-0022-5.
89. Beaudart C, McCloskey E, Bruyere O, et al. Sarcopenia in daily practice: assessment and management. *BMC Geriatr.* 2016;16(1):170. https://doi.org/10.1186/s12877-016-0349-4.
90. Dent E, Lien C, Lim WS, et al. The Asia-Pacific Clinical Practice Guidelines for the Management of Frailty. *J Am Med Dir Assoc.* 2017;18(7):564–575. https://doi.org/10.1016/j.jamda.2017.04.018.
91. Bray NW, Smart RR, Jakobi JM, Jones GR. Exercise prescription to reverse frailty. *Appl Physiol Nutr Metab.* 2016;41(10):1112–1116. https://doi.org/10.1139/apnm-2016-0226.
92. Melov S, Tarnopolsky MA, Beckman K, Felkey K, Hubbard A. Resistance exercise reverses aging in human skeletal muscle (Wenner P, ed.). *PLoS One.* 2007;2(5):e465. https://doi.org/10.1371/journal.pone.0000465.
93. Abate M, Di Iorio A, Di Renzo D, Paganelli R, Saggini R, Abate G. Frailty in the elderly: the physical dimension. *Eura Medicophys.* 2007;43(3):407–415. http://www.ncbi.nlm.nih.gov/pubmed/17117147. Accessed July 10, 2018.
94. Chou CH, Hwang CL, Wu YT. Effect of exercise on physical function, daily living activities, and quality of life in the frail older adults: a meta-analysis. *Arch Phys Med Rehabil.* 2012;93(2):237–244. https://doi.org/10.1016/j.apmr.2011.08.042.
95. Centers for Disease Control and Prevention. Physical Activity for Everyone: Guidelines: Older Adults | DNPAO. http://www.cdc.gov/physicalactivity/everyone/guidelines/olderadults.html.
96. Cameron ID, Murray GR, Gillespie LD, et al. Interventions for preventing falls in older people in nursing care facilities and hospitals. *Cochrane Database Syst Rev.* 2010;(1): CD005465. https://doi.org/10.1002/14651858.CD005465.pub2.
97. Fisher JP, Steele J, Gentil P, Giessing J, Westcott WL. A minimal dose approach to resistance training for the older adult; the prophylactic for aging. *Exp Gerontol.* 2017;99:80–86. https://doi.org/10.1016/j.exger.2017.09.012.
98. Silva NL, Oliveira RB, Fleck SJ, Leon AC, Farinatti P. Influence of strength training variables on strength gains in adults over 55 years-old: a meta-analysis of dose-response relationships. *J Sci Med Sport.* 2014;17(3):337–344. https://doi.org/10.1016/j.jsams.2013.05.009.
99. Danilovich MK, Conroy DE, Hornby TG. Feasibility and impact of high-intensity walking training in frail older adults. *J Aging Phys Act.* 2017;25(4):533–538. https://doi.org/10.1123/japa.2016-0305.
100. Weening-Dijksterhuis E, de Greef MH, Scherder EJ, Slaets JP, van der Schans CP. Frail institutionalized older persons: a comprehensive review on physical exercise, physical fitness, activities of daily living, and quality-of-life. *Am J Phys Med Rehabil.* 2011;90(2):156–168. https://doi.org/10.1097/PHM.0b013e3181f703ef.
101. Tsaih P-LL, Shih Y-LL, Hu M-HH. Low-intensity task-oriented exercise for ambulation-challenged residents in long-term care facilities: a randomized, controlled trial. *Am J Phys Med Rehabil.* 2012;91(7):616–624. https://doi.org/10.1097/PHM.0b013e3182555de3.
102. White NT, Delitto A, Manal TJ, Miller S. The American Physical Therapy Association's top five choosing wisely recommendations. *Phys Ther.* 2015;95(1):9–24. https://doi.org/10.2522/ptj.20140287.

103. Granacher U, Gollhofer A, Hortobagyi T, et al. The importance of trunk muscle strength for balance, functional performance, and fall prevention in seniors: a systematic review. *Sports Med.* 2013;43(7):627–641. https://doi.org/10.1007/s40279-013-0041-1.
104. Liguori I, Russo G, Coscia V, et al. Orthostatic hypotension in the elderly: a marker of clinical frailty? *J Am Med Dir Assoc.* 2018;19(9):779–785. https://doi.org/10.1016/j.jamda.2018.04.018.
105. Bonecutter R. *How to get up from the floor after a fall – MacGyver Style!.* http://homeability.com/how-to-get-up-from-the-floor-macgyver-style/. Accessed August 1, 2018.
106. McMinn J, Steel C, Bowman A. Investigation and management of unintentional weight loss in older adults. *BMJ Br Med J.* 2011;342:d1732. https://doi.org/10.1136/bmj.d1732.
107. Vellas B, Villars H, Abellan G, et al. Overview of the MNA–its history and challenges. *J Nutr Health Aging.* 2006;10(6):456–463; discussion 463–465. http://www.ncbi.nlm.nih.gov/pubmed/17183418. Accessed July 10, 2018.
108. Ruscin JM, Page RL, Yeager BF, Wallace JI. Tumor necrosis factor-α and involuntary weight loss in elderly, community-dwelling adults. *Pharmacotherapy.* 2005;25(3):313–319. https://doi.org/10.1592/phco.25.3.313.61607.
109. Stajkovic S, Aitken EM, Holroyd-Leduc J. Unintentional weight loss in older adults. *CMAJ.* 2011;183(4):443–449. https://doi.org/10.1503/cmaj.101471.
110. Morley JE, Silver AJ. Nutritional issues in nursing home care. *Ann Intern Med.* 1995;123(11):850. https://doi.org/10.7326/0003-4819-123-11-199512010-00008.
111. Gordon MM, Bopp MJ, Easter L, et al. Effects of dietary protein on the composition of weight loss in post-menopausal women. *J Nutr Health Aging.* 2008;12(8):505–509. http://www.ncbi.nlm.nih.gov/pubmed/18810296. Accessed July 10, 2018.
112. Fougère B, Morley JE, Little MO, de Souto Barreto P, Cesari M, Vellas B. Interventions against disability in frail older adults: lessons learned from clinical trials. *J Nutr Health Aging.* 2018;22(6):676–688. https://doi.org/10.1007/s12603-017-0987-z.
113. Abizanda P, López MD, García VP, et al. Effects of an oral nutritional supplementation plus physical exercise intervention on the physical function, nutritional status, and quality of life in frail institutionalized older adults: the ACTIVNES Study. *J Am Med Dir Assoc.* 2015;16(5):439.e9–439.e16. https://doi.org/10.1016/j.jamda.2015.02.005.
114. Deutz NEP, Bauer JM, Barazzoni R, et al. Protein intake and exercise for optimal muscle function with aging: recommendations from the ESPEN Expert Group. *Clin Nutr.* 2014;33(6):929–936. https://doi.org/10.1016/j.clnu.2014.04.007.
115. Cruz-Jentoft AJ, Landi F, Schneider SM, et al. Prevalence of and interventions for sarcopenia in ageing adults: a systematic review. Report of the International Sarcopenia Initiative (EWGSOP and IWGS). *Age Ageing.* 2014;43(6):748–759. https://doi.org/10.1093/ageing/afu115.
116. Kojima G, Avgerinou C, Iliffe S, Walters K. Adherence to Mediterranean diet reduces incident frailty risk: systematic review and meta-analysis. *J Am Geriatr Soc.* 2018;66(4):783–788. https://doi.org/10.1111/jgs.15251.
117. Kelaiditi E, Jennings A, Steves CJ, et al. Measurements of skeletal muscle mass and power are positively related to a Mediterranean dietary pattern in women. *Osteoporos Int.* 2016;27(11):3251–3260. https://doi.org/10.1007/s00198-016-3665-9.
118. Talegawkar SA, Bandinelli S, Bandeen-Roche K, et al. A higher adherence to a Mediterranean-style diet is inversely associated with the development of frailty in community-dwelling elderly men and women. *J Nutr.* 2012;142(12):2161–2166. https://doi.org/10.3945/jn.112.165498.
119. Silva R, Pizato N, da Mata F, Figueiredo A, Ito M, Pereira MG. Mediterranean diet and musculoskeletal-functional outcomes in community-dwelling older people: a systematic review and meta-analysis. *J Nutr Health Aging.* 2018;22(6):655–663. https://doi.org/10.1007/s12603-017-0993-1.
120. Lo Y-L, Hsieh Y-T, Hsu L-L, et al. Dietary pattern associated with frailty: results from nutrition and health survey in Taiwan. *J Am Geriatr Soc.* 2017;65(9):2009–2015. https://doi.org/10.1111/jgs.14972.
121. Voelker R. The Mediterranean diet's fight against frailty. *JAMA.* 2018;319(19):1971. https://doi.org/10.1001/jama.2018.3653.
122. Berdot S, Bertrand M, Dartigues J-F, et al. Inappropriate medication use and risk of falls—a prospective study in a large community-dwelling elderly cohort. *BMC Geriatr.* 2009;9:30. https://doi.org/10.1186/1471-2318-9-30.
123. Swiecicka A, Eendebak RJAH, Lunt M, et al. Reproductive hormone levels predict changes in frailty status in community-dwelling older men: European male ageing study prospective data. *J Clin Endocrinol Metab.* 2018;103(2):701–709. https://doi.org/10.1210/jc.2017-01172.
124. Dalton JT, Barnette KG, Bohl CE, et al. The selective androgen receptor modulator GTx-024 (enobosarm) improves lean body mass and physical function in healthy elderly men and postmenopausal women: results of a double-blind, placebo-controlled phase II trial. *J Cachexia Sarcopenia Muscle.* 2011;2(3):153–161. https://doi.org/10.1007/s13539-011-0034-6.
125. Lee P-H, Lee Y-S, Chan D-C. Interventions targeting geriatric frailty: a systemic review. *J Clin Gerontol Geriatr.* 2012;3(2):47–52. https://doi.org/10.1016/J.JCGG.2012.04.001.
126. Brady TJ, Murphy L, O'Colmain BJ, et al. A meta-analysis of health status, health behaviors, and health care utilization outcomes of the chronic disease self-management program. *Prev Chronic Dis.* 2013;10:120112. https://doi.org/10.5888/pcd10.120112.
127. Franek J. Self-management support interventions for persons with chronic disease: an evidence-based analysis. *Ont Health Technol Assess Ser.* 2013;13(9):1–60. http://www.ncbi.nlm.nih.gov/pubmed/24194800. Accessed October 20, 2018.
128. Cramm JM, Twisk J, Nieboer AP. Self-management abilities and frailty are important for healthy aging among community-dwelling older people; a cross-sectional study. *BMC Geriatr.* 2014;14(1):28. https://doi.org/10.1186/1471-2318-14-28.
129. Jonker AAGC, Comijs HC, Knipscheer KCPM, Deeg DJH. Benefits for elders with vulnerable health from the Chronic Disease Self-MANAGEMENT PROGRAM (CDSMP) at short and longer term. *BMC Geriatr.* 2015;15:101. https://doi.org/10.1186/s12877-015-0090-4.
130. Spoorenberg SLW, Wynia K, Uittenbroek RJ, Kremer HPH, Reijneveld SA. Effects of a population-based, person-centred and integrated care service on health, wellbeing and self-management of community-living older adults: a randomised controlled trial on Embrace (Evans CJ, ed.). *PLoS One.* 2018;13(1):e0190751. https://doi.org/10.1371/journal.pone.0190751
131. Chan D-CD, Tsou H-H, Yang R-S, et al. A pilot randomized controlled trial to improve geriatric frailty. *BMC Geriatr.* 2012;12(1):58. https://doi.org/10.1186/1471-2318-12-58.
132. Apóstolo J, Cooke R, Bobrowicz-Campos E, et al. Effectiveness of interventions to prevent pre-frailty and frailty progression in older adults. *JBI Database Syst Rev Implement Reports.* 2018;16(1):140–232. https://doi.org/10.11124/JBISRIR-2017-003382.
133. Bland MD, Birkenmeier RL, Barco P, Lenard E, Lang CE, Lenze EJ. Enhanced medical rehabilitation: effectiveness of a clinical training model (Danzl M, Etter N, eds.). *Neuro*

Rehabilitation. 2016;39(4):481–498. https://doi.org/10.3233/NRE-161380.

134. Lenze EJ, Host HH, Hildebrand MW, et al. Enhanced medical rehabilitation increases therapy intensity and engagement and improves functional outcomes in postacute rehabilitation of older adults: a randomized-controlled trial. *J Am Med Dir Assoc*. 2012;13(8):708–712. https://doi.org/10.1016/j.jamda.2012.06.014.
135. Frieswijk N, Steverink N, Buunk BP, Slaets JPJ. The effectiveness of a bibliotherapy in increasing the self-management ability of slightly to moderately frail older people. *Patient Educ Couns*. 2006;61(2):219–227. https://doi.org/10.1016/J.PEC.2005.03.011.
136. Schoberer D, Leino-Kilpi H, Breimaier HE, Halfens RJ, Lohrmann C. Educational interventions to empower nursing home residents: a systematic literature review. *Clin Interv Aging*. 2016;11:1351–1363. https://doi.org/10.2147/CIA.S114068.
137. Sherrington C, Fairhall N, Kirkham C, et al. Exercise and fall prevention self-management to reduce mobility-related disability and falls after fall-related lower limb fracture in older people: protocol for the RESTORE (Recovery Exercises and STepping On afteR fracturE) randomised controlled trial. *BMC Geriatr*. 2016;16(1):34. https://doi.org/10.1186/s12877-016-0206-5.
138. Clemson L, Cumming RG, Kendig H, Swann M, Heard R, Taylor K. The effectiveness of a community-based program for reducing the incidence of falls in the elderly: a randomized trial. *J Am Geriatr Soc*. 2004;52(9):1487–1494. http://www.blackwell-synergy.com/links/doi/10.1111/j.1532-5415.2004.52411.x/abs.
139. Fried LP. Geriatrics Care | Geriatric Resources | Online events | Updates - Geriatrics Care Online. American Geriatrics Society. https://geriatricscareonline.org/FullText/B023/B023_VOL001_PART001_SEC004_CH023. Accessed June 19, 2018.
140. Young J. *Physio 14: Catch frailty early, before it leads to a crisis. Chartered Society of Physiotherapy*. http://www.csp.org.uk/news/2014/10/14/physio-14-catch-frailty-early-it-leads-crisis. Published 2014. Accessed July 10, 2018.
141. Yang Y. Is old age depressing? Growth trajectories and cohort variations in late-life depression. *J Health Soc Behav*. 2007;48(1):16–32. https://doi.org/10.1177/002214650704800102.
142. Rogers NT, Marshall A, Roberts CH, Demakakos P, Steptoe A, Scholes S. Physical activity and trajectories of frailty among older adults: evidence from the English Longitudinal Study of Ageing (Ginsberg SD, ed.). *PLoS One*. 2017;12(2):e0170878. https://doi.org/10.1371/journal.pone.0170878.
143. da Silva V, Tribess S, Meneguci J, et al. Time spent in sedentary behaviour as discriminant criterion for frailty in older adults. *Int J Environ Res Public Health*. 2018;15(7):1336. https://doi.org/10.3390/ijerph15071336.
144. Kehler DS. The impact of sedentary and physical activity behaviour on frailty in middle-aged and older adults. *Appl Physiol Nutr Metab*. 2018;43(6):638. https://doi.org/10.1139/apnm-2018-0092.
145. Blodgett J, Theou O, Kirkland S, Andreou P, Rockwood K. Frailty in relation to sedentary behaviours and moderate-vigorous intensity physical activity. *Rev Clin Gerontol*. 2014;24(4):239–254. https://doi.org/10.1017/S0959259814000124.
146. Overbeek A, Rietjens JAC, Jabbarian LJ, et al. Low patient activation levels in frail older adults: a cross-sectional study. *BMC Geriatr*. 2018;18(1):7. https://doi.org/10.1186/s12877-017-0696-9.
147. Puts MTE, Toubasi S, Andrew MK, et al. Interventions to prevent or reduce the level of frailty in community-dwelling older adults: a scoping review of the literature and international policies. *Age Ageing*. 2017;46(3):383–392. https://doi.org/10.1093/ageing/afw247.
148. Fieo RA, Mortensen EL, Rantanen T, Avlund K. Improving a measure of mobility-related fatigue (the mobility-tiredness scale) by establishing item intensity. *J Am Geriatr Soc*. 2013;61(3):429–433. https://doi.org/10.1111/jgs.12122.
149. Gardiner PA, Mishra GD, Dobson AJ. Validity and responsiveness of the FRAIL Scale in a longitudinal cohort study of older Australian women. *J Am Med Dir Assoc*. 2015;16(9):781–783. https://doi.org/10.1016/j.jamda.2015.05.005.
150. Morley JE, Malmstrom TK, Miller DK. A simple frailty questionnaire (FRAIL) predicts outcomes in middle aged African Americans. *J Nutr Health Aging*. 2012;16(7):601–608. http://www.ncbi.nlm.nih.gov/pubmed/22836700. Accessed June 19, 2018.
151. Reuben DB, Siu AL. An objective measure of physical function of elderly outpatients. The physical performance test. *J Am Geriatr Soc*. 1990;38(10):1105–1112.
152. Brown M, Sinacore DR, Binder EF, Kohrt WM. Physical and performance measures for the identification of mild to moderate frailty. *J Gerontol Med Sci*. 2000;55A(6):M350–M355.

CHAPTER

14

Management of the Acutely Ill and Medically Complex Older Patient

Chris L. Wells, Martha Townsend

OUTLINE

INTRODUCTION

The population of older adults is the fastest-growing age group within the United States and represents a substantial segment of health care expenditures. Physical inactivity and a sedentary lifestyle are major contributors to disease and disability in this population subgroup.[1] In 2017, there were 47.8 million people aged 65 and older, according to the U.S. Census Bureau, accounting for nearly 15% of the population.[2] This becomes more alarming when almost 20% of those between 65 and 75 years of age and 28% over 75 years report fair to poor health, which places an enormous burden on society.[3] Forty percent of hospital admissions today are for people over 60 years of age, with only 30% recovering to their preadmission functional status within 1 year.[4] The most common admitting diagnoses are still related to cardiovascular disease including heart failure, myocardial infarction, and dysrhythmias as well as pneumonia and sepsis.[5]

When considering working with this population, the physical therapist must recognize the need to address a complex medical history and be aware of the interplay between each body system. Psychological and mood states as well as cognitive and social factors can also influence the presentation of the patient and the outcome of therapy. It is important to examine each to identify the complexity of the problem, determine a proper diagnosis and prognosis, and develop a comprehensive plan of care that incorporates an understanding of the impact of medical comorbidity on function. The plan of care will be based on a thorough evaluation and may address multiple impairments and medical deficits to improve the patient's functional mobility, health and well-being, and, ultimately, quality of life.

There are many reasons that have led to the need for the physical therapist to acquire the necessary skills to recognize, examine, and determine the proper plan of care when working within the health care system today (Box 14.1). As a result of advances in medical management, people are living longer. As our population ages, mortality rates and medical complexity also increase substantially. A study conducted by the National Institute of Aging on postmenopausal women diagnosed with breast cancer is a good example of the increasing number of comorbidities. Of the 1800 women involved in this study, only 7% did not have any other documented disease. Forty-nine

BOX 14.1 The Impact of Comorbidity

It is commonplace for clinicians to focus their attention on the primary diagnosis or obvious impairments and functional limitations. Many clinicians fail to consider the other systems of the body, how they interact and affect the primary complaint and thus affect the rehabilitation outcome. Even with a healthy, aging individual, the multiple systems of the body are declining in function. This decline may not be substantial enough to cause an overt dysfunction or failure until another stressor is added.

Consider the following case: Suppose an 88-year-old healthy, very physically active woman undergoes an aortic valve replacement. The operation goes well except the patient experiences a slight decline in contractility of the myocardium in the first 24 hours postoperation. The physical therapist may tend to only be concerned with the heart when performing the examination initially after surgery.

However, her decrease in cardiac output leads to hypotension. The consequences of hypotension are a decrease in perfusion to the brain and kidneys. The patient's body cannot tolerate this deviation from homeostasis and the result is a clinically significant decline in mental status and acute renal failure. Along with the fluid retention from the renal failure and cardiac impairment, the patient becomes delirious and is sedated.

These complications prolong the time her respiratory system is supported by a mechanical ventilator. She experiences a ventilator-acquired pneumonia and a partial bowel obstruction due to immobility. The stress and trauma contribute to temporary insulin glucose dysfunction, which in turn delays wound healing. Weakness and multiple joint pains develop that further complicate the ability to mobilize this patient and successfully wean her from the ventilator. The end result of this cascade of events after weeks in the intensive care unit is that the patient undergoes a tracheotomy and percutaneous endoscopic jejunostomy and will be discharged to a subacute skilled nursing facility for ventilator weaning and rehabilitation.

percent had 1 to 3 comorbidities, 34% had 4 to 6 comorbidities, and 9% had 7 to 13 comorbidities at the time of the cancer diagnosis.[6] In a more recent study that examined the comorbidities of patients with arthritis from 2013 to 2015, it was reported that the older adult has a prevalence of 31%, 47%, and 49% for obesity, diabetes, and cardiac disease, respectively.[7]

Regardless of the clinical setting, it is vital that the physical therapist recognize signs and symptoms that do not fit within the authorized scope of practice and identify "yellow flags" and "red flags" to make appropriate referrals with the ultimate goal to improve the well-being and health of the client. The purpose of this chapter is to summarize the knowledge and skills a physical therapist needs to demonstrate to complete a thorough screening to provide proper care for the older adult patient in an acute care setting, work effectively with an older individual in an acute phase of illness in other settings such as the outpatient primary care clinic, and respond appropriately to the individual with medical comorbidities in any setting. The goals of the examination and evaluation are to develop a proper plan of care, make appropriate discharge recommendations, and facilitate discharge planning. This is done by completing a thorough examination of the patient, putting primary and secondary diagnoses in proper perspective for the impact on function, establishing a prognosis, and formulating a comprehensive intervention plan. This process begins with gathering information in a thorough and systematic fashion from medical and health records and through communication with other health care members and caregivers as well as a comprehensive interview of the patient. Implementation of the plan of care will depend on the particular setting and the time frame for implementing the proposed plan of care and discharge recommendations if the patient will be going to another facility or type of residence.

REVIEW OF SYSTEMS

The information-gathering process, also referred to as a *review of systems*, is typically initiated when the physical therapist receives a prescription or request for consultation or a patient enters the physical therapist's office, and can extend to the patient or family interview. The review of systems is a method of systematically screening the major organ systems to determine if the patient has certain symptoms that may make intervention inappropriate, lead the therapist to make a medical referral for further testing, or provide specific interventions or education. In the acute care setting, this process is shared by the medical team, of which the physical therapist is an integral part as the physical therapist's recommendations may add to this review to improve medical care and outcomes. For the outpatient or home care therapist the review of systems becomes a more critical process because the practice is more autonomous and the therapist has less access to the medical team. The reader is referred to Table 14.1 for an example of a review of systems form that shows what can be included in the medical review and places where the physical therapist may contribute to the screening process based on the facility's practice, particular medical services, and type of clientele. Asking about the relative duration of symptoms or condition may help prioritize the systems review. The case described in Box 14.2 illustrates the implications of completing a thorough review of systems.

This request for a physical therapist's evaluation may be very generic or may include pertinent information about the reason for the consult and indicate any restrictions or precautions. If the consult is generic, the therapist should determine if there are any restrictions, or contraindications to care, such as out-of-bed status or weight-bearing precautions. There is typically a differential diagnosis list and a working medical diagnosis that can help to guide the physical therapist to develop a therapy-specific differential list that can help prioritize the examination. The presenting signs and symptoms associated with a chronic disease such as heart failure and obstructive lung disease may be helpful for the physical therapist to document and understand. This information may lead the physical therapist to educate the patient on proper self-monitoring with the goal that the patient will seek medical assistance prior to the need for admission to the emergency department. Typically, there

TABLE 14.1 Review of Systems: Key Items to Obtain and Consider

Item	Relevance
Admitting complaint	Can the symptoms be used to measure activity intolerance or effectiveness of intervention?
Primary diagnosis	How does severity and medical responsiveness affect physical therapist's intervention, discharge planning, patient–family education, and services to prevent readmission?
Secondary diagnosis	How does severity and medical responsiveness complicate the physical therapy plan of care?
Past medical history	How do RELEVANT comorbidities affect the physical therapy plan of care, discharge, and services to prevent readmissions?
Medical/surgical plan	How do these plans affect the physical therapy plan to restore function and prepare for discharge?
Risk of iatrogenic effects	What are the physical therapist's interventions that contribute to reducing the adverse effects of hospitalization and critical illness?
Medications	What medications impact hemodynamic stability and effective activity tolerance?
Psychosocial	What resources does the patient have to assist with discharge planning? What barriers are impeding discharge?

BOX 14.2 The Implications of Review of Systems

Consider a patient with coronary artery disease (CAD). It is very common for patients to self-limit themselves to avoid symptoms, so their answers to questions such as "Are you presently experiencing chest discomfort with exertion or excessive fatigue after exertion?" may be negative, but follow that up to include "Over the past year have you noticed a decrease in the activities that you are willing to do, such as going on community outings, vacuuming, etc., or an increase in the time it takes for you to complete regular daily activities?"

Case: A 72-year-old man presents with excessive fatigue, clumsiness, and a recent fall. On the review of systems, the patient reports an increase in fatigue, inability to mow his lawn without taking rest breaks, and a decreased frequency in urination. He reports being treated for hypertension and has been experiencing this clumsiness for about 2 months. Fatigue is such a nondescript symptom and can be caused by multiple pathologies. The physical therapist puts forth other questions to determine if the fatigue is related to pathologies such as cardiac or renal disease, diabetes, or cancer. The patient revealed that he has been limiting his activity level to avoid shortness of breath with exertion. He reported tightness in the waist of his pants and that he is more comfortable sleeping in his recliner chair. With this information, the therapist knew to complete a thorough examination of the cardiovascular system, including heart and lung sounds, inspection for pitted edema, and jugular vein distention. With the findings of these tests, the therapist discussed with the medical team concerns for uncompensated heart failure.

These types of time-based questions are important to ask when screening for cardiovascular, metabolic, and oncologic conditions. The review of systems should lead the therapist to formulate and prioritize the examination to eventually determine a plan of care that may include recommendations for further medical evaluation and interventions.

is a comprehensive list of medical diagnoses and/or conditions that reflect the known past history of the patient. Caution should be used when taking this list literally as the diagnoses and conditions may have resolved and/or be no longer active. When documenting the diagnoses in the physical therapy record, only those that are relevant to the episode of care need to be listed to assist with clarity. To follow we describe some key areas of the review-of-system process that should be included in preparation of the examination of the patient.

Admission or Reason for Visit

Patients with acute conditions are not always in a hospital setting. Increasingly, physical therapists are part of primary care teams in the outpatient setting or providing acute care services in the patient's own home or other residential setting. If a medical or health record is available prior to the initial clinical encounter, the admission or intake section of the record may contain several important documents that can be reviewed prior to the physical therapist's initial examination. These documents may include the method of admission, information from any emergency medical service field treatment, emergency room evaluations and initial testing procedures, the referring physician's evaluation for planned admissions to an inpatient setting, or the patient's reason for the primary care or outpatient visit. An emergency department report typically concludes with a working differential diagnosis list and a medical problem list. The primary history and physical (H&P) that is usually completed by the admitting service may also be found among these documents. It is extremely helpful to review this data source to the degree it is available because it commonly contains the admitting diagnosis and summary of what led up to the admission, the patient's chief complaint, and past medical/surgical history. The H&P also typically contains family history, social history, risk factors, a medication list, allergies, medical summary, and plan of care. The working medical problem list for an older adult may be extensive owing to multiple comorbidities, and therefore, it is important to review all available information to fully understand the patient's medical status to prepare the appropriate physical therapy evaluation. The therapist needs to prioritize the list of medical issues and comorbidities in a manner that reflects the largest impact on functional recovery for discharge. Prioritizing this list should guide the physical therapist's evaluation and intervention and aid in making recommendations that go beyond the care being provided during this current encounter. Table 14.1 provides a list of suggested key items that a physical therapist should glean from the review of systems to proceed safely to the examination phase. These key items may change based on the patient population.

The therapist should review the medical or health record not only to glean information pertaining to physical therapy but also to understand what other services have been or should be consulted, what diagnostic tests have been requested, and what medications or other treatments have been prescribed. All services typically enter a contact note that describes their contribution to the patient's care. It is important to keep up to date as to who has been treating the patient, any changes in medical status, operative notes, tests that may have been done, and updates on the medical plan. The physical therapist needs to ensure that the physical therapy plan of care is consistent with the medical plan, which can be very complex when the patient has multiple comorbidities. There may also be reports from other health professionals, social workers, psychologists, and case managers that may be important to assist the therapist during formulation of a plan of care or discharge recommendations.

Laboratory Values

The analysis of blood work is critical to fully appreciate the medical status of the patient. Serum enzymes can be examined to determine cellular damage including myocardial injury and infarct. Blood lipids can determine the patient's risks for vascular disease, and the coagulation profile reveals the body's ability to clot. The complete blood count (CBC) examines such factors as hemoglobin (cells that contain iron used for oxygen transport), hematocrit (the proportion of blood that is red blood cells [RBCs]), RBCs, white blood cells (WBCs), and platelet counts. The body's ability to regulate the cellular pH through respiratory and renal function can be determined by examining the arterial blood gases (ABGs). Finally, electrolyte levels can be examined through blood analysis. See Table 14.2 for clinical laboratory studies.[8–13]

Complete Blood Count. The CBC is one of the most common laboratory studies performed and can be used to aid in the formulation of a diagnosis, to assess medical treatment response, and to monitor recovery. The physical therapist can obtain a wealth of information from examining the CBC and should check routinely to make sure the patient is medically stable. A decline in activity tolerance or mental alertness may be related to a decrease in hemoglobin or an infection with a variable change in WBCs.

The CBC contains the analysis of WBCs with respect to both total number and differentiation of cells that will provide the therapist with information about the body's response to an infectious disease. An elevation in total WBCs, which is referred to as leukocytosis, may be due to a bacterial infection, with urinary tract and pulmonary infections leading the incidence of infections in older adults. This is significant, because with age, the chance of these infections progressing to bacteremia increases, as does mortality.[14] Leukocytosis can also be evidence of leukemia or stress related to trauma and inflammation. Leukopenia, or low WBC levels, may be caused by bone marrow depression, acute viral infections, or alcohol abuse. Differentiation of WBCs can further determine the underlying problem: Neutrophils will be elevated in the presence of bacterial or fungal infections, eosinophils are elevated in allergic responses, and lymphocytes are elevated in viral infections. With altered WBCs, the therapist needs to monitor vital signs to ensure an infection has not caused tachycardia or hypotension, which may lead the therapist to change or hold the session.

The second group within the CBC is RBC count and differentiation. The count examines the number of actual RBCs. This information is valuable because the RBCs reflect the oxygen-carrying capacity of the blood that supports cellular activity. If the RBC count is too high, known as polycythemia vera, there is a significant risk of blood clot formation and a subsequent loss of perfusion to tissues. If the RBC count is too low, also known as anemia, then there are insufficient RBCs to adequately supply tissue with oxygen, particularly in the presence of cardiac or pulmonary dysfunction, which can lead to tachycardia, desaturation, and angina.

Part of the RBC study is the quantification of hemoglobin and hematocrit. Hemoglobin is the oxygen-carrying component of the RBC and reflects the ability of the body to sufficiently promote gas exchange to regulate pH. Hematocrit is the measure of the number of RBCs within the blood compared to the total volume of blood and is represented as a percentage. These two numbers are very important to monitor when working with patients in general but especially when working with the older patient. The incidence of anemia is high within the older adult population, with the leading causes being from a nutritional deficiency (including gastrointestinal bleeding), anemia of chronic disease, and anemia from an unexplained cause. Anemia can be the underlying cause and a contributing factor to fatigue, disability, change in cognitive function, and limited activity intolerance. Patients with anemia in the presence of coronary artery disease (CAD) may experience angina, particularly with exertion, and if the coronary disease is extensive, the anemia may lead to heart failure (HF).[15] The therapist needs to understand the patient's clinical presentation of myocardial ischemia such as the patient describing exertion chest tightness, difficulty swallowing, and dyspnea. The therapist should also be monitoring for signs and symptoms like activity intolerance, peripheral edema, progressive dyspnea, and increasing use of pillows to sleep, all of which would suggest heart failure.

Ten percent of people older than age 65 years suffer from anemia, increasing to 20% in those 85 years and older.[16] Anemia is defined by the World Health Organization as a hemoglobin concentration of <120 g/L in women and <130 g/L in men.[17] However, gastrointestinal bleeding is not the only cause of anemia and it is important to determine the actual cause to ensure proper medical treatment. Other causes of anemia, for example, iron, folate, and vitamin B_{12} deficiencies; renal insufficiency;

TABLE 14.2 Clinical Laboratory Studies[8–13]

	Chemistry	
	Reference	**Function**
Sodium (Na)	136–144 mmol/L	Regulates water balance, regulates acid–base balance, membrane integrity, nerve impulse
Potassium (K)	3.7–5.2 mmol/L	Intracellular fluid osmolality, maintenance of resting membrane potential, glucose deposition in liver and skeletal muscles
Chloride (Cl)	96–106 mmol/L	Resting membrane potential, osmotic pressure regulation, extracellular enzymatic reactions
Carbon dioxide (CO_2)	20–29 mmol/dL	Acid–base balance
Anion gap	8–14 mEq/L	Measurement of the acid–base balance
Blood urea nitrogen (BUN)	7–20 mg/dL	Byproduct of protein breakdown, reflection of kidney function: glomerular filtration and urine concentration capacity
Creatinine (Cr)	0.8–1.4 mg/dL	Waste product of body's protein metabolism, reflects long-term glomerular function
BUN/creatinine	10:1–20:1	BUN/Cr ratio >18–20 indication of dehydration
Glomerular filtration rate	60–89 mL/min/ 1.72 m^2	Estimate of how much blood passes through the kidneys in 1 minute
Glucose	70–99 mg/dL	Reflects carbohydrate metabolism
Calcium (Ca)	9–10.5 mg/dL	Bone and teeth health, enzymatic cofactor for blood clotting, plasma membrane stability and permeability
Ionized calcium	1.15–1.29 mmol/L	Free-flowing calcium that is not attached to protein
Magnesium (Mg)	1.8–2.6 mg/dL	Intracellular enzymatic reactions, protein synthesis, neuromuscular excitability
Phosphate (Ph)	2.3–3.7 mg/dL	Intra- and extracellular anion buffer, energy substrate
Total protein	6.3–7.9 g/dL	Rough measurement of albumin and globulin proteins
Albumin	3.9–5 g/dL	Protein synthesized by liver, protein found in blood
Prealbumin	20–90 mg/dL	Protein synthesized by liver that is source for amino acids for other protein production. Short-term measure of nutritional status
Bilirubin total	0.3–1.9 mg/dL	Yellowish pigment from heme (red blood cell) metabolism found in liver bile, test of liver/gallbladder function
Bilirubin (direct)	0–0.3 mg/dL	Is bilirubin attached to another molecule before being released in bile?
Aspartate transaminase (serum glutamine-oxaloacetic transaminase)	10–34 units/L	Enzyme from liver or muscle cells released upon injury
Alanine transaminase (serum glutamic pyruvic transaminase)	8–37 units/L	Enzyme from liver or muscle cells released upon injury
Cortisol	7–9 A.M.: 4.2–38.4 μg/dL 4–6 P.M.: 1.7–16.6 μg/dL	Hormone produced by adrenal cortex that increases blood glucose and liver stores of glycogen in response to stress
Lipase	10–150 units/L	Enzyme that metabolizes dietary lipids
Amylase	27–131 units/L	Enzyme that metabolizes dietary carbohydrates
Lactate dehydrogenase	100–190 units/L	Five enzymes in various organs that are responsible for conversion of pyruvate and lactate. Specific enzyme markers can identify type of cellular damage
Complete Blood Count		
	Reference	**Function**
White blood cell (WBC) count	4.5–11.0 K/μL	Leukocytes, cells of the immune system
Red blood cell (RBC) count	4.0–5.7 K/μL	Erythrocytes, cells that have gas-carrying capacity
Hemoglobin (Hgb)	12.6–17.4 g/dL	O_2/CO_2-carrying capacity protein of the RBC
Hematocrit	37%–50%	Percentage of a given volume of blood that is occupied with erythrocytes
Mean corpuscular volume	80–96 fL	Average RBC volume
Mean corpuscular hemoglobin concentration	32–36 g/dL	Average concentration of Hgb in the RBC
Platelet	153–367 K/μL	Small cell that contributes to clotting

Continued

TABLE 14.2 Clinical Laboratory Studies[8–13]—cont'd

		Chemistry
	Reference	Function
Blood Gases		
	Reference	
Arterial		
pH	7.35–7.45	
$PaCO_2$	32–48 mmHg	
PaO_2	83–100 mmHg	
Bicarbonate (HCO_3^-)	22–26 mEq/L	
Oxygen saturation	94%–99%	
Venous		
pH	7.32–7.44	
$PvCO_2$	38–54 mmHg	
PvO_2	35–45 mmHg	
HCO_3^-	22–26 mEq/L	
Oxygen saturation	60%–80%	
Urinalysis		
	Function	
Urine specific gravity	1.002–1.030	
pH	4.5–8.0	
WBC	0–5/hpf	
RBC	0–2/hpf	
Urine is also examined for presence of color, blood, protein, ketones, glucose, and nitrates		
Coagulation		
	Reference	
Prothrombin time	12.8–14.6 s	
Partial thromboplastin time	25–38 s	
International normalized ratio	0.8–1.2	
Blood Lipid Profile		
	Reference	
Total cholesterol	<200 mg/dL	
High-density lipoproteins	M: >43 mg/dL F: >33 mg/dL	
Low-density lipoproteins	<100 mg/dL	
Triglycerides	<140 mg/dL	

anemia of chronic inflammation; and unexplained anemia, can be further worked up by analyzing the differentiation of RBCs or indices.[16] This set of tests looks at the size of the average RBC, otherwise known as the mean corpuscular volume (MCV). The mean corpuscular hemoglobin (MCH) and mean corpuscular hemoglobin concentration (MCHC) examine the amount and concentration of hemoglobin in an average RBC, respectively. These tests can aid in the diagnosis of what type of anemia the patient has and, therefore, allow the medical team to prescribe the best intervention.

Platelets, which are small cells that aid in clotting and the release of growth factors, are also measured when a CBC is ordered. When the endothelium is damaged, collagen is released into the bloodstream. When the platelets come in contact with the collagen, the platelets are then activated to form a clot to repair the injured area. Platelets also release platelet-derived growth factors and tissue growth factor-β, which contribute to cellular repair and regeneration. A reduction in platelets, otherwise known as thrombocytopenia, can be caused by chemotherapy, a large blood transfusion, or implantation of mechanical heart valves among many other reasons. Also, heparin-induced thrombocytopenia can result from the use of heparin postsurgically or with deep vein thrombosis (DVT) prophylaxis. Thrombocytosis, elevation of platelet count, is less common but is associated with iron-deficient or hemolytic anemia, cancer, or inflammatory or infectious processes such as inflammatory bowel disease and tuberculosis.

Electrolytes. The study of electrolytes, specifically sodium, potassium, chloride, carbon dioxide, creatinine, blood urea nitrogen (BUN), calcium, and magnesium, reveal the state of the cellular function. Sodium and potassium are key to maintaining cellular membrane potential, and carbon dioxide is used to assist in the analysis of the body's acid–base balance. Chloride level is used for further analysis of acid–base balance through the calculation of the anion gap. Creatinine and BUN reflect renal function and the efficiency of glomerular function. BUN is commonly elevated in the presence of heart or renal failure, and low levels of BUN are associated with starvation, dehydration, and liver failure. Electrolyte analysis is very important because the risk of death from chronic kidney disease increases with age, especially in patients with concurrent cardiovascular disease.[18]

Calcium levels can also be analyzed to identify parathyroid dysfunction, malnutrition, and chronic renal disease. Abnormalities in calcium level are related to hyperparathyroidism; malignancy such as metastatic breast, lung, or renal cancer; and immobility. Magnesium contributes to various cellular activities such as muscle and nerve function, assisting in the maintenance of normal cardiac rhythm, bone strength, and health status of the immune system. Abnormally low magnesium levels, or hypomagnesemia, can be related to alcoholism, chronic diarrhea, hemodialysis, and cirrhosis. Renal failure, adrenal disease, and dehydration can cause hypermagnesemia (elevated magnesium levels).

Electrolyte abnormalities are common, and corrections for a toxic or deficient state are important to restore normal cellular function. See Table 14.3 for causes and signs and symptoms of electrolyte abnormalities.[8–10] In older adults, conditions of malnutrition, dehydration, adverse effects of medications, decline in organ function, and increased risk of infections and cancers increase their risk for electrolyte imbalances. Sodium levels may be in constant variability in the presence of heart failure. Hypernatremia is associated with cardiac decompensation and the patient may present with confusion, muscle dysfunction, and decreased activity tolerance. Hyponatremia is commonly associated with diuretics and the patient can present with similar clinical findings. A study by Oliveira et al. reported that 29.1% of the 240 hospitalized older adult patients they studied were considered malnourished. Of those, 13.7% had hypertension, 15.7% had diabetes, 12.8% had some form of cancer, and 15.7% had the sequelae of stroke.[19]

Serum Enzymes and Markers. Serum enzymes and markers are used to assist in the diagnosis of diseases such as cancer or medical events like myocardial infarction, congestive heart failure, or liver dysfunction. Serum enzymes can also show muscle tissue breakdown in the event of trauma or rhabdomyolysis, as noted by an elevation of creatinine kinase (CK) levels. The therapist can review these lab values to obtain an appreciation of the extent of tissue involvement or dysfunction as well as the phase of the event. For example, the evolution of a myocardial infarction can be identified by monitoring the enzymes and marker values and whether these numbers are trending up or down based on serial analysis. Progressive functional training and strengthening should not be resumed until the CK levels start decreasing and cellular pH is within normal range. Cardiac enzyme studies are used to make the diagnosis of myocardial injury or myocardial infarction. There are several specific cardiac enzyme studies that can be analyzed: creatinine phosphokinase–MB isoenzymes, lactic dehydrogenase, troponin, and myoglobin. These enzymes are released at variable rates, so serial studies are needed to determine the peak level, extent of cellular injury and necrosis, and recovery rate. See Table 14.4 for cardiac enzymes and diagnosis for myocardial cellular injury.[10]

Coagulation Profile. The coagulation profile of the patient will indicate the ability of the patient's blood to clot, particularly important for the individual receiving anticoagulation therapy as a treatment for conditions such as atrial fibrillation, mechanical heart valves or devices, DVT, pulmonary embolism (PE), or trauma. Anticoagulation levels that are considered therapeutic will vary depending on reason for coagulation, previous medical history, physician preferences, and institutional policies. The therapist needs to know the therapeutic level, medical goal, and any functional mobility precautions or restrictions. An increased risk of thrombus formation also increases risk for stroke, pulmonary emboli, and other embolic activity. Patients whose coagulation levels are too high are at risk for bleeding, so the therapist should monitor these patients for edema, ecchymosis, limitations in limb range of position, pain, and neurologic changes in the case of a cerebral bleed when there is a drop in hematocrit >3% to 5% and hemoglobin is <7.0. Patients on anticoagulation therapy in the presence of infection or other causes of physiological stress may develop a coagulopathy and be at risk for bleeding.

When a patient has been recently diagnosed with a DVT or PE, it is important for the physical therapist to consult with the medical team regarding the plan of care. The medical plan typically includes the administration of some anticoagulation medication. Today it is common for mobilization to continue after the initiation of the medication and not wait until the medication has reached its therapeutic level. Mobility has been shown not to increase the risk of a PE. It is important for the therapist to have this conversation with the medical team because if the DVT is proximal in the femoral or iliac veins or appears unstable upon Doppler study, the patient may need to be placed on bed rest or restricted activities until a certain therapeutic range has been reached or a certain number of days has passed. The physical therapist should monitor any patient who is on anticoagulation therapy by monitoring the prothrombin, partial prothrombin, or international normalized ratio (INR) anticoagulation level to ensure therapeutic range and modify the therapy session if the patient is hyper-anticoagulated and thus at high risk of bleeding.[20]

TABLE 14.3 Causes and Clinical Signs and Symptoms of Electrolyte Abnormalities[8–10]

Electrolyte	Causes	Clinical Symptoms
Calcium	Increased: Hyperparathyroidism, large consumption of calcium and vitamin D, cancer, immobilization, Paget disease	Asymptomatic, constipation, nausea, vomiting, abdominal pain, loss of appetite, thirst, and dehydration
	Decreased: Hypoparathyroidism; osteomalacia; decreased intake of dairy products; decreased vitamin D intake	Nonspecific central nervous system signs (e.g., mild diffuse brain disease mimicking depression, dementia, or psychosis), tetany or latent neuromuscular irritability; cardiac arrhythmias and heart block; osteoporosis; hypertension
Magnesium	Increased: Mg consumption in presence of renal failure, antacids, or laxative overdose	Weakness, low blood pressure, respiratory distress, asystole
	Decreased: Dietary depletion; renal loss; gastrointestinal (GI) disorders, including vomiting, diarrhea, and malabsorption syndrome; alcoholism; primary defect in renal tubular reabsorption; GI disorders that impair absorption, such as Crohn disease	Nonspecific, neuromuscular irritability and muscle weakness; arrhythmias; increased sensitivity to cardiac glycosides; hypertension; atherosclerosis; loss of appetite; nausea; vomiting; numbness; tingling; muscle contractions and cramps; seizures (sudden changes in behavior caused by excessive electrical activity in the brain); personality changes; abnormal heart rhythms; coronary spasms
Potassium	Increased: Renal failure, use of potassium-sparing diuretics, acidosis, cell damage, dehydration, uncontrolled diabetes, Addison disease, syndrome of inappropriate antidiuretic hormone (SIADH), pneumonia, sepsis, shock, potassium supplements in presence of renal failure	Asymptomatic, bradyarrhythmias
	Decreased: Decreased intake of potassium during acute illness, nausea, and vomiting; increased renal loss; hypomagnesemia; hematologic disorders; certain antibiotics or diuretics; diarrhea (including the use of too many laxatives, which can cause diarrhea); diseases that affect the kidney's ability to retain potassium (e.g., Liddle syndrome, Cushing syndrome, hyperaldosteronism, Bartter syndrome, Fanconi syndrome), eating disorders (such as bulimia); sweating	Fatigue; confusion; muscle weakness and cramps; frank paralysis; breakdown of muscle fibers (rhabdomyolysis); atrial and ventricular ectopic beats; atrial and ventricular tachycardia; ventricular fibrillation; sudden death; atrioventricular conduction disturbances
Phosphorus	Increased: Rare unless in presence of renal dysfunction, hypoparathyroidism; diabetic ketoacidosis, crush injuries, rhabdomyolysis, severe infections, ingestion of large amounts	Asymptomatic, severe arteriosclerosis (angina, poor peripheral perfusion, changes in multiple sclerosis), increased risk of myocardial infarction, stroke and peripheral artery disease, severe itching
	Decreased: Deficiency rare because it is so readily available in the food supply; decreased intake and impaired intestinal absorption of phosphate; vomiting; acidosis; alcoholic ketoacidosis	Anorexia; muscle weakness; osteomalacia; rhabdomyolysis; hemolytic anemia; impaired leukocyte and platelet function; progressive encephalopathy; coma; death
Chloride	Increased: Dehydration, multiple myeloma, kidney dysfunction, metabolic acidosis, hyperparathyroidism, pancreatitis, anemia, prolonged diarrhea, respiratory alkalosis, salicylate toxicity, alcohol abuse, congestive heart failure (CHF)	Rare, changes in mental status, confusion, malaise, bradyarrhythmias, hyperventilation, stupor, muscle twitching, weakness, nausea, vomiting, diarrhea
	Decreased: Fluid loss (e.g., excessive sweating, vomiting, or diarrhea); diuretics	Dehydration; loss of potassium in the urine; alkalosis
Sodium	Increased: Dehydration, hyperaldosteronism, CHF, hepatic failure, severe vomiting/diarrhea, steroid administration, intake or use of high-protein and nutrient-dense products without enough fluid, diabetes insipidus, Cushing disease, glycosuria, hypervolemia	Hypertension, mental status changes, confusion, thirsty, seizures, coma
	Decreased: Use of low-sodium nutritional supplements; vomiting; diarrhea; GI suction; renal disorders; diuretic therapy; burns; CHF; use of diuretics; kidney diseases; liver cirrhosis; sweating	Delirium and confusion; hallucinations; depressed sensorium; depressed deep tendon reflexes; hypothermia; Cheyne-Stokes respiration; pathologic reflexes; convulsions; fatigue; headache; irritability; loss of appetite; muscle spasms or cramps; muscle weakness; nausea and vomiting

TABLE 14.4 Cardiac Enzymes[10]

Enzyme	Normal	Rise	Peak	Return	Abnormal
Creatine phosphokinase (CPK)	5–75 mU/mL	2–8 h	12–36 h	3–4 h	Total ≥200
Lactate dehydrogenase (LDH)	100–225 units/mL	12–48 h	3–6 days	8–14 days	Total ≥170, ≥100 LDH + 40% CPK
CPK-MB	0%–3%	4 h	18–24 h		Total ≥200 with MB ≥4% or total <200 with MB ≥10 units
Troponin	<0.2 μg/mL	4–6 h	24 h	>10 days	>1.5

It is important to look for signs and symptoms of clotting and participate in preventive care for DVT and PE. For DVT, the signs and symptoms may include peripheral edema (typically unilateral), venous distention, and pain; for PE, the patient may present with shortness of breath, abnormal breath sounds, and oxygen desaturation. In those cases where the PE is of a clinically significant size, the patient can suffer from respiratory failure. The use of sequential compression pumps, lower extremity exercises, and increasing the patient's activity level are key for the prevention of DVT and PE development. The American Physical Therapy Association sponsored the development of the clinical practice guide for DVT management with clinical recommendations that the physical therapist should review with the patient's medical team.[20]

Blood Lipids. The examination of the patient's blood lipid profile helps to risk-stratify the patient for cardiovascular disease. Knowing that lipid profile is elevated can be helpful in determining how to focus part of the interview process to complete the risk for cardiovascular disease. This information can guide the therapist to screen the patient for common signs and symptoms associated with cardiovascular disease and determine what tests and measures should be completed to further evaluate the patient for disease and dysfunction.[21] Vital signs should be monitored at rest as well as during exertion to determine if the patient has sufficient exercise tolerance or if further medical evaluation is necessary because of an abnormal vital signs response to exercise. Because cardiovascular disease is a multisystem disease, patients with abnormal blood profiles are at risk for further declines in cerebral function as well as being at risk for cerebral vascular events.[22] Further screening includes the Trails A and B test, counting backward by 7, and the Stroop test.[23] Results may give the therapist further documentation that cerebral function is impaired or has changed from previous admissions. Data on peripheral perfusion testing and skin inspection as well as tolerance to exertion may help to characterize any clinical hypothesis that a functional limitation is related to peripheral arterial disease.[24] Finally, by the therapist appreciating the patient's blood profile along with evaluating for other risk factors, the therapist can determine the patient's risk level for a cardiovascular event and how to safely prescribe an exercise program, initiate patient education on risk reduction and prevention, and make appropriate referrals.[25]

Special Tests. Serum glucose levels examine the body's ability to utilize glucose for cellular activity through the production of adenosine triphosphate (ATP). Hyperglycemia (elevated blood sugar) is generally associated with diabetes mellitus (DM); however, patients without a history of DM could present with elevated glucose levels in the acute care setting that may be related to physiological stress from trauma or surgery, steroid use, or alterations in medications. Hypoglycemia (low blood sugar) is associated with alcoholism, adverse medication reactions, treatment for hyperglycemia, and critical illnesses related to liver or pancreatic disease.

Serum glucose, glycosylated hemoglobin (HbA_{1c}), and routine blood glucose testing are very important for the therapist to examine prior to intervention. If the patient's glucose is elevated, >250 mg/dL, or low, <70 mg/dL, the body does not have the ability to utilize glucose as an energy substrate for exercise. Modifications in therapy will need to be implemented to shorten the duration of functional activities to avoid adverse effects of immobility and further metabolic stress.

Other tests such as serum total protein, including albumin and globulin levels, contribute information about acid–base balance, clotting, immune response, and blood and tissue osmotic pressure. Albumin is very important to maintaining vascular pressure, with low albumin related to significant edema, poor functional outcomes, and high mortality. The prealbumin level reflects current nutritional status and can be helpful in examining the effectiveness of nutritional interventions or to document further progression of the catabolic state.[26] For the acute care therapist, attending to albumin, total protein, and prealbumin levels will reveal the level of protein stores, state of malnutrition, or responsiveness to nutritional intervention. This factor may greatly influence the patient's ability to make gains in therapy and may directly impact functional outcomes.[27,28] The therapist should discuss with the provider when there is poor progression in strength and functional recovery to determine if adjustments need to be made to improve albumin and total protein consumption.

Arterial Blood Gases. The sampling of arterial blood is used to determine the oxygenation state and the acid–base balance, specifically the concentration of hydrogen ions of the body. The pulmonary and renal systems regulate acids, such as carbonic and lactic acids, respectively. The renal system is also the principal regulator of bicarbonate (HCO_3^-), which is the major base of the body.

The partial pressure of oxygen (PaO_2) declines with age. This is the result of the combination of a reduction in the elasticity of the musculoskeletal system, a decrease in muscle fibers, a decrease in the alveolar gas exchange surface area, and a decrease in the responsiveness of the central nervous system. These natural changes lead to a decline in PaO_2, which normally ranges from 80 to 100 mmHg from childhood to middle adulthood, by declining approximately 1 mmHg per year after the age of 60 years or can be calculated by $PaO_2 = 109 - 0.43 \times \text{age}$.[20] It is important to keep this calculation at hand because physical therapists commonly participate in the pulmonary care of patients and supplemental oxygen prescriptions. For a patient who is 75 years old, it would be perfectly normal to have a PaO_2 of 73 to 77 mmHg and show no signs of desaturation or respiratory decompensation.

To examine the acid–base balance, the physical therapist should first look at the pH using 7.4 as the normal level. If the pH is <7.4, the patient is in an acidotic state, and any level >7.4 is considered an alkalotic state. The physical therapist should next examine the partial pressure of carbon dioxide ($PaCO_2$), with 40 mmHg as the reference point, with a value higher or lower being acidotic and alkalotic, respectively. Finally, the therapist also needs to look at the HCO_3^- level, with a value >24 being alkalotic and <24 being acidotic. To determine whether the disorder is respiratory or metabolic, it is as simple as determining if the $PaCO_2$ or the HCO_3^- matches the same state as the pH. If $PaCO_2$ is consistent with the pH, meaning if both $PaCO_2$ and pH are acidotic or alkalotic, then the patient is suffering from a *respiratory* acidotic or alkalotic state. However, if HCO_3^- matches the pH, then there is a *metabolic* acidosis or alkalosis. See Table 14.5 for causes and signs and symptoms of acid–base disorders.[8–10] See Table 14.6 for an example of respiratory acidosis and Table 14.7 for an example of metabolic alkalosis.

Arterial blood gases further quantify the body's response to acid–base imbalance. The renal and pulmonary systems compensate for these imbalances by altering $PaCO_2$ (lungs) for metabolic disorders and HCO_3^- (kidneys) for respiratory disorders. In the case of a respiratory disorder where the HCO_3^- is still within the normal range, the body has not begun to compensate, and therefore it is referred to as an absent compensation. If the pH and HCO_3^- are both outside the normal ranges, this is referred to as a partial compensation. Finally, if the pH has been brought back into the normal range, the acid–base balance would be referred to as a compensated condition. The compensatory description is the same for metabolic disorders as well.

Understanding the basics of ABG analysis is important for the acute care therapist for several reasons. First, understanding what diseases or disorders may lead to a

TABLE 14.5 Causes and Signs and Symptoms of Acid–Base Imbalances[8–10]

	Cause	Signs/Symptoms
Respiratory acidosis	Central nervous system (CNS) injury to respiratory center (traumatic brain injury [TBI], tumor, cerebrovascular accident), airway obstruction, pulmonary disease, respiratory muscle weakness (Guillain-Barré syndrome, myasthenia gravis, spinal cord injury), flail chest, metabolism (sepsis, burns), CNS depressant drugs (barbiturates, sedatives, narcotics, anesthesia)	Hypoventilation, hypercapnia, headache, visual disturbances, coma, confusion, anxiety, restlessness, drowsiness, deep tendon reflex, hyperkalemia, ventricular fibrillation
Metabolic acidosis	Uncontrolled diabetes mellitus, starvation, renal failure, acetylsalicylic acid (ASA) overdose, prolonged stress or physical stress, hypoxia, severe diarrhea, ethanol abuse, metabolic/ethanol ketoacidosis, lactic acidosis	HCO_3^- deficit, headache, hyperventilation, mental dullness, deep respiration, stupor, coma, hyperkalemia, arrhythmias, muscle twitching/weakness, nausea/vomiting/diarrhea, malaise
Respiratory alkalosis	Hypoxemia (emphysema, pneumonia, acute respiratory distress syndrome), stimulation of CNS (sepsis, ammonia, ASA overdose, TBI, tumor, excessive exercise or stress, severe pain), hyperventilation, hepatic encephalopathy, congestive heart failure, pulmonary embolism, impaired lung disease (internal pancreatic fistulae, ascites, scoliosis, pregnancy)	Hypocapnia, tachypnea, lightheadedness, numbness/peripheral tingling, tetany, convulsions, diaphoresis, muscle twitching, hypokalemia, arrhythmias
Metabolic alkalosis	Loss of hydrochloric acid, loss of potassium, diarrhea, exercise, ingestion of alkaline substances, steroids, diuresis, nasogastric suctioning, peptic ulcer disease (PUD), massive blood transfusion	HCO_3^- excess, hypoventilation, mental confusion and agitation, dizziness, peripheral numbness, muscle twitching, tetany, convulsions, hypokalemia, arrhythmias

TABLE 14.6 Example of Respiratory Acidosis

	Actual Value	Normal Range	Reference Value	Acidotic/ Alkalotic
pH	7.24	7.35–7.45	7.4	Acidotic
PaO_2	74 mmHg	80–100 mmHg		
$PaCO_2$	67 mmHg	35–45 mmHg	40 mmHg	Acidotic
HCO_3^-	27 mEq/L	22–26 mEq/L	24 mEq/L	Alkalotic

TABLE 14.7 Example of Metabolic Alkalosis

	Patient	Normal Range	Reference	Acidotic/ Alkalotic
pH	7.5	7.35–7.45	7.4	Alkalotic
PaO_2	77 mmHg	80–100 mmHg		
$PaCO_2$	48 mmHg	35–45 mmHg	40 mmHg	Acidotic
HCO_3^-	37 mEq/L	22–26 mEq/L	24 mEq/L	Alkalotic

disruption of pH should guide the physical therapist to tailor the evaluation process, particularly owing to the pulmonary system compensation. Knowing the associated signs and symptoms of the four basic categories of acid–base imbalance will aid the physical therapist in detecting medical changes and will alter the other health care team members' concerns. Finally, the degree of compensation should be considered when developing a current treatment plan or deciding if there is a need to hold therapy for the day.

Electrocardiogram

There are many changes that can happen in the electrical cardiac cycle with aging. By 60 years of age, there is a decrease in the number of cells in the sinoatrial node and this number continues to decline with age, leading to a slowing of the intrinsic heart rate. Also noted is a left shift of the QRS axis from stiffening of the left bundle branch and left ventricular hypertrophy seen in patients with long-standing hypertension who may also exhibit a decrease in the amplitude of the T-wave.[29]

Even if the physical therapist is not familiar with reading an electrocardiogram (ECG), there are a few things to keep in mind when working with patients. First, when looking at an ECG strip, one should note that immediately after the QRS complex, a large vertical spike that represents ventricular depolarization, the ventricles should contract. If the therapist palpates the peripheral pulse, there should be a pulse that is felt after each QRS seen on the ECG. For some individuals with impaired heart muscle or an abnormal contraction like a premature ventricular contraction (PVC), the pulse may be faint or even absent. Without an ECG, the therapist can compare the heart rate heard with auscultation with the peripheral pulse.

It is also important to remember that the time the heart contracts is the period of the highest myocardial oxygen consumption or demand. If the patient's heart rate is high, then there is a possibility that the coronary blood flow cannot keep up with demand and the patient may experience dysrhythmias and angina. Angina is defined as a discomfort that is experienced above the waist that is not associated with any musculoskeletal or neuromuscular dysfunction. Angina is commonly experienced substernal with or without radiation down the left upper extremity, but it is extremely important that the physical therapist does not forget that there are many patients who do not present with classic symptoms, especially women and patients with diabetes, and who may report pain in the jaw, back, and right upper extremity or gastrointestinal discomfort.

Another point to remember about the ECG is that the time between QRS complexes is the time that the ventricles fill to send blood into the coronary arteries for myocardial perfusion. When the heart rate is high, there is a reduction in ventricular filling time that can reduce the forward flow of blood, particularly when the myocardial tissue is not able to compensate. There is also a reduction in myocardial perfusion time that may lead to angina.

There are other dysrhythmias that are associated with diseases such as hypertension and coronary disease. Hypertension is associated with myocardial left ventricular hypertrophy.[30] Over time, this may lead to enlargement of the left atrium because more blood is being held in the cardiac chambers at the end of contraction. The enlargement of the left atrium is associated with irritability of the atrial tissue and an abnormal control of rhythm, atrial fibrillation (Fig. 14.1). The classic presentation of atrial fibrillation is an unpredictable, irregular heart rate. The patient may become symptomatic if the rate becomes too fast and the heart cannot meet the oxygen demand or the myocardium cannot compensate for the lower volume of blood delivered to the ventricles for circulation throughout the body. The patient may report angina, fatigue, shortness of breath, and dizziness, and changes in mentation may be noted.

Arrhythmias generated from the ventricles, PVCs, are also common with aging but are benign when the dysrhythmia is less than 8 beats per minute (bpm) and the patient's heart can compensate for the premature contractions. Another ventricular dysrhythmia with an increased incidence among older adults is referred to as a bundle branch block (BBB) (Fig. 14.2), which, again, may also

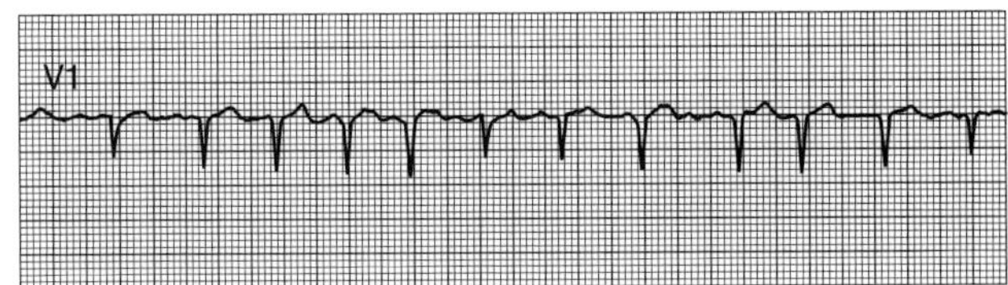

FIG. 14.1 Example of atrial fibrillation.

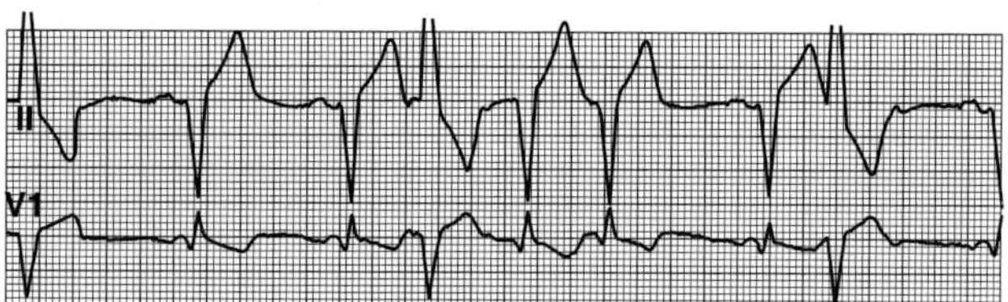

FIG. 14.2 Example of premature ventricular contractions and bundle branch blocks in leads II and V1.

be benign, but in the presence of depressed myocardial dysfunction may lead to signs and symptoms including fatigue, decreased activity tolerance, and shortness of breath.

It is important to know the patient's history of dysrhythmias and current ECG rhythm. If equipment permits, monitoring the rate, rhythm, and regularity during activities will allow the therapist to document any changes along with any signs and symptoms during activity. Patients with a history of dysrhythmias may have a temporary or permanent pacemaker or an automatic implantable coronary defibrillator. For the patient with a temporary pacemaker, the physical therapist should understand what the underlying rhythm is and the patient's heart function (myocardial perfusion and contractility function). The physical therapist should make sure that the temporary pacer wires are secured, to reduce risk of disconnection during mobilization. For the patients with an internal defibrillator, it is important to know at what heart rate level the device will deliver a shock to the patient. The physical therapist needs to monitor these patients and avoid exercising beyond this heart rate level to avoid unwarranted shocks.

Surgical and Medical Procedural Reports

The therapist may alter the examination process after the surgical reports are reviewed. The surgical reports should reveal the specificity of the procedure and identify any associated precautions and restrictions. This information may also assist the physical therapist in working with the surgeon or primary care physician in establishing mobility guidelines with the goal of protecting the surgical site to promote healing and allow the patient to achieve the highest level of function and possibly avoid the iatrogenic complications related to immobility such as pressure sores, pneumonia, and DVTs.

Summary. The medical review, when possible, is a crucial step in initiating the examination as it provides vital information about the patient's past and present medical status. Understanding the effects of chronic diseases should also assist the therapist in prescribing a comprehensive exercise prescription and care plan based on the expected course of the disease and its impact on functional mobility. At the end of the medical record review process, the physical therapist should be able to formulate a clinical picture of the patient in preparation for the examination process, prioritize the anticipated deficits to address, decide what possible education the patient should receive, and determine the need for possible referrals and probable discharge recommendations.

Beyond the medical record review, the physical therapist should discuss the patient's situation with other members of the medical team as available. The members of the team will have information that may not be contained within the medical record at the time of the physical therapist consult. The therapist should also extend the information gathering to include the family or caregiver and patient.

Interview

Within the review of systems, the physical therapist should question the patient for specific factors related to age, occupation, and other behaviors that may indicate increased risk for specific conditions. The reader is directed to Table 14.8 for an example of a form to assess a review of symptoms that can be helpful in deciding what

TABLE 14.8 Example of a Review of Symptoms

Indicate whether condition has been present in the last 1 month and 3 months		
1 month	**3 months**	
		Cognitive/Mood State
		Decreased ability to recall current events
		Decreased ability to remember past events
		Decrease in short-term memory
		Decreased ability to concentrate
		Decreased ability to focus in a busy room
		Decreased ability to complete a task
		Increase in tripping or falling
		Increase in making mistakes
		Difficulty falling asleep

TABLE 14.8	Example of a Review of Symptoms—cont'd
1 month	**3 months**	

1 month	3 months	
		Difficulty staying asleep
		Wakes up coughing
		Wakes up short of breath
		Wakes up anxious
		Wakes up with pain
		Feeling depressed
		Feeling anxious
		Stopped participating in usual activities
		Stopped traveling out into the community
		Prefers to stay at home
		Prefers to be alone
		More irritable or quicker to being angry
		Feeling of forgetfulness
		General
		Increased fatigue
		Experiencing fever or chills
		Unplanned weight loss
		Change in voice or prolonged sore throat
		Increase in thirst or appetite
		Decreased appetite
		Body aches or malaise
		Dizziness or lightheadedness
		Changes in smell
		Changes in hearing, ringing in ears
		Dental pain, mouth sores
		Sweet odor to breath
		Brittle hair or nails
		Any lumps or masses
		Temperature intolerance (heat or cold)
		Muscles and Nerves
		Joint pain, swelling, or redness
		Increase in incidence of headaches
		Change in vision or hearing
		Difficulty finding words or speaking clearly
		Muscle soreness, weakness
		Numbness, tingling
		Dizziness or vertigo
		Decrease in coordination, feeling clumsy
		Pain radiating into arms or legs
		Restlessness, or tremors
		Decreased memory
		Loss of consciousness
		Muscle cramps
		Bones and Skin
		Joint swelling or stiffness
		Muscle pain or weakness
		Significant loss of body height
		White and painful fingers or toes
		Change in appearance of nails
		Skin discoloration
		Open wounds
		Skin rashes or itching

Continued

TABLE 14.8	Example of a Review of Symptoms—cont'd	
1 month	**3 months**	
		Moles or skin marks that have changed in size or color
		Changes in hair (loss, additional growth, brittle)
		Heart and Blood Vessels
		Chest pain, pressure, heaviness, or tightness
		Irregular pulse (heart rate speeds up, slows down, and skips beats)
		Legs ache with walking or stair climbing
		Edema in feet or legs
		Weight gain despite loss of muscle
		Fatigue
		Shortness of breath at rest or during activity
		Avoidance of usual activities
		Discoloration or painful feet or legs
		Swelling in one leg or arm
		Any pain that goes away when you rest
		Changes in heart rate or blood pressure
		Persistent cough
		Bleeding
		Pulmonary
		Shortness of breath
		Persistent cough
		Chest wall pain
		Clubbing of finger and toe nails
		Productive cough, increase in sputum production
		Abdomen
		Changes in appetite or taste
		Difficulty swallowing
		Abdominal pain
		Sense of bloating, gas
		Changes in bowel behavior
		Incontinence of bowel or bladder
		Changes in color or consistency of stool
		Indigestion or heartburn
		Nausea, vomiting, diarrhea
		Changes in urination pattern, stream, or color
		Pain or burning with urination
		Needing to urinate at night
		Hesitation or urgency to urinate
		Gender
		Decrease in sexual interest or activity
		Pain with sexual activity
		Female
		Changes in menstrual cycle
		Vaginal discharge
		Possibility of pregnancy
		Spotting or bleeding
		Irregular moods
		Changes in breast shapes, lumps or masses, painfulness
		Male
		Impotence
		Testicular pain
		Penile discharge
		Genital lesion

BOX 14.3 Common Risk Factors Associated with Four Common Medical Issues in the Older Adult[31–33]

Type 2 Diabetes	Cancer	Osteoporosis	Coronary Artery Disease
Obesity	Being overweight or obese	Age	Obesity
Hypertension	Excessive alcohol use	Family history	Smoking
Hypercholesterolemia	Excessive sun exposure	Low body weight	Hypertension
Race (African American)	Inactivity	Race (Caucasian, Asian)	Dyslipidemia
Genetics		Menopause	Impaired fasting glucose
Inactive or sedentary lifestyle	Others specific to each cancer	History of fractures	Family history
Glucose intolerance	Tobacco use	Diet	Sedentary lifestyle

to examine and identify symptoms that would suggest referrals to other providers for diagnosis and management. Box 14.3 demonstrates some of the risk factors for type 2 diabetes, cancer, and osteoporosis.[31–33] A risk factor that is particularly important to address because of the relevance to physical therapy is an inactive or sedentary lifestyle. Because an inactive lifestyle is a strong risk factor for most chronic diseases such as arthritis, CAD, diabetes, frailty, and so forth, collecting a physical activity history can reveal an opportunity for patient education. Asking specific questions such as "Do you exercise and what kind (including frequency and duration)?", "How many hours do you sit per day?", or "How often do you leave your home?" is one way to get at this important risk factor.

The most well-established risk factor screening is for CAD. Risk factors include the causative factors of smoking, diabetes, and hypertension; predisposing factors include obesity, inactivity, abnormal lipid profile, and family history. Other factors to consider include age, gender, and stress (see Box 14.4 for risk factors for CAD).[25] After establishing how many risk factors the patient exhibits, the physical therapist should determine if the patient is experiencing pain or discomfort above the waist that cannot be attributed to a musculoskeletal or neuromuscular dysfunction, shortness of breath at rest or with mild exertion, dizziness or syncope, orthopnea or paroxysmal nocturnal dyspnea, lower extremity edema, palpitations or tachycardia, claudication, known heart murmur, and/or unusual fatigue.[25] Finally, once all the risk factors are determined, the physical therapist can determine the risk level of a cardiac event during exertion. Box 14.5 lists the American College of Sports Medicine's (ACSM's) risk stratification categories.[25]

The process of risk-stratifying patients for heart disease and other diseases, even in the acute care setting, can aid the therapist in determining what components of the examination should be completed to determine safe activity tolerance parameters. Risk-stratifying followed by testing can guide the therapist to prescribe an appropriate exercise prescription, home exercise program, and education to progress exercise tolerance and function.

Risk factor stratification is a very important process for the therapist to complete for each patient. After the physical therapist has stratified a patient for the likelihood of

BOX 14.4 Risk Factors for Coronary Artery Disease[25]

Positive Risk Factors	Defining Criteria
Family history	Myocardial infarction, coronary revascularization, or sudden death before 55 years of age in father or other male first-degree relative or before 65 years of age in mother or other female first-degree relative
Smoking	Current cigarette smoker or those who quit within the previous 6 months
Hypertension	Systolic BP $\geq$140 mmHg, or diastolic BP $\geq$90 mmHg, confirmed on at least two consecutive occasions, or on hypertensive medication
Dyslipidemia	Low-density lipoprotein >130 mg/dL, high-density lipoprotein <40 mg/dL, on lipid-lowering medications, total cholesterol >200 mg/dL
Impaired fasting glucose	Fasting blood glucose $\geq$100 mg/dL confirmed by measurements on at least two separate occasions
Obesity	Body mass index >30 kg/m^2, or waist girth >102 cm for men and >88 cm for women, or waist/hip ratio $\geq$0.95 for men and $\geq$0.86 for women
Sedentary lifestyle	Not participating in a regular exercise program or not meeting the minimal physical activity recommendations from the U.S. Surgeon General's Report

Modified from American College of Sports Medicine.

BOX 14.5 American College of Sports Medicine Risk Stratification Categories[25]

Low risk	Men younger than age 45 years and women younger than age 55 years who are asymptomatic and meet no more than one risk factor
Moderate risk	Men age 45 years or older and women age 55 years or older or those who meet two or more risk factors
High risk	Individuals with one or more signs and symptoms or known cardiovascular, pulmonary, or metabolic disease

having cardiovascular or pulmonary disease or the likelihood of the patient experiencing medical difficulty during exercise, this information can be used to direct the examination and patient education and give appropriate referrals to physicians, program centers, or other health care professionals.

SYSTEMS REVIEW

Mental Status

Assessing the mental status of a patient can be difficult in the presence of acute and chronic medical conditions, and in the older adult population this can be more of a challenge because of the increased incidence of dementia and Alzheimer disease. Changes in mental state may be associated with a variety of factors, including metabolic disturbances, coexisting comorbidities, medications, and environmental conditions.[34] From a metabolic state, the therapist must recognize that hypoxemia, anemia, hyperglycemia, electrolyte imbalances, malnutrition, and dehydration are contributing factors to changes in mental status. Polypharmaceutical use in the older adult population is very common and has been associated not only with increased risk of falls[35] but also with altered mental status and delirium.[36] The therapist should not overlook the use of alcohol and over-the-counter or illicit drug use when gathering information during the evaluation. The National Council on Alcoholism and Drug Dependence reported that substance abuse is on the rise with older adults, from 2.5 million in 2015 to over 6 million in 2030. The reasons are multifactorial including depression, financial restraints, and polypharmacy.[37] Finally, the therapist needs to recognize the effects of surgery and general anesthesia, the physical stress associated with surgery, the patient's environment, and the use of restraints and medical equipment, such as Foley catheters, as contributing factors to a decline in mental status.

Delirium, also referred to as an acute organic brain syndrome, acute organic mental disorder, or acute confusional state, is a syndrome defined as an acute decline in mental status associated with transient changes that, in many cases, are reversible and sometimes preventable. The patient typically presents with fluctuations in levels of alertness, inability to attend to a task, perceptual disturbance, visual hallucinations, and a decline in cognitive skills such as learning, processing, and problem solving. Delirium may also be associated with changes in mood state such as withdrawal or agitation and combativeness.[34,38,39] There are three states of delirium: the hyperactive state in which the patient is restless and agitated; the hypoactive state in which the patient is lethargic and withdrawn; and a mixed state in which the patient's behavior fluctuates between the hyperactive and hypoactive states.[39] The patient with hypoactive delirium is often undiagnosed because the medical team misinterprets the patient's behavior as depression or fatigue.[40] Delirium is often misdiagnosed as dementia in the older adult patient, which can lead to high mortality rates, longer lengths of stay in medical facilities, and poorer functional outcomes. Of note, there is a higher incidence of delirium in patients who have a baseline of dementia.[38]

Delirium is a significant issue when working with the older adult, particularly those in an institutional setting (acute care hospital, subacute hospital, or a long-term care facility), because of its high incidence and impact on medical and functional outcomes. The therapist should be aware of the features of delirium. This syndrome typically has an acute onset of inattention, disorganized thinking, change in the level of consciousness, disorientation, decreased memory, perceptual disturbances, and altered sleep–wake cycles. In the intensive care units (ICUs), the prevalence of delirium is higher and is associated with longer ICU stays, lower vent-free days, and higher mortality and morbidity rates, and there is a higher discharge rate to long-term care facilities for those with delirium.[38,44] Recently, the American Association of Critical Care Nursing and the Society of Critical Care Medicine has made recommendations for the evaluation and reduction of delirium through addressing pain, reducing sedation, avoiding medications like benzodiazepine, and promoting early mobilization.[42] The entire medical team including the physical therapist needs to improve the patient experience to address modifiable risk factors such as providing patients their glasses and hearing aide; sufficient pain management, nutrition, and hydration; proper sleep; and physical and cognitive activity.[43,44]

Consequently, the therapist should contribute by reporting changes in mentation by completing a delirium assessment tool like the Confusion Assessment Method[41] for the ICU (CAM-ICU), assist with pain management and cognitive retraining, and promote early rehabilitation to improve morbidity and mortality and decrease health care costs associated with delirium.

Dementia may sometimes be separate or intertwined with delirium, which can complicate the evaluation and intervention process and significantly affect outcomes. Dementia is a syndrome of gradual onset and progressive decline of cognitive function. It is a common disorder in older adults that progresses with each decade of life. Alzheimer disease and cerebral vascular insufficiency are the two more common causes of dementia, with Alzheimer disease accounting for 50% to 60% of all cases.[45] There are a variety of standardized instruments that are used to screen and evaluate for dementia, such as the Folstein Mini Mental Status Exam. Chapter 19 has specific details related to evaluation of delirium and dementia.

Vital Signs

Every therapist, regardless of the practice setting and type of patient population treated, should be evaluating the patient's resting vital signs and response to exertion. Even in the acute care setting where the patient's vitals are routinely monitored, the therapist can provide valuable information about the patient's tolerance to upright postures, functional mobility, and activity tolerance. This information can assist in medical decision making, including medication prescription and surgical management.

Heart Rate. The therapist should begin with an assessment of resting HR. It is helpful if the patient can give you an estimate of what his or her HR and blood pressure (BP) typically are to establish a baseline. In the assessment of the pulse and heart rate, the therapist should appreciate the rate, regularity, and quality. When assessing regularity, the therapist is assessing the equal and consistent beat of the pulse. Regularity is defined as having fewer than six interruptions in the rhythm in 1 minute. If the pulse is regular, the rate can be calculated by counting the number of beats within 15 seconds and then multiplying that number by 4 to calculate the heart rate per minute. If the rate is irregular, the therapist should count the number of beats throughout the entire minute. For some patients who have an irregular pulse and those patients with a history of left ventricular dysfunction, the therapist should verify the palpatory rate with the auscultatory rate. The auscultatory rate can be taken over the left anterior chest wall, around the second intercostal space, where the closure of the aortic valve can clearly be heard. Finally, the therapist should appreciate the quality, or how well the pulse is felt upon palpation. A pulse that is described as bounding is very difficult to obstruct, whereas a thready pulse is weak and easily obstructed and is, at times, rapid. Probable causes of a bounding pulse include exercise, fever, anxiety, arrhythmia, volume overload, and hypertension. A thready pulse is associated with dehydration, arrhythmias, aortic stenosis, ketoacidosis, and shock.

The therapist should also consider what is referred to as heart rate reserve (HRR), how much the heart can increase its rate from the resting value to respond to demand. HRR reflects the heart's ability to increase cardiac output. The physical therapist may infer how much activity the patient can tolerate from this calculation (Box 14.6). Heart rate reserve can be calculated by subtracting the resting HR from the maximal (predicted or actual) HR. Predicted maximal HR can be estimated by using the formula: $208 - (0.7 \times \text{age})$. This formula is more accurate than the $220 - \text{age}$ formula, which underestimates maximal heart rates in older adults. Actual maximal HR would be available and more favorable if the patient had undergone some form of exercise test.

BOX 14.6 Application of Heart Rate Reserve

Two patients who are 70 years of age have similar medical histories and functional abilities. They are admitted to the hospital with pneumonia. Each have a predicted maximal heart rate (HR) of 150 bpm. The first patient's resting HR is 70 bpm, which gives him a heart rate reserve (HRR) of 80 bpm. The second patient has a resting HR of 120 bpm and therefore an HRR of 30 bpm. The physical therapist should expect the first patient to have a higher activity tolerance than the second patient because the first patient's heart rate is more able to compensate during exertion before reaching maximum HR.

Heart rate reserve can also be used to determine what percent of predicted or actual maximal heart rate is the patient's resting heart rate. This is calculated by dividing the patient's resting heart rate by the predicted heart rate. This is helpful information when determining if the patient is appropriate to treat and to what extent. HRR and percent of predicted work can be useful tools to manage your case load and formulate a safe and effective exercise prescription.

Blood Pressure. The patient's tolerance or medical stability cannot be completely assessed without examining the blood pressure and its response to activity. All health care professionals should assess their patients for hypertension and make appropriate referrals for medical management. The physical therapist is in a unique position to contribute to the health and well-being of patients by not only assessing for hypertension but also screening for exertional hypertension, which also has been linked to higher risk of suffering a cardiovascular event.

The incidence of hypertension (HTN) rises with age, so it is very important to screen BP with every patient. Hypertension is an independent risk factor for cardiovascular and renal disease. In 2017 the American College of Cardiology and the American Heart Association changed the recommendation of the management of high blood pressure to start at 130/80 instead of the previous recommendation of 140/90. Normal blood pressure is defined as a systolic pressure of <120 mmHg and a diastolic pressure of <80 mmHg.[46] It is well known that the incidence of elevated blood pressure increases with age. In the Johns Hopkins Precursors study reported by Whelton et al., 0.3% of white male medical students developed hypertension at age 25, 6.5% at age 45, and 37% at age 65.[47] While this study used the 140/90 value as the definition of hypertension, the new guidelines change the incidence of hypertension to 46% of the adult population in the United States.[48] The Joint National Committee on Prevention, Detection, Evaluation, and Treatment of High Blood Pressure is urging the health care field to focus on treating HTN with the goal being to decrease the incidence of CAD, stroke, and renal disease.[49] Not only can the therapist document the presence of HTN and make the proper referral for medical management, but also he or she can also assess the effectiveness of antihypertensive medications. Evaluation for HTN should be assessed on at least two to three consecutive sessions,[25] and if the patient is found to have either resting or exercise HTN, he or she should be referred for medical management.[49] See Table 14.9 for the classification of HTN.

Pulse Pressure. Pulse pressure is the difference between systolic and diastolic blood pressure. Pulse pressure can be easily assessed by the clinician and has significant predictive value in cardiovascular disease. Pulse

TABLE 14.9 Classification of Hypertension

	Systolic Blood Pressure (mmHg)		Diastolic Blood Pressure (mmHg)
Normal	<120	and	<80
Elevated	120–129	and	< 80
Hypertension			
Stage 1	130–139	or	80–89
Stage 2	140–179	or	>90
Hypertensive crisis	≥180	and/or	≥120

pressure examines cardiovascular compliance—the ability of the arteries to vasoconstrict and vasodilate to circulate blood to properly meet activity demands. Pulse pressure is calculated by subtracting diastolic blood pressure from systolic pressure. With age there is a decrease in compliance of the aorta and small arteries, which leads to an elevation of systolic pressure and a decline in diastolic pressure, causing an increase in pulse pressure. Pulse pressure can also be elevated with exercise, aortic insufficiency, and atherosclerosis, and when a patient has an elevated intracranial pressure, whereas it will narrow in the presence of aortic stenosis, HF, and pericarditis. As pulse pressure widens, there is an increase in the incidence of cardiovascular disease. Generally, a normal pulse pressure at rest is approximately 40 mmHg. A study conducted by Weiss et al. found that an increased pulse pressure in very old hospitalized patients was a predictor of higher mortality,[50] and therefore, when pulse pressure exceeds 60 mmHg, a medical referral should promptly be made.

Orthostatic Hypotension. Orthostatic hypotension is defined as a decrease in systolic BP by 20 mmHg or a drop by 10 mmHg with a reflexive increase in HR with transitional movements, such as moving from supine to sit or sit to stand. The incidence of orthostasis increases 20% in community-dwelling people older than age 65 years and has been reported to be as high as 50% in frail older adults living in nursing homes.[51] There are many causes of orthostatic hypotension in the acute care environment, including adverse effects of medications, dehydration, anemia, arrhythmias, immobility, sepsis, adrenal insufficiency, and autonomic dysfunction related to diseases like diabetes, Parkinson disease, and central nervous system impairments.[52]

The most common symptoms experienced in orthostatic hypotension are lightheadedness, dizziness, weakness, syncope, and angina. Some clients may experience visual and speech deficits, confusion, and changes in cognitive function. It is difficult to utilize symptoms as an indication of orthostasis, because the complexity of the older adult patient's medical history and presentation may be related to various issues. Therefore, it is critical that the therapist screen the patient's BP with postural changes to rule out orthostatic hypotension whether or not symptoms are present as the patient may be at risk for falls, fractures, myocardial infarction, and cerebral injuries. To thoroughly rule out orthostasis, the client should be monitored before and after medications, before breakfast, after meals, and before bed.[51] Assessing blood pressure within the first minute of standing is the most sensitive for identifying orthostatic hypotension.[53]

Response to Exertion. Blood pressure assessment at rest and during exertion is key to assessing exercise tolerance and assisting in medication prescription. A physical therapist can have a major impact on a person's health care by assessing the patient's blood pressure during exertion, which few other practitioners do, so that a hypertensive blood pressure response to activity can be documented and appropriately treated.

During the examination process, the therapist should monitor the patient's vital signs with activity to determine if the client is having an appropriate HR and BP response to a given workload. It should be noted that patients taking β-blocker medications will have some HR and BP response, although blunted, to an increase in workload. In these situations, it can be helpful to look at an activity chart to determine the patient's estimated metabolic equivalent level (MET level) to examine the relationship between vital signs and workload.[54] There should be an expectation that HR and BP and perception of work should rise with demand. In general, HR should increase 10 to 12 bpm and systolic BP should increase 10 to 12 mmHg per MET level in the absence of medications that will lead to a blunted response.

To complete the assessment of response to exertion, the therapist should take note of the vital sign response during the recovery phase. There should not be any immediate increase in HR upon stopping exercise, which would suggest that the patient is experiencing a reflexive cardiac response to venous pooling or orthostasis. However, within the first minute of recovery, depending on conditioning, there should be a significant decrease in systolic BP and HR. The rate of HR recovery is often indicative of deconditioning and has been linked to mortality and morbidity related to cardiovascular disease. Heart rate recovery of fewer than 12 beats in 1 minute of walking recovery following submaximum exercise is associated with poor prognosis, and a rate of HR recovery fewer than 42 beats at 2 minutes into recovery after a submaximal exercise test in older adults is associated with an increased mortality rate from a cardiovascular event.[25,55]

Rate Pressure Product. Rate pressure product (RPP) represents an estimate of myocardial oxygen consumption and should increase as workload increases. Using the HR and BP data that were recorded at rest and during various activities performed, the therapist can calculate the RPP by multiplying the HR with the systolic blood pressure. Using the systolic blood pressure at rest and then again with activity, you can calculate the increase in oxygen demand with any activity. Any total value >10,000 indicates an increased risk for heart disease. This can be valuable when working with a patient who has a history of coronary disease and the therapist wants to assess for myocardial limitations to exertion. Rate pressure product is also known as the anginal threshold because once the oxygen demand during exertion exceeds the coronary artery's ability to carry sufficient blood and oxygen to the myocardium, ischemia begins. At this point the client will most likely become symptomatic, with varying upper body complaints of discomfort or shortness of breath. The point of imbalance between oxygen supply and demand can be predicted by examining the RPP. The therapist can use this information to document a hypothesized cause of symptoms, document the MET level where symptoms appear, monitor the progression of the disease, and progress the rehabilitation plan in a patient with known disease. This information can also be helpful in making a referral for medical workup and to design a safe exercise program below the anginal threshold.

Pulmonary Function

During the interview and examination process the therapist should also note the respiratory rate and breathing pattern. The average resting adult respiratory rate ranges from 12 to 20 breaths per minute. The inspiratory-to-expiratory ratio should be 1:2. When the ratio becomes closer to 1:1, it may indicate hyperventilation, reducing PaO_2, possibly associated with anxiety or a metabolic problem such as uncontrolled diabetes, alcohol abuse, or a restrictive pulmonary disease. A ratio that reaches 1:3 or greater (hypoventilation, which increases the $PaCO_2$) can be associated with obstructive lung diseases like asthma, chronic bronchitis, and emphysema. Hypoventilation can lead to hypoxemia. The therapist should document the patient's ability to increase the depth and rate of breathing with an increase in exertion. There should be an expansion of the chest wall in all cardinal planes and the therapist should see initiation and expansion of the upper abdominal wall during inspiration, indicating diaphragmatic function. The patient should also be able to speak approximately 12 to 15 syllables per breath at rest. Oxygen saturation at rest and during exercise with a pulse oximeter should be documented. For people with light complexion, a saturation value >93% at rest is normal and these values should not decrease with exercise, whereas that number increases to 95% for darker-skinned people.[56] It should be noted that pulse oximeter accuracy decreases significantly in darker-pigmented patients, especially with saturation values of <80%.[57] A value of <90% at rest or during exercise is abnormal, and a value <88% indicates the need for supplemental oxygen in darker-skinned people.[58] If the therapist notes deviations in these respiratory factors, further investigation of the cardiopulmonary system is warranted to determine why the patient is demonstrating signs of hypoxia, and you should discuss your findings with the patient's provider. The physical therapist must recognize the limits of the pulse oximeter, which include inaccuracies in the reading and the fact that the device is measuring the percentage of existing hemoglobin to carry oxygen. Depending on the quality of the device, there may be as much as a 5% to 6% error rate, which becomes more inaccurate for patients who have atrial fibrillation or other highly irregular dysrhythmias, or when the oxygen saturation rates drop below 90%.[59] In a study by Seifi et al.[60], it was shown that there is variability among probe location, with earlobe placement being the most accurate. Oxygen is a medication and the therapist needs an order from the provider to change the amount delivered. It is advisable for the therapist to have facility guidelines that allow the therapist to titrate oxygen level to the patient's needs during exercise. Once the therapist has determined how much oxygen the patient requires during exercise, then a new oxygen prescription should be ordered by the provider.

Auscultation

As part of the assessment, the therapist should listen to the heart and lungs, both at rest and during exercise. Many therapists are unfamiliar and feel uncomfortable with their auscultation skills, but the only way to begin to feel more confident is to listen to the chest walls of many patients. Not only is auscultation an important examination skill to rule out cardiopulmonary disease or dysfunction, but also it is important to assess the heart and lungs during exercise prescription as it may reveal a reason for exercise intolerance. The authors encourage every therapist to listen to everyone's chest wall to build his or her skills. There are multiple heart and lung sounds posted on the internet to provide examples of various sounds for independent learning.

When listening to basic heart sounds, the therapist should first assess the quality of valvular closure. If the valves are functioning properly, there should be a nice crisp and definitive sound. The best place to listen to the atrioventricular valves (tricuspid and mitral) is in the fifth intercostal space, adjacent to the sternum and left midclavicular line, respectively. Then the therapist should place the diaphragm over the second intercostal space just right of the sternum to hear the aortic valve the loudest. If the therapist does not hear a crisp, strong closure at rest or hears a sound that appears or worsens with exercise, the provider should be notified. Listen in the second intercostal space left of the sternum to assess the pulmonic valve. The sound of the atrioventricular and semilunar valves closing is referred to as the normal heart sounds, S1 and S2. Next the therapist should place the bell of the stethoscope back over the mitral valve area. The therapist should vary the pressure between the bell and chest wall to hear low-pitched sounds. When the therapist presses the bell lightly on the chest wall, low-pitched sounds can be heard, and when the therapist then presses the bell firmly, the low-pitched sound disappears. The appearance of an additional sound may indicate an atrial or ventricular gallop, S4 and S3. If a harsh straining, a lush sound, or a low-pitched sound is heard at rest, worsens with exercise, or appears with exercise, the therapist should seek further assessment for the patient. Murmurs may be appreciated either during the systolic or diastolic phase of the cardiac cycle. Systolic murmurs can be heard between S1 and S2 and are associated with semilunar valve stenosis or atrioventricular valve incompetence. Diastolic murmurs are associated with atrioventricular valve stenosis or semilunar valve incompetence. See Fig. 14.3 for a diagram of the heart sounds. A stenotic valve sounds harsh or strained, whereas an incompetent valve has a lush or swish-like sound. Some abnormal sounds may be benign, but most sounds are associated with a valvular problem or a dysfunction of the myocardium for the older adult and must be further investigated.[61] Finally, a leathery rubbing sound heard over the chest wall that persists when the patient holds his or her breath could possibly be a pericardial friction rub and should be further worked up. A pericardial rub is associated with friction between the pericardium and myocardium and is associated with inflammation or fluid within the pericardium. It is very helpful if the therapist informs the physician if the sound worsens or appears with exertion, because many times the patient is examined only at rest by the medical team.

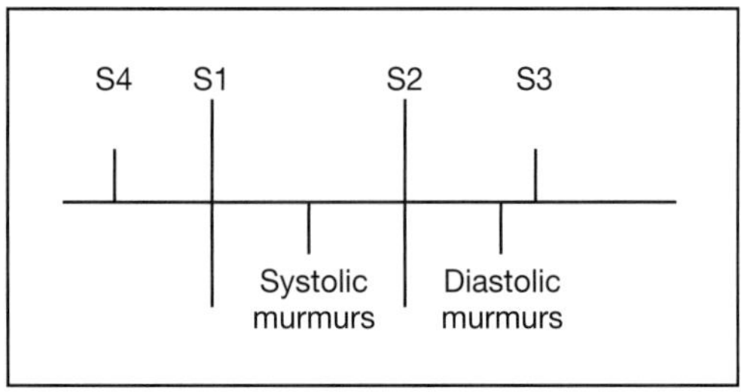

FIG. 14.3 Heart sounds.

The therapist should then listen to each major section of the lung, anteriorly, laterally, and posteriorly. At rest, the patient should be instructed to breathe slightly deeper than normal, in and out through the mouth. Refer to Fig. 14.4 for general guidelines for auscultation sites and Table 14.10 for a brief description of types of lung sounds and associated causes.[62–64] The therapist should appreciate a gentle rustling sound that is louder the closer the therapist places the stethoscope to the main bronchus.[65] The therapist should not normally hear any wheezing or crackling sounds, as this can be indicative of lung disease. Lung sounds should be assessed at rest and during exercise to once again assess for cardiopulmonary disease and exercise intolerance.

Nutritional Status and Physical Appearance

Prealbumin level reflects the current nutritional status for patients in the acute or subacute recovery phase of an illness. Monitoring these levels is critical to adjusting nutritional and fluid needs. There are many reasons a patient may not be making the expected gains with rehabilitation, and the physical therapist must consider that malnutrition can be one of those causes and work with clinical dietary staff to ensure that sufficient nutrition and calories are being provided to account for the rehabilitation process. Simple strategies such as encouraging fluid intake before, during, and after treatment; monitoring the color of urine; or documenting uneaten meals will help the medical team respond in a timely and appropriate way.

The therapist needs to recognize the association between proper nutrition, body composition, and activity tolerance to progress in rehabilitation.[66,67] The therapist can refer to U.S. government websites for nutritional recommendations for the older adult[68,69] and work closely with a consulting clinical dietician and provider to ensure that the older adult is getting sufficient and quality nutrition to maximize recovery.

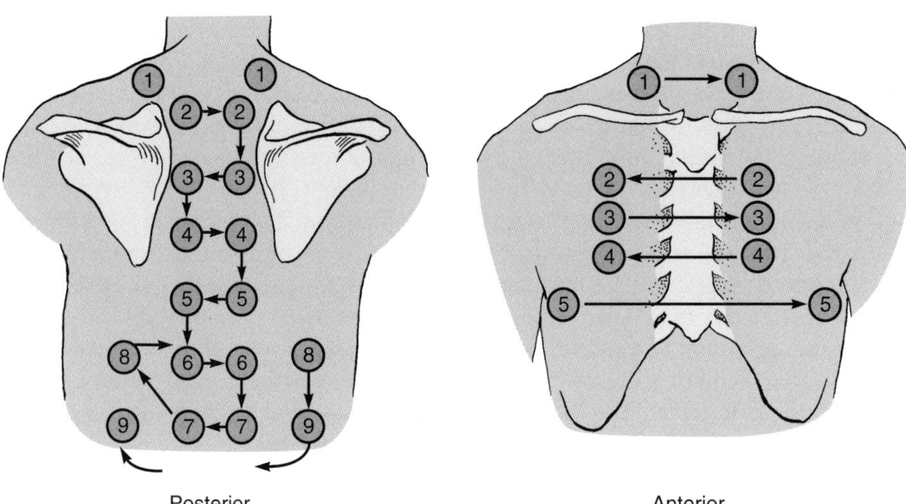

FIG. 14.4 Lung auscultation sites. *(From deWit SC, et al: Medical-Surgical Nursing: Concepts and Practice, ed 3, St. Louis, 2017, Elsevier.)*

TABLE 14.10 Lung Sounds[62–64]

Normal Breath Sounds		
	Description	**Location**
Bronchial	Loud, high-pitched sound with a shorter inspiratory than expiratory duration with a pause between each phase of ventilation	Heard normally adjacent to the sternum
Bronchovesicular	Softer version of bronchial sounds, except are continuous throughout ventilation	Normally heard between the scapulae from T3 to T6 and at the costosternal border of intercostal space (ICS) 2 and 3
Vesicular	Low-pitched, muffled sound Inspiratory sound is louder, longer, and higher in pitch than expiration	Normally heard in the peripheral lung fields
Adventitious Sounds		
	Description	**Dysfunction**
Crackles (rales): inspiratory	May be heard throughout respiratory cycle Heard in the early inspiratory phase Heard in the late inspiratory phase	Associated with fluid or secretion retention Associated with opening of proximal airways Atelectasis, pulmonary edema, fibrosis, or compression of lung tissue from a pleural effusion
Crackles (rales): expiratory	A rhythmic sound Nonrhythmic sound	Associated with opening of more proximal airways Associated with fluid and secretions in large airways
Wheezes: High pitched	A continuous, constant pitch of varying durations Inspiratory Expiratory	Suggestive of rigid airways, bronchospasm, foreign-body partial obstruction, or stenosis Reflects unstable airways that have collapsed; associated with airway obstruction
Wheezes: Low pitched (rhonchus)	Low-pitched, continuous sound Expiratory	Associated with obstruction of airway, commonly thick secretions Reflects unstable airways, airway obstruction
Pleural friction rub	Course, grating, leathery sound from the pulmonary system	Inflammation

There are many reasons the older individual is susceptible to malnutrition, and this type of screening should be part of the physical therapist evaluation, even in the acute care setting. However, the patient's nutritional status may not be assessed or addressed during the hospital stay by the medical team unless a complication arises or the patient has diverted from the expected medical pathway. Common factors that adversely influence nutritional status may include poor dentition, limited income, depression, cognitive impairments, chronic diseases, decreased ability to smell, and altered taste, particularly from medications.

In general, a decrease in activity level and decline in muscle mass likely account for the decrease in basal metabolic rate and a need for a lower caloric intake, but if the individual was active prior to admission, his or her dietary needs may be equal to that of a young adult's.[70] There are many reasons the older adult would require an increase in dietary needs, such as increasing protein and total calories in the presence of an infection, wounds, or stress. The therapist can refer to Table 14.11 for caloric and vitamin recommendations for the older adult.[71–74]

Energy requirements for the older adult can be difficult to determine because of complex medical histories, including HF, renal dysfunction, and different types of cancer. A specialized diet recommendation from a registered clinical dietician may be warranted. It is important to discuss a clinical dietary referral with the referring physician and the patient to ensure the best health and wellness results and to account for the calories spent during rehabilitation.

Observing the client's appearance can generally provide the clinician with valuable information of general health and well-being. The appearance of the patient's skin and fingernails can reveal the presence of pathology. The detection of body or oral odors can suggest diseases such as uncontrolled diabetes, dental abscesses, or pulmonary infections. Body odors and appearance may also suggest alcohol and tobacco abuse, incontinence, and organ dysfunction. Appearance may also suggest the need for a social work consult for referral to community resources and services. See Table 14.12 for signs of nutrient deficiencies that may affect body appearance[72–75] and refer to the American Dietary Association (http://www.eatright.org) or the U.S. Department of Health and Human Services (http://www.hhs.gov) for further information and dietary recommendations.

Older adults are at an increased risk of wound development and complications because of the age-related changes in skin, decreased arteriovenous health, decreased

TABLE 14.11 General Dietary Recommendations for the Older Adult[71–74]

	Recommendations		
	Female	Male	Cellular Function
Calories	1600	2000	
Carbohydrates	130 grams 45%–65% of total calories Using complex carbohydrates, not simple sugars Presence of infections, wounds, catabolic stress: additional 25–30 kcal/kg/day		Supports cell division, leukocyte function, and fibroblast activation
Dietary fiber	22.4 grams	28 grams	
Protein	46 grams 10%–35% of total calories May need to be increased 1.25 g/kg in the healthy active adult Presence of infections, wounds, catabolic stress: 1.6–2.0 kcal/kg/day	56 grams 10%–35% of total calories May need to be increased 1.25 g/kg in the healthy active adult Presence of infections, wounds, catabolic stress: 1.6–2.0 kcal/kg/day	Supports new protein synthesis, cell proliferation, tissue regeneration, inflammatory and immune function
Fats	20%–35%* of total calories 20%–35% of total daily caloric intake*		Builds new cell membranes. Adjust to make food palatable to avoid deficiencies or anorexia
Saturated fats	<10% of total calories		
Cholesterol	<300 mg/day		
Trans fats	Minimal to none		

*May need to be higher to support hormone and bile production.

TABLE 14.12 Signs and Symptoms of Nutritional Deficiency[72–75]

	Signs and Symptoms	Abnormalities
Hair	Dull, dry, lack of natural shine Thin, sparse, loss of curl	Protein deficiency, essential fatty acid deficiency Zinc deficiency
Eyes	White ring around eyes Pale eye membrane Night blindness, dry membranes, dull cornea Redness and fissures of eyelid corners	Hyperlipidemia Vitamin B_{12} deficiency, folic acid and/or iron deficiency Vitamin A deficiency, zinc deficiencies
Lips	Redness and swollen Soreness, swollen, bleeding	Niacin, riboflavin, or iron deficiencies Riboflavin deficiency
Tongue	Sores, swollen Soreness, burning	Folic acid and niacin deficiency Riboflavin deficiency
Taste	Diminished taste	Zinc deficiency
Face	Loss of skin color, dark cheeks and eyes, scaling of skin around nostrils Hyperpigmentation	Protein energy deficiency, niacin, riboflavin deficiencies Niacin deficiency
Neck	Thyroid enlargement	Iron deficiency
Nails	Fragile, banding Spoon shaped	Protein deficiency Iron deficiency
Skin	Slow wound healing Scaliness Dryness, rough Lack of subcutaneous fat, bilateral edema	Zinc deficiency Biotin deficiency Abnormal vitamin A levels Protein energy deficiency
Muscles	Weakness Wasted appearance Calf tenderness, absent patella reflex Peripheral neuropathies Muscle twitch Muscle cramps	Phosphorus and potassium deficiency Protein energy deficiency Thiamine deficiency Folic acid and thiamine deficiencies Abnormal magnesium levels Decreased chloride, sodium deficiency
Bones	Demineralization	Calcium, phosphorus, and vitamin D deficiency
Nerves	Listlessness Decreased sensation, proprioception, depression, and decrease in cognitive function Seizures, behavioral disruption, memory loss	Protein deficiency Thiamine, vitamin B_{12} deficiency Magnesium and zinc deficiencies

activity, cardiovascular disease, and an increase in the incidence of malnutrition. Szewczyk et al. described a study that examined the nutritional status in older adults with or without venous wounds and reported that 48% of the participants were malnourished or at risk for malnutrition.[26]

Each phase of wound healing requires the proper nutrition in a sufficient nutrient distribution to promote healing. Even a brief period of malnutrition, reflected in prealbumin levels, may occur early on in a hospital stay and can delay granulation tissue and collagen formation.[75] It has been reported that as many as 62% of hospitalized older individuals are protein deficient with low prealbumin and albumin levels. Malnutrition doubles the risk of developing pressure ulcers and increases mortality in the older adult.[26] The therapist should keep in mind that many obese patients have low albumin and prealbumin levels and are at equal or greater risk for ulcers and other associated complications from malnutrition than their normal-weight counterparts.

Body Weight/Body Composition

As part of the patient's nutritional status, the patient's body composition should be considered. The relationship between body weight, composition, and function in older adults is a very complex matter. More research is needed to further understand how factors such as body mass index (BMI) as calculated by weight (kg)/height $(m)^2$, fat mass, and lean muscle mass contribute to function, morbidity, and mortality. The research is inconsistent depending on the subjects, medical status, and variables measured. One finding that appears to be consistent is that a BMI <19 is associated with an increase in mortality in hospitalized patients as well as older adult community dwellers. It has been suggested that under health stress, such as infections, hip fractures, or cancer, the older adult patient has fewer energy stores to combat the catabolic state that the patient's body is experiencing.[78] It also appears that patients with a BMI between 30 and 38 who are older than age 60 years, and more significantly in patients older than age 75 years, have an equal mortality rate when compared to age-matched subjects with normal BMI (20 to 25).[67,78] BMI, however, provides limited information for the clinician to truly assess the patient's body composition as well as mortality and morbidity rate. Additionally, BMI does not speak to the percentage of body weight that is fat versus lean muscle, a factor that may affect function.

Protein deficiency along with a reduction in activity can lead to sarcopenia, which is defined as a progressive impairment of muscle function due to loss of skeletal muscle mass that occurs with advancing age.[79] Sarcopenia is associated with an increase in disability and mortality.[80] Sarcopenia is also commonly associated with a low BMI, but it has been documented that there is a group of older, obese individuals that also have been diagnosed with sarcopenia. These individuals have a lower muscle mass of the lower extremities and pelvic girdle than individuals with obesity or individuals of normal weight without sarcopenia. Patients with the combination of obesity and sarcopenia have a decrease in physical function when compared to individuals with sarcopenia and normal BMI.[67] With this in mind, it is important to obtain objective data on strength and function such as grip strength, timed chair rise test, or the short physical performance battery.

Cachexia is a syndrome of metabolic wasting with subsequent loss of skeletal muscle that cannot be fixed by increasing protein intake or even diet alone. In the presence of severe cachexia strength training does not appear to improve function, although some research is now showing that physical activity can help by reducing inflammation, improving erythropoiesis, and increasing bone mineral density, which all contribute to reducing the effects of cachexia and improving overall physical function.[81]

Another factor the therapist needs to consider when working with older adults is body fat deposition. With aging, there is a reduction in subcutaneous fat and an increase in visceral fat accumulation. There is also a reduction in muscle mass along with an increase in total fat mass.[82] This change in body fat deposition and composition is associated with an increase in morbidity and mortality.

Waist circumference is an independent risk factor of metabolic syndrome[83] and can easily be obtained in the clinical setting. Waist circumference can also show higher areas of fat deposition in the elderly. Women and men with a waist circumference >35.5 inches (88 cm) and 39.5 inches (99 cm), respectively, have an increased risk of cardiovascular disease. BMI and waist circumference can be used to assist the therapist in stratifying the risk of diseases such as diabetes, hypertension, and cardiovascular disease.[83] The authors suspect that nutritional status and body composition are not commonly assessed or considered when working with the older adult patient, but these factors have significant consequences to the rehabilitation process. It has been documented that older adults have a significant reduction in neuromuscular recruitment and muscle mass that was not recovered with rehabilitation after a 2-week period of immobility when compared to a young group of subjects with a similar prior level of activity.[67] More recently there has been an increased focus on muscle mass, nutrition, and function in hospitalized patients. Several studies have shown that an older adult can lose up to 35% to 40% of their muscle mass while hospitalized with a critical illness and more than 50% fail to recover to baseline functional levels.[85] For this reason the therapist needs to consider how the level of protein stores and current nutritional status, presence of sarcopenia, and prior level of function will impact the recovery of muscle performance and functional outcomes.[86]

According to the National Health Statistics reports, the five main causes of hospitalization among older adults are

CAD, HF, pneumonia, urinary tract infections (UTIs)/sepsis, and dizziness/falls.[87,88] Of late, hospital admissions for adults older than age 65 years continue to rise, despite the downward trend among those younger than age 65 years. Forty percent of hospital admissions are of patients over the age of 60 years, and more than 40% will suffer a new activities of daily living (ADL) or instrumental activities of daily living (IADL) limitation, while only 50% recover to their preadmission level of function, which leads to a higher level of institutionalization and mortality.[3,4] With heart disease being the leading cause of death in the United States, it is important to risk-stratify your patients and evaluate and educate them to optimize health. Although the other main causes for admission are also prevalent, they may be the sequelae to heart disease once an older adult is admitted to the hospital. The following section will cover all these topics in more detail.

Coronary Artery Disease

Coronary artery disease is the leading cause of morbidity and mortality in the older adult, with the highest incidence between the ages of 65 and 84 years.[89] One out of every four deaths is related to heart disease and 80% of all deaths related to CAD are in individuals older than age 65 years.

There is a wealth of research linking risk factors to the development of atherosclerosis, and there are gender and age differences that the clinician should be aware of when developing the exercise prescription and care plan. Cardiac risk factors in the young-old (age 75 years or younger) appear similar to those of middle-aged adults and include diabetes and smoking. Elevated low-density lipoproteins (LDLs) and total cholesterol are independent risk factors associated with CAD for individuals younger than age 75 years; however, this risk is lower after the age of 85 years. A low level of high-density lipoproteins (HDLs) along with elevated total cholesterol carries a higher risk for CAD in women than men.[90] The incidence of systolic hypertension increases with age along with the various changes that affect arterial function. With age, there is an increase in arterial stiffness and wall thickness that leads to a decrease in the compliance of the arteries and arterioles. There is also endothelial dysfunction that leads to an increase in substances that cause vascular constriction as well as the increase in leukocytes and platelet adherence and migration.[91,92] Untreated HTN leads to left ventricle hypertrophy, which happens to be an independent factor of CAD in the older adult. Left ventricular hypertrophy then results in a decrease in the compliance of the heart to allow for proper filling and ejection, and a subsequent increase in oxygen demand of the myocardium.[92] These changes increase the risk of myocardial ischemia and cellular loss, potentially evolving into HF.

Aging is also associated with an increase in inactivity and obesity, which are also clear risk factors for CAD, but there is a decreased link to mortality for the older adult in comparison to the younger adult.[67,93] The increase in obesity with aging is due to a reduction in activity level, excessive caloric intake, a decrease in muscle mass, and lower basal metabolic rates. Obesity is linked to chronic diseases such as diabetes, cancer, and atherosclerosis and is associated with an increase in functional impairments.[93,94] According to a study by Abdelaal et al., obesity is also linked to an increased mortality affecting life expectancy.[94] Besides inactivity being linked to obesity, inactivity is also associated with a reduction in muscle mass, activity intolerance, and functional limitations.[95] The reduction in muscle mass is independently a predictor of higher mortality rates in older adults.[96]

Coronary artery disease compromises the blood flow to the myocardium. An imbalance between oxygen supply and demand initially results in myocardial ischemia and may lead to myocardial necrosis if the imbalance is not resolved. Angina in the older adult typically does not present itself with the normal symptoms. After the age of 74 years, patients commonly report signs and symptoms including general weakness, dyspnea, fatigue, syncope, and a decrease in mental status, and there is no gender difference in presentation and common reports.[97] Angina can be classified as stable or unstable. Stable angina refers to typical or predicted symptoms upon exertion over time for patients with a diagnosis of CAD. Unstable angina means there is a progression in symptoms with exertion or the patient is experiencing angina at rest.

If CAD progresses to the point where blood flow to the myocardium becomes significantly compromised, the patient is at risk for acute coronary syndrome (ACS) or a myocardial event. The risk of ACS can be from a severe imbalance of oxygen demand and supply during exertion or a further decrease in perfusion. Acute coronary syndrome refers to unstable angina, non-ST elevation myocardial infarction (NSTEMI), or ST-elevation myocardial infarction (STEMI). With ACS in the older adult, there is a reduction in incidence of ST-segment elevation, from 85% of patients younger than age 65 years to less than 35% in patients older than age 84 years. There is also an increase in respiratory failure, syncope, and stroke associated with myocardial infarction and an increase in mortality rates for the older adult.[97,98]

Exercise testing and cardiac catheterization are the principal procedures used to diagnose CAD. During graded exercise testing, the clinician attempts to induce myocardial ischemia and observe the onset of angina along with changes in the 12-lead ECG for diagnostic testing purposes. The pattern of ECG changes on the 12-lead ECG can determine the wall that is underperfused. (For example, ECG changes in leads II and III and augmented aVF leads suggest inferior wall impairment.) Box 14.7 lists the signs and symptoms of CAD. The gold standard for CAD diagnosis is cardiac catheterization, which examines the patency of the coronary arteries. Cardiac enzymes will be very important for diagnostic purposes and to

BOX 14.7 Signs and Symptoms of Coronary Artery Disease

Vitals	• Varies; dependent on degree and stability of coronary artery disease/acute coronary syndrome (ACS) • Heart rate and blood pressure will typically be elevated at time of ACS • Pulse rate may become irregular • Tachypnea associated with pulmonary edema, anxiety, and pain
Auscultation	• Rales associated with pulmonary edema • S3 and S4 cardiac sounds associated with contractility dysfunction
Palpation	• Apical pulse will shift to left with left ventricular hypertrophy • Peripheral edema, jugular vein dysfunction with heart failure
Arterial blood gases	• Varies
Observation	• ↑ Work of breathing • Facial distress
Exercise tolerance	• Reduction in tolerance • Reports of angina • ST-segment depression with ischemia • ST-segment elevation with cell injury

determine extent of injury. Clinical findings upon examination will vary depending on the degree of CAD and its stability.

Heart Failure

Heart failure develops when cardiac output cannot meet the metabolic needs of the body. Heart failure typically is associated with a functional or structural defect such as valvular disease, CAD, or hypertrophic cardiomyopathy.[98] There are approximately 5.7 million individuals in the United States who have been diagnosed with HF, and half of those will die within 5 years of diagnosis.[99] The prevalence of HF increases with age, with 10.3% of individuals aged 65 to 74 years versus 20.7% of those aged 85 years and older; 960,000 individuals are diagnosed with HF annually, and approximately 300,000 individuals die annually with the primary diagnosis of HF.[98,99]

The most common cause of HF is ischemic left ventricular dysfunction secondary to CAD, with hypertension as the second-leading cause.[100] More recently it has been recommended that heart failure be classified by the function of the left ventricle, heart failure with reduced left ventricular function (HFrEF) or heart failure with preserved left ventricular function (HFpEF). Heart failure with reduced left ventricular function is also referred to as systolic failure, where the ejection fraction is low. The heart's inability to relax to allow for sufficient filling, the impairment with HFpEF, is commonly referred to as diastolic failure. Providers can also describe HF as heart failure with borderline function (HFpHF, borderline), where the left ventricular ejection fraction is 41% to 49% and the prognosis is similar to HFpLV. Likewise, HF can be described as heart failure with improving function (HFpLV, improved with serial testing documenting improvements in function). In clinical practice clinicians are still referring to heart failure as right ventricular or left ventricular failure. In most cases, individuals have components of both ventricular dysfunction or both phases of cardiac cycle (systolic and diastolic) dysfunction.

In HFrEF, the left ventricular wall, which typically begins in a hypertrophic state owing to the presence of HTN, progressively dilates to enlarge the chamber. This dilated state initially aids in contractility by increasing the stretch of the myocardium but over time leads to further myocardial dysfunction and insufficient ejection of blood into the systemic circulation to meet the body's demands. The ejection fraction, percentage of end-diastolic volume ejected per beat, which is normally 50% to 70%, is depressed to less than 40% with systolic dysfunction. In HFpEF or diastolic dysfunction, the left ventricle EF is normal, although it accounts for at least 50% of HF in the older adults.[100–102] However, with diastolic dysfunction, the ventricle walls thicken with a normal or slightly smaller chamber size and reduce the myocardium's ability to relax to allow sufficient filling. Heart failure with normal EF is commonly associated with chronic HTN with left ventricular hypertrophy.[96,102]

Clinically, the signs and symptoms of HF are associated with the type of dysfunction: Either the myocardium is causing insufficient filling of the ventricles leading to an increase in venous blood volume or the ventricular contraction is unable to sufficiently eject the blood forward into the arterial circulation. See Box 14.8 for a list of the signs and symptoms of HF. In general, the most

BOX 14.8 Signs and Symptoms Associated with Heart Failure

Right Ventricle	Left Ventricle
Diastolic Dysfunction	***Diastolic Dysfunction***
Jugular vein distension	Dyspnea
Liver engorgement	Tachypnea
Peripheral edema	Cough
	Wheezing
	Rales
	S3 abnormal heart sound
	Systolic murmur
	Hypoxemia
	Orthopnea
Systolic Dysfunction	***Systolic Dysfunction***
Dyspnea	Fatigue
Desaturation	Angina
Cyanosis	Activity intolerance
Tachypnea	Exertional dyspnea
Hypoxia	Narrow pulse pressure
	Decreased mental status
	Decreased urination
	Cool, pale, diaphoresis

common symptoms related to HF are fatigue, shortness of breath, and decreased physical capacity. The clinician needs to recognize that most patients present with a mixture of signs and symptoms because HF typically affects the function of both ventricles.

To clinically assess diastolic dysfunction of the right ventricle, the physical therapist should inspect for pitting edema, commonly of the lower extremities. It is important to document not only the score but also the degree of edema. In the pitting edema scale, a 0 means no pitting edema noted and goes up to a 4, which means the pitted impression remains for longer than 30 seconds. Venous engorgement can also be assessed by examining jugular vein distention. The external jugular vein should rarely be noticeable while the patient breathes comfortably in the sitting position. If the vein is very prominent while the patient is sitting or is distended more than 3 cm above the horizontal line level to the sternal angle with the patient reclined to 45 degrees, it is positive for right ventricle dysfunction. The clinical findings for diastolic dysfunction of the left ventricle are commonly found upon assessment of the pulmonary system, with dependent rales consistent with interstitial edema, and a nonproductive cough with high-pitched wheezing. Often, there is an additional low-pitched heart sound, S3, which can be heard over the left chest wall using light contact of the bell of the stethoscope. The patient may also report orthopnea, or the need to have the upper body elevated while in the supine position secondary to an inability to lay completely flat without progressive shortness of breath. This is most commonly experienced at night and may suggest the level of decompensation.

Patients with systolic dysfunction of the right ventricle commonly present with pulmonary symptoms like dyspnea, desaturation, and tachypnea. Systolic dysfunction of the left ventricle is associated with fatigue and a decrease in activity tolerance, and therefore it is important that the physical therapist complete an assessment of muscular, cardiovascular, and pulmonary endurance, and monitor vitals including pulse rate and regularity during activity and at the peak exercise stage as well as during the recovery phase.

Pneumonia

Pneumonia is an acute inflammation of the lungs caused by a bacterial, viral, or fungal pathogen. The normal defense mechanism of the respiratory system, a mucociliary blanket of macrophages, fails to keep the lower respiratory tract sterile, causing an accumulation of exudate in the small bronchioles and alveoli. The inflammatory process is then activated, along with the immune response, causing localized edema. A vicious cycle develops between the immune response and the infectious growth. With an increase in alveolar edema, the immune cells' ability to phagocytize the invader will be impaired. The collection of edema, RBCs, and WBCs will consolidate, leaving the lung tissue unable to perform ventilation and perfusion. This infection can also spread to other segments of the lungs as well as to the pleural space and pericardium.[103] Pneumonia is the sixth-leading cause of death for community-dwelling individuals and the second-leading type of hospital-acquired infection behind urinary tract infections in patients between the ages of 64 and 85 years, and the second-leading diagnosis for individuals older than age 85 years.[104–106] Pneumonia can be classified by the infectious agent (bacterial, viral, fungal) or by the environment (community, hospital, ventilator associated) in which the patient became infected with the agent that produces the pneumonia. The type of classification can aid the provider in the pharmacologic intervention. Pneumonia can also be classified as the environment in which the individual contracted the infection. This system allows health care professionals to identify specific interventions to treat, minimize, and prevent the common characteristics of the environmental setting.

Community-acquired pneumonia (CAP) is an infection that occurs while the patient is living out in the community or the infection manifests itself within the first 72 hours after hospitalization. CAP has an incidence rate of 8.4 cases per 1000 for individuals between the ages of 60 and 69 years, and 48.5 cases per 1000 for individuals older than age 90 years.[107] Hospital-acquired pneumonia (HAP) as defined by the American Thoracic Society is pneumonia that is acquired while the individual is in the hospital or a resident of some other type of institutional care facility, or an individual who has been exposed to a family member with a multidrug resistance.[108] Approximately 8% to 10% of all hospital admissions involve an HAP for the older adult population, which accounts for roughly 50% of all diagnoses of sepsis and is associated with a 33% mortality rate.[109,110]

The typical clinical presentation for pneumonia includes a fever and a productive cough with sputum production that is usually yellowish, green, or rust colored. The patient may also present with dyspnea, tachycardia, tachypnea, and hypoxemia. Typically, there may be an elevated WBC count, but this is not always seen in the older adult. In most cases, a positive sputum culture will identify the infectious agent. Diagnosis is made based on symptoms and a positive finding of infiltrates or consolidation on chest x-ray. There may be reports of chest wall pain, pleuritis, hemoptysis, or dyspnea, and if sufficient lung tissue is affected by the pneumonia with or without an underlying pulmonary disease, the patient may desaturate at rest or with exertion. The older adult, however, may present with more atypical signs and symptoms, including a change in mental status, anorexia, decrease in function and activity tolerance, falls, incontinence, and an elevated HR.[111,112] The physical therapist should be on the alert for the presence of pneumonia within 30 days of hospital discharge and when the symptoms described previously occur.

There are multiple factors about the age-related changes to the pulmonary system that explain the higher incidence of pneumonia with advanced age. In the upper airway, there is a natural reduction in mucociliary function and oropharyngeal clearance, increasing the risk of aspiration. In the lower airways, there is also a decrease in the cellular and humoral immune response and phagocytosis.[108] These changes reduce the ability of the bronchial system to immobilize pathogens and clear the airways. Older adults also are more susceptible to pneumonia after surgery secondary to the depressive effects of anesthesia and the number and severity of comorbidities.[107]

Aspiration has been clearly identified as a common contributing factor to the development of pneumonia. Aspiration is associated with malnutrition, tube feeding, contracture of cervical extensor muscles, and use of depressant medications.[103] Other events have also been linked to aspiration, including dysphagia due to loss of dentition, poor dental hygiene, decreased saliva production, and weakening of the muscles of mastication. Aging is associated with a delay in the neural processing needed to perform the proper swallowing sequence and decreased sensation of the oral cavity. Finally, there is an increased incidence of aspiration in the presence of Parkinson disease, cerebral vascular accident, gastroesophageal reflux disease, connective tissue disorders, and Alzheimer disease.[103,107]

Once the patient has been treated for acute pneumonia, it is important for the physical therapist to objectively assess activity tolerance through some form of exercise test (e.g., the 6-minute walk test or a bike or treadmill test). These data can be used to ensure stable vitals with exertion, rule out desaturation, and document activity tolerance so the rehabilitation plan can be appropriately prescribed. See Box 14.9 for clinical evaluation findings associated with pneumonia in the older adult.

BOX 14.9 Clinical Evaluation Findings Associated with Pneumonia

Vitals	Tachycardia Tachypnea Hypotension Dyspnea Desaturation
Auscultation	Diminished normal breath sounds Rales Low-pitched wheezes in presence of thick secretions High-pitched wheezes (associated with aspiration) Bronchial breath sounds (associated with consolidated pneumonia)
Palpation	Increased tactile fremitus Dull percussion over consolidation Possible ↓ chest wall excursion
Arterial blood gases	↓ PaO_2 Possible altered $PaCO_2$
Observation	↑ Work of breathing Facial distress Cyanosis
Temperature	Fever

BOX 14.10 Reasons Patients Have an Increased Risk of Urinary Tract Infection[117–119]

Female sex	Urinary obstruction
Prolonged catheterization	Kidney stones
Errors in catheter care	Enlarged prostate
Weakened pelvic floor musculature	Alzheimer disease
Diabetes	Parkinson disease
Multiple sclerosis	History of neurogenic bladder
Spinal cord injuries	History of stroke

Urinary Tract Infections

Urinary tract infections are the second most common type of infection among older adults behind respiratory infections and have become a major clinical issue regardless of current health and mobility status, place of residence (home or nursing home), or number of comorbidities.[113] UTIs account for one-third of all infections found in nursing home residents and fortunately have a significantly lower mortality rate than those with pneumonia.[114,115] With age, there are a multitude of reasons that can put a person at risk of developing a UTI including comorbidities that affect the bladder's nerve supply (diabetes, multiple sclerosis, and spinal cord injuries), urinary flow obstructions from kidney stones and tumors, prolonged catheter use, and weakened pelvic floor musculature from pregnancy in women and enlarged prostate in men.[116] Patients with Alzheimer disease, Parkinson disease, a stroke history, or neurogenic bladders may also not fully empty their bladder and are prone to UTIs.[117] Box 14.10 lists common comorbidities that increase the older adult's susceptibility for a UTI.[117–119]

The urinary tract is usually sterile, except for the most distal portion of the urethra.[119] The urinary tract is designed to prevent the spread of bacteria with the outflow of urine; however, with age, physical and functional changes increase the risk of bacteria in the urinary tract that can lead to an infection. Urinary tract infections primarily start in the lower portion of the urethra. If untreated, an infection of the urethra can affect other structures of the urinary system such as the bladder, ureters, or kidneys.

According to Liang, urinary stasis is the primary contributor to UTIs in the older adult.[117] In older women, there is a decrease in the strength of the pelvic floor musculature from prior pregnancies and a change in estrogen levels that contribute to urinary stasis and incontinence. Older men, on the other hand, have decreased bladder emptying due to obstruction secondary to benign prostatic hypertrophy.[119] Regardless of the reason for decreased urine flow, bacterial colonization is the result of urinary stasis. Also, the change in the normal vagina flora in women and bacterial prostatitis in men contributes to recurrent infections.

Having an indwelling catheter is another risk factor in the development of a UTI. Hazelett et al.,[120] in a retrospective study, determined that 73% of patients who received an indwelling catheter in the emergency department were 65+ years old. Of those patients, 28% were diagnosed with a UTI during their hospital stay; however, 59% of those were diagnosed in the emergency department and therefore prior to receiving the catheter. This study suggests that many of the older patients with catheters who are diagnosed with a UTI may, in fact, have had the UTI prior to receiving the indwelling catheter. This is somewhat contrary to common belief, but it demonstrates that older adults do not present in the same manner as their younger counterparts.[120] There are many types of bacteria that can cause UTIs in noncatheterized patients. However, the bacteria are usually a single isolate of *Escherichia coli*, *Proteus*, or *Klebsiella*. However, in patients with chronic indwelling catheters, the bacteria are usually polymicrobial of *E. coli*, *Proteus*, *Providencia*, *Enterococcus*, *Pseudomonas*, and *Enterobacter*.[116]

Symptoms such as pain with urination, increased frequency, persistent urge to urinate, and hematuria, which are typically used to diagnose a UTI in the younger population, cannot necessarily be used with the older adult because of the changes mentioned earlier. For example, an older male with prostatic hypertrophy may have difficulty urinating, strong and sudden urges to urinate, pain, and hematuria. These are also all symptoms of a UTI; therefore, it is difficult to determine the diagnosis of UTI in the presence of other genitourinary comorbities.[121]

Diagnosis of a UTI in the younger population requires 10^5 colony-forming units (CFUs)/mL with associated symptoms as described earlier.[118] Diagnosis can be made in older adults with a bacterial colony count of 10^2 or 10^3 CFUs if they are also symptomatic.[117] However, with older patients, diagnosis is not that easy as they frequently present without symptoms or have UTI symptoms such as decreased urine flow, which can be a symptom of prostatic hypertrophy. Frequently, the first symptom that is noted is acute confusion. Other symptoms are a sudden functional decline, anorexia, and delirium. It is important to diagnose a UTI early in the older patient because it can quickly spread to the kidneys and to the blood, causing sepsis. Juthani-Mehta reports that diagnostic criteria for nursing home residents who do not have a catheter include having three of the following clinical signs or symptoms: (1) a fever of 100.4°F or greater; (2) new or change in burning of urination, frequency, or urgency; (3) new flank or suprapubic pain; (4) change in color, consistency, or cloudiness of urine; and (5) change in mental or functional status.[119] For nursing home residents who have catheters, two of the following characteristics must be present: (1) fever as noted earlier, (2) new flank or suprapubic pain, (3) change in the characteristic (cloudiness, consistency) of urine, and (4) change in mentation or functional status.[119]

The physical therapist needs to consider the presence of a UTI during the evaluation and treatment process and with any change in mentation because for the older patient with a UTI, acute delirium and decline in mobility may be transient and not appropriately represent the patient's true functional status. The therapist will need to constantly reassess function and needs to make the most appropriate modification to the treatment plan as the infection is medically treated. A thorough discussion of bladder issues in older adults occurs elsewhere in this text.

Sepsis

Recently *sepsis* was redefined as a "life-threatening organ dysfunction caused by a deregulated host response to infection."[122] In lay terms it means that sepsis is a life-threatening condition that occurs when the body's response to an infection actually injures the body's own tissues and organs.[122] Septic shock is a subset of sepsis where the individual is additionally suffering from circulatory dysfunction as defined by requiring vasopressors to maintain a mean arterial pressure of >65 mmHg and metabolic abnormalities defined as a lactate level of >18 mg/dL that further increase the risk of mortality.[123] Patients who become septic usually present with hypotension and a fever >101.3°F and have an elevated heart rate >90 bpm, a respiratory rate >20 breaths per minute, and a probable or confirmed infection from cultures. It is critical to recognize the signs of sepsis because it is associated with a high mortality rate; the incidence is on rise, which is likely related to the aging population; and survivors of sepsis can suffer prolonged psychological, cognitive, and functional deficits, referred to as post–intensive care syndrome (PICS). If sepsis is not diagnosed and the source of the infection not identified, it can progress to severe sepsis or septic shock. Box 14.11 lists the signs and symptoms of sepsis, severe sepsis, and septic shock.[123–125]

Many older adults have multiple comorbidities, making diagnosis of sepsis difficult as the clinical picture

BOX 14.11 Signs and Symptoms of Sepsis, Severe Sepsis, and Septic Shock[123–125]

Sepsis	Severe Sepsis	Septic Shock
• Fever >101.3°F • Heart rate >90 beats per minute • Respiratory rate >20 breaths per minute • Probable or confirmed infection	• Mottled skin • ↓ Urine output • Mental status change • ↓ Platelet count • Respiratory difficulties • Changes in cardiac function	• All signs of severe sepsis • Extremely low blood pressure

may represent infections of other systems.[123] Diagnosis of sepsis is important as there are many conditions that can mimic sepsis, including hemorrhage, PE, myocardial infarction, pancreatitis, diabetic ketoacidosis, and diuretic-induced hypovolemia, just to name a few. It is important to get a blood culture that might determine the underlying bacterial infection that needs to be treated. However, a CBC is not always helpful because results may mimic the aforementioned conditions, which are not technically sepsis. Along with urinalysis, intravenous lines should also be cultured to fully rule out the source. A computed tomography scan is important to rule out pneumonia and PE.[124]

OTHER MEDICAL ISSUES

There are a multitude of reasons an older adult might present with a decline in function and health. Following is a brief description of medical issues that may compromise the older adult's health, result in a decline in function, or lead to further medical complications contributing to increased morbidity and mortality rates.

Dizziness

Dizziness is a common complaint of the older adult. The root cause of dizziness can be difficult to determine because it can be caused by multiple etiologies, including vestibular, visual, or proprioceptive system dysfunctions.[126] It is very important to determine the cause because treatment varies greatly depending on the system involved. A study by Uneri and Polat determined that the most common causes of dizziness in older adults are benign paroxysmal positional vertigo, vestibulopathy (an abnormality of the vestibular apparatus), migraine vestibulopathy, and migraines.[127]

Acute dizziness is among the most common causes for adults visiting the emergency department.[128–130] However, emergency departments are not very accurate in diagnosing dizziness.[131] To ensure proper diagnosis, appropriate screening and testing is of the utmost importance. There are many diagnostic procedures that can be performed, including a thorough physical examination, provocation studies, and neurologic, visual, vestibular, cardiac, and psychiatric examination. The patient report will assist in ascertaining a clear picture of the symptoms and precipitating events.

Vertigo, the most common cause of dizziness among the older adult population, is defined as the abnormal sensation of movement that is brought on by certain positions. There are many causes of vertigo, including trauma, idiopathic, and inner ear diseases. Box 14.12 lists some of the common causes of vertigo. Diagnosis of vertigo can be easily made, as nystagmus is commonly seen in the eyes.[127,131,132] The direction of eye movement is indicative of the part of the inner ear that is affected.[131] It is important to assess the direction as horizontal nystagmus is generally indicative of peripheral vertigo; however, vertical nystagmus can be a sign of a central cause and is usually more serious.[132] Vertigo can be a symptom of basilar artery migraine, so migraines also need to be ruled out as the cause.[132] Patients with vertigo will often report a "spinning" sensation. Balance is dependent on sensory cues and vestibular function, both central and peripheral. Therefore, inner ear problems and gait disturbances affect balance and increase the risk of falls.

BOX 14.12 Common Causes of Vertigo[127,131,132]

Idiopathic	Otosclerosis
Trauma	Sudden sensorineural hearing loss
Ear diseases	Central nervous system disease
Chronic otitis media	Vertebrobasilar insufficiency
Vestibular neuronitis	Acoustic neuroma
Meniere disease	Cervical vertigo

Near syncope, or fainting, is often related to cardiovascular disease rather than to a peripheral or central nervous system disorder. If syncope is present, a search for a cardiac etiology should be initiated. An ECG and a Holter ambulatory cardiac monitor are obtained to evaluate for rhythm disturbances. Syncope also requires a careful physical examination and an echocardiogram to determine if there are blood flow abnormalities. Faintness during standing or bowel movements may relate to orthostatic hypotension or to a Valsalva maneuver, respectively.

Inability to describe symptoms may be related to dementia or psychiatric disorders. Individuals with dementia may be trying to describe the confusion they experience and not true dizziness. An evaluation for depression, anxiety, and dementia may be included in the differential diagnosis, if symptoms are difficult to describe. Finally, iatrogenic postural hypotension that causes positional dizziness is more common in older adults than in younger adults because of the increased prevalence of polypharmacy. Medications are always implicated initially as causative agents, until proven otherwise. These include antihypertensive agents, diuretics, and drugs that cause sedation.

With age, there are many changes that happen to balance, perception, and sensation as well as neurologic and skeletal functioning. Chronic illnesses like diabetes can also contribute to sensory deficits.[127] Polypharmacy and orthostatic hypotension are also common causes and can be differential diagnoses for dizziness. Whatever the cause, dizziness is a precursor to falls, which can be life-threatening for the older adult. Proper examination and treatment of dizziness can aid in reducing the incidence of falls and the morbidity and mortality from them.

Dehydration

Dehydration is a widespread problem in the older adult and directly increases rates of morbidity and mortality. Dehydration is a costly individual and societal problem.

Nearly 40% of all hospitalization admissions in older adults are associated with dehydration but may go unrecognized.[133,134]

There are many reasons the older adult is susceptible to dehydration. First, there is a blunted thirst mechanism, which leads to a decreased desire to drink.[135] Second, there is a reduction in total body fluid with the reduction in muscle mass and an increase in body fat. Also, a decrease in renal function that concentrates the urine prevents the body from retaining enough fluid to avert dehydration. Finally, physical and mental decline also can lead to dehydration.[135]

Dehydration is categorized by the relationship between free water and sodium and can be caused by many factors. Hypertonic dehydration occurs when there is a greater loss of water when compared to sodium loss. This type of dehydration is more common in the presence of infection or exposure to hot environmental temperatures. In isotonic dehydration, there is an equal loss of water and sodium, and vomiting and diarrhea are the two most common causes. Hypotonic dehydration is caused by a greater loss of sodium than water. The use of diuretics is the most common cause of hypotonic dehydration, and hypotonic dehydration is the most common cause of dehydration in the older adult.[136] The most significant laboratory abnormality is sodium imbalance and should be carefully monitored.

There are multiple risk factors associated with dehydration, including advanced age; being of the female gender, because of the higher percentage body fat; and a BMI <21 and >27. Individuals with dementia, history of stroke, urinary incontinence, infections, use of steroids, polypharmaceutical use, and decrease in functional independence also have an increased risk of dehydration.[134]

Presenting symptoms of dehydration may include confusion, lethargy, rapid weight loss, and functional decline, all of which will interfere with rehabilitation goals. Therefore, the physical therapist is in a good position to monitor for dehydration and alert the medical team to the emergence of this syndrome. See Box 14.13 for the signs and symptoms of dehydration.

BOX 14.13 Signs and Symptoms of Dehydration

Examination	Clinical Signs and Symptoms
Interview	• ↓ Cognitive function and mental status
Observation	• Dry mucosa
Palpation	• ↓ Skin turgor
Vitals	• Tachycardia
	• ↓ Blood pressure
	• Orthostatic hypotension
	• Weight loss in short time, <1 kg/day
Jugular vein distention	• In supine, nonappreciable external jugular vein
Function	• ↓ Muscle strength, balance, and function

Metabolic Syndrome

Metabolic syndrome is characterized as a cluster of no fewer than three cardiovascular risk factors that are strongly associated with myocardial infarction. Risk factors from the National Cholesterol Education Program Adult Treatment Panel III Report include increased abdominal fat, high levels of triglycerides, low levels of HDLs, HTN, and an elevated level of fasting plasma glucose.[137] The International Diabetes Foundation definition criteria are slightly different, with abdominal circumference being >94 cm for men and >80 cm for women, and fasting glucose level >100 mg/dL.[137,138] See Box 14.14 for specific criteria, which may differ according to source.[137–139]

It is estimated that around 30% of the U.S. population has metabolic syndrome,[137] which increases their morbidity and mortality from a cardiovascular event including stroke, myocardial infarction, and HF. Metabolic syndrome was also referred to as syndrome X, but the term *insulin resistance syndrome* (IRS) is more recently used to label this clinical issue.[137,138]

Aging is associated with an increased incidence of obesity due to a reduction in activity level, a decrease in muscle mass, and an increase in visceral fat mass.[25,84] The link between obesity and metabolic syndrome, or IRS, is not fully understood, but obesity is associated with increases in free fatty acids and triglycerides and an increase in inflammatory cytokines that is also linked to IRS.[139] Visceral adipocytes produce resistin, proinflammatory substances, interleukin-6, tumor necrosis factor, and plasminogen activator inhibitor-1, which promotes the development of insulin resistance as well as HTN and dyslipidemia.[138,140]

Insulin resistance and abdominal obesity appear to be predictors for the development of metabolic syndrome. Insulin resistance occurs when the cells become less sensitive and eventually resistant to insulin, which leads to the inability of glucose to be absorbed by the cells. A vicious cycle develops with higher levels of glucose that leads to the release of more insulin. With the elevated release of free fatty acids, there is a reduction of glucose oxidation

BOX 14.14 Clinical Criteria for Metabolic Syndrome[137–139]

Risk Factors	Criteria
Abdominal obesity	
Men	>102 cm
Women	>88 cm
Triglycerides	≥150 mg/dL (1.69 mmol/L)
High-density lipoprotein (HDL)	
Men	>40 mg/dL (1.04 mmol/L)
Women	>50 mg/dL (1.30 mmol/L)
Blood pressure	
Systolic	>130 mmHg
Diastolic	>85 mmHg
Fasting glucose	>110 mg/dL

and glucose transport inducing liver production of LDLs that elevates triglycerides and lowers HDL levels.[137] With the increase in free fatty acids, the liver is stimulated to produce more LDLs, release more triglycerides, and lower HDL levels.[137,138]

With obesity and the normal effects of aging, there is an increase in HTN. There is a further increase in the incidence of HTN with a BMI >27 in people older than 40 years.[141] Older adults are among one of the high-risk groups for a cardiovascular event along with African Americans.[142]

Finally, there is an increase in incidence of type 2 diabetes and cardiovascular events in older adults with IRS. It is estimated that 29 million older adults will be diagnosed with type 2 diabetes by 2050.[140] Diabetes itself is defined as a fasting glucose level >126 mg/dL, or a 2-hour postprandial glucose level >200 mg/dL after a 75-g glucose load, or symptoms of diabetes plus casual plasma glucose concentration of 200 mg/dL.[137] Prediabetes is defined as having a fasting plasma glucose level between 100 and 125 mg/dL and a 2-hour postprandial glucose between 140 and 199 mg/dL. Diabetes is an independent risk factor for the older adult suffering a serious cardiovascular event and increases mortality and morbidity rates.[25] The reader is directed to review the Coronary Artery Disease and Heart Failure sections within this chapter for the consequences of cardiovascular risk factors including obesity, HTN, dyslipidemia, and glucose–insulin dysfunction.

PREVENTION

The stratification process is a crucial step in disease prevention and in assessing the risk of experiencing a medical event during exercise or exertion. Every physical therapy plan should address prevention, starting with the initial examination and evaluation regardless of clinical setting. It is important that the therapist completes a thorough interview to determine the level of prevention the therapist should address for the primary and secondary diagnoses.

The ultimate goal of prevention is to optimize health and decrease functional limitations and impairments. All members of the team should address prevention and that, ultimately, should lead to the reduction in health care utilization and costs. The three levels of prevention are primary, secondary, and tertiary.

- *Primary*: focuses on instilling healthy behaviors and reducing risk factors by intervening prior to the biological signs of a disease. An example of primary prevention for CAD would be to instruct your client to eat well, avoid smoking, exercise routinely to control blood pressure, and control weight to minimize risk of diabetes. Another example may be the initiation of a weight training program for an older adult patient to improve muscle strength for the prevention of osteoporosis.
- *Secondary*: the pathology or disease is present, but intervention is focused on behavior modification to manage the disease. The goal is to control progression of the disease, improve strength, avoid loss of function, and minimize or eliminate pain. In treating clients already diagnosed with CAD, the physical therapist would educate them on the reduction or elimination of risk factors (see Box 14.4), activities to reduce blood pressure and cholesterol levels, importance of monitoring for diabetes, and management of the disease by percutaneous coronary intervention.
- *Tertiary*: the patient has a disease and is also afflicted with dysfunction associated with that disease including a decrease in activity tolerance and function. The focus of tertiary prevention is on functional mobility and education of signs or symptoms of the disease and the prevention of further deterioration.[143] An example of tertiary prevention while caring for a patient with HF due to CAD would be to manage the cardiac dysfunction, protect renal function, medicate to improve cardiac function, control food and fluid intake, and introduce job simplification and energy conservation techniques.

If we consider CAD the leading cause of deaths in the United States, the United Kingdom, and Europe, 83% of deaths related to ischemic heart disease involve patients older than age 65 years and the mortality rates continue to rise substantially after 75 years of age. In the geriatric population, there is a shift in the significance of typical risk factors with a reduction in the incidence of smoking and diabetes, and an increase in hypertension, sedentary lifestyle, and obesity.[144]

It should be very common for physical therapists in all settings to address risk factor modifications for patients with known cardiac disease or HF, with the goal to minimize functional limitations and decrease hospitalizations. An example of prevention across the spectrum: Primary prevention could focus on prevention of osteoporosis and diet to maintain proper weight and maintain muscle mass. Secondary prevention may include strength, aerobic exercise, and functional training to minimize skeletal muscle atrophy, promote airway clearance to minimize the effects of atelectasis, and provide proper nutrition to promote general health to avoid exacerbation of HF. Tertiary prevention may focus on functional training and education about signs and symptoms of HF, including progressive exercise intolerance, fatigue, and shortness of breath. Prevention in the young older adult, aged 65 to 75 years, may focus on primary or secondary prevention, including fitness, weight management, smoking cessation, and encouragement for routine lipid profiles and fasting glucose testing. In the older-old, aged 85 years or older, prevention may focus on fitness and function, hypertension control, and weight management. In any prevention program, the therapist will need to consider the age of the patient, as advanced age is associated with an increase in comorbidities.

SUMMARY

Clinical management of the health and function of the older adult is complex. It should be the common goal of all professional practitioners in geriatric health care to treat illnesses and promote optimal health. There have been two shifts in geriatric health care: an increasing attention to wellness and prevention for the older adult, and acutely ill patients are being seen by the physical therapist outside the traditional acute care hospital. The physical therapist needs a basic understanding of the common medical diagnoses that lead older adults to seek medical care and how these diagnoses affect function and quality of life. Physical therapy intervention should consist of constant screening for signs and symptoms that suggest medical concerns, adjusting rehabilitation goals to minimize functional limitations and physical impairments, education, and healthy lifestyles. Finally, the therapist needs to be an active member of the older adult's health care team to maximize health care services and ultimately maximize quality of health and outcomes.

REFERENCES

1. Heckman GA, McKelvie RS. Cardiovascular aging and exercise in healthy older adults. *Clin J Sports Med.* 2008;18(6):479–485.
2. Facts for Features: Older Americans Month: May 2017. U.S. Census Bureau. https://www.census.gov/newsroom/facts-for-features/2017/cb17-ff08.html. Updated August 3, 2018. Accessed October 25, 2018.
3. Ortman JM, Velkoff VA, Hogan H. *An aging nation: the older population in the United States: United States Census Bureau; 2014.* Current Population Reports, P25-1140, http://tinyurf.com/n54vw9e. Accessed 30 March 2015.
4. Bodilsen AC, Klasen HH, Petersen J, et al. Prediction of mobility limitations after hospitalization in older medical patients by simple measures of physical performance obtained at admission to the emergency department. *PLoS One.* 2016;11(5). e0154350.
5. HCUP Fast Stats. Healthcare Cost and Utilization Project (HCUP). November 2017. Rockville, MD: Agency for Healthcare Research and Quality. http://www.hcup-us.ahrq.gov/faststats/national/inpatientcommondiagnoses.jsp. Updated November 14, 2017. Accessed March 28, 2018.
6. Yancik R, Wesley MN, Ries LA, et al. Effect of age and comorbidity in postmenopausal breast cancer patients aged 55 years and older. *JAMA.* 2001;285(7):885–892.
7. Centers for Disease Control and Prevention. Arthritis. https://www.cdc.gov/arthritis/data_statistics/comorbidities.htm. Updated February 22, 2018. Accessed March 29, 2018.
8. Thomas V, Jones E. *The Merck manual of geriatrics.* 3rd ed. Merck & Co; 2000–2006. http://www.merck.com/mkgr/mmg/home.jsp. Accessed 11 November 2018.
9. MedlinePlus. Bethesda, MD: National Library of Medicine (US). http://medlineplus.gov/lab-tests/. Accessed November 11, 2018.
10. American Association of Clinical Chemistry. Lab tests online. http://www.labtestsonline.org. Accessed January 19, 2019.
11. Blood test results: CMP Explained. International Waldenstrom's Macroglobulinemia Foundation. https://www.iwmf.com/sites/default/files/docs/bloodcharts_cmp(1).pdf. Accessed October 22, 2018.
12. FDA. Blood serum chemistry – normal values. Investigations Operations Manual 2015. Appendix C. https://www.fda.gov/downloads/iceci/inspections/iom/ucm135835.pdf. Accessed October 22, 2018.
13. American College of Physicians. Laboratory Values. https://annualmeeting.acponline.org/sites/default/files/shared/documents/for-meeting-attendees/normal-lab-values.pdf. Accessed October 22, 2018.
14. Lee CC, Chen SY, Chang IJ, et al. Comparison of clinical manifestations and outcome of community-acquired bloodstream infections among the oldest old, elderly, and adult patients. *Medicine.* 2007;86(3):138–144.
15. Penninx BW, Pahor M, Cesari M, et al. Anemia is associated with disability and decreased physical performance and muscle strength in the elderly. *J Am Geriatr Soc.* 2004;52:719–724.
16. Guralnik JM, Eisenstaedt RS, Ferrucci L, et al. Prevalence of anemia in persons 65 years and older in the United States: evidence for a high rate of unexplained anemia. *Blood.* 2004;104(8):2263–2268.
17. Zaks GJ, Westenorp RG, Knook DL. The definition of anemia in older persons. *JAMA.* 1999;281(18):1714–1717. Pubmed PMIP:10328071.
18. Jassal SV. Clinical presentation of renal failure in the aged: chronic renal failure. *Clin Geriatr Med.* 2009;25(3):359–372.
19. Oliveira MR, Fogaca KC, Leandro-Merhi VA. Nutritional status and functional capacity of hospitalized elderly. *Nutr J.* 2009;8:54–62.
20. Hillegass E, Puthoff M, Frese EM, et al. The role of physical therapists in the management of individuals at risk for or diagnosed with venous thromboembolism – an evidence-based clinical practice guideline. *Phys Ther.* 2016;96(2):143–166.
21. Kannel WB, Wolf PA. Framingham study insights on the hazards of elevated blood pressure. *JAMA.* 2008;300(21):2545–2547.
22. Luckson M. Hypertension management in older people. *Br J Community Nurs.* 2009;15(1):17–21.
23. Troyer AK, Leach L, Strauss E. Aging and response inhibition: normative data for the Victoria Stroop test. *Aging Neurol Cogn.* 2006;13:20–35.
24. Anderson JD, Epstein FH, Meyer CH, et al. Multifactorial determinants of functional capacity in peripheral arterial disease. *J Am Coll Cardiol.* 2009;54(7):628–635.
25. Thompson WR, Gordon NF, Pascatello LS. *American College of Sports Medicine's Guidelines for Exercise Testing and Prescription.* 10th ed. Philadelphia: Wolters Kluwer/Lippincott Williams & Wilkins Health; 2017.
26. Szewczyk MT, Jawien A, Kedziora-Kornatowska K, et al. The nutritional status of older adults with and without venous ulcers: a comparative, descriptive study. *Ostomy Wound Manage.* 2008;54(9):36–40, 42.
27. Mizrahi EH, Flessig Y, Blumstein T. Admission albumin levels and functional outcomes of elderly hip fracture patients: is it that important? *Aging Clin Exp Res.* 2007;19(4):284–289.
28. Dziedzic T, Slowik A, Szczudlik A. Serum albumin level as a predictor of ischemic stroke outcomes. *Stroke.* 2004;35(6):e156–e158.
29. Physiopedia. Age related changes in cardiovascular system. https://www.physio-pedia.com/Age_related_changes_in_cardiovascular_system. Accessed May 2, 2018.
30. Jones SA, Boyett MR, Lancaster MK. Declining into failure: the age-dependent loss of the L-type calcium channel within the sinoatrial node. *Circulation.* 2007;115:1183–1190.
31. American Heart Association. Understanding Your Risk for Diabetes. http://www.heart.org/HEARTORG/Conditions/More/Diabetes/UnderstandYourRiskforDiabetes/Understand-Your-Risk-for-Diabetes_UCM_002034_Article.jsp#.Wvl31WeWyUk. Updated January 29, 2018. Accessed May 14, 2018.

32. Khan N, Afaq F, Mukhtar H. Lifestyle as risk factor for cancer: evidence from human studies. *Cancer Lett.* 2010;293(2): 133–143. https://doi.org/10.1016/j.canlet.2009.12.013.
33. National Osteoporosis Foundation. Are you at risk? https://www.nof.org/preventing-fractures/general-facts/bone-basics/are-you-at-risk/. Accessed May 14, 2018.
34. Marcantonio ER. Delirium in hospitalized older adults. *N Engl J Med.* 2017;377:1456–1466.
35. Dhalwani NN, Fahami R, Sathanapally H, Seidu S, Davies MJ, Khunti K. Association between polypharmacy and falls in older adults: a longitudinal study from England. *BMJ Open.* 2017;7(10). e016358.
36. Karandikar YS, Chaudhari SR, Dalal NP, Sharma M, Pandit VA. Inappropriate prescribing in the elderly: a comparison of two validated screening tools. *J Clin Gerontol Geriatr.* 2013;4:109–114.
37. National Council on Alcoholism and Drug Dependence. Alcohol, drug dependence and seniors. https://www.ncadd.org/about-addiction/seniors/alcohol-drug-dependence-and-seniors. Updated June 26, 2015. Accessed on May 2, 2018.
38. Inouye SK, Westendorp RG, Saczynski JS. Delirium in elderly people. *Lancet.* 2014;383:911–922.
39. Hosker C, Ward D. Hypoactive delirium. *BMJ.* 2017;357: j2047.
40. De la Cruz M, Fan J, Yennu S, et al. The frequency of missed delirium in patients referred to palliative care in a comprehensive cancer center. *Support Care Cancer.* 2015;23: 2427–2433.
41. Wei LA, Fearing MA, Sternberg EJ, et al. The confusion assessment method: a systematic review of current usage. *J Am Geriatr Soc.* 2008;56:823–830.
42. Barr J, Pandharipande PP. The pain, agitation, and delirium care bundle: synergistic benefits of implementing the 2013 Pain, Agitation, and Delirium Guidelines in an integrated and interdisciplinary fashion. *Crit Care Med.* 2013;41(9 Suppl 1): S99–115.
43. Tabet N, Howard R. Pharmacological treatment for the prevention of delirium: review of current evidence. *Int J Geriatr Psychiatry.* 2009;24:1037–1044.
44. Teale E, Young J. Multicomponent delirium prevention: not as effective as NICE suggest? *Age Ageing.* 2015;44:915–917.
45. Adelman AM. Initial evaluation of the patient with suspected dementia. *Am Fam Physician.* 2005;71:1745–1750.
46. Carey RM, Whelton PK. Prevention, detection, evaluation and management of high blood pressure in adults: synopsis of the 2017 American College of Cardiology/American Heart Association Hypertension Guideline. *Ann Intern Med.* http://annals.org/aim/fullarticle/2670318/prevention-detection-evaluation-management-high-blood-pressure-adults-synopsis-2017. Updated March 6, 2018. Accessed May 15, 2018.
47. Whelton PK, Carey RM, Aronow WS. 2017 ACC/AHA/AAPA/ABC/APhA/ASH/ASPC/NMA/PCNA guideline for the prevention, detection, evaluation, and management of high blood pressure in adults: executive summary: a report of the American College of Cardiology/American Heart Association Task Force on Clinical Practice Guidelines. *Hypertension.* 2018;71:1269–1324.
48. American College of Cardiology. New ACC/AHA High Blood Pressure Guidelines lower definition of hypertension. http://www.acc.org/latest-in-cardiology/articles/2017/11/08/11/47/mon-5pm-bp-guideline-aha-2017. Updated November 13, 2017. Accessed May 15, 2018.
49. Pickering TG, Hall JE, Appel LJ. Recommendations for blood pressure measurement in humans and experimental animals. Part 1: blood pressure measurement in humans. A statement of professional and public education of the American Heart Association Council on High Blood Pressure Research. *Hypertension.* 2005;45:142–161.
50. Weiss A, Boaz M, Beloosesky Y, et al. Pulse pressure predicts mortality in elderly patients. *J Gen Intern Med.* 2009;24(8): 893–896.
51. Gupta V, Lipsitz L. Orthostatic hypotension in the elderly: diagnosis and treatment. *Am J Med.* 2007;120:841–847.
52. Griswold ME, Heiss G, Selvin E. Association of history of dizziness and long-term adverse outcomes with early vs later orthostatic hypotension assessment times in middle-aged adults. *JAMA Intern Med.* 2017;177(9):1316–1323. https://doi.org/10.1001/jamainternmed.2017.2937.
53. Ricci F, De Caterina F, Fedorowski A. Orthostatic hypotension. *J Am Coll Cardiol.* 2015;66(7):848–860.
54. Ainsworth BE, Haskell WL, Whitt MP, et al. Compendium of physical activities: an update of activity codes and MET intensities. *Med Sci Sports Exerc.* 2000;32(9 Suppl) S498–S50.
55. Cole CR, Foody JM, Blackstone EH, et al. Heart rate recovery after submaximal exercise testing as a predictor of mortality in a cardiovascular healthy cohort. *Ann Intern Med.* 2000;132 (7):552–553.
56. Jubran A. Pulse oximetry. *Intensive Care Med.* 2004;30: 2017–2020.
57. Feiner JR, Severinghaus JW, Bickler PE. Dark skin decreases the accuracy of pulse oximeters at low saturation: the effects of oximeter probe type and gender. *Anesth Analg.* 2007;105 (6 Suppl):S18–S23.
58. Kallstrom TJ. AARC Guideline. Oxygen therapy for adults in the acute care facility: 2002 revision and update. *Respir Care.* 2002;47(6):717–720.
59. Van de Louw A, Cracco C, Cerf C, et al. Accuracy of pulse oximetry in the intensive care unit. *Intensive Care Med.* 2001;27(10):1606–1613.
60. Seifi S, Khatony A, Moradi G, Abdi A, Najafi F. Accuracy of pulse oximetry in detection of oxygen saturation in patients admitted to the intensive care unit of heart surgery: comparison of finger, toe, forehead and earlobe probes. *BMC Nursing.* 2018;17:15.
61. Schindler DM. Practical cardiac auscultation. *Crit Care Nurs.* 2007;30(2):166–180.
62. Ferns T, West S. The art of auscultation: evaluating a patient's respiratory pathology. *Br J Nurs.* 2008;17(12):772–777.
63. Moore T. Respiratory assessment in adults. *Nurs Stand.* 2008;21(49):48–56.
64. Kennedy S. Detecting changes in the respiratory status of ward patients. *Nurs Stand.* 2007;21(39):42–46.
65. Pastercamp H, Wodicka GR, Kraman SS. Effect of ambient respiratory noise on the measurement of lung sounds. *Med Biol Eng Comput.* 1999;37(4):461–465.
66. Suetta C, Hvud LG, Justesen L. Effects of aging on human skeletal muscle after immobilization and retraining. *J Appl Physiol.* 2009;107(4):1172–1180.
67. Rolland Y, Lauwers-Cames V, Christini C, et al. Difficulties with physical function associated with obesity, sarcopenia and sarcopenic-obesity in community dwelling elderly women: the EPIDOS study. *Am J Clin Nutr.* 2009;89(6) 1895-1890.
68. U.S. Department of Agriculture. Older adults. https://www.choosemyplate.gov/older-adults. Updated August 9, 2017. Accessed May 22, 2018.
69. Older individuals. Nutrition.gov. https://www.nutrition.gov/subject/life-stages/seniors. Updated May 1, 2018. Accessed May 1, 2018.
70. Drewnowski A, Evans WJ. Nutrition, physical activity and quality of life in older adults: summary. *J Gerontol Series.* 2001;2:89–94.
71. Appendix 7. Nutritional Goals for Age-Sex Groups Based on Dietary Reference Intakes and Dietary Guidelines Recommendations. Dietary Guidelines for Americans

2015-2020. https://health.gov/dietaryguidelines/2015/guidelines/appendix-7/. Accessed April 5, 2018.
72. Tufts University. Food guide pyramid for older adults. http://enews.tufts.edu/stories/777/2003/11/10/TopNutritionGuide. Updated November 10, 2003. Accessed April 5, 2018.
73. U.S. Department of Health and Human Services. Dietary guidelines for Americans. http://www.health.gov/dietaryguidelines/dga2018/document/default.htm. Accessed April 5, 2018.
74. U.S. Department of Agriculture. 2005 Dietary guidelines for Americans. http://www.health.gov/dietaryguidelines/dga2017/document/html/chapter2.htm. Accessed April 5, 2018.
75. Garcia AD, Thomas DR. Assessment and management of chronic pressure ulcers in the elderly. *Med Clin North Am.* 2006;90(5):925–944.
76. Bouillanna O, Dupont-Belmont C, Hay P, et al. Fat mass protects hospitalized elderly persons against morbidity and mortality. *Am J Clin Nutr.* 2009;90(3):505–510.
77. Barclay L. Overweight elderly have similar mortality to normal weight elderly. *J Am Geriatr Soc.* 2010;58:234–241.
78. Cawthon PM, Fox KM, Gandra SR, et al. Do muscle mass, muscle density, strength, physical function similarly influence risk of hospitalization in older adults. *J Am Geriatr Soc.* 2009;57(8):1411–1419.
79. Bianchii L, Abete P, Bellelli G, et al. Prevalence and clinical correlates of sarcopenia, identified according to the EWGSOP definition and diagnostic algorithm in hospitalized older people: the GLISTEN Study. *J Gerontol Med Sci.* 2017;72(11):1575–1581.
80. Chevalier S, Saoud F, Gray-Donald K, et al. The physical functional capacity of frail elderly persons undergoing ambulatory rehabilitation is related to their nutritional status. *J Nutr Health Aging.* 2008;12(10):721–726.
81. Hardee JP, Counts BR, Carson JA. Understanding the role of exercise in cancer cachexia therapy. *Am J Lifestyle Med.* 2019;13(1):46–60.
82. Woodrow G. Body composition analysis techniques on the aged adult: indications and limitations. *Curr Opin Clin Nutr Metab Care.* 2009;12(1):8–14.
83. American College of Sports Medicine. *ACSM's Guidelines for Exercise Testing and Prescription.* 10th ed. Baltimore, MD: Wolters Kluwer Health/Lippincott Williams & Wilkins; 2018.
84. Lopez-Candales A, Hernandez Burgos PM, Hernandez-Suarez DF, Harris D. Linking chronic inflammation with cardiovascular disease: from normal aging to the metabolic syndrome. *J Nat Sci.* 2017;3(4):e341.
85. Puthucheary ZA, McPhail MJ, Hart N. Acute muscle wasting among critically ill patients—reply. *JAMA.* 2014;311(6):622–623.
86. Needham DM, Wang W, Desai SV, et al. Intensive care unit exposures for long term outcomes research: development and description of exposures for 150 patients with acute lung injury. *J Crit Care.* 2007;22(4):275–284.
87. Pfunter A, Wier LM, Stocks C. Most frequent conditions in U.S. hospitals, 2010. HCUP. https://www.hcup-us.ahrq.gov/reports/statbriefs/sb148.pdf. Updated January 2013. Accessed October 23, 2018.
88. HCUP Fast Stats – Most Common Diagnoses for Inpatient Stays: Age 65-74 Years. https://www.hcup-us.ahrq.gov/faststats/NationalDiagnosesServlet?year1=2015&characteristic1=24&included1=0&year2=&characteristic2=0&included2=1&expansionInfoState=hide&dataTablesState=hide&definitionsState=hide&exportState=hide. Published 2015. Updated November 2017. Accessed October 23, 2018.
89. Centers for Disease Control and Prevention. Division for Heart Disease and Stroke Prevention. https://www.cdc.gov/dhdsp/data_statistics/fact_sheets/fs_heart_disease.htm. Updated August 23, 2017. Accessed April 23, 2018.
90. Aslam F, Haque A, Lee LV, et al. Hyperlipidemia in the older adults. *Clin Geriatr Med.* 2009;25:591–606.
91. Lakatta EG, Wang M, Najjar SS. Arterial aging and subclinical arterial disease are fundamentally intertwined at macroscopic and molecular levels. *Med Clin North Am.* 2009;93:583–604.
92. Murphy BP, Dunn FG. Hypertension and myocardial ischemia. *Med Clin North Am.* 2009;93:681–695.
93. Lang IA, Llewellyas DJ, Alexander K, et al. Obesity, physical function and mortality in the older adult. *J Am Geriatr Soc.* 2008;56(8):1474–1478.
94. Abdelaal M, le Roux CW, Docherty NG. Morbidity and mortality associated with obesity. *Ann Transl Med.* 2017;5(7):161.
95. DeFrances CJ, Podgornik MN. *2004 National Hospital Discharge Survey. Advance data from vital and health statistics; no. 371.* Hyattsville, MD: National Center for Health Statistics; 2006.
96. Jacobson C, Marzlin K, Webner C. *A Comprehensive Resource Manual and Study Guide for Clinical Nurses. Cardiovascular Nursing Practice.* Burien, WA: Cardiovascular Nursing Education Association; 2007.
97. Kyriakides ZS, Kourouklin S, Kontaras K. Acute coronary syndrome in the elderly. *Drugs Aging.* 2007;24(11):901–912.
98. Grady KL. Management of heart failure in older adults. *J Cardiovasc Nurs.* 2006;21(5S):S10–S14.
99. Centers for Disease Control and Prevention. Heart Failure Fact Sheet. https://www.cdc.gov/dhdsp/data_statistics/fact_sheets/fs_heart_failure.htm. Updated January 8, 2019. Accessed January 19, 2019.
100. Yancy LW, Jessup P, Bozkurt B, et al. 2013 ACCF/AHA guidelines for the management of heart failure. *Circulation.* 2013;128(16):e240–e327.
101. Hunt SA, Abraham WT, Chin MH, et al. Focused update incorporated into the ACC/AHA 2005 Guidelines for the diagnosis and management of heart failure in adults: a report of the American College of Cardiology Foundation/American Heart Association Task Force on Practice Guidelines: developed in collaboration with the International Society for Heart and Lung Transplantation. *Circulation.* 2009;119(14):e391–e479.
102. Maeder MT, Kaye DM. Heart failure with normal left ventricular ejection fraction. *J Am Coll Cardiol.* 2009;53(11):905–918.
103. Cabre M. Pneumonia in the elderly. *Curr Opin Pulm Med.* 2009;15. 223-222.
104. Wuerth BA, Bonnewell JP, Wiemken TL. Trends in pneumonia mortality rates and hospitalizations by organism, United States, 2002-2011. *Emerging Infections Dis.* 2016;22(9):1624–1629.
105. McNabb B, Isakow W. Probiotics for the prevention of nosocomial pneumonia: current evidence and opinions. *Curr Opin Pulm Med.* 2008;14:168–175.
106. Kharana P, Litaker D. The dilemma of nosocomial pneumonia: what primary care physicians should know. *Cleve Clin J Med.* 2000;67(1):25–41.
107. Chong CP, Street PR. Pneumonia in the elderly: a review of the epidemiology, pathogenesis, microbiology, and clinical features. *South Med J.* 2008;101(11):1141–1146.
108. Donowitz GR, Cox HL. Bacterial community-acquired pneumonia in older patients. *Clin Geriatr Med.* 2007;23:515–534.
109. Cunha BA. Hospital-acquired pneumonia (nosocomial pneumonia) and ventilator-associated pneumonia. https://emedicine.medscape.com/article/234753-overview#a4. Updated May 23, 2017. Accessed April 23, 2018.
110. Burton LA, Price RP, Barr KE. Hospital acquired pneumonia incidence and diagnosis in older patients. *Age Ageing.* 2016;45(1):171–174.

111. Medina-Walpole A, Katz P. Nursing home-acquired pneumonia. *J Am Geriatr Soc.* 1999;47:1005–1015.
112. Hoarse Z, Lim S. Pneumonia: update on diagnosis and management. *Br Med J.* 2006;323:1077–1080.
113. Nicolle LE. Urinary tract infections in the elderly. *Clin Geriatr Med.* 2009;25:423–436.
114. Genao L, Buhr GT. Urinary tract infections in older adults residing in long-term care facilities. *Ann Long Term Care.* 2012;20(4):33–38.
115. Rowe TA, Juthani-Mehta M. Urinary tract infection in older adults. *Aging health.* 2013;9(5):10.2217. https://www.ncbi.nlm.nih.gov/pmc/articles/PMC3878051/.
116. WebMD Medical Reference. Understanding urinary tract infections—the basics. http://www.webmd.com/a-to-z-guides/understanding-urinary-tract-infections-basics. Accessed January 19, 2019.
117. Liang SY, Mackowiak PA. Infections in the elderly. *Clin Geriatr Med.* 2007;23:441–456.
118. Urinary Tract Infection (UTI). Mayo Clinic. https://www.mayoclinic.org/diseases-conditions/urinary-tract-infection/symptoms-causes/syc-20353447. Updated Jan 30, 2019. Accessed July 26, 2019.
119. Juthani-Mehta M. Asymptomatic bacteriuria and urinary tract infection in the older adult. *Clin Geriatr Med.* 2007;23:585–594.
120. Hazelett SE, Tsai M, Gareri M, Allen K. The association between indwelling catheter use in the elderly and urinary tract infection in acute care. *BMC Geriatr.* 2006;6:15–21.
121. Mayo Clinic. Benign prostatic hyperplasia (BPH). https://www.mayoclinic.org/diseases-conditions/benign-prostatic-hyperplasia/symptoms-causes/syc-20370087. Updated September 28, 2018. Accessed December 30, 2018.
122. Singer M, Deutschman CS, Seymour CW, et al. The Third International Consensus Definitions for Sepsis and Septic Shock (Sepsis-3). *JAMA.* 2016;315(8):801–810. https://doi.org/10.1001/jama.2016.0287.
123. DeGuadio AR, Rinaldi S, Chelazzi C, Borracci T. Pathophysiology of sepsis in the elderly: clinical impact and therapeutic considerations. *Curr Drug Targets.* 2009;10:60–70.
124. Cunha BA. Sepsis, bacterial. http://emedicine.medscape.com/article/234587-overview. Updated May 22, 2017. Accessed January 19, 2019.
125. Mayo Clinic. Sepsis symptoms. http://www.mayoclinic.com/health/sepsis/DS01004. Updated November 16, 2018. Accessed December 30, 2018.
126. Jung JY, Kim JS, Chung PS, et al. Effect of vestibular rehabilitation on dizziness in the elderly. *Am J Otolaryngol.* 2009;30(5):295–299.
127. Uneri A, Polat S. Vertigo, dizziness and imbalance in the elderly. *J Laryngol Otol.* 2008;122:466–469.
128. Jung I, Kim J-S. Approach to dizziness in the emergency department. *Clin Exp Emerg Med.* 2015;2(2):75–88.
129. Hain TC. Dizziness in the emergency department. https://dizziness-and-balance.com/practice/approach/emergency.html. Updated February 4, 2017. Accessed January 20, 2019.
130. Kerber KA, Meurer WJ, West BT, Fendrick AM. Dizziness presentations in U.S. emergency departments, 1995-2004. *Acad Emerg Med.* 2008;15(8):744–750.
131. Li JC. Neurologic manifestations of benign positional vertigo. https://emedicine.medscape.com/article/1158940-overview. Updated July 23, 2018. Accessed December 30, 2018.
132. Benson AG. *Migraine-associated vertigo.* http://emedicine.medscape.com/article/884136-overview Updated January 18, 2019. Accessed January 19, 2019.
133. Labuguen RH. Initial evaluation of vertigo. *Am Fam Physician.* 2006;73(2):244–251.
134. Mentes J. Oral hydration in older adults. *Am J Nurs.* 2006;106(6):39–49.
135. El-Sharkawy AM, Watson P, Neal KR, et al. Hydration and outcome in older patients admitted to hospital (The HOOP prospective cohort study). *Age Ageing.* 2015;44(6):943–947.
136. Schols JM, Degroot CP, van der Cammen TJ, Olde Rikkert MG. Preventing and treating dehydration in the elderly during periods of illness and warm weather. *J Nutr Health Aging.* 2009;13(2):150–158.
137. Grundy SM, Cleeman JL, Daniels DR, et al. Diagnosis and management of the metabolic syndrome. An American Heart Association/National Heart and Lung and Blood Institute scientific statement: executive summary. *Crit Pathw Cardiol.* 2005;4(4):198–203.
138. Lechleitner M. Obesity and the metabolic syndrome in the elderly—a mini review. *Gerontology.* 2008;54(5):253–259.
139. International Diabetic Federation. Metabolic syndrome: driving CVD epidemic. https://www.idf.org/e-library/consensus-statements/60-idfconsensus-worldwide-definitionof-the-metabolic-syndrome.html. Accessed December 30, 2018.
140. Bechtold M, Palmer J, Valtos J, et al. Metabolic syndrome in the elderly. *Curr Diabetes Rep.* 2006;6:64–71.
141. American Diabetes Association. How to tell if you have pre-diabetes. http://www.diabetes.org/diabetes-basics/prevention/pre-diabetes/how-to-tell-if-you-have.html. Updated November 21, 2016. Accessed December 30, 2018.
142. Basile J. New therapeutic options in patients prone to hypertension: a focus on direct renin inhibition and aldosterone blockade. *Am J Med Sci.* 2009;337(6):438–444.
143. Gordon RS. Operational classification of disease prevention. *Public Health Rep.* 1983;98(2):107–109.
144. Alexander KP, Newby K, Cannon CP. Acute coronary care in the elderly, Part 1: non-ST segment elevation acute coronary syndromes: a scientific statement for healthcare professionals from the American Heart Association Council on Clinical Cardiology: in collaboration with the Society of Geriatric Cardiology. *Circulation.* 2007;115 2549–2469.

CHAPTER 15

Impaired Joint Mobility in Older Adults

Kevin Chui, Sheng-Che Yen, Tzurei Chen, Cory Christiansen

OUTLINE

INTRODUCTION

Joint mobility is a direct determinant of posture and movement, influencing activity and participation for all individuals. As a person ages, changes occur in joint mobility that can influence overall health and function. Thus, joint mobility is an important component of evaluation, diagnosis, and plan-of-care development for older adults. The purposes of this chapter are to (1) summarize current evidence of age-associated changes in joint mobility and (2) examine implications of impaired joint mobility for clinical management of older adult patients/clients.

As presented elsewhere, optimal aging is reflected by the capacity to participate in life with consideration of the interactions among many aspects of health. Isolating the influence of aging from other determinants of health, such as disease, environment, and other biopsychosocial characteristics of a person, is not possible. As a result, the unique health characteristics of each individual must be kept in mind as a context for considering the associations of aging and joint mobility. An understanding of typical age-associated changes in joint mobility will serve as one component of a larger knowledge base to guide physical therapists in optimizing health and function for older adults. A conceptual framework for interactions among the numerous factors for health and function in regard to age-related joint mobility impairment is presented in Fig. 15.1.

The chapter consists of two primary sections. First presented are age-associated changes in joint mobility. Second, pertinent aspects of patient/client management are considered in view of the numerous interacting factors that contribute to impaired joint mobility in older adults.

JOINT MOBILITY WITH AGING

Operationally defined, joint mobility is the capacity of a joint to move passively, taking into account the joint surfaces and surrounding tissue.[1] Interactions between muscle, tendon, ligament, synovium, capsule, cartilage, and bone at a joint create the unique aspects of joint mobility. Because of the direct association between structure and function, joint mobility is directly influenced by changes in any of the related tissues. Distinct physiological change occurs in joint structures and tissues over the life span. The result of the structural changes can include joint

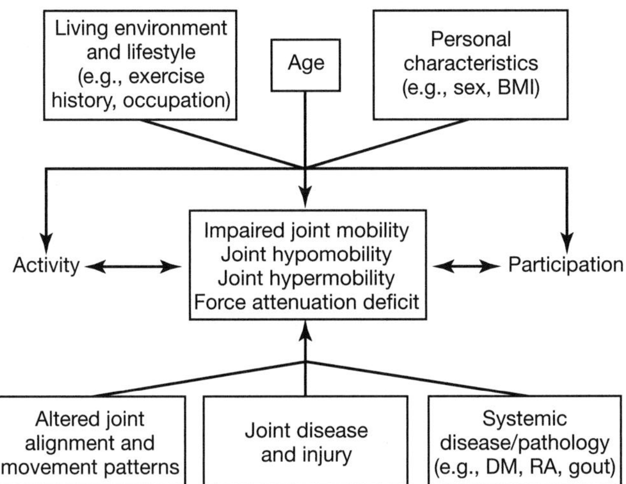

FIG. 15.1 Interaction of factors contributing to impaired joint mobility.

impairment, activity limitation, and participation restriction.

As will be seen, even for people who are aging successfully, changes in joint mobility occur. Although impairment of joint mobility is not concomitant with aging, the possibility of joint problems is a prominent consideration for physical therapists working with older adults. Illustrating the significance of impaired joint mobility in older adults is the increasing prevalence of reporting chronic joint symptoms that occurs as people age. For example, it has been reported by the Centers for Disease Control and Prevention (CDC) that 58.8% of individuals aged 65 years or older self-report arthritis or chronic joint symptoms, compared with 42.1% of people aged 45 to 64 years (Table 15.1).[2] Furthermore, 49.6% of individuals aged 65 years or older were diagnosed by a doctor or other health professional with arthritis, rheumatoid arthritis, gout, lupus, or fibromyalgia, compared with 29.3% of people aged 45 to 64 years.[3] And of those diagnosed by a doctor or other health professional, 44.0% of individuals aged 65 years or older and 44.5% of individuals aged 45 to 64 years will present with activity limitations attributed to their diagnosis.

Connective Tissue Changes

Connective tissue is the primary structural component of all joints, providing a mechanical framework dictating the structural and functional characteristics of individual joints. Musculoskeletal changes occur as we age owing to alterations in normal biological responses that lead to impaired tissue function, independent of pathology.[4] However, connective tissue aging is also influenced by factors unique to each individual, such as level of physical activity, pathology, segmental alignment, and prior injury.

All connective tissue structures of a joint (e.g., ligaments, joint capsule, and cartilage) consist of cellular, protein, and glycoconjugate components within an extracellular matrix. The unique configuration and composition of these components dictate the unique function of each structure. General age-associated changes in cellular and extracellular composition of connective tissue are presented in this chapter and summarized in Box 15.1. The majority of evidence for these changes is based on research on cartilage and bone in weight-bearing joints (e.g., knee, hip, and intervertebral) because of the comparatively large amount of study on those structures.

BOX 15.1 Generalized Age-Associated Changes in Connective Tissue

Molecular
Increased structural protein cross-linkages
Decreased proteoglycan size
Fragmentation of collagen

Cellular
Decreased proliferation
Altered control of apoptosis
Decreased response to growth factors
Altered response to loading

Connective Tissue Structures
Increased stiffness
Decreased water content
Decreased strength
Decreased cross-sectional area and volume

TABLE 15.1 Arthritis and Chronic Joint Symptom Prevalence in the United States

	Self-Reported Arthritis/ Chronic Joint Symptoms*		Doctor-Diagnosed Arthritis†		Arthritis-Attributable Activity Limitation†	
Age (Years)	**Percent**	**95% CI**	**Percent**	**95% CI**	**Percent**	**95% CI**
18–44	19.0	18.5–19.4	7.1	6.8–7.5	39.4	37.0–41.8
45–64	42.1	41.5–42.8	29.3	28.6–30.0	44.5	43.1–45.8
≥65	58.8	58.0–59.7	49.6	48.6–50.5	44.0	42.8–45.2

CI, confidence interval.
*From Prevalence of self-reported arthritis or chronic joint symptoms among adults—United States, 2001. *MMWR Morb Mortal Wkly Rep.* 2002;51(42):948–950.
†Barbour KE, Helmick CG, Boring M, Brady TJ. Vital signs: prevalence of doctor-diagnosed arthritis and arthritis-attributable activity limitation — United States, 2013–2015. *MMWR Morb Mortal Wkly Rep.* 2017;66:246–253.

Cellular Level. Fibroblasts, the basic connective tissue cells, actively produce the extracellular matrix unique to each joint structure. For example, chondroblasts and osteoblasts are differentiated fibroblasts found in cartilage and bone, respectively. As people age, these cells demonstrate decreased proliferation (i.e., cellular senescence) and altered control of apoptosis (i.e., programmed cell death).[5,6] The reduction in cell divisions appears to be related to a preset number of cell divisions (i.e., replicative senescence) as well as altered responsiveness of tissue to exposure to stressful environmental agents over time (i.e., stress-induced premature senescence). The result of decreased proliferation and altered regulation of apoptosis is a decrease in effective maintenance of tissue homeostasis. Another cellular change noted with age is decreased response to circulating growth factors, such as hormones and cytokines.[7] This change in cellular communication processes results in altered ability for repair and maintenance of connective tissue structures. In addition, older connective tissue cells may be less responsive to adaptations with loading. In young individuals, cyclic physiological loading typically stimulates tissue synthesis. In contrast, Plumb et al.[8] observed that cyclic loading of articular cartilage from older adults depressed, rather than stimulated, cartilage synthesis.

Molecular Level. Glycoconjugates are molecules of carbohydrate bonded to other compounds, such as protein and lipid. Forms of these molecules serve various functions in connective tissue, including cell-to-cell communication and cross-linkages between proteins. The presence of glycoconjugates in connective tissue is also critical for maintaining fluid content of the tissue, because of the highly negative charge of some of these molecules that serves to bind water.[9] The ability of connective tissue to retain water is diminished with aging as the content of glycoconjugates, particularly proteoglycan aggregates of the extracellular matrix, significantly decreases.[10] In addition, there is an increase in glycoconjugate degradation and a decrease in synthesis that further contribute to decreased fluid content and connective tissue degeneration.

Collagen, the primary structural protein of connective tissue, also changes across the life span. The unique structure of collagen molecules allows them to provide significant resistance to tensile load. Collagen molecules are arranged in fibrous strands with unique orientations that dictate the mechanical functions of the various joint structures. For example, obliquely oriented collagen fibers within the annulus fibrosus of the intervertebral disc are arranged in perpendicular directions for successive layers. This arrangement allows the disc to respond to compressive, tensile, and torsional loads between vertebrae through tension created in the collagen fibers.

Age-associated changes in collagen include fragmenting of collagen strands and a declining rate of collagen turnover.[11]

Related to these changes is an increased formation of cross-links between collagen molecules. In part, the cross-links result from the formation of specific glycoconjugates, known as advanced glycation end-products (AGEs). Interaction of the fragmented collagen and AGEs create intermolecular collagen cross-links.[12] Mechanically, increased cross-linkages alter the biomechanical function of the collagen structures by increasing stiffness and possibly decreasing the ability to absorb mechanical energy.[11] In addition, the cross-linkages may make structures more brittle, resulting in higher rates of structural damage in response to cyclic loading (i.e., decreased resistance to tissue fatigue). Another connective tissue protein is elastin, which typically functions in conjunction with collagen to return structures to their original shape after deformation.[13] Elastin also demonstrates age-associated cross-linkages related to AGE production. The result, similar to collagen, is an increase in stiffness.

Change in Joint Structures

Joint structures can be categorized as chondroid, fibrous, and bony. Chondroid structures are of cartilaginous make-up and include articular cartilage, menisci, labra, and fibrocartilaginous discs. Fibrous structures include the ligaments and tendons that surround the joint (i.e., extra-articular) as well as ligaments within the joint boundaries (i.e., intra-articular). The other primary fibrous structure is the joint capsule of diarthroses, which defines the border between intra- and extra-articular structures. Bone creates the structural segments that move relative to one another at the articulations. The bones also disperse force and provide structure to the joints. Each of these categories of joint structures is directly influenced by the cellular and molecular changes described earlier.

Chondroid Structures. The majority of evidence for changes in chondroid structures with age comes from examination of articular cartilage and the intervertebral disc. The primary function of these structures is to disperse loads between segments and promote joint mobility by decreasing friction.[14] As with all joint structures, there is no clear distinction between typical aging and pathology of chondroid structures. One factor complicating this delineation is the influence of loading history.

Although it is known that moderate levels of intermittent joint loads promote articular cartilage health, excessive compression impacts and torsion loads are known to create damage.[15] Indication of the negative influence of excessive loading on articular cartilage is the increased incidence of osteoarthritis (OA) in individuals involved in sports[16] and occupations[17] with high levels of traumatic (e.g., contact and collision) and static joint loading. Once articular cartilage becomes damaged, the capacity to heal is limited and initial injury may progress to the development of cartilage lesions (i.e., cartilage fibrillation).[18] The limited intrinsic healing response consists of lesion repair to the original hyaline cartilage with production of matrix molecules or fibrocartilage. The result of increased matrix molecules and fibrocartilage is tissue with inferior wear (load dispersion and friction-reducing) characteristics.

A histologic change specific to articular cartilage is increased calcification over time. Calcification of articular cartilage has been shown to occur independent of osteoarthritic changes, indicating that it is a typical response to aging.[19] Calcification, along with cellular and molecular changes described in the previous section, leads to decreased osmotic pressure in articular cartilage. Decreased hydration compromises the viscoelastic properties and load-absorbing capacity of the cartilage.[20]

Distinct changes specific to the intervertebral disc also occur over time.[21] The nucleus becomes more fibrous and less gel-like and the annulus becomes less organized. As a result, delineation of annulus and nucleus is diminished in older adults.[22] Cracks/lesions may also develop in the annulus and nucleus.[23] Decreased water content is also noted in the intervertebral discs and is associated with reduced disc height.[21] The loss of disc height can lead to the chronic pathological condition referred to as spinal stenosis, a major cause of pain and disability for older adults. Change of the intervertebral disc also alters surrounding structures. For example, the diarthrodial facet joints may experience greater loads,[22] and elasticity of the ligamentum flavum may decrease because of decreasing tensile forces over time.[14]

Fibrous Structures. Information regarding the influence of aging on fibrous structures is relatively limited. As suggested earlier, the vast majority of evidence for age-associated changes of connective tissue structures is based on studies of cartilage and bone. In typical function, fibrous structures absorb and transfer some level of tensile load, based on collagen content. Although orientation and composition of tissue components vary between fibrous structures and between joints, the overarching similarities in response to aging are increased stiffness and reduced elasticity.[13,24] For example, there is evidence that histopathological abnormalities (e.g., collagen fiber disorganization) in the anterior cruciate ligament increase in prevalence with age.[25]

Bone

Bony change is both directly and indirectly related to joint mobility. Directly, changes in bone can influence the joint surfaces to alter joint mechanics. Indirectly, fractures and other bony structural change can alter joint alignment and function with possible secondary influences on joint mobility.

Subchondral bone is the layer of dense bone directly under the articular cartilage providing support to the articular surface. There is indication that the thickness and density of subchondral bone tend to decrease with advancing age, although this is not uniform at all joint surfaces. For example, Yamada et al.[26] examined 140 knee specimens from a wide age range of donors (17 to 91 years) and found that thickness and density of the tibial subchondral bone declined with age, whereas no significant change was noted at the femoral condyles. The authors postulated that dispersion of loads during normal function may create a differential response to subchondral bone structure between the femur and tibia.

It is well established that osteopenia is prevalent with aging, because of increased osteoclast and decreased osteoblast activity, leading to increased risk of osteoporosis.[27,28] Typically, bone acts along with cartilage to absorb and disperse forces transferred between body segments. As a result of osteopenia, the ability of bone to absorb loads is compromised. Corresponding to the problem of decreased load absorption by bone is decreased load dispersion in other joint structures and impaired neuromuscular function, both of which result in increased bone loading. The combination of lowered threshold for loading and increased load demand results in an increased risk of bone fracture with aging.

Fractures can alter joint mobility in a variety of ways, such as disrupting circulation to joint structures, altering loading patterns, and decreasing available range of motion. In addition, pain associated with fractures can be a major problem, interfering significantly with an individual's activity and participation. It is well documented that fractures are common and devastating injuries in older adult populations, particularly among older women.[29] Common fracture locations that influence joint mobility in older adults are the proximal femur (i.e., hip fractures), pelvis, distal radius, and vertebrae.

Whole Joint Changes

Physiological and mechanical interactions between tissues create interdependence such that any change in one structure has direct consequences on the composition and function of other structures. At the level of the whole joint, changes include decreased joint space, increased laxity, altered dispersion of loads, and altered joint moments of force. Over time, the unloading of surrounding tissues and joint structures that provide tensile support, because of decreased joint space, may predispose the joint to decreased range of motion. However, change in mobility varies among joint complexes, with some joints having relatively little change in comparison to others.

Functionally, joint changes are reflected by age-associated changes seen in kinematics both at the segmental level (i.e., osteokinematics) and between joint surfaces (i.e., arthrokinematics). Motion of one segment relative to another is considered osteokinematic motion and can be quantified with measurement of joint ranges of motion as well as angular velocities and accelerations. In comparison, arthrokinematics describes movement of joint surfaces in relation to one another. Research examining both osteokinematic and arthrokinematic motions of older adults compared to younger adults has revealed some general trends. This chapter provides information on individual joint kinematics without broader application in regard to functional task performance. Chapter 9 provides examples of changes in joint kinematics and the effects on the functional task of walking.

Range of Motion. Joint range of motion (ROM) decreases with increasing age, although nonuniformly among joints, and is often direction specific within a given joint. Generally, active and passive motion both decrease, with active ROM tending to decline more than passive. The differing response of active and passive motion indicates the influence of neuromuscular changes in addition to the structural changes of the joint. In addition, passive ROM measures are typically independent of the individual's effort and motivation, whereas active ROM may be influenced by either of these variables.

Motion of the axial skeleton has been examined relative to age in numerous studies. As an example, Fig. 15.2 provides a graphic representation of data from a study by Malmstrom et al.[30] that examined changes of cervical motion across decades for a total of 120 participants. This figure illustrates the fact that change in movement with age is direction specific. For the cervical spine, gradual decline in ROM is seen beyond the age of 30, with extension and lateral flexion demonstrating the greatest decline.[31,32] Cervical transverse rotation and flexion are typically limited to a lesser extent than other motions, with some indication that upper cervical rotation may be less affected than lower segments.[33]

Examinations of thoracic and lumbar motion reveal extension to be most limited in older adults, with minimal or no age-dependent decline in rotation.[34,35] Bible et al.[36] examined maximum sagittal lumbar motion using radiographic measures from 258 participants ranging in age from 18 to 50 years and found age to be the most

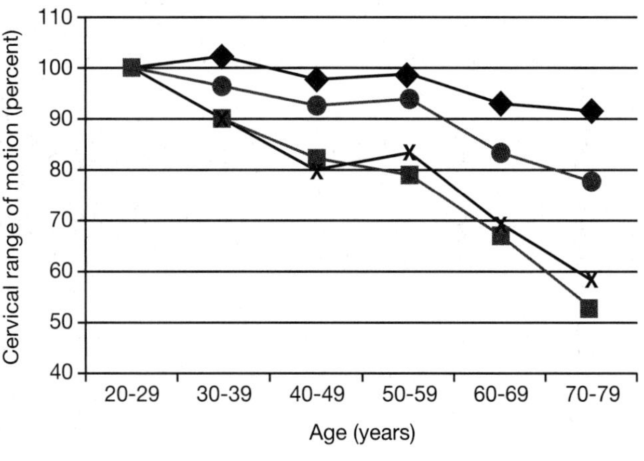

FIG. 15.2 Cervical spine range-of-motion values across the life span. *(Data from Malmstrom EM, Karlberg M, Fransson PA, et al. Primary and coupled cervical movements: the effect of age, gender, and body mass index. A 3-dimensional movement analysis of a population without symptoms of neck disorders. Spine. 2006;31[2]: E44–E50.)*

significant predictor of decreased ROM. In addition, statistical analysis indicated that declines in motion were seen independent of degenerative change.[36] Beyond 50 years of age, data indicate a continued trend for motion decline. For example, Troke et al.[34] examined 400 participants ages 16 to 90 years and found a linear decline in trunk motion with the following approximate percentages of motion reduction across the span of ages: 77% for extension, 50% for flexion, 44% for lateral flexion, and no change in rotation.

Research examining lower extremity ROM in older adults is common, with much consideration being directed toward the relationship between locomotor function and joint kinematics. Declines in joint motion occur at the hip[37] and foot/ankle[38] joint complexes, whereas knee motion, in the absence of pathology, remains relatively consistent across the life span.[39] At the hip, sagittal plane motion is primarily influenced. In this plane of motion, hip flexion is typically well maintained as people age.[39] However, extension ROM has been shown to decrease by more than 20% (decline from 22 to 17 degrees) when comparing individuals 25 to 39 and 60 to 74 years of age.[40] It has been postulated that reduced hip extension seen with aging may directly relate to decreased walking speed in older adults, especially those with sedentary lifestyles.[37,41] Decreased ankle sagittal plane motion is also seen with aging, particularly in the direction of dorsiflexion.[42] Although strength of ankle dorsiflexion is postulated to account for a major portion of decline in ankle motion during function, the presence of progressive decreases in passive ROM indicates causes other than muscle strength alone.

Compared to the lower extremity and trunk, there is relatively less influence of age on upper extremity joint ROM. The shoulder complex is most influenced, with flexion and external rotation being the primary motions affected.[32,43] Movement of the shoulder complex involves glenohumeral, scapulothoracic, and spinal segment interaction.[44] As such, the increased thoracic kyphosis typically seen with age can play a significant role on the amount of motion available at the shoulder. At the elbow and wrist, no age-associated declines in motion have been noted in the absence of disease.[32,45]

Arthrokinematics. Arthrokinematic motions include glide, spin, roll, compression, and distraction of joint surfaces relative to one another. The connective tissue changes previously described can potentially alter arthrokinematics through such mechanisms as increased fibrous structure stiffness, decreased chondroid structure volume and viscoelasticity, and altered bone structure. Although isolated arthrokinematic motions cannot be performed volitionally, limitations can have a direct influence on joint mobility. For example, glenohumeral abduction includes inferior glide of the humeral head in relation to the glenoid fossa. In the case of adhesive capsulitis, a disease more common with age progression, the joint capsule does not allow sufficient laxity. The increased tightness of the joint capsule alters arthrokinematics, reducing inferior glide during activities requiring glenohumeral abduction.[46] Reduced inferior glide may lead to symptoms of shoulder impingement. This example of joint capsule change demonstrates how impaired joint mobility can have direct consequence on arthrokinematics and osteokinematics, leading to activity limitation.

Force Transmission. Kinetic implications of joint mobility relate to force transmission within joint structures and between body segments. It has already been noted that connective tissue structures demonstrate altered capacity to transmit tensile and compressive loads in older adults. These alterations can result in increased demands on specific regions within joints, possibly leading to disease. For example, areas of articular cartilage breakdown are found in specific regions of joints.[47] These areas of breakdown may be correlated with areas of altered contact pressures and can lead to the degenerative changes in cartilage.[48] Additionally, age-related tissue changes can limit the ability of joint structures to heal and a cascade can ensue, leading to greater impairment.

Joint structural changes can also indirectly influence the moment of force (i.e., torque) demands on joints. Changes in posture are predictable over the life span. The changes in posture relate to alterations in joint alignment and mobility. As a consequence of alignment change, static and dynamic demands on joints are altered. A specific example is the typical increase in thoracic kyphosis seen even in successfully aging adults.[49] This change increases the moment arm between the line of action of gravity and mediolateral axes of rotation for the thoracic spine segments. As a result, increased kyphosis will create a larger flexion demand moment on the thoracic joints during daily standing and sitting activities (Fig. 15.3). If these changes in joint mobility and alignment are not corrected, greater neuromuscular activation is needed to compensate or further joint impairment will occur.

Any joint structural change can influence the linear and angular effects of forces. A physical therapist, equipped with foundational knowledge in mechanics and joint anatomy, can determine how changes in joint structure will alter kinetic qualities of each specific joint. Because joints work to produce motion in segmental systems, subtle changes at one joint can have significant alterations in demands at other joints.

Influence on Activity and Participation

Postural control during activities such as walking, position transfers, and reaching are known to decline with age. Among the multiple factors related to these

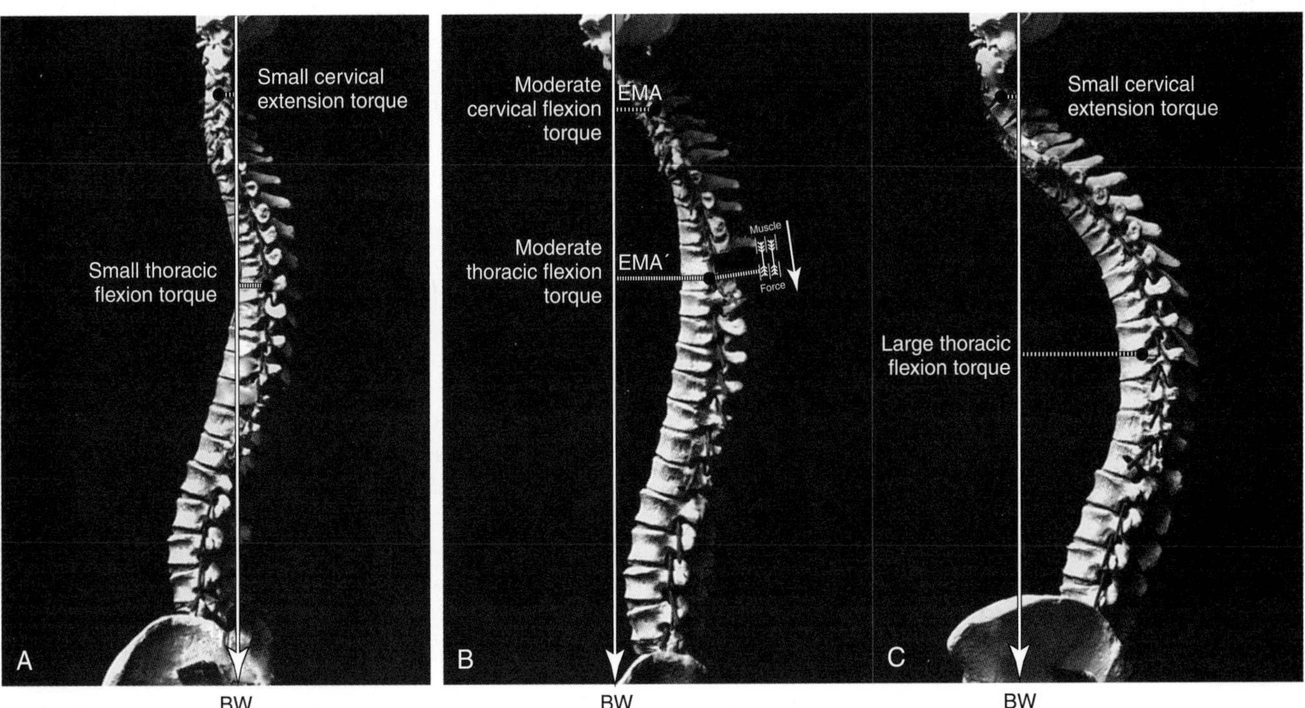

FIG. 15.3 Model showing the orientation of the force line of gravity from body weight (BW, *arrow*) at the cervical and thoracic spines. **A** through **C** show a progression in severity of kyphosis. Each model demonstrates the mediolateral axis at the midpoint of the thoracic and cervical regions (*dark circles*) and the associated external moment arms (*hatched lines*). **A,** Patient with ideal standing posture and normal thoracic kyphosis. BW creates a small cervical extension torque and a small thoracic flexion torque. **B,** Patient with moderate thoracic kyphosis. BW creates a moderate cervical and thoracic flexion torque. *EMA'*, external moment arm at the thoracic spine midpoint; *EMA*, external moment arm at cervical spine midpoint; *IMA*, internal moment arm for back extensor muscular force. **C,** Patient with severe thoracic kyphosis. BW causes a small cervical extension torque and a large thoracic flexion torque.

alterations in activity is change in joint mobility. Changes in joint mobility have significant activity- and participation-related consequences for older adults, as evidenced by correlations such as cartilage thinning with patient-identified disability[50] and intervertebral disc degeneration with back pain.[51] A specific example of joint mobility association with activity is the relationship of ankle mobility and balance. Menz et al.[52] examined foot and ankle risk factors in older adults. In their 12-month prospective study, fallers (41% of the sample) had significantly less ankle mobility, hallux valgus severity, and tactile sensitivity of the first metatarsophalangeal joint.

Impaired joint mobility has also been implicated as a factor in walking limitations. For example, Kerrigan et al.[53] observed gait speed to be decreased between older adults who reported frequent falls compared to "nonfallers" of the same age. In addition, smaller hip extension displacements were observed for individuals reporting falls. The difference in hip motion during gait was the only variable noted to be significantly different between the groups when analyzing any of the 10 joint kinematic variables tested.

Age-associated activity limitation often culminates in decreased participation in life events. The relationship also works in the opposite direction, with changes in activity and participation leading to more sedentary lifestyles and secondary changes to joint structure and function (see Fig. 15.1). Because of the interdependent nature of these factors, it is important that changes in joint mobility are identified and addressed in older adult patients/clients presenting with all types of diagnoses. The second section of this chapter focuses on the process of patient/client management with specific attention to the role of joint mobility.

JOINT EXAMINATION

All older adult patients/clients require consideration of joint mobility as a result of the integral role of joints in health and function. Beyond typical age-related changes, there are many joint conditions with a higher prevalence in older adults (see Table 15.1), such as osteoarthritis, rheumatoid arthritis, polymyalgia rheumatica, and gout.[3] In addition, the age-adjusted prevalence in women (23.5%, 95% confidence interval [CI] = 23.1 to 24.0) was significantly higher than in men (18.1%, 95% CI = 17.6 to 18.6).[3] Examination of the patient/client allows the therapist to determine the relative influence of joint mobility on the presenting activity limitations.

Joint mobility examination is incorporated in the comprehensive examination and should not be viewed as an independent process. Specific lines of questions included in the history and observations from the systems review will determine the extent to which further examination of joint mobility is indicated. If evidence of joint impairment is provided by specific tests and measures, the impairment can be targeted through remediation, compensation, or prevention strategies. Throughout this process, joint mobility is considered in the context of complete patient/client management.

History

A thorough history interview is a key component in the examination of the patient/client. Knowledge gained from the history is critical in determining possible influence of impaired joint mobility on the presenting problems. Included in the history interview are questions regarding activity limitations, participation restrictions, symptom characteristics, activity history, previous joint impairments, family history of joint disease, and living environment.

Activity and participation. It is important to begin the history interview by first identifying activity limitations and participation restrictions. This process clarifies the needs and functional goals of the patient/client. In addition, identifying problems with activity and participation focuses the examination by providing a context for determining how impaired joint mobility may be contributing to the presenting problems. Clear identification of these functional problems will also help in the process of determining appropriate outcomes measures.

It is possible for an older adult to have impaired joint mobility that does not influence the presenting functional problem. Although it is important to consider nonsymptomatic joint impairment for preventive reasons, focusing on impairments not related to the presenting problem can distract from the examination and care planning process. Determining the relative influence that impaired joint mobility has on functional problems can only be done if the activity limitations and participation restrictions are clear to the therapist.

Symptoms. If an individual relates chronic symptoms, development of compensatory movements over time should be suspected. In these cases, the original symptoms as well as the most recent symptoms are important to consider. Altered movement patterns in response to impaired joint mobility can eventually lead to secondary problems. Understanding compensation helps the therapist to develop hypotheses for both original symptoms and symptom progression. It is also of interest to link routine activity change, such as new exercise participation, to symptoms. Knowledge of temporal onset of symptoms is necessary to make this determination.

Behavior of symptoms, such as timing and duration, can indicate the type of joint mobility problem. For example, symptoms of stiffness related to OA are often increased after periods of stationary postures (e.g., upon getting out of bed) and last for short periods (e.g., <30 minutes) after movement is initiated. In contrast, morning stiffness common with rheumatoid arthritis typically lasts for periods >30 minutes.[54] In another example, a patient/client may indicate lower extremity pain during periods of standing and walking that resolves shortly after sitting. One reason for this type of symptom behavior can be neurogenic intermittent claudication related to lumbar spinal stenosis.[55]

Occupation/Activity. Information on joint loading and movement history is provided with knowledge of occupational and leisure activity. Loading history of joints is known to be an important influence on joint mobility in older age, often linked to impairment. For example, a recent review of occupational risk factors reported that heavy physical workload was the most common risk factor for OA, Other risk factors include kneeling, regular stair climbing, crawling, bending, whole body vibration, and repetitive movements.[56] In a population-based study, after adjusting for age and other physical workload factors, heavy physical work had the highest hazard ratios when examining disability retirement secondary to hip OA for both men and women 30 to 60 years old.[57] Lack of physical activity is also of interest, as it has been shown that older age is associated with sedentary lifestyle, which is in turn associated with chronic disease. In fact, data from the CDC Behavioral Risk Factor Surveillance System from 2014 indicates that 25.4%, 26.9%, and 35.3% of adults aged 50 to 64, 65 to 74, and 75 or older, respectively, engage in no leisure-time physical activity.[58] In a large sample of older adults, when compared to intermediate and high levels of physical activity, those that engaged in low physical activity were more likely to have commonly diagnosed chronic conditions, report lower self-rated physical health, use seven or more prescription drugs, and have lower health literacy.[59] A recent review summarizes evidence on how the body maladapts to insufficient physical activity, how physical inactivity is the primary cause of most chronic diseases, and how physical activity can prevent against chronic conditions.[60] Hagströmer and Franzén further describe the relationship by physical activity (a key concept within physical therapy) and health, provide recommendations for physical activity, and explain how to assess physical activity.[61] It is well accepted that joint structures, along with all other biological tissues, will adapt to the amount of physical stress applied to them.[62] Adaptive response of chronically low activity can decrease the tolerance of joint structures to loading. Combined with the typical age-associated joint changes, activity reductions play a key role in joint mobility impairment and threshold for joint injury.

Health Condition/Injury/Surgery. The importance of information regarding disease history cannot be overstated. For joint function, comorbid conditions are often significant factors. Endocrine, neuromuscular, cardiovascular, pulmonary, and musculoskeletal pathology can be linked to systemic conditions that significantly influence joint function. An example is the association of musculoskeletal impairments (e.g., impaired joint mobility) with diabetes mellitus, a common endocrine disease affecting older adults.[63] The high glucose and insulin levels in patients with diabetes are associated with increased cross-linkage formation in connective tissue structures that can compound the age-associated changes discussed earlier in this chapter.[64] Joint mobility impairments that occur as complications of diabetes include adhesive capsulitis of the glenohumeral joint[65] and diabetic cheiroarthropathy, which affects the hands (thickening of skin and limited joint mobility).[66]

Joint loading is also influenced by history of health condition, injury, and surgery. Perhaps the most common health condition associated with atypical joint loading is obesity. History of obesity is a known risk factor for developing OA and related to remission and disease activity of rheumatoid arthritis.[67] Additionally, injury and surgery are often closely related to joint loading through movement and posture compensations. Knowledge of the history of such factors related to joint loading also provides insight into the incidence of degenerative joint change later in life. Murphy et al.[68] performed a longitudinal examination (mean time from baseline to follow-up of 6 years) for knee OA in 1739 people (mean age at baseline 61 years) and found the lifetime risk of symptomatic knee OA was 44.7%. The two factors found to significantly increase the risk of knee OA were the presence of obesity and history of knee injury, which increased the lifetime risk to 60.5% and 56.8%, respectively.

Family History. Studies have demonstrated increased likelihood of joint-specific diseases in older adults resulting from genetic predisposition. OA,[69] gout,[70] rheumatoid arthritis,[71] and systemic lupus erythematosus[72] are all examples of joint pathologies linked to genetic influence. Knowledge of family disease history alerts the physical therapist to early signs of problems and potential relevant interventions. Even patients/clients presenting without joint impairment can benefit from preventive intervention if family history, in combination with other findings, indicates high potential for future joint mobility problems.

Living Environment. Discussion of living environment is integral when gathering information on activity limitations and participation restrictions. Living environments, including both home and community, are unique to each individual. Items such as stair height, chair types, and flooring determine the varying degrees of joint mobility necessary for routine activity.

Based on a recent review of several clinical practice guidelines, the Academy of Geriatric Physical Therapy recommends a home hazard assessment, including modification/correction and follow-up, for older people with a history of falls or those at risk for falls.[73] Even if the therapist does not perform a home visit, information regarding environmental aspects of living can be ascertained through the history interview. Identified environmental concerns can be directly assessed further in the home or simulated in clinical settings. Identification of environmental conditions also allows the potential of targeting environmental modification with intervention.

Systems Review

It is evident that joint mobility should be considered in the complete context of a person's health and function and not solely as a musculoskeletal issue. Joint mobility influences, and is influenced by, multisystem interactions. For example, pulmonary function can be altered by joint mobility of the thorax and spinal column. Study of sternocostal synarthroses reveals increased cartilage calcification and ossification with aging.[74] These sternocostal changes, in conjunction with decreased intervertebral disc height and elasticity, may lead to pulmonary dysfunction by creating increased work of breathing.[75] Such interactions between systems are a primary reason for performing a systems review, as recommended in the *Guide to Physical Therapist Practice*.[1]

Another benefit of the systems review is increased examination efficiency. Selection of focused tests and measures is generated by combining history information with findings of the review. For example, consider a 70-year-old man presenting with symptoms of pain at the posterolateral deltoid region of the shoulder. During the interview, he also reveals a history of chronic lateral elbow pain that has been treated ineffectively in the past as lateral epicondylitis. During the systems review, gross assessment of cervical motion reveals that extension and ipsilateral side flexion reproduce pain symptoms at both the elbow and shoulder. Based on this preliminary information, cervical spine joint mobility would be of primary interest for further examination.[76]

Tests and Measures

Selection of appropriate tests and measures for an older adult with impaired joint mobility requires consideration of health and functional status of the individual, practicality of administration for a given clinical setting, and clinometric properties of the measure.[77] These considerations continually change because each patient has a unique presentation, methods for established tests and measures evolve, clinometric properties are defined with research over time, and new tests and measures emerge. Considering these dynamic aspects, a "cookbook" recipe approach with a specific list of tests and measures for all patients/clients is not reasonable. However, a categorical framework for the selection of tests and measures can be followed and applied to the current state of knowledge. In this section, a guide for a comprehensive approach to tests and measures, applicable to patients with impaired joint mobility, is provided.

The four primary types of tests and measure categories are listed in Box 15.2. Combining results of these four categories of measures allows for quantification of all levels of potential dysfunction: impairments, activity limitations, and participation restrictions (as defined by the International Classification of Functioning, Disability, and Health[78,79]). Considering the intimate interaction between these levels of dysfunction, a comprehensive battery of tests and measures is needed to fully quantify the impact of altered joint mobility.

BOX 15.2 Four Major Types of Tests and Measure Categories to Consider When Assessing Joint Mobility

- Observational task analysis
- Self-report measures of activity and participation
- Performance-based measures of activity
- Joint-specific mobility testing

Observational Task Analysis. A suggested first step in the implementation of tests and measures is observational analysis of the specific functional task(s) identified as problematic by the patient.[80] Observational task analysis can guide the formation of hypotheses, considering impaired joint mobility as a potential cause of activity limitation. In addition, observational task analysis may allow the physical therapist to identify appropriate quantitative tests and measures to further the examination. Procedures for observing and analyzing must be systematic for the process to be effective. Systematic analysis is improved if the therapist has a strong working knowledge of the movement mechanics required for the task, as well as sufficient practice observing and analyzing the given task.[81]

Methods for performing observational task analyses are outlined in various frameworks for patient/client examination.[82] Much of the published work on observational task analysis is rooted in the analysis of walking gait, particularly in relation to the practice of neuromuscular physical therapy. Although observational gait analysis procedures have been published and used in the clinic for many years, reliability for identifying altered joint movements or deviations in posture is poor to moderate.[81,83,84] Considering this lack of established reliability, observational task analysis should be used cautiously, with emphasis on guiding selection of other tests and measures, rather than being used independently for diagnosing or quantifying impaired joint mobility. For example, impaired knee mobility ROM is a potential cause for lack of full knee extension at initial contact during gait. Observed absence of full knee extension, during task analysis, should suggest that valid and reliable measures of knee motion be performed.

Self-Report Measures of Activity and Participation. In addition to direct observation of task performance, patient self-report measures can be used to gather information during the examination. These measures document the patient's perspective of activity performance, which provides different information than direct observation. Valid self-report measures inform the therapist regarding the influence of domains such as pain and psychological functioning on activity limitations. Many self-report measures also allow for gathering information regarding the patient's restrictions in regard to life participation.

Impaired mobility of a given joint will directly influence a specific region of the body: the spine, upper extremities, or lower extremities. Region specificity is a characteristic of a great number of standardized self-report measures. A benefit of having numerous region-specific self-report measures available is the ability to gather information to assess interaction between regional joint mobility impairment and perceived function.

Visit the Rehabilitation Measures Database (https://www.sralab.org/rehabilitation-measures),[85] scroll down to the "Search" feature, open the dropdown menu for "Assessment Type," and apply the "Patient Reported Outcomes" filter to your search. Other filters that can be used include "Area of Assessment," "Population," "Body Cost," and "Cost." A practical problem of having numerous region-specific measures is deciding which measure is most appropriate for a given patient. To provide assistance with the process of selecting self-report measures for the patient with impaired joint mobility, further discussion of these measures is provided in the Outcomes section of this chapter.

Performance-Based Measures of Activity. Observational task analysis and patient self-report measure(s) provide the physical therapist information that allows for selection of appropriate performance-based activity measures. In contrast to self-report, performance-based measures quantify activity while minimizing the patient/client's perception of the performance. An individual's perceptions of activity limitations and participation restrictions are important aspects in every examination. Supplementary to understanding the patient/client's perception in relation to health and function is the ability to directly quantify performance of specific activities. Quantification of actual tasks through performance-based measures provides unique information that will be used, in light of the other examination information, to further evaluate the interaction of impaired joint mobility and other presenting problems of the patient/client.

The quantification of activity, if based on valid and reliable measures, allows the therapist to describe patient/client progression over the course of intervention as well as document outcomes. Similar to self-report measurement, there are a large number of standardized performance-based measures available. Visit the Rehabilitation Measures Database (https://www.sralab.org/rehabilitation-measures),[85] scroll down to the "Search" feature, open the dropdown menu for "Assessment Type," and apply the "Performance Measure" filter to your search. Selection of appropriate performance-based measures is guided in part by determining the daily tasks most likely to be influenced by the joint impairment. As pointed out earlier, the tasks most influenced are determined by the patient/client history and results of the self-report measure(s). Once an activity category is determined, selection of specific performance-based measures can be made. Discussion of selecting activity measures is addressed in the Outcomes section of this chapter.

Joint-Specific Mobility Testing. Targeted examination of older adults with suspected impairment of joint mobility also includes joint-specific mobility testing. Joint-specific mobility is typically examined through measurement of joint ROM, muscle–tendon unit (MTU) extensibility, and segmental mobility. These measures provide the final pieces of information needed to guide formation of the clinical hypotheses required to develop a plan of care.

Established goniometer and inclinometer measurement methods are utilized to clinically quantify joint ROM.[86] Quantification of joint ROM allows for comparison of a given individual's joint ROM with established normative values for people of similar age and gender. Joint ROM values can also be compared between the right and left sides to document the amount of asymmetry for a given patient/client. Visit the Rehabilitation Measures Database (https://www.sralab.org/rehabilitation-measures),[85] scroll down to the "Search" feature, open the dropdown menu for "Area of Assessment," and apply the "Range of Motion" filter to your search.

Another aspect of joint mobility that can be quantified by measurement of joint ROM is MTU extensibility. Extensibility refers to the ability of an MTU to lengthen. If an MTU crosses multiple joints, it may limit joint mobility when the position of the joints creates maximal lengthening of the muscle. To measure the maximal length of an MTU, standardized joint positioning has been established to account for all joints that are crossed by the MTU.[87]

The final component commonly included in examination of joint-specific mobility is segmental mobility testing. Segmental mobility refers to the accessory joint movement that is not under volitional control. As stated previously, the amount of accessory movement at a joint is expected to change with age because of joint structure changes. The difficulty in implementing clinical tests of segmental mobility is the low level of reliability and lack of established validity for the tests. For example, poor levels of interrater reliability are seen with spine segmental mobility testing, regardless of specific advanced training of the therapist.[88–91] In addition, a consensus on the best rating scale to use and the validity of grading in relation to joint mobility is currently lacking. As a result, it is recommended that segmental mobility testing be used as a qualitative guide for selection of quantitative measures such as joint ROM, valid instrumented tests for mobility of specific joints, and other joint- and region-specific special tests.

EVALUATION AND DIAGNOSIS

The evaluation process incorporates all examination results, including information from the history, systems review, and tests and measures, into a complete clinical impression of the patient/client presentation.[1] For example, a period of immobility, reduced knee mobility for biking, vehicular trauma, edema, and the inability to self-care due to stiffness and pain are examples of clinical indications for testing and measuring joint integrity and mobility. Arriving at the clinical impression requires critical analysis by the therapist to determine the potential causes of the patient/client's presenting problems. In assessing causes of the presenting problems, the suspected role of impaired joint integrity and mobility will be identified. Once joint mobility has been identified as an impairment, determining an appropriate diagnostic classification is possible. In addition, impaired joint mobility may be a secondary component of other diagnoses. For example, consider an older adult presenting with impaired hip mobility that limits walking. If this individual seeks intervention after a proximal femur fracture, "impaired joint mobility, muscle performance, and range of motion associated with hip fracture" is an appropriate diagnostic classification. In contrast, consider the patient who presents with hip mobility impairment in addition to several other ipsilateral symptom manifestations from a cerebral vascular accident. In this case, the musculoskeletal diagnostic classification of the hip is secondary to a primary neuromuscular diagnosis. Such distinctions in diagnostic classification serve to clarify the therapist's clinical impression to the patient/client, other health care providers, and reimbursement sources.

Once the diagnosis is clarified, the influence of joint integrity and mobility impairment on patient/client prognosis can be determined, considering the expected time required to achieve an optimal outcome.[1] In the absence of other impairments, the prognosis is favorable for remediating age-associated joint mobility impairment within a short (e.g., 4- to 6-week) time period. Basic factors common to older adults that often complicate prognosis include chronicity of impairment, level of physical activity, and high level of comorbidity. In patients with one or more of these additional factors, prognosis determination can be challenging. The process of identifying diagnostic categories, previously performed to arrive at a clinical impression, can also be a significant help in forming the prognosis. Factors such as the patient/client goals and perceptions, medical management of disease processes, family support, financial considerations, and cognition must also be considered. Being able to effectively incorporate all factors related to prognosis requires practice and experience in working with older adults.

The plan of care should include considerations specifically related to the identified joint integrity and mobility impairment. Strategies for addressing joint mobility impairment should be outlined, including the general intervention categories. The intervention approach will also be reflected in the specific intervention goals. Although it is reasonable to have goals specific to impaired joint mobility, they should be written in terms of the activity limitations or participation restrictions identified in the examination (see Box 15.3). The activity- and participation-based goals will reflect the functional relevance of the joint mobility problem.

BOX 15.3 Writing Patient Goals to Include Activity Limitation or Participation Restriction

A. Incorrect: Incomplete patient goal statement
The patient/client will increase hip extension range of motion (ROM) to 20 degrees within 4 weeks of intervention.

B. Correct: Inclusion of target activity in patient goal statement
The patient/client will increase hip extension ROM to 20 degrees to enable walking with a symmetrical gait pattern within 4 weeks of intervention.

INTERVENTION

Three primary intervention approaches for older adults with problems related to joint mobility impairment are remediation, compensation, and prevention. Education, therapeutic exercise, and manual therapy techniques can be valuable remediation interventions for individuals with functional limitations related to joint mobility. For these same individuals, compensatory interventions such as use of assistive devices can also be of value. For individuals who have not yet developed symptoms or functional difficulties, the interventions mentioned may be used to help prevent onset or progression of problems associated with joint impairment.

As will be presented later, favorable responses to remediation of impaired joint mobility have been seen in body structure and function, activity performance, and participation for older adults. In particular, exercise and increased physical activity can effectively reverse much of the detrimental influence of aging in regard to activity limitations and participation restriction.[92–97] However, age-associated changes in joint structure and function are seen even in people who are active, asymptomatic, or disease-free.[98–101] As a result, compensation and prevention strategies must also be considered as approaches to intervention. In this section of the chapter, patient/client education, therapeutic exercise, manual intervention techniques, and assistive/adaptive devices and equipment will be discussed in relation to remediation, compensation, and prevention of joint mobility impairment for the older adult.

Patient/Client/Society Education

One of the most beneficial interventions for addressing impaired joint mobility is patient/client education. Education for modifying lifestyle in terms of activity and exercise is known to be helpful for older adult populations and can be an important component of preventive, compensatory, and remediation intervention. A randomized controlled trial found that multidisciplinary education of patients with rheumatoid arthritis (RA) significantly improved compliance with their home exercise program and leisure physical activity at 6 months.[102] A narrative review suggests that education for patients with OA of the hip should include activity modification, exercise, methods to reduce loads on arthritic joints including weight reduction, and posture as part of conservative treatment.[103] Similarly, the Hip Pain and Mobility Deficits—Hip Osteoarthritis Clinical Practice Guideline also recommends the combination of patient education including activity modification, exercise, weight reduction (when overweight), and unloading arthritic joints with exercise and/or manual therapy.[104] A meta-analysis on the effectiveness of patient education revealed significant reductions in pain and improvement of function following education of patients/clients with OA and RA.[105] Lastly, in a paper in the *Journal of Orthopaedic and Sports Physical Therapy*, Mintken et al. discuss the importance of educating society (including physicians and other referral sources) about physical therapy as an evidence-based, nonpharmaceutical, and conservative (nonsurgical) alternative for pain management to help solve the opioid epidemic.[106] An example of compensatory activity modification relates to patients/clients with lumbar spinal stenosis. The result of spinal stenosis is a decrease in the spinal canal space, often producing radiating symptoms (termed *intermittent neurogenic claudication*). Changing upright postures to control lumbo-pelvic flexion, such as walking uphill or using an assistive device to shift the upper body position anteriorly, can greatly reduce symptoms by increasing the spinal canal space. In addition, avoiding prolonged overhead activities and prolonged axial loading may help control symptoms.[107] Education provided to make these activity changes may make as large an impact on function as any other intervention for these patients/clients. In most cases, patient/client daily activity will have the greatest impact on determining the success of the intervention.

Therapeutic Exercise

There is evidence that targeted therapeutic exercise, such as stretching and strengthening, can improve joint mobility. However, many intervention studies with older adults include several simultaneous modes of exercise, predominantly combinations of stretching, strengthening, endurance training, and balance training. Joint mobility has been shown to improve with multiple-mode exercise programs, although the amount and location of improvement is program specific. For example, recent meta-analyses found that exercise for OA can reduce finger[108] and knee[109] joint stiffness. The primary mode of exercise targeting impaired joint mobility is stretching.

Stretching Exercise. Stretching exercises for arthritic conditions have been endorsed in clinical practice guidelines by a number of professional organizations including the Academy of Orthopedic Physical Therapy (of the American Physical Therapy Association [APTA]),[104] the American Academy of Orthopedic Surgeons,[110] and the Royal College of Physicians.[111] In addition, the Ottawa Panel endorses stretching exercises to improve stiffness (grade C+) and range of motion (grade A) in the management of hip OA.[112] Researchers have demonstrated the usefulness of isolated stretching, static stretching particularly, for improving joint mobility of older adults.[113–116] Feland et al.[117] examined stretch duration and found that straight leg raise stretches held for 15, 30, or 60 seconds were effective for increasing the combined motion of hip flexion and knee extension for older adults with initially impaired hamstring extensibility. The suggestion by these authors is that the longer the hold of stretch, up to 60 seconds, the greater the ROM benefit. In general, studies using >15 seconds of stretch have identified improvements in joint mobility.[117]

Of particular importance in terms of stretching is that joint mobility increases are linked to improved activity performance. For example, walking performance is known to improve in older adults after stretching of the hip flexors and ankle plantar flexors.[113,115,116] Trends of improved gait speed and kinematics have been noted after static stretching even for community-dwelling, active older adults without participation restriction.[113,116]

Strengthening Exercise. Strengthening exercises for arthritic conditions have been endorsed in clinical practice guidelines by a number of professional organizations including the Academy of Orthopedic Physical Therapy (of the APTA),[104] the American Academy of Orthopedic Surgeons,[110,118] the Department of Veterans Affairs/Department of Defense,[119] the Royal College of Physicians,[111] and the Royal Australian College of General Practitioners.[120] In addition, the Ottawa Panel endorses strengthening exercises to improve stiffness (grade A) and range of motion (grade A) in the management of hip OA.[112] Muscle strengthening influences joint mobility through indirect mechanisms. An indirect link between muscle strength and joint mobility has been demonstrated through the contribution of muscle to joint loading and control of motion.[121] Muscle–tendon units typically serve as a primary mechanism for attenuating load transmission across joints by absorbing energy in activities such as walking. Impaired muscle function associated with aging diminishes this capacity to absorb loads and may result in increased loading of other joint structures, possibly leading to negative changes. Some evidence to support the influence of muscle function on prevention of impaired joint mobility is the link seen between muscle weakness and onset of knee OA[122]; however, a causal relationship has not been definitively established.

Strengthening exercise has been shown to influence joint mobility in older adult populations. For example, Fatouros et al.[123] demonstrated that individuals (mean age 70.6 years) not previously active in an exercise program gained shoulder, elbow, hip, and knee ROM after interventions including resistance and endurance training in the absence of stretching. This finding indicates that joint mobility improvement can be achieved partly as a result of improved muscle function.

Strengthening also influences joint mobility by loading the joint structures. Dynamic loading can stimulate growth of joint connective tissue structures, such as articular cartilage and bone.[124] For instance, Roos and Dahlberg[125] studied knee articular cartilage of patients/clients (mean age 45.8 years) who had previously undergone partial medial meniscectomy. After 4 months of progressive resistance training, there was noted improvement in glycoconjugate, specifically glucosaminoglycan, content in the articular cartilage of the postsurgical knees. Continued examination specific to the influence of resistance exercise on cartilage and other joint structures in older adults is needed.

Combined Exercise Interventions. Several studies that include older adult participants across various levels of fitness and health status have examined the effect of combined exercise interventions (e.g., stretching, endurance exercise, resistance exercise, and functional activity) on joint mobility, with positive results.[126–130] For example, Brown et al.[131] examined sedentary men and women older than age 78 years and found an increase in trunk, hip, and ankle mobility following 3 months of combined resistance, endurance, and stretching exercise. In another study, Thompson and Osness,[132] using a program including resistance, flexibility, and functional training (three times a week for 8 weeks), found no significant increases in hip motion for older adult golfers. It is obvious that findings from such studies are difficult to compare because of the multiple interventions and lack of targeted impairments. Although improvements in joint mobility result from such multimode exercise programs, it is not possible to determine which aspect of the program has the greatest influence on joint mobility.

Other Forms of Exercise Related to Joint Mobility. Other forms of exercise that influence joint mobility include stabilization, tai chi, and yoga. These forms of exercise can theoretically indirectly influence joint mobility by improving motor control. These exercises have limited evidence in relation to remediation or prevention of joint mobility impairment in older adults. Although evidence in research literature is limited, there are indications that all three of these exercise types may benefit joint mobility.

Stabilization exercises are designed to selectively target coactivation of muscles and provide joint stability. Most of the research on stabilization exercises has been based on the spine. In relation to the lumbar spine, it has been concluded that stabilization exercises may improve pain and function in individuals with chronic low back pain, including older adults.[133–135] Tai chi, a Chinese form of mind–body exercise that has gained popularity in use among older adults across the world, has been linked to improving balance, muscle function, and life participation and reducing risk of falls.[136–138] In addition to these benefits, there has also been research indicating that older adults with impaired joint mobility can benefit from tai chi. For example, tai chi exercise has been shown to improve self-report of pain, stiffness, and physical function for older adults with diagnosed OA of the knee.[139–141] Yoga is a traditional Indian form of exercise combining resistance, balance, and flexibility exercises. Initial studies have shown yoga to be an appropriate and simple-to-learn activity for older adults that can improve joint mobility.[142–145] For example, DiBenedetto et al.[146] examined walking in older adults before and after 8 weeks of participation in a yoga exercise program. Participants in the yoga program demonstrated increased hip joint extension during walking along with increased stride length and a trend toward improved walking speed.

Manual Intervention Techniques

Historically, use of manual joint mobilization and manipulation has been approached with much caution when working with older adults. The typical changes to joint connective tissue structures, leading to generalized weakening, has been the primary cause for concern. Although it is important to use caution when dealing with joint structures weakened with age, age is not a contraindication to joint mobilization and manipulation. Studies of joint mobilization and manipulation interventions for aging and older adults have been summarized and indicate favorable results, especially when combined with therapeutic exercise.[147–153] Hoeksma et al.[154] demonstrated specific joint mobilization and manipulation combined with stretching to be superior to exercise alone for remediation of joint impairment in individuals with hip OA. The improved outcome measures for the manual intervention group were patient subjective assessment, visual analog scale reporting for pain, hip ROM, and Harris Hip Score. In a recent meta-analysis, manual therapy improved short- and long-term measures of pain and function in people with hip OA.[155] In addition, the combination of manual therapy with exercise also improved pain and function in the short term.

Joint mobilization has also been examined for people diagnosed with lumbar stenosis.[107,156] In a randomized clinical trial, two groups of patients/clients (mean age of 69.5 years) with magnetic resonance imaging evidence of lumbar spinal stenosis were treated for 6 weeks with one of two intervention regimens.[157] One group received lumbar flexion exercise and treadmill walking, and the other lumbar mobilization, hip mobilization, partial body weight–supported treadmill walking, stretching, and resistance exercise. Although both treatment groups demonstrated improvement, a significantly greater increase in Global Rating of Change Scale scores and walking tolerance was seen in the group receiving joint mobilization. However, the obvious differences in intervention beyond joint mobilization make it difficult to determine the direct influence of joint mobilization.

In relation to older adults with osteoporosis, the use of manual intervention techniques is controversial. For individuals with spinal osteoporosis, grade V mobilization (i.e., manipulation) has been contraindicated based on concerns for fracture risk.[158] In a survey of Canadian physical therapists by Sran and Khan,[159] 91% of the respondents reported concerns with using manual therapy for patients/clients with osteoporosis. For the same respondents, 45% have used manual therapy with this population. However, data to support the use of joint mobilization and manipulation for older adults with osteoporosis is insufficient.[160] One published case report of a patient/client with osteoporosis found that treatment including grade III and grade IV joint mobilization to thoracic and cervicothoracic regions, respectively, resulted in improvement in scores in pain level, quality of life, and function questionnaires.[161] In a study examining postmenopausal women with thoracic kyphosis, the intervention group that received manual mobilization (grade not specified), exercise, and taping demonstrated a significant reduction in their kyphosis.[162] In a different study that examined people with osteoporotic vertebral fracture, the intervention group that received manual mobilization (grade not specified), exercise, and taping demonstrated significant improvements in pain (with movement and at rest) and function.[163] All three of these studies reported that participants had no serious adverse effects from the interventions.[161–163] In addition, it has been shown that anteroposterior mobilization forces are typically well below the level of force required to induce fracture in osteoporotic bones.[164] Substantially more research is needed before clear-cut recommendations can be made regarding the use of mobilization techniques for patients/clients with osteoporosis.

Assistive/Adaptive Devices and Equipment

Assistive and adaptive devices can be used as compensatory or preventive approaches to protect joint structure and assist with load transfer across joints. Devices such as canes and walkers are useful components to physical therapy intervention for individuals with joint mobility impairment. For example, Kemp et al.[165] analyzed knee forces during walking in a group of 20 people (mean age 65 years) with medial knee osteoarthritis. Their finding was a mean decrease in peak knee adduction moment with cane use in the hand contralateral to the symptomatic knee. However, variability among patients/clients illustrated that technique in use of the cane is important. The suggestion is that proper training and evaluation of assistive device use is needed to ensure that patients/clients are benefiting.

Braces designed to alter joint alignment have also been used with older adults. Findings indicate that alignment can be altered and joint loading decreased across painful areas of osteoarthritic joints. A recent systematic review concluded that valgus unloading braces are effective at reducing pain secondary to medial compartment knee OA.[166] A similar meta-analysis found that soft braces improved pain and function in people with knee OA.[167] There is also evidence that use of unloading braces for older adults with knee osteoarthritis can result in improved functional outcomes: decreased muscle co-contraction during walking and stair climbing,[168] decreased gait asymmetry,[169] and increased step length and gait speed.[170]

Footwear can also influence loading of lower extremity joints in older adults during walking.[171] Selection of appropriate footwear, designed to strategically cushion and support, may be a simple way to provide immediate relief of symptoms by decreasing loads across lower extremity joints. Additionally, shoe orthotics may improve lower extremity alignment and bring about changes in joint loading.[172]

OUTCOMES

Observation of task performance, self-report measures of activity and participation, performance-based activity measures, and joint mobility measures from the initial examination guide the development of the patient/client's intervention goals. The design of the intervention, remediation, compensation, or prevention dictates which outcome measures are most appropriate. The outcome measures chosen can be focused at the level of impairment, activity limitation, or participation restriction. Often, self-report measures of activity and participation or performance-based measures of activity are most appropriate as the primary outcome measures because they can effectively quantify how function is influenced by the impairments and may also assess different aspects of function.[173] In cases of prevention intervention, direct joint mobility measures may be most appropriate for quantifying outcome.

As mentioned previously in the Tests and Measures section, selection of specific instruments is based on individual characteristics of the patient/client with joint impairment, practicality of administering the test/measure, and clinometric properties of the test/measure. The selection process is complicated by the large number of self-report and performance-based tests and measures available for use in the clinic. This section provides some recommendations of specific tests and measures appropriate for an older adult with impaired joint mobility that has negatively influenced activity or participation. Despite the perceived benefits of using standardized outcome measures (e.g., enhanced communication with patients and payers, direction with the plan of care, and enhanced thoroughness of the examination), physical therapists still underutilize outcome measures for a variety of reasons (e.g., confusing and difficult for patients to complete, and time-consuming for patients and therapists).[174]

Self-Report Outcome Instruments

Self-report or patient-reported measures that are specific to a given region of the body, though not directly measuring joint mobility impairment, can be helpful to determine patient/client activity limitations and participation restrictions related to a given joint impairment. For example, a patient/client with impaired cervical joint mobility can be given a self-report measure designed specifically to measure his or her perception of function related to the cervical spine. A recent overview of systematic reviews summarized clinometric properties, including reliability, validity, and responsiveness, of eight patient-reported outcome measures. Key findings include the following: Internal consistency from high-quality evidence was reported for the Neck Disability Index and the Copenhagen Neck Functional Disability Scale, and test–retest reliability and construct validity from high-quality evidence was only reported for the Copenhagen Neck Functional Disability Scale.[175]

With respect to low back pain syndromes, a great number of self-report measures have been developed.[176] Zanoli et al.[177] identified 92 instruments designed to evaluate pain, function, disability, health status, and patient satisfaction in relation to low back impairment. In relation to older adult patients/clients with chronic low back problems, the Roland-Morris Disability Questionnaire (RMDQ) and Oswestry Disability Index (ODI) are two of the most established and commonly used measures for pain, function, and disability. The RMDQ and ODI have established validity for measuring the effects of low back pain across a wide range of ages, including older adults,[178] and their use has been endorsed by the Low Back Pain Clinical Practice Guideline from the Academy of Orthopaedic Physical Therapy.[179]

A variety of questionnaires are also available for assessing function of upper extremity joints.[180–182] Some of the most widely used instruments, with validity, reliability, and responsiveness in measuring function in older adult populations, are the Western Ontario Osteoarthritis of the Shoulder Index (WOOS), the Western Ontario Rotator Cuff Index (WORC), the Rotator Cuff Quality of Life Questionnaire (RC-QOL), the American Shoulder and Elbow Surgeons (ASES) score, the Australian/Canadian Osteoarthritis Hand Index (AUSCAN), and the Disabilities of the Arm, Shoulder, and Hand Questionnaire (DASH). As indicated by the titles, elbow-specific measures have been generally less emphasized than shoulder and wrist. In addition, the specific type of impairment (e.g., rotator cuff injury) is a key determinant for questionnaire selection.

Gummesson et al.[183] selected 11 items from the 30-item DASH to determine if a shorter version would be valid and reliable for use with clinical populations. In their study of 105 participants (age range 18 to 83 years), they found outcomes of the 11-item scale to be highly similar to the full 30-item DASH. The conclusion is that the 11-item QuickDASH can replace the DASH while maintaining the established validity and reliability of the original questionnaire. Considering the practicality of time efficiency, the QuickDASH is recommended as a clinical tool for older adults with impaired mobility of upper extremity joints. For individuals with specific pathology, such as a rotator cuff tear or shoulder osteoarthritis, the pathology-specific questionnaires mentioned previously may be more appropriate.

Functional status related to lower extremity joint impairments can also be captured using self-report measures. Various reviews have compared the clinometric properties and usefulness of lower extremity measures.[184–190] Common clinical measures with research evidence based on older adult populations are the Lower Limb Core Score, Functional Ankle Disability Index (FADI), Functional Ankle Ability Measure (FAAM), Knee Injury and Osteoarthritis Outcome Score (KOOS), Oxford Knee Score, Western Ontario and McMaster Universities Osteoarthritis Index (WOMAC), Harris Hip Score (HHS), Hip Disability and Osteoarthritis Outcome Score (HOOS), and Lower Extremity Functional Scale (LEFS). As with the upper extremity measures, many lower extremity self-report measures are highly specific to joint and pathology. The WOMAC, HOOS, LEFS, and HHS are endorsed by the Hip Pain and Mobility Deficits—Hip Osteoarthritis Clinical Practice Guideline.[104]

Performance-Based Outcome Instruments

As stated previously, standardized quantitative measurement of common functional tasks adds to the information gained from self-report measures by providing information on functional performance without direct influence of the patient perceptions. The selection of an appropriate performance-based outcome instrument is based on the daily tasks that are problematic, in addition to the other considerations of appropriateness for a given patient/client, practicality, and clinometric properties. Tasks such as walking, reaching, and transitioning between postures are common targets for quantification with performance-based measures, based on the common need for these activities during daily living. The specific activities that will be measured as outcomes depend on the findings of the initial exam and the goals of the intervention.

Suggested performance-based measures of specific activities for older adults with impaired joint mobility include the functional reach test, timed up and go test, five times sit-to-stand test, 6-minute walk test, stair climb test, and gait speed. These measures are recommended based on their appropriateness for use with older adult populations, clinical practicality, and established clinometric properties.[191–199] The measures must be able to capture the activity limitation that has been linked to impaired joint mobility. However, there is a need to further establish which measures are best for given impairments of joint mobility. For example, Terwee et al.[200] reviewed the clinometric properties of 26 performance-based measures for individuals with hip or knee osteoarthritis. The conclusion of the authors, based on the need for establishing adequate validity and reliability, was that no consensus can yet be made on what activity measures are most appropriate for patients/clients with hip or knee osteoarthritis.[200]

There are numerous other performance-based measures that may be indirectly linked to joint mobility. A comprehensive review of all performance-based measures of activity is not in the scope of this chapter. For more information on performance-based measures related to specific activities, the reader is referred to Chapter 7 (Ambulation) of this text.

This section of the chapter has provided some recommendations on specific outcome measures for patients with joint mobility impairment. It is important to keep in mind that joint mobility is only one part of the larger picture of a given patient/client's health and function. Perspective of the larger picture must be maintained to practically apply the appropriate tests and measures. An outcome measure that is appropriate, based on all impairments, limitations, and restrictions, is ideal. However, it is impractical to capture the complete health and functional status of an individual with a single test or measure. Applying a reasoned approach to outcome selection will allow for a feasible number of tests and measures to be selected that can be performed in a reasonable time span to best capture the health and function of an older adult with impaired joint mobility.

SUMMARY

The health and function of older adults can be greatly influenced by impaired joint mobility. Age-associated decline in joint mobility can occur in the absence of disease or as a result of an interaction of disease processes. Any impairment of joint mobility can be linked to activity limitation and restricted participation, which often results in older adults presenting to a physical therapist for treatment. The therapist can effectively identify joint mobility impairments through systematic examination. Once identified, impaired joint mobility can be addressed as a component of the comprehensive patient/client plan of care. Therapists and patients/clients can be encouraged that an appropriate plan of care can effectively restore joint mobility and promote successful aging.

REFERENCES

1. American Physical Therapy Association. *Guide to Physical Therapist Practice.* 3rd ed. American Physical Therapy Association; 2016.
2. Prevalence of self-reported arthritis or chronic joint symptoms among adults—United States, 2001. *MMWR Morb Mortal Wkly Rep.* 2002;51:948–950.
3. Barbour KE, Helmick CG, Boring M, Brady TJ. Vital signs: prevalence of doctor-diagnosed arthritis and arthritis-attributable activity limitation—United States, 2013–2015. *MMWR Morb Mortal Wkly Rep.* 2017;66:246–253.
4. Roberts S, Colombier P, Sowman A, et al. Ageing in the musculoskeletal system. *Acta Orthop.* 2016;87:15–25.
5. Toh WS, Brittberg M, Farr J, et al. Cellular senescence in aging and osteoarthritis. *Acta Orthop.* 2016;87:6–14.
6. Florencio-Silva R, Sasso GR da S, Sasso-Cerri E, et al. Biology of bone tissue: structure, function, and factors that influence bone cells. *Biomed Res Int.* 2015;421746:1–17.
7. Morley JE, Baumgartner RN. Cytokine-related aging process. *J Gerontol A Biol Sci Med Sci.* 2004;59:924–929.
8. Plumb MS, Treon K, Aspden RM. Competing regulation of matrix biosynthesis by mechanical and IGF-1 signalling in elderly human articular cartilage in vitro. *Biochim Biophys Acta.* 2006;1760:762–767.
9. Gu W, Zhu Q, Gao X, et al. Simulation of the progression of intervertebral disc degeneration due to decreased nutritional supply. *Spine.* 2014;39:1411–1417.
10. Jorgensen AEM, Kjaer M, Heinemeier KM, et al. The effect of aging and mechanical loading on the metabolism of articular cartilage. *J Rheumatology.* 2017;44:410–417.
11. Freemont AJ, Hoyland JA. Morphology, mechanisms and pathology of musculoskeletal ageing. *J Pathol.* 2007;211: 252–259.
12. Saito M, Marumo K. Collagen cross-links as a determinant of bone quality: a possible explanation for bone fragility in aging, osteoporosis, and diabetes mellitus. *Osteoporos Int.* 2010;21:195–214.
13. Barros EM, Rodrigues CJ, Rodrigues NR, et al. Aging of the elastic and collagen fibers in the human cervical interspinous ligaments. *Spine J.* 2002;2:57–62.
14. Raj PP. Intervertebral disc: anatomy-physiology-pathophysiology-treatment. *Pain Pract.* 2008;8:18–44.
15. Griffin TM, Guilak F. The role of mechanical loading in the onset and progression of osteoarthritis. *Exerc Sport Sci Rev.* 2005;33:195–200.
16. Driban JB, Hootman JM, Sitler MR, et al. Is participation in certain sports associated with knee osteoarthritis? A systematic review. *J Athl Train.* 2017;52:497–506.
17. Jensen LK. Knee osteoarthritis: influence of work involving heavy lifting, kneeling, climbing stairs or ladders, or kneeling/squatting combined with heavy lifting. *Occup Environ Med.* 2008;65:72–89.
18. Gomoll AH, Minas T. The quality of healing: articular cartilage. *Wound Repair Regen.* 2014;22:30–38.
19. Lotz M, Loeser RF. Effects of aging on articular cartilage homeostasis. *Bone.* 2015;51:241–248.
20. Kurutz M. Age-sensitivity of time-related in vivo deformability of human lumbar motion segments and discs in pure centric tension. *J Biomech.* 2006;39:147–157.
21. Vo NV, Hartman RA, Patil PR, et al. Molecular mechanisms of biological aging in intervertebral discs. *J Orthop Res.* 2016;34:1289–1306.
22. Cassinelli EH, Kang JD. Current understanding of lumbar disc degeneration. *Operat Tech Orthop.* 2000;10:254–262.
23. Haefeli M, Kalberer F, Saegesser D, et al. The course of macroscopic degeneration in the human lumbar intervertebral disc. *Spine.* 2006;31:1522–1531.
24. Sargon MF, Doral MN, Atay OA. Age-related changes in human PCLs: a light and electron microscopic study. *Knee Surg Sports Traumatol Arthrosc.* 2004;12:280–284.
25. Hasegawa A, Otsuki S, Pauli C, et al. Anterior cruciate ligament changes in the human knee joint in aging and osteoarthritis. *Arthritis Rheum.* 2012;64:696–704.
26. Yamada K, Healey R, Amiel D, et al. Subchondral bone of the human knee joint in aging and osteoarthritis. *Osteoarthritis Cartilage.* 2002;10:360–369.
27. Liberman D, Cheung A. A practical approach to osteoporosis management in the geriatric population. *Can Geriatr J.* 2015;18:29–34.
28. Catalano A, Martino G, Morabito N, et al. Pain in osteoporosis: from pathophysiology to therapeutic approach. *Drugs Aging.* 2017;34:755–765.

29. Black DM, Rosen CJ. Clinical practice. Postmenopausal osteoporosis. *N Engl J Med.* 2016;374:254–262.
30. Malmstrom EM, Karlberg M, Fransson PA, et al. Primary and coupled cervical movements: the effect of age, gender, and body mass index. A 3-dimensional movement analysis of a population without symptoms of neck disorders. *Spine.* 2006;31(2):E44–E50.
31. Demaille-Wlodyka S, Chiquet C, Lavaste JF, et al. Cervical range of motion and cephalic kinesthesis: ultrasonographic analysis by age and sex. *Spine.* 2007;32:E254–E261.
32. Doriot N, Wang X. Effects of age and gender on maximum voluntary range of motion of the upper body joints. *Ergonomics.* 2006;49:269–281.
33. Castro WH, Sautmann A, Schilgen M, et al. Noninvasive three-dimensional analysis of cervical spine motion in normal subjects in relation to age and sex. An experimental examination. *Spine.* 2000;25:443–449.
34. Troke M, Moore AP, Maillardet FJ, et al. A normative database of lumbar spine ranges of motion. *Man Ther.* 2005;10:198–206.
35. Troke M, Moore AP, Maillardet FJ, et al. A new, comprehensive normative database of lumbar spine ranges of motion. *Clin Rehabil.* 2001;15:371–379.
36. Bible JE, Simpson AK, Emerson JW, et al. Quantifying the effects of degeneration and other patient factors on lumbar segmental range of motion using multivariate analysis. *Spine.* 2008;33:1793–1799.
37. Nonaka H, Mita K, Watakabe M, et al. Age-related changes in the interactive mobility of the hip and knee joints: a geometrical analysis. *Gait Posture.* 2002;15:236–243.
38. Menz HB. Biomechanics of the ageing foot and ankle: a mini-review. *Gerontology.* 2015;61:381–388.
39. Escalante A, Lichtenstein MJ, Dhanda R, et al. Determinants of hip and knee flexion range: results from the San Antonio Longitudinal Study of Aging. *Arthritis Care Res.* 1999;12:8–18.
40. Roach KE, Miles TP. Normal hip and knee active range of motion: the relationship to age. *Phys Ther.* 1991;71:656–665.
41. Anderson DE, Madigan ML. Healthy older adults have insufficient hip range of motion and plantar flexor strength to walk like healthy young adults. *J Biomech.* 2014;47(5): 1104–1109.
42. Scott G, Menz HB, Newcombe L. Age-related differences in foot structure and function. *Gait Posture.* 2007;26:68–75.
43. Escalante A, Lichtenstein MJ, Hazuda HP. Determinants of shoulder and elbow flexion range: results from the San Antonio Longitudinal Study of Aging. *Arthritis Care Res.* 1999;12:277–286.
44. Ludewig PM, Reynolds JE. The association of scapular kinematics and glenohumeral joint pathologies. *J Orthop Sports Phys Ther.* 2009;39:90–104.
45. Chaparro A, Rogers M, Fernandez J, et al. Range of motion of the wrist: implications for designing computer input devices for the elderly. *Disabil Rehabil.* 2000;22:633–637.
46. Lin JJ, Lim HK, Yang JL. Effect of shoulder tightness on glenohumeral translation, scapular kinematics, and scapulohumeral rhythm in subjects with stiff shoulders. *J Orthop Res.* 2006;24:1044–1051.
47. Carter DR, Beaupre GS, Wong M, et al. The mechanobiology of articular cartilage development and degeneration. *Clin Orthop Relat Res.* 2004;(427 Suppl):S69–S77.
48. Russell ME, Shivanna KH, Grosland NM, et al. Cartilage contact pressure elevations in dysplastic hips: a chronic overload model. *J Orthop Surg Res.* 2006;1:6.
49. Kado DM, Huang MH, Karlamangla AS, et al. Factors associated with kyphosis progression in older women: 15 years' experience in the study of osteoporotic fractures. *J Bone Mineral Res.* 2013;28(1):179–187.
50. Garstang SV, Stitik TP. Osteoarthritis: epidemiology, risk factors, and pathophysiology. *Am J Phys Med Rehabil.* 2006;85:S2–S11. quiz S2–S4.
51. Luoma K, Riihimaki H, Luukkonen R, et al. Low back pain in relation to lumbar disc degeneration. *Spine.* 2000;25:487–492.
52. Menz HB, Morris ME, Lord SR. Foot and ankle risk factors for falls in older people: a prospective study. *J Gerontol Med Sci.* 2006;61A(8):866–870.
53. Kerrigan DC, Lee LW, Collins JJ, et al. Reduced hip extension during walking: healthy elderly and fallers versus young adults. *Arch Phys Med Rehabil.* 2001;82:26–30.
54. Majithia V, Geraci SA. Rheumatoid arthritis: diagnosis and management. *Am J Med.* 2007;120:936–939.
55. Markman JD, Gaud KG. Lumbar spinal stenosis in older adults: current understanding and future directions. *Clin Geriatr Med.* 2008;24:369–388.
56. Yucesoy B, Charles LE, Baker B, et al. Occupational and genetic risk factors for osteoarthritis: a review. *Work.* 2015;50:261–273.
57. Solovieva S, Kontio T, Viikari-Juntura E. Occupation, physical workload factors, and disability retirement as a result of hip osteoarthritis in Finland, 2005-2013. *J Rheumatol.* 2018;45:555–562.
58. Watson KB, Carlson SA, Gunn JP, et al. Physical inactivity among adults aged 50 years and older - United States, 2014. *MMWR Morb Mortal Wkly Rep.* 2016;65:954–958.
59. Musich S, Wang SS, Hawkins K, et al. The frequency and health benefits of physical activity for older adults. *Popul Health Manag.* 2017;20:199–207.
60. Booth FW, Roberts CK, Laye MJ. Lack of exercise is a major cause of chronic diseases. *Compr Physiol.* 2012;2:1143–1211.
61. Hagströmer M, Franzén E. The importance of physical activity and health for physical therapy. *Phys Ther Rev.* 2017;22: 116–123.
62. Mueller MJ, Maluf KS. Tissue adaptation to physical stress: a proposed "Physical Stress Theory" to guide physical therapist practice, education, and research. *Phys Ther.* 2002;82:383–403.
63. Mueller MJ. Musculoskeletal impairments are often unrecognized and underappreciated complications from diabetes. *Phys Ther.* 2016;96:1861–1864.
64. Burner TW, Rosenthal AK. Diabetes and rheumatic diseases. *Curr Opin Rheumatol.* 2009;21:50–54.
65. Juel NG, Brox JI, Brunborg C, et al. Very high prevalence of frozen shoulder in patients with type 1 diabetes of ≥45 years' duration: the Dialong Shoulder Study. *Arch Phys Med Rehabil.* 2017;98:1551–1559.
66. Cherqaoui R, McKenzie S, Nunlee-Bland G. Diabetic cheiroarthropathy: a case report and review of the literature. *Case Rep Endocrinol.* 2013;257028:1–3.
67. Liu CJ, Chang WP, Araujo de Carvalho I, et al. Effects of physical exercise in older adults with reduced physical capacity: meta-analysis of resistance exercise and multimodal exercise. *Int J Rehabil Res.* 2017;40:303–314.
68. Murphy L, Schwartz TA, Helmick CG, et al. Lifetime risk of symptomatic knee osteoarthritis. *Arthritis Rheum.* 2008;59: 1207–1213.
69. Zengini E, Finan C, Wilkinson JM. The genetic epidemiological landscape of hip and knee osteoarthritis: where are we now and where are we going? *J Rheumatol.* 2016;43:260–266.
70. Dalbeth N, Choi HK, Terkeltaub R. Review: gout: a roadmap to approaches for improving global outcomes. *Arthritis Rheum.* 2017;69:22–34.
71. Mankia K, Emery P. Preclinical rheumatoid arthritis: progress toward prevention. *Arthritis Rheum.* 2016;68:779–788.
72. Sanz I. New perspectives in rheumatology: may you live in interesting times: challenges and opportunities in lupus research. *Arthritis Rheum.* 2017;69:1552–1559.

73. Avins KG, Hanke T, Kirk-Sanchez N, et al. Management of falls in community-dwelling older adults: clinical guidance statement from the Academy of Geriatric Physical Therapy of the American Physical Therapy Association. *Phys Ther.* 2015;95:815–834.
74. Lau A, Oyen ML, Kent RW, et al. Indentation stiffness of aging human costal cartilage. *Acta Biomater.* 2008;4:97–103.
75. Sharma G, Goodwin J. Effect of aging on respiratory system physiology and immunology. *Clin Interv Aging.* 2006;1: 253–260.
76. Wainner RS, Fritz JM, Irrgang JJ, et al. Reliability and diagnostic accuracy of the clinical examination and patient self-report measures for cervical radiculopathy. *Spine.* 2003;28:52–62.
77. VanSwearingen JM, Brach JS. Making geriatric assessment work: selecting useful measures. *Phys Ther.* 2001;81: 1233–1252.
78. Jette AM. Toward a common language for function, disability, and health. *Phys Ther.* 2006;86:726–734.
79. World Health Organization. *International Classification of Functioning, Disability and Health: ICF.* Geneva, Switzerland: World Health Organization; 2001.
80. Schenkman M, Deutsch JE, Gill-Body KM. An integrated framework for decision making in neurologic physical therapist practice. *Phys Ther.* 2006;86:1681–1702.
81. Brunnekreef JJ, van Uden CJ, van Moorsel S, et al. Reliability of videotaped observational gait analysis in patients with orthopedic impairments. *BMC Musculoskelet Disord.* 2005;6:17.
82. The Pathokinesiology Service & the Physical Therapy Dept. *Observational Gait Analysis.* Downey, CA: Rancho Los Amigos Research and Education Institute; 2001.
83. Hickey BW, Milosavljevic S, Bell ML, et al. Accuracy and reliability of observational motion analysis in identifying shoulder symptoms. *Man Ther.* 2007;12:263–270.
84. Silva AG, Punt TD, Johnson MI. Reliability and validity of head posture assessment by observation and a four-category scale. *Man Ther.* 2010;15:490–495.
85. Rehabilitation Measures Database. https://www.sralab.org/rehabilitation-measures.
86. Norkin CC, White DJ. *Measurement of Joint Motion: A Guide to Goniometry.* 5th ed. Philadelphia: FA Davis Company; 2017.
87. Kendall FP, McCreary EK, Provance PG, Rodgers MM, Romani WA. *Muscles: Testing and Function with Posture and Pain.* 5th ed. Baltimore, MD: Lippincott Williams & Wilkins; 2005.
88. Cleland JA, Childs JD, Fritz JM, et al. Interrater reliability of the history and physical examination in patients with mechanical neck pain. *Arch Phys Med Rehabil.* 2006;87:1388–1395.
89. Johansson F. Interexaminer reliability of lumbar segmental mobility tests. *Man Ther.* 2006;11:331–336.
90. Schneider M, Erhard R, Brach J, et al. Spinal palpation for lumbar segmental mobility and pain provocation: an interexaminer reliability study. *J Manipulative Physiol Ther.* 2008;31:465–473.
91. Hicks GE, Fritz JM, Delitto A, et al. Interrater reliability of clinical examination measures for identification of lumbar segmental instability. *Arch Phys Med Rehabil.* 2003;84: 1858–1864.
92. Waller B, Ogonowska-Słodownik A, Vitor M, et al. The effect of aquatic exercise on physical functioning in the older adult: a systematic review with meta-analysis. *Age Ageing.* 2016;45: 593–601.
93. Liu Y, Hazlewood GS, Kaplan GG, et al. Impact of obesity on remission and disease activity in rheumatoid arthritis: a systematic review and meta-analysis. *Arthritis Care Res.* 2017;69:157–165.
94. Yeun YR. Effectiveness of resistance exercise using elastic bands on flexibility and balance among the elderly people living in the community: a systematic review and meta-analysis. *J Phys Ther Sci.* 2017;29:1695–1699.
95. Straight CR, Lindheimer JB, Brady AO, et al. Effects of resistance training on lower-extremity muscle power in middle-aged and older adults: a systematic review and meta-analysis of randomized controlled trials. *Sports Med.* 2016;46:353–364.
96. Chase J-AD, Phillips LJ, Brown M. Physical activity intervention effects on physical function among community-dwelling older adults: a systematic review and meta-analysis. *J Aging Phys Act.* 2017;25:149–170.
97. Hortobágyi T, Lesinski M, Gäbler M, et al. Effects of three types of exercise interventions on healthy old adults' gait speed: a systematic review and meta-analysis. *Sports Med.* 2015;45:1627–1643.
98. Ahmed MS, Matsumura B, Cristian A. Age-related changes in muscles and joints. *Phys Med Rehabil.* 2005;16: 19–39.
99. Wang J, Yang X. Age-related changes in the orientation of lumbar facet joints. *Spine.* 2009;34:596–598.
100. Bonsell S, Pearsall AW, Heitman RJ, et al. The relationship of age, gender, and degenerative changes observed on radiographs of the shoulder in asymptomatic individuals. *J Bone Joint Surg Br.* 2000;82:1135–1139.
101. Gensburger D, Ariot M, Sornay-Rendu E, Roux JP, Delmas P. Radiographic assessment of age-related knee joint space changes in women: a 4-year longitudinal study. *Arthritis Care Res.* 2009;61:336–343.
102. Mayoux-Benhamou A, Quintrec JSGL, Ravaud P, et al. Influence of patient education on exercise compliance in rheumatoid arthritis: a prospective 12-month randomized controlled trial. *J Rheumatol.* 2008;35:216–223.
103. Cibulka MT, Woehrle J. Conservative treatment options for osteoarthritis of hip. *Topics Geriatr Rehabil.* 2013;29: 227–238.
104. Cibulka MT, Bloom NJ, Eneski KR, et al. Hip pain and mobility deficits—hip osteoarthritis: revision 2017. *J Orthop Sports Phys Ther.* 2017;47:1–37.
105. Superio-Cabuslay E, Ward MM, Lorig KR. Patient education interventions in osteoarthritis and rheumatoid arthritis: a meta-analytic comparison with nonsteroidal antiinflammatory drug treatment. *Arthritis Care Res.* 1996;9:292–301.
106. Mintken PE, Moore JR, Flynn TW. Physical therapist's role in solving the opioid epidemic. *J Orthop Sports Phys Ther.* 2018;48:349–353.
107. Backstrom KM, Whitman JM, Flynn TW. Lumbar spinal stenosis-diagnosis and management of the aging spine. *Man Ther.* 2011;16:308–317.
108. Østerås N, Kjeken I, Smedslund G, et al. Exercise for hand osteoarthritis. *Cochrane Database Syst Rev.* 2017;(1): CD010388.
109. Li Y, Su Y, Chen S, et al. The effects of resistance exercise in patients with knee osteoarthritis: a systematic review and meta-analysis. *Clin Rehabil.* 2016;30:947–959.
110. Jevsevar DS. *Treatment of Osteoarthritis of the Knee: Evidence-Based Guideline.* 2nd ed. *J Am Acad Orthop Surg.* 2013;21(9):571–576.
111. National Collaborating Centre for Chronic Conditions (UK). *Rheumatoid Arthritis: National Clinical Guideline for Management and Treatment in Adults.* London: Royal College of Physicians (UK); 2009.
112. Brosseau L, Wells GA, Pugh AG, et al. Ottawa panel evidence-based clinical practice guidelines for therapeutic exercise in the management of hip osteoarthritis. *Clin Rehabil.* 2016;30: 935–946.
113. Zotz TGG, Loureiro APC, Valderramas SR, Gomes ARS. Stretching – an important strategy to prevent musculoskeletal aging: a systematic review and meta-analysis. *Topics Geriatr Rehabil.* 2014;30(4):246–255.

114. Johnson E, Bradley B, Witkowski K, et al. Effect of a static calf muscle-tendon unit stretching program on ankle dorsiflexion range of motion of older women. *J Geriatr Phys Ther.* 2007;30:49–52.
115. Gajdosik RL, Vander Linden DW, McNair PJ, et al. Effects of an eight-week stretching program on the passive-elastic properties and function of the calf muscles of older women. *Clin Biomech (Bristol, Avon).* 2005;20:973–983.
116. Christiansen CL. The effects of hip and ankle stretching on gait function of older people. *Arch Phys Med Rehabil.* 2008;89:1421–1428.
117. Feland JB, Myrer JW, Schulthies SS, et al. The effect of duration of stretching of the hamstring muscle group for increasing range of motion in people aged 65 years or older. *Phys Ther.* 2001;81:1110–1117.
118. American Academy of Orthopaedic Surgeons. *Management of Osteoarthritis of the Hip Evidence-Based Clinical Practice Guideline.* Rosemont, IL: Academy of Orthopaedic Surgeons; 2017.
119. U.S. Department of Veterans Affairs. In: *VA/DoD Clinical Practice Guidelines for the Non-Surgical Management of Hip & Knee Osteoarthritis (OA).* 2014. https://www.healthquality.va.gov/guidelines/CD/OA/.
120. The Royal Australian College of General Practitioners. *Guideline for the Management of Knee and Hip Osteoarthritis.* 2nd ed. East Melbourne, Vic: RACGP; 2018.
121. Herzog W, Longino D, Clark A. The role of muscles in joint adaptation and degeneration. *Langenbecks Arch Surg.* 2003;388:305–315.
122. Bennell KL, Hunt MA, Wrigley TV, et al. Role of muscle in the genesis and management of knee osteoarthritis. *Rheum Dis Clin North Am.* 2008;34:731–754.
123. Fatouros IG, Taxildaris K, Tokmakidis SP, et al. The effects of strength training, cardiovascular training and their combination on flexibility of inactive older adults. *Int J Sports Med.* 2002;23:112–119.
124. Zehnacker CH, Bemis-Dougherty A. Effect of weighted exercises on bone mineral density in postmenopausal women. A systematic review. *J Geriatr Phys Ther.* 2007;30:79–88.
125. Roos EM, Dahlberg L. Positive effects of moderate exercise on glycosaminoglycan content in knee cartilage: a four-month, randomized, controlled trial in patients at risk of osteoarthritis. *Arthritis Rheum.* 2005;52:3507–3514.
126. Reid DA, McNair PJ. Effects of a six week lower limb stretching programme on range of motion, peak passive torque and stiffness in people with and without osteoarthritis of the knee. *N Z J Physiother.* 2011;39:5–12.
127. Crowley L. The effectiveness of home exercise programmes for patients with rheumatoid arthritis: a review of the literature. *Phys Ther Rev.* 2009;14:149–159.
128. Rao S, Riskowski JL, Hannan MT. Musculoskeletal conditions of the foot and ankle: assessments and treatment options. *Best Pract Res Clin Rheumatol.* 2012;26:345–368.
129. Vlieland TPMV, Ende CHVD. Nonpharmacological treatment of rheumatoid arthritis. *Curr Opin Rheumatol.* 2011;23:259–264.
130. Paskins Z, Kamath SN, Hassell AB. Management of inflammatory arthritis in older people. *Rev Clin Gerontol.* 2010;20:42–55.
131. Brown M, Sinacore DR, Ehsani AA, et al. Low-intensity exercise as a modifier of physical frailty in older adults. *Arch Phys Med Rehabil.* 2000;81:960–965.
132. Thompson CJ, Osness WH. Effects of an 8-week multimodal exercise program on strength, flexibility, and golf performance in 55- to 79-year-old men. *J Aging Phys Act.* 2004;12:144–156.
133. Lewis JS, Hewitt JS, Billington L, et al. A randomized clinical trial comparing two physiotherapy interventions for chronic low back pain. *Spine.* 2005;30:711–721.
134. Tomanova M, Lippert-Gruner M, Lhotoska L. Specific rehabilitation exercise for the treatment of patients with chronic low back pain. *J Phys Ther Sci.* 2015;27:2413–2417.
135. Kim M, Kim M, Oh S, et al. The effectiveness of hollowing and bracing strategies with lumbar stabilization exercise in older adult women with nonspecific low back pain: a quasi-experimental study on a community-based rehabilitation. *J Manipulative Physiol Ther.* 2018;41:1–9.
136. Lui PP, Qin L, Chan KM. Tai chi chuan exercises in enhancing bone mineral density in active seniors. *Clin Sports Med.* 2008;27:75–86.
137. Song R, Ahn S, So H, et al. Effects of t'ai chi on balance: a population-based meta-analysis. *J Altern Complement Med.* 2015;21:141–151.
138. Kumar A, Delbaere K, Zijlstra GAR, et al. Exercise for reducing fear of falling in older people living in the community: Cochrane systematic review and meta-analysis. *Age Ageing.* 2016;45:345–352.
139. Song R, Lee EO, Lam P, et al. Effects of tai chi exercise on pain, balance, muscle strength, and perceived difficulties in physical functioning in older women with osteoarthritis: a randomized clinical trial. *J Rheumatol.* 2003;30:2039–2044.
140. Brismee JM, Paige RL, Chyu MC, et al. Group and home-based tai chi in elderly subjects with knee osteoarthritis: a randomized controlled trial. *Clin Rehabil.* 2007;21:99–111.
141. Mat S, Tan MP, Kamaruzzaman SB, et al. Physical therapies for improving balance and reducing falls risk in osteoarthritis of the knee: a systematic review. *Age Ageing.* 2015;44:16–24.
142. Chen KM, Chen MH, Hong SM, et al. Physical fitness of older adults in senior activity centres after 24-week silver yoga exercises. *J Clin Nurs.* 2008;17:2634–2646.
143. Chen KM, Tseng WS. Pilot-testing the effects of a newly-developed silver yoga exercise program for female seniors. *J Nurs Res.* 2008;16:37–46.
144. Youkhana S, Dean CM, Wolff M, et al. Yoga-based exercise improves balance and mobility in people aged 60 and over: a systematic review and meta-analysis. *Age Ageing.* 2016;45:21–29.
145. Cheung C, Wyman JF, Resnick B, Savik K. Yoga for managing knee osteoarthritis in older women: a pilot randomized controlled trial. *BMC Complement Altern Med.* 2014;14:2–18.
146. DiBenedetto M, Innes KE, Taylor AG, et al. Effect of a gentle Iyengar yoga program on gait in the elderly: an exploratory study. *Arch Phys Med Rehabil.* 2005;86:1830–1837.
147. Masaracchio M, Ojha H, MacDonald CW, et al. Thoracic spine manual therapy for aging and older individuals. *Top Geriatr Rehabil.* 2015;31:188–198.
148. Yen SC, Chui KK, Markowski A, et al. Lumbar spine manual therapy for aging and older adults. *Top Geriatr Rehabil.* 2015;31:199–202.
149. Chui KK, Yen SC, Wormley ME, et al. Shoulder manual therapy for aging and older adults—part 1: subacromial impingement syndrome. *Top Geriatr Rehabil.* 2015;31:217–224.
150. Chui KK, Yen SC, Wormley ME, et al. Shoulder manual therapy for aging and older adults—part 2: adhesive capsulitis. *Top Geriatr Rehabil.* 2015;31:225–231.
151. Denninger TR, Lingerfelt WP. Knee manual therapy for aging and older adults. *Top Geriatr Rehabil.* 2015;31:203–210.
152. Tudini F, Chui KK, Grimes J, et al. Cervical spine manual therapy for aging and older adults. *Top Geriatr Rehabil.* 2016;32:8–105.
153. MacDonald CW. Hip manual therapy for aging and older adults. *Top Geriatr Rehabil.* 2016;32:106–113.
154. Hoeksma HL, Dekker J, Ronday HK, et al. Comparison of manual therapy and exercise therapy in osteoarthritis of the hip: a randomized clinical trial. *Arthritis Rheum.* 2004;51: 722–729.

155. Sampath KK, Mani R, Miyamori T, et al. The effects of manual therapy or exercise therapy or both in people with hip osteoarthritis: a systematic review and meta-analysis. *Clin Rehabil.* 2016;30:1141–1155.
156. Rademeyer I. Manual therapy for lumbar spinal stenosis: a comprehensive physical therapy approach. *Phys Med Rehabil Clin N Am.* 2003;14:103–110.
157. Whitman JM, Flynn TW, Childs JD, et al. A comparison between two physical therapy treatment programs for patients with lumbar spinal stenosis: a randomized clinical trial. *Spine.* 2006;31:2541–2549.
158. Ernst E. Chiropractic spinal manipulation for back pain. *Br J Sports Med.* 2003;37:195–196. discussion 6.
159. Sran MM, Khan KM. Physiotherapy and osteoporosis: practice behaviors and clinicians' perceptions—a survey. *Man Ther.* 2005;10:21–27.
160. Gronholz MJ. Prevention, diagnosis, and management of osteoporosis-related fracture: a multifactorial osteopathic approach. *J Am Osteopath Assoc.* 2008;108:575–585.
161. Sran MM, Khan KM. Is spinal mobilization safe in severe secondary osteoporosis? A case report. *Man Ther.* 2006;11: 344–351.
162. Bautmans I, Arken JV, Mackelenberg MV, et al. Rehabilitation using manual mobilization for thoracic kyphosis in elderly postmenopausal patients with osteoporosis. *J Rehabil Med.* 2010;42:129–135.
163. Bennell KL, Matthews B, Greig A, et al. Effects of an exercise and manual therapy program on physical impairments, function and quality-of-life in people with osteoporotic vertebral fracture: a randomized, single-blind controlled pilot trial. *BMC Musculoskelet Disord.* 2010;11:36–47.
164. Sran MM, Khan KM, Zhu Q, et al. Failure characteristics of the thoracic spine with a posteroanterior load: investigating the safety of spinal mobilization. *Spine.* 2004;29:2382–2388.
165. Kemp G, Crossley KM, Wrigley TV, et al. Reducing joint loading in medial knee osteoarthritis: shoes and canes. *Arthritis Rheum.* 2008;59:609–614.
166. Gohal C, Shanmugaraj A, Bedi A, et al. Effectiveness of valgus offloading knee braces in the treatment of medial compartment knee osteoarthritis: a systematic review. *Sports Health.* 2018;10:500–514.
167. Cudejko T, Esch MVD, Leeden MVD, et al. Effect of soft braces on pain and physical function in patients with knee osteoarthritis: systematic review with meta-analyses. *Arch Phys Med Rehabil.* 2018;99:153–163.
168. Al-Zahrani Y, Liu A, Herrington L, et al. The use of valgus knee brace on muscle cocontraction during walking and stair climbing in individuals with medial knee. *Osteoarthr Cartilage.* 2016;24:809.
169. Schmalz T, Knopf E, Drewitz H, et al. Analysis of biomechanical effectiveness of valgus-inducing knee brace for osteoarthritis of the knee. *J Rehabil Res Dev.* 2010;47:419–429.
170. Maleki M, Arazpour M, Joghtaei M, et al. The effect of the knee orthoses on gait parameters in medial knee compartment osteoarthritis: a literature review. *Prosthet Orthot Int.* 2014;40:193–201.
171. Shakoor N, Lidtke RH, Sengupta M, et al. Effects of specialized footwear on joint loads in osteoarthritis of the knee. *Arthritis Rheum.* 2008;59:1214–1220.
172. Telfer S, Lange MJ, Sudduth ASM. Factors influencing knee adduction moment measurement: a systematic review and meta-regression analysis. *Gait Posture.* 2017;58:333–339.
173. Bean JF, Ölveczky DD, Kiely DK, et al. Performance-based versus patient-reported physical function: what are the underlying predictors? *Phys Ther.* 2011;91:1804–1811.
174. Jette DU, Halbert J, Iverson C, et al. Use of standardized outcome measures in physical therapist practice: perceptions and applications. *Phys Ther.* 2009;89:125–135.
175. Bobos P, Macdermid JC, Walton DM, et al. Patient-reported outcome measures used for neck disorders: an overview of systematic reviews. *J Orthop Sports Phys Ther.* 2018;48: 775–788.
176. Resnik LL. Guide to outcome measurement for patients with low back pain syndromes. *J Orthop Sports Phys Ther.* 2003;33:307–318.
177. Zanoli G, Stromqvist B, Padua R, et al. Lessons learned searching for a HRQoL instrument to assess the results of treatment in persons with lumbar disorders. *Spine.* 2000;25: 3178–3185.
178. Roland M, Fairbank J. The Roland-Morris Disability Questionnaire and the Oswestry Disability Questionnaire. *Spine.* 2000;25:3115–3124.
179. Delitto A, George SZ, Dillen LV, et al. Low back pain clinical practice guidelines linked to the International Classification of Functioning, Disability, and Health from the orthopaedic section of the American Physical Therapy Association. *J Orthop Sports Phys Ther.* 2012;42:A1–57.
180. Kirkley A, Griffin S, Dainty K. Scoring systems for the functional assessment of the shoulder. *Arthroscopy.* 2003;19:1109–1120.
181. Dziedzic KS, Thomas E, Hay EM. A systematic search and critical review of measures of disability for use in a population survey of hand osteoarthritis (OA). *Osteoarthrit Cartilage.* 2005;13:1–12.
182. Roy JS, Esculier JF. Psychometric evidence for clinical outcome measures assessing shoulder disorders. *Phys Ther Rev.* 2011;16:331–346.
183. Gummesson C, Ward MM, Atroshi I. The shortened disabilities of the arm, shoulder and hand questionnaire (QuickDASH): validity and reliability based on responses within the full-length DASH. *BMC Musculoskelet Disord.* 2006;7:44.
184. Garratt AM, Brealey S, Gillespie WJ. Patient-assessed health instruments for the knee: a structured review. *Rheumatology (Oxford).* 2004;43:1414–1423.
185. Eechaute C, Vaes P, Van Aerschot L, et al. The clinimetric qualities of patient-assessed instruments for measuring chronic ankle instability: a systematic review. *BMC Musculoskelet Disord.* 2007;8:6.
186. Marx RG. Knee rating scales. *Arthroscopy.* 2003;19:1103–1108.
187. Johanson NA, Liang MH, Daltroy L, et al. American Academy of Orthopaedic Surgeons lower limb outcomes assessment instruments. Reliability, validity, and sensitivity to change. *J Bone Joint Surg Am.* 2004;86-A:902–909.
188. Mehta SP, Fulton A, Quach C, et al. Measurement properties of the lower extremity functional scale: a systematic review. *J Orthop Sports Phys Ther.* 2016;46:200–217.
189. Kivlan BR, Martin RL. Functional performance testing of the hip in athletes: a systematic review for reliability and validity. *Int J Sports Phys Ther.* 2012;7:402–412.
190. Smith MV, Klein SE, Clohisy JC, et al. Lower extremity-specific measures of disability and outcomes in orthopaedic surgery. *J Bone Joint Surg Am.* 2012;94:468–477.
191. Perera S, Mody SH, Woodman RC, et al. Meaningful change and responsiveness in common physical performance measures in older adults. *J Am Geriatr Soc.* 2006;54:743–749.
192. Anemaet WK, Moffa-Trotter ME. Functional tools for assessing balance and gait impairments. *Top Geriatr Rehabil.* 1999;15:66–83.
193. Lin CC, Whitney SL. Quantification of static and dynamic balance while maintaining and changing body position. *Top Geriatr Rehabil.* 2012;28:17–26.
194. Bohannon R. Measurement of sit-to-stand among older adults. *Top Geriatr Rehabil.* 2012;28:11–16.
195. Ohtake PJ. Field tests of aerobic capacity for children and older adults. *Cardiopulmonary Phys Ther J.* 2005;16:5–11.

196. Nightingale EJ, Pourkazemi F, Hiller CE. Systematic review of timed stair tests. *J Rehab Research Develop*. 2014;51:335–350.
197. Lusardi MM. Using walking speed in clinical practice: interpreting age-, gender-, and function-specific norms. *Top Geriatr Rehabil*. 2012;28:77–90.
198. Fritz SL, Peters DM, Greene JV. Measuring walking speed: clinical feasibility and reliability. *Top Geriatr Rehabil.* 2012;28:91–96.
199. Chui K, Hood E, Klima D. Meaningful change in walking speed. *Top Geriatr Rehabil.* 2012;28:97–103.
200. Terwee CB, Mokkink LB, Steultjens MP, et al. Performance-based methods for measuring the physical function of patients with osteoarthritis of the hip or knee: a systematic review of measurement properties. *Rheumatology (Oxford).* 2006;45:890–902.

CHAPTER 16

Impaired Muscle Performance in Older Adults

Robin L. Marcus, Paul Reidy, Paul LaStayo

OUTLINE

INTRODUCTION

Hallmarks of aging include progressive and, in the very old, profound changes in health, body composition, and functional capacity. The age-related loss of muscle, coined *sarcopenia* in 1989, is no longer simply considered another term to describe muscle atrophy associated with disuse and inactivity. The muscle wasting associated with sarcopenia can be a contributing factor to an older individual's deteriorating functional status and can manifest itself in deficits in mobility and metabolic function. With that, the definition of sarcopenia has expanded to include a loss of muscle strength (and power) and functional quality. Because the relationship between muscle decline and physical function decline is nonlinear, the clinical deficits in function may not manifest until a critical level of sarcopenia is reached. Initiating muscle interventions well before signs of functional decline manifest can build muscle reserve and delay the older individual's eventual functional limitations and disabilities. Moreover, metabolic deficits stemming from sarcopenia have been linked to age-related hormonal changes that affect the muscle hypertrophic response and function, thus increasing the importance of optimizing muscle structure and function in all older individuals. Individuals suffering muscle loss in combination with excess fat are classified as having sarcopenic obesity and may be at increased risk of functional decline and mortality. Finally, the prevalence of sarcopenia, while increasing in parallel with an increasing aging population, remains highly variable depending on the operational definition of the term. When criteria incorporate lean mass with strength and/or physical performance, estimates range from 1% to 13% of adults aged 65 years and older.

The purpose of this chapter is to review the consequences associated with sarcopenia in an aging population and collate the studies describing ways physical therapists can counter the associated adverse changes. It is not possible to assign the specific contribution to sarcopenia stemming from aging alone, decreased levels of physical activity, or the impact of comorbid conditions, but it is fair to characterize the adverse muscle and functional consequences as being compounded by all of these factors. With that, a primary focus of this chapter is placed on resistance exercises that have proven to be robust countermeasures in the face of all of these contributors to sarcopenia; this is also supplemented with descriptions of the benefit of protein intake relative to exercise as an additional important consideration when attempting to combat sarcopenia.

CONSEQUENCES OF SARCOPENIA

The loss of skeletal muscle mass is accompanied by the loss of muscle strength, rate of force development, and muscle power. Sarcopenia contributes to deficits in mobility, a decline in functional capacity, and a reduction in skeletal muscle oxidative capacity. These muscle impairments, in combination with a greater fat mass, contribute to the greater risk of falling, frailty, and the development of comorbid conditions such as insulin resistance or type 2 diabetes that adversely impact health.

Muscle mass represents the protein reserve of the body. Sarcopenia leads to a decline in protein reserves that makes it more difficult to meet the increased protein synthesis demands that occur with disease or injury, which then leads to a worsening of the sarcopenia. The negative balance between protein synthesis and muscle protein breakdown is the primary cause of skeletal muscle loss in the elderly. Frailty may be the result of the convergence of the metabolic vicious loop of sarcopenia with neuromuscular and nutritional impairments. Fig. 16.1 displays this metabolic vicious loop and a hypothesized path to frailty.

The following sections characterize the age-induced changes in muscle structure, function, and metabolism that typify sarcopenia.

Changes in Muscle Structure and Function Associated with Aging

Muscle Atrophy and Weakness. The loss of muscle mass and strength with aging, hallmarks of sarcopenia, is undeniable, though great variability exists between individuals at any given age or level of health. At some point in the aging process skeletal muscle loss with aging is inevitable; however, losses are disproportionally greater and have a more profound adverse effect on older adults when coupled with chronic systemic diseases (e.g., heart failure, chronic obstructive pulmonary disorder [COPD], cancer, etc.). A recent quantitative report[1] exposes this accelerated loss of muscle with chronic disease while also recalibrating the losses associated solely with aging as they may have been overestimates. Therefore, the current focus on muscle weakness as the key component of sarcopenia rather than loss of muscle mass is important to consider, though lean tissue losses should not be ignored.

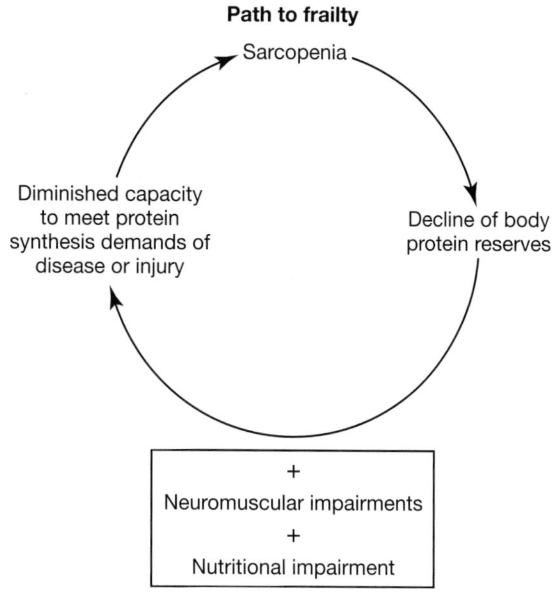

FIG. 16.1 Path to frailty.

On average muscle loss accelerates with advancing age, with annual atrophy rates upward of 1% after age 70. The age at which the decline in muscle mass begins, however, is quite variable, with ages ranging from 27 to 60 years.[2] The mechanisms underlying lean tissue loss are multivariate and only partially understood. Certainly, reduced muscle use and dietary intake of protein can contribute, though chronic inflammation, mitochondrial dysfunction, oxidative stress, and anabolic resistance have been implicated as well. It is muscle weakness, however, that is linked to physical disability and adverse health outcomes more so than muscle size. Specifically, data from a large prospective cohort of older adults indicates that the decrease in muscle strength is more rapid than the loss of muscle mass—with the latter explaining only ~6% of the former.[3] Moreover, maintaining or gaining muscle mass does not prevent aging-related decreases in muscle strength.[4] In a nationally representative sample (>8000 individuals) of older adults, the odds of experiencing a progressive disability in activities of daily living was two times higher in those who are weak.[5] Estimates of a per annum decrease in strength of 1.5% have been reported, though decrements in muscle power output of ~3% per year are more impactful because producing force quickly is more important than maximal force capabilities.[6]

Highlighted next are a few key mechanisms underlying the loss of mass and strength, and Box 16.1 summarizes the typical muscle changes observed in older adults. In general, the loss of muscle mass is exchanged by gains in fat mass, with the lower limb muscle groups undergoing the most atrophy. Increased fat infiltration has been associated with abnormal metabolic consequences[7–9] and, more recently, with both muscle strength[10] and mobility limitations in older adults[11,12] and those with diabetes.[13] The muscle fiber is also characterized by specific type II atrophy, fiber necrosis, fiber type grouping, and a reduction in type II muscle fiber satellite cell content.[14,15] The more powerful myosin heavy chain (MHC) IIa (fast-twitch) muscle fibers undergo greater atrophy than the less powerful MHC I (slow twitch) muscle fibers.[15–19] The potential recovery of muscle mass following disuse is also more impaired in predominantly fast, compared to slow, muscles.[20] The slowing of muscle contractile

BOX 16.1 Typical Muscle Changes with Aging

Whole Muscle Changes
- Decreased muscle mass, replaced by increased fat mass
- Decreased muscle strength (particularly lower extremities)
- Slowing of muscle contractile properties and rate of force development
  - Reduced rate of cross-bridge cycling
  - Alterations on excitation and contraction coupling
  - Increased compliance of muscle's tendinous attachment

Muscle Fiber Changes
- Type II (fast twitch) atrophy more than type I (slow twitch)
- Fiber necrosis
- Fiber type grouping
- Reduction in type II muscle fiber satellite cell content

Reversibility of These Changes
Exercises that overload atrophied and weak muscles can partially reverse "typical" age-related muscle changes.

properties can be ascribed to a reduced rate of cross-bridge cycling,[21,22] alterations on excitation and contraction coupling,[23,24] and an increased compliance of the muscle's tendinous attachment, which collectively can reduce the rate of force development.[25] When considering the clinical impact of these collective changes, physical therapists must recognize that although a complete reversal is unlikely, mitigation of these changes through interventions is very likely. Specifically, skeletal muscle is amenable to change if the correct stimuli are applied. For example, an exercise program that overloads atrophied and weak muscle should enhance muscle size, strength, and power (see the Muscle Countermeasures for Older Individuals section).

Impaired Regeneration of Muscle and the Progressive Denervation/Reinnervation Process. A primary mechanism attributed to the development of sarcopenia in those aged 60 to 65 years and older is a progressive denervation and reinnervation process involving the alpha motor neurons. A 50% decline in available motor neurons[15,26–28] and a diminished number and availability of satellite cells[29,30] that parallel the age-related temporal changes in muscle size and strength have been noted. Fiber type grouping also characterizes aging as remaining alpha motor neurons enlarge their own motor unit territory. When coupled with the reduction in alpha motor neurons and motor units, a reduced motor coordination and strength results,[30] which may underlie age-related mobility impairments. In addition, muscle fiber regeneration is impaired more in type II fibers than type I in large part owing to the degradation of the myogenic satellite stem cells.[31] Compounding these age-related losses are reports of substantially lower basal mixed, myofibrillar, or mitochondrial muscle protein synthesis rates in older adults versus younger ones.[32–34] However, studies that have failed to reproduce these findings and show little or no differences in basal muscle protein synthesis rates may reflect why skeletal muscle responses in rehabilitation settings vary in older adults.[35–37]

Deficits in Absolute and Specific Force Generation. Consistent with the current interpretation of sarcopenia, older individuals become weaker over time. These strength deficits, however, do not necessarily match the magnitude of atrophy that has occurred. In part, this may be explained by the fact that muscle generally becomes weaker even if atrophy is avoided, which suggests that force production, separate from muscle atrophy, also is impaired with aging. Deficits in specific contractile force production (force normalized to muscle cross-sectional area) with aging has been described repeatedly in the literature.[38,39] That is, when the maximum isometric force (for aged mice and rats) is normalized to the smaller muscle fiber cross-sectional area, a significant deficit in specific force remains unexplained by atrophy.[40] The deficit in specific force has been shown to be a widespread phenomenon involving fast- and slow-twitch fibers in different muscles. This has been reported in humans with significant differences noted in specific force in single-skinned muscle fibers between younger and older men.[41,42] Interestingly, however, single muscle fiber contractile function is preserved in older humans in the presence of significant alterations at the whole muscle level. Currently, this discrepancy in the literature has not been resolved, but in general the consensus remains that both absolute and specific force production are adversely affected with aging. Mechanisms have been proposed that might explain the skeletal muscle weakness associated with aging; however, whether the losses of specific and absolute force share common mechanisms is not known. It appears that the age-related impairment in muscle force is only partially explained by the loss in muscle mass. Therefore, the loss in both specific and absolute forces contributes to the muscle weakness measured in older adult and in animal models of aging. This global weakness of muscle underscores the need for effective countermeasures that increase not only the size of the muscle but also the functional ability of muscle.

Muscle Activation Deficits. The declining force production abilities with aging occur at a faster rate than the decline in muscle mass; hence, neural alterations are also thought to contribute to muscle weakness by reducing central drive to the agonist muscles and by increasing coactivation of the antagonist muscles.[43] Researchers have attempted to quantify the contribution of impaired voluntary drive to the decline in muscle force using superimposed electrical stimulation during maximal voluntary contractions and by recording surface electromyographic activity. Although reduced voluntary activation of agonist muscles and increased coactivation of antagonist muscles have been reported with advancing age, such changes are not supported by all studies.[44] Clinically, when encountering older patients with an apparent inhibition/co-contraction of their muscle(s), a detailed assessment of other potential contributors (e.g., pain and central or peripheral nervous system disorder) should be performed. After therapeutically addressing these other contributors, a cautious yet progressive resistance exercise program can be initiated, with or without supplemental neuromuscular electrical stimulation, in an attempt to reverse the muscle activation deficits.

Deteriorating Muscle Quality and Metabolism. A reduction in muscle "quality" due to infiltration of fat and other noncontractile material such as connective tissue, coupled with changes in muscle metabolism, also contribute to the deteriorating muscle condition and advancing frailty with age.[45,46] In addition, oxidative damage accumulated over time is thought to lead to mitochondrial DNA mutations, impaired mitochondrial function, muscle proteolysis, and myonuclear apoptosis. Collectively, these impairments are thought to play additional and prominent roles in the age-associated loss of function.

Changes in Metabolic Function Associated with Aging

Whole body resting metabolic rate (RMR) demonstrates considerable variability based on age, sex, and obesity status; however, the RMR of older adults does appear lower than that of younger adults.[47] This change is linked with age-associated decreases in metabolically active whole-body fat-free mass; however, whether this change is due solely to loss of fat-free tissue is currently a topic of debate. Even after correcting for differences in body composition, RMR remains significantly lower in older than younger adults[48]; thus, reductions in metabolically active mass (including muscle)[49] as well as declines in specific metabolic rates of tissues likely contribute to the overall age-related decline in RMR.

Altered Endocrine Function and Its Consequences. Box 16.2 lists age-related hormone changes commonly linked to sarcopenia, including insulin, growth hormone, insulin-like growth factor I (IGF-I), estrogens, testosterone, parathyroid hormone (PTH), and vitamin D. There is significant controversy as to the effects of these changes on skeletal muscle mass and strength, though the following synopsis reflects current thinking.

Insulin, the main postprandial hormone, is a critical regulator of protein metabolism in muscle, and its anabolic action is essential for protein gain and muscle growth. Lack of insulin, such as that seen in individuals with type 1 diabetes, is associated with substantial muscle protein mass wasting.[50] Both cross-sectional and longitudinal studies show an accelerated loss of muscle mass when compared with non-insulin-resistant individuals.[51] Progressive insulin resistance is commonly reported in older adults, yet aging itself does not appear to be an independent predictor of insulin sensitivity when adiposity and fat distribution are accounted for.[52] It is becoming increasingly well accepted that obesity, fat distribution, and physical inactivity have even more significant influence on insulin action than does advanced age. See Distefano and Goodpaster[53] for a recent review on this topic.

Growth hormone (GH) and IGF-I have each been implicated as potential contributors to sarcopenia, and both are frequently deficient in older adults. Although GH has been reported to lower fat mass, increase lean tissue mass, and improve lipid profiles, a systematic review of 31 studies representing 18 unique study populations that compared healthy older adults who were GH treated to a non–GH-treated control sample concluded that GH treatment in healthy older adults is not supported by a robust evidence base.[54] Further, this review revealed that GH supplementation is associated with substantial adverse events including joint pain and soft tissue edema in the healthy older adults and should not be recommended for use in this population. IGF-I, a growth factor that stimulates skeletal muscle protein synthesis and inhibits protein degradation, plays a critical role in signaling a hypertrophic response in aging skeletal muscle. This role is recognized by activating satellite cell differentiation and proliferation, and increasing protein synthesis in existing fibers.[55,56] Although there appears to be consensus regarding the role of IGF-I in improving muscle mass, the effects on muscle strength and function are equivocal.

Epidemiologic studies suggest that estrogens prevent muscle loss, though clinical trials have not found a relationship between hormone replacement therapy (HRT)—sometimes referred to as estrogen replacement therapy (ERT)—and increased muscle mass.[57] Moreover, the data on the relationship between estrogens and muscle strength are equivocal, as HRT has been shown to be associated with increased muscle strength in some studies[57] but not in all.[58] The association of estrogen with strength improvements does not seem to be supported by an anabolic effect, as estrogens indirectly decrease the level of serum free testosterone and this should have a negative impact on muscle mass. Epidemiologic studies also suggest a relationship between low levels of testosterone and loss of lean muscle, strength, and function in older adults. Further, studies support the hypothesis that low levels of testosterone result in lower protein synthesis and loss of muscle mass.[59] Results from a recent systematic review and meta-analysis indicate that testosterone replacement therapy (TRT) increases total body fat-free mass (FFM) and total body strength in men when both

BOX 16.2 Aging-Associated Changes in Endocrine Function Linked to Sarcopenia

- Increased insulin resistance
- Decreased growth hormone
- Decreased insulin-like growth factor (IGF-I)
- Decreased estrogen and testosterone
- Vitamin D deficiency
- Increased parathyroid hormone (PTH)

transdermal and intramuscular TRT were examined combined and individually when compared to placebo.[60] Moreover, the effect sizes for intramuscular TRT are consistently larger than transdermal administration with percentage improvements three to five times greater. This review suggests that intramuscular TRT results in reliable improvements in FFM and muscle strength in older men.

Vitamin D deficiency is common in older adults. Declining 25-hydroxyvitamin D (25-OHD) levels are also associated with low muscle mass,[61] low muscle strength,[62] poor physical performance,[63,64] and increased risk for falls in older individuals.[65,66] In ambulatory individuals older than age 65 years, a vitamin D deficiency (<10 ng/mL) indicates that individuals may be more than twice as likely to be sarcopenic than those at higher vitamin D levels (>20 ng/mL) based on both muscle weakness and muscle mass loss. In a similar population, those with the lowest mean values of 25-OHD (14 ng/mL) performed worse (3.9%) on the sit-to-stand test and 8-meter walk test (5.6%) than those with higher mean levels (42 ng/mL), even after adjustment for age, sex, ethnicity, body mass index (BMI), number of comorbid conditions, use of an assistive device, or activity level. In addition, a meta-analysis concludes that vitamin D supplementation in older adults with stable health may reduce the risk of falls by more than 20%.[67] These associations may be explained by the observations that vitamin D may influence muscle protein turnover through reduced insulin secretion, and low levels of vitamin D have been shown to decrease muscle anabolism. Because of the strong associations between vitamin D and sarcopenia, it is recommended that older individuals be screened for vitamin D deficiency, and if found to be <30 ng/mL, vitamin D supplements should be considered; however, a recent meta-analysis failed to identify an effect of vitamin D supplementation on muscle mass or muscle power and only a small positive impact on muscle strength.[69]

Consistent with the positive associations observed between low levels of vitamin D and age, elevated levels of PTH are also commonly seen in older adults both independently[70,71] and in combination with vitamin D deficiency.[72,73] Evidence linking elevated PTH to sarcopenia is found in the positive associations between higher PTH levels and falls in nursing home residents[74] and between higher PTH levels and grip strength and muscle mass in community-dwelling older persons.[61] Further, studies of patients with hyperparathyroidism demonstrate not only impaired muscle function but also improved muscle function following treatment.[75,76] Despite these findings, the question of whether hyperparathyroidism is a primary cause of muscle structural and functional impairments remains unanswered as low vitamin D levels stimulate PTH production. PTH may influence muscle directly through impaired energy production, transfer and utilization, muscle protein metabolism, or altering calcium concentrations, or indirectly through the production of proinflammatory cytokines. Vitamin D supplementation, as well as increased exposure to sunlight, will help to normalize vitamin D status and, indirectly, PTH levels as well.

Cytokines and Adiposity. Aging, as well as several chronic medical conditions (COPD, heart disease, cancer, diabetes) that are prevalent with increasing age, is associated with a gradual increase in the production of proinflammatory cytokines (responsible for accelerating inflammation and regulating inflammatory reactions), chronic inflammation, and loss of lean body mass. Although it is currently unknown whether cytokines predict the occurrence of sarcopenia, recent evidence suggests that chronic inflammation is an important contributor to sarcopenia.[77] Associations between elevated levels of tumor necrosis factor-α (TNF-α), interleukin 6 (IL-6), C-reactive protein (CRP) muscle mass, and muscle strength have been reported.[78–80]

Several hypotheses have been put forward as potential explanations of how inflammation contributes to sarcopenia.[81] One hypothesis is that increased proinflammatory cytokines contribute to an imbalance between muscle protein synthesis and breakdown, with the net result favoring protein breakdown. A second hypothesis is that inflammation increases activation of the protein-degrading ubiquitin–protease pathway. Finally, inflammation is accompanied by a decrease in IGF-I, and TNF-α in particular may stimulate muscle loss through the activation of the apoptosis pathway.

Additional evidence implicating an inflammatory role in sarcopenia is found in the link between obesity and inflammation.[82,83] Sarcopenic obesity is a condition that combines excess adiposity with loss of lean tissue. Specific definitions of sarcopenic obesity vary; however, Baumgartner first defined this phenotype as appendicular skeletal muscle mass adjusted for stature (ASM/Ht^2), that is, −2 standard deviations (SD) below the mean of a young population (<7.26 kg/m^2 in men and <5.45 kg/m^2 in women) and percentage body fat greater than the median or >27% in men and 38% in women.[85] Using the most conservative measure (ASM/Ht^2) as the benchmark, sarcopenic obesity occurs in 2% of older adults up to age 70 years and up to 10% of those older than age 80 years.[84,85] Although not clearly established, the relationship between sarcopenic obesity and increased fatty infiltration of skeletal muscle has been reported.[86,87] This finding is especially interesting in light of the significant associations reported between fatty infiltration of muscle and decreased strength, physical function, and future risk of a mobility limitation. Motor unit recruitment is also reduced in the presence of muscle fatty infiltration, and increased fatty acids in muscle fibers result in abnormal cellular signaling. Taken together, the current evidence suggests a role for fat mass in the etiology and pathogenesis of sarcopenia. Alternatively, because sarcopenia occurs regardless of adiposity changes with aging, it may be that the associated chronic low-level inflammatory state that is associated with aging itself, and not just obesity, could lead to accelerated muscle loss in older adults.

Mitochondrial Dysfunction. The role of mitochondrial dysfunction in sarcopenia remains controversial, in part owing to differences in study methodology and factors inherently associated with aging like adiposity and physical activity. The aging-associated damage to muscle mitochondrial DNA (mtDNA) may reduce the rate of muscle cell protein synthesis and adenosine triphosphate (ATP) synthesis and ultimately may lead to the death of muscle fibers and loss of muscle mass. Further studies are needed to more fully determine the extent to which mitochondrial dysfunction is responsible for age-associated muscle loss. For a recent review of this topic see Calvani et al.[88] Consistent with other metabolic changes that are seen with aging, because these mitochondrial abnormalities have also been shown to be at least partially reversible with exercise[89,90] and delayed in highly active older adults, these abnormalities may also be the result of inactivity. However, recent evidence identifying mitochondrial abnormalities and dysfunction in older adult subjects across species[91,92] suggests that the mitochondrial changes seen in older humans are not due to decreased physical activity alone. The clinical importance of the early reports of improved mitochondrial gene transcription (the first step of gene expression—the process by which DNA instructions are converted into a functional product)[93] and function[89,90] as a result of exercise training suggests that this research area should be closely monitored by physical therapists.

Apoptosis. Apoptosis may represent the link between mitochondria dysfunction and loss of muscle in older adults. Research on animal models strongly suggests that apoptosis plays a key role in age-related loss of muscle, and that aged muscle has a different apoptotic response to disuse than younger muscle. Age-related loss of myocytes via apoptosis has been suggested to be a key mechanism behind the muscle loss associated with human aging[94] as well, though this evidence is preliminary. Recent data demonstrate that physical exercise can mitigate skeletal muscle apoptosis in aged animals. These basic science considerations should prompt the clinician to consider exercise as not only a counter to loss of physical fitness and function but also, perhaps, a mode of slowing down the apoptotic pathways underlying sarcopenia. Readers are referred to an excellent review[95] on this topic.

Diseases and Conditions Associated with Skeletal Muscle Decline. Sarcopenia is specifically defined as the *age-related* loss of skeletal muscle mass and strength. Independent of age, however, muscle loss is also a primary impairment that is associated with a variety of disease states. Box 16.3 lists diseases and conditions common in older adults that are associated with skeletal muscle decline. Each of these diseases and conditions can potentially influence the progression of age-related skeletal muscle decline. Cachexia is a hallmark impairment in cancer, COPD, and congestive heart failure (CHF); increased inflammatory levels are present in arthritis, cancer, COPD, CHF, diabetes, metabolic syndrome, kidney disease, and stroke; and all are often accompanied by a sedentary lifestyle. Disease-related inactivity in these individuals then becomes a secondary factor that contributes to the equation of muscle loss.

BOX 16.3 Diseases and Conditions, Common in Older Adults, Associated with Skeletal Muscle Decline

- Diabetes
- Metabolic syndrome
- Chronic obstructive pulmonary disease (COPD)
- Cancer
- Congestive heart failure (CHF)
- Arthritis
- Kidney disease
- Stroke
- Parkinson disease

Influence of Genetics. Genetic epidemiologic studies suggest that between 36% and 65% of an individual's muscle strength and up to 57% of his or her lower extremity performance can be explained by heredity.[68,96–98] Moreover, several genetic factors have been identified that contribute to muscle mass and strength.[99,100] As more information concerning the gene expression patterns surrounding sarcopenia becomes available, future treatment strategies can be expected to be aimed at these gene targets.

MUSCLE COUNTERMEASURES FOR OLDER INDIVIDUALS

Our understanding of the aging process of muscle is influenced by many factors, including genetic variation and differences in socioeconomic, health care and nutritional status, and, crucially, the physical activity status of older adults that is often characterized as sedentary. Older adults are more sedentary than any other age group, and sedentariness may have more damaging consequences in this group.[101] There is a dearth of high-quality research on interventions to reduce sedentary time in older adults. A recent international consensus statement[102] reveals an inability to evaluate the clinical impact of reducing sedentary time in older adults but advocates that interventions should target the environment as well as individual behavior change. Consensus was not reached on whether interventions that focus on physical activity or on sedentary time specifically will be more effective for reducing sedentary time; however, recommendations include educating older adults to reduce total sedentary time, break up prolonged periods of sedentary time, and move more. Because of the complex interaction between aging and a concomitant decline of physical activity, the drivers of age-related changes in muscle remain largely unknown,[103] though a recent study of a highly active subset of the general population of older adults found little evidence of age-related muscle changes across the age range studied (55 to

79 years). This comprehensive assessment of the physiologic structure and function of the vastus lateralis muscle of master cyclists provides evidence that typical muscle degradation with age is eliminated in highly active older adults.[104] The impact of physical activity and the avoidance of sedentariness, while requiring further study on dosage and implementation, should be encouraged in this population.

Resistance Exercise

Resistance exercise training can predictably and effectively combat sarcopenia (whereas pharmacologic interventions cannot) as it positively impacts almost all of the mechanisms known to grow muscle and improve strength. See the excellent review article by Law et al.[105] for additional details. The concept of resistance training in older adults is not unlike that in younger adults: providing muscles with an overload stimulus will lead to an improvement in the muscle's force-producing capability, thus helping to mitigate sarcopenia. Adaptive changes that result from resistance training include improved muscle strength and power, enhanced levels of mobility, a hypertrophic response, and improved muscle composition. The optimal magnitude of the overload stimulus that induces these changes in older adults, however, is not clear. Further, both increased habitual physical activity and nutritional supplementation are also alluring potential countermeasures for sarcopenia.

Resistance training for individuals aged 65 years and older induces predictable increases in muscle strength, muscle power, and mobility function in community-dwelling older persons, nursing home residents, and hospitalized older adults. Significant improvements in strength and mobility function have also been reported in individuals 80 years of age and older. Several review papers on this topic[106–110] have successfully cataloged these beneficial adaptations and ingrained the notion that resistance exercise for older individuals is effective. Evidence of this has existed as early as 1998 in the American College of Sports Medicine Position Stand on Exercise and Physical Activity for Older Adults, where resistance training is recommended as an important component of an overall fitness program. Increases in muscle size, though in absolute terms less than that seen in younger individuals, are also a by-product of resistance training programs in older individuals. Regardless, the ability to increase muscle size with resistance training appears to remain intact, at least through the seventh decade,[111,112] but may diminish after age 80 years.[113,114] Because the increases in muscle strength and power that occur in older adults oftentimes exceed that expected with the muscle size improvements, the variable of muscle quality or force produced per unit of muscle mass has gained recent interest. Increased muscle quality from resistance training is a common finding among older adults, and in men there appears to be no difference in young versus old, though there is some evidence that older women may have a blunted response relative to younger women.[115] Just as changes in muscle composition (increased fatty infiltration) have been shown to accompany aging, resistance training has also been recently found to be associated with maintenance or return of skeletal muscle, specifically in the legs, to a more youthful composition.[116,117] Box 16.4 highlights some of the key resistance exercise considerations discussed in the upcoming pages.

Dosage Considerations for Resistance Exercise. For these positive adaptations to take place, resistance exercise can be performed at different intensities, at different frequencies per week, and at different volumes per session. Resistance training with loads that range from 20% of the maximum weight that an individual can lift (one-repetition maximum [1RM]) to greater than 80% 1RM has resulted in significant gains in muscle strength, muscle power, and mobility in older individuals.[106,111,118–120] There is evidence that older individuals who train with loads at or below 50% of the 1RM can improve their strength, stair-climbing ability, gait speed, and balance to a level equivalent to those exercising with higher-intensity exercise.[113,121,122] Despite this, recent guidelines from the American College of Sports Medicine recommend resistance training with a minimum of moderate (5 to 6 on a 1-to-10 scale) intensity.[123] Further, a recent systematic review by Liu and Latham[108] suggests that high-intensity strength training results in greater improvements in lower extremity strength compared to low-intensity exercise, based on the studies reviewed. There is evidence suggesting that resistance training that exploits the high-force–producing capabilities of eccentric muscle activity is both feasible and effective for older individuals. Because eccentric resistance training can produce high forces at relatively low energetic costs, eccentrically biased resistance training programs are especially useful in an older population. Reviews in the literature have highlighted the rehabilitation potential of eccentric exercise[124] and the potential benefits of chronic eccentric exercise and the older adult. Although the literature lacks a

BOX 16.4 Evidence-Supported Suggestions for Resistance Training with Older Adults

- Resistance exercise—against sufficient load—can increase muscle strength and power, even in the very old
- Effective exercise options:
  - Intensities >50% of one-repetition maximum (1RM), performed two to three times per week, with one to three sets per exercise session
  - Intensities >60% 1RM, performed one to two times per week, with one to three sets per exercise session
  - For individuals older than age 80 years, resistance exercise one time per week at high intensity (70% to 80% 1RM) may add benefit
  - Eccentric resistance exercise at high intensity is particularly beneficial for older adults

clear distinction of what constitutes the ideal intensity dosage for resistance exercise in older adults, the findings that older individuals respond positively to a variety of different intensities suggest that aging muscle is responding to resistance training with both neural and structural adaptations.

Training frequencies of one, two, or three times per week have all resulted in strength improvements. When older individuals train with greater loads (at or above 1RM), there is evidence that training at a lower frequency (one time per week) at this higher intensity[125] induces improvements in strength and neuromuscular performance that are similar to those achieved with a two- and even three-times-per-week training frequency. As well, training at higher intensities may result in greater sustainability of the strength gains. Although exercise volume has not been studied extensively in older adults, it appears that gains in muscle power, strength, and physical functioning[122,126] in older adults may be achieved with less exercise volume (either lower frequency per week or less overall volume per week, e.g., one set vs. three sets) than that required by younger adults.

Overall, it appears that maximum benefit relative to strength, power, and mobility function from resistance training in older adults can be achieved with intensities >50% of 1RM, performed two to three times per week, with one to three sets per exercise session.[106,107,109,110] The available literature suggests that maximizing volume is more important than frequency; hence, if frequencies of one or two times per week are used, intensity should be progressively increased to 60% to 80% of 1RM. As well, if muscle size improvements (hypertrophy) are the primary goal of a training program, higher overall intensities of >60% 1RM[127] and higher volume are recommended. When considering resistance training for individuals older than age 80 years, it may be particularly effective to exercise less frequently (one time per week), at higher relative intensities, to optimize the sustainability of strength gains while not exhausting the older individual's energy reserves. Older individuals should be monitored closely for adverse reactions to resistance training. Although there are risks to participation in a resistance training program, the evidence is strong that physical activity, of which resistance training can be considered a subset, significantly reduces the age-associated risk of chronic disease, with the benefits outweighing the risks of participation.[123]

Adaptations in Muscle Strength and Mobility Levels with Resistance Exercise. Without a doubt, older individuals who participate in at least 6 to 12 weeks of resistance training will improve their strength and mobility function. A 2009 systematic review reporting on 73 exercise trials with 3059 participants revealed that progressive resistance training had a large positive effect on muscle strength; thus, there is overwhelming evidence that older adults can substantially increase strength following resistance training.[108] Strength improvements range from 25% to well over 100%. However, the influence of age on the capacity to increase strength is complex, as some studies report the same response in older versus younger individuals,[128–131] whereas others report a blunted response in the old.[132–135] There are also other variables that affect the strength response. The effects of age may be influenced by gender, duration of training, or muscle groups investigated.

Resistance training improves not only strength but also functional abilities in older adults.[108] This review revealed modest improvements in gait speed (24 trials, 1179 participants, mean difference [MD] = 0.08 m/s; 95% confidence interval [CI], 0.04 to 0.12) and a moderate to large improvement for getting out of a chair (11 trials, 384 participants, standardized mean difference [SMD] = −0.94; 95% CI, −1.49 to −0.38). Data from 12 trials that assessed the timed up-and-go test revealed that participants of resistance training programs took significantly less time to complete this task (MD = −0.69 second; 95% CI, −1.11 to −0.27). In addition, time to climb stairs, available from only eight trials, favored the resistance training groups, but was quite heterogeneous, and there were small but nonsignificant improvements for balance in the resistance-trained groups.

Adaptations in Muscle Power with Resistance Exercise. Resistance training that specifically targets muscle power (40% to 70% of 1RM, "as fast as possible") has a significant impact on physical functioning as well as muscle power production and muscle strength. Leg muscle power—the ability to generate force rapidly—is a strong predictor of both self-reported functional status[136] and falls[137] in older adults, and it accounts for a large percentage of the variance in physical functioning in older individuals.[138] Leg muscle power is especially important when considering that muscle power declines more sharply than strength in older individuals. Previous literature suggests that 4 to 16 weeks of power training results in robust (100% to 150%) improvements in leg muscle power in both healthy[127,128,139,140] and impaired[123] older individuals. Although some authors have reported a dose–response relationship with power training, more recent evidence[141] suggests that the gains in leg muscle power resulting from a three-times-per-week, 12-week high-velocity power training regimen were not only similar to more traditional slow-velocity strength training but also less than power improvements reported previously by other authors.[139] This may be because previous authors have studied healthier populations,[118,139] or self-reported performance measures only, where the recent study measured actual performance in more disabled individuals. There may not be a clear advantage for power training over high-force slow-velocity resistance training with respect to physical function, power production, or strength enhancement. However, it does appear that power training in older individuals is well tolerated and can counteract the age-related decline in neuromuscular function that is customarily observed with aging. Power training may be especially efficacious when considering that it may be performed in a shorter time per session and that fewer sessions per week may be necessary to capitalize on the associated improvements.

Adaptations in Muscle Size and Composition with Resistance Exercise. The impact of resistance training on muscle hypertrophy, an expected outcome in the young, is less predictable in older individuals, especially those older than age 80 years. Early studies suggested that older muscle responded to resistance training with a robust hypertrophic effect, but more recently that assertion has been challenged. Slivka et al.[114] recently reported limited muscle plasticity in men aged 80 years or older after 12 weeks of resistance training at 70% of 1RM. Older women (mean age 85 years) have also been reported to have a blunted hypertrophy response at both the whole muscle and fiber level.[135] This limited hypertrophic response may or may not be important clinically as muscle size has been reported to be less influential than muscle power and strength on functional mobility. However, considering that cross-sectional area is an important variable in the muscle power equation (force = mass × acceleration, power = force × velocity), it may be prudent to recommend individuals begin resistance training prior to age 80 to realize the maximal hypertrophic response.

Although sarcopenia is a well-accepted characteristic of normal aging, aging muscle is also associated with an increase in fat infiltration.[142] The effects of resistance training on altering muscle composition in older individuals is only now beginning to be investigated.

Both the total amount of muscle and its composition appear to be critical to overall health. Low body mass has been linked with sarcopenia, and sarcopenia with frailty. Resistance training, therefore, is an important mode of rehabilitation (vs. aerobic training) for increasing muscle mass and enhancing muscle strength and power. This is especially important when taken in the context of older individuals with limited muscle energetic reserves secondary to comorbid conditions that often accompany aging. Further research should attempt to define the critical variables for improving muscle mass in older adults, and specifically in those older than 80 years of age.

Nutritional Intake as a Countermeasure for Sarcopenia

In addition to decreased physical activity, inadequate protein intake may also contribute to sarcopenia. Although resistance exercise training can partially attenuate the negative effects of a low-protein diet by improving protein efficiency to obtain positive muscular adaptations,[143] its effectiveness is blunted in the presence of inadequate protein intake. Thus, inadequate protein intake in a malnourished older individual is a barrier to building muscle mass and strength even when the individual is participating in a resistance training program. Nutritional intake, like exercise, is a modifiable countermeasure that may help to minimize loss of lean muscle tissue and muscle strength in older adults, though there is significant controversy as to the amount, quality, and timing of protein supplementation in this population. The weighted opinion in the field is that, for resistance exercise to stimulate muscle hypertrophy, there must be a positive energy balance and adequate protein intake. To achieve a positive protein balance, muscle protein synthesis (MPS), stimulated by resistance exercise and by protein intake, must be greater than muscle protein breakdown. The accumulation of these acute periods of positive protein balance will result in increased muscle fiber protein content and, finally, in increased muscle cross-sectional area. Several studies support the ability of dietary protein to acutely stimulate MPS in older adults.[36,144] However, there is no current consensus on the amount of protein intake that is necessary for the maintenance of muscle mass, strength, and metabolic function in older adults, or whether the current recommendations of 0.8 g/kg/day for all adults are adequate for older individuals.[145] Although very-high-protein diets (>45% energy) have been associated with adverse events,[146] diets containing a moderate amount of protein (20% to 35% energy) do not appear to be associated with poor health outcomes.[147] Current literature suggests that moderately increasing daily protein intake to 1.0 to 1.3 g/kg/day may enhance muscle protein anabolism and mitigate some of the loss of muscle mass associated with age.[148] Moderate protein intake (30 g, the equivalent of 4 ounces of lean meat) at any one meal need not exceed 113 g. More information on adequate protein consumption and nutritional information for older adults can be found at http://fnic.nal.usda.gov. Although there is little evidence linking high-protein intakes with impaired kidney function in healthy men and women, higher protein intake may be contraindicated in individuals with renal disease.[149]

The primary variable affected by resistance exercise appears to be MPS, which is stimulated 40% to 100% over resting rate with exercise.[156,157] There appear to be subtle differences in the ability of different protein sources to promote MPS, and the overall difference between protein sources is negligible if an adequate amount (>25 g) of many of the available high-quality protein sources are consumed.[150] Recent research suggests that essential amino acids stimulate protein anabolism in older adults, in whom nonessential amino acids added to essential amino acids have no additive effect.[151] Currently, it is recommended that all meals for older adults contain a moderate amount of high-quality protein. Timing of protein supplementation does not seem to be as important as evenly spreading the protein across meals (~0.4 g/kg body weight per meal) and possibly consuming protein 2 hours before sleep to maximize the effect of the muscle protein anabolic response.[152] In addition, when older adults experience periods of lower energy intake, a higher protein intake is recommended (>1.2 g/kg/day) to offset the muscle protein breakdown and muscle atrophy.[152] Protein supplementation with resistance exercise training does not enhance muscle hypertrophy or physical function in healthy older adults[153] but may be beneficial when combined with other nutrients, and/or when used in less healthy older adults.[154]

SUMMARY

The muscle structural and functional changes associated with sarcopenia contribute to a greater risk of falling, frailty, and mobility impairment in older adults. Because muscle is critical to both mobility and metabolism, the development of muscle-related comorbid conditions, like insulin resistance and type 2 diabetes, amplifies the clinical impairments associated with muscle loss. Coupled with a variety of other disease states, age-associated loss of muscle mass and strength is compounded by the primary muscle loss that is often associated with cancer, COPD, CHF, arthritis, diabetes, kidney disease, stroke, and Parkinson disease as well as the secondary muscle loss that is accompanied by a disease-imposed sedentary lifestyle. Overarching all of these disease states is a progressive inflammatory and apoptotic milieu that accelerates these impairments and functional limitations. Although the specific mechanisms underlying the development and treatment of sarcopenia have yet to be elucidated, several candidate interventions have been suggested to both prevent and reverse muscle loss. Currently, resistance exercise is the most widely accepted countermeasure that has definitive evidence to mitigate muscle loss in older adults. Nutritional intervention is also a promising therapeutic approach to treating sarcopenia.

REFERENCES

1. Mitchell WK, Williams J, Atherton P, Larvin M, Lund J, Narici M. Sarcopenia, dynapenia, and the impact of advancing age on human skeletal muscle size and strength; a quantitative review. *Front Physiol.* 2012;3:260.
2. Kyle UG, Genton L, Hans D, Karsegard L, Slosman DO, Pichard C. Age-related differences in fat-free mass, skeletal muscle, body cell mass and fat mass between 18 and 94 years. *Eur J Clin Nutr.* 2001;55(8):663–672. https://doi.org/10.1038/sj.ejcn.1601198.
3. Delmonico MJ, Harris TB, Visser M, et al. Longitudinal study of muscle strength, quality, and adipose tissue infiltration. *Am J Clin Nutr.* 2009;90(6):1579–1585.
4. Clark BC, Manini TM. What is dynapenia? *Nutrition.* 2012;28(5):495–503.
5. Duchowny KA, Clarke PJ, Peterson MD. Muscle weakness and physical disability in older Americans: longitudinal findings from the U.S. Health and Retirement Study. *J Nutr Health Aging.* 2018;22(4):501–507.
6. Reid KF, Pasha E, Doros G, et al. Longitudinal decline of lower extremity muscle power in healthy and mobility-limited older adults: influence of muscle mass, strength, composition, neuromuscular activation and single fiber contractile properties. *Eur J Appl Physiol.* 2014;114(1):29–39. https://doi.org/10.1007/s00421-013-2728-2.
7. Elder CP, Apple DF, Bickel CS, et al. Intramuscular fat and glucose tolerance after spinal cord injury—a cross-sectional study. *Spinal Cord.* 2004;42:711–716.
8. Goodpaster BH, Krishnaswami S, Resnick H, et al. Association between regional adipose tissue distribution and both type 2 diabetes and impaired glucose tolerance in elderly men and women. *Diabetes Care.* 2003;26:372–379.
9. Yim JE, Heshka S, Albu J, et al. Intermuscular adipose tissue rivals visceral adipose tissue in independent associations with cardiovascular risk. *Int J Obes (Lond).* 2007;31:1400–1405.
10. Goodpaster BH, Carlson CL, Visser M, et al. Attenuation of skeletal muscle and strength in the elderly: the Health ABC Study. *J Appl Physiol.* 2001;90:2157–2165.
11. Visser M, Kritchevsky SB, Goodpaster BH, et al. Leg muscle mass and composition in relation to lower extremity performance in men and women aged 70 to 79: the Health, Aging and Body Composition Study. *J Am Geriatr Soc.* 2002;50:897–904.
12. Visser M, Goodpaster BH, Kritchevsky SB, et al. Muscle mass, muscle strength, and muscle fat infiltration as predictors of incident mobility limitations in well-functioning older persons. *J Gerontol A Biol Sci Med Sci.* 2005;60:324–333.
13. Hilton TN, Tuttle LJ, Bohnert KL, et al. Excessive adipose tissue infiltration in skeletal muscle in individuals with obesity, diabetes mellitus, and peripheral neuropathy: association with performance and function. *Phys Ther.* 2008;88:1336–1344.
14. Miljkovic N, Lim JY, Miljkovic I, Frontera WR. Aging of skeletal muscle fibers. *Ann Rehabil Med.* 2015;39(2):155–162.
15. Lexell J. Human aging, muscle mass, and fiber type composition. *J Gerontol A Biol Sci Med Sci.* 1995;50(Spec No):11–16.
16. Frontera WR, Hughes VA, Lutz KJ, et al. A cross-sectional study of muscle strength and mass in 45- to 78-yr-old men and women. *J Appl Physiol.* 1991;71:644–650.
17. Faulkner JA, Larkin LM, Claflin DR, et al. Age-related changes in the structure and function of skeletal muscles. *Clin Exp Pharmacol Physiol.* 2007;34:1091–1096.
18. Lexell J, Taylor CC, Sjostrom M. What is the cause of the ageing atrophy? Total number, size and proportion of different fiber types studied in whole vastus lateralis muscle from 15- to 83-year-old men. *J Neurol Sci.* 1988;84:275–294.
19. Hwee DT, Bodine SC. Age-related deficit in load-induced skeletal muscle growth. *J Gerontol A Biol Sci Med Sci.* 2009;64:618–628.
20. D'Antona G, Pellegrino MA, Adami R, et al. The effect of ageing and immobilization on structure and function of human skeletal muscle fibres. *J Physiol.* 2003;552:499–511.
21. Hook P, Sriramoju V, Larsson L. Effects of aging on actin sliding speed on myosin from single skeletal muscle cells of mice, rats, and humans. *Am J Physiol Cell Physiol.* 2001;280:C782–C788.
22. Hunter SK, Thompson MW, Ruell PA, et al. Human skeletal sarcoplasmic reticulum $Ca2^+$ uptake and muscle function with aging and strength training. *J Appl Physiol.* 1999;86:1858–1865.
23. Payne AM, Zheng Z, Gonzalez E, et al. External Ca^{2+}-dependent excitation–contraction coupling in a population of ageing mouse skeletal muscle fibres. *J Physiol.* 2004;560:137–155.
24. Narici MV, Maganaris CN. Adaptability of elderly human muscles and tendons to increased loading. *J Anat.* 2006;208:433–443.
25. Doherty TJ, Vandervoort AA, Brown WF. Effects of ageing on the motor unit: a brief review. *Can J Appl Physiol.* 1993;18:331–358.
26. Edstrom E, Altun M, Bergman E, et al. Factors contributing to neuromuscular impairment and sarcopenia during aging. *Physiol Behav.* 2007;92:129–135.

27. Essen-Gustavsson B, Borges O. Histochemical and metabolic characteristics of human skeletal muscle in relation to age. *Acta Physiol Scand.* 1986;126:107–114.
28. Gibson MC, Schultz E. Age-related differences in absolute numbers of skeletal muscle satellite cells. *Muscle Nerve.* 1983;6:574–680.
29. Carosio S, Berardinelli MG, Aucello M, et al. Impact of ageing on muscle cell regeneration. *Ageing Res Rev.* 2011;10(1):35–42.
30. Hepple RT, Rice CL. Innervation and neuromuscular control in ageing skeletal muscle. *J Physiol.* 2016;594(8):1965–1978.
31. Verdijk LB, Gleeson BG, Jonkers RA, et al. Skeletal muscle hypertrophy following resistance training is accompanied by a fiber type-specific increase in satellite cell content in elderly men. *J Gerontol A Biol Sci Med Sci.* 2009;64:332–339.
32. Hasten DL, Pak-Loduca J, Obert KA, et al. Resistance exercise acutely increases MHC and mixed muscle protein synthesis rates in 78-84 and 23-32 yr olds. *Am J Physiol Endocrinol Metab.* 2000;278:E620–E626.
33. Rooyackers OE, Adey DB, Ades PA, et al. Effect of age on in vivo rates of mitochondrial protein synthesis in human skeletal muscle. *Proc Natl Acad Sci U S A.* 1996;93: 15364–15369.
34. Yarasheski KE, Welle S, Nair KS. Muscle protein synthesis in younger and older men. *JAMA.* 2002;287:317–318.
35. Katsanos CS, Kobayashi H, Sheffield-Moore M, et al. A high proportion of leucine is required for optimal stimulation of the rate of muscle protein synthesis by essential amino acids in the elderly. *Am J Physiol Endocrinol Metab.* 2006;291:E381–E387.
36. Paddon-Jones D, Sheffield-Moore M, Zhang XJ, et al. Amino acid ingestion improves muscle protein synthesis in the young and elderly. *Am J Physiol Endocrinol Metab.* 2004;286: E321–E328.
37. Volpi E, Sheffield-Moore M, Rasmussen BB, et al. Basal muscle amino acid kinetics and protein synthesis in healthy young and older men. *JAMA.* 2001;286:1206–1212.
38. Delbono O. Molecular mechanisms and therapeutics of the deficit in specific force in ageing skeletal muscle. *Biogerontology.* 2002;3:265–270.
39. Gonzalez E, Delbono O. Age-dependent fatigue in single intact fast- and slow fibers from mouse EDL and soleus skeletal muscles. *Mech Ageing Dev.* 2001;122:1019–1032.
40. Brooks SV, Faulkner JA. Skeletal muscle weakness in old age: underlying mechanisms. *Med Sci Sports Exerc.* 1994;26:432–439.
41. Frontera WR, Hughes VA, Fielding RA, et al. Aging of skeletal muscle: a 12-yr longitudinal study. *J Appl Physiol.* 2000;88:1321–1326.
42. Frontera WR, Suh D, Krivickas LS, et al. Skeletal muscle fiber quality in older men and women. *Am J Physiol Cell Physiol.* 2000;279:C611–C618.
43. Christou EA. Aging and variability of voluntary contractions. *Exerc Sport Sci Rev.* 2011;39(2):77–84.
44. Klass M, Baudry S, Duchateau J. Voluntary activation during maximal contraction with advancing age: a brief review. *Eur J Appl Physiol.* 2007;100:543–551.
45. Marcus RL, Addison O, LaStayo PC. Intramuscular adipose tissue attenuates gains in muscle quality in older adults at high risk for falling. A brief report. *J Nutr Health Aging.* 2013;17(3):215–218.
46. Moore AZ, Caturegli G, Metter EJ, et al. Difference in muscle quality over the adult life span and biological correlates in the Baltimore Longitudinal Study of Aging. *J Am Geriatr Soc.* 2014;62(2):230–236.
47. McMurray RG, Soares J, Caspersen CJ, McCurdy T. Examining variations of resting metabolic rate of adults: a public health perspective. *Med Sci Sports Exerc.* 2014;46 (7):1352–1358.
48. Krems C, Luhrmann PM, Strassburg A, et al. Lower resting metabolic rate in the elderly may not be entirely due to changes in body composition. *Eur J Clin Nutr.* 2005;59: 255–262.
49. He Q, Heshka S, Albu J, et al. Smaller organ mass with greater age, except for heart. *J Appl Physiol.* 2009;106:1780–1784.
50. Tessari P, Biolo G, Inchiostro S, et al. Effects of insulin on whole body and forearm leucine and KIC metabolism in type 1 diabetes. *Am J Physiol.* 1990;259:E96–E103.
51. Park SW, Goodpaster BH, Lee JS, et al. Excessive loss of skeletal muscle mass in older adults with type 2 diabetes. *Diabetes Care.* 2009;32(11):1993–1997.
52. Lalia AZ, Dasari S, Johnson ML, et al. Predictors of whole-body insulin sensitivity across ages and adiposity in adult humans. *J Clin Endocrinol Metab.* 2016;101(2):626–634.
53. Distefano G, Goodpaster BH. Effects of exercise and aging on skeletal muscle. *Cold Spring Harb Perspect Med.* 2018;8(3): a029785.
54. Liu H, Bravata DM, Olkin I, et al. Systematic review: the safety and efficacy of growth hormone in the healthy elderly. *Ann Intern Med.* 2007;146:104–115.
55. Chen Y, Zajac JD, MacLean HE. Androgen regulation of satellite cell function. *J Endocrinol.* 2005;186:21–31.
56. Fryburg DA. Insulin-like growth factor I exerts growth hormone- and insulin-like actions on human muscle protein metabolism. *Am J Physiol.* 1994;267:E331–E336.
57. Jacobsen DE, Samson MM, Kezic S, et al. Postmenopausal HRT and tibolone in relation to muscle strength and body composition. *Maturitas.* 2007;58:7–18.
58. Taaffe DR, Newman AB, Haggerty CL, et al. Estrogen replacement, muscle composition, and physical function: the Health ABC Study. *Med Sci Sports Exerc.* 2005;37:1741–1747.
59. Galvao DA, Taaffe DR, Spry N, et al. Exercise can prevent and even reverse adverse effects of androgen suppression treatment in men with prostate cancer. *Prostate Cancer Prostatic Dis.* 2007;10:340–346.
60. Skinner JW, Otzel DM, Bowser A, et al. Muscular responses to testosterone replacement vary by administration route: a systematic review and meta-analysis. *J Cachexia Sarcopenia Muscle.* 2018;9(3):465–481.
61. Visser M, Deeg DJ, Lips P. Low vitamin D and high parathyroid hormone levels as determinants of loss of muscle strength and muscle mass (sarcopenia): the Longitudinal Aging Study Amsterdam. *J Clin Endocrinol Metab.* 2003;88:5766–5772.
62. Zamboni M, Zoico E, Tosoni P, et al. Relation between vitamin D, physical performance, and disability in elderly persons. *J Gerontol A Biol Sci Med Sci.* 2002;57:M7–M11.
63. Wicherts IS, van Schoor NM, Boeke AJ, et al. Vitamin D status predicts physical performance and its decline in older persons. *J Clin Endocrinol Metab.* 2007;92:2058–2065.
64. Bischoff-Ferrari HA, Dietrich T, Orav EJ, et al. Higher 25-hydroxyvitamin D concentrations are associated with better lower-extremity function in both active and inactive persons aged > or =60 y. *Am J Clin Nutr.* 2004;80:752–758.
65. Szulc P, Munoz F, Marchand F, et al. Role of vitamin D and parathyroid hormone in the regulation of bone turnover and bone mass in men: the MINOS study. *Calcif Tissue Int.* 2003;73:520–530.
66. Bischoff-Ferrari HA, Dietrich T, Orav EJ, et al. Positive association between 25-hydroxyvitamin D levels and bone mineral density: a population-based study of younger and older adults. *Am J Med.* 2004;116:634–639.
67. Bischoff-Ferrari HA, Dawson-Hughes B, Willett WC, et al. Effect of vitamin D on falls: a meta-analysis. *JAMA.* 2004;291:1999–2006.
68. Reed T, Fabsitz RR, Selby JV, et al. Genetic influences and grip strength norms in the NHLBI twin study males aged 59-69. *Ann Hum Biol.* 1991;18:425–432.
69. Beaudart C, Buckinx F, Rabenda V, et al. The effects of vitamin D on skeletal muscle strength, muscle mass, and muscle power:

a systematic review and meta-analysis of randomized controlled trials. *J Clin Endocrinol Metab.* 2014;99(11): 4336–4345.
70. Prince RL, Dick I, Devine A, et al. The effects of menopause and age on calcitropic hormones: a cross-sectional study of 655 healthy women aged 35 to 90. *J Bone Miner Res.* 1995;10: 835–842.
71. Need AG, Horowitz M, Morris HA, et al. Vitamin D status: effects on parathyroid hormone and 1, 25-dihydroxyvitamin D in postmenopausal women. *Am J Clin Nutr.* 2000;71: 1577–1581.
72. Lips P. Vitamin D deficiency and secondary hyperparathyroidism in the elderly: consequences for bone loss and fractures and therapeutic implications. *Endocr Rev.* 2001;22:477–501.
73. Souberbielle JC, Cormier C, Kindermans C, et al. Vitamin D status and redefining serum parathyroid hormone reference range in the elderly. *J Clin Endocrinol Metab.* 2001;86: 3086–3090.
74. Stein MS, Wark JD, Scherer SC, et al. Falls relate to vitamin D and parathyroid hormone in an Australian nursing home and hostel. *J Am Geriatr Soc.* 1999;47:1195–1201.
75. Joborn C, Joborn H, Rastad J, et al. Maximal isokinetic muscle strength in patients with primary hyperparathyroidism before and after parathyroid surgery. *Br J Surg.* 1988;75:77–80.
76. Kristoffersson A, Bostrom A, Soderberg T. Muscle strength is improved after parathyroidectomy in patients with primary hyperparathyroidism. *Br J Surg.* 1992;79:165–168.
77. Chhetri JK, de Souto Barreto P, Fougere B, Rolland Y, Vellas B, Cesari M. Chronic inflammation and sarcopenia: a regenerative cell therapy perspective. *Exp Gerontol.* 2018;103:115–123.
78. Cesari M, Kritchevsky SB, Baumgartner RN, et al. Sarcopenia, obesity, and inflammation—results from the Trial of Angiotensin Converting Enzyme Inhibition and Novel Cardiovascular Risk Factors study. *Am J Clin Nutr.* 2005;82:428–434.
79. Schaap LA, Pluijm SM, Deeg DJ, et al. Inflammatory markers and loss of muscle mass (sarcopenia) and strength. *Am J Med.* 2006;119:526.e9–526.e17.
80. Visser M, Pahor M, Taaffe DR, et al. Relationship of interleukin-6 and tumor necrosis factor-alpha with muscle mass and muscle strength in elderly men and women: the Health ABC Study. *J Gerontol A Biol Sci Med Sci.* 2002;57: M326–M332.
81. Jo E, Lee SR, Park BS, Kim JS. Potential mechanisms underlying the role of chronic inflammation in age-related muscle wasting. *Aging Clin Exp Res.* 2012;24(5):412–422.
82. Yudkin JS, Kumari M, Humphries SE, et al. Inflammation, obesity, stress and coronary heart disease: is interleukin-6 the link? *Atherosclerosis.* 2000;148:209–214.
83. Ryan AS, Nicklas BJ. Reductions in plasma cytokine levels with weight loss improve insulin sensitivity in overweight and obese postmenopausal women. *Diabetes Care.* 2004;27: 1699–1705.
84. Davison KK, Ford ES, Cogswell ME, et al. Percentage of body fat and body mass index are associated with mobility limitations in people aged 70 and older from NHANES III. *J Am Geriatr Soc.* 2002;50:1802–1809.
85. Baumgartner RN. Body composition in healthy aging. *Ann N Y Acad Sci.* 2000;904:437–448.
86. Baumgartner RN, Wayne SJ, Waters DL, et al. Sarcopenic obesity predicts instrumental activities of daily living disability in the elderly. *Obes Res.* 2004;12:1995–2004.
87. Goodpaster BH, Park SW, Harris TB, et al. The loss of skeletal muscle strength, mass, and quality in older adults: the health, aging and body composition study. *J Gerontol A Biol Sci Med Sci.* 2006;61:1059–1064.
88. Calvani R, Joseph AM, Adhihetty PJ, et al. Mitochondrial pathways in sarcopenia of aging and disuse muscle atrophy. *Biol Chem.* 2013;394(3):393–414.
89. Kent-Braun JA, Ng AV, Young K. Skeletal muscle contractile and noncontractile components in young and older women and men. *J Appl Physiol.* 2000;88:662–668.
90. Jubrias SA, Esselman PC, Price LB, et al. Large energetic adaptations of elderly muscle to resistance and endurance training. *J Appl Physiol.* 2001;90:1663–1670.
91. Fridovich I. Mitochondria: are they the seat of senescence? *Aging Cell.* 2004;3:13–16.
92. Barazzoni R, Short KR, Nair KS. Effects of aging on mitochondrial DNA copy number and cytochrome c oxidase gene expression in rat skeletal muscle, liver, and heart. *J Biol Chem.* 2000;275:3343–3347.
93. Melov S, Tarnopolsky MA, Beckman K, et al. Resistance exercise reverses aging in human skeletal muscle. *PLoS One.* 2007;2:e465.
94. Dupont-Versteegden EE. Apoptosis in muscle atrophy: relevance to sarcopenia. *Exp Gerontol.* 2005;40:473–481.
95. Siu PM. Muscle apoptotic response to denervation, disuse, and aging. *Med Sci Sports Exerc.* 2009.41(10):1876–1886.
96. Carmelli D, Reed T. Stability and change in genetic and environmental influences on hand-grip strength in older male twins. *J Appl Physiol.* 2000;89:1879–1883.
97. Huygens W, Thomis MA, Peeters MW, et al. Linkage of myostatin pathway genes with knee strength in humans. *Physiol Genomics.* 2004;17:264–270.
98. Arden NK, Spector TD. Genetic influences on muscle strength, lean body mass, and bone mineral density: a twin study. *J Bone Miner Res.* 1997;12:2076–2081.
99. Silventoinen K, Magnusson PK, Tynelius P, et al. Heritability of body size and muscle strength in young adulthood: a study of one million Swedish men. *Genet Epidemiol.* 2008;32: 341–349.
100. Mascher H, Tannerstedt J, Brink-Elfegoun T, et al. Repeated resistance exercise training induces different changes in mRNA expression of MAFbx and MuRF-1 in human skeletal muscle. *Am J Physiol Endocrinol Metab.* 2008;294:E43–E451.
101. Colley RC, Garriguet D, Janssen I, Craig CL, Clarke J, Tremblay MS. Physical activity of Canadian adults: accelerometer results from the 2007 to 2009 Canadian Health Measures Survey. *Health Rep.* 2011;22(1):7–14.
102. Dogra S, Ashe MC, Biddle SJH, et al. Sedentary time in older men and women: an international consensus statement and research priorities. *Br J Sports Med.* 2017;51(21):1526–1532.
103. Harridge SD, Lazarus NR. Physical activity, aging, and physiological function. *Physiology (Bethesda).* 2017;32 (2):152–161.
104. Pollock RD, O'Brien KA, Daniels LJ, et al. Properties of the vastus lateralis muscle in relation to age and physiological function in master cyclists aged 55-79 years. *Aging Cell.* 2018;17(2):e12735.
105. Law TD, Clark LA, Clark BC. Resistance exercise to prevent and manage sarcopenia and dynapenia. *Annu Rev Gerontol Geriatr.* 2016;36(1):205–228.
106. Galvao DA, Newton RU, Taaffe DR. Anabolic responses to resistance training in older men and women: a brief review. *J Aging Phys Act.* 2005;13:343–358.
107. Hunter GR, McCarthy JP, Bamman MM. Effects of resistance training on older adults. *Sports Med.* 2004;34:329–348.
108. Liu CJ, Latham NK. Progressive resistance strength training for improving physical function in older adults. *Cochrane Database Syst Rev.* 2009;(3):CD002759.
109. Phillips SM. Resistance exercise: good for more than just grandma and grandpa's muscles. *Appl Physiol Nutr Metab.* 2007;32:1198–1205.

110. Suetta C, Magnusson SP, Beyer N, et al. Effect of strength training on muscle function in elderly hospitalized patients. *Scand J Med Sci Sports*. 2007;17:464–472.
111. Frontera WR, Meredith CN, O'Reilly KP, et al. Strength conditioning in older men: skeletal muscle hypertrophy and improved function. *J Appl Physiol*. 1988;64:1038–1044.
112. Godard MP, Williamson DL, Trappe SW. Oral amino-acid provision does not affect muscle strength or size gains in older men. *Med Sci Sports Exerc*. 2002;34:1126–1131.
113. Kryger AI, Andersen JL. Resistance training in the oldest old: consequences for muscle strength, fiber types, fiber size, and MHC isoforms. *Scand J Med Sci Sports*. 2007;17: 422–430.
114. Slivka D, Raue U, Hollon C, et al. Single muscle fiber adaptations to resistance training in old (>80 yr) men: evidence for limited skeletal muscle plasticity. *Am J Physiol Regul Integr Comp Physiol*. 2008;295:R273–R280.
115. Hakkinen K, Alen M, Kallinen M, et al. Neuromuscular adaptation during prolonged strength training, detraining and re-strength-training in middle-aged and elderly people. *Eur J Appl Physiol*. 2000;83:51–62.
116. Marcus RL, Smith S, Morrell G, et al. Comparison of combined aerobic and high-force eccentric resistance exercise with aerobic exercise only for people with type 2 diabetes mellitus. *Phys Ther*. 2008;88:1345–1354.
117. Taaffe DR, Henwood TR, Nalls MA, et al. Alterations in muscle attenuation following detraining and retraining in resistance-trained older adults. *Gerontology*. 2009;55: 217–223.
118. de Vos NJ, Singh NA, Ross DA, et al. Optimal load for increasing muscle power during explosive resistance training in older adults. *J Gerontol A Biol Sci Med Sci*. 2005;60:638–647.
119. Kalapotharakos VI, Michalopoulou M, Godolias G, et al. The effects of high- and moderate-resistance training on muscle function in the elderly. *J Aging Phys Act*. 2004;12:131–143.
120. Ades PA, Ballor DL, Ashikaga T, et al. Weight training improves walking endurance in healthy elderly persons. *Ann Intern Med*. 1996;124:568–572.
121. Hakkinen K, Pakarinen A, Kraemer WJ, et al. Selective muscle hypertrophy, changes in EMG and force, and serum hormones during strength training in older women. *J Appl Physiol*. 2001;91:569–580.
122. Vincent KR, Braith RW, Feldman RA, et al. Resistance exercise and physical performance in adults aged 60 to 83. *J Am Geriatr Soc*. 2002;50:1100–1107.
123. Chodzko-Zajko WJ, Proctor DN, Fiatarone Singh MA, et al. American College of Sports Medicine position stand. Exercise and physical activity for older adults. *Med Sci Sports Exerc*. 2009;41:1510–1530.
124. LaStayo P, Marcus R, Dibble L, Frajacomo F, Lindstedt S. Eccentric exercise in rehabilitation: safety, feasibility, and application. *J Appl Physiol*. 1985;116(11):1426–1434.
125. Hunter GR, Wetzstein CJ, McLafferty CL Jr, et al. High-resistance versus variable-resistance training in older adults. *Med Sci Sports Exerc* 2001;33:1759–1764.
126. Galvao DA, Taaffe DR. Resistance exercise dosage in older adults: single- versus multiset effects on physical performance and body composition. *J Am Geriatr Soc*. 2005;53:2090–2097.
127. Kumar V, Selby A, Rankin D, et al. Age-related differences in the dose-response relationship of muscle protein synthesis to resistance exercise in young and old men. *J Physiol*. 2009;587:211–217.
128. Hakkinen K, Newton RU, Gordon SE, et al. Changes in muscle morphology, electromyographic activity, and force production characteristics during progressive strength training in young and older men. *J Gerontol A Biol Sci Med Sci*. 1998;53:B415–B423.
129. Holviala JH, Sallinen JM, Kraemer WJ, et al. Effects of strength training on muscle strength characteristics, functional capabilities, and balance in middle-aged and older women. *J Strength Cond Res*. 2006;20:336–344.
130. Joseph LJ, Davey SL, Evans WJ, et al. Differential effect of resistance training on the body composition and lipoprotein-lipid profile in older men and women. *Metabolism*. 1999;48:1474–1480.
131. Newton RU, Hakkinen K, Hakkinen A, et al. Mixed-methods resistance training increases power and strength of young and older men. *Med Sci Sports Exerc*. 2002;34:1367–1375.
132. Lemmer JT, Hurlbut DE, Martel GF, et al. Age and gender responses to strength training and detraining. *Med Sci Sports Exerc*. 2000;32:1505–1512.
133. Macaluso A, De Vito G, Felici F, et al. Electromyogram changes during sustained contraction after resistance training in women in their 3rd and 8th decades. *Eur J Appl Physiol*. 2000;82:418–424.
134. Petrella JK, Kim JS, Tuggle SC, et al. Age differences in knee extension power, contractile velocity, and fatigability. *J Appl Physiol*. 2005;98:211–220.
135. Raue U, Slivka D, Minchev K, et al. Improvements in whole muscle and myocellular function are limited with high-intensity resistance training in octogenarian women. *J Appl Physiol*. 2009;106:1611–1617.
136. Foldvari M, Clark M, Laviolette LC, et al. Association of muscle power with functional status in community-dwelling elderly women. *J Gerontol A Biol Sci Med Sci*. 2000;55: M192–M199.
137. Skelton DA, Kennedy J, Rutherford OM. Explosive power and asymmetry in leg muscle function in frequent fallers and non-fallers aged over 65. *Age Ageing*. 2002;31:119–125.
138. Bean JF, Kiely DK, Herman S, et al. The relationship between leg power and physical performance in mobility-limited older people. *J Am Geriatr Soc*. 2002;50:461–467.
139. Earles DR, Judge JO, Gunnarsson OT. Velocity training induces power-specific adaptations in highly functioning older adults. *Arch Phys Med Rehabil*. 2001;82:872–878.
140. Ferri A, Scaglioni G, Pousson M, et al. Strength and power changes of the human plantar flexors and knee extensors in response to resistance training in old age. *Acta Physiol Scand*. 2003;177:69–78.
141. Reid KF, Callahan DM, Carabello RJ, et al. Lower extremity power training in elderly subjects with mobility limitations: a randomized controlled trial. *Aging Clin Exp Res*. 2008;20:337–343.
142. Gallagher D, Kuznia P, Heshka S, et al. Adipose tissue in muscle: a novel depot similar in size to visceral adipose tissue. *Am J Clin Nutr*. 2005;81:903–910.
143. Castaneda C, Gordon PL, Uhlin KL, et al. Resistance training to counteract the catabolism of a low-protein diet in patients with chronic renal insufficiency. A randomized, controlled trial. *Ann Intern Med* 2001;135(11):965–976.
144. Volpi E, Mittendorfer B, Wolf SE, et al. Oral amino acids stimulate muscle protein anabolism in the elderly despite higher first-pass splanchnic extraction. *Am J Physiol*. 1999;277:E513–E520.
145. Paddon-Jones D, Short KR, Campbell WW, et al. Role of dietary protein in the sarcopenia of aging. *Am J Clin Nutr*. 2008;87:1562S–1566S.
146. Allen LH, Oddoye EA, Margen S. Protein-induced hypercalciuria: a longer term study. *Am J Clin Nutr*. 1979;32:741–749.
147. Hayashi Y. Application of the concepts of risk assessment to the study of amino acid supplements. *J Nutr*. 2003;133: 2021S–2024S.
148. Campbell WW, Trappe TA, Wolfe RR, et al. The recommended dietary allowance for protein may not be

adequate for older people to maintain skeletal muscle. *J Gerontol A Biol Sci Med Sci.* 2001;56:M373–M380.

149. Friedman AN. High-protein diets: potential effects on the kidney in renal health and disease. *Am J Kidney Dis.* 2004;44:950–962.
150. van Vliet S, Burd NA, van Loon LJ. The skeletal muscle anabolic response to plant- versus animal-based protein consumption. *J Nutr.* 2015;145(9):1981–1991.
151. Volpi E, Kobayashi H, Sheffield-Moore M, et al. Essential amino acids are primarily responsible for the amino acid stimulation of muscle protein anabolism in healthy elderly adults. *Am J Clin Nutr.* 2003;78:250–258.
152. Morton RW, Traylor DA, Weijs PJM, Phillips SM. Defining anabolic resistance: implications for delivery of clinical care nutrition. *Curr Opin Crit Care* 2018;24(2):124–130.
153. Morton RW, Murphy KT, McKellar SR, et al. A systematic review, meta-analysis and meta-regression of the effect of protein supplementation on resistance training-induced gains in muscle mass and strength in healthy adults. *Br J Sports Med.* 2018;52(6):376–384.
154. Liao CD, Tsauo JY, Wu YT, et al. Effects of protein supplementation combined with resistance exercise on body composition and physical function in older adults: a systematic review and meta-analysis. *Am J Clin Nutr.* 2017;106(4):1078–1091.
155. Symons TB, Vandervoort AA, Rice CL, et al. Effects of maximal isometric and isokinetic resistance training on strength and functional mobility in older adults. *J Gerontol A Biol Sci Med Sci.* 2005;60:777–781.
156. Phillips SM, Tipton KD, Aarsland A, et al. Mixed muscle protein synthesis and breakdown after resistance exercise in humans. *Am J Physiol.* 1997;273:E99–E107.
157. Biolo G, Maggi SP, Williams BD, et al. Increased rates of muscle protein turnover and amino acid transport after resistance exercise in humans. *Am J Physiol.* 1995;268: E514–E520.

CHAPTER

17

Impaired Motor Control and Neurologic Rehabilitation in Older Adults

Catherine E. Lang, Marghuretta D. Bland

OUTLINE

INTRODUCTION

Human beings have the capacity to execute an enormous repertoire of movements. Our movement repertoire spans typical daily activities such as sitting, transfers, and walking as well as a multitude of specialized capabilities such as dancing, piano playing, and skiing. Compared to young children, adults and older adults typically use only a fraction of many possible movements. Each movement, regardless of its purpose, can be thought of as a concert of complex muscle actions. Like the notes and instruments in a musical concert, each muscle used in the movement must be turned on *just the right amount* and *at just the right time* to produce a coordinated movement. Some muscles provide the melody (agonist and antagonist muscles), while other muscles play on in the background (preparatory and/or supporting muscle activity). The brain and spinal cord are the instruments that play this beautiful concert of muscle actions. Impairments in motor control are the result of breakdowns within and between these instruments.

This chapter opens with a discussion of the most common motor control impairments seen in adults and their neural mechanisms. The chapter is organized around motor control impairments rather than neurological medical diagnoses. Medical diagnoses associated with each impairment are included within impairment categories. Next, examination and interpretation of findings related to impaired motor control are covered at the impairment and activity limitation levels. The chapter then discusses the issues relevant to making prognoses and human movement system diagnoses in adults with impaired motor control and concludes with information on intervention and treatment for these impairments. Discussion and examples in this chapter often emphasize movement control in people with stroke because stroke is the most common cause of motor control impairments in older adults. Particular attention is placed on upper limb movement control as other chapters provide detailed discussion of lower limb and trunk considerations related to balance, mobility, and gait. Motor control impairments in adults are usually a result of a disease or health condition and not a result of the normal aging process. From the perspective of the authors, motor control impairments in older adults are not fundamentally different from motor control impairments in younger adults. What may or may not differ with older adults are the movement goals a person wants to achieve and the health status of the body with which they are trying to achieve them (e.g., other existing comorbidities).

COMMON MOTOR CONTROL IMPAIRMENTS

Motor control is the ability to regulate or direct movements.[1] The field of motor control is focused on studying

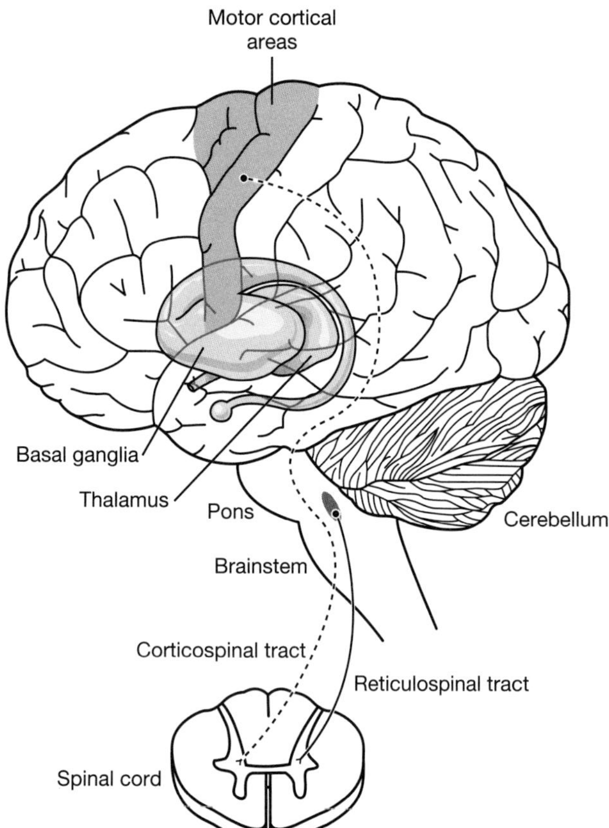

FIG. 17.1 Overview of the neural structures responsible for control of movement. The corticospinal system is made up of the motor cortical areas, corticospinal tract, and spinal cord.

movement and the neural control of movement. Neural control of movement involves the cooperation of numerous structures within the nervous system. Fig. 17.1 provides a simplified overview of the critical neural structures associated with motor control. The motor cortical areas include the primary motor cortex and nonprimary cortical motor areas, such as the premotor and supplementary motor areas. These areas work together to plan and execute voluntary movements. They communicate with the spinal cord and muscles via the corticospinal tract. The corticospinal tract makes both direct (monosynaptic) and indirect (di- or polysynaptic) connections to spinal motoneurons controlling muscles of the trunk and limbs. The reticulospinal tract assists the corticospinal tract in communicating movement information from subcortical structures to the spinal cord. Spinal cord circuitry includes peripheral afferents (sensory neurons), interneurons, and motoneurons that work in concert with the descending motor commands to produce movement. The major role of the cerebellum is coordination and correction of movement. The basal ganglia focuses the selection of desired movements and inhibits competing movements. Sensory information about the body and environment is used in a feedforward manner to plan movements and as feedback about recent or ongoing movements. This overview provides a foundation from which to examine motor control impairments.

BOX 17.1 Major Motor Control Body Structure and Functional Impairments

Motor System Impairments
Paresis
Abnormal tone
Fractionated movement deficits
Ataxia
Hypokinesia

Sensory System Impairments
Somatosensory loss
Perceptual deficits

Motor control impairments in older adults result from medical conditions of the central nervous system (CNS) that preferentially affect this population, such as stroke or Parkinson disease. Box 17.1 lists the major motor and sensory system impairments contributing to motor control deficits.

Fig. 17.2 is a conceptual model of how motor control impairments contribute to activity limitations and participation restrictions in adults. More often than not, patients have multiple motor control impairments, as represented by gray, overlapping circles. The CNS condition will determine the prognosis for recovery from the motor control impairments. Motor control impairments can directly limit activities and restrict participation. The direct activity limitations associated with motor control impairments also lead to additional, secondary impairments that further affect activity and participation. For example, decreased endurance may develop in the presence of paresis when the patient has difficulty ambulating or participating in general exercise programs. Furthermore, the presence of comorbid impairments can further compound an older adult's movement problems. The ovals representing secondary and comorbid impairments are large, representing the idea that these are the targets that may be most amenable to change with rehabilitation. The onset of motor control impairments together with preexisting comorbid impairments such as muscle weakness and pain in older persons can easily push them down the "slippery slope" to loss of independence with daily activities.

Paresis

The most common motor impairment is paresis. Paresis is the reduced ability to volitionally activate the spinal motoneurons. Total paresis is called plegia, reflecting a complete inability to volitionally activate the motoneurons. In the clinical examination, paresis manifests as weakness during movement in gravity-eliminated positions, against gravity, and/or against manual resistance. Paresis can result from a wide range of neurologic conditions, such as stroke, multiple sclerosis, cerebral palsy, amyotrophic lateral sclerosis, traumatic brain injury, Guillain–Barré syndrome, peripheral neuropathy, polio, postpolio syndrome, and spinal cord injury. The medical condition will

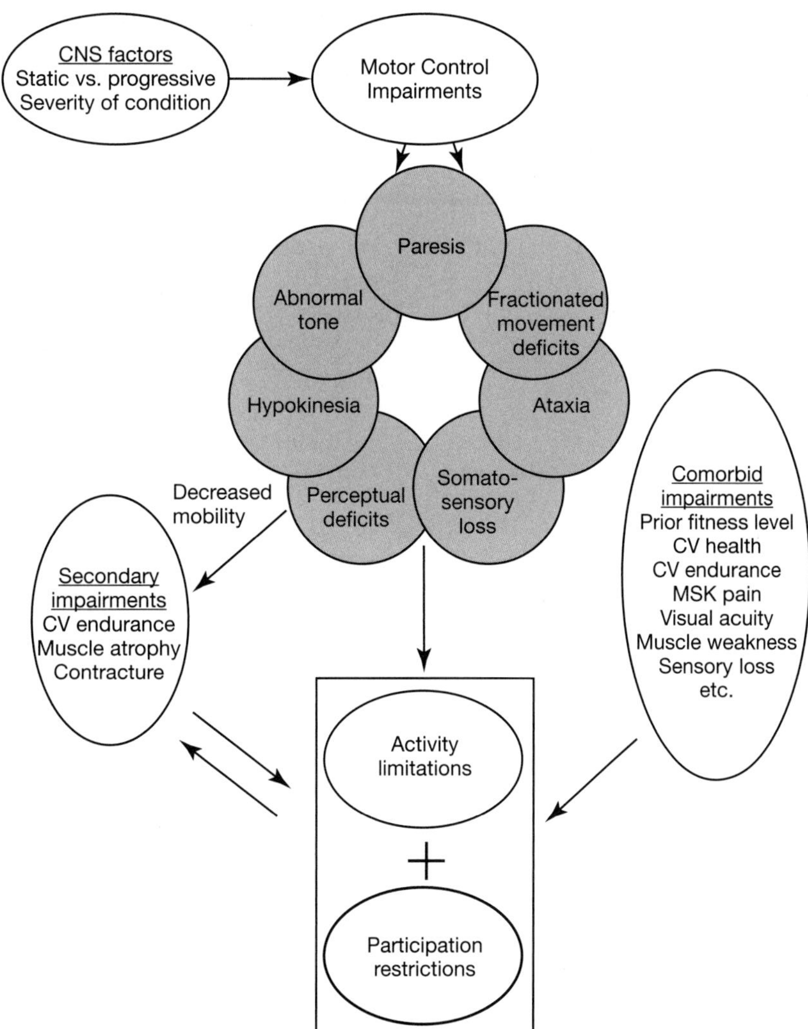

FIG. 17.2 Conceptual model of how motor control impairments lead to activity limitations and participation restrictions of movement. Patients typically have multiple motor control impairments, represented by the gray, overlapping circles. The central nervous system (CNS) condition will determine the prognosis for recovery. Motor control impairments directly limit activities and restrict participation. Decreased mobility can lead to secondary impairments that further affect activity and participation. Comorbid impairments can further compound movement problems. The large ovals representing secondary and comorbid impairments indicate that these may be the areas most amenable to change with rehabilitation. *CV,* cardiovascular; *MSK,* musculoskeletal.

determine the distribution of paresis and other accompanying motor control impairments. A number of prefixes are used with the terms *paresis* or *plegia* to define their distribution. Although most of what we know about paresis comes from studies of stroke, the neural mechanisms underlying paresis are the same regardless of what causes it.

Paresis can be largely considered a problem of movement execution.[2] The primary mechanism underlying paresis is damage to the corticospinal system, that is, the motor cortical areas, the corticospinal tract, and the spinal cord (schematically drawn in Fig. 17.1). Fig. 17.3 illustrates how the disruption of corticospinal system input alters the activation of motor units, the activation of muscles, the activation of sets of muscles, and the ability to move.[3] Together, the changes in the ability to volitionally activate motor units, muscles, and sets of muscles can explain much of the observed alterations and compensatory movement patterns seen in people with paresis. For example, the diminished ability to sufficiently activate the hip and knee extensor muscles when moving from sit to stand often results in increased time to complete the transfer, multiple attempts, and the use of compensatory strategies. Likewise, the common observation in the person poststroke of hip circumduction on the affected side during the swing phase of gait is a compensatory action due to the failure to activate hip flexors and ankle dorsiflexors with sufficient speed and appropriate timing. For upper limb movements, paresis results in slower, less accurate, and less efficient reaching and grasping movements.[4,5]

The distribution and severity of paresis will affect the ability to move. Individuals with more mild paresis will have movements that appear to be normal or near normal. Individuals with more severe paresis, or plegia, may not be able to move at all. Paresis of the upper limbs results in

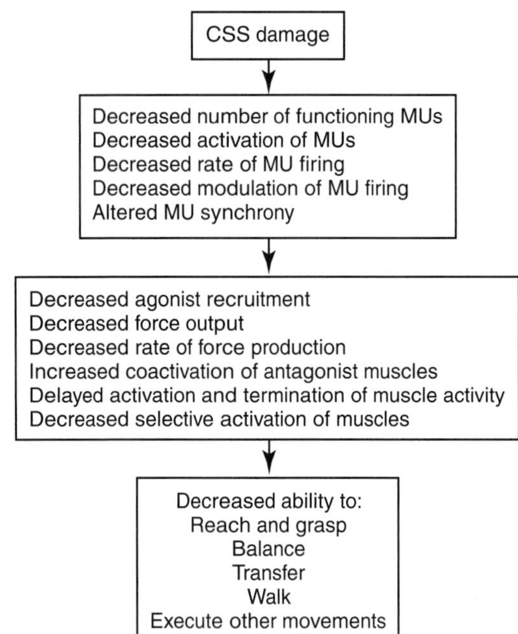

FIG. 17.3 Schematic of relationships between corticospinal system (CSS) damage, motor unit (MU) activity, muscle activity, and movement. Damage to the CSS results in numerous impairments at the MU level (second box). MU impairments in turn lead to muscle activation impairments. Finally, the muscle activation impairments manifest as activity limitations in many movements of interest to physical therapists.

limitations with activities such as bathing, dressing, grooming, and feeding. Paresis of the trunk and lower limbs results in limitations with transfers, balance, gait, and stair climbing. Even mild paresis can limit an older athlete's ability to participate in sport and recreational activities at prior levels of performance. In the presence of other comorbidities that commonly occur with age, the manner in which paresis affects functional activity can often be magnified (see Fig. 17.2). For example, an older adult with osteoarthritis may already have weakened quadriceps muscles due to pain that has led to decreased mobility. If this individual has a stroke, osteoarthritis-related muscle weakness combined with stroke-related paresis compounds the difficulty generating sufficient forces at sufficient rates, even in the less affected lower limb (ipsilateral to the lesion) for functional activities such as climbing stairs.

Abnormal Tone

Abnormal muscle tone is another common motor control impairment. Muscle tone itself is the resistance of muscle to passive elongation or stretch. Muscle tone is a result of inertia, the intrinsic biomechanical stiffness of the muscle and connective tissue, and the residual muscle contraction. There is a broad range of normal muscle tone seen in healthy individuals. Abnormal muscle tone can be divided into two major categories: hypotonicity and hypertonicity.

Hypotonicity is reduced muscle tone. Flaccidity is the extreme case of hypotonicity, where there is a complete loss of muscle tone. Clinically, hypotonicity is apparent as a decreased resistance to passive movement and a decreased or absent stretch reflex response. The limbs move easily and the joints are often hyperextensible. Hypotonicity is seen in a variety of conditions such as peripheral nerve damage, polio, and degenerative neuromuscular diseases and acutely after stroke affecting the corticospinal system or cerebellum. The mechanism underlying hypotonicity is a decreased or absent neural drive to the muscle.[6] In the case of peripheral nerve damage, the muscle may have lost its innervations or be only partially innervated. In the cases where hypotonicity is due to central nervous system damage, it is the spinal motoneurons that are damaged or have lost their major excitatory inputs (i.e., corticospinal connections).

Hypertonicity is increased muscle tone. Clinically, hypertonicity is apparent as increased resistance to passive movement and an increased stretch reflex response. The limbs are harder to move and it may not be possible to move the limb through its full range of motion. Like paresis, hypertonicity is seen in a variety of conditions that cause damage to the central nervous system, such as stroke (typically, hypotonicity is seen first and then hypertonicity develops after the first few days or weeks), spinal cord injury, traumatic brain injury, multiple sclerosis, and cerebral palsy.

Hypertonicity is largely a result of loss of supraspinal inhibition to the spinal cord. An often-forgotten fact about the corticospinal tract is that 40% of it arises from the parietal lobe, and these fibers are primarily inhibitory.[2] When the parietal lobe and/or the corticospinal tract are damaged, then a major source of spinal inhibition is missing. Without this inhibition, the response to afferent input (e.g., input from muscle spindles, cutaneous receptors) is abnormally large. This manifests as increased resistance as a muscle is stretched and even greater increases when the muscle is stretched quickly.

Spasticity is a special type of hypertonicity that has been the subject of considerable attention by rehabilitation clinicians and researchers. Spasticity is defined as a velocity-dependent resistance to passive movement. The resistance is often stronger in one direction than the other (e.g., greater during passive elbow extension vs. flexion). Spasticity is to be differentiated from rigidity by the fact that rigidity is not velocity dependent (e.g., resistance is the same regardless of the speed of passive movement) and is less likely to be directionally dependent (e.g., feels the same during flexion and extension). Unlike spasticity, which arises from corticospinal system damage, rigidity is believed to stem from altered basal ganglia pathology.[7] Rigidity is commonly seen in patients in the later stages of Parkinson disease and in patients with dystonias. The clinical management of rigidity is generally part of the pharmacologic management of the underlying medical condition.

A particularly challenging aspect of spasticity is that it varies within individuals on a day-to-day basis and on a movement-by-movement basis.[8] Factors such as body position, temperature, and the recent history of movement at that segment influence the degree of spasticity. For example, when repeatedly stretching spastic muscles at a given joint, one often feels less resistance with later movements than with earlier ones. The variability in spasticity makes it hard to assess and manage clinically.

It is critical to appreciate that hypertonicity is rarely seen by itself (see Fig. 17.2). It is typically part of a collection of impairments, paresis being one of them. The underlying health condition causing the corticospinal system damage will affect the severity and pattern of hypertonicity. For example, people with spinal cord injury often experience greater levels of spasticity than people with stroke. In stroke, the severity of the spasticity matches reasonably well to the severity of paresis.[9] Patients with more severe paresis have more severe spasticity, whereas patients with mild paresis have minimal or no spasticity. From a neuroanatomical perspective, this is logical because both paresis and hypertonicity are a product of corticospinal system damage. Although hypertonicity (or spasticity) is often correlated with the degree of activity limitation, it is now generally agreed that it is not causal to the activity limitations. The best evidence for this comes from studies of botulinum toxin to treat spasticity. The major conclusion from this collection of studies is that botulinum toxin reduces spasticity in the injected muscles but does not improve functional capabilities.[10]

Fractionated Movement Deficits

Fractionation of movement is a critical part of our ability to use our limbs, particularly the arms and hands, for many different movements.[11] A reduced ability to isolate or fractionate movement will severely limit the ability to perform daily functional tasks. A variety of central nervous system pathologies affecting the corticospinal system result in fractionated movement deficits, including stroke, traumatic brain injury, spinal cord injury, multiple sclerosis, and cerebral palsy. Fractionated movement deficits can also result from less common movement disorders affecting the basal ganglia, such as dystonia (discussed separately later).

Clinically, the ability to fractionate movement can be seen when asking the patient to move one segment in isolation and keep other, adjacent segments still. Assessment of fractionation is most common at the fingers, where patients are asked to touch the tip of the thumb to the tip of each of the other fingertips. Loss of fractionated movement also occurs at more proximal segments. This can be assessed by asking patients to flex the shoulder alone or knee alone and observing what else moves. Fractionated movement deficits can be seen as they flex other joints distal and proximal to the target joint at the same time. This reduction in fractionated movement, particularly in patients with stroke, is the same as the abnormal movement synergies described many years ago by Brunnstrom.[12] Like hypertonicity, the degree of fractionated movement deficit is related to the degree of weakness. Patients with more severe paresis and hypertonicity have less ability to fractionate movement, and people with more mild paresis and minimal hypertonicity can make well-fractionated movements.[9]

The cause of fractionated movement deficits is damage to the corticospinal system resulting in a decreased ability to selectively activate muscles.[2,3] The corticospinal system is the neural substrate that affords humans the ability to execute their extensive repertoire of movements.[13] With damage to this system, the ability to turn on one muscle or a specific set of muscles at just the right time and just the right amount is altered. For example, when turning on the shoulder flexor muscles to reach for an object, the shoulder abductor, elbow flexor, and forearm pronator muscles and finger flexor muscles turn on as well.[14,15] Likewise, in the lower limb, attempting to plantarflex the ankle may result in simultaneous extension at the knee and hip. As with paresis, fractionated movement deficits result in limitations with activities of daily living and mobility.

A different form of fractionated movement deficits is seen in people with dystonia. Dystonias appear as sustained, involuntary muscle contractions producing abnormal postures.[16] People with dystonia may have a primary dystonia or a secondary dystonia that results from an injury at birth, stroke, as side effect of antipsychotic medications, or other central nervous system pathology. This form of fractionated movement deficit is generally a result of pathology to the basal ganglia and its associated structures. The basal ganglia are a collection of large, functionally diverse nuclei located deep within the cerebral hemispheres (see Fig. 17.1). With respect to movement control, the direct pathway through the basal ganglia is thought to focus the selection of the desired motor plan, while the indirect pathway is thought to inhibit selection of undesired motor plans.[7,17]

A general systems-level hypothesis is that dystonias are caused by an underactive indirect basal ganglia pathway, resulting in reduced inhibition of the thalamus and the inability to suppress unwanted muscle activity. Thus, people with dystonia have fractionated movement deficits because many sets of muscle are turned on nearly all of the time.

Ataxia

Ataxia is a lack of coordination between movements and/or body parts.[18] The term *ataxia* has often been applied broadly to refer to any movement that is even somewhat uncoordinated. It is more correctly applied to specific movements (e.g., ataxic gait) that have the characteristic features of dysmetria. Dysmetria comes in two forms: hypermetria, or overshooting the intended target, and hypometria, or undershooting the intended target. People with ataxia tend to make hypermetric movements when trying to move quickly and hypometric movements when trying to move slowly.[19] Hyper- and hypometric movements are most easily seen in movements such as reaching and stepping. Overshooting or undershooting an intended posture with the trunk can also be seen when trying to control balance. When deciding if ataxia is present, it is important not to confuse ataxia with observed coordination problems that arise from paresis and/or fractionated movement deficits. When ataxia is present, the person will still have the capability to move quickly (although may not choose to) and the ataxia will typically look worse at faster movement speeds.

Ataxia results from damage to the cerebellar inputs, outputs, and/or cerebellar structures themselves (see Fig. 17.1). The spinocerebellar atrophies are a group of degenerative, progressive disorders whose major symptom is ataxia. People with other neurologic conditions such as stroke or multiple sclerosis can also have ataxia if the neurologic damage affected the cerebellum, its inputs, or its outputs. In rare cases, large-fiber peripheral neuropathies can result in a type of sensory ataxia that worsens when visual information is not available to assist in movement control.[20]

A major role of the cerebellum is to predict the sensory and motor consequences of movements to generate coordinated actions of multiple segments.[21,22] One way it does this is by predicting and then controlling for rotational forces generated from the movement of one segment on another segment.[21] People with ataxia have difficulty controlling these rotational movement-generated forces such that movements are largely influenced by the rotational forces and not by the intended muscle actions. For example, overshooting a target during fast reaching is largely due to the uncontrolled rotational forces generated at the shoulder and elbow.[19] Likewise, during walking, abnormal knee joint flexion during swing may be due to poorly controlled rotational forces generated by the movement of lower limb segments.[23] Many people with ataxia learn to compensate by moving slowly. Slower movements result in reduced rotational forces because these forces are velocity and acceleration dependent. Many different activities can be limited by ataxia. The most salient of these, the ones that most often bring people to physical therapy, are limitations in gait and balance. It is the gait deficits that are most immediately obvious to clinicians and families, but interestingly, the gait deficits are often due to difficulties in controlling balance during gait.[24]

Hypokinesia

Hypokinesia is a primary motor control impairment associated with Parkinson disease, other parkinsonian-like conditions, and sometimes dementia. It is characterized by slow movement (bradykinesia) or no movement (akinesia). In Parkinson disease, hypokinesia co-occurs with tremor at rest and with rigidity.[7] Hypokinesia is caused by basal ganglia damage and, in Parkinson disease, with loss of the dopaminergic cells in the substantia nigra pars compacta. The general hypothesis underlying hypokinesia is that there is an overactive indirect basal ganglia pathway, resulting in nearly constant thalamic inhibition, and the inability to select the desired motor plan.[7] Clinically, hypokinesia appears as frequent muscle co-contraction where there is difficulty turning off the muscles that are not needed and turning on the muscles that are needed to execute a particular movement. These muscle problems lead to a flexed-forward posture with instability and a slow, shuffling gait. People with hypokinesia have difficulty getting started with movement and can freeze during movement.[7] The major upper limb movement complaint is tremor and small, sometimes illegible, handwriting (termed micrographia). Postural instability, gait deficits, tremor, and micrographia will worsen with disease progression and as pharmacologic management of the disease becomes less effective.

Somatosensory Loss

Somatosensory loss is a common impairment in older adults often resulting in altered motor control. Beyond normal aging, abnormal somatosensory loss can occur in many of the same conditions named previously, such as stroke, spinal cord injury, traumatic brain injury, and multiple sclerosis. Abnormal somatosensory loss can be peripheral or central in origin. If it is from peripheral nerve damage, then the pattern of somatosensory loss will follow the distribution of the damaged nerve, root, or branch. If it is from central nervous system damage, then its distribution will be determined by the underlying condition. Somatosensory loss comes from damage anywhere along the pathways from the somatosensory receptors up through the somatosensory cortical areas in the cerebrum.

The major consequence of somatosensory loss on motor control is that ongoing monitoring of movement is less effective. The somatosensory system provides rapid, ongoing feedback about the consequences of movement.[25–27] For example, cutaneous receptors on the fingertips can provide feedback that a glass full of water is slipping. This information results in increased excitation of neurons at the spinal cord and cortical levels, resulting in an increased grip force that rapidly stops the glass from slipping. The visual system can partially, but not totally, compensate for the lack of somatosensation when planning movements.[28,29] In the glass-of-water example, somatosensory loss means that the person would detect that the glass was slipping only *if* visual attention was focused on the object. But by the time the slip was detected visually and acted upon, the glass might have dropped. Thus, people with somatosensory loss need to rely heavily on the visual system to plan and monitor movements. Their movements are slow, a compensatory response to adjust for the slower visual feedback, and are worse in poor vision or visually distracting conditions. Although somatosensory loss can occur in isolation, it is usually accompanied by one or more of the other motor control impairments discussed in this chapter.

Perceptual Deficits

Perceptual deficits are another sensory impairment that often results in significant motor control problems. One of the most common perceptual deficits seen in older adults is hemispatial neglect after stroke.[30] Because this is primarily managed by occupational therapists, the reader is referred to Corbetta[30] for an extensive review. Another perceptual deficit, pusher syndrome, is a challenging perceptual deficit encountered and treated by physical therapists.[31,32] Medical conditions causing pusher syndrome include stroke, traumatic brain injury, and in some instances dementia or brain tumors.[31,32] People with pusher syndrome due to stroke or brain injury push with the unaffected extremities toward the affected side. Although the specific mechanisms remain unclear, a current hypothesis explaining pusher syndrome is that these patients have a distorted perception of body orientation with respect to gravity despite intact visual and vestibular inputs.[31] The pushing to the affected side and the resistance to correction may be a compensatory control strategy to correct for a sensory and perceptual mismatch. Fortunately, the brain seems to be able to adjust with experience (therapy), because pusher syndrome generally diminishes with time over the first 1 to 2 months after stroke.[33] If pusher syndrome occurs owing to a degenerative condition or persists beyond 1 to 2 months after a specific brain insult, then the prognosis for functional independence is poor.

The most common characteristics seen in patients with pusher syndrome are self-selected body posture tilted toward the affected side, abducted and extended limbs on the unaffected side pushing toward the affected side, and resistance to passive correction of the abnormal posture. This behavioral phenomenon is distinctly different from other balance impairments seen in older adults with stroke or traumatic brain injury, where the presence of paresis and its accompanying reduction in the ability to activate muscles at the right time and right amount results in an inability to maintain the body in upright posture in sitting or standing. Pusher syndrome can occur in sitting, standing, walking, or even supine (resistance to rolling to the nonparetic side). In more severe cases, the person will be unable to maintain independent sitting. In milder cases, the deficit will only appear during walking.

In stroke, pusher syndrome is often accompanied by hemispatial neglect of the affected side of the body, aphasia, paresis, and somatosensory loss.[31,34] Interestingly, pusher syndrome often co-occurs with perceptual deficits such as neglect if the right cerebrum is damaged, or with aphasia if the left cerebrum is damaged.[31,34] Additionally, the paresis in these patients is typically severe. From a physical therapy perspective, the salient feature in patients with pusher syndrome is that the resistance to sitting upright with support and resisting postural corrections is often a more significant contributor to functional deficits than arm and leg paresis.

EXAMINATION OF PATIENTS WITH IMPAIRED MOTOR CONTROL

The examination of motor control impairments requires a somewhat different conceptual approach than examination for musculoskeletal problems. This is because motor control impairments most commonly appear in groups versus in isolation. For example, a person with stroke is more likely to have paresis, hypertonicity, and fractionated movement deficits than they are to have paresis alone. When performing a musculoskeletal examination, much of the effort is focused on muscle length, muscle strength, and specific mobility tests to determine the impairments contributing to the musculoskeletal problem. When performing a neurologic examination, the impairment assessments are differently detailed (e.g., testing muscle groups vs. individual muscles) such that the focus is on determining which of the impairments present are contributing to the loss of movement activity.[35] Much of the examination is devoted to observation and assessment of functional movements. In addition to judging the capability to execute a movement, observational analysis is necessary to determine how impairments may be either associated with or contributing to the functional deficits.

Physical therapists have traditionally placed a strong emphasis on assessment of impairments. As a result, examination forms contain fields for numerous impairment measures. For example, many forms include fields for manual muscle testing of every muscle group of the upper and lower limbs as well as every somatosensory modality at four or more locations on each limb. Most motor control impairments stem from central nervous system damage, where testing every muscle and every somatosensory modality is generally unnecessary and a waste of time. (Note that there are exceptions to this as in the uncommon cases of geriatric spinal cord injury where detailed sensorimotor testing will be critical.) The anatomy and physiology of the motor and somatosensory cortical and subcortical systems are such that central nervous system damage typically affects many muscles, segments, and often limbs. For example, one would never see a person with stroke who has isolated paresis to the left hip abductors, but instead would see paresis affecting all the hip, knee, and ankle muscles on the left side. Likewise, one would never see a person with stroke with loss of light touch sensation only to one finger or only to the shoulder. The loss of light touch sensation would be present across that upper limb and would coexist with loss of other somatosensory modalities (e.g., proprioception). The patterns of motor control impairments therefore allow physical therapists to efficiently evaluate key impairments that are critical for safety, prognosis, and diagnosis (see Lang and colleagues[36] for a description and rationale for a standardized assessment battery for stroke). Shorter examinations reduce the testing burden on the patient and the therapist, and permit more time for education and treatment.

The physical therapy examination has two important goals: (1) to determine the initial level of impairment, activity, and participation so that future progress can be measured, that is, outcome assessment, and (2) to determine the underlying movement system problem, that is, the movement system diagnosis. Some items on the exam may serve one goal or the other, whereas other items might serve both goals. Table 17.1 lists and briefly describes each recommended test, specifies the motor impairment addressed by each test, and highlights salient issues related to each test. The first section of Table 17.1 describes the objective tests used to determine the presence and severity of motor control impairments. The second section of Table 17.1 provides a list of movements for observational analyses. Often movement analysis can be done during the administration of a standardized assessment.

Evaluation of paresis is critical because paresis is most often the impairment causing loss of function.[37–39] Manual muscle testing is an easy way to evaluate paresis. Conceptually, manual muscle testing indirectly measures the ability to volitionally activate spinal motoneuron pools at a given segment. A major debate in the physical therapy community over the years has been whether or not one can reliably test strength in the presence of fractionated movement deficits. In people with stroke, paresis and fractionated movement deficits coexist and severity is highly

TABLE 17.1 Recommended Clinical Tests to Assess the Presence, Severity, and Functional Consequences of Motor Control Impairment

Test	Description (Range of Scores)	Impairment Assessed	Comments, Interpretations, Judgments*
Objective Tests of Motor Control Impairments			
Motricity Index[40]	Test uses standard MMT of three specific UE and three specific LE segments to create UE and LE scores of overall paretic deficit. UE segments: shoulder abduction, elbow flexion, pinch grip LE segments: hip flexion, knee extension, ankle dorsiflexion Range = 0–100 points	Paresis	A benefit of this is that it yields both standard MMT scores that are useful in communicating with other professionals and an overall limb score that is useful in communicating with patients and families.
Modified Ashworth Scale[75]	Test uses passive range of motion of multiple UE and LE segments at varying speeds. Range = 0–4 points	Spasticity	There is rarely a need to assess all segments because the degree of spasticity covaries across segments (Lang et al., unpublished observations). For the UE, the best choice is the elbow because if spasticity is present, it will be most easily felt at the elbow.
Finger–thumb opposition	Patient is asked to touch the thumb to the tips of each finger rapidly. Score based on clinical judgment of performance of movement as unable, impaired, or normal.	Fractionated movement deficits	This may be unnecessary because it is possible to determine the presence/absence of fractionated movement deficits by observation of Motricity Index items.
Finger-to-nose[76]	Patient is asked to touch the examiner's finger, then touch his or her own nose ~10 times rapidly. Score based on clinical judgment of performance of movement as unable, impaired, or normal.	Ataxia	Recommended that this test be skipped if Motricity Index measures indicate more than mild paresis. If given to people with moderate–severe paresis, then coordination deficits are secondary to the paresis.
Rapid alternating movements	Patient is asked to rapidly pronate and supinate the forearm for 10–20 sec. Score based on clinical judgment of performance of movement as unable, impaired, or normal.	Ataxia	Recommended that this test be skipped if AROM and/or Motricity Index measures indicate more than mild paresis. If given to people with moderate–severe paresis, then coordination deficits are secondary to the paresis.
Light touch sensation	Patient is lightly touched on fingertips/foot–ankle. If affected unilaterally, sensations can be compared to other side. Scores: present, impaired, or absent	Somatosensation	Recommend scoring as present, impaired, or absent. Loss of light touch sensation often signals loss of other somatosensory modalities, making it less important to test the others.

TABLE 17.1 Recommended Clinical Tests to Assess the Presence, Severity, and Functional Consequences of Motor Control Impairment—cont'd

Test	Description (Range of Scores)	Impairment Assessed	Comments, Interpretations, Judgments
Unstructured Mesulam[77,78]	Patient marks all the target symbols on a standard test form. More symbols missed on one side of the paper vs. the other indicates neglect. A large overall number of missed symbols may indicate general attentional deficits. Range = 0–30 left–right misses	Perceptual deficits (neglect)	Neglect may be observed during functional movements and formally tested afterward or, more commonly, assessed by occupational therapy.
Burke lateral propulsion test[79]	Patient is rated on degree of pushing in five testing positions: supine rolling, sitting, transferring, standing, and walking. Higher scores indicate more severe deficits. Range = 0–17	Perceptual deficits (pushing)	Recommend administering after the observational assessment of posture if warranted.
Observational Analyses of Movement to Detect Motor Impairments[35]			
Observation of in-hand manipulation	Place a pencil in the patient's palm. Ask him or her to manipulate it for writing. Clinical judgment of if and how impairments from standardized tests influence functional task	Paresis Fractionated movement deficits	Recommended for higher-level patients. Note if there is sufficient movement and if the finger movement is fractionated.
Observation of posture	Patient is asked to sit (feet supported, no UE support) and stand quietly with eyes open. Clinical judgment of if and how impairments from standardized tests influence functional task.	Perceptual deficits	This is included as an assessment for perceptual deficits and is not intended as a formal assessment of postural control. Perceptual deficits are present if posture is not grossly at midline, pushes strongly to one side, and/or resists corrections to midline. Patients with just paresis and no perceptual deficits will not push or resist correction to midline.
Observation of sit to stand	Patient is asked to come to standing from bedside or chair without UE support. Clinical judgment of if and how impairments from standardized tests influence functional task.	Paresis Hypokinesia Perceptual deficits	*Paresis*: cannot lift bottom out of chair, cannot extend hips/knees to stand, rapidly falls if support is removed, performance degrades with fatigue. *Hypokinesia:* limited or slow preparatory movements, falls slowly if support is removed, freezes during attempt. *Perceptual deficits:* shifts toward weaker side, pushes away from midline, resists correction to midline.
Observation of gait	Patient is asked to walk ~10 m, turn around, and come back. Assistance is provided as needed. Clinical judgment of if and how impairments from standardized tests influence functional task.	Paresis Fractionated movement deficits Ataxia Hypokinesia	*Paresis:* lateral trunk bending, hip/trunk flexion, knee hyperextension, leg circumduction, minimal dorsiflexion, performance degrades with fatigue. *Fractionated movement deficits:* stiff leg, movements of UE(s) when trying to step with LE. *Ataxia:* variable foot placement in both A-P and M-L directions, variable line of progression, limited change in performance with corrections or fatigue. *Hypokinesia:* limited or slow preparatory movements, slowness initiating stepping, freezes during attempt.

*See Academy of Neurologic PT (EDGE) for a comprehensive summary and interpretation of scores: http://www.neuropt.org/professional-resources/neurology-section-outcome-measures-recommendations

Note: The measures in the top half of the table are direct impairment assessments. Not all impairments have identified specific tests. The measures on the bottom half of the table are observations of activities where the specific impairments and their contribution to function can be identified.[55] The Comments, Interpretations, Judgments column is intended to highlight salient issues and is not intended as an exhaustive list.

A-P, anterior-posterior; *LE,* lower extremity; *M-L,* medial-lateral; *MMT,* manual muscle testing; *UE,* upper extremity.

correlated.[9] People who cannot move much typically cannot move in isolation, whereas people who can move a lot can make fractionated movements. Thus, an assessment of how much they can activate motor units at a given segment, such as with manual muscle testing, can provide sufficient information about both of these motor control impairments. Standard manual muscle testing in the context of the Motricity Index is a useful way to evaluate paresis.[40] The Motricity Index is one of the preferred tools for patient assessments poststroke and is used widely around the world in research and clinical practice.[41] The benefit of using the Motricity Index[36] is that it allows one to test only three muscle groups per limb, reducing the required testing time. It also does not require equipment or difficult scoring criteria. An older measure, the Fugl-Meyer Assessment,[42] can also assess paresis. This measure is more common in research studies but relatively rare in clinical practice. Both the Motricity Index and the Fugl-Meyer Assessment can quantify global limb impairment. The Motricity Index assesses paresis, whereas the Fugl-Meyer Assessment intermingles the assessment of paresis and fractionated movements. In a busy clinic, the Motricity Index may be most useful because it takes less time to administer (5 vs. 30 minutes) and the manual muscle testing rating scale and definitions are familiar to most clinicians.[36] An additional benefit of the Motricity Index is that the scores are easily understandable to patients and their families—for example, "Your left leg strength is about 30% of your right leg."

A common observation in adults with motor control impairments is that movements are slow. Slowed movement is a consistent finding across neurologic patient populations for a variety of reasons. In patients with paresis, slowness is due to motor unit activation deficits.[3] In patients with ataxia, slowness of movement may be a compensatory technique to minimize the rotational forces generated from the movement of one segment on another segment.[19,21] In patients with somatosensory loss, slowness of movement may also be a compensatory technique, allowing time for accessing the slower visual feedback.[20] In patients with hypokinesia, slowness of movement may be the hallmark feature and a result of the inability to select the desired motor program and turn off other undesired programs.[7] Thus, it is most useful to note the consistencies and/or inconsistencies between observed movement slowness and specific movement impairments versus simply noting that movement slowness is present.

Assessment of outcomes is a key part of the neurologic examination. Recommended tests for assessing functional activity include the Berg Balance Scale, Timed Up and Go (TUG), Walking Speed test (typically over 10 m), the 6-minute Walk Test, Action Research Arm Test, and Canadian Occupational Performance Measure. The first four of these are discussed in Chapter 7, on functional assessment . The last two are particularly useful for assessing upper limb functional activity. The Action Research Arm Test (ARAT)[43,44] is a criterion-rated test with 19 items; the total score ranges from 0 to 57, with higher scores indicating better performance. The Canadian Occupational Performance Measure (COPM)[44,45] is an individualized outcome assessment that allows the person to identify and then measure performance and satisfaction with performance of relevant activities. Performance and satisfaction are rated from 0 to 10, where higher scores are better. Note that these assessments capture capacity for function, which may not be the same as function in daily life outside the clinic or laboratory.[46,47] As with any patient population, outcome measures for the geriatric individual with motor control impairment need to be administered at the time of the initial evaluation and then periodically during the course of treatment to determine patient progress. Outcomes are most appropriately assessed at the activity and participation levels, but it may be useful to assess a few impairment level measures as well. Results from the impairment items can be compared to results from the activity items to confirm or refute the therapist's initial judgment about how the impairments contributed to the activity limitations.

In addition to motor control impairments and functional limitations, the evaluation will need to cover other domains such as cognitive status and living situation, described in other chapters of this book. Lastly, it is important to evaluate secondary, indirect impairments that may arise from the motor control impairments. The presence of motor control impairments will typically lead to decreased mobility (see Fig. 17.2). Moving less results in secondary impairments such as contracture, muscle atrophy, and cardiovascular deconditioning. The presence and severity of secondary impairments will affect the process of selecting the most appropriate treatment and the success of the treatment for an individual patient.

PROGNOSIS AND DIAGNOSIS

The patient's medical diagnosis is only part of the equation in determining the plan of care. The role of the physical therapist is to (1) understand the medical diagnosis, (2) integrate prognosis, and (3) connect assessed impairments and activity limitations to formulate a movement system diagnosis.

Building on the patient examination, prognosis in older adults with motor control impairments is largely a function of the underlying medical condition. It is useful to think about prognosis with regard to the medical condition *and* with regard to the likelihood of possible improvement with rehabilitation intervention. With respect to the medical prognosis, a critical piece of information is whether or not the underlying medical condition is progressive or nonprogressive. Nonprogressive conditions include stroke, spinal cord injury, and traumatic brain injury. Progressive conditions include Parkinson disease, multiple sclerosis, and other degenerative neuromuscular diseases. In nonprogressive conditions, the impairments are more likely to improve early after injury than later

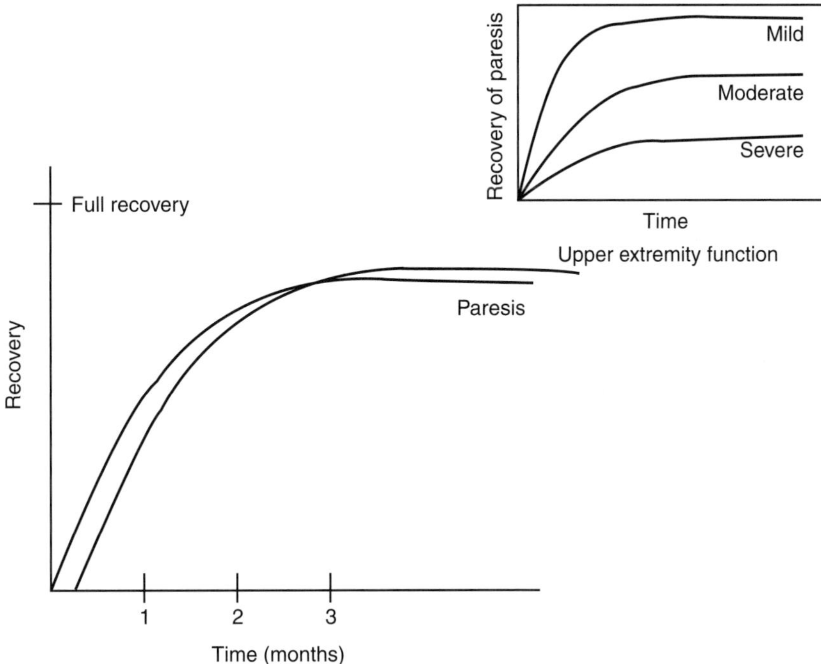

FIG. 17.4 Schematic of the time course of recovery from paresis at the impairment and at the function level, as derived from epidemiologic data after stroke. Recovery of function typically lags recovery of motor deficits by about 1 to 2 weeks, where the shapes of the two recovery curves are very similar. The reason for the lag and the similar shape may be because as the motor ability emerges, movement practice is required to capitalize on the motor recovery and incorporate it into daily function. *Inset:* Those who are most mildly affected will recover more quickly and to a greater extent, whereas those who are more severely affected will recover more slowly and to a lesser extent.

after injury. In progressive conditions, the impairments are expected to worsen over time. The progressive or non-progressive nature of the underlying medical condition is an important factor in selecting appropriate interventions for individual patients.

Epidemiologic data on prognoses are available for most medical conditions. After stroke, recovery of paresis occurs along a predictable time course. Fig. 17.4 illustrates the typical time course of recovery from paresis at the impairment and at the functional activity level, as derived from epidemiologic data after stroke. Most epidemiologic data on stroke recovery are from samples of older adults, with average ages in most samples about 65 years. In general, most motor recovery will occur within the first 3 months.[48,49] The pattern of recovery is similar in older and younger adults with stroke, although older adults (in this study defined as older than age 75 years) are less likely to regain independence with basic activities of daily living and less likely to return to living at home.[50] The reason for limited independence may be the increased number of comorbid impairments present in older adults (see Fig. 17.2). Initial severity of the paretic impairments is the best predictor of eventual motor deficits and function.[51–54] Those with milder deficits recover more quickly and completely, whereas those with more severe deficits recover more slowly and to a much lesser extent (*inset,*Fig. 17.4).[48] For the purpose of predicting recovery of individual patients, the therapist must appreciate that epidemiologic data provide the typical pattern of recovery and that most, but not all, patients will follow a similar time course of changes. There are several consistent predictors of poor outcomes poststroke that are useful to look for when trying to determine prognosis in individuals. First, the more nonmotor impairments there are (e.g., somatosensory loss or visual field loss) that accompany the motor deficits (e.g., paresis, fractionated movement deficit), the less likely a person is to return to functional independence.[55] Second, earlier improvements in motor control impairments indicate that a person is more likely to reach higher levels of independence.[49,56] And third, the presence of any of the following at or after 1 month is associated with poor functional outcomes: no or minimal grip strength, no or minimal shoulder flexion, no or minimal hip flexion against gravity, and assistance needed for sitting.[37,53,57] Recovery of function typically lags recovery of motor deficits by about 1 to 2 weeks, where the shapes of the two recovery curves are very similar.[49] The reason for the lag and the similar shape may be that as the motor ability emerges, movement practice is required to capitalize on the motor recovery and incorporate it into daily function.

Building on the epidemiologic data that is available in combination with the examination results, there are clinical prediction models to assist in determining likelihood of function. The most robust models are available for persons with stroke. For the upper limb, the Predict Recovery Potential 2 (PREP2) model incorporates results of clinical examination (strength) and measures of neural structures (motor evoked potentials) to predict upper limb function at 3 months after stroke.[58,59] The first step is evaluating

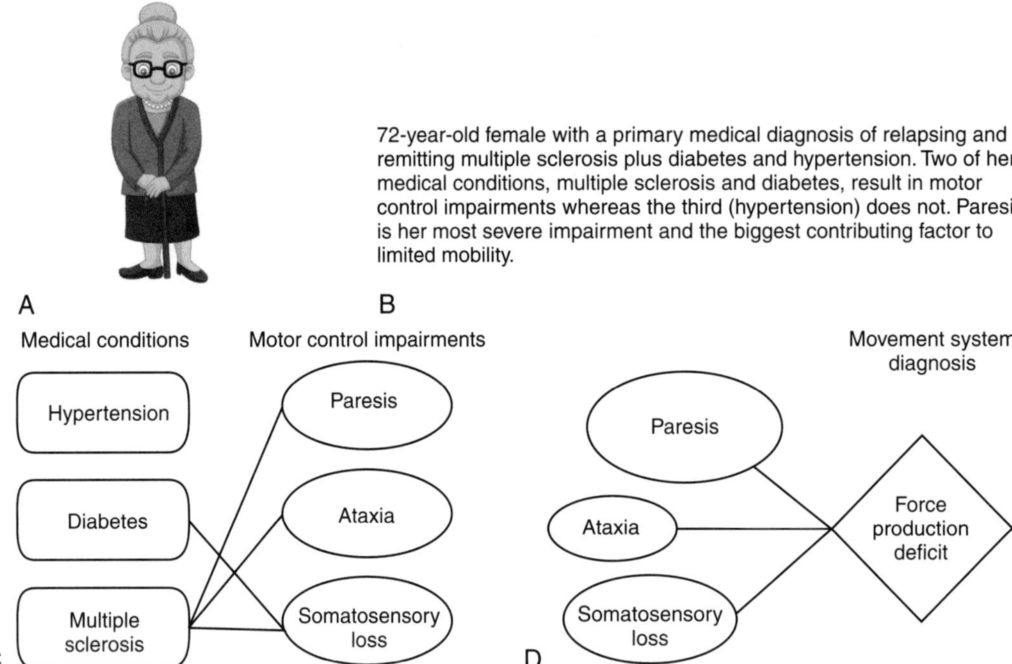
72-year-old female with a primary medical diagnosis of relapsing and remitting multiple sclerosis plus diabetes and hypertension. Two of her medical conditions, multiple sclerosis and diabetes, result in motor control impairments whereas the third (hypertension) does not. Paresis is her most severe impairment and the biggest contributing factor to limited mobility.
A
B
Medical conditions
Motor control impairments
Movement system diagnosis
Hypertension
Diabetes
Multiple sclerosis
Paresis
Ataxia
Somatosensory loss
C
Paresis
Ataxia
Somatosensory loss
Force production deficit
D

FIG. 17.5 Medical conditions, motor control impairments, and movement system diagnosis for a clinical case. **A**, An image of the example. **B**, A description of the clinical example. **C**, A map of the relationships between her medical conditions and her motor control impairments. **D**, A map of how her motor control impairments contribute to her movement system diagnosis. The size of the oval represents the severity of the impairment. The thickness of the line represents the therapist's observations and judgment as to how the impairments contribute to activity limitations and participation restrictions.

upper limb strength at one proximal and one distal muscle group using the common manual muscle testing procedure within the first few days poststroke. The two muscle groups tested on the involved upper limb are the shoulder abductors and the finger extensors, with each muscle group assigned a score of 0 to 5, where 0 = flaccid and 5 = full strength. If at day 3 poststroke a person has a combined muscle strength grade of five or more (sum the scores from the two muscle groups), then that person will likely have an excellent or good upper limb outcome. If the combined strength is less than five, transcranial magnetic stimulation can be used to examine the integrity of the corticospinal tract by eliciting motor evoked potentials in the paretic limb. This in combination with initial stroke severity can predict good, limited, or poor upper limb outcome. For the lower limbs, if at 3 days poststroke a person is able to sit independently for 30 seconds and has a Motricity Index score of $\geq$25 in the involved lower limb, he or she will likely be an independent ambulator at 6 months poststroke.[54] Similarly, the Time to Walking Independently after Stroke (TWIST) algorithm predicts time (6 or 12 weeks) to walking independence or dependence poststroke.[60] If at 1 week poststroke a person has good trunk control (as indicated by being able to roll to each side, sit up, and sit on the edge of the bed with no physical assistance), then he or she will likely be ambulating independently by 6 weeks.[40] If, however, trunk control is poor (as indicated by needing physical assistance to do the aforementioned activities), the presence of hip extensor strength will determine if the person will be independent or dependent with ambulation at 12 weeks poststroke. Use of these models in combination with the medical diagnosis and examination findings can help clinicians to establish a movement system diagnosis and guide the plan of care.

Physical therapists are experts in understanding human movement because of their education in all of the systems that contribute to movement (e.g., musculoskeletal, neurologic, cardiovascular). Although it is outside the scope of physical therapy practice to diagnose the medical condition, it is within the scope of practice to diagnose the movement system problem,[61] that is, diagnosing the impairments in body function and structure that lead to activity limitations of movement.

There is currently only one published set of movement system diagnoses for people with motor control impairments.[35,62] This system was developed from systematic clinical observation and has not been tested empirically. Within this system, there are eight distinct diagnoses related to motor control impairments. The names for the diagnoses (labels) are derived from the impairment believed to be the major contributor to the movement problems.[35] The eight diagnoses within this system and a brief description of each are provided in Table 17.2. A key component of this diagnostic system is that it recognizes that motor control impairments co-occur. Physical therapists determine a diagnosis based on the motor control impairment that is thought to be the *biggest contributor* to the movement dysfunction, instead of having to list diagnoses for all motor control impairments.

TABLE 17.2 Movement System Diagnostic Categories[35] for Motor Control Impairments

Movement System Diagnosis	Primary Movement System Impairment	Description	Relation to Impairments in This Chapter
Movement pattern coordination deficit	Coordination between segments and limbs	Altered timing and sequencing of tasks requiring movement at multiple segments or multiple body parts	No direct match for a specific impairment. The observed movement problems in this diagnostic category often result from very mild paresis, somatosensory loss, or other primary or secondary general immobility.
Force production deficit	Weakness	The origin of the weakness may be central (e.g., paresis) or peripheral (e.g., muscle, neuromuscular junction, nerve).	Paresis
Sensory detection deficit	Sensory loss	Lost sensations can be proprioceptive, visual, and/or vestibular. The lost sensation results in difficulty with movement control.	Somatosensory loss
Sensory selection and weighting deficit	Inability to attend to and weight sensory information	Difficulty with using/choosing incoming sensory information to plan and execute movements	No direct match with any one motor control deficit. The observed movement problems in this diagnostic category can result from sensory loss in one or more modalities. The movement problem is primarily with postural control.
Postural vertical deficit	Altered perception of body orientation/ posture	This is pusher syndrome in stroke, where resistance to postural correction is medial/lateral. In a few conditions, pushing has been observed in the anterior/posterior direction.	Perceptual deficit
Fractionated movement deficit	Inability to make isolated movements	This diagnosis is always associated with central nervous system dysfunction.	Fractionated movement deficit
Hypermetria	Ataxia	This diagnosis is generally associated with damage to the cerebellum or its input/ output structures.	Ataxia
Hypokinesia	Slowness of initiating and executing movement, paucity of movement	Most often associated with Parkinson disease and/or dementia	Hypokinesia

Note: The diagnostic label identifies the major problem resulting in movement dysfunction; it does not mean that other problems are not present. Note that there are a few minor differences in terminology between this system and the way impairments are discussed in this chapter. These differences are detailed in the last column of the table.

As such, the diagnostic system provides a very useful framework to think about how motor control impairments present and might be managed in older adults. The more formal structure is particularly useful for novice clinicians, who are either new to physical therapy or new to treating patients with neurologic dysfunctions. The system supplies a framework for how to treat and manage people falling within each diagnostic category. The management ideas that underlie this framework are discussed in the next sections. Additional research into movement system diagnosis is critically needed, both for persons with and for persons without motor control impairments. Currently, there are a variety of American Physical Therapy Association (APTA) task forces assembled to develop and integrate movement system diagnoses into physical therapy practice, and over the next decades, it is hoped that a variety of research approaches can be used to refine these systems. The challenging aspect of this type of research is that it requires large numbers of patients who are evaluated and treated in a standardized, systematic way.

Fig. 17.4 illustrates a patient with multiple medical conditions and motor control impairments and the relationship between the medical diagnosis, examination findings, prognosis, and movement system diagnosis. The clinician conceptualizes the relationship among medical diagnoses and examination findings to determine the impairments with the greatest impact on the patient's ability to interact with the environment. In this case example, paresis was found to have the greatest influence. Therefore, the movement system diagnosis is "force production deficit." This diagnosis will help the clinician to determine a focus of patient intervention (i.e., improve strength as able).

BOX 17.2 Key Questions to Guide Rehabilitation Prognosis and Treatment Decisions

1. What is the likelihood for motor control changes?
2. What is the likelihood of functional changes?
3. What is the likelihood that a specific intervention is going to change the expected outcome?

Putting it all together, there are three important questions (Box 17.2) to consider with every patient: (1) What is the likelihood for motor control changes? (2) What is the likelihood of functional changes? and (3) What is the likelihood that a specific intervention is going to change the expected outcome? The first question reflects back on the medical condition. Motor control may worsen as in progressive conditions, may stay the same as in chronic nonprogressive conditions, or may improve as in acute/subacute nonprogressive conditions. The second question is partially, but not totally, independent from the first question. In many cases, motor control impairments will not change, but activity limitations and participation restrictions can be lessened. For example, ankle dorsiflexion strength may not change in someone who is 2 years poststroke, but a well-fitted ankle foot orthosis may allow return to community ambulation and volunteer activities. For older adults, there is high personal value placed on resuming participation in activities of interest. Assisting with improving participation can improve quality of life and help to foster optimal aging.

The third question is perhaps the most important and difficult to ponder. As physical therapists, one assumes that interventions will result in better outcomes. In reality though, this assumption is rarely tested in individual patients. For example, it is possible that a patient's gait improves over the course of therapy because he or she must walk to and from the parking lot to receive services and not because of the short time spent practicing gait during therapy. The purpose of asking this third question is not to argue against the value of physical therapy services but to force ourselves to thoroughly examine the value of any possible intervention. Given limited services and busy patient lives, it behooves us to expend services wisely. Trying to answer these three questions about each patient will allow one to make decisions about treatment goals and whether the approach in reaching the goals should be remediation or compensation.

PLAN OF CARE AND REHABILITATION APPROACH

The first, critical decision when deciding on a plan of care to address motor control impairments in adults is to determine whether to use a remedial (also termed restorative) or a compensatory approach for treatment. A remedial approach is aimed at restoring the previously lost motor ability and function. A compensatory approach is aimed at maximizing function within the confines of the limited motor abilities. This major decision is reached by careful consideration of the diagnosis, examination, and prognosis. For example, in an older adult with Parkinson disease, the compensatory approach is usually most appropriate, given that the individual's motor dysfunction is expected to worsen over time. In treating the upper limb poststroke, a remedial approach would be chosen if the individual had a stroke less than 3 months earlier *and* there is voluntary fractionated movement against gravity at several upper limb segments.[10] In contrast, a compensatory approach would be chosen for a patient with minimal or no voluntary fractionated movement, whether early or later poststroke.[10] In the case of the remediation approach with the upper limb, the expectation is that therapy will restore the hand to a reasonable level of dexterity. In the case of the compensatory approach, the expectation is that therapy will teach the person to maintain the health of the limb (i.e., minimize contracture development, edema, and potential hygiene problems) and will permit the hand to be used as an assist or support in daily activities.

Similar to the upper limb, treatment for the lower limb (primarily focused on gait) poststroke follows the same thought process. A remedial approach for gait, where the intent is to restore a relatively normal gait pattern, would be chosen if the individual had a stroke less than 3 months earlier *and* there is sufficient, voluntary, fractionated movement against gravity at multiple lower limb segments. A compensatory approach for gait would be chosen to allow for safe ambulation in the patient with minimal or no voluntary fractionated movement, whether early or later poststroke. In the compensatory approach, therapists will be unconcerned with quality of movement (unless directly affecting safety) and may use assistive devices and/or bracing. By closely monitoring the motor capabilities of each patient, the therapist can determine if the appropriate approach was chosen and can be prepared to adapt approaches if needed.

Once the treatment approach has been decided upon, specific interventions can be chosen. Interventions for impaired motor control should be targeted toward improving function and not targeted at improving impairments in isolation. Support for interventions targeting specific activities and not their underlying impairments comes from the mechanisms underlying motor learning and neuroplasticity, and from clinical rehabilitation research.[10,41,63]

Motor learning is the acquisition, modification, or reacquisition of movement.[1] *Neuroplasticity* is a term indicating that neurons, neural connections, and neural representations are modifiable.[64] Evidence from motor learning and neuroplasticity studies suggests that the experience-dependent changes to the nervous system are unique to the neural structure used during practice.[65–68] The cellular and neural network mechanisms that underlie learning and plasticity are conceptually illustrated in Fig. 17.6. Fig. 17.6A illustrates long-term potentiation, a prerequisite for neural changes associated with learning.

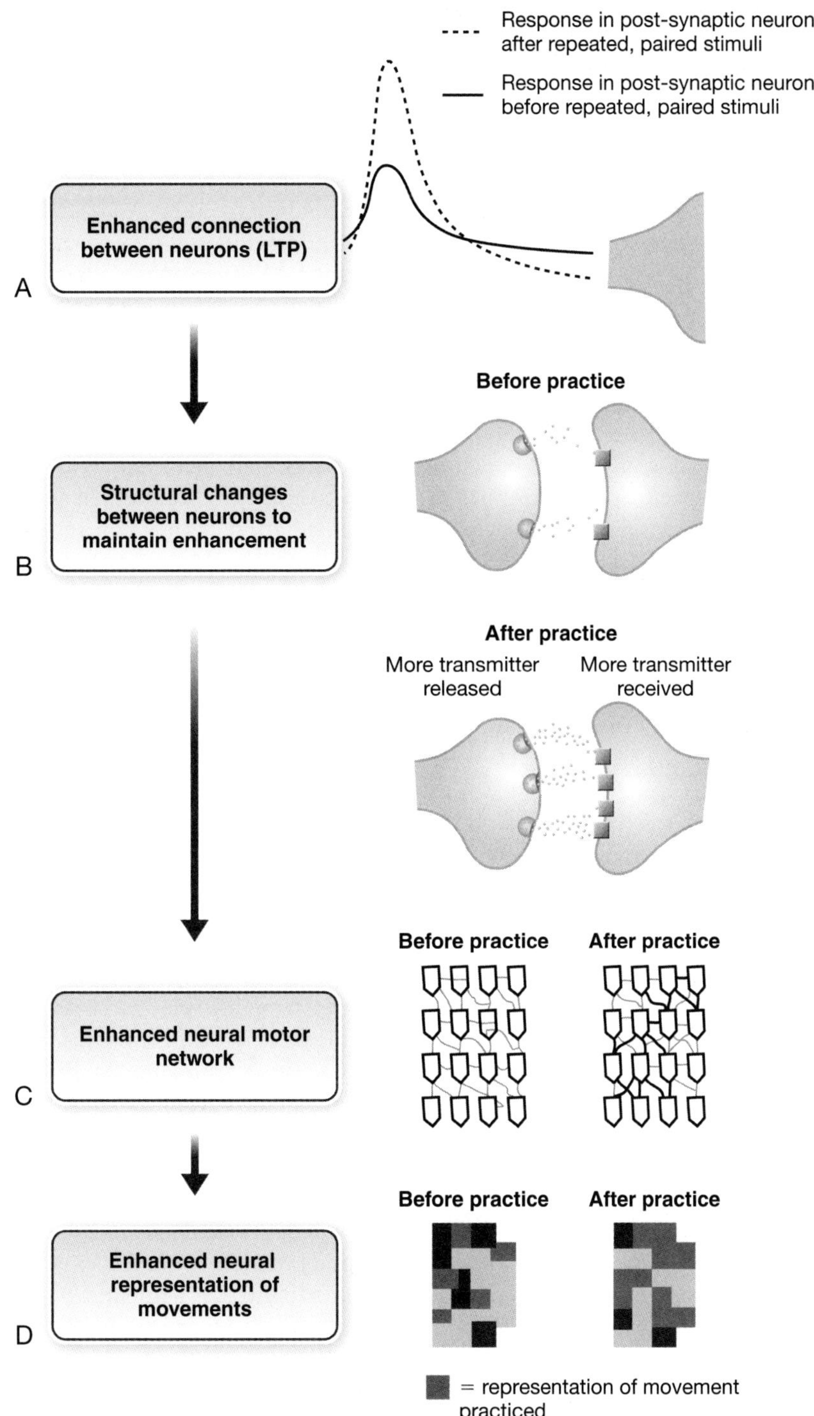

FIG. 17.6 Schematic of neural mechanisms of motor learning/plasticity. **A,** As a new/challenging movement is practiced in a session, the connection between neurons that are fired together is enhanced. **B,** As the movement is practiced over time, structural changes between the two neurons make the enhancement more permanent. **C,** This happens with many neuron pairs across the motor system, such that some connections and combinations of neurons in the network are selectively enhanced via practice. **D,** Neural representations of specific movements (combinations of muscle actions) that are practiced become enhanced. LTP, long-term potentiation.

With long-term potentiation, a neuron's response to input is enhanced by receiving repeated input, as through repeated practice.[69] If the repeated input is sustained, as through practice that is repeated over days and weeks, then the synapse between the presynaptic (input) neurons and the postsynaptic (output) neurons is remodeled (Fig. 17.6B). The remodeling results in structural changes that allow more transmitter to be released from the presynaptic neurons and more transmitter to be picked up by the postsynaptic neurons. This process does not just happen at one neuron or one pair of neurons but across the specific network of neurons used to execute that movement (Fig. 17.6C). Thus, as a movement is practiced, connections within the network that are critical for its execution are enhanced and other connections are left alone or diminished. Lastly, the neural representation of the particular practiced movement is enhanced (Fig. 17.6D), and neural representations of unused movements may be diminished.

The specificity of the neural changes occurring as a result of practice/experience therefore supports the importance of task-specific practice for optimizing function both in intact and in damaged nervous systems. Practice of part of a movement in isolation, such as hip flexion in standing, is unlikely to activate the *exact* same network of neurons that are activated when trying to flex the hip during gait. Tracing the process in Fig. 17.6, if a patient does not start with activating the specific network of neurons needed for the activity of interest, then the network needed for the desired activity will not be enhanced or strengthened. This is the scientific reason that basketball players practice free throws to improve their free-throw percentage and do not practice extending their arms or flexing their wrist only.

Evidence from clinical studies also supports the idea that task-specific training is critical for function. In older adults, practice of balance improves balance but not gait, whereas practice of gait improves gait but not balance.[70,71] In people with stroke, task-specific training is largely considered to be the best way to promote functional recovery.[41] Further support for task-specific training over impairment-based training comes from a recent review of the efficacy of strength training and its effect on function poststroke.[39,41,63] Strength training results in improvements in strength but only results in improvement in function if the strength training is done within the context of the functional task.[39] An excellent practical example of this is practicing sit-to-stand transfers repeatedly and from surface heights that are increasingly difficult. In most patients, this will lead to improved sit-to-stand transfers and to increased quadriceps strength,[72] whereas quadriceps strengthening in the standard seated, non-weight-bearing position may lead to increased quadriceps strength but with little carryover to functional mobility involving quadriceps. Thus, the skills of the physical therapist are needed to appropriately structure the task-specific training to address the movement dysfunction and its underlying impairments.

Let us apply this information to the prior case example. Recall that the primary motor control impairment for this patient was weakness with a movement system diagnosis of *force production deficit*. If the patient's physical therapy goal is to strengthen lower extremity muscles to improve walking speed, then the best way to strengthen his or her quadriceps muscles is to engage those muscles while he or she is walking. Activities such as seated long arc quads, leg presses, or sit-to/from-stand transfers may improve some aspects of impairments but not walking mobility. In addition, if the goal is to improve walking speed versus endurance, then treatment should specifically work to increase walking speed.

Taken all together, the aforementioned literature suggests that interventions should be most often at the activity level and even occasionally at the participation level. This is true whether the selected treatment approach is remediation or compensation. Establishing the movement system diagnosis allows for a focused intervention to be selected. For example, the primary intervention to improve walking is gait training and not exercises to address weight-bearing, weight-shifting, and lower limb strength.[41] If the approach is compensation, such as in a person with the movement system diagnosis of fractionated movement deficit, then the specific treatment will focus on walking safely with whatever gait pattern and assistive devices are deemed appropriate. If the approach is remediation, such as in a person with the movement system diagnosis of force production deficit, then the specific treatment will work on resuming a more normal gait pattern. The role of the skilled physical therapist is to design the therapeutic activities to address the specific goals and to challenge the activity limitations and impairments of each patient.

CURRENT EVIDENCE UNDERLYING IMPAIRED MOTOR CONTROL INTERVENTIONS

It is important to keep in mind that evidence is continually emerging and being refined. The major body of knowledge regarding treatment of motor control impairments comes from people with stroke. Because people with stroke have many of the same motor control impairments as people with other medical conditions, readers may consider the application of these results to others who may have similar motor control impairments but different medical conditions.

Sorting through all the available evidence supporting or not supporting a particular upper or lower limb/mobility intervention is burdensome for a practicing clinician. Clinical practice guidelines[41] and systematic reviews[63] are very helpful but can become outdated quickly. It is our great fortune that an outstanding and current synopsis to guide evidence-based treatment is provided free of charge by the Canadian Partnership for Stroke Recovery. It is called Evidence-Based Review of Stroke Rehabilitation (EBRSR) and is available at http://www.ebrsr.com. The aim of the EBRSR is to provide an up-to-date review of stroke rehabilitation evidence in a clinician-friendly manner, where specific conclusions can be used to guide stroke rehabilitation care.[10] Each of the 22 sections can be downloaded separately in PDF format. The first section provides an introduction to EBRSR and its strong methodology. Each subsequent section deals with a specific area of stroke rehabilitation, including one section on mobility and lower limb interventions and another on upper limb interventions. Other sections focus on aphasia, perception, cognition, depression, and so forth. An important feature of the EBRSR is that it summarizes all the relevant studies, providing clinically relevant conclusions and the level of evidence from which the conclusions are derived. A new edition of the EBRSR is available each year, so that recently published studies are quickly incorporated into the summaries and conclusions. An additional resource for clinical practice guidelines for a variety of neurologic conditions is available from the Academy of Neurologic Physical Therapy website at http://www.neuropt.org/professional-resources/anpt-clinical-practice-guidelines.

As with most rehabilitation evidence, conclusions regarding upper limb and lower limb/gait interventions are hampered by small sample sizes, mixed outcome measures, and differing "control" treatments.[73] Nonetheless, there have been great gains in the available evidence for treating motor control impairments and function.

Considerations for Upper Limb Interventions

Given the limited therapy services and the general emphasis on task-specific training, clinicians are faced with the dilemma of determining what tasks to practice and in which contexts. There are a large number of tasks that are performed by the upper limbs. For example, people generally have a daily grooming routine, which may include five to six tasks, such as brushing teeth, washing the face, brushing hair, shaving, and applying make-up. If one multiplies the number of daily routines by the number of tasks within each routine, the result is an enormous number of tasks within specific contexts that need to be performed by any given individual on a daily basis. It is impossible to practice all tasks in their specific contexts.

There are four essential components of most upper limb movement tasks: reach, grasp, move or manipulate, and release. Almost all functional tasks of the upper limb involve some combination of these four components. What varies across the repertoire of upper limb functional tasks is how the combinations of the components are strung together and the specifics of the component (e.g., direction of reach, type of grasp, manipulative forces required). For example, when eating, a person reaches for the fork, grasps it, manipulates the fork to pick up the food, moves the food and fork to the mouth, returns the fork to the table, and releases the fork. When opening a door, a person reaches forward, grasps the door knob, turns it, pushes the door, and releases the knob. Because most studies of generalization occur in healthy young adults training on highly constrained laboratory tasks, it is unknown how practice and improvement of one functional task (one string of components) might translate or generalize to improvement on other functional tasks in patient populations. The current therapeutic approach is to train a patient on several representative tasks of high interest with the intent that the functional capacity and problem-solving abilities gained on the trained tasks can generalize to other daily tasks. For example, if a patient learns to better manipulate a fork for eating, this may carry over to better handling skills with multiple utensils.

The role of the treating therapist is to select specific upper limb tasks to practice that are functionally important to the patient receiving treatment and that challenge but do not overwhelm the patient's motor abilities. The easiest way to determine which tasks are important to the patient is to ask him or her directly. A more formal way to determine specific tasks for the upper limb is with the Canadian Occupational Performance Measure[45] (COPM, mentioned earlier) or other similar tools. The COPM starts with a semistructured interview and asks the person to identify functional activities that are difficult. Once the patient has identified the tasks he or she is most interested in improving, the therapist and patient can problem-solve together to make sure that the task and goal of being able to do the task are realistic given the patient's motor capacity. For example, consider a 70-year-old woman with a 1-year history of right hemiparesis poststroke. Her motor capabilities include the ability to partially flex the right shoulder against gravity, an upper limb Motricity Index score of 48/100, and an Action Research Arm Test (ARAT) score of 14/57. The score of 14/57 indicates a very basic ability to reach, grasp, and release the easiest objects, without the ability to shape the hand, open the fingers wide, or manipulate objects. Collectively, this information indicates she has and is likely to continue to have limited use of her affected upper limb. If she identifies that she wants to be able to regain normal, dexterous use with her (previously dominant) right hand, then it is critical to have a conversation that helps her identify goals that are more realistic given her prognosis and current motor capabilities. A more realistic set of functional goals for her would focus around learning to use the affected right side as an assist during bilateral tasks, such as securing the jar with the right arm while the left hand opens the jar.

Once a task of interest is identified, the therapist needs to creatively arrange the task to repeatedly challenge, but not overwhelm, the patient's current motor abilities. If the task is too easy, then practice will become rote. If the task is too hard, the patient may quickly become frustrated. A movement task that takes 1 to 2 seconds is probably too easy, whereas a task that takes 30 seconds or more may be too hard. Based on our clinical observations, a useful rule may be to grade the task so that it takes between 6 and 15 seconds to complete a repetition. In our experience, this allows the patient to easily judge success or failure and keeps the patient from getting too frustrated. An example of a task that is of interest to many patients and is easily graded is lifting cans to and from a shelf. This task incorporates the essential components of reach, grasp, move/manipulate, and release. In everyday life, it is similar to many movements needed to function in kitchens, bathrooms, and workshops. The difficulty of the task can be graded up or down by changing can size, can weight, starting location, ending location, and whether or not the patient is sitting or standing while performing the task. With multiple repetitions of a task like this, one can understand how impairments such as decreased motion (change location), strength (change can weight), or endurance (increase the repetitions, have patient stand) can be addressed in a task-specific manner. As the patient improves, the task can be graded up to continually challenge and improve his or her motor capabilities.

In a busy clinic, it is not possible to have the setup and equipment to practice every possible upper limb task. One way to get around this is to have space and materials set aside to practice the most common tasks. For example, a basket or box could be filled with a variety of containers/bottles and their respective lids. Many individuals need to be able to open bottles and containers to prepare food, take medicine, or do self-care activities. The basket can be filled with containers used in daily life, such as medicine bottles, margarine containers, or laundry detergent bottles, that are different sizes and shapes and present various difficulties. The variety of containers will allow variability in how the patient practices, and thereby potentially improve the generalizability of the motor skill to other containers that may be encountered outside of therapy. This is only one example of a useful way to store and use materials for upper limb task-specific practice. Baskets with other themes (e.g., crafts, office work) can be created in therapy clinics to address other common upper limb tasks, based on the needs and interests of the older adults served by that clinic.

Most adults, regardless of age, are motivated to improve their function and are often interested in practicing outside of therapy sessions. This should be strongly encouraged. Similar to within therapy sessions, home programs for the upper limb are most appropriately focused on functional task practice and not on traditional therapeutic exercise. Careful thought in choosing the specific tasks to be practiced at home will permit both impairments and function to be addressed with one or a few activities. If the goal of an older adult is to use the workshop again, then standing or sitting at the workbench while practicing grasping and releasing specific tools may be engaging and motivating for him or her. Many of the materials and tasks created in the clinic can be easily and cheaply recreated in patients' homes (look in recycling bin, workshop, or game closet). As patients practice functional upper limb tasks in their own environments, they often come up with creative and unique solutions to successfully execute activities that are important to them.

The EBRSR[10] section on upper limb interventions reminds us that there are interventions, which are observed routinely in clinics,[74] that have moderate to strong evidence of *minimal or no* benefit. Three interventions that have moderate to strong evidence of no benefit are hand splinting for the reduction of contractures and/or impairments, general stretching and splinting for the reduction of spasticity, and intermittent pneumatic pressure for the reduction of hand edema. Two interventions for the upper limb that have strong evidence showing that they are not superior to conventional physical therapy are neurodevelopmental techniques and electromyographic biofeedback techniques. Other interventions have strong evidence supporting their benefit, but often only for particular circumstances. There is strong evidence that constraint-induced movement therapy is beneficial in people with subacute and chronic stroke who have some active movement of the wrist and hand. There is conflicting evidence, however, that it is beneficial in people with acute stroke. In contrast, there is strong evidence that functional electrical stimulation may be most beneficial for lower-level patients earlier after stroke. Additionally, there is strong evidence that injections of botulinum toxin (Botox) are temporarily beneficial in reducing spasticity but are not beneficial in improving upper limb function. A growing number of emerging interventions are labeled as having uncertain evidence. These include more intensive therapy (additional minutes), sensorimotor training, mental practice, robotic training, virtual reality, transcranial direct current stimulation, and transcranial magnetic stimulation. Uncertainty with evidence stems from either conflicting evidence across studies or insufficient investigations to date.

Considerations for Lower Limb and Gait Task-Specific Interventions

The Mobility and the Lower Extremity section of the EBRSR provides a summary of the evidence of many commonly used physical therapy interventions. A key finding in their analysis is that task-specific gait training improves gait in adults with stroke. Likewise, certain types of balance training improve balance and functional outcomes in adults with stroke. Of importance to most patients with motor control impairments, cardiovascular training can improve physical fitness and function. Critical ingredients for effective cardiovascular treatment are to monitor vital signs and to ensure that cardiovascular training is of the appropriate intensity to stimulate improved fitness. Improved cardiovascular fitness for a person with motor control impairments may provide the person with the endurance needed to make it through their day and to permit participation in meaningful sport or leisure activities. This is a way to lessen activity limitations and participation restrictions by addressing the secondary consequences of motor control impairments. Other interventions for mobility and the lower limb with strong evidence of benefit include ankle–foot orthoses and functional electrical stimulation for those adults with moderate to severe paresis. Interventions with strong evidence of not being superior to overground gait training include neurodevelopmental techniques, teaching/encouraging self-propulsion in a wheelchair, and robotic gait training.

SUMMARY

Major motor control impairments in adults are: paresis, abnormal tone, fractionated movement deficits, ataxia, and hypokinesia. Two additional impairments, somatosensory loss and perceptual deficits, also have important consequences for motor control. Similar motor control impairments can be seen across numerous medical conditions. Most individuals with motor control impairments present with multiple motor control impairments rather than just one. A critical aspect of evaluating adults with motor control impairments is determining which of the motor control impairments are the chief contributors to the loss of activity and which ones make only minor contributions. This step is critical in formulating a movement system diagnosis.

The prognosis of the underlying medical condition is also critical in determining the rehabilitation prognosis in adults with motor control impairments. A crucial role of the physical therapist is to determine how to improve activity and participation in persons whose motor control impairments will stay the same or may worsen. And, a key decision in the treatment of adults with motor control impairments is whether to choose a remedial or a compensatory approach. The approach chosen will guide the plan of care. Task-specific training is the treatment of choice for adults with motor control impairments. Support for interventions targeting specific activities rather than specific impairments comes from the mechanisms underlying motor learning and neuroplasticity, and from clinical rehabilitation research.

An excellent up-to-date synopsis of the current evidence for and against various treatments is Evidence-Based Review of Stroke Rehabilitation (EBRSR) and is freely available from the Canadian Stroke Network at www.ebrsr.com.

ACKNOWLEDGMENTS

Drs. Lang and Bland are supported by National Institutes of Health funds (R01HD068290) to do research that contributed to this chapter. Thanks to Dr. Rita Wong for assistance with editing.

REFERENCES

1. Shumway-Cook A, Woolacott MH. *Motor Control: Translating Research into Clinical Practice*. Philadelphia: Wolters Kluwer; 2017.
2. Sathian K, Buxbaum LJ, Cohen LG, et al. Neurological principles and rehabilitation of action disorders: Common clinical deficits. *Neurorehabil Neural Repair*. 2011;25:21S–32S.
3. Lang CE, Schieber MH. Stroke. In: Nowak DA, Hermsdorfer J, eds. *Sensorimotor Control of Grasping: Physiology and Pathophysiology*. Cambridge: Cambridge University Press; 2009:296–310.
4. Lang CE, Wagner JM, Bastian AJ, et al. Deficits in grasp versus reach during acute hemiparesis. *Exp Brain Res*. 2005;166:126–136.
5. Lang CE, Wagner JM, Edwards DF, Sahrmann SA, Dromerick AW. Recovery of grasp versus reach in people with hemiparesis poststroke. *Neurorehabil Neural Repair*. 2006;20:444–454.
6. Fredericks CM, Saladin LK. Clinical presentations in disorders of motor function. In: Fredericks CM, Saladin LK, eds. *Pathophysiology of the Motor Systems: Principles and Clinical Presentations*. Philadelphia: FA Davis Co.; 1996.
7. Obeso JA, Stamelou M, Goetz CG, et al. Past, present, and future of Parkinson's disease: a special essay on the 200th anniversary of the shaking palsy. *Mov Disord*. 2017;32:1264–1310.
8. Schmit BD, Dewald JP, Rymer WZ. Stretch reflex adaptation in elbow flexors during repeated passive movements in unilateral brain-injured patients. *Arch Phys Med Rehabil*. 2000;81:269–278.
9. Lang CE, Beebe JA. Relating movement control at 9 upper extremity segments to loss of hand function in people with chronic hemiparesis. *Neurorehabil Neural Repair*. 2007;21:279–291.
10. Iruthayarajah J, Mirkowski M, Foley N, et al. Upper extremity motor rehabilitation interventions. Chapter 10 of *Evidence-Based Review of Stroke Rehabilitation*, 19th ed. Toronto, Ont, Canada: Heart and Stroke Foundation of Canada and the Partnership for Stroke Recovery; 2019. http://www.ebrsr.com/evidence-review.
11. Schieber MH. Constraints on somatotopic organization in the primary motor cortex. *J Neurophysiol*. 2001;86:2125–2143.
12. Brunnstrom S. *Movement Therapy in Hemiplegia: A Neurophysiological Approach*. New York: Harper and Row; 1970.
13. Lemon RN, Griffiths J. Comparing the function of the corticospinal system in different species: organizational differences for motor specialization? *Muscle Nerve*. 2005;32:261–279.
14. Miller LC, Dewald JP. Involuntary paretic wrist/finger flexion forces and EMG increase with shoulder abduction load in individuals with chronic stroke. *Clin Neurophysiol*. 2012;123:1216–1225.
15. Dewald JP, Beer RF. Abnormal joint torque patterns in the paretic upper limb of subjects with hemiparesis. *Muscle Nerve*. 2001;24:273–283.
16. Jinnah HA, Teller JK, Galpern WR. Recent developments in dystonia. *Curr Opin Neurol*. 2015;28:400–405.
17. Mink JW. The basal ganglia: focused selection and inhibition of competing motor programs. *Prog Neurobiol*. 1996;50:381–425.
18. Bastian AJ. Mechanisms of ataxia. *Phys Ther*. 1997;77:672–675.
19. Bastian AJ, Zackowski KM, Thach WT. Cerebellar ataxia: torque deficiency or torque mismatch between joints? *J Neurophysiol*. 2000;83:3019–3030.
20. Sainburg RL, Ghilardi MF, Poizner H, Ghez C. Control of limb dynamics in normal subjects and patients without proprioception. *J Neurophysiol*. 1995;73:820–835.
21. Therrien AS, Bastian AJ. Cerebellar damage impairs internal predictions for sensory and motor function. *Curr Opin Neurobiol*. 2015;33:127–133.
22. Bastian AJ, Martin TA, Keating JG, Thach WT. Cerebellar ataxia: abnormal control of interaction torques across multiple joints. *J Neurophysiol*. 1996;76:492–509.
23. Morton SM, Dordevic GS, Bastian AJ. Cerebellar damage produces context-dependent deficits in control of leg dynamics during obstacle avoidance. *Exp Brain Res*. 2004;156(2):149–163.
24. Morton SM, Bastian AJ. Relative contributions of balance and voluntary leg-coordination deficits to cerebellar gait ataxia. *J Neurophysiol*. 2003;89:1844–1856.

25. Johansson RS, Westling G. Roles of glabrous skin receptors and sensorimotor memory in automatic control of precision grip when lifting rougher or more slippery objects. *Exp Brain Res.* 1984;56:550–564.
26. Blakemore SJ, Goodbody SJ, Wolpert DM. Predicting the consequences of our own actions: the role of sensorimotor context estimation. *J Neurosci.* 1998;18:7511–7518.
27. Johansson RS. Dynamic use of tactile afferent signals in control of dexterous manipulation. *Adv Exp Med Biol.* 2002; 508:397–410.
28. Jeannerod M, Michel F, Prablanc C. The control of hand movements in a case of hemianaesthesia following a parietal lesion. *Brain.* 1984;107(Pt 3):899–920.
29. Winges SA, Weber DJ, Santello M. The role of vision on hand preshaping during reach to grasp. *Exp Brain Res.* 2003;152:489–498.
30. Corbetta M. Hemispatial neglect: clinic, pathogenesis, and treatment. *Semin Neurol.* 2014;34:514–523.
31. Karnath HO. Pusher syndrome–a frequent but little-known disturbance of body orientation perception. *J Neurol.* 2007;254:415–424.
32. Karnath HO, Broetz D. Understanding and treating "pusher syndrome.". *Phys Ther.* 2003;83:1119–1125.
33. Babyar SR, Peterson MG, Reding M. Time to recovery from lateropulsion dependent on key stroke deficits: a retrospective analysis. *Neurorehabil Neural Repair.* 2015;29:207–213.
34. Malhotra P, Coulthard E, Husain M. Hemispatial neglect, balance and eye-movement control. *Curr Opin Neurol.* 2006;19:14–20.
35. Scheets PL, Sahrmann SA, Norton BJ. Use of movement system diagnoses in the management of patients with neuromuscular conditions: a multiple-patient case report. *Phys Ther.* 2007;87:654–669.
36. Lang CE, Bland MD, Connor LT, et al. The brain recovery core: building a system of organized stroke rehabilitation and outcomes assessment across the continuum of care. *J Neurol Phys Ther.* 2011;35:194–201.
37. Beebe JA, Lang CE. Absence of a proximal to distal gradient of motor deficits in the upper extremity early after stroke. *Clin Neurophysiol.* 2008;119:2074–2085.
38. Beebe JA, Lang CE. Active range of motion predicts upper extremity function 3 months after stroke. *Stroke.* 2009;40:1772–1779.
39. Bohannon RW. Muscle strength and muscle training after stroke. *J Rehabil Med.* 2007;39:14–20.
40. Collin C, Wade D. Assessing motor impairment after stroke: a pilot reliability study. *J Neurol Neurosurg Psychiatry.* 1990;53:576–579.
41. Winstein CJ, Stein J, Arena R, et al. Guidelines for adult stroke rehabilitation and recovery: a guideline for healthcare professionals from the American Heart Association/American Stroke Association. *Stroke.* 2016;47(6):e98–e169.
42. Fugl-Meyer AR, Jaasko L, Leyman I, Olsson S, Steglind S. The post-stroke hemiplegic patient. 1. A method for evaluation of physical performance. *Scand J Rehabil Med.* 1975;7:13–31.
43. Yozbatiran N, Der-Yeghiaian L, Cramer SC. A standardized approach to performing the action research arm test. *Neurorehabil Neural Repair.* 2008;22:78–90.
44. Lang CE, Bland MD, Bailey RR, Schaefer SY, Birkenmeier RL. Assessment of upper extremity impairment, function, and activity after stroke: foundations for clinical decision making. *J Hand Ther.* 2013;26:104–115.
45. Law M, Baptiste S, McColl M, Opzoomer A, Polatajko H, Pollock N. The Canadian Occupational Performance Measure: an outcome measure for occupational therapy. *Can J Occup Ther.* 1990;57:82–87.
46. Rand D, Eng JJ. Disparity between functional recovery and daily use of the upper and lower extremities during subacute stroke rehabilitation. *Neurorehabil Neural Repair.* 2012;26:76–84.
47. Waddell KJ, Strube MJ, Bailey RR, et al. Does task-specific training improve upper limb performance in daily life poststroke? *Neurorehabil Neural Repair.* 2017;31:290–300.
48. Duncan PW, Lai SM, Keighley J. Defining post-stroke recovery: implications for design and interpretation of drug trials. *Neuropharmacology.* 2000;39:835–841.
49. Jorgensen HS, Nakayama H, Raaschou HO, Vive-Larsen J, Stoier M, Olsen TS. Outcome and time course of recovery in stroke. Part ii: time course of recovery. The Copenhagen Stroke Study. *Arch Phys Med Rehabil.* 1995;76:406–412.
50. Kalra L. Does age affect benefits of stroke unit rehabilitation? *Stroke.* 1994;25:346–351.
51. Kwakkel G, Kollen B, Lindeman E. Understanding the pattern of functional recovery after stroke: facts and theories. *Restor Neurol Neurosci.* 2004;22:281–299.
52. Hendricks HT, van Limbeek J, Geurts AC, Zwarts MJ. Motor recovery after stroke: a systematic review of the literature. *Arch Phys Med Rehabil.* 2002;83:1629–1637.
53. Shelton FN, Reding MJ. Effect of lesion location on upper limb motor recovery after stroke. *Stroke.* 2001;32:107–112.
54. Veerbeek JM, Van Wegen EE, Harmeling-Van der Wel BC, Kwakkel G. Is accurate prediction of gait in nonambulatory stroke patients possible within 72 hours poststroke? The EPOS Study. *Neurorehabil Neural Repair.* 2011;25:268–274.
55. Patel AT, Duncan PW, Lai SM, Studenski S. The relation between impairments and functional outcomes poststroke. *Arch Phys Med Rehabil.* 2000;81:1357–1363.
56. Jorgensen HS, Nakayama H, Raaschou HO, Vive-Larsen J, Stoier M, Olsen TS. Outcome and time course of recovery in stroke. Part I: outcome. The Copenhagen Stroke Study. *Arch Phys Med Rehabil.* 1995;76:399–405.
57. Olsen TS. Arm and leg paresis as outcome predictors in stroke rehabilitation. *Stroke.* 1990;21:247–251.
58. Stinear CM, Barber PA, Petoe M, Anwar S, Byblow WD. The PREP algorithm predicts potential for upper limb recovery after stroke. *Brain.* 2012;135:2527–2535.
59. Stinear CM, Byblow WD, Ackerley SJ, Smith MC, Borges VM, Barber PA. PREP2: a biomarker-based algorithm for predicting upper limb function after stroke. *Ann Clin Transl Neurol.* 2017;4:811–820.
60. Smith MC, Barber PA, Stinear CM. The TWIST algorithm predicts time to walking independently after stroke. *Neurorehabil Neural Repair.* 2017;31:955–964.
61. Norton BJ. Diagnosis dialog: progress report. *Phys Ther.* 2007;87:1270–1273.
62. Scheets PK, Sahrmann SA, Norton BJ. Diagnosis for physical therapy for patients with neuromuscular conditions. *Neurology Report.* 1999;23:158–169.
63. Veerbeek JM, van Wegen E, van Peppen R, et al. What is the evidence for physical therapy poststroke? A systematic review and meta-analysis. *PLoS One.* 2014;9:e87987.
64. Kaas JH. Plasticity of sensory and motor maps in adult mammals. *Annu Rev Neurosci.* 1991;14:137–167.
65. Nudo RJ, Milliken GW, Jenkins WM, Merzenich MM. Use-dependent alterations of movement representations in primary motor cortex of adult squirrel monkeys. *J Neurosci.* 1996;16:785–807.
66. Nudo RJ, Plautz EJ, Frost SB. Role of adaptive plasticity in recovery of function after damage to motor cortex. *Muscle Nerve.* 2001;24:1000–1019.
67. Jones TA. Motor compensation and its effects on neural reorganization after stroke. *Nat Rev Neurosci.* 2017; 18:267–280.
68. Kleim JA, Jones TA. Principles of experience-dependent neural plasticity: implications for rehabilitation after brain damage. *J Speech Lang Hear Res.* 2008;51:S225–S239.

69. Bliss TV, Gardner-Medwin AR. Long-lasting potentiation of synaptic transmission in the dentate area of the unanaesthetized rabbit following stimulation of the perforant path. *J Physiol.* 1973;232:357–374.
70. Shimada H, Uchiyama Y, Kakurai S. Specific effects of balance and gait exercises on physical functioning among the frail elderly. *Clin Rehabil.* 2003;17:472–479.
71. Hornby TG, Holleran CL, Hennessy PW, et al. Variable intensive early walking poststroke (views): a randomized controlled trial. *Neurorehabil Neural Repair.* 2016;30: 440–450.
72. Barreca S, Sigouin CS, Lambert C, Ansley B. Effects of extra training on the ability of stroke survivors to perform an independent sit-to-stand: a randomized controlled trial. *J Geriatr Phys Ther.* 2004;27:59–64.
73. Lohse KR, Pathania A, Wegman R, Boyd LA, Lang CE. On the reporting of experimental and control therapies in stroke rehabilitation trials: a systematic-review. *Arch Phys Med Rehabil.* 2018;99(7):1424–1432.
74. Lang CE, Macdonald JR, Reisman DS, et al. Observation of amounts of movement practice provided during stroke rehabilitation. *Arch Phys Med Rehabil.* 2009;90:1692–1698.
75. Bohannon RW, Smith MB. Interrater reliability of a modified Ashworth scale of muscle spasticity. *Phys Ther.* 1987;67:206–207.
76. Hreib KK, Jones HR. Clinical neurologic evaluation. In: Jones HR, ed. *Netter's Neurology.* Teterboro, NJ: Icon Learning Systems; 2005:2–39.
77. Lowery N, Ragland JD, Gur RC, Gur RE, Moberg PJ. Normative data for the symbol cancellation test in young healthy adults. *Appl Neuropsychol.* 2004;11:218–221.
78. Rengachary J, d'Avossa G, Sapir A, Shulman GL, Corbetta M. Is the Posner reaction time test more accurate than clinical tests in detecting left neglect in acute and chronic stroke? *Arch Phys Med Rehabil.* 2009;90:2081–2088.
79. Koter R, Regan S, Clark C, et al. Clinical outcome measures for lateropulsion poststroke: an updated systematic review. *J Neurol Phys Ther.* 2017;41:145–155.

CHAPTER

18

Aerobic Capacity and the Management of the Patient with Cardiovascular and Pulmonary Limitations

Brady Anderson, Christian Garcia, Lawrence P. Cahalin

OUTLINE

INTRODUCTION

Impaired aerobic capacity, also known as impaired endurance, is a common impairment that can limit participation in functional, occupational, and recreational activities. Even functional tasks that require only a few minutes can be limited by aerobic capacity. Older adults are particularly vulnerable to impaired aerobic capacity owing to anatomic and physiologic changes that occur with aging, a greater propensity for sedentary behaviors, and a greater risk for disease processes that limit the oxygen transport system. In addition, aerobic capacity is directly influenced by the habitual activity pattern of an individual, which may vary across individuals from total inactivity to frequent and intense activity. Any factors that limit habitual physical activity, such as illness, injury, and or travel, will cause adaptations that diminish aerobic capacity. Conversely, any factors that promote habitual physical activity, such as intentional exercise, yard work, and occupation-related physical tasks, will result in adaptations that improve aerobic capacity. In older adults, many physiologic, pathologic, and psychosocial factors can contribute to restricted physical activity. Figure 18.1 depicts the persistent vicious cycle that can be created when sedentary behaviors, chronic disease, and functional dependency interact.

This chapter begins with a brief overview of the factors influencing aerobic capacity in the older adult and then focuses on the most frequently encountered cardiovascular and pulmonary diseases that contribute to impaired aerobic capacity in older adults. Embedded into the discussion of each medical condition is a description of the physical therapist's patient management (examination, evaluation, diagnosis, and interventions) to address decreased endurance and its impact on function. Chapter 3, Physiology of Aging, provides additional insights and details regarding age-related changes in cardiopulmonary and vascular structures and function.

PHYSIOLOGY OF AEROBIC CAPACITY IN OLDER ADULTS

Aerobic capacity reflects the body's ability to take up, deliver, and use oxygen. Many processes are required to ensure that these three steps occur optimally; dysfunction in any part of this oxygen transport system can interfere

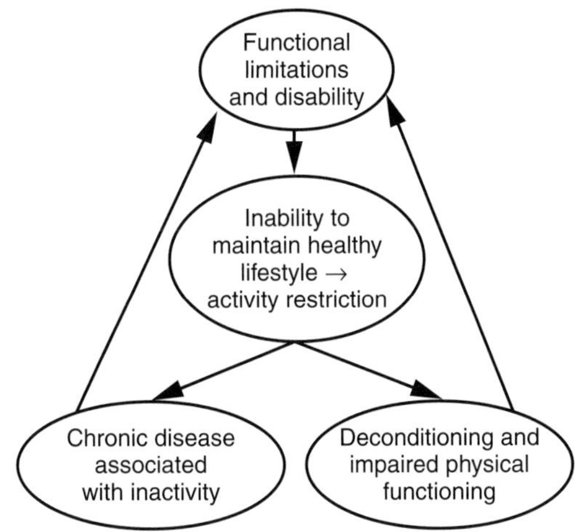

FIG. 18.1 **Cycle created by impaired aerobic capacity**

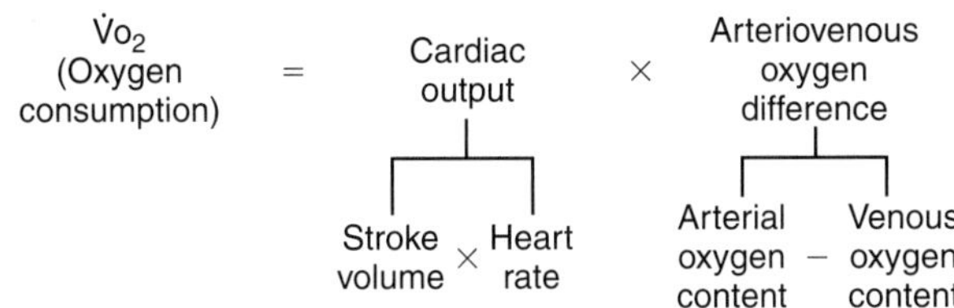

FIG. 18.2 **Parameters that contribute to aerobic capacity as described by the Fick equation.**

with aerobic capacity. Oxygen consumption ($\dot{V}O_2$) is a physiologic measure of how much oxygen the body uses at rest or during activity. Oxygen consumption increases in proportion to intensity of exercise/physical activity and will plateau when maximal ability for oxygen delivery (maximal oxygen consumption [$\dot{V}O_2$ max]) is reached. Maximal oxygen consumption is directly related to aerobic capacity. Increases in maximal oxygen consumption with exercise training reflect improvement in aerobic capacity. The Fick equation, as illustrated in Fig. 18.2, describes the relationship between oxygen consumption as being equivalent to the cardiac output (heart rate × stroke volume) × arteriovenous oxygen difference).[1,2] Dysfunction in one or more of these physiologic processes can lead to impaired aerobic capacity. Each key physiologic variable will be briefly discussed, including how these variables can be altered by aging or pathology, and the potential to adapt chronically to a period of aerobic exercise training.

Heart Rate

During acute aerobic exercise, there is a linear relationship between heart rate and oxygen consumption. At less than 100 beats per minute (bpm), heart rate increases via inhibition of vagal (parasympathetic) tone. As rate approaches 100 bpm, heart rate increases primarily by stimulation of sympathetic tone.[1,2] Maximal heart rate (HRmax) is related primarily to age and for healthy adults across the lifespan can be predicted by the following formula: HRmax = 208 – (0.7 × age).[3] This equation is updated from the widely used HRmax = 220 – age as this was found to underestimate HRmax in older adults and overestimate HRmax in younger adults. In populations with cardiovascular disease, the predictive equations alone are inappropriate when developing exercise prescriptions; a symptom-limited exercise test provides a more accurate and safe estimate of an individual's physiologic limitations.[4]

The age-related reduction in maximal heart rate is thought to be caused by either attenuation of sympathetic drive or decreases in sensitivity and responsiveness of catecholamines.[5] Reduction in maximal heart rate with activity can limit aerobic capacity. Impaired function of the autonomic nervous system, a common finding in older adults with diabetes (autonomic peripheral neuropathy)[6,7] and also following heart transplantation ("denervated heart"),[7a] will decrease heart rate response to activity. Interruption of the autonomic nervous system can also occur with lesions in the central nervous system, such as a stroke or cervical spinal cord injury. Chronotropic disorders in older adults are commonly caused by heart rhythm disturbances such as atrial fibrillation, atrioventricular blocks, and sick sinus syndrome.[2]

With aerobic exercise training, heart rate is lower at rest and during submaximal exercise.[2] Heart rate at rest decreases following aerobic training because of increased parasympathetic activity whereas sympathetic activity declines. Exercise training results in a proportionally lower heart rate at specified submaximal workloads. Therefore, after a period of exercise training, more work can be performed at a lower heart rate. Maximal heart rate tends to be very stable within individuals and is not altered by exercise training. Following a period of aerobic training, the heart rate during recovery from exercise returns to resting levels more quickly.[1]

Stroke Volume

Stroke volume is the difference between the total amount of blood in the ventricles after completely filling (end-diastolic volume) and the amount of blood left behind after ventricular contraction (end-systolic volume). Stroke volume is often described clinically in terms of ejection fraction, which is stroke volume expressed as a percentage of end-diastolic volume. Stroke volume during acute aerobic exercise increases linearly up to intensities of 40% to 60% of maximal oxygen consumption and then plateaus. During aerobic exercise, dynamic skeletal muscle contraction and sympathetic-mediated vasoconstriction facilitate greater venous return and therefore ventricular filling. In addition, myocyte fiber stretching and sympathetic stimulation increase cardiac contractility and ventricular emptying. Both greater ventricular filling and emptying result in increased stroke volume during aerobic exercise.[2]

The evidence to determine whether or not stroke volume is reduced with aging is equivocal.[5] With advanced age (> 80 years), ejection fraction at maximal exercise does appear to decline.[8] Any pathologic process that reduces ventricular filling or emptying will cause a reduction in stroke volume. With less volume of blood filling the ventricles, there is less volume available to pump out and a reduction in preload on the heart. Ventricular filling is reduced when there is a mechanical barrier present, such as cardiac valve dysfunction, heart fibrosis, or hypertrophic myopathy. All of these problems are associated with chronic heart failure, which is a major cause of disability in older adults. Ventricular filling is also impaired when venous return is reduced, commonly owing to a loss of active skeletal muscle pump (e.g., extremity paralysis), dehydration, or impaired autonomic nervous system function (e.g., prolonged bed rest). Ventricular emptying is reduced when cardiac contractility is impaired (e.g., myocardial infarction) or the pressure that the heart has to pump against, referred to as *afterload*, is elevated (e.g., hypertension). All of these cardiac problems, discussed later in this chapter, are common in older adults and therefore often contribute to impaired aerobic capacity.

With aerobic exercise training, stroke volume increases at rest as well as during submaximal and maximal exercise. Following aerobic exercise training, ventricular filling (end-diastolic volume) increases due to an increase in plasma blood volume and more compliant ventricular walls. In addition, ventricular emptying is greater (end-systolic volume) following aerobic exercise training. Ventricular emptying is facilitated by the greater cardiac contractility secondary to enhanced myocyte fiber stretching that occurs during ventricular filling and greater myocyte force production secondary to intrinsic changes and hypertrophy.[1,2]

Cardiac Output

At rest, cardiac output is approximately 5 L/min and, with exercise, can increase up to approximately 20 to 40 L/min. Increases in both stroke volume and heart rate contribute to greater cardiac output during acute aerobic exercise, because cardiac output is the product of heart rate and stroke volume. Oxygen demand is the ultimate stimulus for increasing cardiac output during exercise. Greater cardiac output is needed to increase delivery of oxygen to the working muscles in order to meet the greater oxygen demand of heightened cellular energy metabolism.[1,2]

With aging, maximal cardiac output declines secondary to decreases in heart rate and stroke volume. Any factor that diminishes heart rate or stroke volume response during activity can limit aerobic capacity. A number of pathologic processes can contribute to impairments in cardiac output and therefore aerobic capacity. In addition, deconditioning, dehydration, and bed rest can profoundly diminish cardiac output and aerobic capacity.[2]

Cardiac output does not change significantly at rest or with submaximal exercise. However, at maximal workloads, cardiac output increases significantly following a period of exercise training. This is the result of increases in stroke volume, because heart rate at maximal workloads remains relatively constant. After exercise training, metabolic work capacity (maximal oxygen consumption) is much greater, primarily because of a greater cardiac output.[1,2,8]

Arterial Oxygen Content

Arterial oxygen content is determined by the oxygen-carrying capacity of the blood (hemoglobin concentration and red blood cell count) and oxygen loading in the lungs. Gas exchange at the alveolar–capillary interface is influenced by the time it takes a red blood cell to pass from one end of a capillary to the other end (transit time) and the time it takes for complete saturation of hemoglobin with oxygen in the pulmonary capillary (equilibrium time). Pulmonary capillary transit time at rest and during exercise normally exceeds equilibrium time, which allows for complete hemoglobin saturation. During aerobic exercise, transit time shortens because blood flow rate increases. The pulmonary arterioles normally vasodilate during exercise in order to accommodate the increased cardiac output and maintain adequate time for oxygen loading.

Oxygen loading in the lungs is fairly well preserved during early aging, but decreased oxygen saturation can be seen in the oldest-old (> 85 years).[9] This can be due to slowed oxygen diffusion or less time for oxygen loading across the alveolar–capillary interface. This often occurs with diseases that cause thickening of the alveolar–capillary membrane (e.g., chronic obstructive pulmonary disease) and low partial pressure of alveolar oxygen (e.g., restrictive pulmonary disease). Elevated blood flow rate can occur when there is either inadequate vasodilation or an increase in cardiac output or both. Fast pulmonary arterial flow rates can be caused by destruction of pulmonary capillaries (e.g., emphysema), a functional reduction in arterial conduits (e.g., pulmonary emboli), or increased cardiac output (e.g., renal failure).[1] Aerobic exercise training does not normally change oxygen loading in the lungs, which is typically at full capacity.

Venous Oxygen Content

Venous oxygen content is determined by oxygen delivery, uptake, and use in the peripheral tissues. Oxygen is required for continued regeneration of adenosine triphosphate through oxidative metabolism. During aerobic exercise, the lower venous oxygen content is primarily owing to greater oxygen demand of the working skeletal muscle and diversion of blood to those capillaries, and shunted away from nonmetabolically active tissues resulting in greater oxygen extraction from those capillary beds.[1]

Peripheral oxygen utilization with aging is often impaired by a variety of mechanisms. Pathology that interferes with blood flow, either on a macrovascular level (e.g., peripheral arterial disease) or a microvascular level (e.g., diabetes), can reduce oxygen utilization by peripheral tissues. Also, cellular changes, such as decreased myoglobin and mitochondrial density, can impair use of oxygen for energy production in skeletal muscle. Impaired aerobic capacity because of the loss of skeletal muscle oxidative capacity occurs commonly, associated with deconditioning, peripheral nerve lesions, and central nervous system pathology (e.g., spinal cord injury).

Following a period of aerobic exercise training, venous oxygen levels remain similar to levels measured at rest. At maximal exercise intensities, venous oxygen content may decrease slightly. Lower venous oxygen content with training is owing to greater oxygen extraction at the tissue level and more effective distribution of cardiac output because of increased skeletal muscle capillary density. Skeletal muscle extraction and utilization of oxygen are facilitated by many adaptations, such as increased skeletal muscle capillary density, mitochondrial proliferation, and increased skeletal muscle myoglobin concentrations.

Hypertension

Hypertension (HTN) is a major risk factor for stroke, heart disease, myocardial infarction, and renal disease, among others. Hypertension affects an estimated 64.9% of older adults and is controlled in only 52.5% of these individuals.[10] As depicted in Table 18.1, a recent update by the American College of Cardiology (ACC) and the American Heart Association (AHA) provides guidelines for the prevention, detection, evaluation, and management of high blood pressure (BP) and, notably, lowers the threshold to detect high blood pressure to account for complications that can occur at lower values and to provide an impetus for earlier intervention.[11] Although about 95% of HTN is described as essential, or primary, that is, without definite etiologic cause, several physiologic age-related changes predispose the older adult for its development. Declining performance in peripheral autoregulation (e.g., baroreceptor functioning), humoral and neural systems, as well as changes in the composition of the vasculature and its utilization of vasoactive compounds are all understood to contribute. Secondary HTN (in the remaining 5%) is said to occur in the presence of known causes such renal or endocrine dysfunction.

TABLE 18.1 2017 Updated Guidelines for the Classification of Hypertension

ACC/AHA 2017 Hypertension Guidelines				
Category	Systolic BP (mmHg)		Diastolic (mmHg)	Comparison with JNC 7*
Normal	<120	AND	<80	Same
Elevated BP	120–129	AND	<80	Was classified as Pre-HTN
Stage 1	130–139	OR	80-89	SBP of 140–159 OR DBP of 90–99 mmHg was classified as Stage 1
Stage 2	≥140	OR	≥90	
Hypertensive Crisis	>180	OR	>120	

ACC, American College of Cardiology; *AHA*, American Heart Association; *BP*, blood pressure; *DBP*, diastolic blood pressure; *HTN*, hypertension; *JNC*, Joint National Committee; *SBP*, systolic blood pressure.
*The Seventh Report of the Joint National Committee on Prevention, Detection, Evaluation, and Treatment of High Blood Pressure, 2003.[89]

Known as the "silent killer," mild-to-moderate HTN often goes undetected. Indeed, many adults are not aware that they have the condition, which highlights the importance of screening for its presence in both static and dynamic conditions, across several sessions (owing to diurnal effects), and particularly in the presence of comorbid conditions such as diabetes, left ventricular hypertrophy, and renal insufficiency.

Adequately intense exercise therapy can reduce both systolic and diastolic BP by 5 to 10 mmHg, independent of age. The effects of exercise therapy on vascular structure and function and the autonomic nervous system are both acute and chronic. The acute postexercise hypotension effect observed after a bout of aerobic exercise, in particular, informs current guidelines in their recommendation for near-daily aerobic exercise that may be structured in a continuous or fractionated, moderate- or high-intensity, format.[12–14] Indeed, even exercise durations as short as 15 minutes at low intensities have been found to be effective.[15] The BP-lowering effects of exercise are contingent on adherence to an exercise program. Individuals taking several antihypertensive medications may find it motivating that these medications, along with their side effects, may be contingently lowered given an adequate reduction in BP with exercise. Table 18.2 summarizes current exercise recommendations for individuals with HTN.[16]

In general, individuals with HTN can often demonstrate a relatively faster rate and greater magnitude of rise in systolic BP for a given workload, even if it is controlled at rest (particularly in the setting of renal dysfunction). Formal exercise testing is not necessarily required in controlled HTN; however, it is prudent to consider lighter workload intensities at first in order to assess heart rate and blood pressure responses.

Education regarding dietary modifications, such as limiting sodium, alcohol, saturated fat, and cholesterol intakc, should be emphasized. Because of a propensity for diuretic medication to cause electrolyte imbalance, mindfulness about potassium, calcium, and magnesium levels and side effects (e.g., fatigue, cramping) should be made apparent and supplemented accordingly. Some medications have been found to facilitate physical activity better than others. For example, individuals taking angiotensin-converting enzyme (ACE) inhibitors and angiotensin II receptor blockers to control HTN demonstrated greater exercise tolerance than a comparable group of older adults not on medication.[17] A team-based approach, including the prescribing physician, about current medication regimen may be warranted in such cases.

TABLE 18.2 Exercise Recommendations for Individuals with Hypertension.[16]

Frequency	5–7 days/week	2/3 days/week	>2–3 days/week
Intensity	Moderate intensity (i.e., 40% to 59% VO_2R or HRR, RPE 12–13 on a 6–20 scale)	60% to 70% of 1RM; may progress to 80%. For OA, and novice exercisers, begin with 40% to 50% 1RM	Stretch to the point of feeling tightness or slight discomfort
Time	30 min/day of continuous or accumulated exercise performed; begin with a minimum of 10 min bouts	2–4 sets of 8–12 repetitions for each of the major muscle groups	Hold static stretch for 10–30 s; 2–3 reps of each exercise
Type	Prolonged, rhythmic activities using large muscle groups (e.g., walking, cycling, swimming)	Resistance machines, free weights, and/or body weights	Static, dynamic and/or PNF stretching

1RM, one repetition maximum, *HRR*, Heart Rate Reserve; *OA*, osteoarthritis; *PNF*, proprioceptive neuromuscular facilitation; *RPE*, rate of perceived exertion; *VO_2R*, VO_2 reserve.

TABLE 18.3 Impact of Lifestyle Modification on Reduction of Systolic Blood Pressure (SBP)

Modification	Recommendation	Approximate Reduction in SBP (mmHg)
Physical activity	Engage in regular aerobic physical activity > 30 min/day, most days	4–9
DASH eating plan	Consume diet rich in fruits, vegetables, and low-fat dairy products	8–14
Dietary sodium restriction	Reduce dietary sodium intake to max of 100 mmol/day (2.4 g sodium or 6 g sodium chloride)	2–8
Moderate alcohol consumption	Limit daily consumption to max 1 drink for women or 2 drinks for men	2–4
Weight loss	Maintain normal body weight BMI 12.5–24.9 kg/m^2	5–20 per 10 kg weight loss
Stress reduction	Practice a stress-reduction modality, such as meditation	5
Tobacco cessation	Incorporate cessation modality of choice	2–3 (after 1 week cessation)

BMI, Body mass index. From DASH: Dietary Approaches to Stop Hypertension

Other aspects within the comprehensive management of HTN include stress-management, weight loss, relaxation, smoking cessation, and increasing overall physical activity levels. Table 18.3 summarizes expected outcomes for various nonpharmacologic lifestyle interventions in the treatment of HTN.[18]

COMMON MEDICAL CONDITIONS IMPACTING AEROBIC CAPACITY

Coronary Artery Disease and Myocardial Infarction

Coronary artery disease (CAD) is a progressive disease process whereby a combination of lipid accumulation (atherosis) within and hardening (sclerosis) of the coronary arteries creates conditions of myocardial ischemia. Several major, long-term prospective cohort studies have clearly established many risk factors for CAD (Table 18.4) and its underlying pathogenesis.[19–21] As these studies continue to follow cohorts over time, new findings will continue to emerge. Known, nonmutually exclusive processes include the formation of lesions via an absorption of triglyceride-rich lipoproteins and/or modified low-density lipoprotein (LDL) particles and chronic endothelial injury that together (or separately) predispose the arteries to plaque formation. After significant growth, these plaques, depending on their composition, may rupture and stimulate thrombosis which can lead to embolization, rapid occlusion of the arterial lumen, and/or integration of the thrombus into the plaque, continuing its growth. This progression is known to be phasic and unpredictable with higher-grade lesions tending to advance.[22]

Individuals with underlying CAD often seek initial medical attention owing to angina pectoris, which is the sensation of cardiac ischemia produced by an imbalance between myocardial oxygen supply and demand. As outlined in Table 18.5, angina may be chronic and stable, occurring at predictable workloads (i.e., a certain levels of myocardial oxygen demand) and relieved by resting, reducing the intensity of the activity, and/or taking sublingual nitroglycerin. However, angina may also be described as unstable when it occurs in the absence of demand or at otherwise reduced workloads relative to what normally provokes the imbalance. Unstable angina is a variant manifestation of a condition known as acute coronary syndrome (ACS), which further includes ST-elevation and non–ST-elevation acute myocardial infarctions (AMI). AMIs occur when there is a complete

TABLE 18.4 Risk factors for Cardiovascular Disease

Positive Risk Factors	Defining Criteria
Age	Men ages 45 years or older; women ages 55 years or older
Family history	Myocardial infarction, coronary revascularization, or sudden death before age 55 years in father or other male first-degree relative, or before age 65 years in mother or other female first-degree relative
Cigarette smoking	Current cigarette smoker or those who quit within the previous 6 months or exposure to environmental tobacco smoke
Sedentary lifestyle	Not participating in at least 30 minutes of moderate intensity (40% to 60% VO_2R) physical activity on at least 3 days of the week for at least 3 months
Obesity*	Body mass index $\geq$30 kg/m^2 *or* waist girth >102 cm (40 in.) for men and >88 cm (35 in.) for women
Hypertension	Systolic blood pressure (BP) $\geq$ 140 mmHg and/or diastolic BP $\geq$ 90 mmHg, confirmed by measurements on at least two separate occasions, *or* on antihypertensive medication
Dyslipidemia	Low-density lipoprotein (LDL-C) cholesterol $\geq$ 130 mg/dL (3.37 mmol/L) *or* high-density lipoprotein (HDL-C) cholesterol <40 mg/dL (1.04 mmol/L) *or* on lipid-lowering medication. If total serum cholesterol is all that is available, use $\geq$ 200 mg/dL (5.18 mmol/L)
Prediabetes	Impaired fasting glucose (IFG) = fasting plasma glucose $\geq$ 100 mg/dL (5.50 mmol/L) but <126 mg/dL (6.93 mmol/L) *or* impaired glucose tolerance (IGT) = 2-hour values in oral glucose tolerance test (OGTT) $\geq$ 140 mg/dL (7.70 mmol/L) but <200 mg/dL (11.00 mmol/L) confirmed by measurements on at least two separate occasions
Negative Risk Factors	**Defining Criteria**
High serum HDL cholesterol†	$\geq$ 60 mg/dL (1.55 mmol/L)

*Professional opinions vary regarding the most appropriate markers and thresholds for obesity; therefore, allied health professionals should use clinical judgment when evaluating this risk factor.

†Note: It is common to sum risk factors in making clinical judgments. If HDL is high, subtract one risk factor from the sum of positive risk factors, because high HDL decreases CVD risk.

(Adapted from Thompson WR, Gordon NF, Pescatello LS, eds. ACSM's guidelines for exercise testing and prescription. Philadelphia: Wolters Kluwer/Lippincott Williams & Wilkins, 2010.)

TABLE 18.5 Types of Angina

Type	Description
Stable Angina	Described most commonly as "pressure," "heaviness," "tightness" Develops with a predictable increase in myocardial oxygen demand owing to level of exercise, stress, and/or emotion. Lasts for several minutes and is relieved by rest or nitroglycerin.
Unstable Angina	Similar in symptomatology as stable angina, but with an increase in frequency, duration, and/or intensity. May occur at lower levels of myocardial oxygen demand or at rest. May occur as first experience of angina. Does not result to myocardial damage/necrosis.
Printzmetal or Atypical or Variant Angina	Hypothesized to occur owing to acute coronary artery vasospasm and subsequent decrease in myocardial oxygen supply. Most often occurs at rest (typically in morning) and not associated with level of exertion or increase in myocardial oxygen demand. Relieved by nitroglycerin.
Anginal Equivalents	May result from altered neural processing and include dyspnea, fatigue, and lightheadedness with similar exacerbating and relieving factors as stable angina.
Asymptomatic (silent) Myocardial Ischemia	May occur with any of the above types of angina. Associated with increased age and disease processes that include peripheral neuropathy (e.g., diabetes).

disruption of blood supply to an area of myocardium that leads to a central zone of permanent damage and surrounding areas that remain vulnerable unless rapid perfusion is attained. For this reason, suspicion of ACS always requires immediate medical attention. Diagnosis of ACS depends on a mixture of a history or presentation of ischemic-type chest discomfort, acute and evolutionary changes in electrocardiographic (ECG) tracings, and a rise and fall of serum cardiac enzymes. Via the ECG, they may be classified as transmural (full-thickness) or subendocardial (partial-thickness), or Q-wave or non–Q-wave infarctions. The acute medical management of ACS is characterized by reperfusion, pain control, and prevention of further complications.[23,24]

The acute course and long-term prognosis after myocardial infarction (MI) is largely based on the size and location of the infarction, the subsequent remodeling of the damaged tissue, the incidence of complications, the presence of disease in the other coronary arteries, and comorbid conditions such as diabetes and renal dysfunction. Arrhythmias and hemodynamic instability may be observed along a continuum of post-MI myocardial cell electrical depolarization and contractility derangement. The 6- to 8-week healing process following an MI is characterized by the body's removal of necrotic debris followed by the remodeling of myocardial tissue via the deposition of fibrous, inelastic scar tissue.[25]

Current guidelines remain unsettled about when exercise should optimally commence after an MI. Most cardiac rehabilitation and secondary prevention programs begin at least 4 to 6 weeks after hospital discharge, but several recent studies suggest that earlier initiation may lead to improved remodeling and cardiopulmonary capacity in patients who are clinically stable and without complications.[26] In these patients, who most often have smaller-sized infarcts, the risk of adverse events or complications (e.g., reinfarction) does not appear to be greater when exercise is initiated at 1 week versus 6 weeks post-MI.[27] This is consistent with findings that demonstrate that exercise stress testing is safe and feasible in the majority of patients post-MI 3 days after infarction.[28] In patients with larger infarcts or complicated courses, initiation of exercise may be more safely deferred or otherwise limited to low-level intensities until later phases of healing when the newly laid scar tissue is less vulnerable to stress. A relatively conservative approach is also advised after subendocardial MIs owing to higher observed rates of reinfarction.[25]

Symptom-limited or maximal exercise testing via cardiopulmonary exercise testing that directly measures oxygen uptake (e.g., peak V_{O_2}) alongside other ventilatory indices is the gold-standard examination procedure in the assessment of aerobic capacity and cardiorespiratory fitness. Where ventilatory gas analysis is unavailable, maximal achievable metabolic equivalents (METs) may be estimated with standard exercise tolerance testing (ETT). Here, nonventilatory indices (e.g., heart rate and rhythm, blood pressure) can be visualized and monitored with an electrocardiogram through graded or ramping protocols on treadmills (e.g., Bruce protocol) or cycle ergometers until criteria for termination are met (Box 18.1) and a maximal speed/grade or wattage produced is recorded.

In the older adult, excessive cardiovascular risk and/or orthopedic or neurologic comorbid conditions may limit the safety, validity, or otherwise feasibility of maximal exercise testing. Submaximal ETTs, in their capacity to produce lesser levels of physiologic and biomechanical strain, may be used in the assessment of rate of perceived exertion, HR and rhythm responses, and other key parameters up to predetermined testing end points. The selection of the particular testing modality and protocol should be based on expected levels of exercise capacity

BOX 18.1 Aerobic Exercise Contraindications and Stopping Points

Absolute Exercise Contraindications
- Unstable angina
- Uncontrolled cardiac dysrhythmias causing symptoms of hemodynamic compromise
- Uncontrolled symptomatic heart failure
- Acute or suspected major cardiovascular event (including severe aortic stenosis, pulmonary embolus or infarction, myocarditis, pericarditis, or dissecting aneurysm)
- Acute systemic infection, accompanied by fever, body aches, or swollen lymph glands
- A recent significant change in resting ECG suggestive of ischemia, myocardial infarction, or other acute cardiac event*

Relative† Exercise Contraindications
- Known significant cardiac disease (including left main coronary stenosis, moderate stenotic valvular disease, hypertrophic cardiomyopathy, high-degree atrioventricular block,* ventricular aneurysm)
- Severe arterial hypertension (systolic BP of >200 mmHg or a diastolic BP of >110 mmHg) at rest
- Tachydysrhythmia or bradydysrhythmia*
- Electrolyte abnormalities
- Uncontrolled metabolic disease
- Chronic infectious disease
- Mental or physical impairment leading to inability to exercise safely

Absolute Indications for Terminating Exercise
- Drop in systolic BP of >10 mmHg from baseline despite an increase in workload when accompanied by other evidence of ischemia
- Moderately severe angina (>2/4)
- Increasing nervous system symptoms
- Signs of poor perfusion
- Subject's desire to stop
- Technical difficulty with monitoring equipment
- Sustained ventricular tachycardia*
- ST elevation (+ 1.0 mm) in leads without diagnostic Q-waves*

Relative Indications for Terminating Exercise
- Drop in systolic BP of >10 mmHg from baseline despite an increase in workload in the absence of other evidence of ischemia
- Increasing chest pain
- Hypertensive response (systolic BP of >250 mmHg or diastolic BP of >115 mmHg)
- Fatigue, shortness of breath/wheezing, leg cramps, or claudication
- ST or QRS changes such as excessive ST depression (>2 mm ST-segment depression)*
- Arrhythmias other than sustained ventricular tachycardia (including multifocal premature ventricular contractions (PVCs), triplets of PVCs, supraventricular tachycardia, heart blocks, or bradyarrhythmias)*
- Development of bundle-branch block or intraventricular conduction delay that cannot be distinguished from ventricular tachycardia*

(Adapted from Thompson WR, Gordon NF, Pescatello LS, ed. ACSM's Guidelines for Exercise Testing and Prescription. Philadelphia, PA: Wolters Kluwer/Lippincott Williams & Wilkins, 2010.)

* Assume that ECG monitoring is available.

† Relative contraindications can be superseded if there are benefits.

ECG, Electrocardiogram.

and seek to maximize performance, safety, and congruence with patient-centered values.[29] The Balke and Naughton protocols, for example, utilize relatively gradual increments of exercise demand and may be more appropriate for older adults limited by physiology, comorbid conditions, and/or medications.[30] Where balance or other motor impairments are observed, submaximal cycle ergometers or the 6-minute walk test (which allows for the use of an assistive device) may be used effectively. The use of target heart rates (e.g., 70% of the HR reserve or 85% of the age-predicted maximal HR) in any mode can assess rate of perceived exertion (RPE) and hemodynamic responses at safer workloads, noting, however, that age-predicted estimates of maximal HR demonstrate wide variation and are susceptible to the effects of medications.[31]

Regardless of protocol chosen, any evidence of arrhythmias (or palpitations), ST-segment depression, subjective report of angina (Box 18.2) or its equivalent (e.g., dyspnea), and/or changes in heart sounds (e.g., development of S3 or S4) should be quantified and qualified within documentation in order to facilitate any needed changes in medical management. Threshold data, such as the rate-pressure product (systolic blood pressure multiplied by the heart rate) at the first sign of ischemia (1 of 4 on an angina scale) or other signs of decompensation, can be used to set parameters for further exercise training.[16] Should the individual be on HR-limiting medications (e.g., a beta- or calcium channel blocker), exercise testing should be performed while on that regimen.

Where ECG is not available, the clinician should closely monitor vital signs, subjective reporting of angina (or its equivalent), and signs and symptoms of developing arrhythmias via findings of irregular pulses and/or reports of "palpitations/fluttering." Any increases in arrhythmia(s) with activity, particularly if accompanied by symptoms of hemodynamic instability, such as lightheadedness, warrants termination of testing and follow-up with the medical team for ECG-guided, graded-exercise testing and/or Holter monitoring. Caution must be taken in women and individuals with diabetes owing to their propensity to display atypical symptoms of angina (e.g., dyspnea) or no symptoms at all.

The overall treatment of an individual with CAD (with or without a history of an MI) should emphasize (1) risk factor reduction, (2) exercise training, and (3) self-management. All individuals with diagnosed CAD, angina, or silent ischemia should be referred to cardiac rehabilitation where available and feasible. Existing guidelines for exercise training continue to be refined in regard to frequency, intensity, duration, and type. Current guidance and recommendations for exercise therapy for the older adult with stable angina, post-MI, and postcardiac surgery are summarized in Table 18.6. Shorter, interval-type bouts of exercise are often better tolerated in earlier stages of rehabilitation, and the use of prophylactic nitroglycerin and/or an allotment of time for dedicated warm-up exercise may facilitate coronary vessel dilation and improved oxygen extraction efficiency prior to exercise therapy.

Given the reduced level of physical activity and increased incidence of sarcopenia with CAD and older age, resistance training (RT) should be utilized in *addition* to aerobic training to facilitate improvement in an individual's overall activity level that may be initially limited by low strength, power, and/or muscular endurance. Establishing safe dosages of resistance intensity remains an active area of research because of concerns that lifting weights at higher percentages of an individual's one-repetition maximum (1-RM) may increase cardiac demand and BP to unsafe levels. For this reason, the majority of current guidelines suggest low to moderate intensities (30% to 69% 1-RM); however, future studies seek to identify the efficacy and safety of progressive RT at high to maximal intensities which may actually be safer and more effectual in comparison to lower intensities.[32–34]

Progression of exercise therapy should be based on demonstration of a higher work-rate performance

BOX 18.2 Commonly Used Symptom Scales

Angina Scale
1 = Mild, barely noticeable
2 = Moderate, bothersome
3 = Moderately severe, very uncomfortable
4 = Most severe or intense pain ever experienced

Dyspnea Scale
1 = Light, barely noticeable
2 = Moderate, bothersome
3 = Moderately severe, very uncomfortable
4 = Most severe or intense dyspnea ever experienced

Claudication Scale
1 = Definite discomfort or pain, but only at initial or modest levels (established, but minimal)
2 = Moderate discomfort or pain from which the patient's attention can be diverted (e.g., by conversation)
3 = Intense pain (short of grade 4) from which the patient's attention cannot be diverted
4 = Excruciating and unbearable pain

Rating of Perceived Exertion (RPE)
0 = Nothing at all
1 = Very light
2 = Fairly light
3 = Moderate
4 = Somewhat hard
5 = Hard
6
7 = Very hard
8
9
10 = Very, very hard

TABLE 18.6 Recommendations for Exercise Therapy for the Older Adult with Stable Angina, Post-MI, and Postcardiac Surgery.[90]

Diagnosis	Indication	Contraindications	Recommended Training Program EACPR Position Paper
• Stable Coronary Artery Disease (CAD)	• Percutaneous coronary intervention (PCI)	• Unstable angina pectoris, acute endomyocarditis, or other acute infections • Recent pulmonary artery embolism or phlebothrombosis • Hemodynamically relevant arrhythmia • Critical obstructions of the left ventricular outflow tract	• Medically supervised exercise training programs are recommended for patients with multiple risk factors, and with moderate-to-high risk (i.e., recent heart failure episode) for training initiation and motivation to long-term adherence • Expanding physical activity to include resistance training.

• S/P Myocardial Infarction	• Acute coronary syndrome (STEMI and NSTEMI)	• Postinfarction angina pectoris (owing to incomplete revascularization)
		• Heart failure
		• Contraindications listed under stable CAD
			• Exercise training should be recommended to all patients (supervised or monitored in moderate to high-risk ones). The program should include: at least 30 min, 5 days/week, aerobic exercise
			  • At 70% to 85% of the peak heart rate, or at 70% to 85% of the heart rate at the onset of ischemia (defined as $\geq$ 1 mm of ST depression, in case of asymptomatic exercise-induced ischemia). Prophylactic nitroglycerine can be taken at the start of the training session.
			  • At 50% of the peak heart rate in high-risk patients because of left ventricular dysfunction, coronary disease severity, comorbid conditions, aging
			• Resistance training.

• S/P Cardiac Surgery	• S/P CABG • S/P Valve surgery • S/P Aortic surgery	• Wound infection after sternotomy, harvesting of saphenous veins and/or radial arteries • Respiratory infection (e.g., secondary to sternotomy) • Contraindications listed under stable CAD	• Exercise training can be started early in-hospital • Programs should last 2–4 weeks for in-patient or up to 12 weeks for out-patient settings. • Upper-body training can begin when the sternal wound is stable. • Exercise training should be individually tailored according to the clinical condition, baseline exercise capacity, ventricular function, and different valve surgery (after mitral valve replacement exercise tolerance is much lower than after aortic valve replacement, particularly if there is residual pulmonary hypertension).

CABG, coronary artery bypass graft; *S/P*, status post; *STEMI*, ST-segment elevation myocardial infarction; *NSTEMI*, non-ST-segment elevation myocardial infarction.

Adapted from Table 1 in Gielen S, Laughlin MH, O'Conner C, Duncker DJ. Exercise training in patients with heart disease: review of beneficial effects and clinical recommendations. Progress in Cardiovascular Diseases. 2015;57(4):347–55.

without production of symptoms. Patient education should emphasize safety, including information regarding their individualized anginal symptoms and provoking factors, basic treatment strategies (e.g., rest, nitroglycerin [NTG]), exercise limitations, and medication effects.[16,35]

Aortic Stenosis

The same risk factors for atherosclerosis, namely, dyslipidemia, smoking, and hypertension, among others, may also predispose the aortic valve tissue to endothelial dysfunction, inflammation, and lipid accumulation.[36] Together, these processes lead to a degenerative calcification of the valve's leaflets and a narrowing of the outflow track of blood into the systemic circulation. This increases the pressure the left ventricle must contract against (i.e., afterload) and consequentially promotes a concentric hypertrophy of the ventricular myocardium that initially (and compensatorily) reduces wall stress, but ultimately may lead to conditions that precipitate heart failure and decreased cardiac output.[37]

Aortic stenosis (AS) is a particularly significant clinical finding in the older adult because of the sharp rise in its prevalence in the older adult and the poor prognosis it carries in severe cases. In general, some form of degenerative aortic valve disease (e.g., aortic sclerosis) is estimated to occur in 25% of individuals over 65 years of age. A lesser amount, around 2% to 5%, actually has outflow tract obstruction. Some estimates, however, suggest that as many as one in eight individuals over 75 years of age show moderate to severe AS. Indeed, the epidemiology of AS is complicated by the fact that many patients with severe AS often live asymptomatically owing to comorbid mobility impairments that prevent them from performing activities that would otherwise provoke symptoms. In these cases, the symptoms (and disease state) only manifest in more advanced stages where the 2-year mortality rate is estimated to be 50% to 60% and a 3-year survival rate of less than 30% if left untreated.[38,39] Therefore, the physical therapist has a valuable role in screening for this condition.

The cardinal signs and symptoms of advanced AS are angina, exertional syncope, and heart failure. Therefore, during exercise testing, an observed drop in blood pressure or other hypotensive pressor response (i.e., owing to decreased cardiac output) may argue in favor of significant AS over simple disuse or deconditioning. A medical referral is indicated in this scenario. Sometimes, a "watchful waiting" strategy is employed in patients with severe stenosis who are asymptomatic. In any case of AS, but particularly in more severe cases, each treatment session should be approached with vigilance for signs and symptoms suggesting stenotic progression. Individuals with moderate or severe AS (Table 18.7) should be monitored via echocardiography every 2 to 3 years and 1 to 2 years, respectively. Table 18.8 lists exercise recommendations.[16,35]

Nearly all symptomatic severe cases of AS require aortic valve replacement. The traditional surgical approach has been an open-heart procedure (e.g., via a median sternotomy). However, in the patient at intermediate to high risk, the transcatheter aortic valve replacement procedures has emerged as an increasingly successful alternative.[4] In these patients, who are often of relatively greater age and comorbidity load (i.e., of "high-risk" status), it is particularly important to emphasize the promotion of a healthy lifestyle with cardiac risk factor reduction, patient education and coordination of care, and cardiac rehabilitation. Readmission rates are over 40% in the first year after the procedure owing to both noncardiac causes (e.g., respiratory problems, infections and bleeding events) and cardiac causes (arrhythmias and heart failure).[40]

TABLE 18.7 Degrees of Severity of Aortic Stenosis

Severity	Mean Gradient	Aortic Valve Area
Mild	< 20 mmHg	> 1.5 cm
Moderate	20–40 mmHg	1.0–1.5 cm
Severe	> 40 mmHg	< 1.0 cm

Heart Failure

Heart failure (HF) is a complex clinical syndrome that results in a heart that is unable to provide a sufficient forward output to meet the perfusion and oxygenation requirements of the body's metabolizing tissues. Acute, decompensated heart failure is one of the most common admitting diagnoses in older Americans, resulting in nearly 1 million hospitalizations in 2014.[41] The AHA estimated that, in 2006, 5.1 million people in the United States were living with HF.[42] It is well established that prevalence of HF and left ventricular dysfunction increases sharply with chronological age, from 8 men per 1000 at ages 50 to 69 years to 66 per 1000 at ages 80 to 89 years (women show a similar trend).[43] Predictions suggest the number of cases will increase 2.3-fold by 2040 and triple by 2060.[44]

Broadly speaking, HF can be associated with systolic dysfunction (i.e., where there is impaired cardiac contractile function), diastolic dysfunction (i.e., where there is abnormal filling of the left or right ventricle), or both, or described in terms of whether the dysfunction is primarily occurring in the left or right side of the heart, or both (Tables 18.9 and 18.10, respectively). HF can be

TABLE 18.8 Exercise Recommendations for Individuals with Aortic Stenosis

Degree of Stenosis	Precautions	Mode	Intensity
Mild	Generally not limited	Generally not limited	Avoid reaching symptoms
Moderate	Should consult with cardiologist prior to initiating exercise program	Avoid high dynamic load exercises (e.g., cycling, running, and swimming)	Requires ET to determine safe work levels
Severe, asymptomatic	Should consult with cardiologist prior to initiating exercise program	Avoid high dynamic load exercises (e.g., cycling, running, and swimming)	Requires ET to determine safe work levels, which will generally be low.
Severe, symptomatic	Should receive surgical treatment prior to exercise training.	Avoid high dynamic load exercises (e.g., cycling, running, and swimming)	Requires ET to determine safe work levels, which will generally be low.
Status Post Valve Repair or Replacement	Strongly consider cardiac rehabilitation	Similar to mild degree of stenosis	Similar to mild degrees of stenosis. Use ET to assess proposed peak work levels.

ET, exercise testing

TABLE 18.9 Primary Causes, Etiologic Factors, and Characteristics of Systolic and Diastolic Heart Failure

Systolic and Diastolic Heart Failure			
Systolic		**Diastolic**	
Primary Causes/ Etiologic Factors	**Characteristics**	**Primary Causes/ Etiologic Factors**	**Characteristics**
Decreased contractility Myocardial ischemia Myocardial infarction Cardiomyopathies Valvular disease (e.g., regurgitation) Increased afterload Hypertension Valvular disease (e.g., stenosis)	Decreased ejection fraction Varying signs/symptoms of right or left heart failure Jugular venous distension Crackles S3 heart sound Peripheral edema More frequently male, ages 50–70 years, history of smoking	Decreased compliance and relaxation/filling Ventricular hypertrophy Cardiomyopathy Valvular disease (e.g., stenosis) Pericarditis Tamponade	Preserved, normal, or increased ejection fraction S4 heart sound Crackles Hypertension Renal dysfunction Atrial fibrillation Frequently female, elderly

more specifically categorized as (1) HF with reduced ejection fraction (HfrEF) (EF < 40%) or (2) HF with preserved ejection fraction (HfpEF) (EF < 50%). Regardless of these distinctions, cardiovascular pump performance can be thought of as existing along a continuum where specific signs and symptoms emerge and progress throughout the disease state. Medical treatment across this continuum of dysfunction to failure is based on the results of numerous tests and measures, the utilization of which should form the basis of the physical therapy plan of care.[45]

The initial evaluation and routine assessment of heart failure signs and symptoms (Table 18.11) should reflect the pathophysiologic profile of the disease. A thorough interview should include a comprehensive inquiry into symptoms (e.g., history, exacerbating factors, frequency), accompanying pain (e.g., angina, claudication), presence of orthopnea, paroxysmal nocturnal dyspnea, or fluid retention, and descriptions of activity intolerance (e.g., as within activities of daily living, walking). Owing to their roles as primary etiologic factors within the development of cardiac disease and HF itself, hypertension, arrhythmias, valvular diseases, and CAD with or without a history of MI are frequent findings within established pump dysfunction or failure. Frequently, an individual's current medication profile and/or past medical history will reflect these comorbid factors and should be reviewed and considered within their potential influence on physical therapy intervention.

Frailty and skeletal muscle abnormalities share common biological mechanisms with HF and should be examined as a related causative factor for exercise

TABLE 18.10 Primary Causes, Etiologic Factors, and Common Signs and Symptoms of Left- and Right-Sided Heart Failure

Right and Left Heart Failure			
Right		**Left**	
Primary Causes/ Etiologic Factors	**Common Signs and Symptoms**	**Primary Causes/ Eiologic Factors**	**Common Signs and Symptoms**
Pulmonary hypertension caused by: • Left ventricular pump dysfunction • Emphysema • Pulmonary embolism • Mitral valve disease Tricuspid valve disease Restrictive or hypertrophic cardiomyopathies Myocarditis Right ventricular infarction	"Systemic signs" • Peripheral edema • Pitting edema • Ascites • Jugular vein distension • S3 heart sound • Hepatojugular reflex • Abdominal discomfort/ anorexia	Intrinsic myocardial disease • Atherosclerotic heart disease • Cardiomyopathy Excessive workload on LV • Hypertension • Valvular disease • Arrhythmias	"Breathing signs" • Orthopnea • Paroxysmal nocturnal dyspnea • Exercise intolerance with fatigue and weakness • Pulmonary rales • Dyspnea of exertion • Dry, nonproductive cough in supine • Unexplained mental status changes

TABLE 18.11 Assessment of Signs and Symptoms of Heart Failure

Examination of Heart Failure	
Assessment	**Rationale/Comments**
Symptoms of dyspnea, PND, orthopnea	Excessive fluid in alveoli and interstitium, which may be increasingly provoked in recumbency
Heart or pulse rate and rhythm	Sinus tachycardia or tachyarrhythmia as a result of increased sympathetic tone and, an attempt to increase cardiac output and increase delivery of fluid and oxygen to the periphery. Pulsus alterans may suggest more severe left ventricular dysfunction.
Blood pressure	Hypertension may be present as an etiologic factor.
Respiratory rate and breathing pattern	Rapid and shallow, reflecting poor gas transport, impaired diaphragmatic excursion limitations owing to ascites, ventilatory muscle weakness, orthostatic hypotension, and/or fluid overload in interstitium
Auscultation of heart and lung sounds	S3 in a stiff, noncompliant ventricle and S4 in exaggerated "atrial kicks." Inspiratory rales/crackles owing to alveolar opening in the presence of pulmonary edema, commonly found in bases, but may extend upward in more severe cases. An inferolaterally displaced point of maximal impulse suggests dilated cardiomyopathy.
Observation for signs of fluid overload	Peripheral edema and weight gain may occur owing to decreased fluid excretion in response to falling cardiac output. Jugular venous distension may occur as fluid "backs up" into venous system. Weight gain > 3 lb/day suggestive of decompensation.

PND, Paroxysmal nocturnal dyspnea.

intolerance.[46] The Fried Frailty Index, which consists of five domains (slowness, weakness, low physical activity, exhaustion, and unintentional weight loss), is the most validated tool to examine this syndrome.[47] Single components of the Fried index (e.g., gait speed and hand grip strength, together) may be used as a proxy for the Fried frailty phenotype.[48]

The global benefits of exercise training in patients with stable chronic HF with reduced ejection fraction include improved peak $\dot{V}O_2$, improved quality of life, and decreased all-cause and HF-related hospital admission and hospital days.[49–52] Despite a paucity of studies examining the effectiveness of interventions focused on individuals with HF with preserved ejection fraction, emerging evidence suggests that these individuals can also benefit from exercise training via improvements in exercise capacity, symptom reduction, and quality of life.[53] Exercise training should be based on a symptom-limited or submaximal exercise test.

Electrocardiographic monitoring is not required per se, but it is indicated in individuals with a history of clinically significant dysrhythmias, exertional hypotension, or cardiac arrest. When combined with measurements of expired gases (e.g., to discern peak $\dot{V}O_2$, $\dot{V}e/\dot{V}CO_2$ slope), exercise testing can further provide useful risk stratification and prognostic information. The emphasis of testing should be placed on symptoms and hemodynamics (e.g., pressor and chronotropic responses) and consider that many individuals will demonstrate alterations (e.g., hypotension, dyspnea) within 5 METs. Compared with age-matched healthy individuals, patients with HF exhibit lower peak cardiac output and concomitant reduced exercise tolerance in the order of approximately 30% to 40%. The Naughton treadmill protocol is often used owing to its relatively lower initial work rate and moderate ramping. However, walk tests, such as the 2-, 6-, or 12-minute walk tests, may also be used. Information regarding functional status, exercise tolerance, oxygen consumption, and short- and long-term survival can be estimated from these examinations via a comparison of normative values and derived prediction equations.[29,54] If, however, these examinations are not performed, exercise testing can be based on approximating the peak MET level attained within examination, where functional capacities of 5 to 6 and 4 to 5 METs can be used to categorize patients into pump dysfunction versus failure, respectively.[4]

Table 18.12 summarizes a recent clinical practice guideline update of the levels, grades, and strength of recommendations for various modes of exercise for individuals with HF.[55] Where heart rate and $\dot{V}O_2$ are not realistic to use as indicators, consider utilizing RPE and dyspnea scales (see Box 18.2) that may represent patient limitations more accurately. Reducing exercise intensity to allow for longer durations and slower work rates, introducing more rest breaks, and extending warm-up and cool-down periods are general strategies that may accommodate the exercise-intolerant patient. The overall volume of exercise should be consistently increased over time based on observable adaptive cardiopulmonary responses and decreases in adverse subjective responses (e.g., reports of dyspnea) at specific workloads.

Specific patient education on HF should be included within any plan of care and consist of self-management skills including (1) volume status monitoring, (2) medication adherence, (3) dietary restrictions, and (4) monitoring for signs and symptoms of decompensation. Figure 18.3 shows one common piece of patient education material. A patient-centered, quality-of-life outcome measure, such as the Minnesota Living with Heart Failure Questionnaire, can facilitate directed dialogue with patients about their specific needs, because it illuminates the effects of HF on a patient's daily life and wellbeing.[56]

TABLE 18.12 Exercise Recommendations for Individuals with Heart Failure[55]

Strength of Recommendation	Type	Parameters	Comments
Strong, must include	Aerobic	• Time: 20–60 minutes • Intensity: 50% to 90% of peak $\dot{V}O_2$ or peak work • Frequency: 3–5 times per week • Duration: at least 2–3 months • Mode: treadmill, cycle ergometer, or dancing	• Patient characteristics – Training parameters • Setting • Safety • Adherence
Moderate, should include	Resistance	• Time: 45–60 minutes, 2–3 sets per major muscle group • Intensity: 60% to80% 1-RM • Frequency: 3 times per week • Duration: 8–12 weeks	• Transient musculoskeletal pain that may require adjustment of the exercises performed • Patient preference • Avoid isometrics and valsalva maneuver
Strong, should include	High-intensity, interval-based exercise	• Time: > 35 minutes • Intensity: > 90% to 95% of peak $\dot{V}O_2$ or peak work • Frequency: 2–3 times per week • Duration: 2–3 months • Mode: treadmill or cycle ergometer	• HIIT total weekly exercise doses should be at least 460 kcal, 114 minutes, or 5.4 MET-hours
Strong, should include	Inspiratory muscle training	• Time: 30 min/day • Intensity: > 30% maximal inspiratory pressure (PIMax or MIP) • Frequency: 5–7 days/week • Duration: 8–12 weeks • Mode: Threshold device (or similar)	• Strength vs. endurance? • Intensity? • Patient selection
Strong, should include	NMES for quadriceps, gastrocsoleus	• Current/Frequency: Bi-phasic 10–50 Hz, pulse width 0.2–0.7 msec • On/Off: 2s/4s–10s/50s • Time: 30–60 min/day • Intensity: Strong muscle contraction • Frequency: 5–7 d/week	• Pacemaker precautions • DOMS

DOMS, delayed onset muscle soreness; *HIIT*, high-intensity interval training; *MET*, metabolic equivalent; *NMES*, neuromuscular electrical stimulation.

Atrial Fibrillation

Atrial fibrillation (AF) affects 9% of U.S. adults aged 65 and over, and is predicted to affect 6 to 12 million people by 2050.[57] It is the most common arrhythmia, accounting for one-third of hospital admissions for cardiac rhythm disturbances.[58] Largely a disease of advancing age, it is etiologically related to processes that increase atrial pressures and enlargement, such as heart failure, hypertension, valvular heart disease, CAD, and lung disease, but can also be caused by thyrotoxicosis and excessive alcohol intake. Upon initial detection, AF is classified as first detected AF and subsequently further classified as paroxysmal if self-terminating within seven days. Otherwise, it is classified as persistent. Any unsuccessful attempts made to resolve persistent AF via cardioversion reclassifies the arrhythmia as permanent.

The medical management of AF often utilizes anticoagulation therapy at a minimum and, based on symptoms, may further include rate and/or rhythm control therapies. In asymptomatic cases, it is often sufficient to control the ventricular rate (e.g., with beta-receptor or calcium channel antagonists) alongside anticoagulation therapy. In cases of persistent AF that are refractory to antiarrhythmic therapy or when the arrhythmia is the main factor responsible for acute HF, hypotension, or worsening angina pectoris, cardioversion may be performed after which antiarrhythmics may be used to maintain normal sinus rhythm.[59,60]

The hallmark physical finding of AF is an "irregularly irregular" pulse owing to fast (> 300 atrial discharges/min) and chaotic atrial rates that only intermittently summate to produce AV nodal depolarization. The ECG is characterized by a jagged, fibrillatory baseline instead of P waves, and irregular R-R intervals. Many patients are often asymptomatic when the ventricular rate is less than 100 beats/min, but may feel palpitations, dizziness, and shortness of breath at higher rates owing to the underlying impairment in ventricular filling and cardiac pump function. In general, exercise tolerance in individuals with AF is about 20% lower than age-matched normal individuals, but this may vary daily owing to changes in ventricular response. Indeed, some individuals are observed to

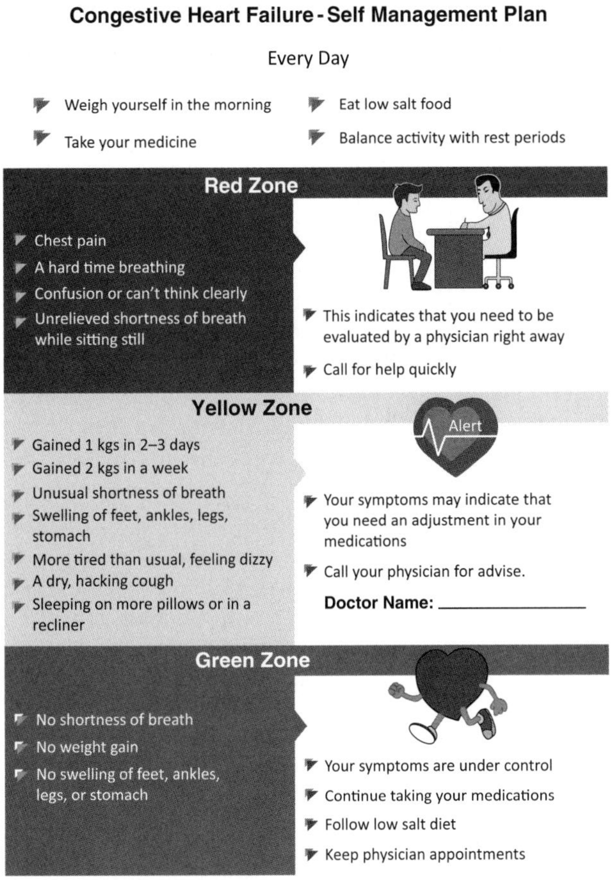

Congestive Heart Failure - Self Management Plan

Every Day

- Weigh yourself in the morning
- Eat low salt food
- Take your medicine
- Balance activity with rest periods

Red Zone

- Chest pain
- A hard time breathing
- Confusion or can't think clearly
- Unrelieved shortness of breath while sitting still

- This indicates that you need to be evaluated by a physician right away
- Call for help quickly

Yellow Zone

Alert

- Gained 1 kgs in 2–3 days
- Gained 2 kgs in a week
- Unusual shortness of breath
- Swelling of feet, ankles, legs, stomach
- More tired than usual, feeling dizzy
- A dry, hacking cough
- Sleeping on more pillows or in a recliner

- Your symptoms may indicate that you need an adjustment in your medications
- Call your physician for advise.

Doctor Name: ______________

Green Zone

- No shortness of breath
- No weight gain
- No swelling of feet, ankles, legs, or stomach

- Your symptoms are under control
- Continue taking your medications
- Follow low salt diet
- Keep physician appointments

FIG. 18.3 Example of patient education material for patients with heart failure.[88] *From Seth S, Vashista S. The Hriday Card: A checklist for heart failure. Journal of the Practice of Cardiovascular Sciences.* 2017;3(1):5.

fluctuate between AF and normal sinus rhythm on a daily basis; therefore, it is important to assess rhythms frequently and use work rate (e.g., METs, watts) and/or RPE instead of heart/pulse rate during exercise or functional mobility training. If pulse rate is used, consider longer samples of measurement to account for irregular rhythms. Overall, individuals with AF are able to exercise safely much like anyone else, but strong considerations of other comorbid conditions, particularly other cardiac conditions, should be made and placed at or near the forefront of plan-of-care rationale.[16] Any suspicion of new-onset AF without an established history should be medically investigated prior to continuing physical therapy.

Peripheral Arterial Disease

The same atherosclerotic processes described in CAD may affect the peripheral arteries to create a supply and demand mismatch and ischemia. Peripheral arterial disease (PAD) has been shown to limit functional mobility, activity levels, and quality of life, and is estimated to occur in 6% in individuals over 60 years of age. The presence of PAD carries a two- to six-fold increase risk of CAD and a four- to five-fold increase risk of strokes.[16,35]

TABLE 18.13 Fontaine Classification System of Peripheral Arterial Disease (PAD)

Stage	History
I	Asymptomatic
IIa	Mild claudication
IIb	Moderate to severe claudication
III	Ischemic rest pain
IV	Tissue loss or ulceration

Adapted from Table 1 in Norgren L, Hiatt WR, Dormandy JA, et al. Inter-society consensus for the management of peripheral vascular disease (TASC II). *J Vasc Surg*. 2007:45:S5–S67

TABLE 18.14 Scores on the Ankle-Brachial Index Associated with the Extent of Arterial Luminal Occlusion

Ankle-Brachial Index (SBP LE/SBP UE)	
> 1.40	Abnormal, suggests incompressible tibial arteries owing to calcification/atherosclerosis, obese lower limb
1.00–1.40	Normal
0.90–0.99	Borderline, acceptable
0.80–0.89	Mild disease: < 0.90 is diagnostic for PA; manage risk factors
0.50–0.79	Moderate disease, seek routine specialist referral
< 0.30	Severe limb disease; seek urgent specialist referral

The severity of PAD can be measured along a continuum of clinical symptoms (e.g., the Fontaine classification, Table 18.13) or more commonly, by the ankle-brachial index (Table 18.14), which compares systolic pressures of the leg and arm to approximate the extent of arterial luminal occlusion.[61,62] Other findings suggestive of advancing disease are dry and shiny skin, hair loss, trophic changes at the nails, muscular atrophy, impaired sensation, and decreased pulses. Although only occurring in around 10% of individuals, intermittent claudication is considered the classic symptom of PAD. A majority of patients will experience some form of adverse symptoms that may limit weight-bearing activity owing to reduced vascular perfusion, skeletal muscle damage, and peripheral nerve changes.[62a]

The reduction of risk factors of atherosclerosis, particularly smoking cessation and increasing physical activity, are mainstay treatments for mild to moderate forms of PAD. The primary goals of exercise testing include obtaining information on maximal pain-free walking distance, overall maximal walking distance, and assessing underlying CAD in order to inform a tailored exercise prescription. Walking tests, such as incremental-ramping treadmill protocols or the 6-minute walk test are the preferred examination modes as they closely approximate actual activity limitation.[35] Sometimes, individuals with

BOX 18.3 General Considerations for Exercise Adaptations for Individuals with Peripheral Arterial Disease

- Interval training may be better tolerated initially
- Non–weight-bearing activity is not as effective as weight-bearing, but can be used to supplement warm-ups.
- Longer warm-up times are useful, particularly in colder environments.
- Sensory considerations and foot care should be emphasized because of the increased risk of peripheral neuropathy.
- Exercise should be progressed in volume first and then in intensity, as tolerated.
- Evidence for the efficacy of unsupervised exercise training (e.g., at-home or within the community setting) is mounting.
- Shifting culture toward technology-driven tele-coaching and tele-monitoring systems, which many patients prefer.[91]

strong claudication symptoms are so normally self-limiting that symptom-limited exercise testing may provide the novel opportunity to unmask covert heart disease (e.g., coronary ischemia). The clinician should, accordingly, perform diligent monitoring of vital signs. An exaggerated BP response to exercise testing, as in general, atherosclerosis, may also occur.[63]

Supervised exercise training for individuals with PAD can provide a supportive environment that encourages the individual to overcome fear of claudication pain and falling,[64] thus increasing the intensity of exercise. Traditional thinking suggests that individuals should exercise to intensities that create moderate to maximally tolerable symptoms (i.e., a 3 of 4 on the claudication scale, Box 18.2), but recent studies suggest that exercising to intensities that provoke only mild symptoms or no symptoms may be equally as effective at improving walking ability.[65] General exercise considerations for individuals with PAD that are consistently identified in the literature are summarized in Box 18.3.

PULMONARY DISEASE

Chronic Obstructive Pulmonary Disease

The Global Initiative for Chronic Obstructive Lung Disease (GOLD), an international collaboration of experts in chronic obstructive pulmonary disease (COPD) originally formulated by the National Heart Lung and Blood Institute, the United States National Institutes of Health, and the World Health Organization, describes COPD as "*a common, preventable, and treatable disease that is characterized by persistent respiratory symptoms and airflow limitation that is due to airway and/or alveolar abnormalities usually caused by significant exposure to noxious particles or gases. The chronic airflow limitation that characterizes COPD is caused by a mixture of small airways disease (e.g., obstructive bronchiolitis) and parenchymal destruction (emphysema), the relative contributions of which vary from person to person. Chronic inflammation causes structural changes, small airways narrowing, and destruction of lung parenchyma. A loss of small airways may contribute to airflow imitation and mucociliary dysfunction, a characteristic feature of the disease.*"[66]

According to the Center for Disease Control (CDC), in the year 2015, there were 15.5 million adults living in the United States with COPD. Approximately 10% of women over 65 years of age and 11% of men over 75 years of age have COPD.[67] The CDC reported 150,350 deaths from COPD (40.3 per 100,000 population), the third most common cause of death in the United States.[68] A significant amount of health care resources are devoted to the management of COPD annually. The total cost of managing COPD in the United States was estimated at $32.1 billion in 2010, and has been projected to rise to $49.0 billion in 2020.[69] As available treatments for COPD have improved, so have the life expectancies of patients with COPD.[70] Medical management of COPD focuses not only on prolonging survival but also on reducing symptoms and the frequency and severity of exacerbations.[66]

COPD represents a cluster of conditions, all of which cause obstruction to airflow within the pulmonary system, and can be present to varying extents in any given patient. Obstruction can result from bronchoconstriction (increased tone or spasm of bronchial smooth muscle), inflammation of the mucosal lining of the airways, degradation of the structural support of the airways, alveolar destruction and over-inflation, and secretion retention. In older adults with COPD, these pathophysiologic changes are then superimposed on what are already considered normal anatomic and physiologic changes owing to the aging process.

The two primary etiologic pathways for the development of airway obstruction are inhalation of foreign matter and genetics. The primary source of inhalation-related COPD is cigarette smoke. Smoke exposure causes a reduction of lung function in a dose-dependent manner. This can be calculated by the number of packs of cigarettes smoked per day multiplied by the number of years of smoking, which is then referred to as "pack years." Other inhalation-related irritants may include various chemicals and environmental pollutants.[71] The genetic contribution to COPD stems from the inheritance of α-1-antitrypsin deficiency, which is a gene that contributes to the maintenance of the structural integrity of alveoli. Deficiency in the α-1-antitrypsin therefore results in the earlier onset of emphysematous changes.

The increased resistance to expiratory airflow caused by these conditions results in a progressively worsening cascade of pathophysiologic changes. Incomplete emptying of the lung results in the trapping of air in distal spaces, which hyperinflates the lungs. Lung hyperinflation affects both the biomechanics of the musculoskeletal contribution to ventilation as well as gas exchange. The rib cage dimensions become increased in the anteroposterior direction, a shape referred to as "barrel chest." The ability of the rib cage to perform excursion in the bucket handle and pump handle motions becomes more limited. This is in addition to the typically observed age-related changes to chest wall and airway compliance. Because of hyperinflation, the diaphragm becomes flattened, affecting its length-tension relationship and reducing its ability to adequately contract and relax. Diaphragmatic muscle fibers shift from type II to type I, sacrificing power and strength for greater endurance, also a shared feature of the aging process.

Inhalation becomes more effortful and an increased contribution is required from the accessory muscles of breathing. The accessory muscles may hypertrophy and shorten, accentuating postural deviations, such as forward head, rounded shoulders, and thoracic kyphosis. The tripod position, as depicted in Figure 18.4, is often used in order to facilitate the actions of the accessory muscles.

Exhalation, normally passive, may require an increased active contribution. Airway clearance is impaired by the change in length-tension relationship of the respiratory muscles along with reduction in power-producing muscle fiber types. Skeletal muscle endurance is reduced owing to a shift from type I to type II muscle fibers, a reduction in mitochondrial density, and a reduction in capillary density. These changes are associated with a decrease in aerobic metabolism and exercise capacity.[72,73]

As COPD is a generic term that describes a cluster of conditions that results in airflow limitation, air trapping, and lung hyperinflation, it is also important to know the most common subtypes of the disease. The two most frequently encountered subtypes are emphysema and chronic bronchitis. Chronic bronchitis is defined as the presence of a chronic productive cough for 3 months in each of two successive years, provided that other causes of chronic mucus production (cystic fibrosis, bronchiectasis, and tuberculosis) have been ruled out. The pathophysiology involves hypertrophy of the submucosal glands and thickening of the airway walls. Mucus hypersecretion typically occurs primarily in the larger airways in early stages of simple bronchitis. As the disease progresses in chronicity and with increasing frequency of exacerbations, the more distal airways are more increasingly affected by the increase in mucus production. Thus, the patient with this subtype presents clinically with dyspnea and a productive cough, and is therefore likely to benefit from interventions to assist with secretion management.

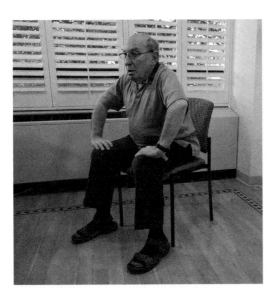

FIG. 18.4 Tripod position often used in order to facilitate the actions of the accessory muscles in individuals with COPD. *(From Yoost BL, Crawford LR. Fundamentals of Nursing: Active Learning for Collaborative Practice, ed 2. St. Louis: Elsevier, 2020.)*

Emphysema is characterized by destruction of alveolar walls and enlargement of air spaces distal to the terminal bronchioles, including the respiratory bronchioles, alveolar ducts, and alveoli. Inhaled foreign matter leads to inflammatory cell recruitment, proteolytic injury (the hydrolysis of proteins by enzymes) to the extracellular matrix, and cell death. In addition, airway walls become perforated and, in the absence of repair, the walls become obliterated and small distinct airspaces appear, changing into larger abnormal airspaces. Bullae, emphysematous spaces larger than 1 cm in diameter, are commonly present in patients with emphysema. Surgical intervention to remove bullae may be indicated.[74] The most common symptoms of emphysema, consistent with the destruction of distal airways and alveolar walls, is dyspnea and a nonproductive cough.

These subtypes can exist together. COPD is best thought along a spectrum that may have overlapping or combining features of more than one subtype. Thus, patients with COPD require individualized interventions according to their specific presentation. Auscultation of the lungs of individuals with obstructive lung disease reveals a prolonged expiratory phase with breath sounds diminished in intensity in all lung fields. In the presence of secretion retention, rhonchi and occasionally localized wheezing may also be heard over affected areas. Mediate percussion of the thorax is often hyperresonant because of lung hyperinflation. Observation of posture may include forward head, rounded shoulders, thoracic kyphosis, and barrel chest along with accessory muscle hypertrophy.

The patient's use of strategies, such as tripod position and pursed lip breathing, should be noted; they are often used during activity or even at rest in the case of severe disease. Cyanosis of the skin and mucosal membranes, a sign of inadequate oxygenation, must also be noted. Oxygenation is further evaluated by pulse oximetry or blood gas analysis. Nail clubbing is not as typical to COPD as compared with other pulmonary diseases (interstitial lung disease, bronchiectasis, lung cancer), but may be evident in some cases. A wide range of chronic pulmonary disease conditions, including COPD, may lead to the development of pulmonary hypertension and right-side heart failure, or cor pulmonale. Failure of the right side of the heart to produce adequate forward flow results in observable jugular venous distention, ascites, lower leg swelling, and the possibility of a third heart sound.

Pulmonary function tests are paramount in the diagnosis of COPD with the forced expiratory volume in one second (FEV_1) and the forced vital capacity (FVC) as the most relevant. Airway obstruction is indicated by a decreasing FEV_1 relative to FVC. During comprehensive testing, these measurements are taken both pre- and post-administration of a bronchodilator. The postbronchodilator ratio of FEV_1/FVC determines whether airflow limitation is present, whereas the postbronchodilator percent predicted value for FEV_1 determines the severity of airflow limitation. The use of bronchodilators also allows the condition to be evaluated for reversibility.[71]

Lung volumes are also altered in patterns that express increased air trapping, which will be exhibited by an increased functional residual capacity (FRC), residual volume (RV), and total lung capacity (TLC), whereas inspiratory capacity (IC) and vital capacity (VC) will be decreased. The diffusing capacity for carbon monoxide (DLCO), when decreased, proportionally indicates the severity of emphysematous changes in the presence of airflow limitation. Chest radiography and computed tomography (CT) may be performed as a part of the differential diagnosis, to exclude the possibility of an alternative cause for the patient's symptoms (e.g., pneumonia, pneumothorax, primary cardiac disease). Smoking cessation is essential to the management of COPD and can slow the rate of deterioration of lung function. The use of medications to reduce airflow limitations, including bronchodilators and anti-inflammatory agents, may help many patients manage their symptoms.

To help prevent respiratory infections, older adults should receive the pneumococcal vaccination as well as an annual influenza vaccination. Respiratory infections may trigger exacerbations of the inflammatory response and worsening of the patients' symptoms. The use of supplemental oxygen is recommended for individuals with stage IV COPD who have resting PaO_2 of 55 mm Hg or lower or an SpO_2 of 88% or less. Oxygen administration may also be used in less severe COPD to improve exercise tolerance or to relieve episodes of acute dyspnea. Hillegass et al.[63], summarizing guidelines released by the Cardiovascular and Pulmonary Section of the American Physical Therapy Association (APTA) in 2014, offer insight into the role of the Physical Therapist in managing patients who have been prescribed supplemental oxygen therapy. These include titrating oxygen therapy to the relevant activity by assessing vital signs, symptoms, and breathing with a target SpO_2 in mind (for example, $\geq$ 90%) that should be stated by the prescribing physician. If the prescription does not state a specific target in this manner, the clinician should contact the referring practitioner for clarification.[63]

The cornerstone of exercise intervention in patients with COPD is endurance training, and the same basic principles of exercise prescription that are applied to healthy older adults can be utilized in older adults with COPD.[75] In general, walking may be preferred over cycling for the functional training effect as well as lower cost and greater accessibility (at least in the case of over ground walking versus treadmill walking). However, patients with COPD may have a higher ventilatory response to walking interventions as compared with cycling, and thus cycling may be preferred in order to minimize sensations of dyspnea, ventilatory fatigue, and the chances of desaturation during exercise.[76] Cycling interventions also allow for the potential to perform single limb exercise training, which allows patients to sustain a high-intensity stimulus to the large muscles of one leg while providing more time before reaching the ventilatory limitation, thereby extending the time exposed to the exercise stimulus. In fact, the training load achieved during one-legged cycling has been shown to be nearly double per leg compared with two-legged cycling.[77] Interval training as compared with continuous training has been shown to reduce symptom scores significantly while maintaining similarly high training loads in patients with COPD.[75]

Specific resistance training for strength should also be considered in older adults with COPD, because endurance-type exercises alone are suboptimal for increasing muscles mass and strength.[75] Box 18.4[78] outlines the general guidelines for prescription of endurance, resistance, and flexibility training for individuals with COPD, which are consistent with the general recommendations for FITT (frequency, intensity, time, type) given to the general population. Flexibility training may also be incorporated, with the therapist keeping in mind the pathophysiologic changes associated with the disease process as well as the aging process, with an emphasis on thoracic mobility and rib cage expansion, as well as awareness of the need to optimize the length-tension relationship of the accessory muscles of breathing.

Also relevant for inclusion in the intervention plan for older adults with COPD are controlled breathing techniques (pursed lip breathing, paced breathing), which should be practiced and mastered while at rest and then integrated into exercise and activity. Specific resistive inspiratory muscle strength training (IMT) alone has been shown to improve inspiratory muscle strength, exercise capacity, and quality of life, as well as decreasing the perception of dyspnea. However, when studied in combination with the exercise training performed as a part of a standard pulmonary rehabilitation program, IMT did not add benefit and the authors of a systematic review concluded that more studies were needed to determine the optimal settings of IMT.[79] IMT protocols reported in available literature are highly variable in terms of frequency, intensity, and duration.[75]

Multiple interventions are used to mitigate the effects of increased secretion production on ventilation, respiration, and aerobic capacity. Breathing strategies that do not require outside equipment or assistance to perform include autogenic drainage, active cycle of breathing,

BOX 18.4 Guidelines for Exercise Interventions in Patients with COPD[78]

	ACSM	ATS/ERS	AACVPR
Endurance exercise			
Modality	Walking and/or cycling	Cycling or walking (ground-based or treadmill)	Walking (treadmill, track, supported walking via walker or wheelchair), cycling, stationary bike, arm ergometry, arm-lifting exercises with/without weights, step exercises, swimming, modified aerobic dance, seated aerobics
Frequency	3 to 5 days per week (minimum)	3 to 5 times per week	3 to 5 times per week
Intensity	Light intensity: 30% to 40% peak work rate Vigorous intensity: 60% to 80% peak work rate Alternative criterion: dyspnea rating 4 to 6 on Borg CR10 scale Light-intensity exercise improves symptoms, health-related quality of life, and performance of ADL Vigorous-intensity exercise optimizes physiologic improvement	> 60% maximal work rate	High intensity (60% to 80% peak work rate)
Duration	No specific recommendation for total length of session. Duration recommendations are based on severity of COPD; individuals with moderate to severe COPD may be able to exercise at a specific intensity for only a few minutes during the initial stages of training and may require intermittent interval training initially	20 to 60 min per session	20 to 60 min per session for 4 to 12 wks
Progression	Individualized on the basis of health and fitness status. These are general guidelines for older adults that may apply Initial: increase duration by 5 to 10 min every 1 to 2 wks during first 4 to 6 wks Thereafter, gradual increase in duration, frequency, and/or intensity	Titrate to symptoms 4 to 6 on Borg scale or 12 to 14 on RPE scale	Options Include titrating to selected RPE level, dyspnea scale rates, or predetermined MET level
Commend	Intermittent training may initially be used until individuals can tolerate longer duration exercise Shorter, intermittent bouts involving vigorous exercise intensity have been reported to decrease symptom ratings	For individuals who cannot tolerate continuous training owing to intolerable symptoms, interval training should be considered	Interval training should be considered for individuals who cannot sustain extended continuous periods of high-intensity exercise Warm-up before and cool-down after exercise
	ACSM	**ATS/ERS**	**AACVPR**
Resistance exercise	Note: The ACSM guidelines do not include specific recommendations (or resistance training and flexibility exercises in patients with COPD but refer to the recommendations for use with older and healthy adults. The following statements reflect those recommendations.	Resistance exercise should follow the same FITT principle exercise prescription for healthy and/or older adults	Not stated
Modality	Emphasize functional activities (e.g., stair-climbing) Free weights, machines with stacked weights or pneumatic resistance, resistance bands	Repetitive lifting of relatively heavy	Weight lifting: hand and ankle weights, free weights, machine weights, elastic resistance, using one's body weight (stair-climbing, squats)

BOX 18.4 Guidelines for Exercise Interventions in Patients with COPD[78]—cont'd

Frequency	≥ 2 d/wk	2 to 3 times per week	Not stated.
Initial intensity	Light intensity: 40% to 50% 1RM Moderate intensity: 60% to 70% 1RM	60% to 70% 1RM or 100% of 8 to 12 RM	Begin with lower weights/resistance and higher repetitions to increase muscle endurance On individual basis, higher weights and fewer repetitions may be indicated to promote strength development
Duration	1 to 4 sets; 8 to 10 exercises; 10 to 15 repetitions to improve muscular strength/endurance	Not stated	Not stated
Progression	Gradual progression increasing resistance and/or repetitions and/or frequency	Increase weight, number of repetitions per set, number of sets per session or reduce rests when individuals can perform 1 to 2 repetitions over the desired number on 2 consecutive sessions	Monitor RPE plus muscle/joint fatigue, soreness, and pain
Comments	Rest 2 to 3 min between sets; use proper techniques for each exercise; move through entire range of motion; use proper breathing technique; exercise each major muscle group using multijoint and single joint exercises	Endurance training is the mainstay of pulmonary rehabilitation. However, resistance exercise will confer greater gains in muscle mass and muscle force and evoke less dyspnea	For osteoporosis: Caution with spine flexion/rotation and heavy weight training For pulmonary hypertension: Low resistance training with paced breathing, aerobic training is acceptable
	ACSM	**ATS/ERS**	**AACVPR**
Upper limb exercise			
Modality	Not stated	Endurance exercise (e.g., arm ergometry) and/or resistance exercise (i.e., free weights and elastic bands)	Task-specific training of muscles involved in functional living
Frequency	Not stated	Not specifically stated, but would be consistent with above recommendations	Not stated
Initial intensity	Not stated	Not stated	Not stated
Duration	Not stated	Not stated	Not stated
Progression	Not stated	Not specifically stated, but would be consistent with above recommendations	Not stated
Comments	Not stated	Improves upper limb function (e.g., strength and performance during upper limb tasks)	Not stated
	ACSM	**ATS/ERS**	**AACVPR**
Flexibility exercise			
Modality	Any physical activity that maintains or increases flexibility using slow movements that involve sustained stretches for each major muscle group	Stretching of major muscle groups	Balance training and stretching to increase range of motion (e.g., modified (yoga for whole-body stretching with coordinated breathing)
Initial intensity	Stretch to point of feeling tightness or slight discomfort	Not stated	Not stated
Duration	10 to 30 s static stretch; holding stretch for 30 to 60 s may increase benefit in older patients	Not stated	Not stated
Progression	30 to 60 s of total stretch for each exercise 2 to 4 repetitions for each exercise	Not stated	Not stated
Frequency	≥ 2 d/wk	2 to 3 times per week	Not stated

BOX 18.4 Guidelines for Exercise Interventions in Patients with COPD[78]—cont'd

Program duration	Not stated	Longer programs are thought to produce greater gains and maintenance of benefits; a minimum of 8 weeks is recommended to achieve a substantial effect	4 to 12 wks
Comments	Series of stretches for each major muscle-tendon group (chest, shoulders, upper and lower back, abdomen, hips, and legs)	No clinical trials to support the inclusion of this component. Nevertheless, it is commonly included in pulmonary rehabilitation programs.	Goal of increasing ROM. Target-specific muscle groups to ensure good posture and proper body mechanicals and minimize joint and muscle injury

AACVPR, American Association of Cardiovascular and Pulmonary Rehabilitation; ACSM, American College of Sports Medicine; ADL, activities of daily living; ATS, American Thoracic Society; COPD, chronic obstructive pulmonary disease; ERS, European Respiratory Society; FITT, frequency, intensity, time, type; MET, metabolic equivalent; RM, repetition maximum; ROM, range of movement; RPE, rating of perceived exertion.
Reprinted with permission.

and the forced expiratory technique. Autogenic drainage typically takes several sessions to teach and learn, whereas the active cycle of breathing and the forced expiratory technique can generally be learned within a single session. Techniques requiring assistive devices vary in scale from simple acapella, flutter, or PEP therapies, to more complex intermittent positive pressure ventilation. Manual techniques may be applied, such as chest percussion, vibration, and shaking.

All of these techniques can be used in conjunction with positioning for bronchial drainage.[4,80] When selecting airway clearance techniques, the patient's preference should be taken into consideration, as well as each individual's specific symptom presentation and pathophysiology. Older adults may have more limited tolerance to head down positions for postural drainage. Osteoporosis is a precaution for manual percussion and vibration over the rib cage. The ability to remember and follow instructions may be affected in older adults with cognitive impairment, and this should be taken into consideration during the educational process.

Asthma

Asthma is characterized by episodic, reversible airway obstruction related to inflammation leading to hyperreactivity within the lungs. Between exacerbations lung function can be relatively normal. Exacerbations, or "asthma attacks," may be triggered by air pollutants, allergens (e.g., pollen, animal dander, food allergies), respiratory infections, exercise, and medication. Medications that have been linked to asthma include nonsteridal anti-inflammatory drugs (NSAIDs), aspirin, nonselective beta blockers, and ACE inhibitors.

Approximately 10% of older adults have a past medical history that includes asthma. It is estimated that as many as 25% of older adults may be undiagnosed with asthma. It often takes 5 years before a diagnosis of asthma is made despite the presence of classic symptoms, and only about one-third of older adults affected by asthma are under appropriate medical care for their condition.[4,81] Thorough history taking and evaluation may facilitate earlier diagnosis and provide clues regarding the severity of the patient's condition. This will help direct appropriate disease management to minimize exacerbations.

An asthma exacerbation is characterized by the onset of shortness of breath, sensations of chest tightness, and wheezing (especially during the expiratory phase), after exposure to a known or unknown trigger. Exacerbations may be avoided by identifying and avoiding asthma triggers, use of bronchodilators (both short-acting and long-acting), and individualized exercise training.[81,82] The benefits of exercise training as well as guidelines for exercise prescription mirror those of the general public, including a beneficial impact on quality of life and overall cardiopulmonary fitness.[82]

Although exercise is an effective intervention for the long-term management of asthma, exercise can also trigger an asthma attack. Exercise-induced asthma (EIA) is thought to be caused by a loss of water or heat from the lower respiratory system. Breathing through the mouth during exercise bypasses the nasal passages that warm and humidify the inspired air. EIA symptoms can occur during or immediately after exercise, or up to 2 to 8 hours after the cessation of exercise. The therapist must be aware of each patient's asthma triggers in order to minimize the risk of exacerbation during exercise while closely monitoring the patient for onset of symptoms.[4]

Physical therapist should understand the role of bronchodilators. Short-acting bronchodilators are commonly referred to as "rescue" medications because of their ability to cause rapid relaxation of airway smooth muscle. The two major classes of short-acting bronchodilators are beta-adrenergic agonists and anticholinergics. Long-acting bronchodilators are used in patients with moderate-to-severe asthma in order to prevent or reduce the frequency of exacerbations. They include beta-adrenergic agonists with longer mechanisms of action (salmeterol, formoterol), corticosteroids (fluticasone, budesonide, beclomethasone), leukotriene receptor antagonists (montelukast), and mast cell stabilizers (cromolyn sodium). Long-acting medications are not useful in managing an acute asthma exacerbation. Long-acting medications are commonly administered via metered dose inhalers (MDIs) or dry powder inhalers (DPIs), which require both a coordinated effort and the ability to generate an effective inhalation to intake each dose. Proper administration of medication with an MDI is facilitated with the addition of a spacer chamber, and one-on-one instruction in its use. Medications may also be delivered via a nebulized solution, which may be appropriate if the patient is having difficulty utilizing an MDI or DPI effectively.

Restrictive Pulmonary Disease

Restrictive pulmonary disease (RPD) is a broad category that includes a vast number of diseases. The common characteristic of all restrictive pulmonary disease types is the reduction of lung volumes owing to decreased compliance of the chest wall and lung tissue. RPD can result from an alteration to any structure within the thorax: from the musculoskeletal components to the parenchyma and the pleura. Additionally, even in the absence of a primary decrease in lung compliance, dysfunction of the neuromuscular system, which affects the ability of the respiratory muscles to generate sufficient force to create the pressure gradients required for adequate air movement and gas exchange, can result in a restrictive lung disease. The hallmark symptom of RPD is dyspnea with a rapid shallow breathing pattern. Dry crackles may be auscultated. The patient is likely to be hypoxemic and, in advanced cases, demonstrate cyanosis and nail clubbing. As in obstructive pulmonary disease, persistent pulmonary dysfunction may lead to pulmonary hypertension and cor pulmonale.[83]

The gold standard for diagnosis of RPD, direct measurement of TLC by body plethysmography or helium/nitrogen wash-outs, are not always available in general clinical practice. Therefore, measurement of FVC via spirometry is the most commonly utilized method to clinically diagnose RPD. The diagnostic criteria for RPD is TLC or FVC values less than 80% of expected for age, sex, and height, while having an FEV_1/FVC ratio that is either normal or closer to 1.[84,85]

Epidemiologic studies have found that between 7% and 13% of the general population has identifiable restrictive pattern deficits. Additionally, it has been estimated that from approximately the age of 30, vital capacity begins to decline in an amount approximating 30 mL a year.[83] Individuals with RPD are at increased risk for all cause and cardiovascular mortality, and also have significant functional impairment and various comorbid conditions, including diabetes, metabolic syndrome, hypertension, stroke, and cardiovascular disease.[86] Some general risk factors for restrictive lung disease that have been identified include age 50 years or older, body mass index (BMI) of 30 or greater, and nonwhite race. Cognitive decline and disability, more common in older adults, can affect the quality of spirometry measurements. More research is needed on the reliability of spirometry scores in the diagnosis of restrictive lung diseases for older adults.[87]

Table 18.15 provides a representative list of the wide range of health conditions that can lead to RPD. Treatment interventions for RPD vary and are dependent on

TABLE 18.15 Categories of Restrictive Lung Disease and Common Precipitating Causes

Restrictive Pulmonary Diseases	
Interstitial Lung Diseases	Pulmonary fibrosis
	Idiopathic pulmonary fibrosis
	Sarcoidosis
	Eosinophilic pulmonary infiltrate
	Bronchiolitis obliterans
	Scleroderma
Connective Tissue Disorders	Rheumatoid arthritis
	Systemic lupus erythematous
	Polymyositis
	Dermatomyositis
Environmental	Pneumoconiosis
	Silicosis
	Asbestosis
Infectious	Bacterial
	Viral
	Fungal

Continued

TABLE 18.15 Categories of Restrictive Lung Disease and Common Precipitating Causes—cont'd

Restrictive Pulmonary Diseases	
Neoplastic	Lung cancer
Cardiovascular	Pulmonary embolism Pulmonary edema
Other Pulmonary	Atelectasis ARDS/ALI
Musculoskeletal	Kyphosis/scoliosis/kyphoscoliosis Ankylosing spondylitis Pectus carinatum/excavatum Diaphragmatic paralysis/paresis Trauma/fractures
Neurologic	Spinal cord injury Cerebrovascular accident Poliomyelitis Amyotrophic lateral sclerosis Guillain-Barre syndrome Myasthenia gravis Tetanus Muscular dystrophy
Immunologic	Goodpasture's syndrome Wegener's granulomatosis
Nutritional/Metabolic	Obesity Diabetes
Pharmaceutical/Chemical	Oxygen Antibiotics Amiodarone Chemotherapy Poisons/toxins Anesthetics/muscle relaxants Cocaine/heroin Talc
Other	Surgery (thoracic and abdominal) Pregnancy Radiation pneumonitis and fibrosis

addressing the cause of the restrictive impairment. In general, older adults with RPD may benefit from the generalized interventions for impaired aerobic capacity, including endurance training, strength training, flexibility training, airway clearance techniques, and breathing exercises with specific respiratory muscle training. It is important to consider the progression of pathologic alterations, as once the lung has undergone fibrotic changes, the pathologic alterations are irreversible and interventions are used with a supportive or compensatory mindset.

SUMMARY

In summary, the impairment of aerobic capacity in older adults is typically related to multiple factors, including age-related physiologic changes, specific pathology, and the ongoing cycle of decreased physical activity and deconditioning. Research has upheld the numerous benefits of aerobic exercise training for healthy older adults as well as for adults with a variety of cardiovascular and pulmonary diseases. The additional components of a comprehensive physical therapy approach to individualized interventions should not be ignored. The understanding of specific pathophysiologic processes of common diseases will help to ensure patient safety during treatment intervention as well as to guide exercise prescription and assessment of exercise tolerance.

REFERENCES

1. Brooks GA, Fahey TD, Baldwin KM. *Exercise Physiology: Human Bioenergetics and Its Applications.* New York, NY: McGraw-Hill; 2005.
2. Ehrman JK, Gordon PM, Visich PS, Keteyian SJ. *Clinical Exercise Physiology.* Champaign, IL: Human Kinetics; 2009.
3. Tanaka H, Monahan KD, Seals DR. Age-predicted maximal heart rate revisited. *J Am Coll Cardiol.* 1;37(1):153–6. 2001.
4. DeTurk WE, Cahalin LP. *Cardiovascular and Pulmonary Physical Therapy: An Evidence-Based Approach.* New York: McGraw-Hill Professional; 2018.
5. Heckman GA, McKelvie RS. Cardiovascular aging and exercise in healthy older adults. *Clin J Sport Med.* 2008;18:479–485.
6. Marwick TH, Hordern MD, Miller T, et al. Exercise training for type 2 diabetes mellitus: impact on cardiovascular risk: a scientific statement from the American Heart Association. *Circulation.* 2009;119:3244–3262.
7. Cade WT. Diabetes-related microvascular and macrovascular diseases in the physical therapy setting. *Phys Ther.* 2008;88: 1322–1335.

7a. Bengel FM, Ueberfuhr P, Schiepel N, et al. Effect of sympathetic reinnervation on cardiac performance after heart transplan tation. *N Engl J Med.* 2001;345:731–738.

8. Tanaka H, Seals DR. Invited review: dynamic exercise performance in Masters athletes: insight into the effects of primary human aging on physiological functional capacity. *J Appl Physiol.* 2003;95:2152–2162.
9. Taylor BJ, Johnson BD. The pulmonary circulation and exercise responses in the elderly. *Semin Respir Crit Care Med.* 2010;31:528–538.
10. Go AS, Mozaffarian D, Roger VL, et al. Heart disease and stroke statistics-2013 update: a Report from the American Heart Association. *Circulation.* 2013;127(1):e6–e245. doi: https://doi.org/10.1161/CIR.0b013e31828124ad.
11. Carey RM, Whelton PK. Prevention, detection, evaluation, and management of high blood pressure in adults: synopsis of the 2017 American College of Cardiology/American Heart Association hypertension guideline. *Ann Intern Med.* 2018;168(5):351–358.
12. Bhammar DM, Siddhartha SA, Glenn AG. Effects of fractionized and continuous exercise on 24-h ambulatory blood pressure. *Med Sci Sports Exerc.* 2012;44(12): 2270–2276.
13. Park S, Rink LD, Wallace JP. Accumulation of physical activity leads to a greater blood pressure reduction than a single continuous session, in prehypertension. *J Hypertens.* 2006;24 (9):1761–1770.
14. Costa EC, Hay JL, Kehler DS, et al. Effects of high-intensity interval training versus moderate-intensity continuous training on blood pressure in adults with pre-to established hypertension: a systematic review and meta-analysis of randomized trials. *Sports Med.* 2018;48(9):1–6.
15. Kessler HS, Sisson SB, Short KR. The potential for high-intensity interval training to reduce cardiometabolic disease risk. *Sports Med.* 2012;42(6):489–509.
16. Moore G, Durstine JL, Painter P. *ACSM's Exercise Management for Persons with Chronic Diseases and Disabilities.* In: *Human Kinetics* ed 4. Champaign, IL: American College of Sports Medicine; 2016.
17. Coelho VA, Probst VS, Nogari BM, et al. Angiotensin-II blockage, muscle strength, and exercise capacity in physically independent older adults. *Journal of Physical Therapy Science.* 2016;28(2):547–552.
18. Lenz TL, DeSimone EM, Pomeroy JM. Implementing lifestyle medicine in hypertensive patients. *U.S Pharmacist.* 2011;36 (2):44–50.
19. Kannel WB, Castelli WP, Gordon T, McNamara PM. Serum cholesterol, lipoproteins, and the risk of coronary heart disease. The Framingham Study. *Ann Intern Med.* 1971;74 (1):1–12. http://annals.org/.
20. Sharrett AR, Ballantyne CM, Coady SA, et al. Coronary heart disease prediction from lipoprotein cholesterol levels, triglycerides, lipoprotein (a), apolipoproteins AI and B, and HDL density subfractions: The Atherosclerosis Risk in Communities (ARIC) Study. *Circulation.* 2001;104(10): 1108–1113.
21. Odden MC, Shlipak MG, Whitson HE, et al. Risk factors for cardiovascular disease across the spectrum of older age: the Cardiovascular Health Study. *Atherosclerosis.* 2014;237(1): 336–342.
22. Stone GW, Maehara A, Lansky AJ, et al. A prospective natural-history study of coronary atherosclerosis. *N Engl J Med.* 201;364(3):226–35.
23. Amsterdam EA, Wenger NK, Brindis RG, et al. 2014 AHA/ACC guideline for the management of patients with non–ST-elevation acute coronary syndromes: a report of the American College of Cardiology/American Heart Association Task Force on Practice Guidelines. *J Am Coll Cardiol.* 2014;64 (24):e139–e228.
24. O'Gara PT, Kushner FG, Ascheim DD, et al. 2013 ACCF/AHA guideline for the management of ST-elevation myocardial infarction: a report of the American College of Cardiology Foundation/American Heart Association Task Force on Practice Guidelines. *J Am Coll Cardiol.* 2013;61 (4):e78–140.
25. Cassady S, Cahalin L. Cardiovascular pathophysiology. In: DeTurk W, Cahalin L. *Cardiovascular and Pulmonary Physical Therapy* ed 3. New York, NY: McGraw-Hill Education/Medical; 2017
26. Garza MA, Wason EA, Zhang JQ. Cardiac remodeling and physical training post myocardial infarction. *World Journal of Cardiology.* 2015;7(2):52–64. https://doi.org/10.4330/wjc.v7.i2.52.
27. Haykowsky M, Scott J, Esch B, et al. A meta-analysis of the effects of exercise training on left ventricular remodeling following myocardial infarction: start early and go longer for greatest exercise benefits on remodeling. *Trials.* 2011;12(1):92.
28. Senaratne MP, Smith G, Gulamhusein SS. Feasibility and safety of early exercise testing using the Bruce protocol after acute myocardial infarction. *J Am Coll Cardiol.* 2000;35(5):1212–1220.
29. Forman DE, Fleg JL, Kitzman DW, et al. 6-min walk test provides prognostic utility comparable to cardiopulmonary exercise testing in ambulatory outpatients with systolic heart failure. *J Am Coll Cardiol.* 2012;60(25):2653–2661.
30. Fletcher GF, Ades PA, Kligfield P, et al. on behalf of the American Heart Association Exercise, Cardiac Rehabilitation, and Prevention Committee of the Council on Clinical Cardiology, Council on Nutrition, Physical Activity and Metabolism, Council on Cardio- vascular and Stroke Nursing, and Council on Epidemiology and Prevention. Exercise standards for testing and training: a scientific statement from the American Heart Association. *Circulation.* 2013;128:873–934.
31. Arena R, Myers J, Kaminsky LA. Revisiting age-predicted maximal heart rate: can it be used as a valid measure of effort? *Am Heart J.* 2016;173:49–56.

32. Gjovaag T, Mirtaheri P, Simon K, et al. Hemodynamic responses to resistance exercise in patients with coronary artery disease. *Med Sci Sports Exerc*. 2016;48(4):581–588.
33. Hollings M, Mavros Y, Freeston J, Fiatarone Singh M. The effect of progressive resistance training on aerobic fitness and strength in adults with coronary heart disease: a systematic review and meta-analysis of randomised controlled trials. *European Journal of Preventive Cardiology*. 2017;24 (12):1242–1259.
34. Xanthos PD, Gordon BA, Kingsley MI. Implementing resistance training in the rehabilitation of coronary heart disease: a systematic review and meta-analysis. *Int J Cardiol*. 2017;230:493–508.
35. Riebe D, Ehrman JK, Liguori G, Magal M. *ACSM's Guidelines for Exercise Testing and Prescription*, ed 10. Philadelphia, PA: Wolters Kluwer; 2018.
36. Novaro GM, Katz R, Aviles RJ, et al. Clinical factors, but not C-reactive protein, predict progression of calcific aortic-valve disease: the Cardiovascular Health Study. *J Am Coll Cardiol*. 2007;50(20):1992–1998.
37. Bhatia N, Basra SS, Skolnick AH, Wenger NK. Aortic valve disease in the older adult. *J Geriatr Cardiol: JGC*. 2016;13 (12):941.
38. Spaccarotella C, Mongiardo A, Indolfi C. Pathophysiology of aortic stenosis and approach to treatment with percutaneous valve implantation. *Circ J*. 2010;75(1):11–19.
39. Zilberszac R, Gabriel H, Schemper M, Laufer G, Maurer G, Rosenhek R. Asymptomatic severe aortic stenosis in the elderly. *JACC Cardiovasc Imaging*. 2017;10(1):43–50.
40. Otto CM, Kumbhani DJ, Alexander KP, et al. Writing Committee. 2017 ACC expert consensus decision pathway for transcatheter aortic valve replacement in the management of adults with aortic stenosis: a report of the American College of Cardiology Task Force on Clinical Expert Consensus Documents. *J Am Coll Cardiol*. 2017;69(10): 1313–1346.
41. Roger VL. Epidemiology of heart failure. *Circ Res*. 2013;113 (6):646–659.
42. Yancy CW, Jessup M, Bozkurt B, et al. 2013 ACCF/AHA guideline for the management of heart failure: a report of the American College of Cardiology Foundation/American Heart Association Task Force on Practice Guidelines. *Journal of the American College of Cardiology*. 2013;62(16):e147–e239.
43. Ho K, Pinsky J, Kannel W, Levy D. The epidemiology of heart failure: the Framingham Study. *J Am Coll Cardiol*. 1993;22(4 Suppl A):6A–13A.
44. Danielsen R, Thorgeirsson G, Einarsson H, et al. Prevalence of heart failure in the elderly and future projections: the AGES-Reykjavík study. *Scand Cardiovasc J*. 2017;51(4):183–189.
45. Gorodeski EZ, Goyal P, Hummel SL, et al. Domain management approach to heart failure in the geriatric patient: present and future. *J Am Coll Cardiol*. 2018;71(17): 1921–1936. https://doi.org/10.1016/j.jacc.2018.02.059.
46. Joseph SM, Rich MW. Targeting frailty in heart failure. Current treatment options in cardiovascular medicine. *Curr Treat Options Cardiovasc Med*. 2017;19(4):31.
47. Fried LP, Tangen CM, Walston J, et al. Frailty in older adults: evidence for a phenotype. *J Gerontol A Biol Sci Med Sci*. 2001;56(3):M146–M157.
48. Lee L, Patel T, Costa A, et al. Screening for frailty in primary care: accuracy of gait speed and hand-grip strength. *Can Fam Physician*. 2017;63(1):e51–e57.
49. Hsu C-Y, Hsieh P-L, Hsiao S-F, Chien M-Y. Effects of exercise training on autonomic function in chronic heart failure: systematic review. *Biomedical Research International*. 2015;591708.
50. Davies EJ, Moxham T, Rees K, et al. Exercise training for systolic heart failure: Cochrane systematic review and meta-analysis. *Eur J Heart Fail*. 2010;12(7):706–715. https://doi.org/10.1093/eurjhf/hfq056.
51. Forman DE, Arena R, Boxer R, et al. Prioritizing functional capacity as a principal end point for therapies oriented to older adults with cardiovascular disease: a scientific statement for healthcare professionals from the American Heart Association. *Circulation*. 2017;135(16):e894–e918.
52. Piepoli MF, Conraads V, Corr U, et al. Exercise training in heart failure: from theory to practice. A consensus document of the Heart Failure Association and the European Association for Cardiovascular Prevention and Rehabilitation. *Eur J Heart Fail*. 2011;13(4):347–357. https://doi.org/10.1093/eurjhf/hfr017.
53. Edelmann F, Gelbrich G, Dngen HD, et al. Exercise training improves exercise capacity and diastolic function in patients with heart failure with preserved ejection fraction: results of the Ex-DHF (exercise training in diastolic heart failure) pilot study. *J Am Coll Cardiol*. 2011;58(17):1780–1791.
54. Cahalin LP, Mathier MA, Semigran MJ, Dec GW, DiSalvo TG. The six-minute walk test predicts peak oxygen uptake and survival in patients with advanced heart failure. *Chest*. 1996;110(2):325–332.
55. Collins S. A Clinical Practice Guideline Update on Chronic Heart Failure. APTA Combined Sections Meeting, 24 February 2018, Hilton Riverside, New Orleans, Louisiana, Educational Session.
56. Kelkar AA, Spertus J, Pierson R. Utility of patient-reported outcome instruments in heart failure. *J Am Coll Cardiol: Heart Failure*. 2016;4(3):165–175.
57. Morillo CA, Banerjee A, Perel P, Wood D, Jouven X. Atrial fibrillation: the current epidemic. *J Geriatr Cardiol*. 2017;14 (3):195–203.
58. Sharma PS, Callans DJ. Treatment considerations for a dual epidemic of atrial fibrillation and heart failure. *Journal of Atrial Fibrillation*. 2013;6(2):740.
59. Alipour P. Chapter 4. Approaches to treatment of atrial fibrillation. In: *Cardiac Arrhythmia*. Telangana, India: AvidScience; 2016:2–39.
60. Amin A, Houmsse A, Ishola A, Tyler J, Houmsse M. The current approach of atrial fibrillation management. *Avicenna J Med*. 2016;6(1):8–16.
61. McDermott MM. Lower extremity manifestations of peripheral artery disease: the pathophysiologic and functional implications of leg ischemia. *Circ Res*. 2015;116(9):1540–1550.
62. Hardman RL, Jazaeri O, Yi J, Smith M, Gupta R. Overview of classification systems in peripheral artery disease. *Seminars in Interventional Radiology*. 2014;31(4):378–388.
62a. Diaz-Guzman E, Mannino DM. Airway obstructive diseases in older adults: from detection to treatment. *J Allergy Clin Immunol*. 2010;126(4):702–709. https://doi.org/10.1016/j.jaci. 2010.08.022.
63. Hillegass E, Fick A, Pawlik A, et al. Supplemental oxygen utilization during physical therapy interventions. *Cardiopulmonary Physical Therapy Journal*. 2014;25:38–49.
64. Wu A, Coresh J, Selvin E, et al. Lower extremity peripheral artery disease and quality of life among older individuals in the community. *J Am Heart Assoc*. 2017;6(1):e004519.
65. Lyu X, Li S, Peng S, Cai H, Liu G, Ran X. Intensive walking exercise for lower extremity peripheral arterial disease: a systematic review and meta-analysis. *J Diabetes*. 2016;8(3): 363–377.
66. Vogelmeier CF, Criner GJ, Martinez FJ, et al. Global strategy for the diagnosis, management and prevention of chronic obstructive lung disease. Report GOLD Executive Summary. *Respirology*. 2017;22:575–601.
67. Akinbami LJ, Liu X. NCHS Data Brief, Number 63. http://www.cdc.gov/nchs/data/databriefs/db63_tables.pdf#2.
68. Croft JB, Wheaton AG, Liu Y, et al. Urban-rural county and state differences in chronic obstructive pulmonary

disease—United States, 2015. *MMWR Morb Mortal Wkly Rep*. 2018;67(7):205–211. https://doi.org/10.15585/mmwr.mm6707a1.
69. Ford ES, Murphy LB, Khavjou O, Giles WH, Holt JB, Croft JB. Total and state-specific medical and absenteeism costs of COPD among adults aged ≥ 18 years in the United States for 2010 and projections through 2020. *Chest*. 2015;147(1):31–45. https://doi.org/10.1378/chest.14-0972.
70. Mapel DW. Improved survival in COPD: reasons for hope. *Thorax*. 2010;65(4):284–285. https://doi.org/10.1136/thx.2009.128330.
71. Deleted in Proof.
72. Gea J, Agusti A, Roca J. Pathophysiology of muscle dysfunction in COPD. *J Appl Physiol*. 2013;114(9):1222–1234. https://doi.org/10.1152/japplphysiol.00981.2012.
73. Alter A, Aboussouan LS, Mireles-Cabodevila E. Neuro-'muscular weakness in chronic obstructive pulmonary disease: Chest wall, diaphragm, and peripheral muscle contributions. *Curr Opin Pulm Med*. 2017;23(2):129–138.
74. Mahmudi-Azer S. Breathing easier: respiratory disease in the older adult. In: *Evidence-Based Geriatric Medicine*. Oxford, UK: Wiley-Blackwell; 2012:43–57. https://doi.org/10.1002/9781118281796.ch4.
75. Spruit MA, Singh SJ, Garvey C, et al. An official american Thoracic Society/European Respiratory Society statement: key concepts and advances in pulmonary rehabilitation. *Am J Respir Crit Care Med*. 2013;188(8):e13–e64. https://doi.org/10.1164/rccm.201309-1634ST.
76. Gloeckl R, Marinov B, Pitta F. Practical recommendations for exercise training in patients with COPD. *Ear Respir Rev*. 2013;22(128):178–186. https://doi.org/10.1183/09059180.00000513.
77. Evans RA, Dolmage TE, Mangovski-Alzamora S, et al. One-legged cycle training for chronic obstructive pulmonary disease: a pragmatic study of implementation to pulmonary rehabilitation. *Ann Am Thorac Soc*. 2015;12(10):1490–1497. https://doi.org/10.1513/AnnalsATS.201504-231OC.
78. Garvey C, Bayles MP, Hamm LF, et al. Pulmonary rehabilitation exercise prescription in chronic obstructive pulmonary disease: review of selected guidelines: an official statement from the American Association of Cardiovascular and Pulmonary Rehabilitation. *J Cardiopulm Rehabil Prev*. 2016;36(2):75–83. https://doi.org/10.1097/HCR.0000000000000171.
79. Beaumont M, Forget P, Couturaud F, Reychler G. Effects of inspiratory muscle training in COPD patients: a systematic review and meta-analysis. *Clin Respir J*. 2018;12(7):2178–2188. https://doi.org/10.1111/crj.12905.
80. Hillegass EA. *Essentials of Cardiopulmonary Physical Therapy*. St. Louis, MO: Elsevier; 2017.
81. Gibson PG, McDonald VM, Marks GB. Asthma in older adults. *Lancet*. 2010;376(9743):803–813. https://doi.org/10.1016/S0140-6736(10)61087-2.
82. Craig TJ, Dispenza MC. Benefits of exercise in asthma. *Ann Allergy Asthma Immunol*. 2013;110(3):133–140, e2. https://doi.org/10.1016/j.anai.2012.10.023.
83. Scarlata S, Pedone C, Fimognari FL, Bellia V, Forastiere F, Incalzi RA. Restrictive pulmonary dysfunction at spirometry and mortality in the elderly. *Respir Med*. 2008;102(9):1349–1354. https://doi.org/10.1016/j.rmed.2008.02.021.
84. Hankinson JL, Odencrantz JR, Fedan KB. Spirometric reference values from a sample of the general U.S. population. *Am J Respir Crit Care Med*. 1999;159:179–187.
85. Pellegrino R, Viegi G, Brusasco V, et al. Interpretative strategies for lung function tests. *Eur Respir J*. 2005;26:948–968.
86. Guerra S, Sherrill DL, Venker C, Ceccato CM, Halonen M, Martinez FD. Morbidity and mortality associated with the restrictive spirometric pattern: a longitudinal study. *Thorax*. 2010;65(6):499–504. https://doi.org/10.1136/thx.2009. 126052.
87. Backman H, Eriksson B, Hedman L, et al. Restrictive spirometric pattern in the general adult population: methods of defining the condition and consequences on prevalence. *Respir Med*. 2016;120:116–123. https://doi.org/10.1016/j.rmed.2016.10.005.
88. Seth S, Vashista S. The Hriday Card: a checklist for heart failure. *Journal of the Practice of Cardiovascular Sciences*. 2017;3(1):5–7.
89. Chobanian AV, Bakris GL, Black HR, et al. The Seventh Report of the Joint National Committee on Prevention, Detection, Evaluation, and Treatment of High Blood Pressure: the JNC 7 Report. *JAMA*. 2003;289(19):2560–2571. https://doi.org/10.1001/jama.289.19.2560.
90. Gielen S, Laughlin MH, O'Conner C, Duncker DJ. Exercise training in patients with heart disease: review of beneficial effects and clinical recommendations. *Prog Cardiovasc Dis*. 2015;57(4):347–355.
91. Cornelis N, Buys R, Fourneau I, Dewit T, Cornelissen V. Exploring physical activity behaviour needs for and interest in a technology-delivered, home-based exercise programme among patients with intermittent claudication. *VASA*. 2018; 47:109–117. https://doi.org/10.1024/0301-1526/a000654.

CHAPTER

19

Cognitive Issues in the Older Adult

Cathy Haines Ciolek, Sin Yi Lee

OUTLINE

INTRODUCTION

Older adults fear cognitive changes more than any other aspect that comes with age. Dementia, the most common cognitive loss with age, occurs across a continuum. As understanding and knowledge about dementia and its impact develops, it is imperative that physical therapists align their knowledge and practice with contemporary evidence. This chapter sets forth what is currently known and understood about dementia and how physical therapy can have an impact on the individual with cognitive issues and how cognitive issues can have an impact on the physical therapy session.

NORMAL COGNITIVE AGING

Cognition is a complex and interwoven series of functions that are responsible for regulating specific behaviors and actions of the human being. The Oxford dictionary defines cognition as "the mental action or process of acquiring knowledge and understanding through thought, experience and the senses."[1] The *Diagnostic and Statistical Manual of Mental Disorder*, 5th Edition (DSM-V) details six domains of cognitive function, including Learning and Memory, Language, Complex Attention, Executive Function, Perceptual-motor Function, and Social Cognition.[2] These cognitive domains are defined in Table 19.1.

TABLE 19.1 DSM-V Cognitive Domains

DSM-V Cognitive Domain	Example
Complex Attention	Sustained attention, selective attention, and information processing speed
Executive Function	Planning, decision-making, working memory, responding to feedback, inhibition, and mental flexibility
Learning and Memory	Free recall, cued recall, semantic and autobiographical long-term memory
Language	Object naming, word finding, fluency, and syntax
Perceptual-motor Function	Visual perception, perceptual-motor coordination
Social Cognition	Recognition of emotions, behavioral regulation, and understanding societal context

Data from American Psychiatric Association. DSM-5 Task Force. *Diagnostic and Statistical Manual of Mental Disorders: DSM-5.* American Psychiatric Association; 2013.

Cognition, as most other human biological systems, has a continuum of function from exceptional performance to disease. As we age, subtle cognitive changes occur that are considered normal. Aspects of cognition that remain relatively stable with age include some aspects of memory, language, and social cognition.[3, 4] Implicit memory, defined as the "unconscious influence of previously encountered information on subsequent performance, is often stable with age or shows only slight age-related changes (Table 19.2).[3] Thus, physical therapists should expect that patients with normal cognition will express appropriate emotion, accurately remember their past, process current information, and make appropriate decisions that align with their past experiences and current value system.

However, other domains of cognition, such as processing speed, encoding of information into episodic memory,[3] short-term memory, and executive functioning, show gradual and linear declines throughout the lifespan.[5] Research has noted little accelerated decline in the later decades in these cognitive functions. Age differences are also demonstrated by a reduced learning ability, retrieval of both nonverbal and verbal information[4] and reduction in cognitive flexibility.[6] Therefore, in the absence of pathology, an older person may demonstrate slower processing time, the need for more rehearsal to encode information into long-term memory, a decreased ability to multi-task and difficulty finding alternate methods of problem solving when their "usual" method is compromised. These areas are discussed below.

Memory

The three main interrelated components of memory are sensory, short-term, and long-term memory (further described in Table 19.2). The process of remembering begins with a sensory event that is seen, heard, experienced, or felt, called *sensory memory*. Sensory memory

TABLE 19.2 Types of Memory

Memory	Subset	Definition	Changes with Age	Location
Sensory	Iconic (visual) Echoic (auditory) Haptic (touch)	Input from the 5 senses; can be ignored or perceived and transferred to short memory in <1 second.	Stable except for sensory impairment that may occur with age. (e.g., visual or hearing loss)	Initial input to sensory areas of the brain and then processed by hippocampus
Short-term (or working memory)		Limited capacity Temporary recall Processed in 10–15 seconds long-term storage or decay	Stable, but may require more effort to encode before decay.	Prefrontal cortex
Long-term	**Implicit** (or procedural)	Subconscious influence of previously encountered information on subsequent performance Automatic, rote	Stable (e.g., remains intact until late in a cognitive disease state)	Cerebellum, putamen, caudate nucleus, and motor cortex
	Explicit (or declarative) **Semantic**	Structured facts, meanings, concepts, and knowledge	Gradual and linear decline across lifespan; primarily associated with encoding and retrieval	Prefrontal and temporal cortex
	Explicit (or declarative) **Episodic**	Autobiographical of events, contextual knowledge, and associated emotions	Gradual and linear decline across lifespan primarily associated with encoding and retrieval.	Hippocampus connects various sensory areas of the brain to create an "episode" that is consolidated to one event

is very brief, lasting a portion of a second. If attended to (most sensory experiences never make it any farther), the sensory memory is encoded into short-term memory. Sensory memory reaches short-term memory through attention or focus. Short-term memory involves a combination of short-term storage and executive processes.[7] Short-term memory is quite limited, generally only holding five to nine items at a time. To transfer (encode) short-term memory items into long-term memory, encoding in the form of rehearsal or repetition must happen. Encoding is an effortful process and includes memorization. Repetition is the key to moving items from short-term memory into long-term memory.

There are several implications for physical therapists regarding memory processing. For example, getting a patient's attention through a sensory experience, such as touch, may enhance focus. Eliminating distractions (i.e., reducing too much sensory input) will also enhance the person's ability to retain the items needed in short-term memory. Finally, opportunities for repetition will help the brain encode the information into long-term memory.

Long-term memory can be subdivided into implicit (subconscious) and explicit (conscious) memory. Implicit memory involves procedural tasks and actions that are retained through motor learning and are considered rote. These implicit memories are generally maintained through activity (tying one's shoes, standing from a chair), but can degrade without practice or use (e.g., jumping). Explicit memory includes episodic (i.e., autobiographical memory) and semantic memory (i.e., facts and words). Older adults experience difficulties with episodic memory, reduction in the efficiency of working memory processes, as well as increased response times on memory tasks.[7] Neuroimaging studies indicate small differences in processing speed between younger and older adults for simple tasks and greater latency for complex tasks that require older adults to supplement with different neural resources.[7] This reinforces greater attention and effort required for complex memory tasks in normally aging adults and why dedicated time for patient education should be separated from functional training.

Executive Functioning

Executive functioning (or ability) involves complex behavior that combines memory, intellectual capacity, and cognitive planning. Activities of executive functioning include planning, active problem-solving, short-term memory, anticipating possible consequences of an intended course of action, initiating an activity, and being able to monitor the effectiveness of one's behavior.[8] Executive functioning is also an important factor for self-reported and observed performance of complex, independent activities of daily living (IADLs), such as managing money and medications.[9, 10] Short-term memory is the center of executive functioning; it incorporates complex attention, strategy formation, and interference control. It can be affected in conditions such as Parkinson disease where dopamine depletion can lead to a slowing down of processing speed.[11]

The interesting aspect of executive functioning is its relationship to motor function. Although there is evidence of a mild decline of executive functioning with normal aging, executive functioning declines are greater when a neurologic disorder, such as a cerebrovascular accident or dementia, is also present. Executive functioning is characterized by a decrease in planning ability, working memory, inductive reasoning, and ability to modify and update working memory.[12] For example, intact executive functioning can serve as a fall prevention measure by minimizing behavior that jeopardizes safety despite motor or sensory impairment.[13] Conversely, executive dysfunction should trigger the therapist's awareness of the risk for falls.[13] Indeed, fall risk in community-dwelling older adults is associated with reduced executive functioning including dual tasking when walking.[14] Additionally, challenges in executive function limit will result in difficulty with self-assessment to accurately reflect knowledge of performance indicators required for motor learning.

Language

Language ability remains intact with normal aging with vocabulary ability sustained over time. However, some features of language do show small declines in later aging (in the 70th decade). These include visual confrontation naming (identifying an object and naming it) and word generation to a category (e.g., animal names starting with A).[15]

Complex Attention

Simple attention shows only a slight decline in late life; however, more complex tasks show a more noticeable age-related change.[15] Selective attention (the ability to focus on specific information in the environment while ignoring less relevant information) and divided attention (multi-tasking simultaneously) do show declines in older adults compared with younger adults.[15] As with memory processing, the environment should be evaluated for optimal learning to minimize distractions or to increase distractions if the goal is to challenge the divided attention system during gait or other tasks.

Social Cognition

Social cognition involves self-behavioral regulation, along with the ability to understand the mental states of others and societal expectations. One study found that older adults were often challenged when they had to assess another person's emotional state or when having to discern the accuracy or falseness of another's statements.[16] This decline in insight may be why some older adults are more susceptible to abuse, neglect, and exploitation.

However on a positive note, some research has noted a "positivity affect" compared with younger adults where the older adult can recall more positive information than negative.[17]

Perceptual-motor Function

Processing speed for both cognitive activities and motor responses begins to decline gradually starting in the third decade. [15] Although gradual, this change in processing can result in challenges across other cognitive domains as well as in function. The impact on balance regulation and the ability to identify a loss of balance and create the appropriate motor response after a trip or slip is one example.

STRUCTURAL CHANGES IN THE BRAIN

Research suggests that normal structural changes in the aging brain may explain some, but not all, of the differences in brain activity between older and younger adults. Plaques and tangles, present in both healthy and diseased brains, are the waste products that fill up the spaces between neurons (amyloid plaques) and form inside the neuron (tangles) (Fig. 19.1). Both senile neuritic plaques and neurofibrillary tangles may be seen in cognitively intact aged individuals, but they are generally less extensive than seen in individuals with dementia of the same age. Moreover, as we age, there is a decline in gray and white matter structures and volume in the brain, especially in the frontal lobes. Such structural decline can prove significant. For example, reduction in hippocampal volume and integrity of white matter in the corpus callosum of older adults are correlated with declining memory performance.[18] In addition, volume decline in gray matter in older adults is suggested to result, not from cell death, but from lower synaptic densities in the older population.[19] If you consider that larger synaptic densities increase the range of neuronal communication, this may explain the increased processing time and loss of cognitive flexibility previously described. Age-related decline has also been found in the human striatum, a brain area that has extensive connections to the prefrontal cortex and is responsible for a large proportion of dopamine production, therefore affecting dopamine-dependent circuitry and its related cognitive processes. Dopamine concentration, transporter availability, and dopamine D2 receptor density decline with age.[3] These changes, along with the aging synapse, make the aging brain more susceptible to pathology such as Parkinson disease and Alzheimer disease.

Cognition should be viewed as a spectrum with normal cognitive changes consisting of a gradual slowing of processing, short-term memory's inability to handle the same quantity as a younger person, and greater need for enhanced rehearsal and retrieval. Some older individuals will demonstrate no observable slowing, whereas others will demonstrate noticeable changes, but still be

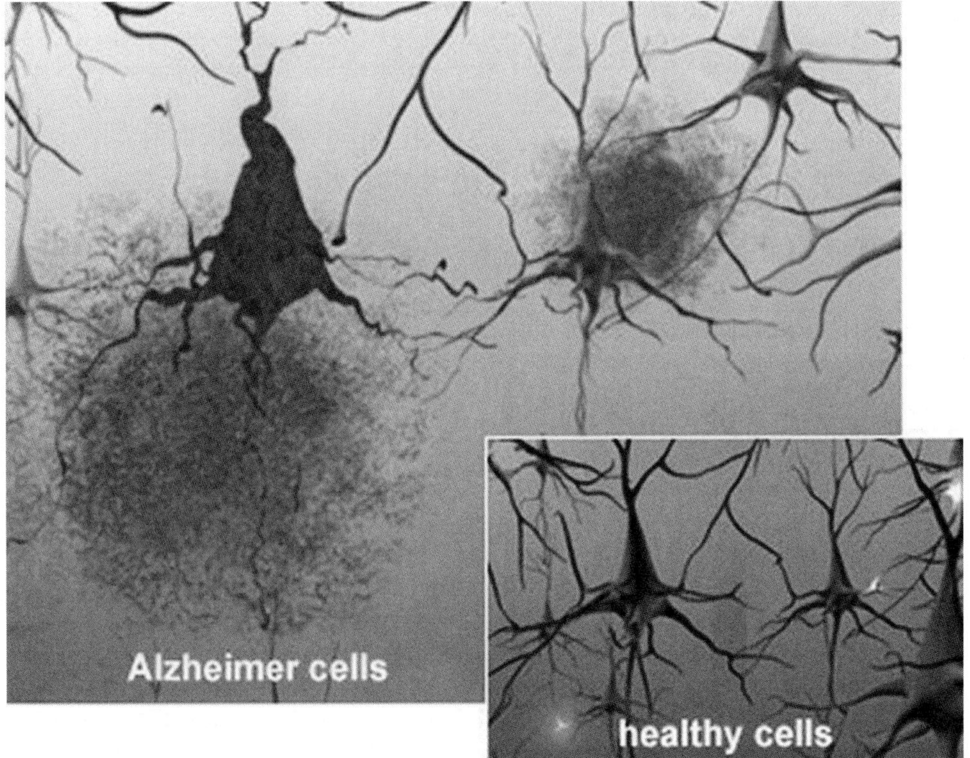

FIG. 19.1 Plaques and Tangles of Alzheimer Disease https://www.alz.org/espanol/about/brain/10.asp. *Image courtesy of the National Institute on Aging/National Institutes of Health.*

considered within the standard of normal. It is when these changes become more pronounced and interfere with functioning that pathology may be suspected.

DELIRIUM

Definition, Epidemiology, and Clinical Presentation of Delirium

Delirium is a clinical syndrome characterized by disturbed consciousness, cognitive function, or perception. Hospitalized older adults are most at risk for this extremely common and serious condition. Delirium develops in 2% to 50% of older people on general medicine wards and increases with increasing severity of illness.[20] For example, delirium develops in up to a half of older adults postoperatively, especially following hip fracture and vascular surgery.[21] In the intensive care unit, delirium occurs in up to 80% of older adults.[20] The key features of delirium are listed in Box 19.1.

The differentiation of delirium and dementia is crucial, because their assessment and clinical management are distinct.[22] Care must be taken not to diagnose dementia in the presence of delirium and that delirium should not be diagnosed when symptoms can be "better accounted for by a preexisting, established, or evolving dementia."[22] In situations where there is clinical uncertainty in distinguishing between delirium and dementia, the person should be treated initially for delirium.[23]

Although delirium and dementia share some common characteristics that make them difficult to tell apart, many signs and symptoms can be used to distinguish between them (Table 19.3).[22] For example, in delirium, the type, number, and severity of symptoms vary and fluctuate throughout day and night-time, often within minutes. Another feature is disturbance of the sleep–wake cycle, which results in agitation at night and drowsiness during the day.

Types of Delirium

The three main types of delirium are hyperactive, hypoactive, and mixed delirium. Hyperactive delirium is probably the most easily recognized type, with symptoms such as restlessness (e.g., pacing), agitation, and rapid mood changes or hallucinations. Hypoactive delirium is observed as inactivity or reduced motor activity, sluggishness, abnormal drowsiness, or seeming to be in a daze. It is important to note that hypoactivity is often mistaken for dementia, resulting in delayed or missed opportunities for therapeutic intervention.[24] Many individuals are likely to experience a fluctuating course known as mixed delirium, with a mixture of both the hyper- and hypoactive variants. Delirium is linked to adverse consequences, including an average increase of 8 days in the hospital, worse physical and

BOX 19.1 Key Features of Delirium

1. Disturbance of attention and awareness
2. Disturbance develops over a short period of time 3.
3. Additional disturbance in cognition (e.g., memory deficit, disorientation)
4. Disturbances in 1 and 3 that are not better explained by another preexisting, established, or evolving neurocognitive disorder, and do not occur in the context of a severely reduced level of arousal, such as coma
5. Evidence from the history, medical examination, and laboratory findings that the disturbances are caused by the physiologic consequences of another medical condition, substance intoxication, or withdrawal

TABLE 19.3 Differentiating Delirium and Dementia[22]

	Delirium	Dementia
Onset	Abrupt, although initial loss of mental clarity can be subtle	Insidious and progressive
Duration	Hours to days (although can be prolonged in some cases)	Months to years
Attention	Reduced ability to focus, sustain, or shift attention is a hallmark feature that occurs early in presentation.	Normal, except in severe dementia
Consciousness (i.e., awareness of the environment)	Fluctuating (thus assessment at multiple time-points is necessary); reduced level of consciousness and impaired orientation	Generally intact
Speech	Incoherent and disorganized; distractible in conversation.	Ordered, but development of anomia or aphasia is possible
Cause	Underlying medical condition, substance intoxication, or side-effect of drugs	Underlying neurologic process
Other features	Hyperactive, hypoactive, and mixed forms	Symptoms vary depending on underlying pathology

Reprinted with permission from Elsevier (Fong TG, Davis D, Growdon ME, Albuquerque A, Inouye SK. The interface between delirium and dementia in elderly adults. Lancet Neurol. 2015;14(8):823–832.)

cognitive recovery at 6 and 12 months, and increased time in institutional care. Patients diagnosed with delirium in the hospital have an overall high morbidity because of a high risk of dehydration, malnutrition, falls, continence problems, and pressure sores. They also have higher 1-year mortality rates (35% to 40%) and higher readmission rates.[25] Although delirium is considered a short-term temporary problem, evidence indicates it may persist in about one-third of individuals.[26] The presence of delirium is associated with persistent and clinically meaningful impairment of functional recovery for up to 18 months.[27] Cognitive decline after delirium is accelerated in older adults who have undergone surgery.[28] In addition, delirium is a strong independent predictor of cognitive impairment within 3 years of being discharged from the hospital.[29] Finally, there is an increased risk for worsening cognitive decline over a one- and five-year period in those with Alzheimer disease who developed delirium during hospitalization versus those who did not.[30, 31]

Pathophysiology and Risk Factors of Delirium

Structural changes, including cortical atrophy, ventricular dilatation, and white matter lesions, identified by neuroimaging, can be predictors of delirium, perhaps providing a clue to why dementia and delirium are so closely related.[32] The pathophysiology of delirium is thought to be partly owing to neurotransmitter disturbances with imbalances in the central cholinergic and adrenergic pathways. For example, elevated levels of inflammatory cytokines, such as serum interleukin (IL-6 and IL-8), have been found in hospitalized older adults who develop delirium,[33] with similar elevations in patients after hip fracture,[34] hence, one prominent hypothesis for delirium pathogenesis is that it is precipitated by pathologically elevated cortisol occurring with acute stress from illness or surgery.[35] Evidence of increased dopaminergic signaling has been detected in the cerebrospinal fluid (CSF) of patients with delirium.[35] Elevated CSF levels of S100B, which is a biomarker of central nervous system damage derived largely from astrocytes, were reported in patients with hip fracture with delirium, compared with those without delirium.[36]

Delirium is usually multifactorial in older adults. The development of delirium in an older individual depends on the complex relationships between the predisposing vulnerability of the person, as well as exposure to insults to the body system.[37] For example, in older adults with underlying dementia or with existing comorbid conditions, a seemingly benign insult, such as an upper respiratory tract infection, can result in the development of delirium. However, in older adults who are healthy and less vulnerable, it may take a severe insult, such as major surgery or prolonged stay in the ICU, to develop delirium. Thus, the more predisposing risk factors for delirium present, the more vulnerable the older person is. Potential predisposing risk factors for delirium include vision impairment (being without one's usual eyewear), hearing impairment (being without the usual hearing aid), functional mobility impairment, cognitive impairment, existence of comorbid conditions, and a history of delirium.[37] Other risk factors for delirium include the use of psychoactive drugs, infection, surgery, physical restraints, and use of bladder catheter.[37] All these risk factors can result in decreased mobility and sensory deprivation, so providing early mobility and a variety of appropriate sensory stimulation(s), both directly and through the environment, can help prevent and or minimize the effects of delirium.

Prevention and Management of Delirium

Prevention is the key to managing delirium, because no convincing evidence indicates that pharmacologic intervention is effective.[37] Drug treatment should be used as a last resort, and only for those patients at risk to themselves or others. Prevention of delirium is directly related to the risk factors for delirium. At least 30% to 40% of delirium cases are preventable.[38] As delirium is a life-threatening condition, particularly for older adults, time is of essence. The cause of the delirium should be ascertained, and appropriate steps taken to remediate the cause as soon as possible. Hence, the initial management should focus on three simultaneous priorities: (1) maintaining patient safety, (2) searching for the causes of the delirium episode, and (3) managing the delirium symptoms.[37] For example, the management of hypoxia, hydration, and nutrition; minimizing the time spent lying in bed; and walking are important steps to preventing and treating delirium.

Drugs are an important risk factor and may be the sole factor in 12% to 39% of cases of delirium.[39] The most common drugs associated with delirium are psychoactive agents, such as benzodiazepines; narcotic analgesics, such as morphine; and drugs with anticholinergic effects. Many drugs have anticholinergic effects and, whenever possible, should be discontinued in patients who are at risk for developing delirium.[40]

The original evidence-based multicomponent intervention program targeted to delirium risk factors is the Hospital Elder Life Program (HELP), a widely known international program in Germany and the Netherlands.[36] The HELP utilizes an interdisciplinary team and trained volunteers to implement practical strategies to reduce the risk of developing delirium. It has been shown to be cost effective and successful in preventing delirium and functional decline.[41,42] High effectiveness of these multicomponent nonpharmacologic strategies in the prevention of delirium and falls was demonstrated by a recent systematic review of 14 studies, 9 of which involved HELP adaptations or included at least some evidence-based interventions from HELP.[38] This review found a greater than 50% odds reduction in delirium prevention and a greater than 60% reduction in falls related to delirium. Notably, 12 of the 14 studies included exercise interventions designed to enhance mobility. Table 19.4 lists nonpharmacological interventions found to be effective.[38]

TABLE 19.4 Evidence-based Nonpharmacologic Delirium Prevention Interventions

Risk Factors	Interventions
Cognition/Orientation	Cognitive stimulation activities Orientation board with names of care team members and daily schedule Orienting communication
Early Mobility	Ambulation or active range-of-motion exercises Minimizing the use of immobilizing equipment
Hearing	Portable amplifying devices and special communication techniques, with daily reinforcement Ear wax clearing as needed
Sleep–wake Cycle Preservation	Warm milk or herbal tea, relaxation tapes or music, and back massage Unit-wide noise reduction strategies and schedule adjustments to allow uninterrupted sleep
Vision	Visual aids (glasses, magnifying lenses) and adaptive equipment (large illuminated telephone keypads, large print books, fluorescent tape on call bell), with daily reinforcement of their use
Hydration	Encourage fluids Feeding assistance and encouragement during meals

Hshieh TT, Yue J, Oh E, et al. Effectiveness of multicomponent nonpharmacological delirium interventions: a meta-analysis. *JAMA Intern Med*. 2015;175(4):512–520. https://doi.org/10.1001/jamainternmed.2014.7779. Erratum in: *JAMA Intern Med*. 2015;175(4):659.

Physical restraints should be avoided because they tend to increase agitation and may cause injury. Sensory deprivation is a known risk factor for delirium. To reduce sensory deprivation, any orienting stimulation, such as introducing familiar pictures, a family member's presence, the patient's favorite pillow or blanket, and familiar music and sounds may help. Finally, because of the inherent risk factors of hospitalization, early discharge to home-based medical management is associated with significantly reduced incidence of delirium.[43]

DEMENTIA

Dementia is considered a public health priority by the World Health Organization (WHO) to improve the care and quality of life for people with dementia and their caregivers.[44] Because dementia is related to increased age, the rising health and social care needs of the large and rapidly growing numbers of older adults has huge implications for rehabilitation professionals. It is, therefore, crucial for us to understand how cognitive decline and dementia have an impact on the lives of older adults and caregivers, and shape how rehabilitation programs or services should be delivered. Not only will this facilitate the rehabilitation process better, but it will also lead to the meaningful design and implementation of evidence-based rehabilitation programs, chronic disease self-management strategies, health care services, and policies that will support their integration into society.

Definition of Dementia

Dementia can be defined as a clinical syndrome of cognitive and functional decline,[45] usually of a chronic or progressive nature. The diagnosis of dementia is based on a careful history with a semistructured interview, detailed medical and neurologic examination, as well as neurocognitive testing. Under the DSM-V criteria,[2] dementia was named a major neurocognitive disorder, although the term dementia is still used clinically. The cognitive deficits must be sufficiently severe to cause impairment in occupational or social functioning and must represent a decline from a previously higher level of functioning to be diagnosed as a major neurocognitive disorder.[46]

The four most common subtypes of dementia, listed in Table 19.5 in order of frequency, are Alzheimer disease (AD) (41%) vascular dementia (VaD) (32%), dementia with Lewy bodies (DLB) (8%) and frontotemporal dementia (FTD) (3%).[44] Mixed pathologies are more commonly seen than "pure" pathologies; for example in one study, approximately 50% of individuals with dementia also had vascular changes and 65% had other neurodegenerative conditions, such as DLB.[47] Among individuals with onset of dementia before 60 years of age, FTD is a common subtype, particularly among men. Compared with VaD, AD typically occurs at a later age with the prevalence increased as the number of very old persons increases.

Epidemiology

Prevalence. The total number of people with dementia is projected to almost double every 20 years, to 82 million in 2030 and 152 million in 2050.[48] The exponential rise in the population with dementia can be attributed to population growth and demographic aging. Global regional prevalence varies from 4.6% in Central Europe to 8.7% in North Africa and the Middle East. Estimated prevalence is higher in East Asia and Africa. Of all people with dementia, 58% live in countries currently classified by the World Bank as low- or middle-income countries. This proportion is estimated to increase to 63% in 2030 and 69% in 2050.[49]

In the United States, 5.7 million people of all ages are living with AD in 2018 (0.2 million are under the age of 65), thus, 10% (1 in 10) individuals age 65 and older has AD. Of those who have AD, 81% are age 75 and older. These numbers are widely recognized as underestimates because a large number of people are underdiagnosed and underreported.[50]

More women than men have AD or other dementias. Almost two-thirds of Americans with AD are women. Although the chief explanation for this disparity is that

TABLE 19.5 Subtypes of Dementia and their Distinguishing Features[46]

Form of Dementia	Memory	Language	Executive function	Visuospatial	Behavior	Motor symptoms
Alzheimer Dementia	Early, short term loss is greater than long term	Poor list generation	Preceded by memory loss	Early topographic disorientation	Socially inappropriate, late agitation, misidentification	Late onset
Vascular dementia	Variable	Aphasia if cortex is involved	Variable	Variable	Apathy or depression	Focal findings depending on lesion site; mild bradykinesis if basal ganglia involved
Dementia with Lewy Bodies	Fluctuating alertness, memory spared	Slower	Impaired	Impaired	Hallucinations, bizarre delusions	Worse with antipsychotics
Frontal-temporal dementia	Reduced concentration is greater than short term memory loss	Unrestrained, but empty. Aphasia may antedate dementia.	Early decline	Spared	Early disinhibition, hypochondriasis, affective disorders, mania	Infrequent motor neuron disease

women on average live longer than men, the survival bias is also posited as an explanation. The Framingham Heart Study suggests that because men in middle age have a higher rate of death from cardiovascular disease than women in middle age, men who survive beyond age 65 may have a healthier cardiovascular risk profile and thus apparent lower risk for dementia than women of the same age. Thus, those men living to a very old age may be the healthiest men and therefore at a low risk of developing AD.[51]

Societal Cost of Dementia

Prioritizing rehabilitation strategies and efforts to improve the lives of people with dementia and their caregivers will not be possible without a proper understanding of the societal costs of dementia and how they impact families, and health and social care systems. Societal cost is calculated based on the estimated prevalence of dementia, cost of illness, and amount of informal care that exists in different countries and regions of the world.[52] The total global societal costs of dementia have increased from $604 billion in 2010[44] to $818 billion in 2015, and is estimated to climb to $1 trillion by 2018.[49] About 70% of the global societal costs of dementia occur in only two WHO regions, North America (mainly US) and Western Europe.[44]

The difference in expenditures for dementia in different countries is related to the type of formal versus informal care provided and available.[53] In low- and middle-income countries, the formal social care sector is practically nonexistent, which means that the responsibility of caring for people with dementia falls primarily on unpaid informal caregivers where informal care costs predominate. In contrast, for high-income countries, the direct costs of care in the community by paid social care professionals account for nearly half of all costs. Across the globe, rehabilitation professionals must seek ways to maximize the function and quality of life of people with dementia and of their caregivers, through building capability beyond trained professionals, but also through the empowerment of lay-extenders, volunteers, and the community at large.

Mild Cognitive Impairment (MCI)

Mild cognitive impairment (MCI) is a category of altered cognition that was developed by Petersen et al.[54] at the end of the 1990s, to address the gap between normal and dementia-type pathologic cognitive changes. Under DSM-V criteria, MCI is now termed as a mild neurocognitive disorder.[2] The prevalence of MCI in individuals older than 65 is 15% to 20%.[50] People with MCI have more memory problems than normal for people their age, but their symptoms are not as severe as those of people with AD. For example, they do not experience the personality changes or other problems that are characteristic of AD. People with MCI are still able to carry out their normal daily activities and function is largely preserved. Signs of MCI include losing things often, forgetting to go to events or appointments, and having more trouble coming up with words than other people of the same age.

The criteria of MCI continue to evolve as research continues to reveal important features and associations of MCI. Fig. 19.2 summarizes these widely accepted criteria. MCI is considered to characterize core criteria of the earliest symptomatic stages of several cognitive disorders.[55]

The clinical evaluation of MCI is based on a patient's, patient's informant, or physician's cognitive concern. This cognitive concern should reflect a change in the person's cognitive performance, such as increased forgetfulness of recently experienced events, appointments, visits of

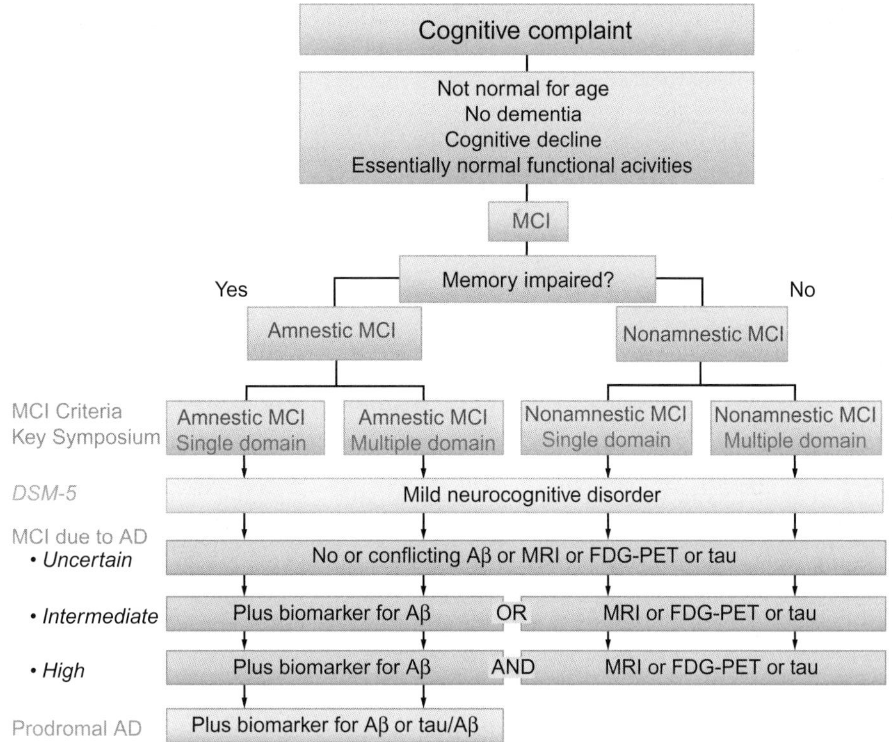

Temporal evolution of criteria for mild cognitive impairment (MCI) and prodromal Alzheimer disease (AD). *DSM-5 = Diagnostic and Statistical Manual of Mental Disorders, Fifth Edition;* NIA-AA = National Institute on Aging–Alzheimer's Association.

FIG. 19.2 Criteria of mild cognitive impairment continuum (Minneap Minn). 2016 Apr; 22(2): 404–418. doi: [https://doi.org/10.1212/CON.0000000000000313]

friends or conversations; and repeating oneself more than usual. The clinical examination should differentiate between memory concerns and changes that reflect attention or concentration. Screening instruments, such as the Montreal Cognitive Assessment or the Short Test of Mental Status, can be useful, but are not sufficient to establish a diagnosis. However, the results of these screening tools may indicate further neuropsychiatric testing is needed. One of the primary purposes of clinical examination is to confirm or eliminate the diagnosis of dementia. The most sensitive marker for MCI is difficulty in performance of IADLs, such as shopping and managing finances.[56]

The progression from MCI to dementia is still under debate and may relate to the type of MCI (e.g., amnesic or nonamnesic). Amnesic MCI, when memory is impaired but other cognitive functions are spared, is considered the prestage of dementia of the Alzheimer type. Nonamnesic type is seen when memory remains intact, but one or more other cognitive abilities are significantly impaired. Neuroimaging, such as MRI and tau PET, amyloid PET, and FDG-PET scans, is aiding the research on the risk of progression to dementia. For example, medial temporal lobe atrophy on MRI tends to predict such progression and those with a positive amyloid PET are likely to experience progression rapidly.[57] Additionally, carriers of the apolipoprotein E4 (APOE4) genotype are more likely to progress rapidly. However, physical therapists should be aware that not all individuals with MCI will progress to dementia; stability and reversion rates are being studied to help determine what factors may be involved.[58]

Currently no accepted pharmacologic treatments exist for MCI or for delaying its progression to dementia. However, some studies indicate that exercise, particularly aerobic exercise, may be effective at reducing the rate of progression from MCI to dementia and will be discussed later in this chapter.[59]

Alzheimer Disease

The most common form of dementia is Alzheimer disease, and it is associated with advancing age. Neuropathologic changes may precede clinical symptoms by as much as 20 years.[60] Memory decline is the earliest and predominant symptom. Amyloid plaques and neurofibrillary tangles are the most common pathologic changes associated with the development of AD (see Fig. 19.1). Amyloid plaques are protein fragments known as B-amyloid peptides mixed with additional proteins, remnants of neurons, and bits and pieces of other nerve cells.[61] Neurofibrillary tangles are abnormal collections of a protein called tau.

Although tau is required for healthy neurons, in AD, tau clumps together, causing neurons to fail and die. The presence of B-amyloid and tau proteins activates chronic inflammation.

Synaptic connections permit the flow of information from one neuron to another or to the end organ via neurotransmitters (acetylcholine). Inadequate levels of acetylcholine are associated with AD.[62] Reduced synaptic density is postulated to be one of the causes of the significant atrophy in the inferior prefrontal cortex of individuals with AD.[3] The volume loss in the entorhinal cortex, an important relay between the hippocampus and association cortices, adversely affects the hippocampus, critical for encoding.[3] Episodic memory, especially retrieval, is frequently affected. The entorhinal cortex also demonstrates volume declines in individuals with MCI, compared with healthy older adults.

Brain-derived neurotrophic factor (BDNF), a neurotrophin, has been linked to AD and other neurologic disorders.[63] Within the brain, nerve growth factors (neurotrophins) play a vital role in neuronal growth, development, and survival. They are important signaling molecules that regulate the synapse and lead to learning and memory. The inhibition of BDNF and another neurotrophic factor, neural growth factor (NGF), stimulates the molecular events typical of the AD process.[63] Amyloid beta (Aβ), the plaque lesions present in the brain in individuals with AD, is increased in a deprived BDNF and NGF neural environment. The interruption of the BDNF and NGF signaling sets up the toxic mechanisms that induce the death and loss of neurons, which in turn cause brain tissue atrophy.[64]

The earliest clinical symptom is difficulty in remembering recent conversations, names, or events. Apathy and depression are also early symptoms. Later symptoms include impaired communication, disorientation, confusion, poor judgment, behavioral changes, and ultimately difficulty speaking, swallowing, and walking.[50] Differential characteristics of AD and various other dementia types are listed in Table 19.5.

Vascular Dementia

Vascular dementia or vascular cognitive impairment is classified under the DSM-V as an organic mental disorder, with the essential feature of underlying cardiovascular disease.[2] It often coexists with AD and dementia with Lewy bodies. It is estimated that 50% of those with AD have pathologic evidence of silent strokes.[50] VaD with AD is the most common mixed type of dementia.

Risk factors for vascular dementia are similar to risk factors for cardiovascular disease, such as hypertension, history of smoking, hypercholesterolemia, and diabetes mellitus.[65] Ischemic brain damage and cognitive loss result from the cerebrovascular disease, usually through vascular stroke(s). Multi-infarct dementia is a type of vascular dementia that is the result of the additive effects of small and large infarcts that produce a loss of brain tissue. The risk for dementia is significantly higher in someone who has had a stroke. The rate of cognitive decline for VaD is similar to that for AD and life expectancy of VaD is shorter than that of AD. Treatment consists of blood pressure control and prevention of further strokes.

Slowed processing speed, impaired judgment, or impaired ability to make decisions, plan, or organize (executive function) is more likely to be the initial symptom, as opposed to the memory loss associated with the initial symptoms of AD. In addition to changes in cognition, people with vascular dementia can have difficulty with motor function, especially slow gait and poor balance. The location, number, and size of the brain injuries determine whether dementia will result and how an individual's' thinking and physical functioning will be affected. Focal neurologic deficits may include weakness, visual field cuts, and symmetric reflexes if the injury lies within the motor-sensory networks. Extrapyramidal signs, including gait disturbances or bradykinesia, are associated with lesions in the basal ganglia. As the frontal-subcortical circuit structures are very vulnerable to perfusion changes, people with VaD are more likely to be apathetic and depressed, instead of being agitated or psychotic.[66] In general, compared with people with AD, memory impairment is more variable, less severe, and more likely to respond to cueing. In addition, with small artery disease, diminished executive function is characteristic, whereas aphasia, apraxia, and neglect are common with involvement of larger arteries.

Dementia With Lewy Bodies

People with DLB have some of the same symptoms common in AD, but they are more likely to have initial or early symptoms of sleep disturbances, well-formed visual hallucinations, and gait slowness or imbalance or other parkinsonian movement features. These features, as well as early visuospatial impairment, may occur in the absence of significant memory impairment.

The symptoms of DLB are caused by the build-up of Lewy bodies, accumulated bits of alpha-synuclein protein, inside the nuclei of neurons in the cortex that controls particular aspects of memory and motor control.[67] Researchers do not know exactly why alpha-synuclein accumulates into Lewy bodies or how Lewy bodies cause the symptoms of DLB, but they do know that alpha-synuclein accumulation is also linked to Parkinson disease (PD), multiple system atrophy, and several other disorders, which are referred to as the "synucleinopathies."[68] Although people with DLB and PD have Lewy bodies, the onset of the disease is marked by motor impairment in PD and cognitive impairment in DLB. The brain changes of DLB alone can cause dementia, but people with DLB may have coexisting AD. The diagnostic criteria for DLB based on the latest DLB consortium[67] are listed in Table 19.6.

TABLE 19.6 Criteria for the Clinical Diagnosis of Probable or Possible Dementia With Lewy Body[67]

Clinical Feature	Description
Essential	Progressive cognitive decline sufficient to interfere with daily function
Core	Fluctuating cognition, alertness, and attention
	Recurrent visual hallucinations (well-formed and detailed)
	REM sleep behavior disorder
	One or more cardinal features, of parkinsonism (bradykinesia, tremor, or rigidity)
Supportive	Severe sensitivity to antipsychotics
	Postural instability, falls
	Syncope
	Severe autonomic dysfunction
	Hypersomnia or hyposomnia
	Anxiety, apathy, depression

Frontemporal Lobe Dementia

Frontemporal lobe dementia has emerged as a group of dementias caused by progressive nerve cell loss in the brain's frontal lobes or its temporal lobes, inherited in a third of all cases. This nerve cell damage leads to loss of function in these brain regions, causing deterioration in behavior and personality, language disturbances, or alterations in muscle or motor functions.[69] FTD used to be called Pick's disease after Arnold Pick, a physician who first described a patient with distinct symptoms affecting language. Corticobasal degeneration, amyotrophic lateral sclerosis (ALS), and progressive supranuclear palsy are included in the group of disorders involving the protein tau. FTD is the second most common cause of dementia (after Alzheimer disease) in people under age 65.[69] The clinical presentation is insidious with age of onset between 45 and 70 years of age. The estimated duration of the disease was 3 to 17 years. In all the FTDs, there is mild to moderate frontal lobe atrophy. Microscopically, this degenerative process consists of cortical microvacuolation and an increase in astrocytes with neurons showing atrophy with striking loss of synapses.

Compared with individuals with AD, those with FTD commonly exhibit an impairment of executive function, are less disoriented, but have more difficulty with problem solving. They have memory impairment owing to retrieval and organizational problems associated with their frontal lobe deficits. Most of these people demonstrate a lack of concentration. Unlike those with AD, individuals with FTD have relatively preserved abilities in their memory and spatial orientation. Problems with spatial orientation, for example getting lost in familiar places, is more common in AD than FTD. However, their lack of insight may be profound, leading to risk-taking and unsafe practices. The most common early symptoms of FTD are listed in Table 19.7.[69]

TABLE 19.7 Common Early Symptoms of Frontotemporal Dementia[69]

Early symptoms	Description
Disinhibition	Behaviors that are socially inappropriate, impulsive, careless, or exhibit poor judgment and lack of consideration of consequences
	Poor manners, lack of social decorum and an absence of any sense of embarrassment are characteristic.
	May also be irritable, superficially jocular and euphoric, or depressive
Apathy	Inertia, disinterest, social withdrawal, and/or a lack of engagement, drive, or motivation.
Lack of empathy	Self-involvement, diminished interpersonal warmth, loss of sympathy for others, and/or lack of regard for the effect of the individual's behaviors on the feelings of others
Repetitive, stereotyped or perseverative behaviors	Simple movements or speech patterns, or more complex rituals and compulsions
Substantial changes in food preferences and eating habits	A shift to over-consumption of sweets and carbohydrates, binge eating, gluttony, and substantial weight gain
	Hyperorality may include mouthing of nonfood objects

Data from Schildkrout B. Frontotemporal Dementia: a brain disease that challenges difinitions of mental illness. Psychiatr Times. 2017;34(8):1–5.

COGNITIVE SCREENING AND ASSESSMENT TOOLS

Medical Assessment for Dementia

The assessment of any cognitive disorder begins with a medical history to determine the precise features of cognitive loss. The medical history should include the patient and the patient's caregiver and/or family members to form an accurate picture of the concern. Questions about past medical history, such as falls, head trauma, hypertension, heart disease, diabetes, vitamin deficiencies, or thyroid disorder, and alcohol use and substance exposure, should be asked to identify reversible causes of cognitive changes. Medications should be reviewed for relevance and appropriate dose.[70] A comprehensive physical and neurologic examination performed by the health care team should include a check for focal weakness, gait impairment, language impairment, and extrapyramidal signs (rigidity, tremor, bradykinesia) to aid in the differential diagnosis. A gross assessment of functional status includes questions about bathing, dressing, toileting, transferring, as well as intermediate activities (e.g., managing finances, medications, cooking, shopping) to determine the degree of loss. Finally, an evaluation of mental status for attention, immediate and delayed recall, remote memory, executive function, and depression should be conducted.

Biomarkers, biological factors that can be measured to indicate the presence of a disease or risk of developing a disease, are being extensively researched for associations with dementias.[50] Biomarkers, such as the amount of beta-amyloid in the brain as shown by positron-emission tomography (PET) imaging, levels of certain proteins in fluid (e.g., levels of beta-amyloid and tau in the cerebrospinal fluid and levels of particular groups of protein in the blood), and level of glucose metabolism in the brain as shown on PET imaging using the radiotracer fluorodeoxyglucose, are used to diagnosis various forms of dementia; however, these tests are prohibitively expensive and routinely not available. Research is ongoing for a routine blood test that can diagnosis AD.[50] Other types of neuroimaging may aid in the differential diagnosis of dementia, such as computed tomography (CT) or MRI. These tests may reveal cerebral atrophy, focal brain lesions (cortical strokes, tumors, subdural hematomas), hydrocephalus, or periventricular ischemic brain injury.

Physical therapists have a role in both screening and further assessment of cognitive function because it will often have an impact on the physical therapy plan of care. For example, in direct access situations the physical therapist may be the first person to note cognitive changes or the only health care professional providing care. When cognitive screening indicates further testing, such as in a sudden change in cognitive symptoms or an undiagnosed suspicion of cognitive deficits, the patient should be referred to the patient's medical practitioner for a comprehensive evaluation.

Screening Tools

The Alzheimer's Association recommends three screening tools for clinicians in primary care settings, which are easy to administer by nonphysicians, quick (< 5 minutes), have excellent psychometric properties, free from education and cultural bias, and free from copyright.[71] These recommended screening tools are described next.

Mini-Cog. The Mini-Cog is a simple three-step test with recitation of three words, a clock drawing, and then recall of three original words.[72] Several three-word sets allow for repeated testing, if needed. A simple scoring method for the Mini-Cog is described in Fig. 19.3. A total score of 3, 4, or 5 indicates a lower likelihood of dementia, but does not rule out some degree of cognitive impairment.[73] A cut score of less than 4 of 5 indicates the need for further testing.[69] The Mini-Cog is readily available online. The use of graphic instructions has been shown to decrease administration time and increase accuracy of scoring and it is available online.[74]

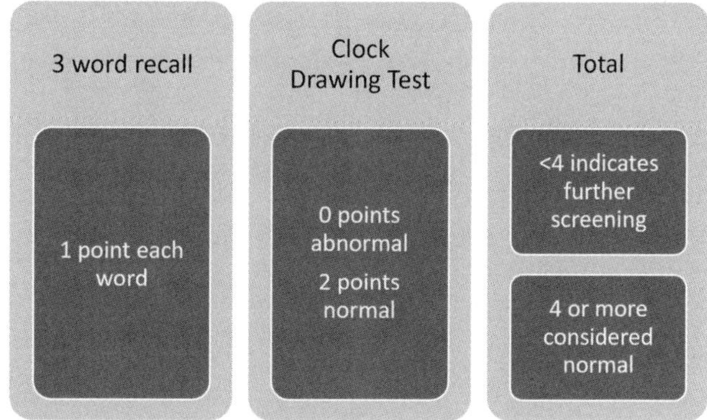

FIG. 19.3 Mini-Cog Scoring Criteria. A score of less than 4 of a possible 5 indicates the need for further testing.[72]

General Practitioner Assessment of Cognition (GPCOG). The GPCOG is a paper or online tool that can be given directly to the patient or to the patient's informant. It takes 4 minutes to administer. It includes both recall items (stated name/address and the date) and the clock drawing test. Each correct answer scores one point for a total possible score of 9. A score of 9 indicates no significant cognitive impairment and further testing is not required. A score between 5 and 8 triggers the informant interview to obtain further information. A score from 0 to 4 indicates cognitive impairment that requires further cognitive testing.[75] The informant version has a possible total of 6 with higher scores indicating less impairment. If the score is 0 to 3 on the informant version, cognitive impairment is indicated requiring further cognitive testing.[76]

Memory Impairment Screening (MIS). The MIS is a brief screening tool readily available online consisting of the introduction of four words read aloud followed by asking the patient to identify into which category the word fits.[77] This second part helps determine the patient's understanding of the word. The third part is a free recall of the four words approximately 2 to 3 minutes later, during which a distracting task is administered. Each word recalled without any cues (free recall) is given 2 points or, if recalled with a categorical cue, given 1 point. A score of 5 to 8 indicates no cognitive impairment, whereas a score of 4 or less indicates possible cognitive impairment and the need for further testing.[77]

Assessment Tools

Although there are many additional tools in neuropsychiatry for assessing cognitive changes and performance, the following tools are arguably those most likely to be encountered and utilized in clinical practice. These each have good psychometric properties for dementia. They are used in everyday practice and freely available, except for the Mini-Mental Status examination, which is proprietary, but included below because it has long been considered the "gold standard" of cognitive assessment.

Mini-Mental State Examination. The Mini-Mental State Examination (MMSE) first developed by Folstein in 1975, has become the most recognized tool for assessing an individual's cognitive state.[78] It assesses six areas of cognitive ability for a maximal score of 30 points. Owing to its moderate sensitivity (79%), but higher specificity (95%) with a cut-off score of 27, it does help determine if a cognitive impairment exists, but not what specific type.[79] The MMSE is proprietary and because of this and other reasons, such as its education bias, other tests are being used more widely in clinical practice.

The Montreal Cognitive Assessment. The Montreal Cognitive Assessment (MOCA) was initially developed as a test for mild cognitive impairment, but has also been determined to match qualities of the MMSE.[80] It assesses seven areas of cognition for a total possible score of 30 points. A score of 25 or less is indicative of cognitive impairment. This test is easy to administer in about 10 minutes and has been translated into many languages.[81] Training and forms are available online.[82]

Saint Louis University Mental Status. The Saint Louis University Mental Status (SLUMS) examination, available free and online,[83] was designed to identify early dementia and mild neurocognitive disorders.[84] The SLUMS contains 11 items of orientation, short-term memory, calculations, the naming of animals, the clock drawing test, and recognition of geometric figures. It takes approximately 7 minutes to administer. Scores range from 0 to 30. Scores of 27 to 30 are considered normal in a person with at least a high school education. Scores between 21 and 26 suggest mild neurocognitive disorder and scores between 0 and 20 indicate dementia. For those with less than a high school education, normal scores are between 25 and 30, scores between 20 and 24 indicate mild neurocognitive disorder and scores of 19 or less indicate dementia.

Trail Making Test. The Trail Making Test (TMT) is a freely available, timed, neuropsychological test that involves visual scanning and working memory. The TMT has two parts; the TMT-A (rote memory) and TMT-B (executive functioning).[85] In each test the participant is asked to draw a line between 24 consecutive circles that are randomly arranged on a page. The TMT-A uses all numbers, whereas the TMT-B alternates numbers and letters, requiring the patient to switch between numbers and letters in consecutive order. The TMT is scored by how long it takes to complete the test. The time includes correction of errors prompted by the examiner. If the person cannot complete the test in 5 minutes, the test is discontinued. An average score for TMT-A is 29 seconds and a deficient score is greater than 78 seconds. For TMT-B, an average score is 75 seconds and a deficient score is greater than 273 seconds. Norms have been established based on age and education.[86] This test has been shown to be useful to indicate if a road test is required to determine continued safe driving ability.[87]

Staging Progression of Dementia

Several methods of staging dementia have been attempted, but application is complicated by the various dementia presentations and trajectories of the different subtypes of dementia. The clinician may encounter various staging criteria including the Clinical Dementia Rating Scale (CDR), the Global Deterioration Scale (GDS) and its subpart the Functional Assessment Staging (FAST). A recent systematic review found the CDR to be the best current evidenced-based scale measure.[88] Knowing the more basic level of mild, moderate, or severe symptoms is generally going to be sufficient to direct interventions for people with dementia. A brief comparison of these staging methods is available in Table 19.8.[89] Although staging may assist in communication between health care professionals and for family education about typical progression, it is important to remember that not all forms of dementia follow the same pathway or timeline and each person needs to be assessed individually for current functional and cognitive abilities.

TABLE 19.8 Comparison of Dementia Staging Scales[89]

Dementia Level	CDR Stage	GDS/FAST Stage	Functional Characteristic	MMSE Score
Normal	0	1	No deficits	29–30
MCI	0	2	Subjective deficits of memory loss (no functional change)	28–29
Mild	0-0.5	3	Functional deficit only with complex tasks	24–28
Mild	0-0.5	4	IADLs impacted	19.20
Moderate	1	5	ADLs impacted, able to contribute to process with assistance	15
Moderate/ Severe	2	6 (a-e)	ADLs severely impacted, limited ability to assist Onset of incontinence	1–9
Severe	3	7(a-f)	Dependent for ADL Limited to no interaction	0

Data from Reisberg B, Jamil IA, Khan S, et al. Staging Dementia. Third Edit. (Abou-Saleh MT, Katona C LE, Kumar A, eds.). Wiley-Blackwell; 2010.

MANAGEMENT

Pharmacology

The primary use of pharmacologic interventions is to slow the decline of cognitive function and maintain physical function for as long as possible. The U.S. Food and Drug Administration (FDA) has approved two types of medications for Alzheimer disease and Lewy-Body dementia: cholinesterase inhibitors and memantine.[90] However, currently no medications demonstrate they can reverse or halt the symptoms of dementia. Vascular dementia currently does not have any FDA-approved medications for maintaining cognitive function. A more thorough discussion of drug therapy for cognitive disorders is contained in the pharmacology chapter of this text.

Person-Centered Dementia Care

Health care has evolved from a paternalistic approach with providers knowing best, to a more holistic and person-centered approach.[91] The stigma of dementia and challenges of applying therapeutic interventions with this population has created a "therapeutic nihilism" where even clinicians who may have adopted person-centered care principles feel there is not value to providing such care for people with dementia.[92] Evidence indicates that many people with dementia may still be visualized as "subhuman" or lacking "personhood" by health care professionals.[93, 94]

The concepts of person-centered care (PCC) play an important role for all older adults, but particularly for people with dementia. PCC includes components of care that are holistic, individualized, respectful, and empowering. The Institute of Medicine first addressed person-centered care when addressing quality of health care as "care that is respectful and responsive to individual patient preferences, needs, and values, and ensuring that patient values guide all clinical decisions."[95] More recently Morgan defined PCC as "... a holistic approach to the delivery of respectful and individualized care, allowing negotiation of care and offering choice through a therapeutic relationship in which persons are empowered to be involved in health decisions."[96] Specific regulations for long-term care facilities that accept federal money describe person-centered care as "... *focus on the resident as the locus of control and support the resident in making their own choices and having control over their daily lives.*"[97]

In the United States concepts of person-centered dementia care have evolved as the medical community adopted a more biopsychosocial approach to care. Built from the work of Kitwood in the 1990s,[98] individuals with dementia are recognized as self-actualized people rather than as "less than" what they previously had been.[99] Moving away from strict medicalization of illness to a broader focus on enhancing the person's remaining skills, supports the evolving regulations for many care facilities to promote personal choice and involvement in care. A shift from a deficit approach in the medical model to a strengths-based approach is being integrated into practice and research.

Practice recommendations for person-centered dementia care are listed in Table 19.9.[100] These recommendations are applicable to physical therapy practice in any setting. In practical terms, the physical therapist who practices in a skilled nursing facility must be aware of the residents' care plans and participating with the interdisciplinary team in their development. For physical therapists in other settings, patient-centered dementia care can be practiced by working together to create the person's goals, respecting what they can do, and advocating for autonomy whenever possible. Communication is an

TABLE 19.9 Person-Centered Care Practice Recommendations[100]

Person-Centered Care Practices	Description
Know the person living with dementia	It all starts with knowing the person, their preferences and individual likes/dislikes. If you have access to social services materials, these often help describe some pieces. Other tools like the Preferences for Everyday Living Inventory (PELI) can assist in providing this information if the person cannot share it themselves.
Recognize and accept the person's reality	Validation provides comfort, may ease fear and promote empathy and improved communication.
Identify and support ongoing opportunities for meaningful engagement	Beyond preplanned activities, engagement must be purposeful and reflect the preferences listed above. For the patients, using their music preferences can encourage participation in therapy.
Build and nurture authentic, caring relationships	All relationships should be built on dignity and respect; when you know the person beyond the disease, a deeper more authentic relationship develops.
Create and maintain supportive community for individuals, families, and staff.	Respecting individual differences and needs creates a community that welcomes all.
Evaluate care practices regularly and make appropriate changes.	Continual assessment of care practices and adoption of tools as they develop.

important aspect in patient-centered care and is described next.

Communication Strategies. Person-centered approaches, such as positive communication that focuses on the person as an individual with unique needs and that recognize their abilities, is known to set the stage for positive interactions. Alternatively, a focus on the individual with dementia's deficits has been shown to impede interaction and reduce the individual's sense of personhood.[101]

Table 19.10 describes several strategies to use in managing the presenting memory difficulties while enhancing learning and affirming and showing respect for the person.[102] Applying these strategies will require flexibility, depending on the stage of dementia. For example, a person who has a recent hip fracture and is in an early stage of dementia will be more capable of learning, able to interact and participate in a skilled program, and require little adaptation on the part of the therapist. However, a person in the middle stages of dementia will require a more function-based approach with shorter, simple instruction, and likely will benefit from a greater emphasis on caregiver training and utilization of implicitly retained motor functions.

Attention must be paid to body language and tone because words can be a small portion of perceived communication. The therapist must be mindful that emotional memory of an encounter may be maintained even if the encounter itself is unable to be recalled.[103] The popular axiom "They may not remember you, but they will remember how you made them feel" is quite accurate. In the "Positive Approach to Care" program, use of spatial boundaries are important to create first a visual, then verbal, and lastly a physical connection.[104] For example, be sure to approach from the front and establish eye contact prior to verbal introductions or touching the person. This approach is supported by literature on mindfulness that indicates care partners promote well-being through a multi-sensory approach.[105] The typical physical therapist position for guarding techniques (slightly behind, out of visual field) may require adaptation, such as standing to the person's side after approach while maintaining hand-in-hand contact. The "Hand In Hand" series of videos and support guides is a useful resource. Released in 2013, they were provided free to every nursing home in the United States. It includes modules specific to positive communications and remains available on the Center

TABLE 19.10 Strategies to Manage Memory Difficulties[102]

	Visual	Auditory	Tactile
SENSORY MEMORY			
Problems with registration, recognition, and identification	➢ Approach the person from the front, in his or her visual field. ➢ Smile.	➢ Use calm, positive, unhurried speech ➢ State the person's name and yours to increase sense of familiarity.	➢ Use touch to reassure. ➢ Use touch to guide, lead, redirect, and prompt desired behaviors.
Strategies to support sensory memory	➢ Present objects or written cues to focus attention on communication topic. ➢ Provide contextual and environmental cues; use colors, highlighting, enlargement, pictures, drawings, symbols	➢ User praise and compliments befitting an adult ➢ Hearing aids, assistive listening devices.	➢ Use familiar objects as reminders.
SHORT-TERM, TEMPORARY WORKING MEMORY	➢ Use a variety of modalities to convey information: visual, auditory, tactile cues ➢ Use simple, one-step instructions; wait for evidence of comprehension; support with written cues.		
Problems with encoding/ decoding	➢ Use the same words when repeating instructions and support with written cues. ➢ Use encouraging, nondirective language: "Let's go take a shower;" "Let's find out what's happening over there."		
Strategies to enhance encoding of information	➢ Incorporate training, rehearsal, and repetitive practice to ensure learning of desired information.		
LONG-TERM (SEMANTIC, EPISODIC, and PROCEDURAL MEMORY):	➢ Use written, visual, color, auditory, and tactile cues to enhance access to information. ➢ Use personal objects, pictures, memory books, familiar music, and smells to trigger associations. ➢ Use a variety of external memory aids to store important information for later retrieval.		
Problems with retrieval	➢ Use two-choice questions: "Do you want coffee or orange juice?" ➢ Avoid yes/no questions: "Do you want to take a shower?" "Would you like some help with that?"		
Strategies to facilitate information retrieval	➢ Establish and maintain routines.		

Modified from Bourgeois MS. "Where is my wife and when am I going home?" The challenge of communicating with persons with dementia. *Alzheimers Care Q.* 2002;3(2):141.

for Medicare and Medicaid Service website for download.[106]

Learning and Education Strategies. It is important to remember that a diagnosis of dementia does not mean the person is incapable of learning. However, people with dementia learn differently and require different training methods to enhance learning.[107] For example, people with dementia benefit more from implicit/procedural learning methods,[108] which is consistent with studies of memory showing procedural memory is retained until the late stages of dementia. Also, people with dementia benefit most when learning under constant practice conditions.[109] Therefore, to promote performance, people with dementia benefit from blocked practice without variation (same environment, same steps, same tools) that builds on the familiar (relevancy) and consistent sequencing in mass practice (frequent training with minimal rest). Practice in a similar environment to the eventual performance is also important, because there is poor carryover to or from unfamiliar environments. The kind of feedback most effective for patients with dementia has not been conclusively demonstrated, but it may be that both knowledge of results and knowledge of performance may place too much of a cognitive load on the individual.[108] However, verbal praise seems to be effective, even in the late stages of dementia. Practice under errorless learning conditions may also have some benefit, but the results are equivocal.[110] Errorless learning involves creating a training environment in which the person displays no effort to recall steps of the task and is protected from making mistakes during practice through cues, such as hand-over-hand training, verbal, or tactile cues.

The STOMP (Skill-building through Task Oriented Motor Practice) program was developed to improve ADL performance and delay ADL decline in patients with dementia by combining training methods that have shown promise.[107] The STOMP program consists of highly structured, task-oriented training through massed practice and errorless learning paradigms. The protocol for people with an MMSE score of greater than 10 and less than 25 is based on Taub's learned nonuse theory and the constraint induced movement therapy protocol. The protocol[111] consists of 3-hours/day, 5 times per week for 2 weeks and focuses on three individual and/or family-generated occupational goals (ADL or IADLs). Using the learning methods described above, improvement of function was seen up to 90 days after intervention.[107]

Positive Risk Management. Adopted within the United Kingdom Department of Health, positive risk management is the balance of known risks to physical, mental, and emotional health of an activity or intervention weighed against the risk of not intervening.[111] It is the recognition that a focus on the person's physical safety is often the primary concern of the health care professional, but this may fail to address the mental and emotional risks and impact on well-being.[112] See Box 19.2 for an example of applying the concepts of positive risk management. These are reflected in a growing awareness of relational autonomy and how social, economic, and cultural factors need to be assessed with the individual and others who may be impacted.[113] As physical therapists who are often called on to assess the risk of falling, wandering, discharge location, and other challenging activities, we must recognize that decisions must involve the entire team (including the individual and family) who come to the table with varied personal and professional risk aversion levels.[114]

Issues of Behavior Expression. In 1999, the International Psychogeriatric Association released a definition of Behavioral and Psychological Symptoms of Dementia (BPSD) as "Symptoms of disturbed perception, thought content, mood, or behavior that frequently occur in patients with dementia."[115] Observed behavioral expression symptoms can include physical aggression, wandering, shadowing, restlessness, and sexual disinhibition. Psychological symptoms are based on interview and include anxiety, depressive mood, hallucinations, and delusions. Four categories for subdividing behaviors include psychosis, mood, agitation, and behavioral dyscontrol.[116] Others have included specific items, such as sleep disturbance, apathy, and eating disorders.[117]

The prevalence of at least one symptom of BPSD in people over the course of dementia is estimated at over 95%.[117] Table 19.11 lists the most common behavior expressions by dementia type. These expressions are a major source of burden for care partners of people with dementia and are frequently cited as a reason for admission to long-term care.[115] They are frequently treated with medications that often have untoward effects on function and mood, and thus are a last-resort intervention.

The process of root cause analysis can offer insights into stressors that may be causing behavioral expressions.[118] The most common categories of stressors are related to personal, care partner, and environmental factors.[119] Issues associated with unmet personal needs (physical such as the need to use the bathroom, emotional such as needing a purpose, or psychological such as needing comfort) may be exhibited as nonverbal expressions. Other personal factors include a change in medical status, such as an infection or delirium, and premorbid personality characteristics. Care partner factors are often related to approach and expectations. People with dementia benefit when they are included in ADLs, but this often requires increased time and patience which is challenging to even the most devoted care partners. Similarly, mismatched expectations (e.g., thinking the person can or should do more or less than they are capable of at that time) can lead to frustration of one or both parties. Environmental factors also contribute to stressors when they create excessive noise and use passive engagement and variable routines.

Assessment tools for behavioral expressions exist that physical therapists may encounter and utilize as part of

BOX 19.2 Case Example: Positive Risk Management

At the morning meeting, the nursing staff is asking for a bed/chair alarm to be implemented for Mrs. Jones—a resident of your skilled nursing facility.

Mrs. Jones, 88, who has dementia, completed a course of physical therapy after hip fracture 1 month ago and is full weight-bearing. At discharge her Berg Balance Score (BBS) was 42/56 and she used a walker. The physical therapist's (PT's) recommendation was that she walk with supervision. Noting PT's recommendation, nursing updated the care plan to state: Mrs. Jones should ambulate with walker and a staff person for supervision.

The CNS staff is frustrated as Mrs. Jones wants to walk "all the time." She repeatedly tries to stand but they do not have a staff person available to help her walk every time she attempts to get up. Thus, the staff "encourages" Mrs. Jones to sit down and would like an alarm to help her remember that she "shouldn't be walking alone". Her daughter is frustrated because her mother loved to walk and often took long walks in the woods alone prior to her dementia progressing.

Positive risk management helps reframe the issue to look at the issue from several perspectives. From a physical perspective there is an increased risk of falls as determined by the BBS and history of falls.

Perspective	Walking without staff		Restricting walking and/or use of alarm	
	Negative	**Positive**	**Negative**	**Positive**
Mrs. Jones physical	Potential for falls or injury	Sustain strength, walking	Loss of strength, walking skills, cardiovascular health	None/alarm does not reduce falls
Emotional/ mental	Potential falls or injury	Less frustrated, anxious	Learned helplessness, anxiety, decreased communication	None
Mrs. Jones' daughter	Worries about falls	Feels mom would accept the risk Pleased with staff focus on her needs	Dislikes the alarm Frustrated with staff	None
Staff	Worries about workload if fall occurs	Staff can provide general (facility) level supervision	Less likely to check in, wait for alarm Anxiety "running" to alarm	False comfort
Facility administration	Potential falls	Person-centered Negotiated risk	Alarm coded as restraint-impacts quality rating	None
Other residents	Potential hazard to others	More time for care if staff not having divided attention	Noise from alarm may irritate other residents	None

Each of the positive and negative "risks" to members of the community (in this case the skilled nursing facility) need to be reviewed and weighed, and no one person/department can make the decision in isolation.

TABLE 19.11 Most Common BPSD Expressions by Dementia Type[118]

	Alzheimer Disease	Frontotemporal	Vascular	Mixed	Lewy Body Dementia
Hallucinations and delusions					X
Agitation/aggression	X	X		X	X
Depression/dysphoria	X		X	X	X
Anxiety			X		X
Apathy	X	X	X	X	X
Irritability	X	X	X	X	X
Aberrant motor		X			
Sleep disorder	X	X		X	X
Appetite and eating disorder		X			X

Data from Mukherjee A, Biswas A, Roy A, Biswas S, Gangopadhyay G, Das SK. Behavioural and Psychological Symptoms of Dementia: Correlates and Impact on Caregiver Distress. Dement Geriatr Cogn Dis Extra. 2017;7(3):354–365.

the interdisciplinary team. The Cohen-Mansfield Agitation Inventory assesses up to 29 observed behavioral expressions that care partners may encounter.[81] Behavioral Pathology in Alzheimer's Disease Rating Scale (BEHAVE-AD) measures more categories of disruptive behaviors, but also requires additional time.[81] The Cornell Scale for Depression in Dementia has been validated for use in people with dementia and can be used in those individuals who have depression coexisting with dementia.[81] The Behavioral Dyscontrol Scale assesses the ability to regulate complex motor and behavioral tasks by the frontal lobe and its impact on ADLs.[120] These assessment tools categorize some expressions that are observed in people with dementia; however, it remains uncertain if some of these behavioral expressions are caused by dementia or merely are expressions of unmet needs in the only way remaining to the individual.[121]

There is a growing understanding that by medicalizing these behavioral expressions as BPSD, health care professionals may have contributed to the significant increase in unnecessary antipsychotic use in nursing homes in the United States.[122] It is essential to remain aware of the role of environmental triggers and utilize root cause analysis to assess any behavioral responses.

Exercise and Mobility Management

Exercise in Prevention of Cognitive Impairment. Over the years the evidence for aerobic fitness, physical activity, and exercise in the prevention of cognitive impairment has been mounting.[123] The association between regular aerobic exercise and a lower risk for dementia is confirmed in several longitudinal studies.[124–126] It has been found that older adults with poor physical performance (e.g., slower walking speed, poorer chair rise ability) were more likely to develop cognitive impairment.[127, 128] Recent studies have also demonstrated that a long-lasting physically active lifestyle improves executive control and processing speed in older adults, compared with a sedentary lifestyle.[129–131] Regular exercise and physical activity also protect against cardiovascular disease risk factors, such as hypertension, diabetes, and obesity, which may contribute to the development of cognitive impairment.

Actual neurophysiologic changes occur with aerobic exercise, including increased gray matter volume in the hippocampal regions,[132] increased levels of neurotrophic factors such as peripheral BDNF,[133] and increased blood flow to the brain.[134] Indeed, the neurophysiologic mechanisms accounting for this neuroprotective effect of exercise and physical activity have been one of the growing areas of research in the field. In healthy older adults, higher cardiorespiratory fitness is associated with lower rates of age-related decline in gray matter, particularly in the prefrontal, superior parietal, and temporal cortices.[124] The effects of these neurophysiologic findings are reflected in enhancement of cognitive function in both young and older adults, such as memory abilities,[135] efficiency of attentional processes, and executive function.[134] It is important to note that neurotrophic factor, BDNF (released with exercise), may be important in combating age-related brain atrophy and neurodegenerative diseases.[136]

Resistance Exercise. There is also growing evidence about the effect of resistance training on cognition. Research by Liu-Ambrose et al.[137] demonstrated improvement in selective attention and conflict resolution performance among healthy senior women following resistance training over 1 year. Although some evidence also indicates that high-intensity resistance training improved memory performance in older men,[138, 139] other studies were nonconclusive of the impact of resistance training, [140, 141] perhaps because of the inadequate intensity prescribed. However, the Cassilhas et al.[139] study has provided valuable insight into the possible mechanisms on how resistance training benefits cognition. The research team found that serum insulin-like growth factor-1 (IGF-1) levels are higher in the resistance training groups than in the control group, where IGF-1 promotes neuronal growth, survival, differentiation, and improves cognition.

Multimodal Exercise Programs. Apart from physical activity and exercise, interventions that stimulate cognitive activity in a broader sense, as well as cognitive exercises that target specific cognitive functions, demonstrate improved cognitive performance in controlled trials.[142] A combination of both physical and cognitive exercise has been suggested to induce larger functional benefits on cognition, than each activity on its own. One of the newer possible interventions include Exergaming, where researchers have demonstrated a 23% risk reduction in clinical progression to MCI for a cybercylist group (i.e., cycling with virtual reality-enhanced exercise) compared with the traditional stationary bike cycling in a group of older adults living in retirement communities.[143] In addition, the study also revealed that the cybercylist group experienced a higher increase in BDNF, and hence enhanced neuroplasticity compared with the traditional cycling group.[143] In fact, a short-term 8-week memory training program for healthy older adults induced changes in the cortical thickness in the right fusiform and lateral orbitofrontal cortex, which in turn correlated positively with improvement in memory performance in the short term, reiterating the potential for neuroplasticity to occur with cognitive interventions.[144] Cybercycling has been introduced for institutionalized older adults with dementia in the United Kingdom and Norway with staff anecdotally noting a boost in "wellbeing and happiness."[145]

Exercise for Persons With Mild Cognitive Impairment. Strong evidence indicates that persons with various levels of cognitive impairment, including individuals with MCI, benefit from physical activity and exercise.[146] Based on current research, both aerobic and resistance exercise programs were found to benefit this population in both the short and long run.[147,148] Even a single bout of aerobic exercise stimulated noradrenergic activation and enhanced memory consolidation in both older adults with MCI and non-MCI.[149] More importantly, physical activity (including both aerobic and resistive training) demonstrates a sustained impact on cognitive function for at least 12 months after the interventions were discontinued in individuals with reported memory problems.[59] Specifically, a resistance training program twice-weekly for 6 months significantly improved selective attention, associative memory, and regional patterns of functional brain plasticity in individuals with probable MCI.[150]

Multicomponent community-based programs for individuals with MCI also demonstrate important benefits. A 6-month, multicomponent exercise program of biweekly 90-minute sessions involving aerobic exercise, resistance training, and balance and dual task training significantly improved scores on the MMSE and logical memory scores, reducing whole brain cortical atrophy in a subset of participants with amnestic MCI.[151] In addition, low total cholesterol and higher BDNF was associated with improved cognitive scores, suggesting the neurophysiologic underpinnings of the effects of exercise and cognition.[151] The impact of exercise continued over time for the group of participants with amnestic MCI with significant positive effects on general cognitive function, immediate memory, and language ability.[152] A 9-week program of 90 minutes, one time per week, exercise (strength, balance, flexibility, and endurance) and a discussion of behavioral strategies to increase physical activity, improved physical activity, quality of life, and MMSE scores in older adults with MCI.[153] Other forms of exercises, such as tai chi (carried out at least three times per/week) improved global cognitive function, delayed recall, and subjective cognitive complaints in older adults with MCI,[154] although long-term impacts remain to be explored.

Exercise for Persons With Dementia. Several systematic reviews and meta-analyses have examined the effects of stand-alone, community-based exercise programs and those that are a part of multimodal interventions for persons with various levels of cognitive impairment. Importantly, exercise training for persons in all stages of dementia have a positive effect on the physical and functional performance, behavioral measures, and cognitive measures.[155–157] Exercise training is effective in all forms, including endurance, resistance training, multimodal (including both strength and endurance), functional skill training, and mobility training. Interestingly, researchers generally study exercise programs that focus on functional skills and mobility exercises particularly for people with higher severity of dementia, compared with a focus on endurance and/or resistance training for people with mild dementia. Most recently, a systematic review concluded that strong evidence supports the application of physical exercise of all forms in bouts of 60 minutes/day two to three times a week in improving strength, step length, balance, mobility, and walking endurance for persons with mild cognitive impairment and mild to moderate dementia.[146] It is critical to note that strength and endurance outcomes for older adults with cognitive impairment after exercise training are similar to age- and gender-matched older adults.[156] This further emphasizes that older adults with cognitive impairment have significant rehabilitation potential and should not be denied the opportunity to participate in rehabilitation and exercise.

Although evidence for exercise interventions for persons with severe dementia appeared less conclusive, in part because of the paucity of research,[146] some studies have demonstrated positive findings for people with higher severity of dementia. A 12-month multicentered, randomized, controlled trial incorporated a multicomponent exercise program (aerobic, resistance, flexibility, and balance training) for 1-hour per session, twice a week for older adults with dementia living in nursing homes.[158] This study demonstrated significant improvement in walking speed for participants with moderate to severe dementia (mean MMSE 9.7 $\pm$ 6.8) at 6 and 12 months and, although there was a decline in ADL function as measured by the Katz index, it was slower than in those in the control group who did not exercise.[158] Bossers et al.[159] investigated the feasibility of conducting a combined aerobic and resistance training program of moderate intensity for people with moderate to severe dementia in a nursing home with three, 30-minute walking sessions and two progressive strength training sessions (rate of perceived exertion [RPE] "somewhat hard"). The researchers found an improvement in 6-minute walk test, walking speed, quadriceps strength, and balance in the exercise group after the 6-week exercise program. Even shorter multicomponent programs of just 8 weeks (flexibility, strength, balance, and gait exercises) demonstrated a significant improvement in walking speed, stride length, stride frequency, and symmetry index.[160]

The literature also describes evidence-based interventions for older adults with severe dementia who are more functional and activity-based in nature. High-intensity, progressive functional exercise consisting of everyday tasks challenging leg strength, postural stability, and gait in weight-bearing positions for 29 sessions over 3 months yielded significant benefits, such as significant improvement in comfortable gait speed and lower limb strength for people with moderate to severe dementia.[161, 162] A randomized, controlled compared an activity specific exercise program (strength, flexibility balance, and endurance) with a self-paced walking program.[163] The authors found the indivdiuals participitaing in the activity-specific program improved in their transfer and 6-minute walk distance, while the individuals in the self-paced walking group declined. On the other hand, other studies introducing "walk and talk" programs as interventions for residents in long-term facilities with moderate to severe dementia appear to have limited benefit in view of ineffective exercise prescription (e.g., lack of intensity or progression).[164,165] Indeed, it is key to ensure that exercise programs prescribed for people with dementia should be of sufficient intensity and with progression and overload, even for people with moderate to severe dementia.

Based on current evidence where interventions are largely heterogeneous, there is no clear conclusion on whether aerobic or resistance exercises have a preferred benefit for older adults with dementia. As multicomponent exercise programs showed significant benefit for older adults with dementia, it is crucial that the exercise programs be tailored and that they are composed of different forms of exercise, including flexibility, aerobic, resistance, and balance exercises. In addition, functional training has been advocated and found to benefit older adults with dementia.[161,162,166] More importantly, in view of the improvements in outcomes with appropriate intensity, duration with progression, exercise prescription for older adults with dementia should not differ from individuals with normal cognition.

Multimodal Exercise Programs. A combination of both physical and cognitive training programs also benefits people with dementia.[167] Some preliminary evidence suggests that multimodal interventions, including physical exercise (tai chi), cognitive behavioral training, and use of support groups, led to a significant difference in MMSE scores for the intervention versus control group in community-dwelling older adults with mild to moderate dementia.[168] A 12-month institution-based program (98 patients with moderate to severe primary degenerative dementia, across five nursing homes) composed of functional activities, including 40 minutes of ADL training and 30 minutes of games (e.g., bowling), together with 30 minutes of cognitive tasks (e.g., word jumbles, picture puzzles) showed that cognitive function and the ability to carry out ADLs remained stable in the intervention group, but had decreased in the control group.[169] In addition, augmentation of multicomponent cognitive therapy with a physical component, such as aerobic exercise over 6 months, led to a better cognitive function in individuals with moderate to severe dementia, compared with the group who underwent only the cognitive therapy (i.e., activities, such as handicraft, horticulture therapy).[170] Hence, despite the lack of strong evidence in specific recommendations for combined physical and cognitive training, it remains important to consider the inclusion of a cognitive component into the physical activity or exercise programs for individuals with dementia, because they could possibly augment the benefits of exercise.

Gait, Balance, and Falls. A growing body of evidence shows that gait changes may be an early indicator of cognitive changes and may vary by type of dementia.[171–173] Performance in spatiotemporal gait parameters was noted to match the cognitive decline in various stages of dementia, but was more affected in the non-AD than the Alzheimer type.[173] These spatiotemporal changes measured by Gait Mat® were in areas of stride length, stride width, and gait velocity. Poor gait performance was shown to be present between 3 and 9 years before dementia was diagnosed in one systematic review.[171] A more recent prospective study found that changes in motor function that result in gait velocity decline could be noted in serial assessments more than a decade before cognitive decline.[174]

Executive function and dual tasking, the ability to focus on a cognitive task while performing a motor task, has an impact on people with dementia. For example, the cognitive load demands of using an assistive device can slow gait speed owing to split attention needs.[175] Lower gait velocities were recorded in individuals with MCI who were asked to perform specific dual tasks, such as backward counting by 7,[176–178] backward counting by 1,[179,180] and naming animals.[176,177,180]

Although gait changes are associated with dementia, evidence indicates that intervention can be successful in improving gait parameters in this population.[181] Because both physical and cognitive factors affect gait performance, interventions should address both deficits.[181] A systematic review by Zhang et al.[181] found strong evidence that "exercise programs focusing on strength and balance training, especially when combined with functional mobility training, improve gait in people with MCI or dementia."[181] The review also found strong evidence that programs "combining strength and balance training, functional mobility training, and attention and executive function training improve gait."[181]

Balance changes associated with dementia remain an area for more research. A systematic review and meta-analysis showed that increased anterior/posterior and medial lateral sway occurred in static standing for individuals with MCI, but only under eyes-open conditions.[182] Balance was more significantly impaired as measured by the Tinetti Mobility Test and Berg Balance Scale for people with LBD as compared with individuals with Alzheimer disease and Parkinson disease.[183] Executive function demands of maintaining upright posture with mobility were best captured by the Timed Up and Go (TUG)-Dual Task test, reflecting a more significant slowing of performance on the TUG in dual task conditions.[175]

Falls are multifactorial events and a challenge for people with dementia and their care partners. A history of a fall within the previous year is a strong predictor of future falls in all older adults regardless of cognitive status.[184] In addition to the typical issues having an impact on fall risk for older adults, as discussed elsewhere in this text, psychological factors, such as attention-seeking and being verbally disruptive, play a large role in fall risk for people with dementia living in nursing facilities.[185] Caregiver depression and emotional stress was associated with caring for the person who had a higher fall frequency.[185] Sleep disruption as well as sleep medications are key contributors in falls for people with dementia.[186] It should be noted that the use of physical restraints and alarms have not been shown to decrease falls.[187]

Most fall prevention intervention studies exclude people with cognitive impairment, so only limited evidence-based recommendations exist to lower fall risk in this population.[188] A pilot study tested the acceptability of individualized home safety recommendations and exercise to reduce falls that was tailored to cognitive abilities. Results indicated after 10 home visits by an occupational therapist that half (n=5) implemented 50% or more recommendations, 73% (n=8) adhered to some exercises with fewer falls in the intervention group.[189] The Westmead Home Safety Checklist is considered the gold standard for assessing home-based hazards that have an impact on fall risk for older adults.[190] This checklist should be part of a home-based physical therapy assessment because one study found that 44% of people with dementia living at home had outdoors stairs without a railing, among other hazards.[191]

A study of the impact of education on fall risk revealed that people with dementia and their caregivers benefit from having the right information at the right time.[192] These authors found through conducting interviews with people with dementia that a personalized approach and contextual information was needed.[192] For example, a single session of falls prevention education may not be sufficient to meet individual needs. A program that provides education and practice components of stepping strategies together with additional follow-up sessions may be more beneficial.

Assessment of Mobility. The Six Minute Walk Test has excellent test-retest values for people with dementia and has shown validity for exercise capacity.[193] The Timed Up and Go test, as recommended by the American/British Geriatric Society, is an easy-to-use tool for people of varying cognitive abilities.[194] A systemic review by Bossers et al.[193] recommends the Tinetti Mobility Test for measures of balance in older adults with dementia. Additionally, in a small study of nursing home residents with mild to moderate dementia, the Berg Balance Scale has shown excellent relative interrater reliability and internal consistency.[195] Normative scores for people with dementia, along with test administration, are discussed elsewhere in this text.

Activities of Daily Living. Apraxia is the inability to perform a previously learned motor activity, whereas dyspraxia is a discoordination of that activity. Someone in the early stages of Alzheimer disease may display signs of apraxia in dressing, complicated later with loss of a motor plan to don the item (ideomotor changes) and knowing its intended purpose (ideational changes). In late stages of AD, apraxia may be expressed in challenges with eating/swallowing.[196] Buccopharyngeal changes and gait changes (increased stride time and variance) appear earlier and to a greater degree in FTD than in other forms of dementia.[196]

Based on the type of apraxia, specific strategies need to be designed to help improve the performance of a task. For example, if the individual has difficulty with the sequence of brushing teeth, verbal instruction in a stepwise sequence can be used. If the individual has difficulty in recognizing the tools needed for a task, all the equipment can be set up in advance. Others may benefit from simultaneous visual demonstration. Thus, an individual's capacity should be supplemented by the care partner to promote active involvement whenever possible. Using an abilities-focused approach has been demonstrated to improve functional performance and decrease agitation and resident interaction.[197] Montessori principles are being applied to therapeutic interactions and focus on the enhancing the ADL skills the person has retained.[198]

Pain. People with dementia do not report pain spontaneously, or often, even when questioned.[199] In fact, it is believed that as many as 50% of people with dementia may be regularly experiencing pain,[200] and observational studies indicate that pain is undertreated.[201] Because known autonomic responses are altered in people with dementia, traditional physiologic symptoms of pain, such as in increase in heart rate, may not be observed.[201] However, data suggest that chronic pain may result in sensory-affective responses in people with dementia. An increased sensitivity to noxious stimuli (hyperalgesia) and painful response to nonnoxious stimuli (allodynia) may result in pain "behavior" that appears out of proportion to the observer.[202] These behavior expressions are most easily observed during assistance with ADLs that lead to aggressive responses from the person with dementia despite "normal" nonpainful stimuli being provided by the care partner. In FTD there is a described loss of pain consciousness that may be associated with changes in pain processing, so pain may not be expressed, but instead results in a disturbed feeling.[201]

Physical therapists and other health care professionals are taught to assess pain via many tools, most of which rely on a verbal or written self-report from the individual. Health care professionals must also rely on visual observation of facial and behavioral expressions combined to postulate that the person may be in pain. Several studies have demonstrated that nurses are no better than lay observers at visually assessing pain expressions despite their educational preparation.[199,203] The seven components of facial expressions identified, which can indicate pain in people with dementia, that can be discriminated with focused attention and observation, are listed in Box 19.3.[203]

Pain Assessment. Many pain assessment tools exist to address observed pain behaviors, although none have been officially endorsed. The Pain in Advanced Dementia (PAINAD) is a five-item measure with scores that range from 0 to 2 for each item.[204] It covers three of the six American Geriatric Society pain assessment domains.[205] The PAINAD is recommended for its ease of use and its reliability and validity.[206] The Pain Assessment Checklist for Seniors with Limited Ability to Communicate (PACSLAC-II) is an observational scale with 31 behaviors (present or absent) that assesses all 6 of the American Geriatrics Society pain assessment domains (described in Table 19.12).[205] Nursing practice consensus recommends that both the PAINAD and PACSLAC-II tests be

BOX 19.3 Facial Expressions of Pain[203]

- Frowning
- Narrow eyes
- Raised upper lip
- Tightened lip
- Opened mouth
- Frightened expression
- Looking tense

TABLE 19.12 Comparison of American Geriatric Society (AGS) Pain Domains With Assessment Tools

AGS Pain Domains	PAINAD	PACSLAC-II
Facial expressions	x	X
Verbalizations and vocalizations	x	X
Body movements	x	X
Changes in interpersonal interactions		X
Changes in activity patterns or routines		X
Mental status changes		X

PACSLAC-II, Pain Assessment Checklist for Seniors with Limited Ability to Communicate; *PAINAD*, Pain in Advanced Dementia.

used because they assess different components of pain expressions, and combined may offer the best method to identify pain in people with dementia.[207]

Once pain or potential pain has been identified, treatment may be implemented. Additionally, guidelines suggest that if pain findings in people with dementia are ambiguous, the recommendation is to start a trial of pain treatment.[208] The first course of action should be the trial of a nonpharmacologic approach. Using a person-centered care approach that recognizes the individual needs of each person is at the basis of nonpharmacologic interventions.[121] Knowing the person and learning to "read" his or her needs improved with dedicated staffing patterns and it leads to improved care outcomes and employee retention/satisfaction.[209,210] Structured care protocols (e.g., oral care and bathing practices) that may be personalized, but also set a baseline expectation are more effective.[211] Examples of these include the "Bathing Without a Battle" educational program that assesses for the optimal bathing method (singing together, bathing in segments; e.g., one area per day, towel baths),[212] sensory practices that stimulate or enhance calm (e.g., aromatherapy, massage, light), as well as activities that are individualized and engaging (e.g., pet therapy, music, physical activity) can reduce pain behavioral expressions and falls.[213]

If medication is needed, the American Geriatrics Society and British Geriatrics Society recommend that acetaminophen should be the first pharmacologic management for pain in older adults owing to its good safety profile and effectiveness.[214] If pain is neuropathic in origin, medications such as gabapentin are first-line medications for treatment, although specific guidelines for people with dementia need to be developed.[215] Higher intensity medications should be individually assessed because narcotic analgesics have significant side effects and these risks have to be balanced against quality of life.

CAREPARTNER EDUCATION

An effective physical therapist must address not only the patient's needs and environment, but also available support systems and family dynamics in order to implement an individual plan of care. Education and training for the caregiver are essential because management of the patient is heavily dependent on the family support and coping resources.

Psychological health of the caregiver should be a concern to the therapist and is often related to the function of the patient. Although the physical therapist is with the patient for only a few minutes to an hour per day, the caregiver may be with the person every day, all day. Depression, anxiety, and caregiver burden are reported to be much higher among caregivers caring for an individual with dementia compared with caregivers of persons with physical frailty.[216] The increase in these symptoms is owing to the changes in personality, disruptive behaviors, lack of spare time, isolation, and progressive deterioration associated with dementia.[216] Further investigation of spouse involvement reveals female caregivers experiencing a greater degree of negative psychological effects than male caregivers.[217] Fortunately, positive effects of caregiving for persons with dementia have also been demonstrated. These include feeling useful, important, and confident, as well as increased satisfaction in their caregiving role and the ability to provide a good quality of life to a loved one.[53]

The therapist's awareness of the potential for a caregiver to have mental health problems is the first step. Identification of warning signs, such as caregiver denial, anger, depression, exhaustion, or health problems, should be a call for action by the therapist to avoid a complex situation. Studies of the REACH (Resources for Enhancing Alzheimer's Caregiver Health) identify the keys to decreasing caregiving stress (Box 19.4).[218]

Some stress can be avoided by educating the caregiver on the limitations of the patient. Education should minimize unrealistic goals that are translated into demands on the patient that could result in failure, frustration, and sometimes behavior problems. The therapist can assist in identifying patient activities that can be performed successfully. Identification of community support groups for the caregiver should be part of the treatment plan, offering an opportunity for education and emotional assistance. The growth of Memory Cafes allows an opportunity for both the persons with dementia and their care partners to engage in activities for cognitive stimulation in a judgment-free environment. First introduced in the Netherlands, Dr. Bere Miesen started a group to reduce stigma because dementia was not openly discussed.[219] These cafes are designed to meet the needs of those in early stages of dementia who may be losing social engagement and to offer a welcoming community.[220] Numerous sources of information and support groups are also available on the Internet from the Alzheimer's Association, American Geriatric Society, and the National Institute on Aging. Respite care, either in the home, adult day care, or at long-term care facilities, can provide the caregiver the needed time for self-care and enjoyable activities. The reader is also referred to the chapter on caregiving elsewhere in this text for additional information about addressing caregiver stress.

BOX 19.4 Keys to Decreasing Caregiver Stress[218]

- Extensive education regarding strategies to deal with behavioral problems, including role-playing
- Enhance ADL abilities with strategies to reinforce
- Reinforcement with practice, home visits, and phone calls
- Encourage self-care with pleasurable activities and health-promoting behaviors

SUMMARY

In this chapter, we have summarized the normal and pathologic cognitive changes that occur as we age. In addition, we have explored the assessment and management of delirium, mild cognitive impairment, and the different types of dementia. More importantly, we have highlighted and elaborated on the nonpharmacologic interventions for cognitive impairment, especially the role of exercise and physical activity. It is key to make modifications to exercise and physical therapy programs (e.g., communication aspects and appropriate assessment of pain) based on the severity of the dementia. Lastly, we emphasize that caring for people with dementia also involves caring for their caregivers and families. As such, physical therapists play a critical role as strong advocates for person-centered care and rehabilitation, in order to restore and maintain the dignity and quality of life for people with dementia.

REFERENCES

1. Oxford Dictionary. *Cognition | Definition of cognition in English by Oxford Dictionaries.* https://en.oxforddictionaries.com/definition/cognition; 2018. Accessed January 2, 2019.
2. American Psychiatric Association. American Psychiatric Association. DSM-5 Task Force. *Diagnostic and Statistical Manual of Mental Disorders*: DSM-5. American Psychiatric Association; 2013. https://www.appi.org/Diagnostic_and_Statistical_Manual_of_Mental_Disorders_DSM-5_Fifth_Edition. Accessed December 31, 2018.
3. Hedden T, Gabrieli JDE. Insights into the ageing mind: a view from cognitive neuroscience. *Nat Rev Neurosci.* 2004;5(2):87–96. https://doi.org/10.1038/nrn1323.
4. Grady C. The cognitive neuroscience of ageing. *Nat Rev Neurosci.* 2012;13(7):491–505. https://doi.org/10.1038/nrn3256.
5. Reuter-Lorenz PA, Park DC. Human neuroscience and the aging mind: a new look at old problems. *J Gerontol B Psychol Sci Soc Sci.* 2010;65B(4):405–415. https://doi.org/10.1093/geronb/gbq035.
6. Ballesteros S, Nilsson L-G, Lemaire P. Ageing, cognition, and neuroscience: an introduction. *Eur J Cogn Psychol.* 2009;21(2-3):161–175. https://doi.org/10.1080/09541440802598339.
7. Macpherson H, Pipingas A, Silberstein R. A steady state visually evoked potential investigation of memory and ageing. *Brain Cogn.* 2009;69(3):571.
8. Duff K, Schoenberg M, Scott J, Adams R. The relationship between executive functioning and verbal and visual learning and memory. *Arch Clin Neuropsychol.* 2005;20(1):111–122.
9. Grigsby J, Kaye K, Robbins LJ. Behavioral disturbance and impairment of executive functions among the elderly. *Arch Gerontol Geriatr.* 1995;21(2):167–177.
10. Grigsby J, Kaye K, Baxter J, Shetterly SM, Hamman RF. Executive cognitive abilities and functional status among community-dwelling older persons in the San Luis Valley Health and Aging Study. *J Am Geriatr Soc.* 1998;46(5):590–596.
11. Gabrieli JD. Memory systems analyses of mnemonic disorders in aging and age-related diseases. *Proc Natl Acad Sci U S A.* 1996;93(24):13534–13540.
12. de Frias CM, Dixon RA, Strauss E. Characterizing executive functioning in older special populations: from cognitively elite to cognitively impaired. *Neuropsychology.* 2009;23(6):778–791.
13. Rapport LJ, Hanks RA, Millis SR, Deshpande SA. Executive functioning and predictors of falls in the rehabilitation setting. *Arch Phys Med Rehabil.* 1998;79(6):629–633.
14. Richardson JK. Imbalanced: The confusing circular nature of falls research…and a possible antidote. *Am J Phys Med Rehabil.* 2017;96(1):55–59.
15. Harada CN, Natelson Love MC, Triebel KL. Normal cognitive aging. *Clin Geriatr Med.* 2013;29(4):737–752.
16. Moran JM, Jolly E, Mitchell JP. Social-cognitive deficits in normal aging. *J Neurosci.* 2012;32(16):5553–5561.
17. Lantrip C, Huang JH. Cognitive control of emotion in older adults: a review. *Clinical Psychiatry* (Wilmington, Del). 2017;3(1):1–10.
18. Persson J, Nyberg L, Lind J, et al. Structure–function correlates of cognitive decline in aging. *Cereb Cortex.* 2006;16(7):907–915.
19. Morrison JH, Baxter MG. The ageing cortical synapse: hallmarks and implications for cognitive decline. *Nat Rev Neurosci.* 2012;13(4):240–250.
20. Eubank KJ, Covinsky KE. Delirium severity in the hospitalized patient: time to pay attention. *Ann Intern Med.* 2014;160(8):574–575.
21. Whitlock EL, Vannucci A, Avidan MS. Postoperative delirium. *Minerva Anestesiol.* 2011;77(4):448–456.
22. Fong TG, Davis D, Growdon ME, Albuquerque A, Inouye SK. The interface between delirium and dementia in elderly adults. *Lancet Neurol.* 2015;14(8):823–832.
23. National Institute for Health and Clinical Excellence. *Delirium: Prevention, Diagnosis and Management | Guidance and Guidelines* | NICE; 2010. https://www.nice.org.uk/guidance/cg103.
24. Caplan G. Managing delirium in older patients. *Aust Prescr.* 2011;34(1):16–18.
25. Saxena S, Lawley D. Delirium in the elderly: a clinical review. *Postgrad Med J.* 2009;85(1006):405–413.
26. McAvay GJ, Van Ness PH, Bogardus ST, et al. Older adults discharged from the hospital with delirium: 1-year outcomes. *J Am Geriatr Soc.* 2006;54(8):1245–1250.
27. Hshieh TT, Saczynski J, Gou RY, et al. Trajectory of functional recovery after postoperative delirium in elective surgery. *Ann Surg.* 2017;265(4):647–653.
28. Inouye SK, Marcantonio ER, Kosar CM, et al. The short-term and long-term relationship between delirium and cognitive trajectory in older surgical patients. *Alzheimer's Dementia.* 2016;12(7):766–775.
29. Bickel H, Gradinger R, Kochs E, Förstl H. High risk of cognitive and functional decline after postoperative delirium. A three-year prospective study. *Dement Geriatr Cogn Disord.* 2008;26(1):26–31.
30. Fong TG, Jones RN, Marcantonio ER, et al. Adverse outcomes after hospitalization and delirium in persons with Alzheimer disease. *Ann Intern Med.* 2012;156(12):848.
31. Gross AL, Jones RN, Habtemariam DA, et al. Delirium and long-term cognitive trajectory among persons with dementia. *Arch Intern Med.* 2012;172(17):1324–1331.
32. Fong TG, Tulebaev SR, Inouye SK. Delirium in elderly adults: diagnosis, prevention and treatment. *Nat Rev Neurol.* 2009;5(4):210–220.
33. de Rooij SE, van Munster BC, Korevaar JC, Levi M. Cytokines and acute phase response in delirium. *J Psychosom Res.* 2007;62(5):521–525.
34. Van Munster BC, Korevaar JC, Zwinderman AH, Levi M, Wiersinga WJ, De Rooij SE. Time-course of cytokines during delirium in elderly patients with hip fractures. *J Am Geriatr Soc.* 2008;56(9):1704–1709.

35. Maclullich AMJ, Anand A, Davis DHJ, et al. New horizons in the pathogenesis, assessment and management of delirium. *Age Ageing*. 2013;42(6):667–674.
36. Hall RJ, Ferguson KJ, Andrews M, et al. Delirium and cerebrospinal fluid S100B in hip fracture patients: a preliminary study. *Am J Geriatr Psychiatry*. 2013;21(12):1239–1243.
37. Inouye SK, Westendorp RGJ, Saczynski JS. Delirium in elderly people. *Lancet*. 2014;383(9920):911–922.
38. Hshieh TT, Yue J, Oh E, et al. Effectiveness of multicomponent nonpharmacological delirium interventions: a meta-analysis. *JAMA Intern Med*. 2015;175(4):512–520.
39. Alagiakrishnan K, Wiens CA. An approach to drug induced delirium in the elderly. *Postgrad Med J*. 2004;80 (945):388–393.
40. Young J, Inouye SK. Delirium in older people. *BMJ*. 2007;334 (7598):842–846.
41. Leslie DL, Marcantonio ER, Zhang Y, Leo-Summers L, Inouye SK. One-year health care costs associated with delirium in the elderly population. *Arch Intern Med*. 2008;168(1):27–32.
42. Rubin FH, Neal K, Fenlon K, Hassan S, Inouye SK. Sustainability and scalability of the hospital elder life program at a community hospital. *J Am Geriatr Soc*. 2011;59 (2):359–365.
43. Caplan GA, Coconis J, Board N, Sayers A, Woods J. Does home treatment affect delirium? A randomised controlled trial of rehabilitation of elderly and care at home or usual treatment (The REACH-OUT trial). *Age Ageing*. 2006;35(1):53–60.
44. World Health Organization, Alzheimer's Disease International. *Dementia: A Public Health Priority*. Geneva, Switzerland: World Health Organization; 2012.
45. Bouchard RW. Diagnostic criteria of dementia. *Can J Neurol Sci*. 2007;34(Suppl 1):S11–S18.
46. Vicioso BA. Dementia: when is it not Alzheimer disease? *Am J Med Sci*. 2002;324(2):84–95.
47. Kapasi A, DeCarli C, Schneider JA. Impact of multiple pathologies on the threshold for clinically overt dementia. *Acta Neuropathol*. 2017;134(2):171–186.
48. World Health Organization. Dementia. https://www.who.int/news-room/fact-sheets/detail/dementia. Published 2017. Accessed December 29, 2018.
49. Wimo A, Gauthier S, Prince M. *Global Estimates of Informal Care*. Sweden: Huddinge; 2018.
50. Alzheimer's Association. *Alzheimer's Facts and Figures Report*. https://www.alz.org/alzheimers-dementia/facts-figures. Published 2018. Accessed December 29, 2018.
51. Chêne G, Beiser A, Au R, et al. Gender and incidence of dementia in the Framingham Heart Study from mid-adult life. *Alzheimer's Dementia*. 2015;11(3):310–320.
52. Wimo A, Winblad B, Jönsson L. The worldwide societal costs of dementia: estimates for 2009. *Alzheimer's Dementia*. 2010;6 (2):98–103.
53. Roth DL, Fredman L, Haley WE. Informal caregiving and its impact on health: a reappraisal from population-based studies. *Gerontologist*. 2015;55(2):309–319.
54. Petersen RC, Smith GE, Waring SC, Ivnik RJ, Kokmen E, Tangelos EG. Aging, memory, and mild cognitive impairment. *Int Psychogeriatr*. 1997;9(Suppl 1):65–69.
55. Petersen RC. Mild cognitive impairment. *Contnuum (Minneap Minn)*. 2016;22(2, Dementia):404–418.
56. Rodakowski J, Skidmore ER, Reynolds CF, et al. Can performance on daily activities discriminate between older adults with normal cognitive function and those with mild cognitive impairment? *J Am Geriatr Soc*. 2014;62 (7):1347–1352.
57. Weiner MW, Veitch DP, Aisen PS, et al. Impact of the Alzheimer's disease neuroimaging initiative, 2004 to 2014. *Alzheimer's Dementia*. 2015;11(7):865–884.
58. Pandya SY, Clem MA, Silva LM, Woon FL. Does mild cognitive impairment always lead to dementia? A review. *J Neurol Sci*. 2016;369:57–62.
59. Lautenschlager NT, Cox KL, Flicker L, et al. Effect of physical activity on cognitive function in older adults at risk for Alzheimer disease. *JAMA*. 2008;300(9):1027–1037.
60. Villemagne VL, Burnham S, Bourgeat P, et al. Amyloid β deposition, neurodegeneration, and cognitive decline in sporadic Alzheimer's disease: a prospective cohort study. *Lancet Neurol*. 2013;12(4):357–367.
61. Resnick SM, Sojkova J, Zhou Y, et al. Longitudinal cognitive decline is associated with fibrillar amyloid-beta measured by [11C]PiB. *Neurology*. 2010;74(10):807–815.
62. Kumar A, Singh A. Ekavali. A review on Alzheimer's disease pathophysiology and its management: an update. *Pharmacol Rep*. 2015;67(2):195–203.
63. Budni J, Bellettini-Santos T, Mina F, Garcez ML, Zugno AI. The involvement of BDNF, NGF and GDNF in aging and Alzheimer's disease. *Aging Dis*. 2015;6(5):331–341.
64. Matrone C, Ciotti MT, Mercanti D, Marolda R, Calissano P. NGF and BDNF signaling control amyloidogenic route and A β production in hippocampal neurons. *Proc Natl Acad Sci*. 2008;105(35):13139–13144.
65. Hayden KM, Zandi PP, Lyketsos CG, et al. Vascular risk factors for incident Alzheimer disease and vascular dementia. *Alzheimer Dis Assoc Disord*. 2006;20(2):93–100.
66. Levenson RW, Sturm VE, Haase CM. Emotional and behavioral symptoms in neurodegenerative disease: a model for studying the neural bases of psychopathology. *Annu Rev Clin Psychol*. 2014;10:581–606.
67. McKeith IG, Boeve BF, Dickson DW, et al. Diagnosis and management of dementia with Lewy bodies. *Neurology*. 2017;89(1):88–100.
68. Marti MJ, Tolosa E, Campdelacreu J. Clinical overview of the synucleinopathies. *Mov Disord*. 2003;18(S6):21–27.
69. Schildkrout B. Frontotemporal dementia: a brain disease that challenges definitions of mental illness. *Psychiatric Times*. 2017;34(8):1–5.
70. American Geriatrics Society. *Geriatrics Care | Geriatric Resources | Online events | Updates: Geriatrics Care Online*. https://geriatricscareonline.org/FullText/B007/B007_CH004 Published 2018. Accessed December 29, 2018.
71. Alzheimer's Association. *Cognitive Assessment Toolkit*; 2013.
72. Borson S, Scanlan J, Brush M, Vitaliano P, Dokmak A. The mini-cog: a cognitive "vital signs" measure for dementia screening in multi-lingual elderly. *Int J Geriatr Psychiatry*. 2000;15(11):1021–1027.
73. Mini-Cog. Scoring the Mini-Cog© – Mini-Cog©. https://mini-cog.com/mini-cog-instrument/scoring-the-mini-cog/. Accessed November 17, 2017.
74. Tam E, Gandesbery BT, Young L, Borson S, Gorodeski EZ. Graphical instructions for administration and scoring the Mini-Cog: results of a randomized clinical trial. *J Am Geriatr Soc*. 2018;66:987–991.
75. GPCOG | Frequently Asked Questions. http://gpcog.com.au/index/frequently-asked-questions. Published 2018. Accessed November 17, 2018.
76. Brodaty H, Pond D, Kemp NM, et al. The GPCOG: a new screening test for dementia designed for general practice. *J Am Geriatr Soc*. 2002;50(3):530–534.
77. Kuslansky G, Buschke H, Katz M, Sliwinski M, Lipton RB. Screening for Alzheimer's disease: the memory impairment screen versus the conventional three-word memory test. *J Am Geriatr Soc*. 2002;50(6):1086–1091.
78. Carnero-Pardo C. Should the mini-mental state examination be retired? *Neurologia*. 2014;29(8):473–481. https://doi.org/10.1016/j.nrl.2013.07.003. Epub 2013 Oct.

79. Hancock P, Larner AJ. Test Your Memory test: diagnostic utility in a memory clinic population. *Int J Geriatr Psychiatry*. 2011;26(9):976–980.
80. Nasreddine ZS, Phillips NA, Bédirian V, et al. The Montreal Cognitive Assessment, MoCA: a brief screening tool for mild cognitive impairment. *J Am Geriatr Soc*. 2005;53 (4):695–699.
81. Sheehan B. Assessment scales in dementia. *Ther Adv Neurol Disord*. 2012;5(6):349–358.
82. Mocatest.org. MoCA Montreal Cognitive Assessment. https://www.mocatest.org/. Accessed December 31, 2018.
83. Tariq SH, Tumosa N, Chbnall JT, et al. The Saint Louis University Mental Status (SLUMS) | Measurement Instrument Database for the Social Sciences. http://www.midss.org/content/saint-louis-university-mental-status-slums. Accessed December 31, 2018.
84. Tariq SH, Tumosa N, Chibnall JT, Perry MH, Morley JE. Comparison of the Saint Louis University Mental Status Examination and the Mini-Mental State Examination for Detecting Dementia and Mild Neurocognitive Disorder—a pilot study. *Am J Geriatr Psychiatry*. 2006;14(11):900–910.
85. Arbuthnott K, Frank J. Trail Making Test, Part B as a measure of executive control: validation using a set-switching paradigm. *J Clin Exp Neuropsychol*. 2000;22(4):518–528.
86. Tombaugh TN. Trail Making Test A and B: normative data stratified by age and education. *Arch Clin Neuropsychol*. 2004;19:203–214.
87. Papandonatos GD, Ott BR, Davis JD, Barco PP, Carr DB. Clinical utility of the Trail-Making Test as a predictor of driving performance in older adults. *J Am Geriatr Soc*. 2015;63(11):2358–2364.
88. Olde Rikkert MGM, Tona KD, Janssen L, et al. Validity, reliability, and feasibility of clinical staging scales in dementia. *Am J Alzheimers Dis Other Demen*. 2011;26 (5):357–365.
89. Reisberg B, Jamil IA, Khan S, et al. Staging dementia. In: Abou-Saleh MT, Katona CLE, Kumar A, eds. *Principles and Practices of Geriatric Psychiatry*, vol. 3. Hoboken, NJ: Wiley-Blackwell; 2010.
90. Matsunaga S, Kishi T, Iwata N. Combination therapy with cholinesterase inhibitors and memantine for Alzheimer's disease: a systematic review and meta-analysis. *Int J Neuropsychopharmacol*. 2015;18(5):pyu115.
91. Jo Delaney L. Patient-centred care as an approach to improving health care in Australia. *Collegian*. 2018;25(1):119–123.
92. Benbow SM, Jolley D. Dementia: stigma and its effects. *Neurodegener Dis Manag*. 2012;2(2):165–172.
93. Gately M, Trudeau S. Occupational therapy and advanced dementia: a practitioner survey. *J Geriatr Ment Heal*. 2017;4 (1):48.
94. Challen R, Low L-F, McEntee MF. Dementia patient care in the diagnostic medical imaging department. *Radiography*. 2018;24:S33–S42.
95. Committee on Quality Health Care in America, Institute of Medicine. *Crossing the quality chasm: a new health system for the 21st century*. Natl Acad Press. Washington, DC: National Academy Press; 2001.
96. Morgan SS, Yoder L, Morgan S, Yoder LH. A concept analysis of person-centered care. *J Holist Nurs*. 2012;30(1):6–15.
97. Center for Medicare and Medicaid Services. National-Partnership-to-Improve-Dementia-Care-in-Nursing-Homes. https://www.cms.gov/Medicare/Provider-Enrollment-and-Certification/SurveyCertificationGenInfo/National-Partnership-to-Improve-Dementia-Care-in-Nursing-Homes.html. Published 2018. Accessed May 9, 2018.
98. Kitwood TM. *Dementia Reconsidered: The Person Comes First*. Bukingham, England: Open University Press; 1997.
99. Downs M, Lord K. Person-centered dementia care in the community: a perspective from the United Kingdom. *J Geronotol Nurs*. 2017;43(8):11–17.
100. Fazio S, Pace D, Flinner J, Kallmyer B. The fundamentals of person-centered care for individuals with dementia. *Gerontologist*. 2018;58(suppl_1):S10–S19.
101. Savundranayagam MY, Moore-Nielsen K. Language-based communication strategies that support person-centered communication with persons with dementia. *Int Psychogeriatrics*. 2015;27(10):1707–1718.
102. Bourgeois MS. "Where is my wife and when am I going home?": the challenge of communicating with persons with dementia. *Alzheimer's Care Quarterly*. 2002;3(2):132–144.
103. Sabat SR. Implicit memory and people with Alzheimer's disease: implication for caregiving. *Am J Alzheimers Dis Other Demen*. 2006;21(1):11–14.
104. Murphy J. Positive approaches to care: a new look at dementia education. *J Prim Health Care*. 2017;27(1):29–33.
105. Staal J. Mindfulness and therapeutic presence integrated into 24 hour sensory care or elders with dementia. *JSM Alzheimers Dis Relat Dement*. 2016;3(2):1025–1028.
106. Centers for Medicare & Medicaid Services. Hand in Hand: A Training Series for Nursing Homes Toolkit. Hand in Hand: A Training Series for Nursing Homes Toolkit. https://surveyortraining.cms.hhs.gov/pubs/HandinHand.aspx. Published 2015. Accessed May 4, 2018.
107. Ciro CA, Dung Dao H, Anderson M, Robinson CA, Hamilton TB, Hershey Li A. Improving daily life skills in people with dementia: testing the STOMP intervention Model. *J Alzheimers Dis Parkinsonisim*. 2014;04(05):1–10.
108. van Halteren-van Tilborg IADA, Scherder EJA, Hulstijn W. Motor-skill learning in Alzheimer's disease: a review with an eye to the clinical practice. *Neuropsychol Rev*. 2007;17 (3):203–212.
109. Dick MB, Shankle RW, Beth RE, Dick-Muehlke C, Cotman CW, Kean ML. Acquisition and long-term retention of a gross motor skill in Alzheimer's disease patients under constant and varied practice conditions. *J Gerontol B Psychol Sci Soc Sci*. 1996;51(2):P103–11.
110. Clare L, Jones RSP. Errorless learning in the rehabilitation of memory impairment: a critical review. *Neuropsychol Rev*. 2008;18(1):1–23.
111. Taub E, Uswatte G, Mark VW, Morris DM. The learned nonuse phenomenon: implications for rehabilitation. *Eura Medicophys*. 2006;42(3):241–256.
112. Department of Health, Director SCLGCP, Older People and Dementia. Nothing Ventured, Nothing Gained: Risk Guidance for Dementia. London: Department of Health; 2010.
113. Clarke CL, Wilcockson J, Gibb CE, Keady J, Wilkinson H, Luce A. Reframing risk management in dementia care through collaborative learning. *Health Soc Care Community*. 2011;19(1):23–32.
114. Durocher E, Kinsella EA, Ells C, Hunt M. Contradictions in client-centred discharge planning: through the lens of relational autonomy. *Scandinavian Journal of Occupational Therapy*. 2015;22(4):293–301.
115. Dingwall L, Fenton J, Kelly TB, Lee J. Sliding doors: did drama-based inter-professional education improve the tensions round person-centred nursing and social care delivery for people with dementia: a mixed method exploratory study. *Nurse Educ Today*. 2017;51:1–7.
116. Draper B. Behavioral and Psychological Symptoms of Dementia: The IPA Complete Guides to Behavioral and Psychological Symptoms of Dementia (BPSD). Milwaukee, WI: International Psychogeriatric Association; 2012.
117. Proitsi P, Hamilton G, Tsolaki M, et al. A multiple indicators multiple causes (MIMIC) model of behavioural and

psychological symptoms in dementia (BPSD). *Neurobiol Aging*. 2011;32(3):434–442.
118. Mukherjee A, Biswas A, Roy A, Biswas S, Gangopadhyay G, Das SK. Behavioural and psychological symptoms of dementia: correlates and impact on caregiver distress. *Dement Geriatr Cogn Dis Extra*. 2017;7(3):354–365.
119. Kales HC, Gitlin LN, Lyketsos CG. Detroit Expert Panel on Assessment and Management of Neuropsychiatric Symptoms of Dementia. Management of neuropsychiatric symptoms of dementia in clinical settings: recommendations from a multidisciplinary expert panel. *J Am Geriatr Soc*. 2014;62(4):762–769.
120. Belanger HG, Wilder-Willis K, Malloy P, Salloway S, Hamman RF, Grigsby J. Assessing motor and cognitive regulation in AD, MCI, and controls using the Behavioral Dyscontrol Scale. *Arch Clin Neuropsychol*. 2005;20: 183–189.
121. Power GA. *Dementia beyond Disease: Enhancing Well-Being*. Revised Ed. Towson, MD: Health Professions Press; 2016.
122. Gurwitz JH, Bonner A, Berwick DM. Reducing excessive use of antipsychotic agents in nursing homes. *JAMA*. 2017;318 (2):118.
123. Kramer AF, Erickson KI. Effects of physical activity on cognition, well-being, and brain: human interventions. *Alzheimers Dement*. 2007;3(2):S45–S51.
124. Colcombe S, Kramer AF. Fitness effects on the cognitive function of older adults. *Psychol Sci*. 2003;14(2):125–130.
125. Larson EB, Wang L, Bowen JD, et al. Exercise is associated with reduced risk for incident dementia among persons 65 years of age and older. *Ann Intern Med*. 2006;144(2):73–81.
126. Barnes JN. Exercise, cognitive function, and aging. *Adv Physiol Educ*. 2015;39(2):55–62.
127. Waite LM, Grayson DA, Piguet O, Creasey H, Bennett HP, Broe GA. Gait slowing as a predictor of incident dementia: 6-year longitudinal data from the Sydney Older Persons Study. *J Neurol Sci*. 2005;229–230:89–93.
128. Wang L, Larson EB, Bowen JD, van Belle G. Performance-based physical function and future dementia in older people. *Arch Intern Med*. 2006;166(10):1115.
129. Renaud M, Maquestiaux F, Joncas S, Kergoat M-J, Bherer L. The effect of three months of aerobic training on response preparation in older adults. *Front Aging Neurosci*. 2010;11 (2):148.
130. Ballesteros S, Mayas J, Manuel Reales J. Does a physically active lifestyle attenuate decline in all cognitive functions in old age? *Curr Aging Sci*. 2013;6(2):189–198.
131. Ballesteros S, Kraft E, Santana S, Tziraki C. Maintaining older brain functionality: a targeted review. *Neurosci Biobehav Rev*. 2015;55:453–477.
132. Erickson KI, Voss MW, Prakash RS, et al. Exercise training increases size of hippocampus and improves memory. *Proc Natl Acad Sci U S A*. 2011;108(7):3017–3022.
133. Miyamoto T, Hashimoto S, Yanamoto H, et al. Response of brain-derived neurotrophic factor to combining cognitive and physical exercise. *Eur J Sport Sci*. 2018;18(8):1119–1127.
134. Mandolesi L, Polverino A, Montuori S, et al. Effects of physical exercise on cognitive functioning and wellbeing: biological and psychological benefits. *Front Psychol*. 2018;9:509.
135. Hötting K, Röder B. Beneficial effects of physical exercise on neuroplasticity and cognition. *Neurosci Biobehav Rev*. 2013;37(9):2243–2257.
136. Ahlskog JE, Geda YE, Graff-Radford NR, Petersen RC. Physical exercise as a preventive or disease-modifying treatment of dementia and brain aging. *Mayo Clin Proc*. 2011;86(9):876–884.
137. Liu-Ambrose T, Nagamatsu LS, Graf P, Beattie BL, Ashe MC, Handy TC. Resistance training and executive functions. *Arch Intern Med*. 2010;170(2):170–178.
138. Lachman ME, Neupert SD, Bertrand R, Jette AM. The effects of strength training on memory in older adults. *J Aging Phys Act*. 2006;14(1):59–73.
139. Cassilhas RC, Viana VA, Grassman V, et al. The impact of resistance exercise on the cognitive function of the elderly. *Med Sci Sport Exerc*. 2007;39(8):1401–1407.
140. Tsutsumi T, Don BM, Zaichkowsky LD, Delizonna LL. Physical fitness and psychological benefits of strength training in community dwelling older adults. *Appl Human Sci*. 1997;16(6):257–266.
141. Kimura K, Obuchi S, Arai T, et al. The influence of short-term strength training on health-related quality of life and executive cognitive function. *J Physiol Anthropol*. 2010;29 (3):95–101.
142. Bamidis PD, Vivas AB, Styliadis C, et al. A review of physical and cognitive interventions in aging. *Neurosci Biobehav Rev*. 2014;44:206–220.
143. Anderson-Hanley C, Arciero PJ, Brickman AM, et al. Exergaming and older adult cognition. *Am J Prev Med*. 2012;42(2):109–119.
144. Engvig A, Fjell AM, Westlye LT, et al. Effects of memory training on cortical thickness in the elderly. *Neuroimage*. 2010;52(4):1667–1676.
145. BBC News. Dementia patients go "cycling." BBC News. https://www.bbc.com/news/av/health-46634594/care-home-trials-virtual-cycling-trips-for-dementia-patients. Published 2018. Accessed January 1, 2019.
146. Lam FM, Huang M-Z, Liao L-R, Chung RC, Kwok TC, Pang MY. Physical exercise improves strength, balance, mobility, and endurance in people with cognitive impairment and dementia: a systematic review. *J Physiother*. 2018;64(1):4–15.
147. Öhman H, Savikko N, Strandberg TE, Pitkälä KH. Effect of physical exercise on cognitive performance in older adults with mild cognitive impairment or dementia: a systematic review. *Dement Geriatr Cogn Disord Extra*. 2014;38(5–6):347–365.
148. Song D, Yu DSF, Li PWC, Lei Y. The effectiveness of physical exercise on cognitive and psychological outcomes in individuals with mild cognitive impairment: a systematic review and meta-analysis. *Int J Nurs Stud*. 2018;79:155–164.
149. Segal SK, Cotman CW, Cahill LF. Exercise-induced noradrenergic activation enhances memory consolidation in both normal aging and patients with amnestic mild cognitive impairment. *J Alzheimer's Dis*. 2012;32(4):1011–1018.
150. Nagamatsu LS, Handy TC, Hsu CL, Voss M, Liu-Ambrose T. Resistance training promotes cognitive and functional brain plasticity in seniors with probable mild cognitive impairment. *Arch Intern Med*. 2012;172(8):666.
151. Suzuki T, Shimada H, Makizako H, et al. A randomized controlled trial of multicomponent exercise in older adults with mild cognitive impairment. *PLoS One*. 2013;8(4): e61483.
152. Suzuki T, Shimada H, Makizako H, et al. Effects of multicomponent exercise on cognitive function in older adults with amnestic mild cognitive impairment: a randomized controlled trial. *BMC Neurol*. 2012;12(1):128.
153. Logsdon RG, McCurry SM, Pike KC, Teri L. Making physical activity accessible to older adults with memory loss: a feasibility study. *Gerontologist*. 2009;49(S1):S94–S99.
154. Lam LCW, Chau RCM, Wong BML, et al. Interim follow-up of a randomized controlled trial comparing Chinese style mind body (Tai Chi) and stretching exercises on cognitive function in subjects at risk of progressive cognitive decline. *Int J Geriatr Psychiatry*. 2011;26(7):733–740.
155. Heyn P, Abreu BC, Ottenbacher KJ. The effects of exercise training on elderly persons with cognitive impairment and

dementia: a meta-analysis. *Arch Phys Med Rehabil.* 2004;85:1694–1704.
156. Heyn PC, Johnson KE, Kramer AF. Endurance and strength training outcomes on cognitively impaired and cognitively intact older adults: a meta-analysis. *J Nutr Health Aging.* 2008;12(6):401–409.
157. Groot C, Hooghiemstra AM, Raijmakers PGHM, et al. The effect of physical activity on cognitive function in patients with dementia: a meta-analysis of randomized control trials. *Ageing Res Rev.* 2016;25:13–23.
158. Rolland Y, Pillard F, Klapouszczak A, et al. Exercise program for nursing home residents with Alzheimer's disease: a 1-year randomized, controlled trial. *J Am Geriatr Soc.* 2007;55 (2):158–165.
159. Bossers WJR, Scherder EJA, Boersma F, Hortobágyi T, van der Woude LHV, van Heuvelen MJG. Feasibility of a combined aerobic and strength training program and its effects on cognitive and physical function in institutionalized dementia patients. A pilot study. *PLoS One.* 2014;9(5): e97577.
160. Perrochon A, Tchalla AE, Bonis J, Perucaud F, Mandigout S. Effects of a multicomponent exercise program on spatiotemporal gait parameters, risk of falling and physical activity in dementia patients. *Dement Geriatr Cogn Dis Extra.* 2015;5(3):350–360.
161. Rosendahl E, Lindelöf N, Littbrand H, et al. High-intensity functional exercise program and protein-enriched energy supplement for older persons dependent in activities of daily living: a randomised controlled trial. *Aust J Physiother.* 2006;52(2):105–113.
162. Littbrand H, Lundin-Olsson L, Gustafson Y, Rosendahl E. The effect of a high-intensity functional exercise program on activities of daily living: a randomized controlled trial in residential care facilities. *J Am Geriatr Soc.* 2009;57 (10):1741–1749.
163. Roach KE, Tappen RM, Kirk-Sanchez N, Williams CL, Loewenstein D. A randomized controlled trial of an activity specific exercise program for individuals with Alzheimer disease in long-term care settings. *J Geriatr Phys Ther.* 2011;34(2):50–56.
164. Tappen RM, Roach KE, Applegate EB, Stowell P. Effect of a combined walking and conversation intervention on functional mobility of nursing home residents with Alzheimer disease. *Alzheimer Dis Assoc Disord.* 2000;14 (4):196–201.
165. Cott CA, Dawson P, Sidani S, Wells D. The effects of a walking/talking program on communication, ambulation, and functional status in residents with Alzheimer disease. *Alzheimer Dis Assoc Disord.* 2002;16(2):81–87.
166. Hauer K, Schwenk M, Zieschang T, Essig M, Becker C, Oster P. Physical training improves motor performance in people with dementia: a randomized controlled trial. *J Am Geriatr Soc.* 2012;60(1):8–15.
167. Karssemeijer EGA, Aaronson JA, Bossers WJ, Smits T, Olde Rikkert MGM, Kessels RPC. Positive effects of combined cognitive and physical exercise training on cognitive function in older adults with mild cognitive impairment or dementia: a meta-analysis. *Ageing Res Rev.* 2017;40:75–83.
168. Burgener SC, Yang Y, Gilbert R, Marsh-Yant S. The effects of a multimodal intervention on outcomes of persons with early-stage dementia. *Am J Alzheimers Dis Other Demen.* 2008;23 (4):382–394.
169. Graessel E, Stemmer R, Eichenseer B, et al. Non-pharmacological, multicomponent group therapy in patients with degenerative dementia: a 12-month randomized, controlled trial. *BMC Med.* 2011;9(1):129.
170. Kim M-J, Han C-W, Min K-Y, et al. Physical exercise with multicomponent cognitive intervention for older adults with Alzheimer's disease: a 6-month randomized controlled trial. *Dement Geriatr Cogn Dis Extra.* 2016;6(2):222–232.
171. Beauchet O, Annweiler C, Callisaya ML, et al. Poor gait performance and prediction of dementia: results from a meta-analysis. *J Am Med Dir Assoc.* 2016;17(6):482–490.
172. De Cock A-M, Fransen E, Perkisas S, et al. Gait characteristics under different walking conditions: association with the presence of cognitive impairment in community-dwelling older people. *PLoS One.* 2017;12(6):e0178566.
173. Allali G, Annweiler C, Blumen HM, et al. Gait phenotype from mild cognitive impairment to moderate dementia: results from the GOOD initiative. *Eur J Neurol.* 2016;23(3):527–541.
174. Montero-Odasso M, Speechley M. Falls in cognitively impaired older adults: implications for risk assessment and prevention. *J Am Geriatr Soc.* 2018;66(2):367–375.
175. Muir-Hunter SW, Montero-Odasso M. Gait cost of using a mobility aid in older adults with Alzheimer's disease. *J Am Geriatr Soc.* 2016;64(2):437–438.
176. Montero-Odasso M, Muir SW. Simplifying detection of mild cognitive impairment subtypes. *J Am Geriatr Soc.* 2010;58 (5):992–994.
177. Muir SW, Speechley M, Wells J, Borrie M, Gopaul K, Montero-Odasso M. Gait assessment in mild cognitive impairment and Alzheimer's disease: the effect of dual-task challenges across the cognitive spectrum. *Gait Posture.* 2012;35(1):96–100.
178. Maquet D, Lekeu F, Warzee E, et al. Gait analysis in elderly adult patients with mild cognitive impairment and patients with mild Alzheimer's disease: simple versus dual task: a preliminary report. *Clin Physiol Funct Imaging.* 2010;30 (1):51–56.
179. Gillain S, Warzee E, Lekeu F, et al. The value of instrumental gait analysis in elderly healthy, MCI or Alzheimer's disease subjects and a comparison with other clinical tests used in single and dual-task conditions. *Ann Phys Rehabil Med.* 2009;52(6):453–474.
180. Tarnanas I, Laskaris N, Tsolaki M, Muri R, Nef T, Mosimann UP. On the comparison of a novel serious game and electroencephalography biomarkers for early dementia screening. *Adv Exp Med Biol.* 2015;821:63–77.
181. Zhang W, Low L-F, Gwynn JD, Clemson L. Interventions to improve gait in older adults with cognitive impairment: a systematic review. *J Am Geriatr Soc.* 2018;67(2):1–11.
182. Bahureksa L, Najafi B, Saleh A, et al. The impact of mild cognitive impairment on gait and balance: a systematic review and meta-analysis of studies using instrumented assessment. *Gerontology.* 2017;63(1):67–83.
183. Fritz NE, Kegelmeyer DA, Kloos A, et al. Motor performance differentiates individuals with Lewy body dementia, Parkinson's and Alzheimer's disease. *Gait Posture.* 2016;50:1–7.
184. Avin KG, Hanke TA, Kirk-Sanchez N, et al. Management of falls in community-dwelling older adults: clinical guidance statement from the Academy of Geriatric Physical Therapy of the American Physical Therapy Association. *Phys Ther.* 2015;95(6):815–834.
185. Fernando E, Fraser M, Hendriksen J, Kim CH, Muir-Hunter SW. Risk factors associated with falls in older adults with dementia: a systematic review. *Physiother Canada.* 2017;69(2):161–170.
186. Min Y, Kirkwood CK, Mays DP, Slattum PW. The effect of sleep medication use and poor sleep quality on risk of falls in community-dwelling older adults in the US: a prospective cohort study. *Drugs Aging.* 2016;33(2):151–158.
187. Oliver D. David Oliver: Do bed and chair sensors really stop falls in hospital? *BMJ.* 2018;360:k433.
188. Shaw FE. Prevention of falls in older people with dementia. *J Neural Transm.* 2007;114(10):1259–1264.

189. Wesson J, Clemson L, Brodaty H, et al. A feasibility study and pilot randomised trial of a tailored prevention program to reduce falls in older people with mild dementia. *BMC Geriatr*. 2013;13(1):89.
190. Romli MH, Mackenzie L, Lovarini M, Tan MP, Clemson L. The clinimetric properties of instruments measuring home hazards for older people at risk of falling: a systematic review. *Eval Health Prof*. 2018;41(1):82–128.
191. Marquardt G, Johnston D, Black BS, et al. A descriptive study of home modifications for people with dementia and barriers to implementation. *J Hous Elderly*. 2011;25 (3):258–273.
192. Meyer C, Dow B, Hill KD, Tinney J, Hill S. "The right way at the right time": insights on the uptake of falls prevention strategies from people with dementia and their caregivers. *Front Public Heal*. 2016;4:244.
193. Bossers WJR, van der Woude LHV, Boersma F, Scherder EJA, van Heuvelen MJG. Recommended measures for the assessment of cognitive and physical performance in older patients with dementia: a systematic review. *Dement Geriatr Cogn Dis Extra*. 2012;2(1):589–609.
194. Panel on the Prevention of Falls in Older Persons. Summary of the Updated American Geriatrics Society/British Geriatrics Society Clinical Practice Guideline for Prevention of Falls in Older Persons. *J Am Geriatr Soc*. 2011;59(1): 148–157.
195. Telenius EW, Engedal K, Bergland A. Inter-rater reliability of the Berg Balance Scale, 30 s chair stand test and 6 m walking test, and construct validity of the Berg Balance Scale in nursing home residents with mild-to-moderate dementia. *BMJ Open*. 2015;5(9):e008321.
196. Chandra SR, Issac TG, Abbas MM. Apraxias in neurodegenerative dementias. *Indian J Psychol Med*. 2015;37(1):42–47.
197. Wells DL, Dawson P, Sidani S, Craig D, Pringle D. Effects of an abilities-focused program of morning care on residents who have dementia and on caregivers. *J Am Geriatr Soc*. 2000;48(4):442–449.
198. Roberts G, Morley C, Walters W, Malta S, Doyle C. Caring for people with dementia in residential aged care: successes with a composite person-centered care model featuring Montessori-based activities. *Geriatr Nurs (Minneap)*. 2015;36(2):106–110.
199. Lautenbacher S, Niewelt BG, Kunz M. Decoding pain from the facial display of patients with dementia: a comparison of professional and nonprofessional observers. *Pain Med*. 2013;14(4):469–477.
200. Corbett A, Husebo B, Malcangio M, et al. Assessment and treatment of pain in people with dementia. *Nat Rev Neurol*. 2012;8(5):264–274.
201. Guerriero F, Guerriero F, Sgarlata C, et al. Pain management in dementia: so far, not so good. *J Gerontol Geriatr*. 2016;64:31–39.
202. Achterberg WP, Pieper MJC, van Dalen-Kok AH, et al. Pain management in patients with dementia. *Clin Interv Aging*. 2013;8:1471–1482.
203. Lautenbacher S, Walz AL, Kunz M. Using observational facial descriptors to infer pain in persons with and without dementia. *BMC Geriatr*. 2018;18(1):88.
204. Warden V, Hurley AC, Volicer L. Development and psychometric evaluation of the Pain Assessment in Advanced Dementia (PAINAD) Scale. *J Am Med Dir Assoc*. 2003;4(1):9–15.
205. Hadjistavropoulos T, Fitzgerald TD, Marchildon GP. Practice guidelines for assessing pain in older persons with dementia residing in long-term care facilities. *Physiother Canada*. 2010;62(2):104–113.
206. Schofield P. The assessment of pain in older people: UK National Guidelines. *Age Ageing*. 2018;47(suppl_1) i1–i22.
207. Herr K, Bursch H, Ersek M, Miller LL, Swafford K. Use of pain-behavioral assessment tools in the nursing home. *J Gerontol Nurs*. 2010;36(3):18–29.
208. Horgas A, Yoon S, Grall M. Pain management in older adults. In: *Evidence-Based Geriatric Nursing Protocols for Best Practice*. ed 4. New York: Springer; 2012:246–267.
209. Castle N. Consistent staff assignment in Alzheimer's special care units. *Alzheimer's Dement*. 2011;7(4):S292.
210. Roberts T, Nolet K, Bowers B. Consistent assignment of nursing staff to residents in nursing homes: a critical review of conceptual and methodological issues. *Gerontologist*. 2015;55(3):434–447.
211. Scales K, Zimmerman S, Miller SJ. Evidence-based nonpharmacological practices to address behavioral and psychological symptoms of dementia. *Gerontologist*. 2018;58(suppl_1):S88–S102.
212. UNC: The Cecil G. Sheps Center for Health Services Research. Bathing without a Battle. http://bathingwithoutabattle.unc.edu/. Accessed January 1, 2019.
213. Mitchell MD, Lavenberg JG, Trotta R, Umscheid CA. Hourly rounding to improve nursing responsiveness: a systematic review. *J Nurs Admin*. 2014;44(9):464–472.
214. Abdulla A, Adams N, Bone M, et al. Guidance on the management of pain in older people. *Age Ageing*. 2013;42 (Suppl 1):i1–i57.
215. Cruccu G, Truini A. A review of neuropathic pain: from guidelines to clinical practice. *Pain Ther*. 2017;6(Suppl 1):35–42.
216. Cheng S-T. Dementia caregiver burden: a research update and critical analysis. *Curr Psychiatry Rep*. 2017;19(9):64.
217. Pöysti MM, Laakkonen M-L, Strandberg T, et al. Gender differences in dementia spousal caregiving. *Int J Alzheimers Dis*. 2012;2012:162960.
218. Schulz R, Burgio L, Burns R, et al. Resources for Enhancing Alzheimer's Caregiver Health (REACH): overview, site-specific outcomes, and future directions. *Gerontologist*. 2003;43(4):514–520.
219. Lokvig J. *The Alzheimer's or Memory Café : How to Start and Succeed with Your Own Café*. Santa Fe, NM: Endless Circle Press; 2016.
220. McKeown M. Assessment of needs for dementia care partners related to wellness/fitness respite programs. *Health Sciences Student Work*. 2018: 9.

CHAPTER

20

The Management of Post-Surgical Orthopedic Conditions in the Older Adult

Anne Thackeray, Caitlin Miller

OUTLINE

INTRODUCTION

Musculoskeletal conditions are a major source of disease burden worldwide, with back pain as the number one leading cause of years lived with disability.[1] Older adults bear the greatest burden of musculoskeletal diseases. Back pain, arthritis, and fragility fractures are associated with high rates of chronic pain and loss of participation in many common activities.[2] This has a dramatic impact on quality-of-life. Not surprisingly, rates of elective orthopedic surgery are increasing in adults over 65 and even among adults 80 years and older.[3–7]New surgical technique reducing time in surgery, advances in anesthesia, and patient expectations all contribute to the increase in surgeries among older adults.

Costs attributable to surgical management for musculoskeletal conditions in the United States are substantial and individuals over 65 years of age accounting for nearly half of musculoskeletal surgical costs. For musculoskeletal conditions in particular, estimated costs for surgeries secondary to arthritis were $19 billion, for injuries owing to falls costs were $13 billion, and just over $7 billion was spent on surgery and hospital stays for neck and back pain.[8] Despite the increase in health care expenditures, population measures of physical, social, and work limitations are rising.[9] It is imperative that physical therapists recognize and embrace their role in managing musculoskeletal conditions in a way that can reduced the burden to both the individual and society.

Postsurgical management of orthopedic conditions in older adults is highly variable and there is limited research to direct the most appropriate care. Improving perioperative and postoperative rehabilitation holds great potential to improve quality of life and reduce costs for many older adults. Physical therapists must use their specialized and unique skill set to critically assess patient needs, prioritize treatment, and develop innovations that can highlight the value of rehabilitation. This chapter focuses on rehabilitation of the older adult after common fragility fractures, total joint arthroplasties, rotator cuff tears, and spinal surgeries.

HEALTH BEHAVIOR CHANGE

It is important to recognize that many older adults presenting for postsurgical treatment have experienced health challenges for many years. These challenges may range from chronic joint pain and stiffness from osteoarthritis to postural deformities from loss of bone mass. Individuals with these chronic conditions are more likely to report poor overall health, serious psychological distress, and limited social participation.[10,11] A strong relationship exists between painful musculoskeletal conditions and reduced physical activity resulting in functional decline, frailty, reduced well-being, and loss of independence. The result is a downward spiral in health. These effects are even more pronounced with aging.[12] Surgical interventions may reduce pain and allow for greater participation in physical activity and social roles,[13,14] but this is not universal.[15] In fact, most patients do not increase physical activity even after surgical intervention aimed at addressing musculoskeletal pain. Improving health status and function following surgery for orthopedic conditions requires that patients take an active role in rehabilitation, communication with health providers, and make behavioral changes. Increasing routine physical activity is critical in remediating chronic pain and improving well-being.[16] This requires interventions that support physical activity behavior change alongside traditional physical therapy interventions that include mobility and strengthening. Physical therapists must consider how to promote behavior change toward increasing physical activity to improve rehabilitation participation, quality of life, and successful aging.

Essential elements of the physical therapy evaluation and treatment, regardless of the primary diagnosis, include individually tailored interventions to improve movement (exercise, manual therapy), patient education, and cognitive-based interventions that can support sustained changes in physical activity. Although some patients will require additional support from other health professionals, such as rehabilitation psychologists, psychologically informed physical therapy can help many patients improve their participation and function following orthopedic surgeries or injuries. Specific interventions, as shown in Fig. 20.1, include motivational interviewing, shared decision-making, coping and self-management strategies, condition-specific pain education, and finding exercise interventions that are enjoyable and relevant.[17,18] These interventions can enhance adherence to physical therapy interventions and increase physical activity, subsequently improving function and health outcomes.

FRACTURES

Fractures that occur in older adults are either related to a high-energy impact, such as a fall, or low-energy fragility fractures from osteoporosis. Any fracture that results from a fall from a standing height or less is considered a fragility fracture.

Fragility Fractures. As society ages the incidence of fragility fractures is increasing. A global call to action to improve care after fragility fractures was put forth in 2018.[19] This call was the result of multidisciplinary and multiprofessional collaboration from organizations around the world. The statement calls for a systematic approach to fragility fracture to include three recommendations:

1. *Acute multidisciplinary care following major fragility fractures requiring medical care.*

The first objective across providers is to manage preexisting chronic diseases and minimize delirium. This can be done through appropriate pain management and

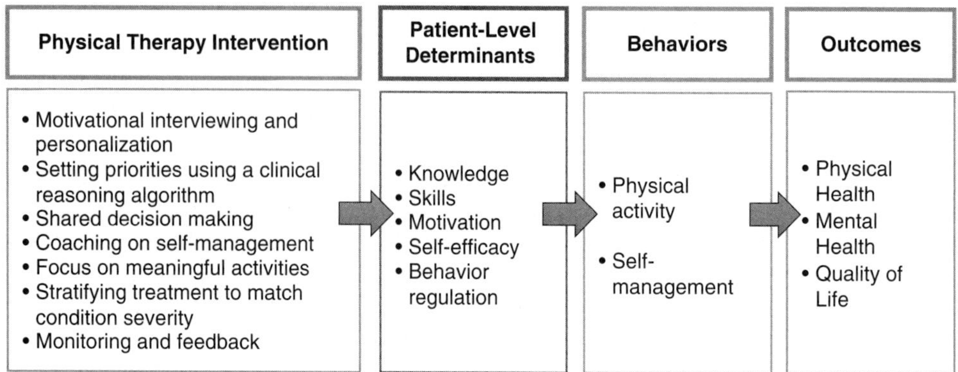

FIG. 20.1 Logic model of change in physical activity behavior.

rapid optimization of fitness for surgery, when indicated. When a fragility fracture is significantly limiting mobility, early surgery can reduce morbidity and mortality. Care managed both by orthopedic and geriatric specialists can result in a shorter time to surgery, decreased length of hospital stay, and lower mortality rates.

2. *Rapid secondary prevention after the first occurrence of all fragility fractures.*

Osteoporosis management and falls prevention are critical after a fragility fracture. Physical therapists are crucial in this stage. Thoughtful assessment and treatment planning by physical therapists can improve bone mass and reduce fall risk.

3. *Ongoing postacute care of people whose ability to function is impaired by major fragility fractures.*

As many as 50% of older adults with a hip fracture fail to recover prefracture ability to walk. Recovery from fragility fractures can be slow and prolonged. It is important for physical therapists to critically evaluate how to support rehabilitation beyond the early stages of recovery.

Although fractures may occur at different sites, many older patients experience common challenges. For example, older adults who fracture their wrist from a fall have a fear of falling similar to individuals who fall and break their hip. Nearly one-half of women with hip, pelvic, or lower limb fracture had not regained prefracture mobility at 1 year after the injury.[20] Individuals report difficulty with bending (hip and vertebral fractures), walking down stairs (hip, ankle, and vertebral fractures), and reaching (vertebral and humeral fractures). These mobility issues can have a negative impact on balance and activity levels. Chronic pain after a fracture and in the later stages of recovery is also a frequent complaint. Rates of chronic pain among older adults with fracture is high, estimated at 43% in vertebral fractures and 42% in hip fractures.[21,22] This pain has a negative impact on return to normal activities, may restrict social participation, and reinforces inactivity. Pain education and cognitive behavioral therapy with a focus on strategies to improve function, even in the persistence of pain, can provide patients with coping strategies and help them achieve their goals. All fractures should prompt clinicians to examine medical management for bone density, strength, and fall prevention.

Hip Fractures

Every year, over 300,000 older adults in the United States are hospitalized because of a hip fracture. Most hip fractures occur owing to a fall from a standing position. Women more often sustain fractures because of the higher prevalence of osteoporosis. Recent studies suggest the incidence of osteoporosis for individuals over 70 years is declining, a trend which may be partially explained by the widespread prescription of bisphosphonate medications, decreasing incidence of tobacco use, awareness of falls, and promotion of active aging.[23] Hip fracture, however, remains a prototypical geriatric condition and can be devastating. Many older adults who have a hip fracture are also managing several different health conditions. It is not uncommon for a patient presenting with a hip fracture to have congestive heart failure, kidney disease, cognitive changes, frailty, or other joint conditions, such as low back pain or knee arthritis.

Risk. Caucasian females aged 85 and older are at the highest risk for a hip fracture.[24] The average age at the time of a hip fracture is 80 years[25] and falling is the most common cause. Patients who have had a hip fracture are 2.5 times as likely to have a subsequent hip fracture caused by a fall when compared with age-matched peers.[26] The major risk factors for a hip fracture, such as polypharmacy, use of assistive devices, and cognitive impairment, are still present following a hip fracture. It is imperative that the physical therapy assessment and treatment planning include a comprehensive fall risk assessment accounting for medication, cognition, nutrition, arthritis, gait and balance, and home safety.[27] Furthermore, an older adult is at greatest risk for a fall in the thirty days following hospital discharge.[28]

Indications for Surgery. Surgery is the intervention of choice for long-term mobility and function after a hip fracture. Without surgery, there are poorer outcomes, including increased mortality.[29] Surgery generally allows for early mobilization which can be critical in this population. The timing of surgery is often dictated by the medical evaluation. Surgery is recommended within 24 hours for medically stable individuals without significant comorbid conditions. Surgery for all other individuals is recommended within 72 hours and is dependent on the ability to stabilize coexisting medical conditions. The benefits of early surgery are associated primarily with reducing complications associated with prolonged bed rest, including skin breakdown, pneumonia, urinary tract infections, deep venous thrombosis, and loss of muscle mass.

Hip fractures are classified as intracapsular (femoral head and neck fractures) and extracapsular (intertrochanteric) as shown in Fig. 20.2. Intracapsular fractures have a higher incidence of avascular necrosis and degenerative changes owing to the tenuous blood supply and thinner periosteum. There is debate as to whether open reduction with internal fixation or arthroplasty is the most appropriate surgical intervention. Internal fixation results in less blood loss or deep wound infection. However, patients treated with arthroplasty had lower reoperation rates and reduced risk of avascular necrosis and nonunion.[30] Screw fixation, with or without a plate, may be sufficient for minimally or nondisplaced fractures of the femoral neck.

Extracapsular fractures are most often treated with internal fixation.[30] These fractures have less risk for blood supply complications, but a higher risk of displacement. Intertrochanteric fractures often result in greater edema

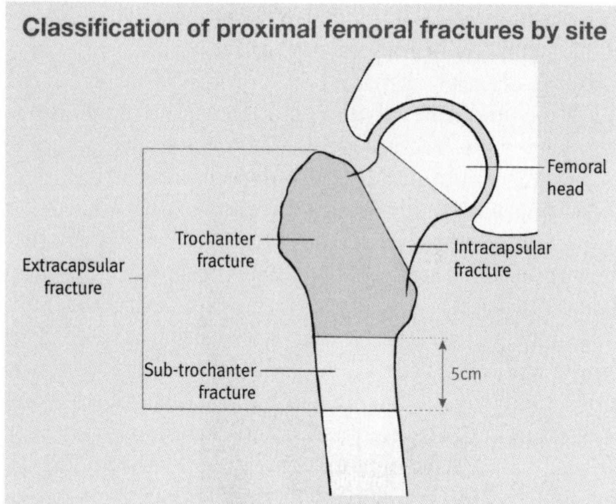

FIG. 20.2 Classifications of hip fracture. *(From Chesser T, Kelly M, et al. Surgery (Oxford), Management of hip fractures in the elderly. Surgery. 2016; 34(9): 440–43.)*

compared with femoral neck fractures. This edema has a significant impact on mobility, postural control, and lower leg strength.[31] Additionally, the numerous muscle attachments in this region can add stress to the bone during movement. In general, mobility is more painful and gait speed is reduced, resulting in a longer recovery and more difficulty returning to prior level of function.

Acute Stage Complications. One or more complication occurs in up to 50% of hip fracture patients.[32] Pain and anemia occur in nearly all patients after hip fracture and affect outcomes by disrupting participation in physical therapy and mobility efforts. Multidisciplinary comanagement approaches that focus on pain management, delirium prevention, early surgery, and aggressive mobilization may maximize patient recovery. In fact, coordinated care in a higher risk population resulted in fewer cardiac and delirium complications than usual care in a lower risk population.[33] Key considerations of pain control, delirium, anemia, mobility, nutrition, catheter management, and pressure ulcer prevention during hospitalization and acute postoperative rehabilitation should be the focus of everyone on the medical team.[34]

Anemia. Anemia is present in approximately half of patients with hip fracture at hospital admission and in 80% to 90% postoperatively.[35] Mild anemia is often defined as hemoglobin levels of less than 120 g/L for women and less than 130 g/dL men.[36] Anemia is related to poor physical performance, falls, frailty, and a decline in cognition.[35,37] The presence of anemia and poor nutritional status may adversely affect functional recovery[38]; therefore, clinicians should be alert to possible signs and symptoms. Clinical presentation can include increased fatigue or exhaustion, pallor, headache and dizziness, and shortness of breath. Symptoms may not be as noticeable in an older adult with chronic anemia and can be difficult to differentiate from other comorbid conditions, making the interpretation of laboratory values important in the diagnosis of anemia. Fatigue is one of the primary factors limiting patient participation in rehabilitation early after hip fracture surgery.[39] Given the very high prevalence of anemia postoperatively, physical therapists must consider anemia a highly probable contributor to this fatigue and work with the medical team on appropriate management, including iron supplementation and nutritional interventions.[36,40] In cases where anemia and associated fatigue persist, physical therapists must reconsider a typical longer and single treatment session to several shorter sessions throughout the day.

Delirium. Delirium is a complex neuropsychiatric syndrome and one of the most frequent complications among older adults when hospitalized. In patients without baseline dementia, delirium occurs in 24% of patients who experience a hip fracture and will persist in nearly 40% of patients after hospital discharge.[41] In those with dementia, over half will experience delirium.[42] Delirium is characterized by a fluctuating course of acute changes in cognition, including confusion, poor attention, incoherent speech, agitation, and altered level of consciousness.[43] Proactive geriatrics consultation and coordinated multidisciplinary care can reduce the onset of delirium and its impact on outcomes.[44,45] This starts with early care planning because once delirium has developed, few interventions appear to reduce the duration or severity of delirium.[46] Multicomponent interventions vary across studies. In general, effective interventions involve multiple strategies and disciplines. Protocols consistently include strategies to address cognition, sleep, fluid and electrolyte balance, pain management, medication management, early removal of urinary catheters, and early mobilization. A well-implemented multicomponent intervention can reduce the occurrence of both delirium and falls by more than 50%.[45] Physical therapists have an active role in preventing delirium. Coordinating care with medical staff to support early mobility is a key component. Providers should also actively challenge cognition. Consider integrating activities to stimulate cognitive processes into the physical therapy treatment. These may include route finding, orientation to date/time/recent events, identifying familiar objects, environmental stimulation, and family participation as shown in Fig. 20.3.[47,48]

Pressure Ulcers. Mobility and education also play key roles in reducing pressure ulcers. An estimated 16% of patients after a hip fracture will develop a stage II or greater pressure ulcer at 7 days with the heel being the most common site. This number increases to 28% at 14 days and 36% at 32 days.[49] Patients at higher risk are those with nutrition complications, worse mobility tolerance, and altered cognition. A key component in ulcer development is the time to surgery. Those receiving surgical intervention within 24 hours have less risk in developing a pressure ulcer.[50] Physical therapists can help to reduce pressure ulcer development by encouraging frequent position changes, assessing the skin for signs of pressure, and assuring patients at high risk use appropriate pressure-relieving overlays and heel protectors.

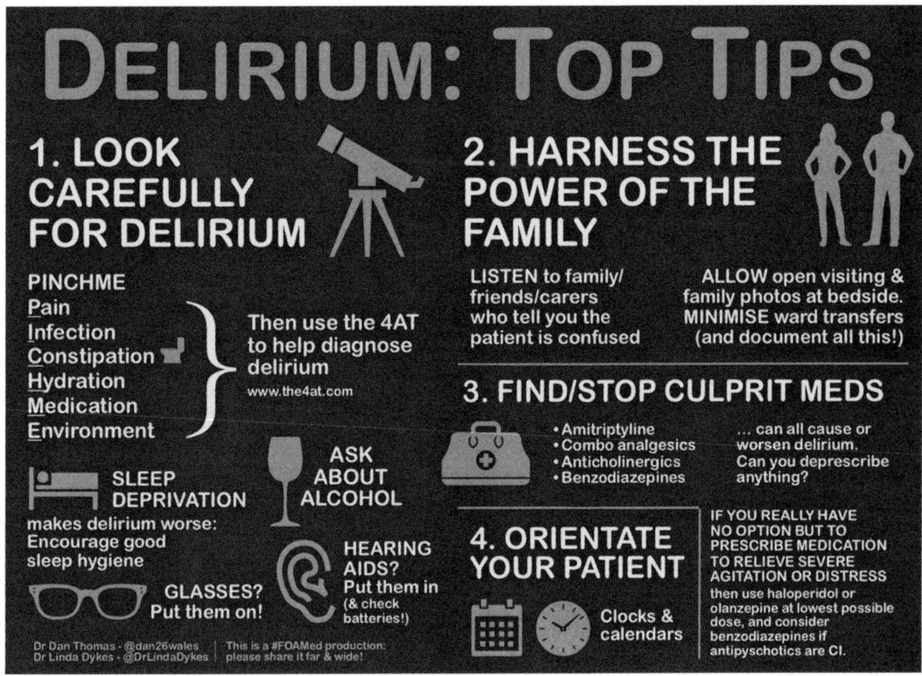

FIG. 20.3 Tips for managing delirium in the hospital. *(Copyright Dr. Linda Dykes. https://www.grepmed.com/images/3642/geriatrics-management-pinchme-delirium-mnemonic-tips-diagnosis Accessed August 4, 2019.)*

Pain Control. Severe pain is common after a hip fracture. Pain from fracture of the hip is often complex and multifactorial, involving muscle spasm, fracture movement, surgical wounds, and psychosocial factors. Effective pain control strategies are essential for improving participation in rehabilitation, and quality of life.[39] Controlling pain can also reduce complications of pneumonia, urinary tract infection, and delirium,[51] which likely can be mediated through improving participation in early mobility. Combining effective pain control, nutrition, and early mobility has a positive impact on clinical outcomes, reducing hospital mortality rates and increasing rates of home discharge.[52] It is important for physical therapists to assess pain routinely, especially in those with cognitive impairment, and determine if pain is inhibiting participation in rehabilitation. In these cases, there are several options for pain management and these options should be discussed with the medical team. During the acute phase of recovery, the most effective pain control programs often use multimodal analgesia, including femoral nerve blocks, systemic acetaminophen, and opiate medications. Timing physical therapy interventions with optimal pain management can help to improve participation.

Survival. One-year mortality rate following a hip fracture is estimated between 12% and 37%.[53–55] In general, men have a higher mortality rate up to one year after hip fracture.[24] Mortality can be the result of the complexity of multiple comorbid conditions contributing to a hip fracture in the first place, but mortality is also associated with how those conditions are managed in the hospital. Individual risk factors include advanced age, preoperative functional status, frailty, cognitive status, cardiovascular and metabolic health, and postoperative complications—sepsis in particular.[55,56] A detailed discussion of sepsis and other postoperative complications is found in the chapter on Management of the Acutely Ill and Medically Complex Older Patient elsewhere in this text.

Post-acute Care Considerations. Femoral neck fractures have a relatively high rate of complications compared with extracapsular hip fractures. In particular, for patients with repaired intracapsular fractures (femoral neck and head), clinicians should consider avascular necrosis as a differential diagnosis in patients with a loss of hip range of motion and an increase in pain at 3 to 6 months postoperatively. Nonunion is a complication of all hip fracture types. A number of factors determine the risk of nonunion, including patient age, bone density, fracture displacement, fracture comminution, reduction quality, and the prosthetic device and its position. Nonunion or loss of reduction can present with groin, hip, or thigh pain that never fully resolves following surgery, or increases after a period of improvement.

Recovery of Function. Many individuals experience severe long-term consequences following a hip fracture. Fewer than half of patients experiencing a hip fracture regain their prior level of ambulation at 1 year and 20% become immobile.[57] At 2 years, more the 80% are unable to walk a block and 90% are unable to climb five stairs.[58] Approximately 50% of patients are unable to live independently. Reduced prefracture functional independence adversely affects recovery following hip fracture.[59] Functional status should be critically monitored to assure patients receive necessary interventions. For patients experiencing a worsening of comorbid conditions and/or experiencing multiple readmissions, it is important to discuss patient goals and desires and address these through alternative approaches, both in institutions and at home.

Prognosis. The recovery timeline varies by domain. Cognition, depression, and independence with daily activities requiring primarily upper extremity function are recovered by about 4 months. Recovery of maximal lower extremity function is not seen until about 12 months post-injury.[72] This timeline may be extended for frail elderly who are still progressing at 12 months. Reliable measurement of function over time (e.g., gait speed, five times sit-to-stand, stair-climbing, Timed Up and Go) can help identify when modifications to the treatment plan may be needed.

Persistent Residual Pain. Between 40% and 50% of patients who experience a hip fracture reported moderate to severe pain at 3 to 6 months. Physical activity and palliative strategies (e.g., heat, cold, massage) may help with pain management. Sudden-onset or worsening pain should prompt further evaluation of new onset musculoskeletal inflammation, such as a trochanteric bursitis versus more severe impairments such as the loss of fixation, dislocation, infection, or osteonecrosis.

Depression and Anxiety. Clinically significant depression develops in 14% to 20% of patients with hip fracture[60] and may adversely affect recovery.[59] This can be triggered by the challenges of recovery and has a circular influence by negatively impacting rehabilitation outcomes. Anxiety is also common—in particular a fear of falling. This fear also has an association with poor rehabilitation outcomes, mobility loss, and institutionalization.[34] A critical part of rehabilitation following a hip fracture is working with patients to improve self-efficacy and a sense of safety. Graded exposure and problem-solving across a variety of environments may be effective interventions for improving confidence in mobility.

Specific Physical Therapy Interventions Following Hip Fracture

Patient Education. Managing expectations can help patients and their caregivers plan for recovery. It is key for patients to understand recovery takes time. Treatment after a hip fracture is prolonged and recovery trajectories are variable. Understanding and anticipating the challenges of recovery can enhance care. Involving the patient in goal-setting and focusing on the patient's goals may help enhance participation. Clear goals and targets for mobility also help patients understand the recovery process and elicit greater participation and patience. Table 20.1 lists general interventions and expectations.

Acute Stage Mobility. The first goal in acute physical therapy is aimed at regaining independence in basic mobility. Three targets for independence include[61]:

- Getting in and out of bed
- Moving from sitting to standing and back from a chair with arms
- Walking with an assistive device

Early ambulation improves functional recovery, reduces mortality rate and the risk of new-onset delirium.[34] Both short- and long-term mortality rates are also associated with early postsurgery ambulatory level.[62] This association is complex, representing comorbid disease severity and the impact of complications on function. The challenge for a physical therapist is to understand what is limiting ambulation and work with the medical

TABLE 20.1 Expected Recovery and Associated Interventions Following Hip Fracture

Stage of Hip Fracture	Acute Rehabilitation (Hospital)	Postacute Rehabilitation	Enduring Stage	
• Approximate duration	• ~7–10 days	• 7 days–3 months	• 3–6 months	• 6 months–1 year
• Primary interventions	• Early weight-bearing • Bed mobility • Lower extremity/quadriceps strengthening • Pain modulation	• Stepping and improving quality of movement to reduce fear of falling • Improve confidence with activity • Improve muscle strength through progressive high-intensity resistance training • Mood/self-efficacy (goal setting, self-monitoring)	• Progressive strengthening tailored toward persisting deficits (e.g., full loading, gluteal weakness) • Advanced balance training	• Support for independent exercise routine • Problem-solving any residual symptoms • Community-based physical activity

• Goals of intervention	• Independent with:
	  • bed mobility
	  • sit to stand
	  • walking with assistive device
	• Cognitive recovery (2–4 months)
			• Prefracture walking ability: 6 months	• 6–9 months: gait and balance recovered
				• 10–14 months lower limb function recovered

team to determine appropriate solutions. Of particular importance is identifying when pain or fatigue is the limiting factor and assuring appropriate management strategies are in place.[39] Some early evidence indicates that three episodes of daily physical therapy can reduce time in the hospital.[63] The research on progressive resisted strengthening within a few days of surgery is less clear.[64]

Outpatient Rehabilitation. Outpatient rehabilitation and home-based interventions can improve performance at 1 to 12 months. Comprehensive outpatient interventions should include interventions to improve balance, flexibility, and movement speed. High-intensity strength training, once the fracture has healed, optimizes physical performance, function, and quality of life.[65] To maximize outcomes, strength training should be designed at an intensity to promote muscle fatigue, typically strengthening at 65% to 100% of a patient's one-repetition maximum.[65–67] Patients continuing with a progressive resisted strength program for up to 6 months after hospitalization demonstrate greater improvements in overall mobility, gait speed, activities of daily living (ADLs) and balance.[68, 69]

Research supporting rehabilitation beyond 6 months is limited and varied in the intervention components examined. In general, programs have encouraged increasing resistance with exercise and functional tasks with evidence of continued improvement in physical activity and mobility up to 1 year after surgery.[66,67,70] This does not all need to be done in the clinic, but can be performed at home with weight vests, hand weights, body weight step-ups, and sit-to-stand repetitions and appropriate, but limited, supervision.[71] Evidenced-informed exercise guidelines, as described in the Chapter 8 on exercise elsewhere in this text, should be utilized for optimal outcomes.

Humeral Fractures

Proximal humeral fractures are the third most common osteoporotic fracture.[73] Despite the prevalence, there is no consensus on the treatment of proximal humeral fractures in older adults. Although an array of surgical approaches including tension bands, pinning, locking plates, and hemiarthroplasty exist, no clear evidence indicates that surgical approaches result in clinically significant improvement in pain and function over conservative care following a humeral fracture (even up to four-part fractures).[74,75] Surgical complication rates are high, estimated between 10% and 29% and include infection, pulmonary embolus, and hardware complications. Rates of reoperation are 16% to 30%. Individuals opting for nonsurgical treatment also may note complications, including nonunion (~20%) and tuberculum malposition (~16%) compromising function and range of motion. Surgery for displaced fractures should consider the patient's level of independence, bone quality, and surgical risk factors.

Following a surgical repair, rehabilitation goals center around improving range of motion in the first 6 to 8 weeks and regaining strength for ADL performance. Low-quality research suggests early mobilization following a proximal fracture tends to minimize disability both in the short term (8 to 16 weeks) and at 1 year.[75] Early mobilization also resulted in fewer physical therapy visits, with independent function achieved at 16 weeks. It is recommended to initiate mobility exercises within the first week of a humeral fracture managed conservatively, but it is unclear if these need to be supervised by a physical therapist. Studies to date suggest self-directed exercise is equally as effective as supervised physical therapy in improving joint mobility and function. Of note, compliance was poorly measured in these studies and is a consideration in treatment planning. Evidence suggests that intensive support can improve general exercise compliance at home,[76] but this has not been examined specifically with individuals following a fracture. Furthermore, some patients will still lack sufficient understanding or motivation to perform the required exercises independently. These patients may improve compliance with increased supervision, monitoring, and feedback.[77]

Wrist Fractures

Distal radial fracture (DRF), which is the second most common fracture among people older than 50 years, occurs after a fall on an outstretched hand from standing height. This prevalence reflects the association between DRF and bone loss from osteoporosis in older people. DRFs are usually treated in outpatient settings with around 20% of patients requiring hospital admission.[78] These fractures are generally closed, involve radial shortening and fragmentation with dorsal displacement. The majority of these fractures are treated nonoperatively with reduction and immobilization, but plate fixation is on the rise.[79]

The majority of patients (84% to 93%) with a DRF can expect good recovery 1 year after injury. Of note, only a quarter of individuals with DRF will be pain-free and without disability. In approximately 7% to 11% of those after DRF, severe pain and moderate to severe disability will persist. Risk stratification may help identify those at higher risk for a poor recovery. Older age, being female, poor bone healing (or having an associated fracture of the ulnar styloid), high initial pain scores, injury compensation at the workplace, and lower socioeconomic status/level of education are associated with poor recovery. In these individuals, physical therapists should perform a more comprehensive assessment examination to understand the source of pain, pain perceptions, coping strategies, and occupation goals in these patients in an effort to reduce their risk of disability. Close monitoring of progress and innovative treatments may also improve prognosis for individuals at higher risk of developing chronic pain and disability.[80]

Secondary displacement of DRFs after closed reduction are not uncommon. Individuals at highest risk for a secondary displacement include women over 60 years of age and fractures with dorsal comminution.[81] Patients with these risk factors should be considered for close monitoring during the course of rehabilitation. A significant lack of progress may indicate instability and warrant further examination by the orthopedic physician. The complication rate after volar plate surgery is estimated at 16.5%. The most common complications are tendon or nerve irritation (5.5%), complex regional pain syndrome (1.6%), and carpal tunnel syndrome (2.8%).[82] Other common complications include persistent neuropathies of the median, ulnar, or radial nerves (one of three patients). Physical therapy interventions may need to be modified to address symptoms arising from these complications.

Initial treatment includes elevation, range-of-motion exercise and exercise of non-immobilized joints to counter swelling and stiffness. There is low quality evidence that hand physical therapy during immobilization has a significant impact on outcomes after immobilization.[78] After immobilization for a conservatively treated fracture, physical therapy has a favorable effect on wrist extension, function, and pain. This benefit appears to be maximized by treatment over 3 to 4 weeks for an average of five visits.[78] In contrast, supervised rehabilitation after volar plate fixation did not improve grip, function, or motion over a progressive home exercise program. In fact, the progressive home exercise program was significantly more effective in improving grip strength and general motion.[83,84] No evidence of benefit has been identified for multiple other modalities such as pulsed electromagnetic field, ice, intermittent pneumatic compression, ultrasound, whirlpool, and dynamic wrist splinting.[78] Of note, the quality of evidence for the use of modalities is very low.

Otherwise healthy individuals with osteopenia or osteoporosis often transition to a physically inactive lifestyle following DRF.[85] Pain, disability, and fear of falling all contribute to this transition. In DRF, as other fractures, it is important to monitor and address losses in physical activity.

Ankle Fractures

Ankle fractures in older adults make up only 8% of patients hospitalized for osteoporosis-related fractures.[86] The most common type of fractures are transsyndesmotic or suprasyndesmotic (often called Weber B or Weber C). Although ankle fractures are less common than other fragility fractures, mobility limitations following the injury can have a dramatic impact on morbidity and mortality. Best outcomes are achieved when open reduction internal fixation and primary closure of the wound is possible (Fig. 20.4).[87] Otherwise, recommended operative techniques after a displaced ankle fracture include the use of locking plates and second stage reconstruction with external fixation.[88] This hardware may allow for modified weight-bearing, but caution is still warranted given balance limitations.

Age (> 80 years), severe systemic disease (ASA >3), and preinjury mobility significantly affect recovery. These factors are associated with an inability to return home following acute management of the fracture and subsequent increased mortality rates. Mortality at one year following an ankle fracture in older adults is between 7% and 23%.[88] This mortality is reflective of low reserves and

TTC nailing technique under image intensifier. Insertion of the guide wire (a), followed by insertion of the nail (b). The TTC nail was locked proximally (c) and distally (d).

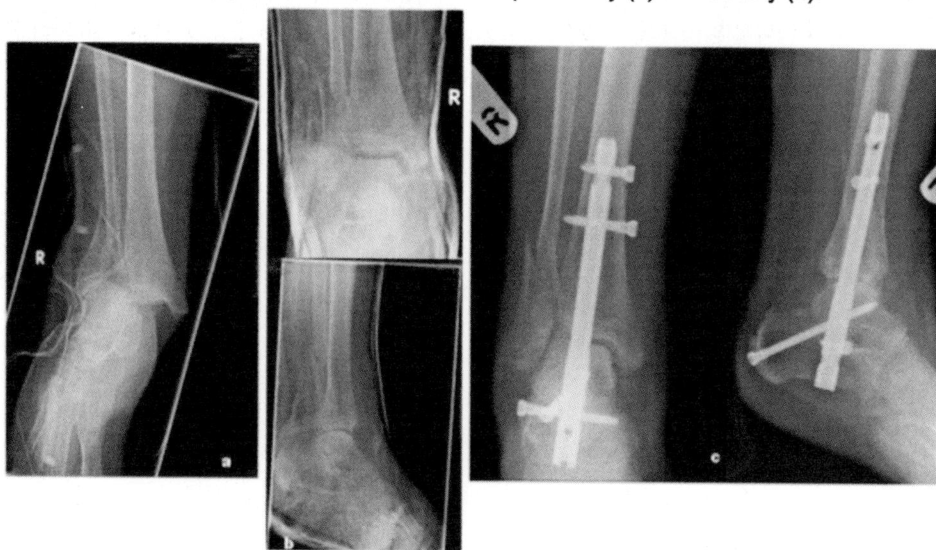

FIG. 20.4 Fragility ankle fracture and repair. A. Anteroposterier (AP) radiograph showing a right ankle fracture-dislocation. B. AP and lateral views after fracture manipulation and reduction. C. AP and lateral radiographs 6 weeks postoperatively. *(From Georgiannos D, Lampridis V, Bisbinas I. Injury. 2017, 48 (2):519–24, © 2017 Elsevier Ltd.)*

health challenges comparable to other fractures seen in older adults.[89]

Major inpatient complications are similar to many acute injuries in older adults, including pulmonary embolism, cardiac arrest, stroke, and infection. The greatest complications for ankle fractures, however, is poor wound healing (10%) and nonunion (5%).[87,88] Perioperative management includes instruction on wound care, transfers, and ambulation options. Early fixation and definitive skin closure improve the options for early mobility.[87] It should still be noted that altered weight-bearing status is a significant challenge for older adults with ankle fractures. Many older individuals do not have the strength to ambulate non–weight-bearing or even partial weight-bearing with crutches or a walker. Early planning may need to include preparing individuals and caregivers for use of a wheelchair, if appropriate.

Around 70% of individuals report they have regained preinjury autonomy by around 7 to 8 months after surgery.[90] Postoperative rehabilitation generally begins after immobilization of the ankle (6 to 8 weeks) and focuses on ankle range of motion, gross lower extremity strengthening, gait and balance training.

Vertebral Fractures

Fractures in the vertebral spine are the most common osteoporotic fracture and thus are a type of fragility fracture. The prevalence of these fractures increases exponentially with age. Vertebral fragility fractures (VFF) are generally compression fractures of the vertebral vertebrae with the anterior body being most susceptible. VFFs can be a result of low-energy trauma to the spine during daily activities such as bending or twisting. Many times these fracture are asymptomatic or patients simply ignore the increase in back pain.[91] This results in some patients never knowing when the fracture occurred. Estimates suggest 30% of the fractures are undiagnosed and less than 10% of patients with VFF are admitted to the hospital.[92] Those admitted to the hospital generally have symptoms that are more difficult to manage (higher pain and disability), are more frail, and have more coexisting comorbid conditions. Of those women with VFF, 30% to 40% develop kyphosis that can evolve into reduced pulmonary function and increased risk of mortality.[93]

Initial management of VFF is conservative care aimed at pain management and activity modification. The primary goal is to resume activity as quickly as possible. Bed rest contributes to further bone loss and rapid loss of muscle mass and is not recommended. The use of oral analgesics may be sufficient for pain control and are the first line of therapy for pain. Hospitalization may be required for intractable pain. Thoracic support and postural braces are often prescribed for patients with the belief they will reduce pain and improve activity tolerance (Fig. 20.5). Yet, few clinical data support the efficacy of bracing in VFF. Physical therapists should be judicious in the use of bracing because of interference with mobility and balance. In general, bracing should provide some relief almost immediately and testing activity before and after bracing may help identify who will benefit. Additionally, many products are difficult to don and doff and can adversely affect balance and mobility. Patients must have the caregiver support to don the brace properly.

The majority of patients with VFF manage well with conservative care. Exercise can be initiated as pain

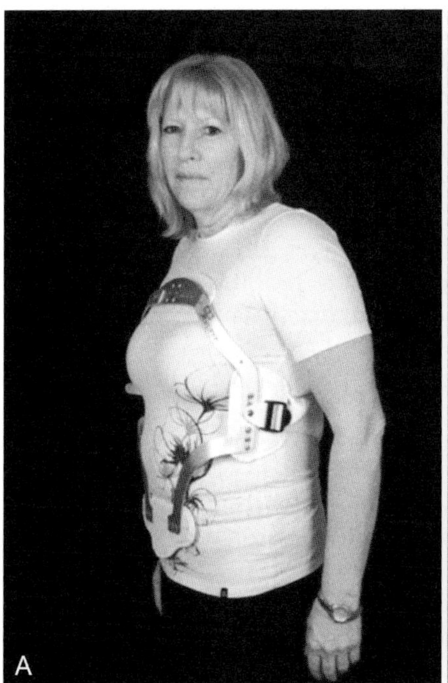

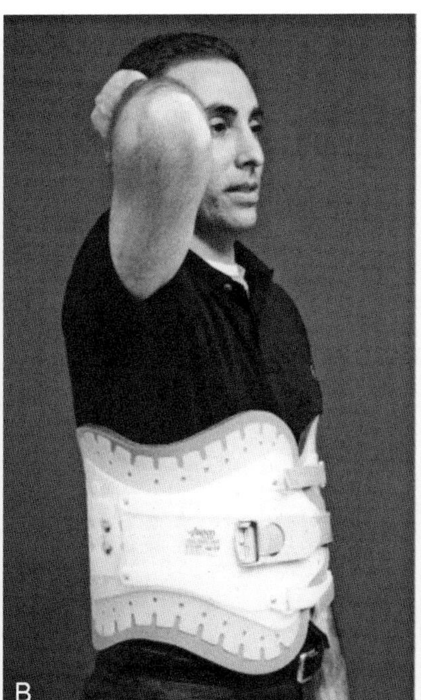

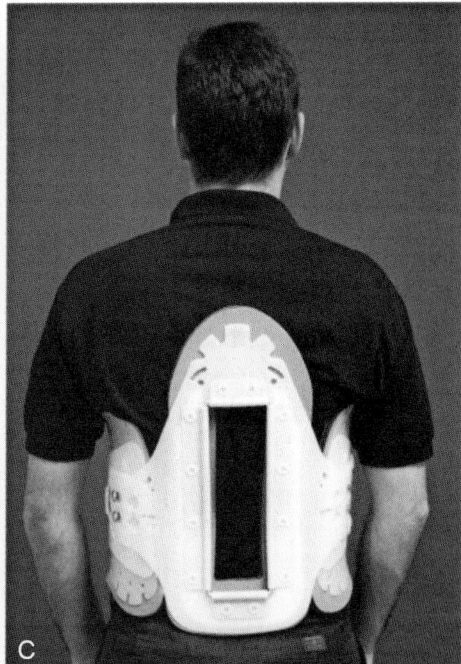

FIG. 20.5 Examples of a thoracolumbar brace. *(From Browner, BD, et al. Skeletal Trauma, ed 5. Philadelphia: Saunders, Elsevier, 2015.)*

diminishes. Patients will often tolerate early exercise intervention in a pool where the spine is unloaded. It is important to progress to land-based exercises to improve bone mass development. Although the optimal exercise intervention has not been identified, progressive resistance exercises for postural muscles to improve upright tolerance and spinal extensor strength appear to have the greatest benefit.[94] Physical therapists should also educate patients and families on the risk of future fractures. A VFF is a warning signal. Vertebral fractures are highly predictive of future fractures and should prompt secondary prevention to improve bone density (e.g., bisphosphonates and resistance training), balance, and environmental safety.[95] High-impact loading is effective in addressing the risk factors for osteoporotic fractures including decreasing the degree of kypohosis.[96,97]

The indications and timing of surgical treatment for vertebral augmentation procedures are controversial. This may be the optimal treatment, however, for patients unable to tolerate movement or where conservative management is unsuccessful. In general, patients are recommended to surgery only after the inability to optimize analgesia (e.g., reporting pain >6/10) and having failed to resume daily activities at 3 to 6 weeks.[98] Vertebral augmentation aims at reducing pain and spinal deformity by restoring vertebral height and may be most effective when performed within 4 months of the fracture incidence. Primary surgical techniques include percutaneous vertebroplasty, percutaneous balloon kyphoplasty, and percutaneous implantation procedures. These techniques involve the percutaneous injection of bone cement under image guidance into the fractured vertebrae to reduce the fracture and, in theory, reduce kyphosis. Complication rate is low (2% to 4%), but complications to consider include site infection, bleeding, pneumothorax, nerve injury from the heat or pressure, and symptomatic cement leakage resulting in anaphylaxis and/or neural injury).[98] Outcomes are similar between types of surgical interventions with symptomatic improvement comparable with conservative management.[99]

Fractures: Summary

Any type of fracture occurring in an older adult is a significant, potentially catastrophic injury. Fragility fractures are especially of concern because of the implications of osteoporosis, reduced activity, and risk for further complications. Management following a fracture demands comprehensive assessment and monitoring for potential complications, such as reduced mobility, reduced nutritional status, depression, and the potential for subsequent fractures. Regardless of the individual restorative program for an individual fracture, focus on addressing preexisting balance issues, sedentary behavior or low physical activity, and fear that may limit mobility is required. Additionally, the therapist should be aware of the patient's bone mineral density and risk for additional fractures to initiate proactive care.

HIP AND KNEE JOINT ARTHROPLASTIES

Total joint arthroplasty is increasingly utilized for management of end-stage osteoarthritis. The most common joints affected, including knee, hip, and shoulder, are covered in this section. Although presented regionally, it is important to remember treatment planning for a patient after should include a global look at preoperative function, postoperative function expectations, social support, and psychological readiness.

Recent changes to the health care system, including Bundled Payments for Care Improvement (2012) and the comprehensive care for joint replacement model implemented in 2016, have caused changes in arthroplasty management. These changes have resulted in decreased hospital length of stay, standardization of arthroplasty implants, and decreased utilization of skilled nursing and inpatient hospital rehabilitation facilities. Increased attention has been placed on the formulation of care process models aimed to determine the appropriate discharge planning for patients. Reimbursement models will continue to evolve and therefore physical therapists treating the older adult need to remain up to date because changes may alter utilization of services in the postacute care timeframe.

Total Knee Arthroplasty

Total knee arthroplasties (TKAs) were the most common surgical procedures performed with 700,100 procedures performed in 2012.[100] It has been projected that this rate of procedures could increase two to five times by the year 2030.[101]

Early Postoperative Considerations. Introduction to the patient with a TKA for the physical therapist can occur along a continuum of care. The patient may participate in preoperative rehabilitation, continue with acute care management, receive home health following hospital discharge, be seen in the outpatient setting or a combination of these settings. The utilization of physical therapy services should be monitored and altered to maximize clinical outcomes without overutilizing visits. The setting itself is not as critical as evaluating the patient as a whole to include postoperative status and procedures performed, social support system, current and previous health status, psychological readiness to participate in therapy, and personal goals for recovery. Although surgeons may have individualized preferences regarding protocols, treatment is best approached from an objective-based criteria framework. For example, if the surgeon has stated in the protocol that individuals may climb stairs in an alternating pattern 4 weeks after surgery, but a patient is presenting with only 70 degrees of flexion, it does not make sense to advise the patient to begin stair-climbing in an alternating pattern when the available range of motion will not allow it. Physical therapists have the ability and skill to evaluate and continually assess function while considering personal factors to best equate rehabilitation goals with an individualized treatment plan.

Early rehabilitation should focus on restoration of range of motion (ROM), managing effusion and inflammation, and normalizing gait. When it comes to short-term goals in the early phase of recovery from TKA, achievement of neutral extension ROM is critical. Full knee extension allows for the proper biomechanics needed to normalize gait pattern. Passive knee extension may be limited by muscle flexibility and/or joint capsule tightness. Inability to meet this goal early may lead to long-term deficits. If early ROM goals of extension or flexion are not met, patients may undergo a manipulation under anesthesia (MUA). Limitation of movement is categorized as mild, moderate, or severe based on flexion ROM (90–100, 70–89, < 70, respectively) or extension ROM (5–10, 11–20, > 20, respectively).[102] The implications of MUA are discussed in the complications section below.

Range of motion improvements can be made with passive, active, or active assisted mobility exercises. Common exercises prescribed in this phase include long sitting heel slides using a strap assist, wall slides in which the patient is supine with feet placed up on wall and allowing gravity to assist the knee into flexion (Fig. 20.6), or seated with passive overpressure from the opposite lower extremity into flexion (Fig. 20.7). Flexion-based activities may also include stationary biking (≈105 degrees required for full revolutions). Patella mobility should be continually assessed and intervention for hypomobility addressed with mobilization and education on self-mobilization techniques. Superior and inferior glides of the patella help improve flexion and extension ROM (Fig. 20.8). Extension-based stretches may include low load long duration stretches, such as sitting with the heel propped on a bolster (may add external weight to thigh and calf) (Fig. 20.9), prone extension hangs (Fig. 20.10), seated hamstring stretches, or standing calf stretching. Exercise selection should incorporate patient tolerance to positioning for the activity (i.e., many patients do not tolerate a prone position secondary to body morphology or a history of low back pain) and dosing should be geared to address specific ROM deficits. Generally a patient will not achieve more ROM than was present preoperatively.

Effusion management includes cryotherapy, compression stockings or sleeves, elevation, and appropriate activity modifications. Education of patients to monitor their effusion in response to their daily activities may be a better indicator than subjective pain levels. It has been shown that effusion in the joint has an indirect relationship to activation of the quadriceps muscle.[103] Arthrogenic muscle inhibition, which occurs as a result of trauma to the knee joint, contributes to inhibition of the quadriceps

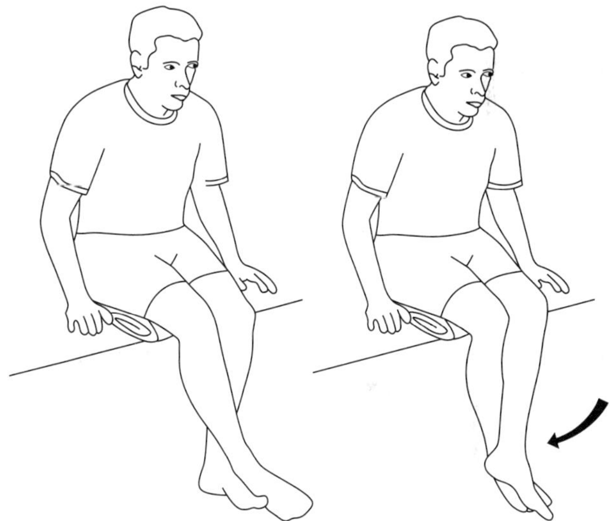

FIG. 20.7 Drop and dangle exercise for knee flexion. *(Copyright © Dr. Robert Marx.)*

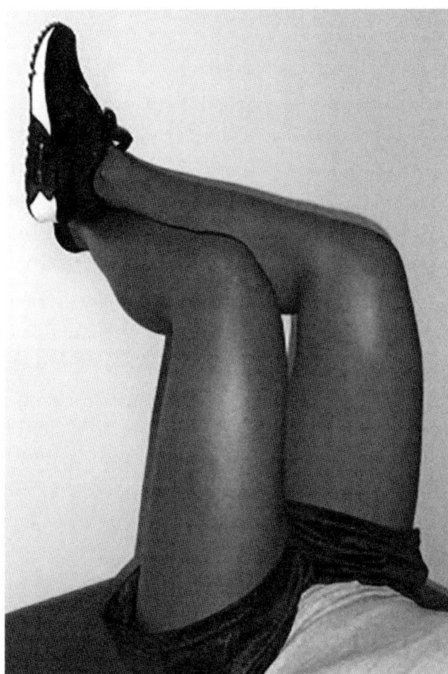

FIG. 20.6 Wall slide exercise for knee flexion. *(From Reider B et al. Orthopaedic Rehabilitation of the Athlete Philadelphia: Saunders, Elsevier, 2015.)*

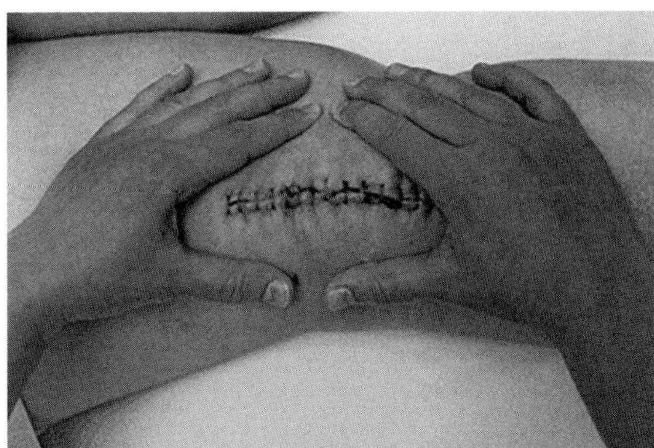

FIG. 20.8 Patellar mobilization. *(From Gokeler A, et al. Physical Therapy for Persistent Pain after Total Knee Replacement. In The Unhappy Total Knee Replacement: A Comprehensive Review and Management Guide. Hirschmann MT, Becker R (Eds). New York. Springer Nature, 2015.)*

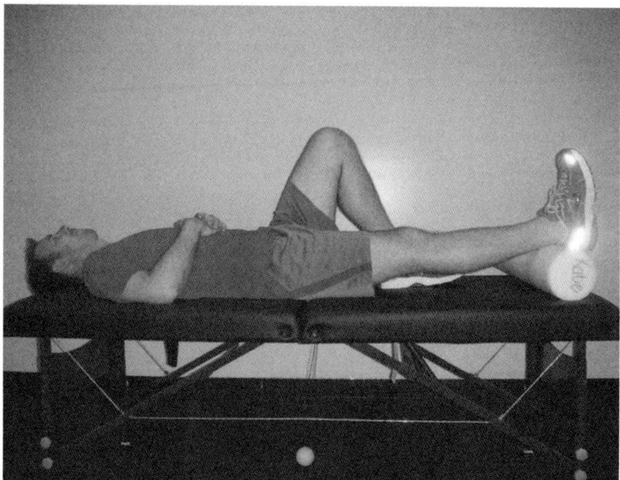

FIG. 20.9 Supine passive knee extension exercise. *(From Reider B et al. Orthopaedic Rehabilitation of the Athlete. Philadelphia: Saunders, Elsevier, 2015.)*

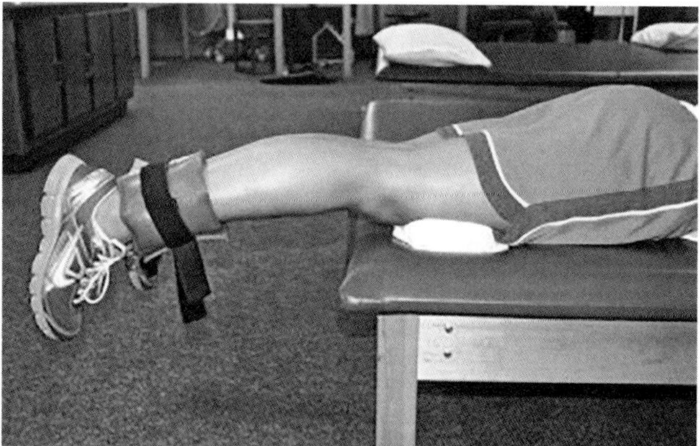

FIG. 20.10 Prone knee extension hangs. *(From Andrews J, et al. Physical Rehabilitation of the Injured Athlete, ed 4. Philadelphia: Elsevier, 2012.)*

muscle. Some patients demonstrate up to 50% to 60% decrease in quadriceps strength from preoperative levels in just 3 to 4 weeks following surgery.[104] Therefore, minimizing effusion in the joint will improve the ability of the quadriceps muscle to contract, leading to improved standing tolerance and a more normalized gait pattern. Flexion ROM will be limited by intraarticular swelling, which can lead to difficulty in movements, such as sit to stand, stair-climbing, or prolonged sitting.

Strengthening activities help to maintain range of motion gains, normalize gait, and improve the ability to perform ADLs. High-intensity exercise is as safe and effective in the early postoperative phase as a low-intensity strengthening program. Rehabilitation can normalize quadriceps strength to preoperative levels at 6 months postsurgery.[105] However the therapist should note that patients undergoing TKA also demonstrate decreased quadriceps strength compared with similar age-matched norms in the presurgical period.[106]

Although the literature has not supported a specific strengthening protocol, quadriceps strengthening is the one most established in current studies. Weakness has been shown to persist after discharge from physical therapy, with asymmetry values up to 20% to 65%. There is also emerging support for rehabilitation efforts to focus on the hip abductor muscles, knowing weakness and functional deficits exists in end-stage knee osteoarthritis.[107] A lack of voluntary muscle activation of the quadriceps contributes more to postoperative weakness than muscle atrophy. Some evidence supports the use of neuromuscular electrical stimulation (NMES) in the acute phase of rehabilitation because it helps to increase quadriceps strength and activation and therefore improves function.[108,109] If possible, initiation of electrical stimulation in the first 48 hours has attenuated quadriceps weakness in the first month with significant improvements in functional outcomes assessment compared with a control group, with differences lasting up to 1 year postoperative.[108] Recommended dosage parameters may vary; however, two times per day, 6 days per week with 40 to 50 Hz, 250 cycles/s, 15 seconds on with a 3-second ramp-up time and 45 seconds of rest for up to 15 cycles leads to improved quadriceps function. Electrodes should be large and placed as shown in Fig. 20.11. Although patient comfort is important, higher intensity as tolerated has been shown to be more beneficial and, therefore, clinicians should opt for large electrodes and utilize rest time and up to 15 cycles to optimize tolerance. Importantly, lower extremity strength deficits may present as balance impairments warranting targeted interventions to minimize fall risk. A 24.2% postoperative fall rate for patients with TKA was reported up to 1 year postoperatively and, although this is less than the average rate for community-dwelling older adults (estimated at 33%),[110,111] it still indicates an area that physical therapy interventions need

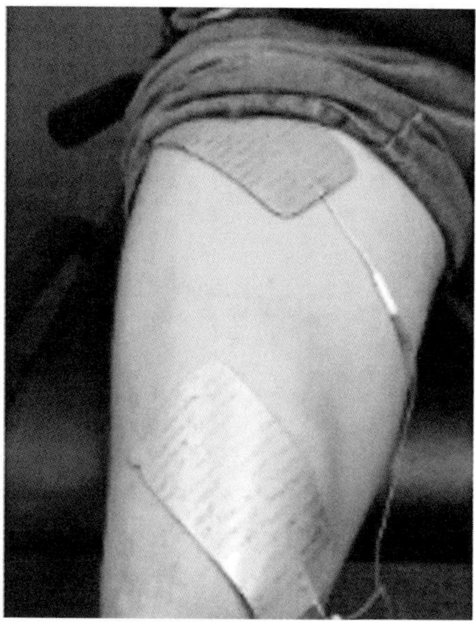

FIG. 20.11 Electrical Stimulation to Quadriceps. *(From https://www.themanual therapist.com/2016/05/5-common-mistakes-for-neuromus cular.html.)*

to address. Although surgery itself leads to decreased fall rates (54.2% of pre-TKA fallers became nonfallers),[111] it is likely this number could be further improved with appropriate and comprehensive rehabilitation. A recent systematic review has demonstrated an improvement in functional mobility and balance in patients after surgical TKA with rehabilitation exercises targeting proprioception, postural control, and coordination.[112]

Long-Term Treatment Considerations. Attention to regaining strength in the surgical limb leads to improved functional mobility as well as minimizing asymmetric movement patterns. Assessment of strength may include isometric or isotonic assessment (e.g. Biodex, KinCom dynamometer, hand-held dynamometer), which can give information about relative limb symmetry or limb symmetry index. Standardized functional assessments represent how range of motion, strength, balance, and motor control are being utilized by the patient. The Chapter 7 on Functional Measures elsewhere in this text provides specific information regarding administration and interpretation of the tests relevant to total joint arthroplasties, including stair climb test, six-minute walk test, timed up and go, 30-second chair stand test, and static and dynamic balance assessments (balance evaluation systems test, Berg balance scale, functional gait assessment). These assessments provide comparisons with standardized normative values as well as serve to guide treatment interventions. Use of these assessments can also help patients establish goals, understand the severity of their impairments, or appreciate their progress by showing them how they compare with age-matched peers.

Prognosis. Patients will frequently rely on input from the treating therapist on when they will return to certain activities. Encouragement should be given for patients to be physically active, however it is important to consider the stress on hardware components. At present, components have an average of 78% to 90% survivorship with lifespans of 10 years up to 20 years.[113,114] This survivorship has not changed in 20 years. It has been suggested that high load, repetitive activities may decrease the longevity of the hardware. *In vivo* prosthetic joint forces are listed in Table 20.2.[115] Although variation of recommendations exist within the literature, 139 surveys obtained at the 2007 annual meeting of the American Association for Hip and Knee Surgeons (AAHKS) revealed that more than 95% of the responses placed no limitations on low-impact activities including level surface walking, stair climbing, level surface bicycling, swimming and golf. Higher impact activities, listed in Table 20.3 show greater variability. It should be noted there is no strong evidence for the recommendations.[116]

High satisfaction levels have been demonstrated following TKA, with most studies showing greater than 80% satisfaction and a small number of studies reported 60% to 80% satisfaction, mostly around the outcome of pain relief.[117] Approximately one in five patients will be dissatisfied with the outcome of surgery.[117] It has also been shown that most functional recovery occurs within the first year of surgery, with no significant improvements made in the second and third years.[118] Quadriceps weakness on the contralateral limb is a predictor of poorer outcomes 3 years following TKA.[119] The American Academy of Orthopaedic surgeons identified strong evidence for less improvement in outcomes for patients with a body mass index of obese and moderate evidence for lower patient-reported outcomes for individuals with chronic pain conditions, and limited evidence for depression/anxiety as a risk factor.[120]

TABLE 20.2 In Vivo Prosthetic Joint Forces by Activity

Activity	Force
Cycling	1.3 × body weight (BW)
Treadmill (walking)	2.05 × BW
Walking on level ground	2.6 × BW
Tennis	3.6 × BW during forehand stroke; 3.1 × BW during backhand stroke
Jogging	4.3 × BW
Golf driving swing	4.5 × BW in leading leg and 3.2 × BW in opposite leg

The most common complications include infection, manipulation under anesthesia, deep vein thrombosis, and pulmonary embolism. Signs of infection warranting contact with the surgeon includes an increase of pain, excessive wound drainage (especially white or yellow drainage), redness around the incision and spreading in size, in addition to reported feelings of fatigue or general malaise. Typically, diagnosis of a deep infection will require aspiration of the joint fluid and appropriate laboratory work-up. Surgical management for deep infection can include retention or replacement of the prostheses, both encompass intravenous antibiotics until cultures are clear. Replacement of the prosthesis requires temporary implantation of an antibiotic impregnated spacer with eventual revision surgery. Better outcomes are observed in infections that are not methicillin resistant.[121]

Treatment of a patient who undergoes revision surgery owing to deep joint infection should be progressed slowly owing to possible deconditioned status. It is likely they will present with greater strength deficits and possible joint stiffness secondary to loss of a functional limb during the infection recovery process. As previously noted, physical therapists have a direct role in management of range of motion to help avoid manipulation under anesthetic or to know when a referral back to the surgeon is appropriate. A recent systematic review determined MUA for postoperative stiffness was efficacious, although the optimal timing remains unclear.[122] It is suggested that if an MUA is indicated, performing MUA within 20 weeks postoperative produces the greatest ROM improvements.[122] Higher complication risks have been identified in patients with

TABLE 20.3 Percentages of Orthopedic Surgeons Recommending Frequency of High-Impact Activities Following a THA and TKA

Activity	Walk Uneven Surfaces	Climbing	Jogging	Sprinting	Cycling Incline	Cycling Off Road	Skiing Groomed	Skiing Difficult	Doubles Tennis	Singles Tennis
Total Hip Arthroplasty										
Unlimited	87.6	53.7	7.3	2.9	75.9	31.6	44.9	5.9	70.1	17.4
Occasional	12.2	25.2	20.9	3.6	20.1	32.4	39.6	10.1	26.6	32.4
Discouraged	0.0	20.6	71.5	93.4	3.6	35.3	14.7	83.7	2.9	50.0
Total Knee Arthroplasty										
Unlimited	83.9	55.1	4.3	1.4	73.2	27.0	43.8	3.7	65.7	10.9
Occasional	15.1	26.6	20.1	4.3	22.3	36.7	39.6	10.1	28.8	28.1
Discouraged	0.7	17.6	75.4	94.2	4.3	35.8	16.1	85.9	5.1	60.6

comorbid conditions such as diabetes (moderate evidence) and cirrhosis/Hepatitis C (limited evidence).[120] Postoperative delirium has been found in up to 10% of patients post-arthroplasty joint and should be monitored by therapists, especially considering the adverse consequences.

Rehabilitation prior to TKA may help to improve outcomes, specifically for range of motion and quadriceps strength. Preoperative ROM is a strong predictor of poor ROM after total knee arthroplasty.[123–125] A preoperative knee flexion of 100 degrees or more was associated with 0.8 fold lower odds ratio of undergoing MUA.[126]

Total Hip Arthroplasty

Total and partial hip arthroplasy surgical procedures were the third most often performed musculoskeletal surgery in 2012 at 468,000 procedures.[100] It is estimated that by 2030 there will be 570,000 primary and 96,700 revision total hip arthroplasty (THAs) performed in the United States annually.[101]

Surgeon preference and specific patient characteristics drive decision-making for the surgical approach performed in THA. Recovery and rehabilitation management will vary depending on the surgical approach, thus making it critical to review operative reports. The three most common approaches include posterior, direct lateral, and anterior (Fig. 20.12). Table 20.4 describes advantages and rehabilitation considerations for each of these approaches.[127]

Early Postoperative Considerations. Maximizing range of motion (within the constraints of surgical precautions), restoring hip abductor strength, normalizing gait, and restoring functional mobility should be the primary focus of early rehabilitation. Range-of-motion exercises should target muscle groups of the lower extremity, including quadriceps, hamstrings, hip external rotators, and hip flexor, as appropriate. It is less common to see postoperative capsule restrictions that become problematic unlike that following knee arthroplasty. However, the chronicity of osteoarthritis prior to surgery may contribute to capsule restrictions that may need to be addressed. To allow for immediate postoperative healing to occur, mobilization to address capsular restrictions should occur after 4 to 6 weeks postoperatively.

Weight-bearing restrictions will vary depending on hardware components and cement versus cementless implants. Most patients will be allowed to weight-bear

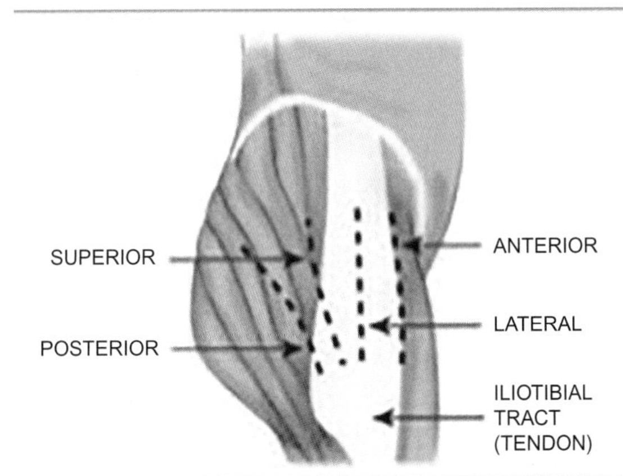

FIG. 20.12 Surgical approach for total hip arthroplasty (THA). *(Copyright © 2019 James W. Pritchett, MD.)*

TABLE 20.4 Total Hip Arthroplasty Approaches and Rehabilitation Concerns

Approach	Description	Rerhabilitation Considerations
Posterior	Traditional approach that provides the best visualization, minimal risk of nerve damage. Used in presence of osteoporosis, obesity, and significant bone deformity. Generally splits the gluteus maximus and excises the tendons of the piriformis, superior and inferior gemelli. Spares the gluteus medius.	No flexion over 90 degrees. No internal rotation. No adduction past midline for 3–6 weeks. Generally difficult to return home immediately because of precautions and amount of surgical dressing.
Anterior (Smith-Peterson)	More technically demanding, requires special surgical table. Risk to lateral femoral cutaneous nerve. Leaves posterior capsule and muscles intact, thus no hip precautions, except maybe to restrict hip extension to neutral. Incision is made between the rectus femoris and tensor fascia latae.	Active and isolated hip flexion can be extremely painful, thus causing activities such as sit-to-supine transition to be very difficult. Overall less pain and faster progression in function and use of assistive device as compared with posterior approach. These patients can manage at home on their own.
Lateral Approach	Low chance of posterior dislocation. More abductor insufficiency (4% to 20% vs. 0 to 16% with posterior approach) because hip abductors are incised.	Patient may limp for 3 or more months secondary to gluteus medius weakness. May need assistive device for 3 or more months postoperatively. Risk of permanent limp.
Superior	Advertised as outpatient procedure or 1-night stay. Avoids incising IT band, but does incise the piriformis tendon. Blood loss is minimal (no transfusions). Dislocations rare.	No precautions. Early return to function. Minimal hospital stay.

as tolerated and therefore gait training should emphasize normal gait pattern with the use of an assistive device, as necessary. Canes or single crutches should be used on the opposite side of the involved limb to decrease load on the involved hip. Strengthening efforts should focus on hip abductors and extensors because they present with weakness secondary to preoperative disuse as well as inhibition from surgery. The hip flexors, extensors, and abductors, as well as knee flexors and extensors, demonstrate 14% to 26% strength loss within the first month of surgery.[128] An exercise program should consider the muscle groups disrupted by the surgical approach. Modifications should be made to adhere to dislocation precautions. Some examples of early mobility and strengthening exercises may include prone quadriceps stretch using a strap for assistance, supine active heel slides, seated hamstring stretch, isometric exercises for the quadriceps and the gluteal muscles, or short arc quadricep extension (Fig. 20.13).

Long-Term Treatment Considerations. Unfortunately, literature regarding the specific type of exercise and appropriate time for intervention remains limited despite the growing incidence of THA surgeries being performed. Two systematic reviews were unable to conclude a specific postoperative protocol owing to low level evidence secondary to low sample size or poor methodology.[129,130] Hip strength deficits are known to persist following surgical intervention and therefore selecting interventions to address weakness as well as normalizing motor patterns will likely lead to improved functional outcomes. Exercise selection for a patient should include attention to targeted muscle group weakness and individualized to their specific impairments. Therapists should also consider the surgical approach performed in allowing adequate recovery time during the protection phase (postoperative weeks 4 to 6). Progressive resistance exercises should begin with lower level maximal voluntary isometric contraction (MVIC) values to ensure appropriate muscle activation patterns. This may then be progressed to higher level exercises performed in more functional positions. A systematic review examined electromyographic findings of common exercises for hip abductors and external rotators in both weight-bearing and non–weight-bearing positions to assist with improved exercise selection. These exercises are listed in Table 20.5.[131,132] Exercise dosage should be provided with the level of activation in mind, generally starting with lower loads and higher repetitions.

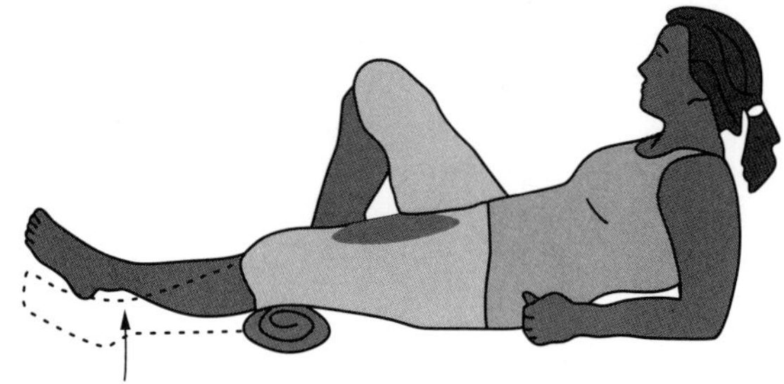

FIG. 20.13 Short arc quad exercise. *(Copyright Elsevier Inc.)*

Prognosis. Total hip arthroscopy is successful in improving outcomes of pain, function, and quality of life from preoperative status.[133] However, it has also been shown that strength deficits may persist up to 1 year following surgery. Patients demonstrate 15% to 25% less strength in the knee extensors and knee flexors compared with age-matched health controls.[128] This weakness highlights the need to encourage patients to continue with physical activity and strengthening activities beyond the scope of time spent formally in the physical therapy clinic. Improved clinical outcomes are anticipated by patients demonstrating higher preoperative Western Ontario & McMaster Universities Osteoarthritis Index (WOMAC)[134] and Hip Harris Score (HHS) outcomes.[135] Poorer outcomes have been associated with the following factors: increased age,[135, 136] female gender,[136,137] high BMI,[136] and increased number of comorbid conditions,[136]. Individuals of older age, females, those with higher BMI, more comorbid conditions, and depression had greater odds for predicted use of an assistive device in a 2- to 5-year follow-up following THA.

Potential complications include deep venous thrombosis, pulmonary embolism, infection, periprosthetic fracture, and dislocation. Dislocation occurs rarely, but varies in rates from 1% up to 15%, depending on the experience of the surgeon, and the approach and size of the prosthetic component.[138–140] Education on avoidance of positions as described in Table 20.4 may help to minimize the dislocation rate; however, it has been suggested that removal of these restrictions does not alter the incidence of dislocation.[141] Higher rates of dislocations occur with surgical revisions. Nerve injury is possible owing to injury from dissection during the surgery, component positioning, or postoperative incision site adhesion (mostly anterior approach). The most commonly injured nerves include superior gluteal, lateral femoral cutaneous, sciatic, and femoral. Typically, the superior gluteal, lateral femoral cutaneous and femoral nerves will all recover, albeit nerve regrowth is slow. Unfortunately, half of patients who suffer injury to the sciatic nerve have persistent disability. Patients need to be educated on how to allow the nerve to rest by avoiding positions of prolonged compression or excessive and ballistic stretching. Delirium following total joint arthroplasty has been reported to occur from 5% to 14%.[142] The short form of the Informant Questionnaire on Cognitive Decline in the Elderly (short IQCODE) has shown to be effective for identifying older adults undergoing total joint replacement at risk of developing delirium. Additionally, avoidance of high-dose opioids, early mobility, and return to familiar environments may all be strategies to help decrease this risk. Periprosthetic fracture occurs at a rate of 0.1% to 4.1% and has similar mortality rates to those of patients with a hip fracture.[143] Identified risk factors include female gender, older than 80 years, THA revision, rheumatoid arthritis, and osteonecrosis. Implant survivorship at 10 to 15 years has been reported to be up to 97.5%.[143] As discussed in the TKA section, recommendations for return to physical activity may vary by surgeon.

TABLE 20.5 Examples of Common Gluteal Exercises and the Associated Level of Activation as Determined by Electromyography

	Gluteus medius	Gluteus maximus
Low-level activation (0 to 20% MVIC)	Variations of the clamshell (no resistance) Monster walks with the band at knees	Monster walks with band at knees/ankle/feet, lateral stepping with band at feet Lateral lunge Bridging on swiss ball Prone plank
Moderate level activation (21% to 40% MVIC)	Clamshell with band at knee Clamshell with 60 degrees hip flexion Lateral stepping with band at foot Standing hip abduction (stance leg) Prone bridge/plank Bridging on stable surface	Lateral step-up with 10% body mass Clamshell with 60 degrees hip flexion
High level activation (41% to 60% MVIC)	Lateral step up Single-limb squat Wall squat Quadruped with contralateral arm and leg lift Unilateral bridge Side-lying hip abduction	Lateral step-up Clamshell with band at knee Transverse lunge Single limb deadlift Quadruped with contralateral arm and leg lift Unilateral bridge Side-lying hip abduction
Very high activation (> 61% MVIC)	Side-lying bridge with dominant leg down Seated hip abduction machine (RPE $\geq$7) Single limb squat	Side-lying bridge with dominant* leg down Standing hip abduction with band at ankle Side-lying hip abduction with 5% BM Seated hip abduction machine (RPE $\geq$ 7) Forward step-up

MVIC, Maximal voluntary isometric contraction; BM, Body mass; RPE, Rate of perceived exertion.
*Gluteus maximus of dominant leg is being exercised

Table 2.3 highlights the results of surveys obtained at the American Association for Hip and Knee Surgeons (AAHKS) at the 2007 annual meeting regarding activity recommendations following hip and knee arthroplasty.[116]

Joint Arthroplasty: Summary

Surgical procedures for total hip and knee arthroplasties often improve quality of life and mobility in older adults with arthritic joint conditions. Physical therapists play a key role in early mobility and monitoring for complications. Early rehabilitation focuses on regaining range of motion (particularly following TKA), strengthening, and supporting patients in resuming physical activity. Performance tests, such as stair-climbing, sit to stand, and gait speed are important to quantify in later stages of recovery and compare against age-matched norms. Patients often report good recovery in daily activities, but may not recognize continued strength and balance deficits.

SHOULDER SURGERIES

Rotator Cuff Repair

Rotator cuff repair surgery is a common procedure with more than 270,000 procedures performed annually in the United States.[144] Four muscles comprise the shoulder's rotator cuff: the supraspinatus, infraspinatus, teres minor, and subscapularis. Critical for providing dynamic stability to the highly mobile shoulder, the musculotendinous junction is susceptible to degenerative tearing.

Tissue healing at the tendon–bone junction begins 3 to 4 weeks after the repair with continued remodeling of scar tissue and tensile strength improving around the 3-month mark. Structural integrity of the repair is vulnerable until at least 6 months after surgery.[145] Therefore, rehabilitation efforts should focus initially on protection, with gradual progression to functional use of the surgical shoulder. Factors affecting the rehabilitation process may include the number of tendons involved, tissue quality, chronicity of tear, and surgical techniques used.

Early Postoperative Considerations. As with any musculoskeletal remodeling process, there are three stages: the protection phase, mobilization, and the strengthening/return to function phase. Each of these phases will be described for rotator cuff repair.

The protection phase occurs up to the first 6 weeks postoperatively. During this time, scar tissue is being formed, which may strengthen the tendon. Protection of the repaired tendon(s) is achieved by use of a sling and avoidance of any *active* range of motion. Considerations for time in the sling includes the number of involved tendons, tissue quality, and tissue mobility. Education on the importance of sling compliance, guidance on donning and doffing of the sling, and home modifications to avoid active use of the surgical arm is key in these first few

TABLE 20.6 Clinical Recommendation for Timeline to Wean from Sling Following Rotator Cuff Repair

Weaning from the Sling	
Day 1	1–2 hours
Day 2	2–4 hours
Day 3	4–6 hours
Day 4	6–8 hours
Day 5	8–10 hours
Day 6	10–12 hours
Day 7	Fully weaned

- Night time use of the sling is dependent on sleeping position and behavior. Individuals who tend to toss and turn may benefit from keeping the sling on at night throughout the weaning process.
- The sling may be useful to wear in the community for up to 2 weeks from the start of the weaning process to protect the shoulder from an unanticipated fall or from people bumping into the surgical shoulder.

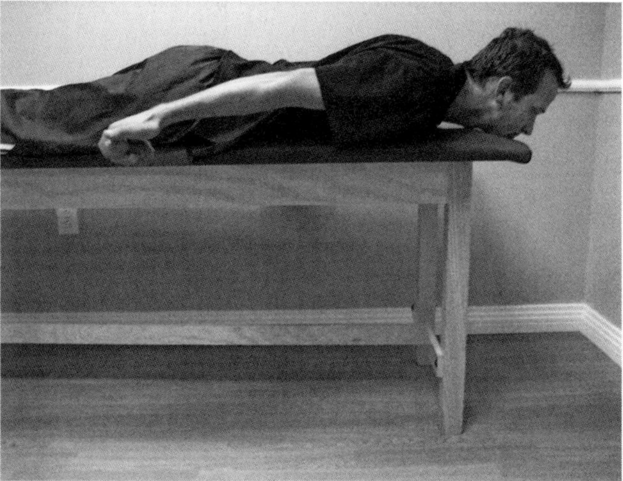

FIG. 20.14 Prone shoulder extension exercise. *(From Giangarra CE, Manske RE. Clinical Orthopaedic Rehabilitation: A Team Approach, ed 4. Philadelphia: Elsevier, 2018.)*

weeks. Weaning from the sling is achieved through a gradual decrease of time spent immobilized. Table 20.6 lists a recommendation for weaning a patient from the sling. The weaning period is described starting from the day of discharged sling use, which will vary based on surgical procedures performed and surgeon preference. Mobilization is achieved through therapist-delivered passive ROM activities and joint mobilizations. The current highest level of evidence suggests that early-motion (passive) movement after rotator cuff repair results in superior postoperative ROM up to 1 year.[146]

The mobilization phase occurs from 6 to 12 weeks postoperatively. Active assisted ROM activities may begin at this time and may include exercises, such as lying supine using a dowel to assist shoulder flexion motion, wall crawls, and shoulder external rotation motion. During this phase it is also beneficial to maintain activation of the scapular stabilizers and this can begin with seated scapular retraction with progression to more challenging positions, such as prone as shown in Fig. 20.14. During this phase, attention should be drawn to scapular mechanics, especially to ensure shoulder forward elevation is returning without overrecruitment of the upper trapezius muscle. Conditioning of the rotator cuff may begin at approximately 8 to 9 weeks postoperatively provided pain and symptoms are well managed. Conditioning of the musculotendinous junction involves low activation of the involved tendon(s) to prepare for strengthening for muscle hypertrophy. This can include side-lying external rotation to neutral or seated/standing external rotation without resistance if the side-lying position is not tolerated, as well as seated/standing active scaption without resistance. It is important to monitor a patient's tolerance to the rehabilitation program. Signs and symptoms of poor tolerance are described in Table 20.7.[145]

Long-Term Treatment Considerations. During the return to function or strengthening phase after 12 weeks postoperative, the tendon may gradually be introduced to resistance and strengthening activities. This phase should be started only if a patient demonstrates ROM that is close to normative ranges as described in Table 20.7.[147] Range of motion and strengthening should be performed with continued attention to proper scapular mechanics. The most effective strengthening exercises for the rotator cuff muscles are described in Table 20.8.[145] It is

TABLE 20.7 Signs and Symptoms of Poor Tolerance during Rotator Cuff Repair Rehabilitation

Symptom	Protection Phase	Mobilization Phase	Return to Function Phase
Pain at rest/night	> 6/10	> 4/10	> 2/10
Range of motion	> 20 degrees behind ROM goals	> 20 degrees behind ROM goals	> 20 degrees behind ROM goals Elevation of ≥140 degrees External rotation at 20 degrees abduction of ≥ 30 degrees External rotation at 90 degrees abduction of ≥75 degrees
Strength			Inability to demonstrate active elevation or gross loss of strength after 8–12 weeks

ROM, Range of motion.

TABLE 20.8 Most Effective Strengthening Exercises for Rotator Cuff

Muscle	Low (0 to 15% MVIC)	Medium (16% to 40% MVIC)	High (41% to 100% MVIC)
Supraspinatus	Supine bar assisted ER Supine self-assisted elevation Pendulum exercise	Pull-assisted elevation Wall walk/slide Active flexion/elevation with elbow straight	Side-lying ER Full can shoulder ABD, prone ER at 90 degrees
Infraspinatus	Supine assisted ER Supine self-assisted elevation Pendulum exercise	Active flexion/elevation, standing ER at 45 degrees of abduction High rows	Standing resisted shoulder extension Side-lying ER Prone ER at 90 degrees
Teres Minor	Standing ER 0 degrees with towel Standing ER scapular plane		Prone ER at 90, side-lying ER High row
Subscapularis	Pulley-assisted elevation, table slide seated row	Upright bar-assisted elevation Upright bar-assisted ER, forward punch	High row IR at 0 degrees of ABD ER at 0 degrees of ABD

ABD, abduction, ER, external rotation, IR, internal rotation, MVIC, maximal voluntary isometric contraction.

recommended that patients demonstrate adequate tolerance to resisted elevation in the scapular plane before attempting overhead strengthening positions.[147]

Prognosis. The size of the tendon tear affects recovery rates, with reports of 6 months in patients with small tears and 18 months in patients with medium tears. Patients with large-to-massive tears showed continuous improvement in strength up to 18 months; however, they did not reach the strength of the contralateral shoulder at final follow-up.[148] It is important to educate patients on the expected rate of recovery and regarding recommendations and the need to continue participation in a home exercise program beyond discharge from formal physical therapy. Additionally, failure rates have been linked to tear size, with 78% of larger tears (> 4 cm) and full thickness tears failing within the first 3 months. (149) Older age has a negative impact on failure rates secondary to reduced blood supply and the presence of osteoporotic bone. (149) However, functional outcomes are good in the majority of failed repairs at 1 year.[149]

Factors shown to affect the risk of a retear include older age, fatty infiltration of the rotator cuff muscles, tear size, concomitant procedures to the long head of the biceps or acromioclavicular joints, as well as the number of tendons involved.[150] Although less supported, some evidence does suggest low bone mineral density negatively affects tendon healing.[151] Regarding clinical outcome scores, patients undergoing rotator cuff repair were older than 65 years, had a lower score on the Medical Outcomes Study, 36-item Short Form and Health Survey Quality of Life tool than those younger than 60 years.[151] Furthermore, 77% of patients with a longer functional recovery time were older than age 60.[151] Other contributing factors to a lower functional outcome and physical quality of life included a history of diabetes or obesity.[151] The risk factors of a hospital readmission following rotator cuff repair include age greater than 80 years, chronic obstructive pulmonary disease, hypertension requiring medication, or an American Society of Anesthesiologist (ASA) classification of 3 or 4. The most common complications associated with readmission are related to cardiovascular (29%), infection (19%), or respiratory (17%) events.[152] Postoperative stiffness occurs in 3% to 10% of individuals 1 year following surgery and more commonly occurs in patients with diabetes, thyroid disorders, acute rotator cuff tears, partial-thickness tears, and adhesive capsulitis.[147]

Total Shoulder and Reverse Shoulder Arthroplasty

Total shoulder arthroplasty (TSA) is indicated to manage end-stage arthritis in the shoulder joint. For individuals with irreparable rotator cuff muscle damage, fractures, or a previously failed TSA where the rotator cuff tendons are deficient, a reverse total shoulder arthroplasty (rTSA) is indicated. Mechanically, TSA without appropriate rotator cuff stabilization leads to persistent superior migration of the humeral head causing component loosening and inferior outcomes. Important differences exist between the surgical procedures that require unique rehabilitation considerations and those that do not. This section will review both procedures, highlighting the important treatment differences. Factors that affect both procedures include preoperative shoulder status, the type of implant used and surgical approach performed, bone quality of the glenoid and humerus, the integrity of the rotator cuff muscles, any concomitant rotator cuff repair, tendon repair, or tendon transfer; and, the overall component stability of the reconstruction.[153] Clinical signs and symptoms should be utilized to move a patient through postoperative phases versus time-based criteria. This ensures activities are appropriate for postoperative healing while also carefully evaluating each patient to progress their program individually at a pace that matches the function of the patient's shoulder with consideration of the previous factors mentioned.

Early Postoperative Considerations. In comparison with arthroplasty in the lower extremity, early treatment revolves around protection and healing. Phase I (0 to 6 weeks) includes immediate postsurgical protection, with patients spending the first 4 to 6 weeks in a sling. Passive ROM may be restored through therapist-assisted movement.

In TSA, the integrity of the rotator cuff musculature and associated rotator cuff repair during the TSA surgery guides passive ROM restrictions. The subscapularis tendon may be repaired, which typically will limit early motion to less than 30 to 40 degrees of external rotation. Some surgical procedures include tenotomy of the subscapularis tendon, which would not have specific motion restrictions.

In rTSA elevation over 90 degrees is discouraged to help minimize strain during tissue healing. The subscapularis tendon may be repaired during rTSA, which could lead to limitations of passive external rotation motion to 30 to 40 degrees. Risk of dislocation occurs in positions of adduction and internal rotation, so avoidance of stretching into internal rotation is not recommended during this phase. The deltoid muscles and periscapular muscles will become the primary glenohumeral movers owing to absent or deficient rotator cuff muscles. Gentle isometrics in this early phase can help maintain integrity of these muscles during the immobilization period.

In phase II (typically 6 to 12 weeks), if passive ROM goals have been achieved, active assisted and active ROM may be initiated for both types of repair. The therapist should monitor the patient for muscular recruitment to avoid compensatory strategies and patterns that may lead to faulty mechanics. Progression of exercises initially should be performed in the supine position to improve tolerance to activities because of a gravity minimized position with progression to seated and standing positions to mimic functional activities more closely. Typically, no restrictions are given for forward elevation in this phase. Some suggested activities include supine positioning using a dowel or wand, wall walking or crawling in which patients uses their fingers and hand to "crawl" up the wall, or overhead pulleys. In the presence of a subscapularis repair, rotational isometrics may begin in the week 8.

Phase III/IV (12+ weeks) will progress strengthening exercises and aim to assist with return to functional activities. Progression to this phase should not begin until active, active-assisted, and passive ROM are full and with minimal pain. A prospective case-control study demonstrated flexion ROM achieved in patients with TSA to be 144 degrees versus 136 degrees in those with rTSA, with external rotation of 53 degrees and 38 degrees, respectively, and abduction 136 degrees and 129 degrees, respectively.[154]

Prognosis. A recent systematic review established that following TSA, the majority of individuals recover within the first year following surgery.[155] Both the TSA and rTSA procedures demonstrate effective pain relief.[154] Return to physical activity, including sports, in this population is high with one systematic review demonstrating 92.6% overall return rate in patients undergoing a TSA, 74.9% in rTSA, and 71.1% in individuals with hemiarthroplasty.[156] The most common sports returned to included swimming, golf, fitness sports, and tennis.[156] A separate systematic review demonstrated rates of return to sports to range from 57.1% to 97.3% in a population of recreational athletes. In nearly all studies in the latter review, the individuals reported playing their desired sport within the 3 months prior to their surgery, an important issue to understand about the cohort that returned to their preferred sport. In the review by Aims et al., individuals with an rTSA demonstrated slightly lower return rates of 60% to 85.5%, which may be attributed to older age or altered mechanics secondary to hardware components.[154] Complication rates between TSA and rTSA have been shown to be similar at 2-year follow-up—15% and 13%, respectively.

Shoulder Surgeries: Summary

Common shoulder surgeries for older adults include rotator cuff repair and joint arthroplasty. It is important to guide patients in what to expect from each respective surgery. Understanding expected recovery times and planning for immobilization are important for both patients and their families. Shoulder replacement procedures can be effective for arthritic conditions with a main goal of pain relief. Reverse total shoulder arthroplasties are the preferred procedure when the rotator cuff musculature cannot be salvaged. In these cases, patients can expect good pain relief, but may not regain full function of the shoulder.

SPINAL SURGERIES

Disorders of the spine can have a considerable impact on function and quality of life. Spinal stenosis is the most common indication for spinal surgery in those older than 65 years.[157] Spinal stenosis is frequently described from an anatomic perspective as a narrowing of the spinal canal (central or foraminal). This is often a result of degeneration of numerous structures, including a loss of disc height, disc herniation, osteophytes, and thickening of the ligamentum flavum. Surgical interventions are generally only recommended after conservative treatments have failed to provide pain relief or improvement in function.

Rates of spinal decompression and elective fusions for symptom reduction are increasing in the older population. From 2004 to 2015 elective lumbar fusion procedures among individuals age 65 and older increased by 73%.[151] Patients with a diagnosis of spondylolisthesis accounted for the majority of these surgeries followed by degenerative scoliosis.[158] The most common surgical technique used was a decompression laminectomy, which involves the removal of the structures compressing the nerve root. Decompression is often performed alongside a spinal fusion when multiple nerve roots are involved, spondylolisthesis is present, or there is significant spinal deformity, such as degenerative scoliosis. In the cervical spine, the primary diagnosis and surgical procedure among older adults is cervical spondylosis with myelopathy treated with fusion procedures.

Surgical rates are increasing partially because of a growing population of older adults, advances in surgical procedures, and an increased demand for continued or improved function with increasing age.[3] Because spine surgery is generally performed only after conservative treatment has failed, it is important to consider both the physiologic and psychological changes that result from prolonged pain. Degenerative changes of the bones, joints, ligaments, and muscles contribute to reduced paraspinal strength and compromised spinal dynamics. Alongside impaired function, these individuals frequently experience anxiety, depression, and a loss of social and recreational participation. Rehabilitation that incorporates the biopsychosocial model is the optimal intervention after surgery to reduce pain and disability.

Indications for Surgery. Rapidly progressing neurologic deficits and/or bladder dysfunction is an indication for urgent surgery. This presentation is rare in spinal conditions owing to degenerative changes. In the absence of rapidly progressing neurologic deficits, there is no consensus regarding the indications and timing for spine surgery. For patients with mild clinical features of myelopathy, close neurologic follow-up to assess for progressive deficits is appropriate. Surgery consultation is recommended for individuals with a higher risk for deterioration of function, including those with severe spinal cord compression on MRI, progressing loss of dexterity, or highly active lifestyles. Most surgery for degenerative spine conditions is performed as an elective procedure after a patient has failed to improve with conservative care.

Prognosis and Treatment Planning

Cervical Spine. Patients undergoing surgery for cervical spondylotic myelopathy can expect significant functional recovery for up to 2 years after surgery. On average, patients report a 50% improvement in function at 1 year and about 60% improvement at 2 years.[159] Smoking status and duration and severity of symptoms all contribute to worse clinical outcomes following surgery. Prognosis is further dependent on the duration and degree of neurologic compression prior to surgery. Conditions, such as foot drop, loss of hand dexterity, and neurogenic bladder, may not recover following surgery. Treatment planning should include methods for accommodating for these impairments, including the prescription of appropriate assistive devices and orthoses.

Lumbar Spine. Medically stable patients appropriate for surgery generally report significant benefit from surgical treatment for lumbar spinal stenosis. Patients can expect a 50% reduction in pain and 55% improvement in function over the first 3 months following surgery.[160] Further changes in pain and function are small, but may continue up to 2 years postoperatively. Complete recovery is uncommon, with back pain being the most recalcitrant complaint. Success and satisfaction after lumbar decompression surgery are highly variable. Patient-level factors influencing a poor recovery include depression, high catastrophizing, lower preoperative mobility and physical activity, and higher preoperative pain intensity. Physical therapists should account for these variables when planning treatment following surgery because recovery time is generally protracted in these patients. Additionally, treatment interventions need to be adapted based on these factors. Psychologically informed physical therapy can change coping strategies, such as catastrophizing, and facilitate changes in physical activity, although the impact in older adults is less well defined.

Complications

Rates of surgical complications in the spine vary by the complexity of the surgical procedure with more complications with increasing levels of fusions as shown in Fig. 20.15.[159,161,162] Early complications include infection, dural tears, and deep venous thrombosis. Physical therapists should monitor patients for a change in status that may be associated with a complication and alert the medical team if noted. Nerve damage is a complication that may not be apparent early in the postoperative period. Sequelae for surgery-related nerve damage are highly variable, depending on the level involved and the extent of the injury to the nerves. The physical therapist can elicit evidence of a nerve injury with a thorough examination and patient interview inquiring about significant changes or loss of function, motor loss, and bowel or bladder changes. Nerve damage may gradually resolve, and improvements may be seen for up to 12 to 18 months after surgery. If little to no recovery is observed in the early phase of recovery, it is important to begin examining ways to accommodate to the impairment. For example, in the patient who exhibits foot-drop following a L3-L4-L5 fusion without resolution over the subsequent 4 weeks of treatment, addressing the foot drop with an ankle-foot orthosis may have a greater impact while continuing to work on facilitation of the tibialis anterior. Using the orthosis may have a significant positive impact on ADLs, gait speed, and quality of life. Longer-term complications (6 months to 1 year) from spine surgery include ongoing or increasing spinal pain, pseudoarthrosis, and delayed infection. Factors, such as loss in ROM owing to muscle spasm or pain or a significant change in status, should prompt a referral back to the surgical team for further work-up. A list of most reported problems following surgery and potential actions are presented in Table 20.9.

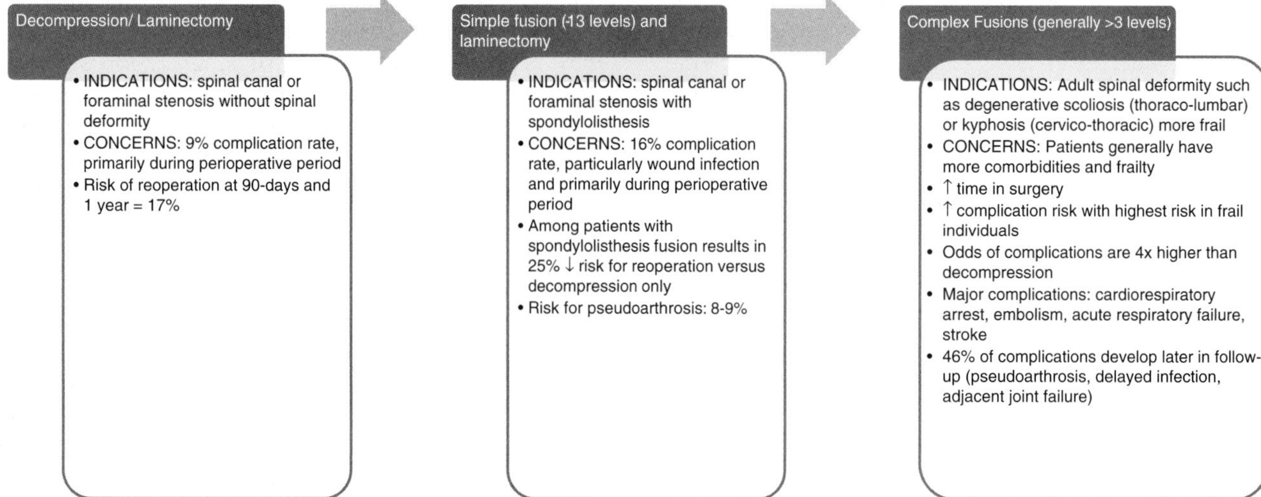

FIG. 20.15 Increasing complexity of spinal surgeries and associated concerns. *(From Yagi M, Fujita N, Okada E, et al. Impact of frailty and comorbidities on surgical outcomes and complications in adult spinal disorders. Spine 2018;43:1259-67. Yavin D, Casha S, Wiebe S, et al. Lumbar fusion for degenerative disease: a systematic review and meta-analysis. Neurosurgery 2017;80:701-15.)*

TABLE 20.9 Postoperative Problems and Related Actions following Spinal Surgeries

Patient Concern	Probable Causes	Recommended Action
Leg pain or arm pain	Neural sensitivity	Can take up to 4 weeks to decrease. Ensure adequate analgesia. Keep exercises pain-free. Decrease walking/exercise times slightly. Progressing activities too quickly or too slowly. Modify positions or pain provoking activities. If persists, refer back to surgical team.
Neurologic deterioration	Possible instability	Review comorbid conditions and preoperative neurologic status for potential alternate causes. Closely monitor and inform surgical team.
Inflamed or weeping wound	Possible infection	Refer to surgical team or primary care physician.
Exercises painful	Poor technique Exercise aggravates neck or back pain	Alter exercise interventions/correct technique, adjust position, load, and/or dose. Ensure exercises are focused and relate to function.
Patient not exercising regularly enough or not following restrictions	Poor patient compliance	Explain importance of good muscle function and posture to avoid flare-ups. Work with patient to identify motivation for improved function and match exercises with meaningful activity.
Persisting back or neck (axial) pain	Common source may be unknown or of mixed origin. Faulty exercise technique or ineffective activity intensity (too little or too much)	Ensure adequate analgesia. Ensure exercises are appropriate and not increasing too quickly or too slowly. Review and modify pain-provoking activities (e.g., reducing prolonged sitting or standing). Reassure it can be common, but also that conditioning postural muscles will help reduce pain.
Headaches	Dural tear (1st 4 weeks) Postural or altered neuropathodynamics Other pathology	If has dural tear during surgery, headaches may be present for up to 2 weeks postoperatively. If onset is after 4 weeks postoperative, assess and treat, if appropriate, otherwise refer.

Many experts debate the appropriateness of surgery for stenosis in the octogenarian population. The research is inconclusive likely owing to substantial selection bias. Opponents argue these individuals are at greater risk for complications, but this is likely confounded by other conditions, such as frailty. In general, rates of fusion are lower in patients over 80 years of age even when patients are diagnostically similar to their younger counterparts.[163] Most patients progressing to surgery have a higher prevalence of multilevel stenosis, severe stenosis, and asymmetric motor weakness. They also have higher rates of hypertension, heart disease, and osteoporosis, but are still likely to tolerate surgery. Between 3% and 5% can expect a major complication (e.g., sepsis, pulmonary embolism), whereas 15% will have a minor complication (e.g., urinary tract infection, deep venous thrombosis, blood transfusion). Factors increasing the odds of a postoperative complication include surgical time longer than 2 hours, instrumentation procedure, lower BMI, and dependent mobility prior to surgery.

Complications unique to cervical spine surgery include dysphagia (laryngeal nerve injury) and C5 palsy.[159] Dysphasia occurs in 1.4% to 4% of individuals having surgery for cervical myelopathy and is more common in anterior approaches. Symptoms may include hoarseness, breathy voice, a weak cough, difficulty swallowing, or the sensation of shortness of breath. Postoperative C5 palsy occurs in approximately 1.4% to 2.4% of patients. Clinical presentation includes motor paresis of the deltoid and/or biceps brachii muscles. Time to onset of the palsy is most commonly day 1, but may not be apparent for up to 2 weeks. Both dysphasia and C5 palsy will recover fully in the majority of patients. Steroid injections, speech therapy, and strengthening may support recovery in recalcitrant cases.[164,165]

Precautions

There are no uniform precautions following spinal surgery. A good relationship with the surgeon performing the surgery will help rehabilitation providers understand the reasoning behind tailored surgical precautions. It also benefits the patient to work on treatment planning in conjunction with the surgeon to assure postoperative advice is congruent across providers. In general, most precautions are founded on the principle of reducing mechanical stress on the surgical site, promoting healing of the bone and surrounding soft tissues, and limiting inflammation. Common restrictions include no lifting greater than 10 to 15 pounds (~5 to 7 kg) and no overhead lifting during the first 10 to 12 weeks following surgery. Surgeon recommendations for other activities, such as end-range motion, running, lifting, and driving a car, are highly variable. Given the paucity of evidence that can help direct these recommendations, physical therapists must be judicious in their recommendations about returning to activities placing high demands on the spine, especially considering the rate of deconditioning that can occur prior to surgery and during the postoperative period.

Mobilization. There is little research to guide clinicians in the use of manual therapy following spine surgery. In general, when selecting rehabilitation interventions following fusion surgery, mobilization at the site of the fusion is never recommended as this is contrary to the purpose of the fusion surgery. Mobilization of the hips or thoracic spine can be performed early in the rehabilitation process (~6-weeks) as patients can be positioned in a neutral lumbar spine to torsional or end-range joint motion placing stress on the fused segments. Following non-fusion procedures, mobilization of the spine can be approached as tolerated by the patient. Pain and/or segmental hypomobility are still the primary indicators mobilization may be appropriate. Dosing of mobilization should be determined by individual patient response and assessed pre- and post-mobilization using pain and movement assessments. High velocity, low amplitude manual therapy techniques (thrust manipulation) may be appropriate in select cases. Clinicians must consider the bone health of the patient and the purpose for selecting this technique. Thrust manipulation specific to the lumbar spine or cervical spine has primarily demonstrated effectiveness in acute conditions. In the majority of older adults, these spine conditions will be chronic and the value of a thrust manipulation is questionable. Thrust manipulation in the thoracic spine for chronic neck pain/conditions or distraction manipulation for hip mobility limitations are effective and safe when indicated. Judicious clinical exam, testing a patient's tolerance through pre-positioning the joint, examining patient preference, and having a clear logic model for the purpose of a thrust manipulation in this population will help clinicians determine if this intervention is appropriate. In the vast majority of cases, mobilization is equally as effective as thrust manipulation and is perceived as safer.[130a]

Treatment Progression

Rehabilitation that enables patients to take charge of their own recovery has been shown to improve medium and long-term outcomes. Important topics of discussion with patients include methods for relaxing and reducing stress, balancing rest and activity, setting activity and walking goals, and creating a personal recovery plan. In addition to addressing the physical impairments present after surgery, the physical therapist becomes a coach.[166] Although this has primarily been studied in the postoperative phase of treatment, emerging evidence indicates that delivering components of these interventions preoperatively may improve early mobility and reduce the need for pain medications.[166a]

Early Postoperative Considerations

Lumbar Spine. During the first week the focus of rehabilitation is on getting in/out of bed, standing, walking, and climbing stairs. No definitive guidelines exist for when these activities should occur. In a survey of orthopedic and neurosurgeons, most agreed sitting, standing, and walking should all be encouraged by postoperative day 1.[167] Active rehabilitation after lumbar spine surgery has a beneficial impact on both pain and function. Planning for physical activity can begin in the hospital and is a key component of postoperative treatment, particularly because many patients do not receive physical therapy for the first 2 to 3 months after hospital discharge. By discharge the patient should:

- Mobilize independently and safely.
- Have a plan for gradually increasing cardiovascular exercise.

- Demonstrate an understanding of neutral spine and how to maintain it during transitions.
- Demonstrate an ability to manage pain using diaphragmatic breathing and relaxation exercises.
- Understand self-management and pacing, particularly with ADLs.

Cervical Spine Surgery. As with lumbar surgery, early postoperative rehabilitation focuses on pain management and the general mobility needed to return home safely. This often includes strategies for and practice of transfers, bed mobility, and negotiating stairs. Pain management strategies can also be encouraged, including the promotion of relaxation, diaphragmatic breathing, and working to keep the shoulders back and relaxed. The majority of patients following cervical surgery will be required to wear a cervical collar. Treatment may include discussions with patients on how to correctly don and doff these collars and adjust for comfort. Additionally, because these collars limit mobility of the cervical spine and alter the center of gravity, physical therapists must work to help patients adapt to changes in the visual field forced by the limited spine motion and to adapt balance strategies. Often this can be simply learning to take more caution with activities, such as stair-climbing using tactile feedback, but sometime may require teaching the family to provide contact-guard assist and verbal cuing. For more frail patients, postoperative physical therapy will continue either at home or in a postacute setting. The focus is still on strengthening and balance training to improve participation in ADLs. This includes extremity strengthening and specific tasks, such as gait and overhead reach.

Postoperative Treatment. Variations in surgical outcomes following spine surgery are caused, in part, by variation in postoperative rehabilitation or the lack thereof. There is wide disparity in recommendations by surgeons with respect to activity levels, return to work, and referrals to physical therapy. Yet, active rehabilitation initiated 4 to 6 weeks postoperatively is more effective at improving function and reducing pain than recommending patients return to normal activity on their own or advised to stay active.[168] Additionally, many patients with spine conditions have experienced long-standing chronic pain and have multiple comorbid conditions that can contribute to functional compromise. Patients express concerns and find it challenging to progress activity while managing multiple comorbid conditions. There is value in supervised active rehabilitation that can identify how to adapt exercises to address adjacent joint impairments, cardiovascular or respiratory limitations, and sensory changes. An effective practitioner will provide the patient with the knowledge and self-efficacy needed to continue active rehabilitation independently over time.

Moderate quality evidence suggests multidisciplinary rehabilitation reduces pain and disability.[169] However, having multiple providers involved in rehabilitation can be costly and difficult for the patient to comply with (e.g., scheduling appointments with multiple providers), thus making it imperative to tailor referrals based on individual needs. The majority of patients can optimize recovery through quality physical therapy with psychologically informed interventions. Key to this is opening the discussion for behavior change. Critical communication skills include active listening, guided questioning, and goal setting. Listening, expressing appreciation for the patient's story and challenges, and presenting optimism toward change create an atmosphere for collaboration with a patient. Examples of ways to open this discussion are included in Box. 20.1. For patients with significant depression, anxiety, or challenges coping, it may be necessary to refer to a rehabilitation psychologist or social worker to complement physical therapy.

BOX 20.1 Building Therapeutic Alliance Around Behavior Change

At first visit, introduce yourself, acknowledge with affirmation, define visit duration, explain expectations and visit flow.

Ask open-ended questions such as:

- *What do you think it would take for you to get better?*
- *Tell me how you feel about exercising right now?*
- *How confident are you that you will be able to consistently do these exercises if you decided to do so?*
- *Where do you see yourself in 3 years in regard to [fill in area they are seeking help for]?*
- *What is your expectation of physical therapy?*
- *If I could flip a switch and remove all your pain, what things that you have given up on would you do again?*
- *If your pain increases, tell me what you plan to do.*

Spinal pain is rarely completely resolved with surgery and a patient's understanding of pain can have an impact on their outcomes. Pain Neuroscience Education (PNE) is one approach that can help improve coping and manage expectations following surgery.[170] PNE aims to help patients understand the biology and psychology of their pain experience from a biopsychosocial perspective.[171] This includes helping patients understand that pain is multifactorial. An example of this explanation might be:

> *"The nervous system is extremely complex. The pathways or nerves carry many different signals to a processing center, primarily the brain. It is much like your computer. Many programs can be running at one time and fairly efficiently. However, if a faulty program triggers an abnormal response in one program, many functions can be affected. Similarly, pain is a normal response in the nervous system. But if it is not addressed, many other systems in your body can have difficulty regulating. Surgery may address some sources of pain but other areas of the nervous system have not yet calmed down. Learning how to switch off or tone down pathways that contribute to a pain experience will be important in recovery. This sensitivity can be reduced with exercise, relaxation techniques, breathing, and mindfulness."*

Cardiovascular exercise, strengthening, and flexibility are critical components of helping patients with chronic spine conditions recover.[172] Exercise has a positive impact on both mental and physical well-being and should be included in every physical therapy session. Addressing trunk muscle dysfunction plays a key role in improving postoperative outcomes. Chronic pain has often contributed to inhibition of spinal stabilizing muscles (multifidi, transversus abdominus, deep neck flexors, spinalis). Compounding the impact on the spine, compression and irritation of the nerve roots often results in weakness of postural support muscles that are designed to help offload spinal forces.

Lumbar Spine. Common impairments following lumbar surgery include weakness in the gluteal muscles limiting pelvic support in weight-bearing and weakness in the hamstrings and plantar flexors limiting propulsion and making stair-climbing difficult. Progressive strengthening of these muscles should include functional strengthening, varying load and velocity demands.[173] Except in cases with extensive fusion (> 5 levels), few patients will note functional loss of mobility in the spine. Resuming functional activity will also depend on regaining mobility throughout the entire spine and hips. Manual therapy of the hip joint and thoracic spine may facilitate this mobility with long-term results dependent on patients using the full range of motion routinely.[174] Nonthrust mobilizations may be safely initiated after 6 weeks. Manual therapy techniques following lumbar surgery generally include nonthrust mobilizations to the hip emphasizing rotation, flexion/extension, and distraction (Fig. 20.16). This can be followed-up with home exercises focused on self-mobilization and stretching (Fig. 20.17). Improving thoracic extension may also improve upright tolerance with walking and overhead reach (Fig. 20.18).

Cervical Spine. By 3-months most patients having cervical spine surgery are cleared for spine mobility and strengthening. Directed active ROM exercise aimed at improving end-range motion of the cervical spine is often sufficient for returning to preoperative mobility levels. One should also assure that a patient has regained full mobility of the temporomandibular joint because jaw opening may be stiff following cervical spine immobilization. Manual therapy interventions may be used for recalcitrant stiffness in regions of the spine distal to the fusion site, such as the thoracic spine (see Fig. 20.18). The majority of rehabilitation will focus on strengthening. This should include exercises for the stabilizers (deep cervical extensors and flexors, Fig. 20.19) and postural stability with upper quadrant strengthening.[175,176] Regaining this strength is an important component of recovery because reduced muscle strength of the posterior cervical muscles is associated with persistent central neck pain following cervical fusion.[177] These exercises often need to be tailored to the individual both for tolerance and positioning because significant thoracic kyphosis can make extension in the lower cervical spine difficult.

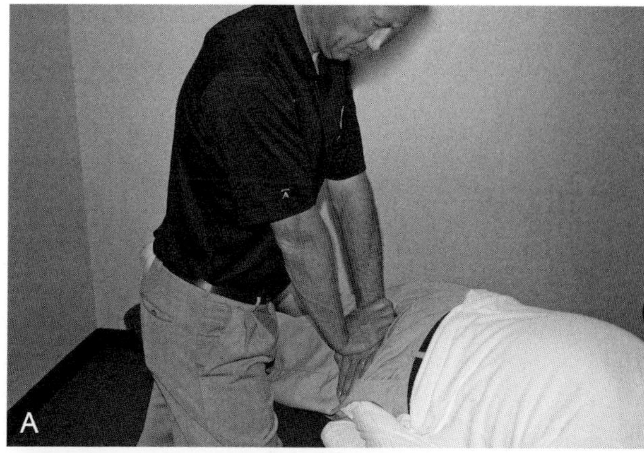

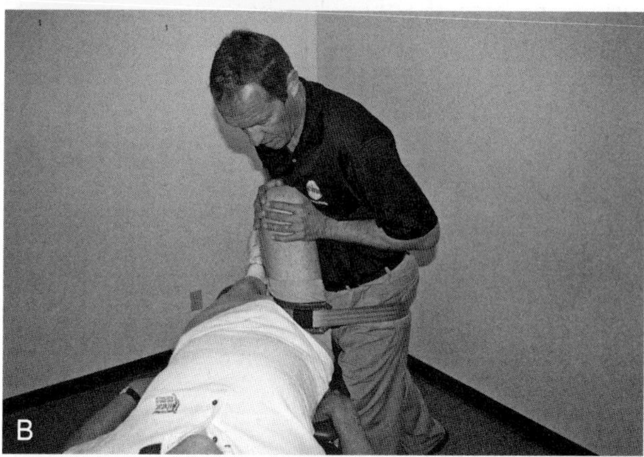

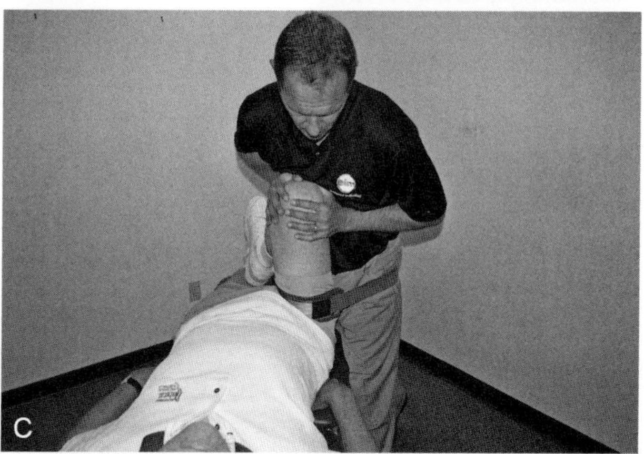

FIG. 20.16 Manual therapy to improve hip mobility (femur on acetabulum). **A**. Prone hip posterior-anterior mobilization. **B**. Supine hip lateral glide. **C**. Supine hip inferior glide. *(From Backstrom KM, Whiman JM, Flynn TW. Lumbar spinal stenosis-diagnosis and management of the aging spine. Man Ther. 2011;Aug 15 (4):308–17.)*

Prognosis. Patients can expect good relief of leg or arm pain and a significant decrease in neck and back pain following spinal surgery. Although axial pain often persists to some degree, most individuals report a significant overall improvement in function. Improvements can continue for up to 18 months postoperatively, particularly for more complex procedures. Milestones and appropriate activities following surgery are presented in Table 20.10.[159,160]

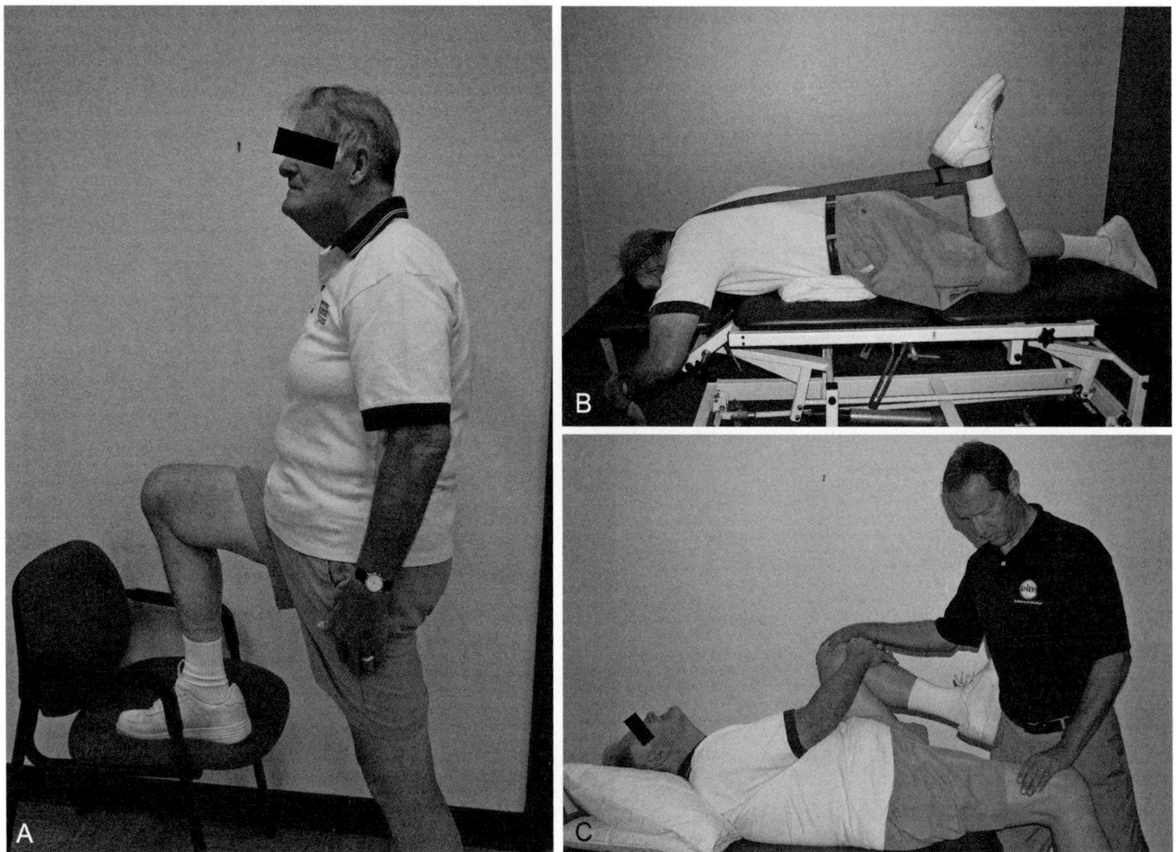

FIG. 20.17 Hip flexibility exercises. A. Iliopsoas self-stretch (left side). **B**. Rectus femoris self-stretch. **C**. Supine manual hip flexor stretch (right side). *(From Backstrom KM, Whiman JM, Flynn TW. Lumbar spinal stenosis-diagnosis and management of the aging spine. Man Ther. 2011;Aug 15 (4):308–17.)*

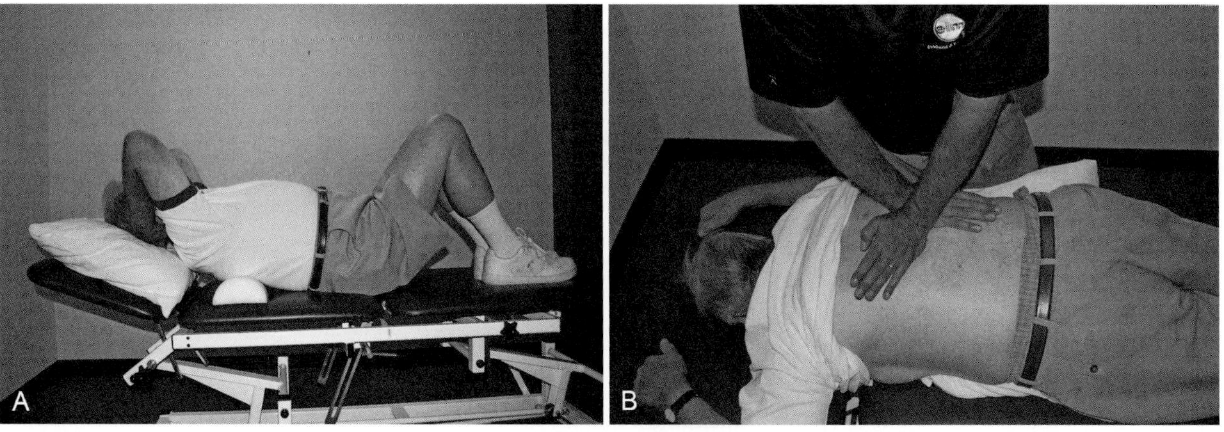

FIG. 20.18 Thoracic mobilizations. A. Thoracic extension self-mobilization. **B**. Prone thoracic mobilization. *(From Backstrom KM, Whiman JM, Flynn TW. Lumbar spinal stenosis-diagnosis and management of the aging spine. Man Ther. 2011; Aug 15 (4):308–17.)*

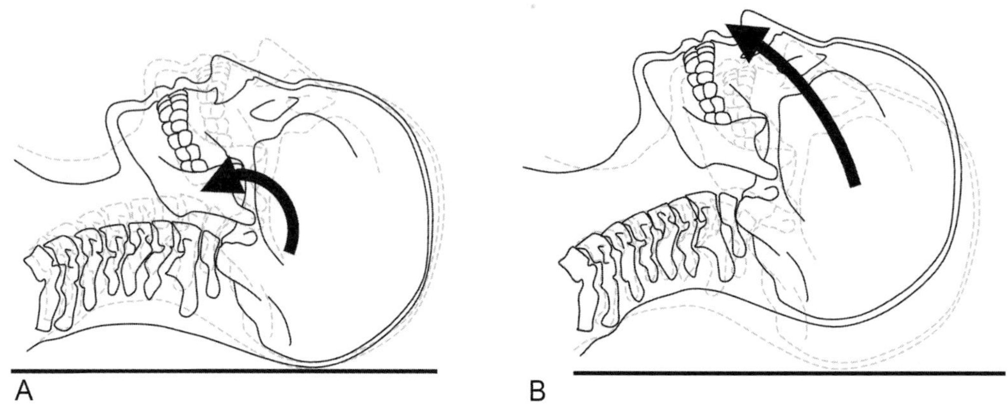

FIG. 20.19 Cervical strengthening exercises. A. Craniocervical-flexion. **B**. Cervical flexion endurance.

Continued

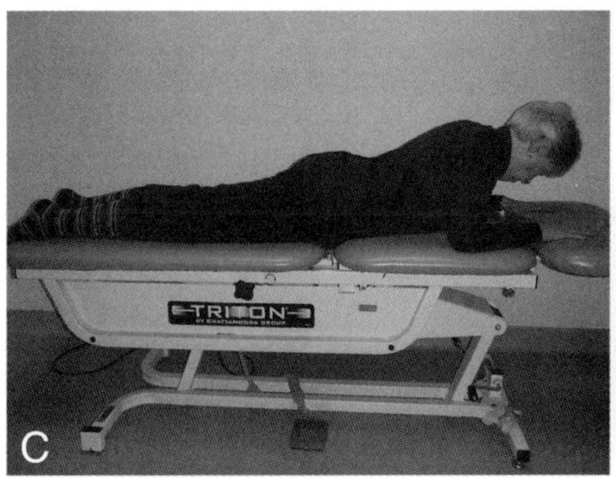

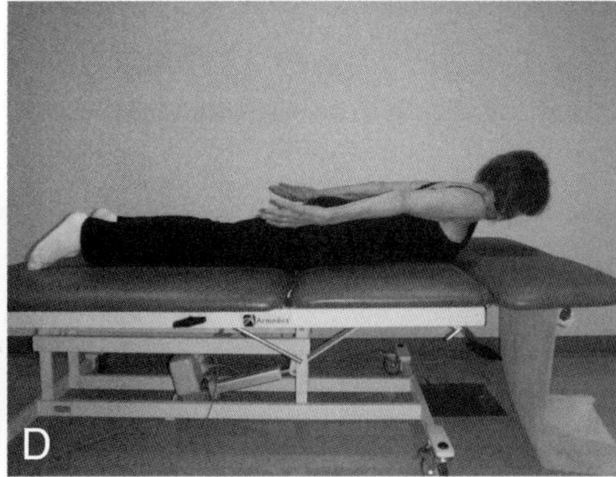

FIG. 20.19, cont'd **C**. Cervical retraction against gravity. **D**. cervical retraction with thoracic extension. *(A and B from O'Leary S, et al. Journal of Pain. 2007;8(11): 832–39, Copyright © 2007 American Pain Society. C and D from Marcus R. Osteoporosis, ed 4. Oxford: Academic Press–Elsevier, 2013.)*

TABLE 20.10 Recommendations for Progression of Activity following Spinal Surgery

	0 to 6 Weeks	6 to 12 Weeks	3 to 6 Months	6 to 12 Months
Expectations	Greatest change in pain/disability. Patient can expect ~50% reduction in both pain and disability by 3 months. Independent with ADLs. Adherent to a routine physical activity program.	Improvements in tasks with higher cardiovascular and mobility demands. Majority of individuals will return to work with modifications. Minimal arm or leg pain.	Improvements in activities with greater spinal loads. Patient is independent in progressive strengthening program.	68% to 70% reduction of pain and disability (from preoperative levels).
Interventions	Gradual pacing of activity. Avoid sustaining activities that increase neural sensitivity > 15–20 min at 4–6 weeks. Log-roll at 4–6 weeks. Pain relief: analgesia, positioning, relaxation and breathing exercises. Education: spine mechanics. Exercises: core stability with a neutral spine, active hip/UE exercises, isometrics. Mobility: transfers, stair safety, walking.	Avoid heavy lifting until 12 weeks or surgeon approval. Progress core and postural stability. Balance and proprioceptive training. Progress functional range of movement. Progress cardiovascular activity (duration or intensity). Walking: increase pace. Stretching/flexibility of adjacent joints. Advice on healing times, smoking, weight, and stress.	Begin progressive spinal loading to increase lifting tolerance. Increase complexity of trunk stabilization (unsteady surfaces, co-contractions). Begin conditioning for sport. Trunk, upper and lower limb conditioning as relevant to patient's goals.	Sport- or task-specific training, as needed.
Milestones	Adequate pain relief. Basic core stability. Building up normal activities. Normal gait. Walk tolerance of 20 min.	Self-managing pain. Good spinal position with transitions, lifting. Cardiovascular tolerance of 30 minutes. Sitting/standing tolerance 15–60 minutes.	Full functional range of motion and strength. Self-management plan for pain and physical activity.	Full return to athletic and work activities.
Failure to meet milestones	Discuss with surgical team Assess and address source of limitation: medical, psychosocial.			

Spinal Surgeries: Summary

Many older adults undergoing surgery for degenerative spinal conditions pursue that option with hope of improving mobility and function. Outcomes are generally favorable, but recovery is enhanced by directed rehabilitation. Limited research supports the optimal rehabilitation program following surgery for degenerative spinal conditions in older adults. Effective rehabilitation interventions include cardiovascular exercise, motor control and strengthening, joint mobilization, flexibility, and patient education. Treatment planning and intervention selection should be individually tailored based on the complexity of impairments and psychosocial contributors to recovery, such as self-efficacy, coping, and social support.

SUMMARY

This chapter has described the indications, surgical procedures, complications, prognosis, and rehabilitation considerations for the regions of the hip, knee, shoulder, and spine. Common themes that apply to all regions is the symbiosis of behavioral and physical interventions to maximize the patient's physical activity and functional outcomes. Consideration of graded and progressive resistive exercise, with consideration of MVIC, is important for optimal outcomes. Generally, surgery should not be denied an older adult on the basis of age. Rather, coexisting conditions have a greater impact on prognosis. Finally, excellent communication with the surgeon and medical team will optimize outcomes and reduce complications.

REFERENCES

1. Murray CJ, Barber RM, Foreman KJ, et al. Global, regional, and national disability-adjusted life years (DALYs) for 306 diseases and injuries and healthy life expectancy (HALE) for 188 countries, 1990–2013: quantifying the epidemiological transition. *Lancet*. 2015;386:2145–2191.
2. Murray CJL, Vos T, Lozano R, et al. Disability-adjusted life years (DALYs) for 291 diseases and injuries in 21 regions, 1990–2010: a systematic analysis for the Global Burden of Disease Study 2010. *Lancet*. 2013;380:2197–2223.
3. Wang MC, Kreuter W, Wolfla CE, Maiman DJ, Deyo RA. Trends and variations in cervical spine surgery in the United States: Medicare beneficiaries, 1992 to 2005. *Spine*. 2009;34:955–961 discussion 62–63.
4. Deyo RA, Mirza SK, Martin BI, Kreuter W, Goodman DC, Jarvik JG. Trends, major medical complications, and charges associated with surgery for lumbar spinal stenosis in older adults. *JAMA*. 2010;303:1259–1265.
5. Yoshihara H, Yoneoka D. Trends in the incidence and in-hospital outcomes of elective major orthopaedic surgery in patients eighty years of age and older in the United States from 2000 to 2009. *J Bone Joint Sur Am*. 2014;96: 1185–1191.
6. Zmistowski B, Padegimas EM, Howley M, Abboud J, Williams Jr. G, Namdari S. Trends and variability in the use of total shoulder arthroplasty for Medicare patients. *J Am Acad Orthop Surg*. 2018;26:133–141.
7. Sloan M, Premkumar A, Sheth NP. Projected volume of primary total joint arthroplasty in the U.S., 2014 to 2030. *J Bone Joint Surg Am*. 2018;100:1455–1460.
8. Dieleman JL, Baral R, Birger M, et al. US spending on personal health care and public health, 1996–2013. *JAMA*. 2016;316: 2627–2646.
9. Martin BI, Turner JA, Mirza SK, Lee MJ, Comstock BA, Deyo RA. Trends in health care expenditures, utilization, and health status among US adults with spine problems, 1997–2006. *Spine*. 2009;34:2077–2084.
10. Theis KA, Murphy L, Hootman JM, Wilkie R. Social participation restriction among US adults with arthritis: a population-based study using the International Classification of Functioning, Disability and Health. *Arthritis Care Res* (Hoboken). 2013;65:1059–1069.
11. Hootman JM, Cheng WY. Psychological distress and fair/poor health among adults with arthritis: state-specific prevalence and correlates of general health status, United States, 2007. *International Journal of Public Health*. 2009;54(Suppl 1):75–83.
12. McPhail SM, Schippers M, Marshall AL. Age, physical inactivity, obesity, health conditions, and health-related quality of life among patients receiving conservative management for musculoskeletal disorders. *Clinical Interventions in Aging*. 2014;9:1069–1080.
13. Ravi B, Croxford R, Austin PC, et al. The relation between total joint arthroplasty and risk for serious cardiovascular events in patients with moderate-severe osteoarthritis: propensity score matched landmark analysis. *BMJ*. 2013;347:f6187.
14. Hassett AL, Marshall E, Bailey AM, et al. Changes in anxiety and depression are mediated by changes in pain severity in patients undergoing lower-extremity total joint arthroplasty. *Reg Anesth Pain Med*. 2018;43:14–18.
15. Arnold JB, Walters JL, Ferrar KE. Does physical activity increase after total hip or knee arthroplasty for osteoarthritis? A systematic review. *J Orthop Sports Phys Ther*. 2016;46:431–442.
16. Tak E, Kuiper R, Chorus A, Hopman-Rock M. Prevention of onset and progression of basic ADL disability by physical activity in community dwelling older adults: a meta-analysis. *Ageing Research Reviews*. 2013;12:329–338.
17. Skolasky RL, Maggard AM, Li D, Riley 3rd LH, Wegener ST. Health behavior change counseling in surgery for degenerative lumbar spinal stenosis. Part I: improvement in rehabilitation engagement and functional outcomes. *Arch Phys Med Rehabil*. 2015;96:1200–1207.
18. de Vries NM, Staal JB, van der Wees PJ, et al. Patient-centred physical therapy is (cost-) effective in increasing physical activity and reducing frailty in older adults with mobility problems: a randomized controlled trial with 6 months follow-up. *Journal of Cachexia Sarcopenia Muscle*. 2016;7: 422–435.
19. Dreinhofer KE, Mitchell PJ, Begue T, et al. A global call to action to improve the care of people with fragility fractures. *Injury*. 2018;49:1393–1397.
20. Pasco JA, Sanders KM, Hoekstra FM, Henry MJ, Nicholson GC, Kotowicz MA. The human cost of fracture. *Osteoporos Int*. 2005;16:2046–2052.
21. Nevitt MC, Ettinger B, Black DM, et al. The association of radiographically detected vertebral fractures with back pain and function: a prospective study. *AnnIntern Med*. 1998;128:793–800.
22. Herrick C, Steger-May K, Sinacore DR, Brown M, Schechtman KB, Binder EF. Persistent pain in frail older adults after hip fracture repair. *J Am Geriatr Soc*. 2004;52: 2062–2068.
23. Brauer CA, Coca-Perraillon M, Cutler DM, Rosen AB. Incidence and mortality of hip fractures in the United States. *JAMA*. 2009;302:1573–1579.

24. Sullivan KJ, Husak LE, Altebarmakian M, Brox WT. Demographic factors in hip fracture incidence and mortality rates in California, 2000–2011. *J Orthop Surg Res*. 2016;11:4.
25. Parker M, Johansen A. Hip fracture. *BMJ*. 2006;333:27–30.
26. Colón-Emeric C, Kuchibhatla M, Pieper C, et al. The contribution of hip fracture to risk of subsequent fractures: data from two longitudinal studies. *Osteoporos Int*. 2003;14:879–883.
27. Stolee P, Poss J, Cook RJ, Byrne K, Hirdes JP. Risk factors for hip fracture in older home care clients. *Journals of Gerontology Series A: Biomedical Sciences and Medical Sciences*. 2009;64:403–410.
28. Wolinsky FD, Bentler SE, Liu L, et al. Recent hospitalization and the risk of hip fracture among older Americans. *Journals of Gerontology Series A: Biological Sciences and Mmedical Sciences*. 2009;64:249–255.
29. van de Ree CLP, De Jongh MAC, Peeters CMM, de Munter L, Roukema JA, Gosens T. Hip fractures in elderly people: surgery or no surgery? A systematic review and meta-analysis. *Geriatric Orthopaedic Surgery & Rehabilitation*. 2017;8:173–180.
30. Parker MJ, Gurusamy K. Internal fixation versus arthroplasty for intracapsular proximal femoral fractures in adults. *Cochrane Database Syst Rev*. 2006; CD001708.
31. Kristensen MT, Bandholm T, Bencke J, Ekdahl C, Kehlet H. Knee-extension strength, postural control and function are related to fracture type and thigh edema in patients with hip fracture. *Clin Biomech*. 2009;24:218–224.
32. Colon-Emeric CS. Postoperative management of hip fractures: interventions associated with improved outcomes. *BoneKEy Reports*. 2012;1:241.
33. Friedman SM, Mendelson DA, Bingham KW, Kates SL. Impact of a comanaged geriatric fracture center on short-term hip fracture outcomes. *Arch Intern Med*. 2009;169:1712–1717.
34. Hung WW, Egol KA, Zuckerman JD, Siu AL. Hip fracture management: tailoring care for the older patient. *JAMA*. 2012;307:2185–2194.
35. Vochteloo AJ, Borger van der Burg BL, Mertens B, et al. Outcome in hip fracture patients related to anemia at admission and allogeneic blood transfusion: an analysis of 1262 surgically treated patients. *BMC Musculoskeletal Disorders*. 2011;12:262.
36. Girelli D, Marchi G, Camaschella C. Anemia in the elderly. *HemaSphere*. 2018;2:e40.
37. Sim YE, Sim SD, Seng C, Howe TS, Koh SB, Abdullah HR. Preoperative anemia, functional outcomes, and quality of life after hip fracture surgery. *J Am Geriatr Soc*. 2018;66:1524–1531.
38. Wyers CE, Reijven PL, Evers SM, et al. Cost-effectiveness of nutritional intervention in elderly subjects after hip fracture. A randomized controlled trial. *Osteoporos Int*. 2013;24:151–162.
39. Munter KH, Clemmesen CG, Foss NB, Palm H, Kristensen MT. Fatigue and pain limit independent mobility and physiotherapy after hip fracture surgery. *Disabil Rehabil*. 2018;40:1808–1816.
40. Goodnough LT, Schrier SL. Evaluation and management of anemia in the elderly. *Am J Hematol*. 2014;89:88–96.
41. Yang Y, Zhao X, Dong T, Yang Z, Zhang Q, Zhang Y. Risk factors for postoperative delirium following hip fracture repair in elderly patients: a systematic review and meta-analysis. *Aging: Clinical and Experimental Research*. 2017;29:115–126.
42. Lee HB, Mears SC, Rosenberg PB, Leoutsakos JM, Gottschalk A, Sieber FE. Predisposing factors for postoperative delirium after hip fracture repair in individuals with and without dementia. *J Am Geriatr Soc*. 2011;59: 2306–2313.
43. Marcantonio ER. Delirium in hospitalized older adults. *N Engl J Med*. 2017;377:1456–1466.
44. Martinez F, Tobar C, Hill N. Preventing delirium: should non-pharmacological, multicomponent interventions be used? A systematic review and meta-analysis of the literature. *Age Ageing*. 2015;44:196–204.
45. Hshieh TT, Yue J, Oh E, et al. Effectiveness of multicomponent nonpharmacological delirium interventions: a meta-analysis. *JAMA*. 2015;175:512–520.
46. Oberai T, Laver K, Crotty M, Killington M, Jaarsma R. Effectiveness of multicomponent interventions on incidence of delirium in hospitalized older patients with hip fracture: a systematic review. *Int Psychogeriatr*. 2018;30: 481–492.
47. Martinez FT, Tobar C, Beddings CI, Vallejo G, Fuentes P. Preventing delirium in an acute hospital using a non-pharmacological intervention. *Age Ageing*. 2012;41:629–634.
48. Martinez F, Donoso AM, Marquez C, Labarca E. Implementing a multicomponent intervention to prevent delirium among critically ill patients. *Critical Care Nurse*. 2017;37:36–46.
49. Baumgarten M, Margolis DJ, Orwig DL, et al. Pressure ulcers in elderly patients with hip fracture across the continuum of care. *J Am Geriatr Soc*. 2009;57:863–870.
50. Hommel A, Bjorkelund KB, Thorngren KG, Ulander K. Nutritional status among patients with hip fracture in relation to pressure ulcers. *Clin Nutr*. 2007;26:589–596.
51. Pedersen SJ, Borgbjerg FM, Schousboe B, et al. A comprehensive hip fracture program reduces complication rates and mortality. *J Am Geriatr Soc*. 2008;56:1831–1838.
52. Liu VX, Rosas E, Hwang J, et al. Enhanced recovery after surgery program implementation in 2 surgical populations in an integrated health care delivery system. *JAMA*. 2017;152: e171032.
53. Panula J, Pihlajamaki H, Mattila VM, et al. Mortality and cause of death in hip fracture patients aged 65 or older: a population-based study. *BMC Musculoskeletal Disorders*. 2011;12:105.
54. LeBlanc ES, Hillier TA, Pedula KL, et al. Hip fracture and increased short-term but not long-term mortality in healthy older women. *Arch Intern Med*. 2011;171:1831–1837.
55. Hu F, Jiang C, Shen J, Tang P, Wang Y. Preoperative predictors for mortality following hip fracture surgery: a systematic review and meta-analysis. *Injury*. 2012;43:676–685.
56. Nijmeijer WS, Folbert EC, Vermeer M, Slaets JP, Hegeman JH. Prediction of early mortality following hip fracture surgery in frail elderly: The Almelo Hip Fracture Score (AHFS). *Injury*. 2016;47:2138–2143.
57. Vochteloo AJ, Moerman S, Tuinebreijer WE, et al. More than half of hip fracture patients do not regain mobility in the first postoperative year. *Geriatrics & Gerontology International*. 2013;13:334–341.
58. Magaziner J, Hawkes W, Hebel JR, et al. Recovery from hip fracture in eight areas of function. *The Journals of Gerontology: Series A*. 2000;55:M498–M507.
59. Beaupre LA, Binder EF, Cameron ID, et al. Maximising functional recovery following hip fracture in frail seniors. *Best Pract Res Clin Rheumatol*. 2013;27:771–788.
60. Cristancho P, Lenze EJ, Avidan MS, Rawson KS. Trajectories of depressive symptoms after hip fracture. *Psychol Med*. 2016;46:1413–1425.
61. Duke RG, Keating JL. An investigation of factors predictive of independence in transfers and ambulation after hip fracture. *Arch Phys Med Rehabil*. 2002;83:158–164.
62. Kristensen MT, Kehlet H. The basic mobility status upon acute hospital discharge is an independent risk factor for mortality up to 5 years after hip fracture surgery. *Acta Orthop*. 2018;89:47–52.

63. Kimmel LA, Liew SM, Sayer JM, Holland AE. HIP4Hips (High Intensity Physiotherapy for Hip fractures in the acute hospital setting): a randomised controlled trial. *Med J Aust.* 2016;205:73–78.
64. Kronborg L, Bandholm T, Palm H, Kehlet H, Kristensen MT. Effectiveness of acute in-hospital physiotherapy with knee-extension strength training in reducing strength deficits in patients with a hip fracture: a randomised controlled trial. *PLOS One.* 2017;12 e0179867.
65. Binder EF, Brown M, Sinacore DR, Steger-May K, Yarasheski KE, Schechtman KB. Effects of extended outpatient rehabilitation after hip fracture: a randomized controlled trial. *JAMA.* 2004;292:837–846.
66. Sherrington C, Lord SR, Herbert RD. A randomized controlled trial of weight-bearing versus non-weight-bearing exercise for improving physical ability after usual care for hip fracture. *Arch Phys Med Rehabil.* 2004;85:710–716.
67. Mangione KK, Craik RL, Palombaro KM, Tomlinson SS, Hofmann MT. Home-based leg-strengthening exercise improves function 1 year after hip fracture: a randomized controlled study. *J Am Geriatr Soc.* 2010;58:1911–1917.
68. Diong J, Allen N, Sherrington C. Structured exercise improves mobility after hip fracture: a meta-analysis with meta-regression. *Br J Sports Med.* 2016;50:346–355.
69. Auais MA, Eilayyan O, Mayo NE. Extended exercise rehabilitation after hip fracture improves patients' physical function: a systematic review and meta-analysis. *Phys Ther.* 2012;92:1437–1451.
70. Sherrington C, Lord SR. Home exercise to improve strength and walking velocity after hip fracture: a randomized controlled trial. *Arch Phys Med Rehabil.* 1997;78:208–212.
71. Latham NK, Harris BA, Bean JF, et al. Effect of a home-based exercise program on functional recovery following rehabilitation after hip fracture: a randomized clinical trial. *JAMA.* 2014;311:700–708.
72. Perracini MR, Kristensen MT, Cunningham C, Sherrington C. Physiotherapy following fragility fractures. *Injury.* 2018;49:1413–1417.
73. Calvo E, Morcillo D, Foruria AM, et al. Nondisplaced proximal humeral fractures: high incidence among outpatient-treated osteoporotic fractures and severe impact on upper extremity function and patient subjective health perception. *J Shoulder Elbow Surg.* 2011;20:795–801.
74. Launonen AP, Lepola V, Flinkkila T, Laitinen M, Paavola M, Malmivaara A. Treatment of proximal humerus fractures in the elderly: a systemic review of 409 patients. *Acta Orthop.* 2015;86:280–285.
75. Handoll HH, Brorson S. Interventions for treating proximal humeral fractures in adults. *Cochrane Database Syst Rev.* 2015; CD000434.
76. Cameron ID, Gillespie LD, Robertson MC, et al. Interventions for preventing falls in older people in care facilities and hospitals. *Cochrane Database of Syst Eev.* 2012;12: CD005465.
77. Room J, Hannink E, Dawes H, Barker K. What interventions are used to improve exercise adherence in older people and what behavioural techniques are they based on? A systematic review. *BMJ Open.* 2017;7: e019221.
78. Handoll HH, Elliott J. Rehabilitation for distal radial fractures in adults. *Cochrane Database Syst Rev.* 2015; CD003324.
79. Mattila VM, Huttunen TT, Sillanpaa P, Niemi S, Pihlajamaki H, Kannus P. Significant change in the surgical treatment of distal radius fractures: a nationwide study between 1998 and 2008 in Finland. *J Trauma.* 2011;71:939–942. discussion 42–3.
80. MacIntyre NJ, Dewan N. Epidemiology of distal radius fractures and factors predicting risk and prognosis. *J Hand Ther.* 2016;29:136–145.
81. Walenkamp MM, Aydin S, Mulders MA, Goslings JC, Schep NW. Predictors of unstable distal radius fractures: a systematic review and meta-analysis. *J Hand Surg [Br].* 2016;41:501–515.
82. Bentohami A, de Burlet K, de Korte N, van den Bekerom MP, Goslings JC, Schep NW. Complications following volar locking plate fixation for distal radial fractures: a systematic review. *J Hand Surg [Br].* 2014;39:745–754.
83. Krischak GD, Krasteva A, Schneider F, Gulkin D, Gebhard F, Kramer M. Physiotherapy after volar plating of wrist fractures is effective using a home exercise program. *Arch Phys Med Rehabil.* 2009;90:537–544.
84. Souer JS, Buijze G, Ring D. A prospective randomized controlled trial comparing occupational therapy with independent exercises after volar plate fixation of a fracture of the distal part of the radius. *J Bone Joint Surg Am.* 2011;93:1761–1766.
85. Edwards BJ, Song J, Dunlop DD, Fink HA, Cauley JA. Functional decline after incident wrist fractures–Study of Osteoporotic Fractures: prospective cohort study. *BMJ.* 2010;341:c3324.
86. Weycker D, Li X, Barron R, Bornheimer R, Chandler D. Hospitalizations for osteoporosis-related fractures: Economic costs and clinical outcomes. *Bone Reports.* 2016;5:186–191.
87. Wijendra A, Alwe R, Lamyman M, Grammatopoulos GA, Kambouroglou G. Low energy open ankle fractures in the elderly: outcome and treatment algorithm. *Injury.* 2017;48:763–769.
88. Schray D, Ehrnthaller C, Pfeufer D, et al. Outcome after surgical treatment of fragility ankle fractures in a certified orthogeriatric trauma center. *Injury.* 2018;49:1451–1457.
89. Della Rocca GJ, Uppal HS, Copeland ME, Crist BD, Volgas DA. Geriatric patients with fractures below the hip are medically similar to geriatric patients with hip fracture. *Geriatric Orthopaedic Surgery & Rehabilitation.* 2015;6:28–32.
90. Gauthe R, Desseaux A, Rony L, Tarissi N, Dujardin F. Ankle fractures in the elderly: Treatment and results in 477 patients. *Orthopaedics & Traumatology: Surgery & Research.* 2016;102:S241–S244.
91. Zeytinoglu M, Jain RK, Vokes TJ. Vertebral fracture assessment: enhancing the diagnosis, prevention, and treatment of osteoporosis. *Bone.* 2017;104:54–65.
92. Cummings SR, Melton LJ. Epidemiology and outcomes of osteoporotic fractures. *Lancet.* 2002;359:1761–1767.
93. Lorbergs AL, O'Connor GT, Zhou Y, et al. Severity of Kyphosis and Decline in Lung Function: The Framingham Study. *The Journals of Gerontology Series A.* 2017;72: 689–694.
94. Giangregorio LM, Papaioannou A, Macintyre NJ, et al. Too Fit To Fracture: exercise recommendations for individuals with osteoporosis or osteoporotic vertebral fracture. *Osteoporos Int.* 2014;25:821–835.
95. Nelson ME, Fiatarone MA, Morganti CM, Trice I, Greenberg RA, Evans WJ. Effects of high-intensity strength training on multiple risk factors for osteoporotic fractures. A randomized controlled trial. *JAMA.* 1994;272:1909–1914.
96. Heinonen A, Kannus P, Sievanen H, et al. Randomised controlled trial of effect of high-impact exercise on selected risk factors for osteoporotic fractures. *Lancet.* 1996;348:1343–1347.
97. Watson SL, Weeks BK, Weis LJ, Harding AT, Horan SA, Beck BR. High-intensity resistance and impact training improves bone mineral density and physical function in postmenopausal women with osteopenia and osteoporosis: The LIFTMOR Randomized Controlled Trial. *J Bone Miner Res.* 2018;33:211–220.
98. Sahota O, Ong T, Salem K. Vertebral Fragility Fractures (VFF)—Who, when and how to operate. *Injury.* 2018;49: 1430–1435.

99. Rodriguez AJ, Fink HA, Mirigian L, et al. Pain, quality of life, and safety outcomes of kyphoplasty for vertebral compression fractures: report of a task force of the american society for bone and mineral research. *J Bone Miner Res*. 2017;32:1935–1944.
100. Fingar KR, Stocks C, Weiss AJ, et al. Most Frequent Operating Room Procedures Performed in U.S. Hospitals, 2003–2012: Statistical Brief #186. 2014 Dec. In: Healthcare Cost and Utilization Project (HCUP) Statistical Briefs [Internet]. Rockville (MD): Agency for Healthcare Research and Quality (US); 2006 Feb. Available from: https://www.ncbi.nlm.nih.gov/books/NBK274246/.
101. Kurtz S, Ong K, Lau E, Mowat F, Halpern M. Projections of primary and revision hip and knee arthroplasty in the United States from 2005 to 2030. *J Bone Joint Surg Am*. 2007;89: 780–785.
102. Kalson NS, Borthwick LA, Mann DA, et al. International consensus on the definition and classification of fibrosis of the knee joint. *Bone Joint J*. 2016;98–b:1479–1488.
103. Pua YH. The time course of knee swelling post total knee arthroplasty and its associations with quadriceps strength and gait speed. *J Arthroplasty*. 2015;30:1215–1219.
104. Mizner RL, Petterson SC, Snyder-Mackler L. Quadriceps strength and the time course of functional recovery after total knee arthroplasty. *J Orthop Sports Phys The*. 2005;35:424–436.
105. Bade MJ, Stevens-Lapsley JE. Early high-intensity rehabilitation following total knee arthroplasty improves outcomes. *J Oorthop Sports Phys Ther*. 2011;41:932–941.
106. Mizner RL, Petterson SC, Stevens JE, Axe MJ, Snyder-Mackler L. Preoperative quadriceps strength predicts functional ability one year after total knee arthroplasty. *J Rheumatol*. 2005;32:1533–1539.
107. Loyd BJ, Jennings JM, Judd DL, et al. Influence of hip abductor strength on functional outcomes before and after total knee arthroplasty: post hoc analysis of a randomized controlled trial. *Phys Ther*. 2017;97:896–903.
108. Stevens-Lapsley JE, Balter JE, Wolfe P, Eckhoff DG, Kohrt WM. Early neuromuscular electrical stimulation to improve quadriceps muscle strength after total knee arthroplasty: a randomized controlled trial. *Phys Ther*. 2012;92:210–226.
109. Stevens-Lapsley JE, Balter JE, Wolfe P, et al. Relationship between intensity of quadriceps muscle neuromuscular electrical stimulation and strength recovery after total knee arthroplasty. *Phys Ther*. 2012;92:1187–1196.
110. Swinkels A, Allain TJ. Physical performance tests, self-reported outcomes, and accidental falls before and after total knee arthroplasty: an exploratory study. *Physiotherapy Theory and Practice*. 2013;29:432–442.
111. Swinkels A, Newman JH, Allain TJ. A prospective observational study of falling before and after knee replacement surgery. *Age Ageing*. 2009;38:175–181.
112. Moutzouri M, Gleeson N, Billis E, Tsepis E, Panoutsopoulou I, Gliatis J. The effect of total knee arthroplasty on patients' balance and incidence of falls: a systematic review. *Knee Surgery, Sports Traumatology, Arthroscopy: Official Journal of the ESSKA*. 2017;25:3439–3451.
113. Rand JA, Trousdale RT, Ilstrup DM, Harmsen WS. Factors affecting the durability of primary total knee prostheses. *J Bone Joint Surg Am*. 2003;85–a:259–265.
114. Sartawi M, Zurakowski D, Rosenberg A. Implant survivorship and complication rates after total knee arthroplasty with a third-generation cemented system: 15-year follow-up. *Am J Orthop*. 2018;47. https://fmc-reg.onecount.net/onecount/login/loginlogout.cgi?gid=36971,36971&return=https%3A%2F%2Fwww.mdedge.com%2Fsurgery%2Farticle%2F197087%2Fknee%2Fimplant-survivorship-and-complication-rates-after-total-knee&brand=edge3&sid=n8thrm139hnsv7c5crpl8a5gb2.
115. D'Lima DD, Patil S, Steklov N, Slamin JE, Colwell Jr. CW. Tibial forces measured in vivo after total knee arthroplasty. *J Arthroplasty*. 2006;21:255–262.
116. Swanson EA, Schmalzried TP, Dorey FJ. Activity recommendations after total hip and knee arthroplasty: a survey of the American Association for Hip and Knee Surgeons. *J Arthroplasty*. 2009;24:120–126.
117. Kahlenberg CA, Nwachukwu BU, McLawhorn AS, Cross MB, Cornell CN, Padgett DE. Patient satisfaction after total knee replacement: a systematic review. *HSS Journal: The Musculoskeletal Journal of Hospital for Special Surgery*. 2018;14:192–201.
118. Zeni Jr. JA, Snyder-Mackler L. Early postoperative measures predict 1- and 2-year outcomes after unilateral total knee arthroplasty: importance of contralateral limb strength. *Phys Ther*. 2010;90:43–54.
119. Farquhar S, Snyder-Mackler L. The Chitranjan Ranawat Award: The nonoperated knee predicts function 3 years after unilateral total knee arthroplasty. *Clin Orthop*. 2010;468:37–44.
120. American Academy of Orthopaedic Surgeons clinical practice guideline on surgical management of osteoarthritis of the knee. American Academy of Orthopaedic Surgeons (AAOS), 2015 (Accessed August 1, 2018, at http://www.orthoguidelines.org/topic?id=1019.)
121. Nakano N, Matsumoto T, Ishida K, et al. Factors influencing the outcome of deep infection following total knee arthroplasty. *The Knee*. 2015;22:328–332.
122. Gu A, Michalak AJ, Cohen JS, Almeida ND, McLawhorn AS, Sculco PK. Efficacy of manipulation under anesthesia for stiffness following total knee arthroplasty: a systematic rReview. *J Arthroplasty*. 2018;33:1598–1605.
123. Harvey IA, Barry K, Kirby SP, Johnson R, Elloy MA. Factors affecting the range of movement of total knee arthroplasty. *J Bone Joint Surg Br*. 1993;75:950–955.
124. Gatha NM, Clarke HD, Fuchs R, Scuderi GR, Insall JN. Factors affecting postoperative range of motion after total knee arthroplasty. *The Journal of Knee Surgery*. 2004;17: 196–202.
125. Kim J, Nelson CL, Lotke PA. Stiffness after total knee arthroplasty. Prevalence of the complication and outcomes of revision. *J Bone Joint Surg Am*. 2004;86-a:1479–1484.
126. Issa K, Rifai A, Boylan MR, Pourtaheri S, McInerney VK, Mont MA. Do various factors affect the frequency of manipulation under anesthesia after primary total knee arthroplasty? *Clin Orthop*. 2015;473:143–147.
127. Petis S, Howard JL, Lanting BL, Vasarhelyi EM. Surgical approach in primary total hip arthroplasty: anatomy, technique and clinical outcomes. *Can J Surg*. 2015;58:128–139.
128. Judd DL, Dennis DA, Thomas AC, Wolfe P, Dayton MR, Stevens-Lapsley JE. Muscle strength and functional recovery during the first year after THA. *Clini Orthop*. 2014;472: 654–664.
129. Di Monaco M, Castiglioni C. Which type of exercise therapy is effective after hip arthroplasty? A systematic review of randomized controlled trials. *European Journal of Physical and Rehabilitative medicine*. 2013;49:893–907. quiz 21–3.
130. Lowe CJ, Davies L, Sackley CM, Barker KL. Effectiveness of land-based physiotherapy exercise following hospital discharge following hip arthroplasty for osteoarthritis: an updated systematic review. *Physiotherapy*. 2015;101: 252–265.
130a. de Luca KE et al. The effectiveness and safety of manual therapy on pain and disability in older persons with chronic low back pain: a systematic review. Journal of Manipulative and Physiological Therapeutics. 2017;40(7): 527–534.
131. Macadam P, Cronin J, Contreras B. An examination of the gluteal muscle activity associated with dynamic hip abduction and hip external rotation exercise: a systematic review. *International Journal of Sports Physical Therapy*. 2015;10:573–591.

132. Reiman MP, Bolgla LA, Loudon JK. A literature review of studies evaluating gluteus maximus and gluteus medius activation during rehabilitation exercises. *Physiotherapy Theory and Practice*. 2012;28:257–268.
133. Ethgen O, Bruyere O, Richy F, Dardennes C, Reginster JY. Health-related quality of life in total hip and total knee arthroplasty. A qualitative and systematic review of the literature. *J Bone Joint Surg Am*. 2004;86–A:963–74.
134. Wang W, Morrison TA, Geller JA, Yoon RS, Macaulay W. Predicting short-term outcome of primary total hip arthroplasty:a prospective multivariate regression analysis of 12 independent factors. *J Arthroplasty*. 2010;25:858–864.
135. Smith GH, Johnson S, Ballantyne JA, Dunstan E, Brenkel IJ. Predictors of excellent early outcome after total hip arthroplasty. *Journal of Orthopaedic Surgery and Research*. 2012;7:13.
136. Singh JA, Lewallen DG. Predictors of activity limitation and dependence on walking aids after primary total hip arthroplasty. *J Am Geriatr Soc*. 2010;58:2387–2393.
137. Griffin DR, Dickenson EJ, Wall PDH, et al. Hip arthroscopy versus best conservative care for the treatment of femoroacetabular impingement syndrome (UK FASHIoN): a multicentre randomised controlled trial. *Lancet*. 2018;391: 2225–2235.
138. Hummel MT, Malkani AL, Yakkanti MR, Baker DL. Decreased dislocation after revision total hip arthroplasty using larger femoral head size and posterior capsular repair. *J Arthroplasty*. 2009;24:73–76.
139. Khatod M, Barber T, Paxton E, Namba R, Fithian D. An analysis of the risk of hip dislocation with a contemporary total joint registry. *Clin Orthop*. 2006;447:19–23.
140. Phillips CB, Barrett JA, Losina E, et al. Incidence rates of dislocation, pulmonary embolism, and deep infection during the first six months after elective total hip replacement. *J Bone Joint Surg Am*. 2003;85-a:20 26.
141. Restrepo C, Mortazavi SM, Brothers J, Parvizi J, Rothman RH. Hip dislocation: are hip precautions necessary in anterior approaches? *Clin Orthop*. 2011;469:417–422.
142. Bin Abd Razak HR, Yung WY. Postoperative delirium in patients undergoing total joint arthroplasty: a systematic review. *J Arthroplasty*. 2015;30:1414–1417.
143. Zhu Y, Chen W, Sun T, Zhang X, Liu S, Zhang Y. Risk factors for the periprosthetic fracture after total hip arthroplasty: a systematic review and meta-analysis. *Scandinavian Journal of Surgery*. 2015;104:139–145.
144. Jain NB, Higgins LD, Losina E, Collins J, Blazar PE, Katz JN. Epidemiology of musculoskeletal upper extremity ambulatory surgery in the United States. *BMC, Musculoskeletal Disorders*. 2014;15:4.
145. Thigpen CA, Shaffer MA, Kissenberth MJ. Knowing the speed limit: weighing the benefits and risks of rehabilitation progression after arthroscopic rotator cuff repair. *Clin Sports Med*. 2015;34:233–246.
146. Saltzman BM, Zuke WA, Go B, et al. Does early motion lead to a higher failure rate or better outcomes after arthroscopic rotator cuff repair? A systematic review of overlapping meta-analyses. *J Shoulder Elbow Surg*. 2017;26: 1681–1691.
147. Thigpen CA, Shaffer MA, Gaunt BW, Leggin BG, Williams GR, Wilcox 3rd RB. The American Society of Shoulder and Elbow Therapists' consensus statement on rehabilitation following arthroscopic rotator cuff repair. *J Shoulder Elbow Surg*. 2016;25:521–535.
148. Shin SJ, Chung J, Lee J, Ko YW. Recovery of muscle strength after intact arthroscopic rotator cuff repair according to preoperative rotator cuff tear size. *Am J Sports Med*. 2016;44:972–980.
149. Abtahi AM, Granger EK, Tashijian RZ. Factors affecting healing after arthroscopic rotator cuff repair. *World Journal of Orthopedics*. 2015;6(2):211–220.
150. Saccomanno MF, Sircana G, Cazzato G, Donati F, Randelli P, Milano G. Prognostic factors influencing the outcome of rotator cuff repair: a systematic review. *Knee Surgery, Sports Traumatology, Arthroscopy: Official Journal of the ESSKA*. 2016;24:3809–3819.
151. Fermont AJ, Wolterbeek N, Wessel RN, Baeyens JP, de Bie RA. Prognostic factors for successful recovery after arthroscopic rotator cuff repair: a systematic literature review. *J Orthop Sports Phys Ther*. 2014;44:153–163.
152. Kosinski LR, Gil JA, Durand WM, DeFroda SF, Owens BD, Daniels AH. 30-Day readmission following outpatient rotator cuff repair: an analysis of 18,061 cases. *The Physician and Sportsmedicine*. 2018;46:466–470.
153. Boudreau S, Boudreau ED, Higgins LD, Wilcox 3rd. RB. Rehabilitation following reverse total shoulder arthroplasty. *J Orthop Sports Phys Ther*. 2007;37:734–743.
154. Kiet TK, Feeley BT, Naimark M, Gajiu T M, Hall SL, Chung TT, et al. Outcomes after shoulder replacement: comparison between reverse and anatomic total shoulder arthroplasty. *J Shoulder Elbow Surg*. 2015;24(2):179–185. https://doi.org/10.1016/j.jse.2014.06.039.
155. Puzzitiello RN, Agarwalla A, Liu JN, et al. Establishing maximal medical improvement after anatomic total shoulder arthroplasty. *J Shoulder Elbow Surg*. 2018;27:1711–1720.
156. Liu JN, Steinhaus ME, Garcia GH, et al. Return to sport after shoulder arthroplasty: a systematic review and meta-analysis. *Knee Surgery, Sports Traumatology, Arthroscopy: Official Journal of the ESSKA*. 2018;26:100–112.
157. Deyo RA, Mirza SK, Martin BI, Kreuter W, Goodman DC, Jarvik JG. Trends, major medical complications, and charges associated with surgery for lumbar spinal stenosis in older adults. *JAMA*. 2010;303:1259–1265.
158. Martin B, Mirza SK, Spina N, Spiker WR, Lawrence B, Brodke DS. Trends in lumbar fusion procedure rates and associated hospital costs for degenerative spinal diseases in the United States, 2004–2015. *Spine*. 2019;44:369–376.
159. Fehlings MG, Tetreault LA, Kurpad S, et al. Change in functional impairment, disability, and quality of life following operative treatment for degenerative cervical myelopathy: a systematic review and meta-analysis. *Global Spine Journal*. 2017;7:53S–69S.
160. Fritsch CG, Ferreira ML, Maher CG, et al. The clinical course of pain and disability following surgery for spinal stenosis: a systematic review and meta-analysis of cohort studies. *European Spine Journal*. 2017;26:324–335.
161. Yagi M, Fujita N, Okada E, et al. Impact of frailty and comorbidities on surgical outcomes and complications in adult spinal disorders. *Spine*. 2018;43:1259–1267.
162. Yavin D, Casha S, Wiebe S, et al. Lumbar fusion for degenerative disease: a systematic review and meta-analysis. *Neurosurgery*. 2017;80:701–715.
163. Rihn JA, Hilibrand AS, Zhao W, et al. Effectiveness of surgery for lumbar stenosis and degenerative spondylolisthesis in the octogenarian population: analysis of the Spine Patient Outcomes Research Trial (SPORT) data. *J Bone Joint Surg Am*. 2015;97:177–185.
164. Gokaslan ZL, Bydon M, De la Garza-Ramos R, et al. Recurrent laryngeal nerve palsy after cervical spine surgery: a multicenter AO Spine Clinical Research Network Study. *Global Spine Journal*. 2017;7. 53S–7S.
165. Thompson SE, Smith ZA, Hsu WK, et al. C5 Palsy After Cervical Spine Surgery: A Multicenter Retrospective Review of 59 Cases. *Global Spine Journal*. 2017;7:64S–70S.

166. Archer KR, Devin CJ, Vanston SW, et al. Cognitive-behavioral-based physical therapy for patients with chronic pain undergoing lumbar spine surgery: a randomized controlled trial. *The Journal of Pain: Official Journal of the American Pain Society*. 2016;17:76–89.

166a. Rolving N, Neilsen CV, Christensen FB, Holm R, Bunger CE, Osetergaard LG. Preoperative cognitive-behavioural intervention improves in-hospital mobilization and analgesic use for lumbar spinal fusion patients. *BMC Musculoskeletal Disorders*. 2016;17:217.

167. van Erp RMA, Jelsma J, Huijnen IPJ, Lundberg M, Willems PC, Smeets R. Spinal surgeons' opinions on pre- and pPostoperative rehabilitation in patients undergoing lumbar spinal fusion surgery: a survey-based study in the Netherlands and Sweden. *Spine*. 2018;43:713–719.

168. McGregor AH, Probyn K, Cro S, et al. Rehabilitation following surgery for lumbar spinal stenosis. A Cochrane review. *Spine*. 2014;39:1044–1054.

169. Kamper SJ, Apeldoorn AT, Chiarotto A, et al. Multidisciplinary biopsychosocial rehabilitation for chronic low back pain: Cochrane systematic review and meta-analysis. *BMJ*. 2015;350:h444.

170. Louw A, Diener I, Landers MR, Puentedura EJ. Preoperative pain neuroscience education for lumbar radiculopathy: a multicenter randomized controlled trial with 1-year follow-up. *Spine*. 2014;39:1449–1457.

171. Nijs J, Paul van Wilgen C, Van Oosterwijck J, van Ittersum M, Meeus M. How to explain central sensitization to patients with 'unexplained' chronic musculoskeletal pain: practice guidelines. *Manual Therapy*. 2011;16:413–418.

172. Madera M, Brady J, Deily S, et al. The role of physical therapy and rehabilitation after lumbar fusion surgery for degenerative disease: a systematic review. *Journal Neurosurgery Spine*. 2017;26:694–704.

173. Backstrom KM, Whitman JM, Flynn TW. Lumbar spinal stenosis-diagnosis and management of the aging spine. *Manual Therapy*. 2011;16:308–317.

174. Whitman JM, Flynn TW, Childs JD, et al. A comparison between two physical therapy treatment programs for patients with lumbar spinal stenosis: a randomized clinical trial. *Spine*. 2006;31:2541–2549.

175. O'Leary S, Falla D, Elliott JM, Jull G. Muscle dysfunction in cervical spine pain: implications for assessment and management. *J Orthop Sports Phys Ther*. 2009;39:324–333.

176. O'Leary S, Cagnie B, Reeve A, Jull G, Elliott JM. Is there altered activity of the extensor muscles in chronic mechanical neck pain? A functional magnetic resonance imaging study. *Arch Phys Med Rehabil*. 2011;92:929–934.

177. Fujibayashi S, Neo M, Yoshida M, Miyata M, Takemoto M, Nakamura T. Neck muscle strength before and after cervical laminoplasty: relation to axial symptoms. *Journal of Spinal Disorders & Techniques*. 2010;23:197–202.

CHAPTER 21

Management of Integumentary Conditions in Older Adults

Alan Chong W. Lee

"All the carnall beauty of my wife is but skin-deep."

Sir Thomas Overbury, "A Wife" (1613)

OUTLINE

INTRODUCTION

Sir Thomas Overbury eloquently stated that physical beauty is superficial and is not important as one of a person's essential qualities in a poem titled "A Wife." A person's essential beauty is influenced by many physical, environmental, and psychosocial factors in life. For example, sun tanning without proper skin protection throughout one's life may lead to permanent damage to the exposed skin and greater risk for skin cancer. Immobility, lack of proper nutrition, and depression in compromised older adults increase risks for pressure-related wound injury. Hence, integumentary and wound management in older adults must address physical, environmental, and psychosocial factors to impact overall quality of life (QOL) in older adults. Therefore, physical therapists must become well suited to identify impairments, activity limitations, and community participation restrictions related to integumentary and wound injury in older adults.

Aging by itself is not a risk factor for impaired integumentary and wound injury. However, older adults may be at risk for integumentary impairments and delayed wound healing owing to slower cellular responses, thinner skin, and harmful habits such as smoking and sedentary lifestyle. Additionally, comorbid conditions more common in older adults are also commonly associated with integumentary and wound impairments (e.g., congestive heart failure, diabetes, vascular disease). These comorbid conditions put older adults at higher risk for integumentary and wound impairments. With diligent preventive care and collaborative practice within geriatric and wound care disciplines, most older adults with conditions that put them "at risk" for integumentary and wound injury can enjoy intact and healthy skin into oldest age.

This chapter begins with a discussion of normal age-related changes in skin and selected skin conditions prevalent in older adults. The chapter continues with a discussion of physical examination related to malnutrition and dehydration impacting the integumentary system. Dermatologic skin cancer screening of older adults will be covered, followed by a discussion of the role of the physical therapist as a member of the health care team. Common categories of integumentary wounds in older adults are presented, each with a distinct etiology and management approach: pressure ulcers, diabetic/neuropathic ulcers, arterial and venous ulcers, atypical inflammatory wounds, and burns. The chapter concludes with recent recommendations from aging and wound healing practitioners addressing QOL in older adults with integumentary and common wound conditions.

AGING-RELATED CHANGES IN THE SKIN

As with other organs in the body, the skin undergoes changes with aging. However, these changes do not typically cross the threshold of impairment. Integumentary-related impairments most typically occur when extrinsic stresses combined with the presence of comorbid health conditions are added to aging. For example, stress to the skin due to immobility and incontinence increases risks for pressure injury.

The skin is composed of two main layers, the epidermis and the dermis, with a basement membrane separating the two layers, totaling 16% of body weight (Fig. 21.1). The epidermis is the thin outermost layer of the skin composed of five sublayers. From deep to superficial, the five sublayers of the epidermis are the stratum germinativum, stratum spinosum, stratum granulosum, stratum lucidum, and stratum corneum. The main functions of the skin are thermoregulation, sensation, moisture elimination, vitamin D synthesis, and protection of deeper structures. The epidermis regenerates every 4 to 6 weeks and does not have a blood supply. With normal aging, the epidermis thins and decreases in density of Langerhans cells. Langerhans cells initiate the immune response when foreign cells are present. Consequently, with decreased thickness and immune function, the epidermis becomes less effective at protecting the body from infection and dehydration.[1,2] The basement membrane is the interface between the epidermis and dermis. The basement membrane is composed of many projections of the dermis into the epidermis. These projections are known as rete pegs and they provide resistance to shearing forces between the epidermis and dermis. The basement membrane also thins with age because of a flattening of the rete pegs, and this increases vulnerability to shear-related insults to the skin.[2–4]

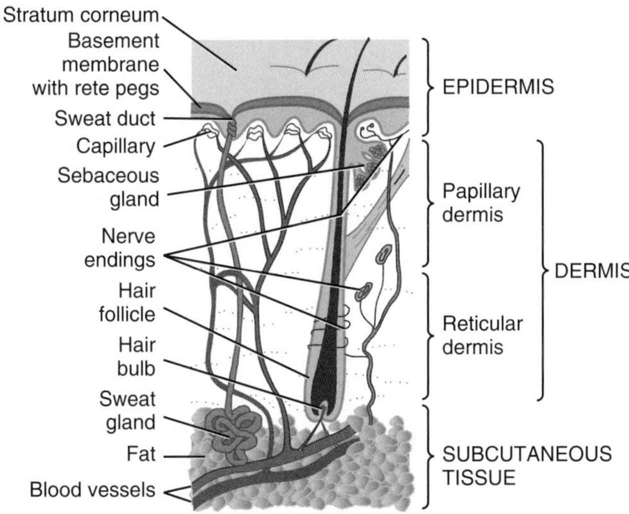

FIG. 21.1 Layers of the skin and its underlying tissue. *(From Goodman CC. Pathology: Implications for the Physical Therapist.* 3rd ed. Philadelphia: Saunders; 2008.)

The dermis is the thick, deeper layer of the skin responsible for structural integrity of the integument. The dermis provides nutrition, hydration, and oxygen to the epidermis via diffusion. The dermis is primarily composed of the protein collagen, which provides tensile strength, and elastin, which allows the skin to stretch. Collagen and elastin are produced by fibroblasts. As fibroblasts decrease with age, so too does the rate of production of collagen and elastin. Elastin fibers become degraded while collagen bundles become disorganized.[2,3,5] The dermis also thins as a normal consequence of aging with fewer blood vessels and nerve endings. As the blood vessels in the skin become thinner, they are more prone to hemorrhages known as senile purpura. Senile purpura is often the site of skin tears, possibly owing to a decrease in pain perception in the area of the purpura.[1,6] Finally, Pacinian and Meissner corpuscles found in the dermis degenerate with normal aging and contribute to decreased perception of light touch and pressure sensation.

Below the dermis is the subcutaneous layer, composed mainly of adipose tissue but also consisting of blood and lymphatic vessels as well as nerves. The subcutaneous layer facilitates regeneration of the dermis by providing blood supply and it also connects the dermis to underlying structures. As with the more superficial layers of the skin, the subcutaneous layer becomes thinner with age and diminishes in its ability to provide mechanical protection and thermal insulation.[1,2] Therefore, all functions of the skin are affected by normal aging. Other lifestyle considerations, particularly sun exposure and cigarette smoking, have an aging effect on skin, including the formation of wrinkles, hyperpigmentation, and change in skin texture. The most significant extrinsic cause of skin degeneration is photo aging, that is, the effect of exposure of the skin to ultraviolet irradiation (Fig. 21.2A). This image of a 64-year-old woman demonstrates the impact of sun damage and aging of the skin with ultraviolet photography. Environmental damage to skin from sunlight is known as dermatoheliosis. The effects of photo aging are seen only in areas exposed to the sun, primarily the face, neck, and hands.[1,7] Dermatoheliosis may produce tough, leathery texture on the skin owing to cross-hatching to the dermis. Age spots, once called "liver spots," are flat, brown spots often caused by years in the sun that show up on areas such as the face, hands, arms, back, and feet, whereas skin tags or flesh-colored growths raised over skin may be found on the eyelids, neck, and body folds (armpits, chest, and groin), especially in women.[8] Cigarette smoking increases the incidence of skin wrinkling in smokers when compared to similarly aged nonsmokers. Although the exact cause for increased wrinkling is unknown, it is believed to be a consequence of the cigarette smoke's toxicity on microvasculature as well as a negative effect on oxidative and enzymatic activity in connective tissue in the dermis.[1,9]

Although the basic wound healing process does not change in older adults, the lower physiological reserve

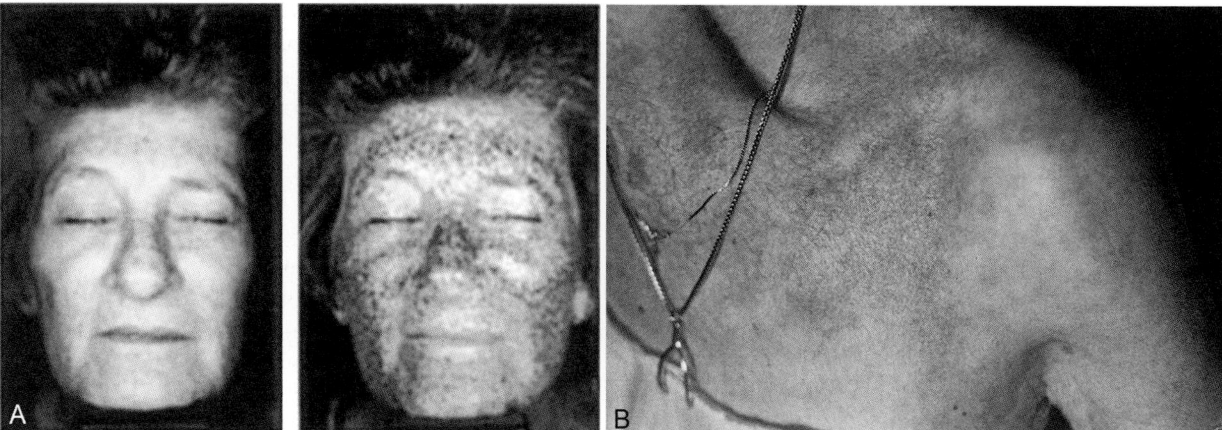

FIG. 21.2 **A,** This 64-year-old beach-community resident's skin chronicles a lifetime of sun exposure. (Photos provided courtesy of David H. McDaniel, MD). **B,** Xerosis. *(From Ignatavicius DD. Medical-Surgical Nursing: Patient-Centered Collaborative Care.* 6th ed. Philadelphia: Saunders; 2009.)

of older adults and the increased prevalence of comorbid conditions associated with delayed wound healing make older adults more susceptible to factors that delay wound healing and increase rates of wound infection.[10] Understanding the overlapping cascade of inflammation, proliferation, and remodeling as the foundation of wound care is essential for practitioners in the field of aging and wound repair.[3] For example, platelets recruit inflammatory cells to form a wound matrix and macrophages to regulate the cytokine environment, assisting proliferative responses and wound closure. Chronic wounds have resident cells that proliferate less and morphologic cellular senescence, resulting in lack of progress in wound healing. Age-related changes in hormonal status affect wound repair and blunt the healing response.[3] Overall, wound healing can be delayed by many factors.[11–13] Some of these factors are intrinsic, meaning they emerge from internal physiological abnormalities that impair effective wound healing. Other factors are extrinsic, meaning they arise from external forces deterring normal healing processes. Box 21.1 provides a list of common intrinsic and extrinsic factors associated with delayed wound healing. It is important to modify extrinsic risk factors to progress through wound healing and repair in older adults.

PHYSICAL SKIN ASSESSMENT

Malnutrition

Older adults are susceptible to a host of intrinsic and extrinsic factors that may lead to malnutrition, leading to an increased risk of developing new wounds and impaired ability to heal existing wounds. For example, changes in the digestive system of older adults include decreased production of digestive enzymes and acids, which leads to decreased absorption of nutrients. Impaired dentition may lead to difficulty with chewing, and dry mouth may lead to difficulty swallowing. Chronic illness or impaired mobility can decrease the ability of older adults to shop, cook, or eat independently. Impaired mental function can suppress appetite, as can many medications, including antidepressants, blood pressure medications, and even over-the-counter medications such as aspirin. Older adults may also have a decreased sense of taste and smell, both of which can significantly decrease appetite. Other extrinsic risk factors for malnutrition in

BOX 21.1 Common Intrinsic and Extrinsic Factors Associated with Impaired Wound Healing

Intrinsic Factors	Extrinsic Factors
Immobility	Tobacco use
Malnutrition	Pressure that impairs circulation in area
Impaired hydration	Desiccation, leading to dryness
Obesity	Presence of necrotic tissue (eschar or slough)
Cachexia	Repetitive trauma causing high shear forces
Infection or colonization	Maceration (typically from incontinence or perspiration)
Edema around the wound (inhibits oxygen and nutrient transport)	Lack of participation in wound plan of care or inappropriate care
Decreased circulatory function	
Decreased respiratory function	
Immunosuppressed state (including use of corticosteroids and NSAIDs)	
Radiation therapy	
Chronic diseases such as:	
Diabetes	
PAD/PVD	
CAD	
Renal failure	
Anemia	
Cancer	

CAD, coronary artery disease; *NSAID,* nonsteroidal anti-inflammatory drug; *PAD,* peripheral arterial disease; *PVD,* peripheral vascular disease.

older adults include low or fixed income, depression, social isolation, and dietary restrictions necessitated by other comorbidities.[14] Older adults may experience a nutritional decline that may delay skin and wound healing. Key nutritional indicators are necessary for optimal wound healing, and malnutrition may impact overall clinical outcomes.

Malnutrition is defined as unintentional weight loss >10% or >5% over the last 3 months or body mass index (BMI) <18.5 kg/m^2.[15] The prevalence of malnutrition in patients at hospital admission is 30% to 55%, and patients may continue to lose weight at discharge, increasing the risk for hospital readmissions.[16] A focused physical assessment by the physical therapist using valid screening tools for assessing malnutrition for older adults can lead to early identification of malnutrition. For example, the Malnutrition Universal Screening Tool (MUST) can be used to screen community-dwelling older adults, and the Mini Nutrition Assessment (MNA) is designed for older adults aged 65 and older.[17] In the screening process, more than two of these six characteristics may identify malnutrition: declining functional status, fluid accumulation, muscle loss, subcutaneous fat loss, unintentional weight loss, and insufficient energy intake.[18] Fat and muscle loss, the most prevalent characteristics for chronic illness-related malnutrition, can be assessed through palpitation of anatomical landmarks to help determine the degree of muscle and/or fat loss.[19] Fat loss is commonly identified by assessing and palpating six anatomical and body regions including the temporal bone, zygomatic arch, triceps, biceps, ribcage, and midaxillary line to the lumbar region. For example, severe fat loss between the midaxillary line and the lumbar region may display prominent ribs with depressions and protruding iliac crest. Subcutaneous fat loss in triceps can be examined by flexing the elbow at 90 degrees and pinching the triceps without the muscle between fingers. Severe fat loss will allow the fingers to nearly approximate while pinching mostly skin.[20] Overall, fat loss is usually more prominent in the upper body. The skilled practitioner may verify if this fat loss is normal for older adults by quantifying the severity and investigating other characteristics such as muscle loss. Typical muscles for identifying muscle loss include the temporalis, pectoralis major, deltoids, trapezius, latissimus dorsi, supraspinatus, infraspinatus, interosseous, quadriceps, and gastrocnemius. For example, assessing both the dorsal and palmar interosseous muscles and thenar region for prominent depressions while the older adult moves the hand or makes an "OK" sign may identify the severity of muscle loss related to nutritional decline. When indicated, referral to the nutritionist and dietitian for optimal nutritional support for older adults must be communicated to the health care team.

Dehydration

Older adults are at greater risk of dehydration than younger people and this can lead to serious health complications including increased time to wound healing. It is generally accepted that the increased risk of dehydration among older adults is not a direct consequence of aging but rather the result of age-associated factors such as increased physical dependence, multiple medical comorbidities, and self-limiting hydration habits.[21,22] Commonly used assessments of dehydration in older adults may include dry mucous membranes, rapid pulse, furrowed tongue, decreased fluid intake, urine color or volume, and feeling thirsty but should not be used alone because combining several symptoms and tests (expressing fatigue, missing drinks between meals) may improve diagnostic accuracy.[23] Furthermore, the commonly accepted test of skin turgor at the sternum is not reliable in older adults because of the previously discussed changes in skin elasticity.[21,23,24] Other measures of dehydration are obtained from lab values, including increased concentration of serum sodium, increased serum osmolality, and increased ratio of blood urea nitrogen to creatinine.[25]

The incidence of xerosis, or dryness of the skin, increases as people age. Xerosis, depicted in Fig. 21.2B, occurs when the moisture level of the stratum corneum is below 10%.[1,26] The precise cause of xerosis is not known; however, age-related changes including water-loss dehydration as well as environmental and genetic factors contribute to the severity of this problem. Xerosis can negatively impact the quality of life for older adults by producing pruritus (itching), burning or stinging, and an uncomfortable sensation of tightness in the skin. As xerosis becomes more severe, it can lead to redness or cracking of the skin.[1] Older adults should be encouraged to keep hydrated and to use a moisturizing lotion to prevent or manage dry skin and moisturize the skin. Overall, a collaborative approach to proper skin assessment and proper education of older adults on optimizing nutrition and hydration are key factors to healthy skin.

Assessment and Prevention

Fragile skin in older adults can be associated with the intrinsic and extrinsic factors in aging-related changes in older adults (see Box 21.1). Older adults describe fragile skin as paper thin skin that can be easily traumatized by falls and lead to skin tears. Approximately one in five falls may result in scrapes, bruises, or blisters. As mentioned earlier, the epidermal proliferative capacity is reduced with aging owing to changes in the basal keratinocyte microenvironment. The flattening of epidermal rete pegs at the epidermis–dermis junction of the skin can contribute to impaired skin integrity in older adults through separation of the epidermis and dermis with shearing, friction, or blunt trauma. In addition, skin structure with increased wrinkling, rough dryness, laxity, and reduced elasticity predispose older adults to skin tears. The etiology of skin tears is multifactorial. For example, cachexia with loss of muscle and fat is common in patients with cancer as well as patients on prolonged anticoagulant therapy and may make them susceptible to skin tears. Anticoagulant medications to treat chronic medical conditions can predispose older adults to skin tears and bruising. However, certain unintentional consequences of drugs or polypharmacy can be remedied by educating older adults about the increased risk of injuring fragile skin. Older adults may experience skin tears anywhere on the body, though the most common locations are the arms and hands, followed by the lower extremities.[1,27] The risk of skin tears increases with dependence in activities of daily living such as requiring assistance with transfer and with the removal of tapes and adhesives from the skin.[1,28] Visual impairment increases the risk of skin tears because of bumping into objects.[1,27,29] Preventing skin tears means protecting the skin from trauma. Older adults should be encouraged to apply lotion twice per day and to wear loose, long-sleeved shirts and pants and skid-free footwear. Avoidance of soaps and lotions containing alcohol and excessive washing with soap, which reduces intrinsic skin lubrication, is also important.[30,31] The environment can be modified to limit risk of skin tears by eliminating superfluous furniture, providing adequate lighting (including nightlights), and padding edges on furniture, wheelchairs, and bedrails.[29,32] Skin tears are commonly underreported in long-term care residents. Hence, practitioners should be educated on classification and types of skin tears (Table 21.1). Although Payne and Martin developed the first classification system, another tool developed in Australia called the Skin Tear Audit Research (STAR) Classification System exists and was reported to be implemented within the United Kingdom.[28] Caregivers should be educated in and assessed for proper transfer technique to prevent friction, shear, or trauma. Protective sleeves to secure dressings should be used instead of applying adhesive tape directly to an older patient's skin.[31,32] In addition, older adult residents with frequent skin tears or mobility issues should have routine skin inspections. Using a universal system to classify skin tears in health care may assist in developing evidence-based guidelines and practice to improve the quality of life and reduce health care burden from skin tears in older adults.

TABLE 21.1 Payne-Martin Skin Tear Classification System

Category	Amount of Tissue Loss	Description
I	Skin tear without tissue loss	Linear type (epidermis and dermis layers separated in an incision-like lesion) Flap type (an epidermal flap that covers the dermis, and wound edges are within 1 mm of separation)
II	Partial tissue loss	Scant tissue loss: <25% epidermal flap lost Moderate to large tissue loss: >25% epidermal flap lost
III	Skin tears with complete tissue loss	Epidermal flap completely gone

(From Baranoski S. Meeting the challenge of skin tears. *Adv Skin Wound Care.* 2005;18[2]:74–75.)

Skin Cancer

Dermatologic skin cancer ABCDE screening[33] as well as calculating older adults' risk of melanoma by using valid tools such as the melanoma risk assessment[34] is available for physical therapists. For example, practitioners should educate older adults to assess their skin regularly for skin cancer in sun-exposed areas, including top of head, posterior neck and ears, tip of nose, upper back, shoulders, and exposed extremities. Suspicious skin areas with (A) asymmetry, (B) irregular borders, (C) dark colors, (D) diameter >0.5 mm, and (E) elevated skin should be screened for skin cancer by a dermatologic specialist in a timely manner. Furthermore, information on the benefits, harms, and description of the evidence on skin cancer screening for health professionals (the PDQ)[35] can be helpful to discern appropriate care for older adults. General practitioners should be aware of free and secure resources to access dermatology specialist consultation through the Internet known as AccessDerm.[36] AccessDerm, with the support of the American Academy of Dermatology (AAD), has provided consultations to underserved patients, which have included diagnoses of a previously undiagnosed melanoma and Kaposi sarcoma. In addition, the AAD provides information on free SPOTme skin cancer screenings in local areas in the United States when users sign up for email alerts on the AAD website.[36]

Skin cancer is common in older adults and increases with age. The three most common types of skin cancer include basal cell carcinoma, squamous cell carcinoma, and melanoma (Fig. 21.3).[33] Although melanoma makes up 4% of skin cancers compared to basal cell (80%) or squamous cell (16%) carcinoma, it is more deadly with rapidly spreading malignancy. Squamous cell carcinoma tends to be scaly, ulcerate, and metastasize, whereas basal

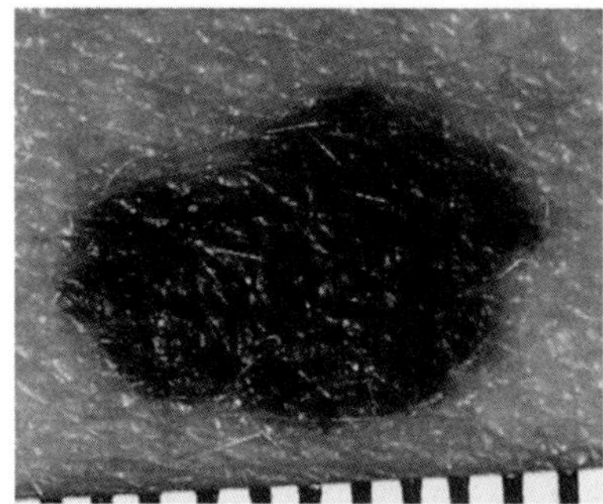

FIG. 21.3 Melanoma. *(From Goodman CC. Pathology: Implications for the Physical Therapist.* 3rd ed. Philadelphia: Saunders; 2008.)

cell carcinoma is shiny, translucent, and rarely metastasizes. For example, squamous cell carcinomas are the most commonly encountered cancer arising from venous leg ulcers and basal cell carcinoma is much rarer.[37] Risk factors for skin cancer include men and women older than age 65 years, patients with atypical moles, patients with more than 50 moles, family history of skin cancer, and a history of severe sunburns. Physical therapists should educate older adults on common skin cancer prevention strategies including wearing protective clothing (long sleeves, wide-brimmed hat, and sunglasses), avoiding excessive sun rays between 10 a.m. and 2 p.m. or seeking shade, using and reapplying water-resistant sunscreen with an SPF >30, using self-tanning products, avoiding tanning beds, and performing regular skin self-exams. The referral of an older adult to a board-certified dermatologist if new or suspicious spots on the skin are detected is imperative.[38] Other AAD recommendations for antiaging skin tips for older adults include preventing dry skin by avoiding bar soaps and bath oil during bathing, avoiding fragrant skin care products, using a humidifier to reduce dry air, wearing gloves for housework and gardening outdoors, wearing skin protective clothing, and examining skin regularly.[39] Therefore, physical therapists can positively influence aging older adults to manage common dermatologic changes and skin integrity conditions. The role of physical therapists is to collaborate with specialists in dermatology and primary care to detect abnormalities in the skin and provide preventive educational strategies with early surveillance of skin risk factors for older adults.

COMMON SKIN CONDITIONS

Candida

Candida, illustrated in Fig. 21.4, is a superficial yeast infection that most commonly affects older adults and the immunocompromised. Candida presents most often in the groin, axilla, or breast folds; affected skin may appear macerated and erythematous with papules and pustules due to prolonged exposure to moisture damage.[1] Standard treatment for candida consists of topical antifungal agents alone or in combination with topical steroids.[1] The most common pathogen is *Candida albicans,* which is involved with moisture-associated skin damage; however, the more serious *C. auris* infection is emerging as a multi-drug-resistant pathogen isolated from fluid and skin samples.

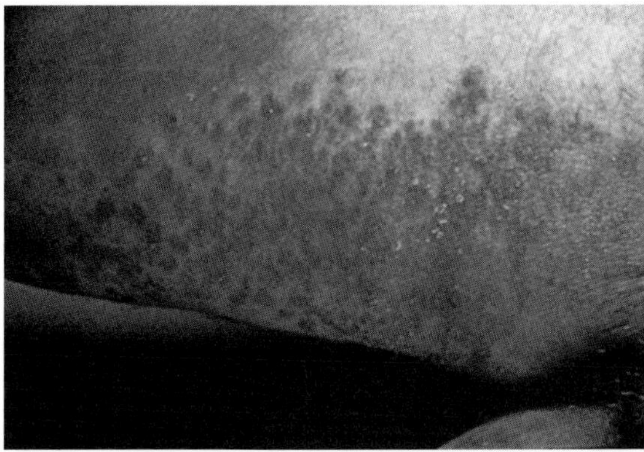

FIG. 21.4 Candida. *(From Paul A. Volberding, MD, University of California San Francisco)*

Cellulitis

Cellulitis, illustrated in Fig. 21.5, is a rapidly spreading infection of the dermis and subcutaneous layer most commonly seen in the face and extremities. Typically, cellulitis occurs in older adults in the presence of edema, obesity, and openings in the skin[1] but can occur at any site where the skin has been broken: cracks, cuts, blisters, insect bites, burns, injection sites, surgical incisions, or catheter insertion sites. The infection can be caused by the normal flora of the skin but may also be caused by exogenous bacteria, most commonly, group A *Streptococcus* or *Staphylococcus.* In older adults, group G *Streptococcus* may occur more frequently with underlying chronic illness.[40] Signs and symptoms of cellulitis include pain, increased warmth, erythema, and edema. When edema is present anywhere in the body, there is a higher risk of cellulitis in that area, and obese people are at highest risk for cellulitis in the folds and rolls of the skin. The prevalence of health care charges from 1998 to 2013 owing to cellulitis was reported to have more than doubled, and admissions for cellulitis are quite seasonal. For example, during the peak month of July, the incidence was 34.8% higher than the baseline month of February in one study.[41] Cellulitis is most commonly treated with oral antibiotics, but in severe

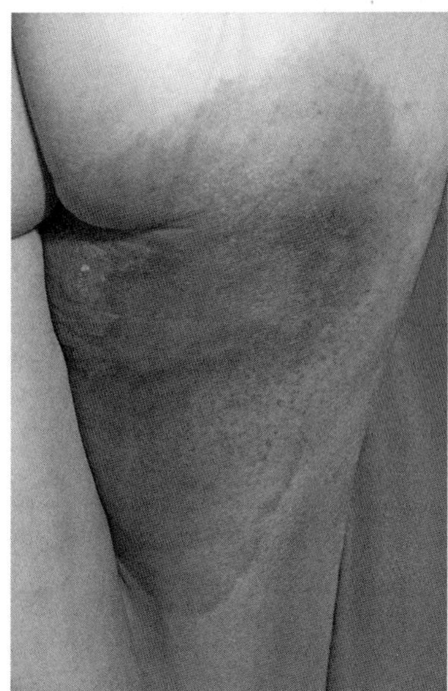

FIG. 21.5 Cellulitis. *(From Gould BE. Pathophysiology for the Health Professions.* 3rd ed. Philadelphia: Saunders; 2006.)

cases, intravenous antibiotics may be considered. Most patients' conditions respond well to these treatments. However, if cellulitis progresses to serious illness by uncontrolled contiguous spread and systemic infection, emergent medical care is necessary to prevent sepsis and potential life-threating illness in older adults.

Herpes Zoster

Herpes zoster, also known as shingles, is illustrated in Fig. 21.6. Herpes zoster results from the reactivation of the varicella zoster virus, which lies dormant in nerve ganglia after chickenpox. Age is one of the most significant risk factors for developing shingles. One study reports that incidence increases with age by a factor of >10, from 0.74 per 1000 person-years in children aged <10 years to 10.1 per 1000 person-years in persons aged 80 to 89 years, with much of the increase beginning at age 40 to 60 years. Approximately 50% of people who live to age 85 years will have experienced zoster.[42] Shingles can be identified by complaints of tingling or pain in a unilateral dermatome followed in 1 to 2 days by erythema and vesicles. The vesicles break down into crusted plaques, and patients remain contagious for chickenpox until all of the vesicles have crusted over. It typically takes 2 to 3 weeks from the initial onset of dermatome pain to the resolution of the zoster plaques.[43] Shingles occurs most commonly in the thoracic, cranial, lumbar, and sacral dermatomes. Once identified, shingles are treated with oral antiviral agents such as valacyclovir and famciclovir to minimize the duration of the disease and incidence of postherpetic neuralgia (PHN).[1,44] Areas of skin affected by vesicles can be treated by topical application of emollients, and PHN symptoms are commonly managed through oral agents such as gabapentin and tricyclic antidepressants.[1] Physical therapists may be involved in the management of PHN and educate older adults about a shingles vaccination. Since 2016, 33.4% of adults aged 60 years and older reported receiving Zostavax, a shingles vaccine in use since 2006. This is an increase from the 31% reported the previous year. In 2018, the Centers for Disease Control and Prevention (CDC) will collect data on vaccination of adults aged 50 years and older using Shingrix (recombinant zoster vaccine) as preferred over Zostavax (zoster vaccine live) for prevention of herpes zoster and related complications.[44] The CDC recommends two doses of Shingrix separated by 2 to 6 months for immunocompetent adults aged 50 years and older.

Scabies

Scabies, illustrated in Fig. 21.7, is very contagious and common to long-term care and other settings where people live in close proximity to each other. The rate of scabies occurrence varies in the recent literature from 0.3% to 46%.[45] Scabies is caused by a mite that lays its eggs in burrows on the skin. In 3 to 4 days the larvae hatch, come to the skin, and repeat the process. Several weeks after the initial infection, itching will be reported as a result of the immune response to the mites and their wastes; once the itch is scratched a secondary infection may result. Scabies infections can be recognized by

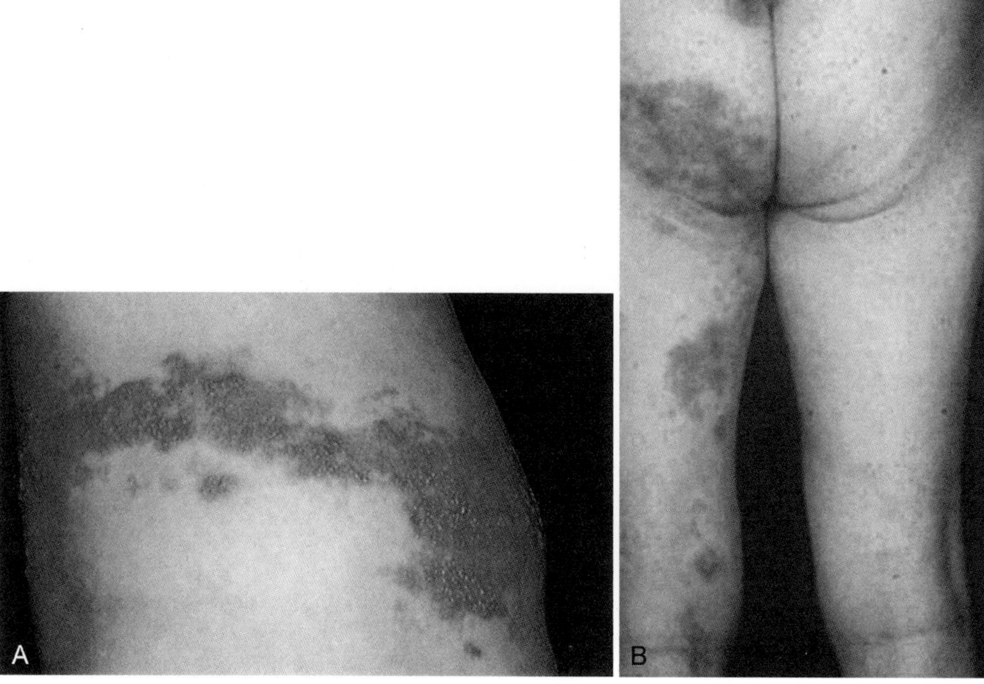

FIG. 21.6 Herpes zoster. *(From Goodman CC. Pathology: Implications for the Physical Therapist.* 3rd ed. Philadelphia: Saunders; 2008.)

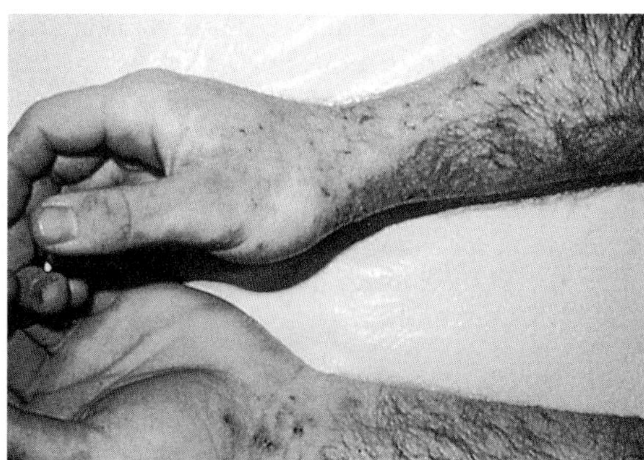

FIG. 21.7 Scabies. *(From Christsensen BL. Adult Health Nursing.* 5th ed. St. Louis: Mosby, 2005.)

excoriation and papules around the groin, abdomen, axillae, and wrists. Scabies often goes undetected in cognitively impaired older adults because of the inability to report symptoms. Treatment for scabies includes a topical scabicide such as permethrin, and all bed linens should be washed in the hottest possible water (i.e., 140°F to 200°F or 60°C to 90°C).[1,46,47]

COMMON WOUND CONDITIONS

According to the U.S. Centers for Medicare and Medicaid Services (CMS), it is estimated that nearly 15% of all Medicare beneficiaries (8.2 million older adults) experienced chronic nonhealing wounds at an annual cost of nearly $32 billion in 2014.[48] Surgical infections were the largest-prevalence category (4.0%) followed by diabetic infections (3.4%). The highest costs occurred for hospital outpatients followed by hospital inpatients.[48] Pressure injury and ulcers across hospitals in 34 states declined from 2011 to 2014,[49] largely owing to early identification and management of pressure injuries. Overall, pressure injury/ulcers, diabetic neuropathic ulcers, and arterial and venous ulcers, discussed next, represent common wound conditions in older adults addressed by physical therapists as part of integumentary care.

Pressure Injury/Ulcer

Pressure injury and ulcers are most common among older adults and are a source of premature mortality in some patients, interfering with functional recovery complicated by pain and infection.[50] Each year, more than 2.5 million people in the United States develop pressure ulcers.[51] In 2008, the CMS announced it would not pay for additional costs incurred for hospital-acquired pressure ulcers.[52] In 2016, the National Pressure Ulcer Advisory Panel (NPUAP) replaced the term *pressure ulcer* with *pressure injury* in the NPUAP injury staging system and added use of Arabic numerals instead of the previous Roman numerals.[53] Box 21.2 provides a description of pressure ulcer staging and additional pressure injury categories. Stage 1 pressure injury is a nonblanchable localized area of intact skin with erythema (redness). In people with darker skin tones, the stage 1 pressure injury may appear differently. Stage 2 pressure injury involves partial-thickness skin loss with exposed dermis. Full-thickness skin loss is classified as stage 3 pressure injury and involves damage extending down to, but not through, underlying fascia with adipose (fat) visible in the ulcer. Stage 4 pressure injury involves full-thickness skin loss penetrating through the fascia, muscle, tendon, ligament, cartilage, or bone in the ulcer.[53]

BOX 21.2 Pressure Ulcer Staging

Stage	Description
Stage 1	Nonblanchable localized area of intact skin with erythema that does not resolve within 30 minutes of complete pressure relief
Stage 2	Partial-thickness skin loss with exposed dermis but no slough, eschar present at this level
Stage 3	Full-thickness skin loss involves fascia with adipose tissue; however, damage does not expose tendon, bone, or joint capsule
Stage 4	Full-thickness skin loss extending through the fascia, muscle, tendon, ligament, cartilage, or bone
Deep-tissue pressure injury	Nonblanchable purple or maroon discoloration of intact skin that may indicate damage to the underlying tissue
Unstageable pressure injury	Ulcers completely covered with slough, eschar, or necrotic debris to the extent that the wound base is not visualized
Medical device–related pressure injury	Generally conforms to the pattern or shape of device and should be staged using the staging system.
Mucosal membrane pressure injury	Pressure injury found on mucous membranes with a history of a medical device in use at the location of the injury; due to the anatomy of the tissue these injuries cannot be staged

Pressure injury develops as soft tissue is compressed from sources of intense and/or prolonged pressure or shearing forces, restricting the blood supply and causing tissue damage. The most common wound locations in older adults are over bony prominences, most notably the sacrum and coccyx, heel, malleolus, trochanter, ischial tuberosity, elbow, knee, scapula, and occiput.[53] However, pressure ulcers may occur in other locations as sources of external pressure compress soft tissues. Examples of these injuries are on the leg where it is pressed against a bed rail or across the thigh where a urinary catheter was pulled tight. Hence, additional pressure injuries occur from medical device–related pressure as well as mucosal membrane pressure found on mucous membranes that is not stageable.[53] Other pressure injuries include unstageable obscured full-thickness skin loss and deep tissue pressure injury. Overall, pressure injury and ulcers are affected by microclimate of the skin and support surface, nutrition, perfusion, comorbidities, and condition of the soft tissue.

Prevention of pressure injury and ulcers in older adults includes assessing risk, providing proper skin care for those at risk, and educating patients.[53] The NPUAP recommends risk assessment tools such as the Norton scale[54] or the Braden scale[55] be used routinely (at admission and at regular intervals thereafter) with at-risk persons to ensure systematic evaluation of individual risk factors. Proper skin care, educational programs, and a rehabilitation program to maintain or improve mobility and activity status are important prevention strategies. Once an ulcer is present, early treatment is critical. In addition, pressure reduction is essential in preventing and treating pressure ulcers. There are many options for wheelchair cushions, mattresses, mattress overlays, positioning aids, and orthotics to assist with off-loading.[56] Recent literature suggests the need for the correct support surface for specific situations to reduce and prevent pressure injuries. For example, a small trial found that sheepskin placed under the legs significantly reduced redness and that profiling beds were better than standard beds in terms of healing existing stage 1 pressure injuries.[56] On the other hand, foam overlays are no longer used for pressure redistribution. Although physical therapists have training in most of these products, advanced training is beneficial in determining the optimal choices for a given patient. Therefore, the physical therapist may wish to consult other physical therapists, an occupational therapist, or a durable medical equipment provider with more experience in that area. Clinical guidelines to prevent and treat pressure ulcers include proper skin and tissue assessment, preventive skin care, prophylactic dressings, early mobilization/repositioning, adequate nutrition, cleansing, debridement, assessment of infection/biofilms, and use of biophysical agents.[57] Nutritional evaluation including serum albumin and prealbumin levels are needed, although decreased levels may reflect production of inflammatory cytokines, not actual nutritional status. In addition, practitioners should educate caregivers not to massage an area at risk over bony prominences while applying moisturizing lotions or creams because this may increase the risk of breakdown. Overall, improvements in continence care through scheduling toileting every 2 hours and use of skin-protectant barrier creams to help maintain skin health and pressure relief are key to reducing pressure injury.[50]

Diabetic Neuropathic Ulcers

Diabetes is a pandemic health care problem affecting 366 million people globally.[58] Diabetic peripheral neuropathy (DPN) is the most common complication with a lifetime prevalence of 50% with diabetes.[58] The pathophysiology of diabetes leading to a series of vascular, immune, sensory, neurological, and orthopedic changes in older adults can lead to neuropathic foot ulcers. Diabetes is the leading cause of nontraumatic lower extremity amputations in the United States, with approximately 5% with foot ulcers each year and 1% requiring amputation. On a large scale, the annual cost of diabetes in the United States in 2012 was $245 billion, and it has been estimated that about 27% of health care costs of diabetes can be attributed to DPN.[58] In addition, atherosclerosis of large and small vessels results in ischemia of the feet. This arterial compromise damages tissue and limits the healing ability, with occlusive events leading to gangrene. Consequently, diabetic neuropathic ulcers have traits in common with arterial insufficiency and pressure injury on weight-bearing skin of both the dorsum and plantar foot. In addition, diabetes impairs the immune system, allowing bacteria to become entrenched more easily in the wound, making infection harder to fight and leading to limited phagocytosis. Consequences of diabetes, such as nephropathy and impaired vision from retinopathy, can complicate the prevention and treatment of diabetic foot ulcers in older adults. Overall, DPN is an important risk factor for skin breakdown, amputation, and reduced physical mobility. The nonenzymatic glycation predisposes ligaments to stiffness, and loss of coordination and sensation lead to mechanical stresses during ambulation.[59]

The diabetic unholy triad affects sensory, autonomic, and motor nerves, and each has sequelae that contribute to diabetic neuropathic ulcers. Sensory neuropathy prevents the older adult from feeling when something is harming the foot. Practitioners quantifiably test sensation with monofilaments (Fig. 21.8). The 5.07 monofilament

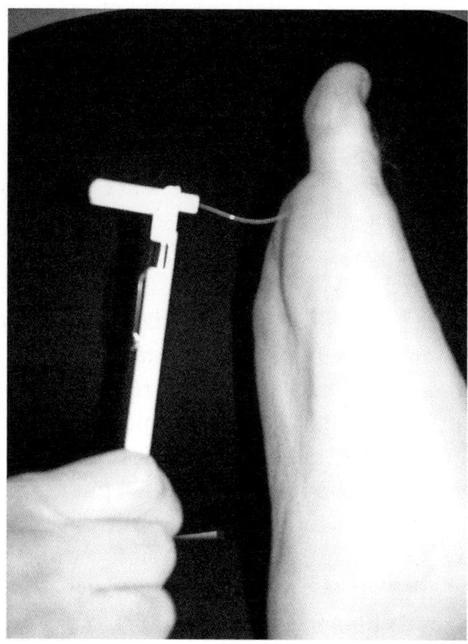

FIG. 21.8 Semmes-Weinstein monofilament test. *(Courtesy of Erica LaPierre, PT, 2009; VNA of CNY, Syracuse, NY.)*

tests for sensitivity to 10 grams of pressure, called protective sensation. This threshold of sensation is only 2% of normal sensation.[60] If a person does not feel 10 grams of force, he or she is more likely to develop an ulceration from pressure from a sock seam or wrinkle, friction from a sandal strap, or even a steel nail through the sole of the shoe. People with diabetes should have their sensation tested with a 5.07 monofilament at least once a year.[61] To maximize the diagnostic value of testing, a three-site test involving the plantar aspects of the great toe, the third metatarsal, and the fifth metatarsal should be used; ankle reflexes are not a reliable way to assess DPN.[62,63] Screening is easily taught and vital in identifying DPN early and can be performed by most health care providers.

Autonomic neuropathy results in reduced perspiration and oil production. The skin on the feet becomes very dry, creating cracking and a route for bacterial entry. Feet with autonomic neuropathy have a greater occurrence of a loss of vasomotor tone, contributing to impaired tissue perfusion.[63] Motor neuropathy leads to muscle atrophy. Musculoskeletal problems arise as structural deformities such as hammertoes then develop from muscle imbalances. Altered foot pressure distribution occurs so that the metatarsal heads press more firmly down onto the walking surface, and the dorsal interphalangeal joints are raised, pressing onto the top of the shoe. The skin breaks down more easily from pressure and friction owing to the skin thinning from arterial insufficiency. The first metatarsal–phalangeal joint stiffens with diabetes, creating a condition called hallux rigidus. Without first metatarsal–phalangeal joint extension, extreme pressure is placed on the plantar hallux, increasing diabetic neuropathic ulcer risk. Diabetes also thins the protective fat pads of the foot, further increasing pressure on the metatarsal heads and the heel.

The prevention and treatment of diabetic neuropathic ulcers must include systemic and local approaches. Metabolic control of diabetes is critical and a key position published by the American Diabetes Association (ADA).[64] Consistent blood sugar control reduces the progression of the diabetic complications. The person's diet must support glycemic control and meet any other needs the person may have, such as proper wound healing. An educational dietary consultation may be necessary to keep tight glycemic control and limit hyperglycemia. Future prospective studies should assess the effect of decreased hemoglobin A1c (HbA1c) levels (the ADA recommends <7%),[64] a reflection of glycemia over 2 to 3 months in the blood, in diabetic wound healing because poor wound healing is associated with hyperglycemia.[65] On the weight-bearing tissue, off-loading is important in relieving pressure for anyone with a foot injury or open sore due to DPN. Non–weight-bearing gait is the best option, yet it is the most difficult to achieve with an older person owing to the strength, balance, and endurance demands. Total contact casting has been considered the gold standard for off-loading, but in recent years, other methods (healing shoe, walking boot, and felt pad) have shown comparable results.[64] Most recently, the evidence for the stress threshold for safe exercise prescription in people with DPN is emerging with proper assessment of all the risk factors in integument, nervous, musculoskeletal, and vascular systems.[66] Although weight-bearing exercise and ambulation with proper foot wear in patients with DPN is recommended, cautionary advice for physical therapists includes special considerations for older adults with DPN to address coexisting medical conditions and functional impairments in hearing, vision, gait, and balance, and limit postural instability and falls in older adults.[66] Overall, physical activity should be encouraged in older adults with DPN with proper screening, assessment, and careful consideration of safety with physical therapist supervision.[66] Lastly, the U.S. Federal Drug Administration (FDA) has issued an ongoing safety review regarding becaplermin (Regranex), a topical recombinant form of human platelet-derived growth factor to treat neuropathic ulcers, owing to a likely increased risk of death from cancer in patients who had used three or more tubes of Regranex, who had a mortality rate five times higher than patients who did not use Regranex.[67]

Arterial and Venous Insufficiency Ulcers

Both arterial and venous insufficiency may manifest in the lower extremity of older adults as ulcerated wounds (Figs. 21.9 and 21.10). According to the American Heart Association (AHA),[68] the risk factors for peripheral arterial disease (PAD) include age >70, history of smoking and/or diabetes, hypertension, stroke, known atherosclerosis and history of claudication, abnormal pulses, obesity, inactivity, and high blood cholesterol. The factors

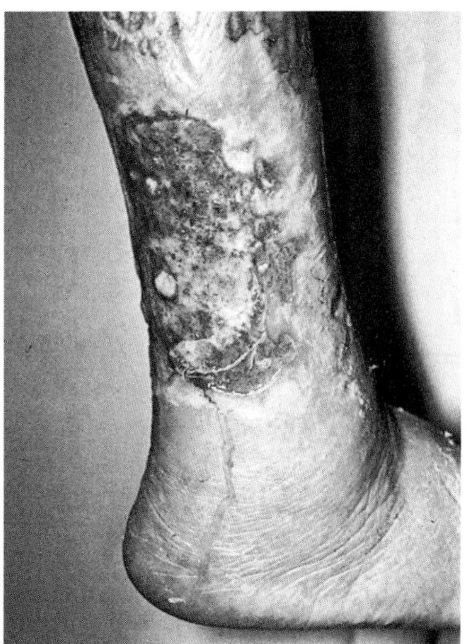

FIG. 21.9 Venous insufficiency ulcer. *(From Kamal A, Brockelhurst JC. Color Atlas of Geriatric Medicine.* 2nd ed. St Louis: Mosby Year Book; 1991.)

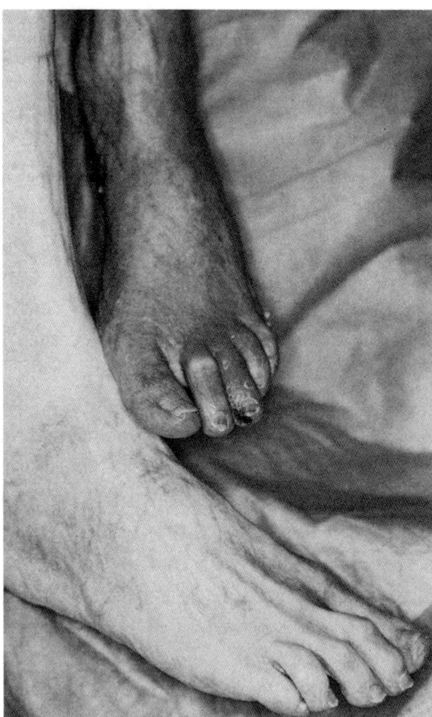

FIG. 21.10 Arterial insufficiency ulcer. *(From Black JM. Medical-Surgical Nursing: Clinical Management for Positive Outcomes.* 8th ed. Philadelphia: Saunders; 2008.)

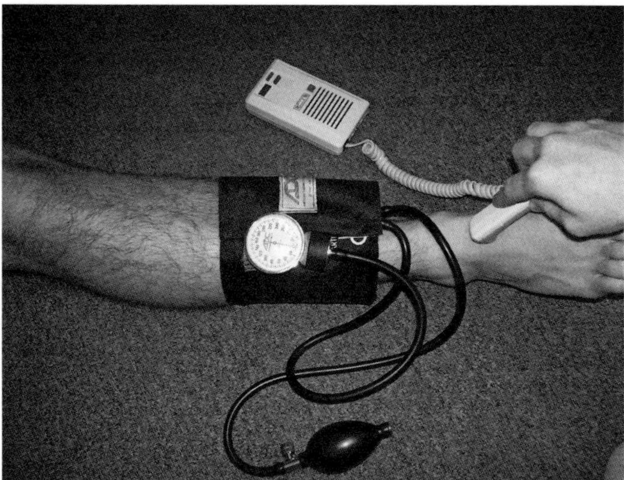

FIG. 21.11 Ankle–brachial index test: blood pressure cuff placement and Doppler ultrasound placement to measure systolic pressure through dorsal pedal pulse. *(Courtesy of Erica LaPierre, PT, 2009; VNA of CNY, Syracuse, NY.)*

leading to venous disease include immobility, ineffective calf muscle pump, venous valve dysfunction from trauma, deep vein thrombosis, and phlebitis.[69] Therefore, common arterial and venous insufficiency leg ulcers occur below the knees.[70] Although most leg ulcers are caused by venous disease alone (72%), arterial insufficiency ulcers are the second most common, ranging from 10% to 30% of lower leg ulcers. Within the venous wounds, 10% to 15% are of mixed arteriovenous etiology with a compromised ankle–brachial index (ABI = 0.5 up to 0.85) (Fig. 21.11).[70] Normal ABI values are between 0.9 and 1.0, and the lower ABI values (<0.5) indicate further compromised arterial insufficiency and difficulty for the wound to heal.[3] Common sites for arterial insufficiency ulcers are over toe joints, under heels, over malleoli, and on anterior shins, whereas venous ulcers occur above the medial and lateral ankles and below the knees.[3] Furthermore, arterial ulcers have minimal drainage with a dry, red wound base, whereas venous ulcers are shallow and have moderate to copious drainage with a yellow gelatinous wound base. Other signs and symptoms of arterial insufficiency ulcer include atrophic skin, diminished or absent pedal dorsal pulses, and pain with activity. Venous insufficiency ulcers tend to have less pain, more edema, and hemosiderin staining due to iron permanently staining the lower calves in a brownish-ruddy color. Table 21.2 provides a differentiation of arterial and venous ulcers.[3]

TABLE 21.2 Wound Differentiation Between Arterial Versus Venous Ulcers

Differentiation	Arterial Ulcers	Venous Ulcers
Location	Tips of or between toes, over the phalangeal heads, or over the lateral malleolus	Near or above medial or lateral malleolus, above malleoli
Drainage	Minimal to slight exudate	Moderate to heavy exudate
Wound margins	Discrete punched out	Irregular borders
Wound appearance	Pale	Hyperpigmentation
Edema	None	Likely
Odor	None	Strong
Pain	Likely	None

(From Gist S, Tio-Matos I, Falzgraf S, Cameron S, Beebe M. Wound care in the geriatric client. *Clin Interv Aging.* 2009;4:269–287.)

The skin relies on steady blood flow from the circulatory system for nourishment, hydration, oxygen, and removal of waste products to remain healthy. In both arterial and venous insufficiency, the systemic circulatory dysfunction manifests itself locally on the lower legs. Simply put, arterial ulcers are due to poor "pipes" in the arterial system, whereas venous ulcers are due to poor "plumbing" in the venous system. For example, arterial insufficiency may cause arteriosclerotic development of plaques that restrict the arterial flow to the body region as well as microthrombi in some of the capillaries in patients with venous leg ulcers. This problem may be located in the small vessels, large vessels, or both. Regardless of the reason for the circulation compromise, the result is the same. Localized ischemia starves the tissue of vital nutrients and oxygen. The tissue begins to necrose, and cells are unable to clear waste products. Therefore, wounds will not heal well owing to poor tissue perfusion. Further, systemic antibiotics will not be able to reach the involved area, so topical treatment may be more appropriate. Prevention and management of arterial insufficiency is crucial for wound healing and preventing recurrence. This includes smoking cessation to slow progression of atherosclerosis and decrease the risk of cardiovascular events, and medical management of the underlying disease (e.g., atherosclerosis, peripheral vascular disease, diabetes, hypertension, hypercholesterolemia). The treatment of arterial ulcers is based on adequate perfusion with risk factor modification and a daily walking program.[70] Compared to the FDA-approved drugs of pentroxifylline (Trental) and cilostazol (Pletal) for promoting blood flow in patients with arterial ulcers or claudication; a supervised exercise program with treadmill or track walking was able to improve the mean change in maximal walking distance greater than the medication alone.[70] To achieve these gains, as the patients improve their walking ability, the exercise workload should be increased to ensure that there is always the stimulus of claudication pain during the workout. As a caution, the practitioner must be watching for the possibility that cardiac signs and symptoms (dysrhythmia, angina, or ST-segment depression) may appear in patients while doing the treadmill or track walking program.[70] Other surgical treatment for arterial ulcers is recommended for patients with rest claudication who are at risk for limb loss.[3] It is the position of the American Physical Therapy Association (APTA) that procedural interventions like sharp selective debridement, which is a component of wound management, is performed exclusively by the physical therapist. Therefore, it would be prudent to review the specific state practice acts with regard to procedural interventions and selected interventions that can be performed by the physical therapist assistant under the direction and supervision of the physical therapist.[71] Lastly, some patients with arterial and venous ulcers (mixed) should wear compression bandages or stockings only with careful and close monitoring by physical therapists.[72]

In venous insufficiency ulcers, the superficial veins, deep veins, or perforator veins may be compromised. Veins have valves that keep the blood flowing in one upward direction. They open for the pulse of blood upward, then close to prevent backflow into a lower segment.[73] Valves may become damaged through thrombophlebitis, deep vein thrombosis, or other trauma. As a result, blood flow becomes bidirectional and downward. Venous hypertension results in vessel bulging, stretching the gaps between vessel wall cells. The microtrauma stimulates leukocyte aggregation, occluding the vessel. Other cells leak from the vessel. Fibrin cuffs form around the vessel wall. The leukocyte occlusion and fibrin cuffs impair perfusion of oxygen from the blood to the tissue. Erythrocytes also leech into the tissue, breaking down to leave iron deposits behind, described earlier as hemosiderin staining. The fluid that escapes from the vessels causes swelling in the lower leg(s). This edema compresses capillaries, further restricting local tissue oxygenation. The gastrocnemius–soleus muscles compress the veins when contracting, and this muscle pump action promotes venous return. Thus, when the muscle pump is insufficient through loss of ankle range of motion, inactivity, or loss of muscle tone, the body is less able to counteract the effects of gravity. Blood can pool in the veins, causing venous hypertension and resulting in vein distention and tissue hypoxia.[73] Without adequate compression to mimic a competent venous system, the underlying problem escalates the condition, worsening the venous insufficiency ulcer.

Venous leg ulcers affect up to 3% of people aged 65 years and older, and these chronic wounds recur at rates of up to 69%.[74] Compression of venous legs must be used for the rest of one's life to reduce the risk of recurrence. Compression stockings at a strength of 30 to 40 mmHg are considered the gold standard of treatment and the most commonly used form of compression to prevent venous insufficiency ulcer recurrence. Compression stockings must be replaced approximately every 6 months, as the elastic degrades and the compressive force weakens. When stockings are worn beyond their lifespan, wounds often recur from the lack of venous support. Older adults with chronic venous insufficiency can further reduce the risk of new ulcerations by elevating the legs and modifying activity (e.g., limiting sitting and standing still) as much as possible while maintaining a prescribed exercise program because gravitational ulcers require elevation.[69] Although managing edema is paramount, venous insufficiency ulcers must be managed with proper moisture-capturing dressings and compression to optimize wound healing for older adults.[75]

Atypical Inflammatory Wounds

Some wounds are created out of inflammatory or autoimmune conditions. Vasculitis is an inflammation of the blood vessels, which may degrade soft tissue and lead to ulcer formation. These exquisitely painful wounds are most commonly located on the lower leg and triggered by underlying infections with palpable purpura. Rheumatoid arthritis can cause leg wounds directly, as well as via small-vessel vasculitis owing to immune complex formation.[76] The inflammation must be halted with medications for the body to progress beyond this phase and begin wound healing. Other wounds are autoimmune in nature. Pyoderma gangrenosum is a poorly understood disease with an unknown etiology, though it is no longer considered to be infectious in origin.[77] It is found almost exclusively in people with a systemic autoimmune disorder, such as Crohn disease, ulcerative colitis, or rheumatoid arthritis. Wounds have an inflammatory appearance and typically enlarge with debridement or other treatments that increase inflammation. These atypical inflammatory wounds present with irregular raised wound margins with round erythema on the legs and chronic wound sites. These atypical wounds may require tissue biopsy and systemic corticosteroids, which necessitates collaborative medical and physical therapy management.

Burns

Aging is associated with delays in thermal sensation, leading to a greater risk of burns, especially while bathing. Animal models in older mice demonstrate slower wound healing from scald wounds[78] owing to limited chemokines as well as comorbid diabetic burn injuries with fewer bone marrow–derived angiogenic cells, diminished hypoxia-inducible factor 1 expression, and dampened homing responses.[79] Older adults, especially those with diabetes with sensory neuropathy, should be encouraged to test water temperature with the hand instead of the more sensory-impaired feet. Even better, turning the water heater to a lower temperature or using safety products (e.g., bath mats, tub thermometers, and color-changing rubber duckies that indicate an unsafe water temperature) may reduce the risk of burns. Burns that extend to large and deep areas of the skin require serious medical attention. Older adults over age 65 have twice the fire death rate as the population as a whole. Adults over age 85 have a fire death rate 3.5 times that of the general population.[80] Older adults may not react as quickly to extinguish a fire or move away from a source of potential burn injury. Furthermore, older adults may take more prescription drugs that may dull the senses and their vision, exposing the individual to risks for fire and burn injury. More importantly, some older adults may have careless attitudes that may increase their risk of experiencing a fire or burn injury. Educating older adults on the leading causes of fire and burns from cooking and scald burn injuries due to faulty electrical wiring, portable heating source, boiling baths, or showers may help alter dangerous attitudes and change unsafe behaviors in older adults. The key to preventing burn injury in older adults is to educate on safety risks and provide resources to older adults.[80] In addition, serious burn injuries should be managed in designated burn centers with available specialty care.[81] Therefore, skin and burn management in older adults must be identified, prevented, and treated in a timely manner by physical therapists.

QUALITY OF LIFE AND FUTURE DIRECTIONS

Older adults who sustain an acute wound injury and who have chronic wounds report physical problems, mental health problems, and cognitive problems.[82] The effect of chronic wounds on quality of life is particularly profound in older individuals.[82] Using the World Health Organization's International Classification of Functioning, Disability, and Health (ICF),[83] physical therapists need to address the profound effect on QOL of acute and chronic wounds because individuals seen in outpatient wound centers have an average of eight comorbid conditions.[82] Recently, exercise has been shown to be paramount in cutaneous wound healing from rodent and human studies.[84] Exercise is a relatively low-cost intervention and it has been shown to speed healing in both aged and obese mice and in older adults.[84] Although little is known about the mechanisms by which exercise speeds wound healing, physical therapists can play a major role in proper supervision of exercise and prevention of harm in older adults with comorbidities and integumentary wound conditions. By addressing the appropriate activity imitations and participation restrictions with proper dosage of exercise and functional activities, physical therapists can assist older adults with improving their QOL and proper wound healing.

Recently, with the health care burden focusing on changing older adults' demographics and chronic medical conditions, key gaps in wound care knowledge and research priorities were addressed by an international meeting of stakeholders in the fields of aging, and wound repair and regeneration in 2015.[82] From this meeting, key research questions and outcomes were generated for future studies[82] (Boxes 21.3 and 21.4). Therefore, it would be prudent for physical therapists to collaborate with a wound care interdisciplinary team to develop appropriate care plans based on research needs and

BOX 21.3 Research Questions for Wound Healing in Older Adults

Category	Research Questions
Epidemiology and quality of life	What is the burden of illness due to chronic wounds in populations of older adults?
	What is the frequency of multiple wounds and recurrent wounds in older adults?
Basic biology of wound healing, chronic wounds, and aging	What causes acute injuries to become chronic wounds?
	How can immune cells in the wound environment, or recruitment of immune cells to the wound, be modulated to harness benefit?
	What strategies can be used to reverse macrophage impairment?
	What factors regulate or activate macrophage phenotypes in wound repair?
	What are the mechanisms underlying endothelial and epidermal stem cell activation and homing to the wound site?
	What are the roles of proliferation and apoptosis in acute versus chronic wounds?
	What are reasons for delayed chemotaxis and lack of neutrophil function in chronic wounds?
	How does neutrophil depletion delay wound closure with advanced age?
	What are the mechanisms for matrix metalloproteinase overproduction with aging in chronic wounds?

(From Gould L, Abadir P, Brem H, et al. Chronic wound repair and healing in older adults: current status and future research. *J Am Geriatr Soc.* 2015;63[3]:427–438.)

BOX 21.4 Potential Outcomes for Clinical Studies of Wound Healing in Older Adults

Synergy between age and comorbidities
Pathology of tissue left behind in the wound
Costs of nonhealing wounds
Goals for healing at the time of wound presentation
Effects of standardized clinical decision support based on electronic medical records
Quality of life
Functional status
Morbidity
Pain
Level of independence
Sepsis
Prevention of amputation and mortality
Palliative care versus healing

(From Gould L, Abadir P, Brem H, et al. Chronic wound repair and healing in older adults: current status and future research. *J Am Geriatr Soc.* 2015;63 [3]:427–438.)

recommendations. By following this chapter's recommendations on skin and wound management for older adults, practitioners can develop solid clinical judgment based on the current evidence and future needs for research in aging and wound healing. Therefore, the carnal beauty of older adults' skin is truly deeper than what meets the eye.

REFERENCES

1. Reddy M. Skin and wound care: important considerations in the older adult. *Adv Skin Wound Care.* 2008;21(9):424–436
2. Farage MA, Miller KW, Elsner P, Maibach HI. Structural characteristics of the aging skin: a review. *Cutan Ocul Toxicol.* 2007;26(4):343–357
3. Gist S, Tio-Matos I, Falzgraf S, Cameron S, Beebe M. Wound care in the geriatric client. *Clin Interv Aging.* 2009;4:269–287
4. Waller JM, Maibach HI. Age and skin structure and function, a quantitative approach (I): blood flow, pH, thickness, and ultrasound echogenicity. *Skin Res Technol.* 2005;11 (4):221–235.
5. Stotts N. Facilitating positive outcomes in older adults with wounds. *Nurs Clin North Am.* 2005;40:267–279.
6. Sanada H, Nakagami G, Koyano Y, Lizaka S, Sugama J. Incidence of skin tears in the extremities among elderly patients at a long-term medical facility in Japan: a prospective cohort study. *Geriatr Gerontol Int.* 2015;15 (8):1058–1063.
7. Ratliff CR, Fletcher KR. Skin tears: a review of the evidence to support prevention and treatment. *Ostomy Wound Manage.* 2007;53(3):32–34.
8. Cordrey R, Lee AC. *Integumentary System: Age-Related Changes and Common Problems.* Madison, WI: Section on Geriatrics of American Physical Therapy Association; November 2006.
9. Skinner AL, Woods A, Stone CJ, Penton-Voak I, Munao MR. Smoking status and attractiveness among exemplar and prototypical identical twins discordant for smoking. *R Soc Open Sci.* 2017;4(12):161076.
10. Sgonc R, Gruber J. Age-related aspects of cutaneous wound healing: a mini-review. *Gerontology.* 2013;59:159–164.
11. Hess CT, Kirsner RS. Orchestrating wound healing: assessing and preparing the wound bed. *Adv Skin Wound Care.* 2003;16(5):246–257.
12. Pittman J. Effect of aging on wound healing: current concepts. *J Wound Ostomy Continence Nurs.* 2007;34(4):412–415.
13. Brown G. Wound documentation: managing risk. *Adv Skin Wound Care.* 2006;19(3):155–165.
14. Mayo Clinic Staff. Malnutrition and seniors: when a relative doesn't eat enough. https://www.mayoclinic.org/healthy-lifestyle/caregivers/in-depth/senior-health/art-20044699. Updated 2018. Accessed April 29, 2018.
15. Cederholm T, Bosaeus I, Barazzoni R, et al. Diagnostic criteria for malnutrition – an ESPEN consensus statement. *Clin Nutr.* 2015;34:335–340.
16. Tappenden KA, Quatrara B, Parkhurst ML, Malone AM, Fanjiang G, Ziegler TR. Critical role of nutrition in improving quality of care. *JPEN J Parenter Enteral Nutr.* 2013;37(4):482–497.
17. Jensen GL, Compher C, Sullivan DH, Mullin GE. Recognizing malnutrition in adults: definitions and characteristics, screening, assessment, and team approach. *JPEN J Parenter Enteral Nutr.* 2013;37(6):802–807.
18. White JV, Guenter P, Jensen G, et al. Consensus statement: Academy of Nutrition and Dietetics and American Society for Parenteral and Enteral Nutrition: characteristics recommended for the identification and documentation of adult malnutrition (undernutrition). *JPEN J Parenter Enteral Nutr.* 2012;36(2):275–283.
19. Gregg D, Hiller L, Fabri P. The need to feed: balancing protein need in a critical ill patient with Fournier's gangrene. *Nutr Clin Pract.* 2016;31(6):790–794.
20. Fischer M, JeVenn A, Hipskind P. Evaluation of muscle and fat loss as diagnostic criteria for malnutrition. *JPEN J Parenter Enteral Nutr.* 2015;30(2):239–248.
21. Mentes J. Oral hydration in older adults: greater awareness is needed in preventing, recognizing, and treating dehydration. *Am J Nurs.* 2006;106(6):40–49.
22. Morgan AL, Masterson MM, Fahlman MM, et al. Hydration status of community-dwelling seniors. *Aging Clin Exp Res.* 2003;15(4):301–304.
23. Clinical symptoms, signs and tests for identification of impending and current water-loss dehydration in older people. Cochrane Review. http://www.cochrane.org/CD009647/RENAL_clinical-symptoms-signs-and-tests-for-identification-of-impending-and-current-water-loss-dehydration-in-older-people. Accessed July 18, 2018.
24. Tricco AC, Antony J, Vafaei A, et al. Seeking effective interventions to treat complex wounds: an overview of systematic reviews. *BMC Med.* 2015;13:89.
25. Posthauer ME. The role of nutrition in wound care. *Adv Skin Wound Care.* 2006;19(1):43–52.
26. Haroun MT. Dry skin in the elderly. *Geriatr Aging.* 2003;6:41–44.
27. Brillhart B. Preventative skin care for older adults. *Geriatr Aging.* 2006;9(5):334–339.
28. Wounds International. Skin tears made easy. http://www.woundsinternational.com/media/issues/515/files/content_10142.pdf. Accessed July 18, 2018.
29. LeBlanc K, Baranoski S. Skin tears: state of the science: consensus statements for the prevention, prediction, assessment, and treatment of skin tears. *Adv Skin Wound Care.* 2011;24(9):2–15.
30. Baranoski S. Skin tears: staying on guard against the enemy of frail skin. *Nursing.* 2000;30(9):41–46.
31. Registered Nurses Association of Ontario. Risk assessment and prevention of pressure ulcers. http://rnao.ca/bpg/guidelines/risk-assessment-and-prevention-pressure-ulcers. Accessed April 27, 2018.

32. Baranoski S. Meeting the challenge of skin tears. *Adv Skin Wound Care.* 2005;18(2):74–75.
33. Loehne HB, Lee AC. The integumentary system. In: Goodman CC, Fuller KS, eds. *Pathology: Implications for the Physical Therapist.* 4th ed. New York: Elsevier; 2015:416–459.
34. National Cancer Institute. Melanoma risk assessment tool. http://www.cancer.gov/melanomarisktool/. Accessed April 29, 2018.
35. National Cancer Institute. Skin cancer screening-for health professionals (PDQ®). http://www.cancer.gov/types/skin/hp/skin-screening-pdq. Accessed April 29, 2018.
36. American Academy of Dermatology. SPOTme skin cancer screenings. https://www.aad.org/public/spot-skin-cancer/programs/screenings. Accessed July 31, 2018.
37. Agullo FJ, Santillan AA, Palladino H, Miller WT. Malignancy in chronic wounds. *Wound Repair Regen.* 2007;15(2):A45.
38. American Academy of Dermatology. Prevent skin cancer. https://www.aad.org/public/spot-skin-cancer/learn-about-skin-cancer/prevent. Accessed May 11, 2018.
39. American Academy of Dermatology. How to care for your skin in your 60s and 70s. https://www.aad.org/public/skin-hair-nails/anti-aging-skin-care/creating-anti-aging-plan/skin-care-in-your-60s-and-70s. Accessed May 11, 2018.
40. Komatsu Y, Okazaki A, Hirahara K, Araki K, Shiohara T. Differences in clinical features and outcomes between group A and group G Streptococcus-induced cellulitis. *Dermatology.* 2015;230(3):244–249.
41. Peterson RA, Polgreen LA, Cavanaugh JE, Polgreen PM. Increasing incidence, cost, and seasonality in patients hospitalized for cellulitis. *Open Forum Infect Dis.* 2017;4(1):ofx008.
42. Center for Disease Control and Prevention. Prevention of herpes zoster. https://www.cdc.gov/mmwr/preview/mmwrhtml/rr5705a1.htm. Accessed July 16, 2018.
43. Scheinfeld N. Infections in the elderly. *Dermatol Online J.* 2005;11(3):8.
44. Center for Disease Control and Prevention. Shingles (Herpes Zoster). https://www.cdc.gov/shingles/surveillance.html. Accessed July 16, 2018.
45. World Health Organization. Scabies. http://www.who.int/lymphatic_filariasis/epidemiology/scabies/en/. Accessed July 16, 2018.
46. Puza CJ, Suresh V. Scabies and pruritus-a historical review. *JAMA Dermatol.* 2018;154(5):536.
47. Gunning K, Pippitt K, Kiraly B, Sayler M. Pediculosis and scabies: treatment update. *Am Fam Physician.* 2012;86(6):535–541.
48. Nussbaum SR, Carter MJ, Fife CE, et al. An economic evaluation of the impact, cost, and Medicare policy implications of chronic nonhealing wounds. *Value Health.* 2018;21(1):27–32.
49. Owens PL, Limcangco R, Barrett ML, Heslin KC, Moore BJ. Patient safety and adverse events, 2011 and 2014. https://www.hcup-us.ahrq.gov/reports/statbriefs/sb237-Patient-Safety-Adverse-Events-2011-2014.jsp?utm_source=AHRQ&utm_medium=EN-616&utm_term=&utm_content=1&utm_campaign=AHRQ_EN5_22_2018. Accessed May 11, 2018.
50. Reddy M, Gill SS, Kalkar SR, et al. Treatment of pressure ulcers. A systematic review. *JAMA.* 2008;300(22):2647–2662.
51. Agency for Healthcare Research and Quality. Preventing pressure ulcers in hospitals. https://www.ahrq.gov/professionals/systems/hospital/pressureulcertoolkit/index.html. Accessed May 17, 2018.
52. Cooper K. Evidence-based prevention of pressure ulcers in the intensive care unit. *Crit Care Nurse.* 2013;33(6):57–66.
53. National Pressure Ulcer Advisory Panel (NPUAP). NPUAP pressure injury stages. http://www.npuap.org/resources/educational-and-clinical-resources/npuap-pressure-injury-stages/. Accessed May 17, 2018.
54. Norton D, Mclaren R, Exton-Smith AN. *An Investigation of Geriatric Nursing Problems in Hospital.* Edinburgh. NY: Churchill Livingstone; 1962.
55. Braden BJ, Bergstrom N. A conceptual schema for the study of the etiology of pressure sores. *Rehabil Nurs.* 1987;12:8–12.
56. McInnes E, Durmville JC, Jammali-Blasi A, Bell-Syer SE. Support surfaces for treating pressure ulcers. *Cochrane Database Syst Rev.* 2011;12:CD009490.
57. National Pressure Ulcer Advisory Panel. Prevention and treatment of pressure ulcers: clinical practice guideline. http://www.internationalguideline.com. Accessed May 11, 2018.
58. Juster-Switlyk K, Smith AG. Updates in diabetic peripheral neuropathy. *F1000Res* 2016;5:F1000.
59. Medscape. Diabetic ulcers. https://emedicine.medscape.com/article/460282-overview. Accessed July 22, 2018.
60. Jeng C, Michelson J, Mizel M. Sensory thresholds of normal human feet. *Foot Ankle Int.* 2000;21:501–504.
61. Conner-Kerr T, Templeton MS. Chronic fall risk among aged individuals with type 2 diabetes. *Ostomy Wound Manage.* 2002;48(3):28–34, 35.
62. Feng Y, Schlosser FJ, Sumpio BE. The Semmes Weinstein monofilament examination as a screening tool for diabetic peripheral neuropathy. *J Vasc Surg.* 2009;50(3):675–682.
63. Al-Geffari M. Comparison of different screening tests for diagnosis of diabetic peripheral neuropathy in primary health care setting. *Int J Health Sci (Qassim).* 2012;6(2):127–134.
64. American Diabetes Association. Standards of medical care in diabetes: 2016. *Diabetes Care.* 2016;39(Suppl 1):S1–S112.
65. Christman AL, Selvin E, Margolis DJ, Lazarus GS, Garza LA. Hemoglobin A1c is a predictor of healing rate in diabetic wounds. *J Invest Dermatol.* 2011;131(10):2121–2127.
66. Kluding PM, Bareiss SK, Hastings M, Marcus RL, Sinacore DR, Mueller MJ. Physical training and activity in people with diabetic peripheral neuropathy: paradigm shift. *Phys Ther.* 2017;97(1):31–43.
67. U.S. Food and Drug Administration. FDA Drug Safety Communication Regranex (becaplermin). http://www.pdr.net/fda-drug-safety-communication/regranex?druglabelid=954&id=5253. Accessed July 22, 2018.
68. American Heart Association. Understand your risk for PAD. https://www.heart.org/en/health-topics/peripheral-artery-disease/understand-your-risk-for-pad#.Vp3JklJPIWs. Accessed July 31, 2018.
69. Etufugh CN, Phillips TJ. Venous ulcers. *Clin Dermatol.* 2007;25(1):121–130.
70. Milani RV, Lavie CJ. The role of exercise training in peripheral arterial disease. *Vasc Med.* 2007;12:351–358.
71. American Physical Therapy Association. Procedural interventions exclusively performed by physical therapists. https://www.apta.org/uploadedFiles/APTAorg/About_Us/Policies/HOD/Practice/ProceduralInterventions.pdf. Accessed on May 25, 2018.
72. Humphreys ML, Stewart AH, Gohel MS, Taylor M, Whyman MR, Poskitt KR. Management of mixed arterial and venous leg ulcers. *Br J Surg.* 2007;94(9):1104–1107.
73. Valencia IC, Falabella A, Kirsner RS, Eaglstein WH. Chronic venous insufficiency and venous leg ulceration. *J Am Acad Dermatol.* 2001;44:401–421.
74. Kapp S, Miller C, Donohue L. The clinical effectiveness of two compression stocking treatments on venous leg ulcer recurrence: a randomized controlled trial. *Int J Lower Extrem Wounds.* 2013;12(3):189–198.

75. Dere K, Opkaku A, Golden A, et al. The 21st century treatment of venous stasis ulcers. *Long-Term Care Interface.* 2006;7:34–37.
76. Jorizzo JL, Daniels JC. Dermatologic conditions reported in patients with rheumatoid arthritis. *J Am Acad Dermatol.* 1983;8:439–457.
77. Ahmadi S, Powell FC. Pyoderma gangrenosum: uncommon presentations. *Clin Dermatol.* 2005;23:612–620.
78. Shallo H, Plackett TP, Heinrich SA, et al. Monocyte chemoattractant protein-1 (MCP-1) and macrophage infiltration into the skin after burn injury in aged mice. *Burns.* 2003;29:641–647.
79. Zhang X, Sarkar K, Rey S, et al. Aging impairs the mobilization and homing of bone marrow-derived angiogenic cells to burn wounds. *J Mol Med.* 2011;89:985–995.
80. American Burn Association. Verification. http://ameriburn.org/quality-care/verification/. Accessed May 11, 2018.
81. American Burn Association. Prevention resources. http://ameriburn.org/prevention/prevention-resources/. Accessed May 23, 2018.
82. Gould L, Abadir P, Brem H, et al. Chronic wound repair and healing in older adults: current status and future research. *J Am Geriatr Soc.* 2015;63(3):427–438.
83. World Health Organization. *The International Classification of Functioning, Disability and Health (ICF).* Geneva, Switzerland: World Health Organization; 2001.
84. Pence BD, Woods JA. Exercise, obesity, and cutaneous wound healing: evidence from rodent and human studies. *Adv Wound Care.* 2012;3(1):71–79.

CHAPTER

22

Management of the Pelvic Floor in Older Men and Women

Cynthia E. Neville

OUTLINE

INTRODUCTION

Pelvic floor disorders are a group of conditions that affect the pelvic floor and include bladder control problems and urinary incontinence (UI), pelvic organ prolapse (POP), bowel control problems, and pelvic pain conditions. Bladder control problems, including urinary incontinence and other lower urinary tract symptoms (LUTS) (e.g., urinary urgency and frequency, nocturia), are prevalent in older adults, affecting around 50% of older women and 25% or more of older men.[1] Urinary urgency and incontinence increase risk of falling in older adults.[2] Functional decline is directly correlated with bladder control problems.[3] Other negative consequences of bladder control problems include decreased work productivity, decreased sexual function,[4] psychosocial problems,[5] decreased quality of life,[6] and negative rehabilitation outcomes, such as increased risk of admission to long-term care.[7] The annual direct and indirect costs of bladder control problems such as overactive bladder in the United States is estimated to exceed $100 billion.[8]

Perhaps because of the changes with age, older adults have the highest prevalence of UI and other LUTS (UI/LUTS) of any group, except for those with specific neurologic diseases.[1] Older women are at greater risk for and have twice the rate of UI and LUTS as men, perhaps because of the effects of vaginal delivery.[9] Vaginal delivery leads to alterations of the anatomy and support structures of the urethra and pelvic organs. UI /LUTS rates are different by setting. For example, upward of 52% of community-dwelling and/or homebound persons over the age of 60 have UI or other LUTS.[10] In long-term care settings, however, 50% to 70% of residents experience UI.[11] UI/LUTS are a common reason for older adults to require long-term care.

UI and LUTS are negative prognostic indicators for rehabilitation outcomes. Therefore, rehabilitation professionals should identify these problems and seek and/or implement appropriate interventions. The prevalence of UI and LUTS indicates that routine screening questions should be included in every history of an older adult. As direct access and primary care professionals, physical therapists have a fiduciary responsibility to provide direct care for the whole person, rather than for a single condition or diagnosis for which the patient seeks care or is referred. Once UI or other LUTS are identified, physical therapists are well qualified to manage this condition and provide education and treatment or to refer the patient with UI or LUTS to another qualified practitioner.

This chapter aims to systematically describe the assessment and intervention options for bladder control problems in older adults that can and should be implemented by all physical therapists. It will discuss the aging of the lower urinary tract (LUT) and the negative impact of bladder control problems on older adults. A review of the normal functions and common dysfunctions of the bladder, lower urinary tract, and pelvic floor muscles is included, as well as a review of the neural control of the LUT and pelvic floor. Explanation and instructions for screening, assessment, and interventions for bladder control problems including UI and other LUTS will prepare the practicing physical therapist to optimize rehabilitation outcomes through the provision of effective evidence-based interventions and/or referral to an appropriate provider for care.

NORMAL BLADDER FUNCTION

Most people take normal bladder function for granted. Normal bladder function means that the bladder will fill, store, and empty on a regular basis. A healthy bladder is pain-free. A healthy bladder does not cause a person to have an overwhelming sensation of the need to urinate, and a healthy bladder never leaks. Adults of any age should be able to sleep through the night without the frequent need to urinate causing waking (nocturia). Bladders should be free of infection and painless during filling, storing, and emptying.[12] The bladder should normally store urine long enough for a person to sit through a concert or a movie for a few hours without having to move to a toilet to empty the bladder. During urination, the healthy bladder will empty completely or normally retain a small postvoid residual volume.

Normal adult bladder function is characterized by cycles of filling with urine, storing of urine, and emptying of urine.[13] The urinary system is made up of the upper and lower tracts. The kidneys and ureters make up the upper urinary tract. The kidneys filter 200 quarts of blood daily to remove excess water and waste products and produce approximately 2 quarts of urine. Urine travels from the kidneys to the bladder through the ureters fairly consistently throughout the day, at about 15 drops per minute. Urine production normally decreases at night but may increase in the aging adult, considered a normal aspect of aging.

The LUT consists of the bladder and urethra (Fig. 22.1). The bladder is a hollow muscular organ, the detrusor muscle, which is lined by mucosa (urothelium) and is sensitive to the volume of urine and its chemical composition. Urine is stored in the bladder until it is emptied through the urethra. During storage, the pressure in the bladder is less than the pressure of the urinary sphincters, which maintain closure of the bladder outlet. Normal functional bladder capacity is 300 to 400 mL of urine.[13] Adults typically store urine for 2 to 5 hours during the day based on the volume and composition of liquid consumed.

Adults who are adequately hydrated empty their bladders approximately five to eight times per day and one time or fewer at night.[12] When the bladder is approximately two-thirds full, a person normally experiences an urge to void. Individuals should be able to defer voiding as needed.[12] The process of emptying the bladder, called urination, is initiated by relaxation of the pelvic floor muscles and the bladder neck. Relaxation of the internal urinary sphincter at the bladder neck and the external urinary sphincter and pelvic floor muscles is promptly

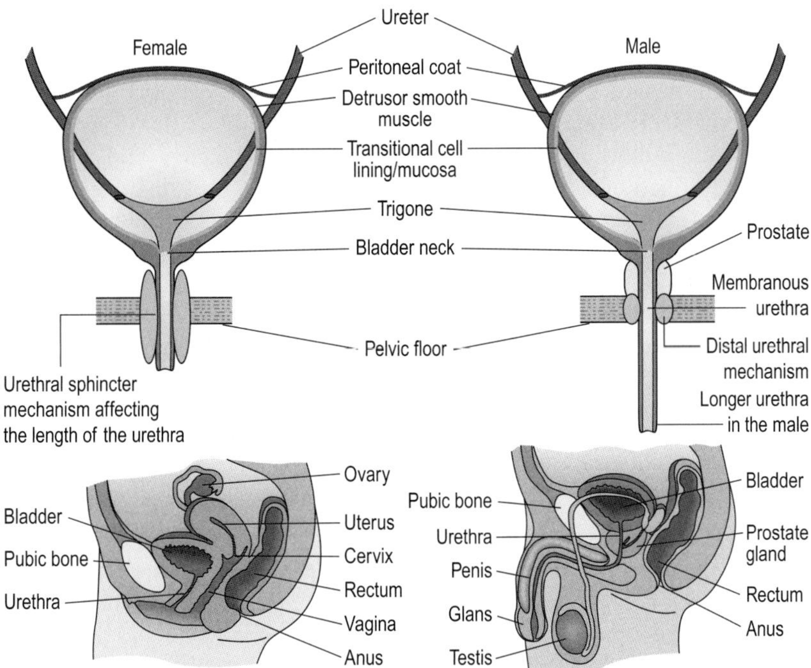

FIG. 22.1 Anatomy of the lower urinary tract in both sexes. *(From Chapple CR. Urodynamics Made Easy. 4th ed. St Louis: Elsevier; 2019.)*

followed by contraction of the detrusor muscle, causing a strong continuous flow of urine and emptying of the bladder called elimination. Bladder emptying is characterized by bladder pressure higher than bladder outlet pressure. The bladder may empty completely, or there may be a residual volume of urine of up to 100 to 200 mL, which may be considered normal.[14]

Neural Control of the Lower Urinary Tract

Bladder control and continence depend on the neural coordination between the bladder, urethra, and pelvic floor muscles (PFMs). Filling and storage of the bladder are mediated by the sympathetic and central nervous systems. As more urine is stored, bladder outlet resistance must increase to maintain continence. For this to occur, bladder afferent nerve endings send information regarding bladder fullness to the dorsal horn of the spinal cord. This information is relayed onto spinal interneurons that activate somatic pudendal and sympathetic hypogastric efferents. Somatic pudendal efferent activation causes contraction of the striated urethral sphincter and increased pelvic diaphragm muscle tone. Coincidentally, activation of sympathetic hypogastric efferents via the hypogastric nerve inhibits detrusor contractions and promotes urethral smooth muscle contraction.[13] Information from bladder stretch receptors is also sent to the pontine continence center, the periaqueductal gray (PAG) matter, and the right anterior cingulate cortex. These areas promote continence by increasing sympathetic efferent activity, bladder compliance, and external urethral sphincter tone; inhibiting parasympathetic activity (activated during voiding); and facilitating pudendal motoneurons.[13] Once a person determines an appropriate time and place to void, afferent signals from the bladder are sent to the PAG matter. The PAG matter coordinates voiding by activating the pontine micturition center (PMC). The PMC activates parasympathetic pelvic efferents to the detrusor via the pelvic nerve, causing the bladder to contract. Coincidentally, sympathetic and somatic efferents to the urethra are inhibited, allowing urethral relaxation and urine flow.[13]

THE PELVIC FLOOR

Bladder control and continence depend on the function of the PFMs, as well as the integrity of anatomic structures that support the pelvic organs and affect urethral pressure. The PFMs include the perineal membrane and levator ani muscles (Fig. 22.2).[15] The perineal membrane is the superficial layer of the PFMs and includes the ischiocavernosus, bulbospongiosus, and superficial transverse perineal muscles. The levator ani group is the deep layer of the PFMs, also known as the pelvic diaphragm. The posterior region consists of the iliococcygeus and coccygeus muscles, which originate from a fibrous band on the pelvic wall called the arcus tendineus levator ani and insert into the central perineal body. Together, they form a relatively flat, horizontal shelf from the pelvic sidewalls on which the pelvic organs rest. The anterior region of the levator ani muscle includes the pubococcygeus and puborectalis muscles. They originate from the pubic bone on either side and form a sling around and behind the rectum. The pubococcygeus muscle attaches to the coccyx via the anococcygeal ligament. It is further delineated into the puboperinealis, pubovaginalis or puboprostaticus/levator prostate, and puboanalis portions. Both the superficial and deep layers of muscle function as a unit during a PFM contraction.

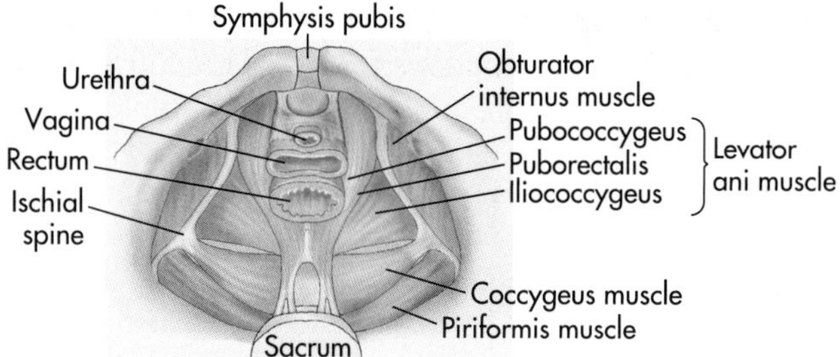

FIG. 22.2 Pelvic floor muscles. *(From Hagen-Ansert SL. Textbook of Diagnostic Sonography. 8th ed. St. Louis, MO: Elsevier; 2018.)*

The three levator ani muscles are tonically active, providing constant support to the pelvic organs.[15] In women, they narrow the urogenital hiatus and draw the urethra, vagina, and rectum toward the pubic bone. In this situation, the supporting connective tissues experience minimal tension. If muscular support is lost, such as denervation from childbirth, deconditioning, or just age, connective tissues can stretch or tear, providing a mechanism for pelvic organ prolapse and/or stress UI. The levator ani muscles can also be contracted voluntarily during abrupt rises in abdominal pressure (as occurs with a cough or sneeze) to stop urine leakage by compressing the urethra against the symphysis pubis or by preventing urethral descent. In both men and women, the striated urethral sphincter plays an important role in continence. It is composed predominately of slow-twitch (type I) muscle fibers. This muscle is constantly active and assists continence during prolonged periods of bladder filling and urine storage.[13]

The anatomic structures of the pelvic ligaments (urethral, cardinal, and uterosacral), endopelvic fascia, and urethral smooth muscle and vascular plexus are important to continence. They maintain anatomic position, which influences organ function. Ligamentous support is integral to the effective functioning of the bladder neck and urethra, as well as the PFMs. Optimal function of the PFMs requires anatomic integrity, motor control, coordination, endurance, power, and mobility of the connective tissue.[16] The pelvic floor muscles have several vital and musculoskeletal functions that are listed in Box 22.1. The PFMs are composed of approximately 30% fast-twitch type II muscle fibers and about 70% slow-twitch type I muscle fibers[13,16] and typically act as a functional unit.[17] The quality of contraction and relative contribution of the different muscle layers may impact voluntary

BOX 22.1 Functions of the Pelvic Floor[20,32,54]

- Bladder control
- Bowel control
- Support of pelvic organs
- Respiration
- Lumbopelvic stability
- Sexual function
- Childbirth

(Livingston[13]; Sapsford et al[20]; Memon and Handa[54])

BOX 22.2 Bladder and Bowel Control Problems Associated with Pelvic Floor Dysfunction

- Urinary incontinence
- Urinary urgency and frequency
- Nocturia
- Incomplete bladder emptying
- Painful urination
- Pelvic organ prolapse
- Fecal incontinence
- Constipation
- Obstructed defecation
- Incomplete bowel emptying
- Painful defecation

control of the pelvic floor. The PFMs contract voluntarily, described as a "squeeze and lift" around the urethra and anus, and the vagina in woman. Magnetic resonance imaging (MRI) studies show approximately 30 degrees of coccyx movement with a maximal concentric contraction of the pelvic floor muscles.[18,19] No other movement of the pelvis or contraction of other muscles (abdominals, gluteal, or adductors) is necessary for the squeeze-and-lift contraction of the pelvic floor muscles. Verbal cueing to engage the contraction around both the anterior (urethral) and posterior (anal) aspects of the PFMs is more effective than cueing only the anterior aspect.[17] In other words, instructing a patient to "squeeze and lift your internal pelvic muscles as if stopping both urine and gas" is most effective at eliciting an effective PFM contraction. Voluntary relaxation occurs after a person stops performing the voluntary contraction. Table 22.1 describes these muscle contractile functions under normal and symptomatic conditions.

Anticipatory control of the pelvic floor involving the involuntary contraction of the PFMs precedes most or all body movement as an automatic co-contraction to increase trunk stability.[20] This should occur automatically in anticipation of increases in intra-abdominal pressure, such as laughing, jumping, coughing, or sneezing. The PFMs maintain position of the bladder neck during increased intra-abdominal pressure.[21] Bladder neck descent may occur if PFM activation is lacking or if anatomic support is compromised. Descent and decompression of the urethra are associated with urine leakage and stress urinary incontinence, and with the eventual development of mixed urinary incontinence. The PFMs must relax to initiate urination. Involuntary relaxation of the PFMs occurs during normal urination, defecation, and vaginal childbirth. Bladder (and bowel) control problems are associated with PFM dysfunctions and are listed in Box 22.2.

BLADDER CONTROL AS A GERIATRIC SYNDROME

Health care providers are often not aware of the individual psychological and social impact of UI/LUTS. Bladder control problems are not similar to having hypertension, which could lead directly to a stroke or heart attack, and death. Instead, UI/LUTS are considered to be a "geriatric syndrome" because many of its risk factors are not directly related to the genitourinary tract. Geriatric

TABLE 22.1 Pelvic Floor Muscle (PFM) Function and Dysfunction

Name of Condition	Description	Symptoms/Diagnosis (Patient Complaints)	Signs/Impairments (Tests, Measures, Observations)
Normal PFM	PFMs are able to contract and relax on command and in response to increased intra-abdominal pressure as appropriate	Normal urinary, bowel, and sexual functioning	Strong or normal voluntary and involuntary contraction Complete relaxation
Underactive PFM	PFMs are unable to contract when needed	Urinary or fecal incontinence, pelvic organ prolapse	Absent or weak voluntary and involuntary PFM contraction Noncontracting PFM
Overactive PFM	PFMs are unable to relax and may contract during functions such as defecation or micturition	Obstructive voiding or defecation (constipation), dyspareunia, pelvic pain	Absent or partial voluntary PFM relaxation Nonrelaxing PFM
Nonfunctioning PFM	No PFM action palpable	Any PFM symptom may be present	Noncontracting, nonrelaxing PFM

syndromes have been defined as "multifactorial health conditions that occur when the accumulated effects of impairments in multiple systems render an older person vulnerable to situational challenges."[22,23] As such, UI and other LUTS are strongly associated with functional decline.[24] The insidious sequalae of bladder control problems are evident in the psychosocial ramifications of fear of an embarrassing incident. As the older person begins to have symptoms that require the use of pads or special garments to avoid embarrassing incidents, the older adult may gradually limit his or her physical and social activities. This limitation may promote deconditioning, a risk for frailty, and a risk for increased infections and falls. It is not uncommon for the older adult to become homebound because of effects of untreated bladder control problems. Elders with UI are twice as likely to feel depressed than those without incontinence.[25] They have higher levels of anxiety and lower scores on quality-of-life measures.[26] Thus, LUTS are associated with embarrassment, stigmatization, social isolation, and depression.[5,27]

Polypharmacy

Another geriatric challenge is polypharmacy that directly and indirectly affects bladder control problems. Medical providers who prescribe pharmaceuticals often prioritize the treatment of other conditions over addressing UI/LUTS, which alters management of LUTS.[28] For example, therapeutic pharmaceutical competition exists such that the treatment for one condition, such as heart failure, may adversely affect a coexisting condition, such as UI.[29] An example of therapeutic competition is when a patient who has heart failure must take a diuretic that iatrogenically contributes to LUTS of urinary urgency, frequency, and incontinence. The presence of certain comorbid conditions and functional impairments listed in Box 22.3 can lead the health care provider to overlook UI/LUTS.[28] Additionally, many pharmaceutical interventions for common comorbid conditions existing in older adults can adversely affect bladder control problems. These drugs are also listed in Box 22.3.

Caregiver Burden

Bladder control problems also can cause a considerable burden on the elder's caregivers.[30] The burden of toileting, dealing with changing and washing clothing and linens, cleaning furniture, and managing irritated skin exposed to urine may become overwhelming. Exposure of the skin and perineum to urine may lead to the development of infections and wounds, requiring further care.[31] All of these factors can lead to incontinence being the "last straw" before a caregiver decides to place his or her loved one or client in a skilled nursing environment, which may explain the relationship between incontinence and institutionalization.[30]

BOX 22.3 Medical Conditions and Drugs That Directly Affect Bladder Function

Medical Conditions
- Congestive heart failure
- Peripheral venous insufficiency
- Renal disease
- Urinary tract infection
- Bladder tumor
- Bladder stones
- Bladder outlet obstruction (prostatic or bladder neck in men; pelvic organ prolapse, bladder neck, or urethra in women)
- Diabetes
- Neurologic conditions
- Radiation therapy

Conditions That Can Precipitate Urinary Incontinence (UI) by Increasing Intra-Abdominal Pressure
- Chronic cough (chronic obstructive lung disease, smoking, asthma, allergies, emphysema)
- Constipation
- Obesity
- Occupation (involving heavy lifting) and/or recreational activities (weight lifting, jogging)

Obstetric History
- Number of pregnancies and deliveries
- Mode of delivery (vaginal vs. cesarean delivery; forceps- or vacuum-assisted vaginal delivery)
- Episiotomy and/or anal sphincter laceration during delivery
- Infant birth weight
- UI/fecal incontinence during or following pregnancy

Gynecologic History
- Menopausal status (including hormone replacement therapy)
- Surgery (hysterectomy, pelvic organ prolapse, and anti-incontinence procedures)

Drugs Adversely Affecting Bladder Control

α-Adrenergic antagonists (α-blockers) for hypertension contract the bladder neck, causing urinary retention and thus overflow urinary incontinence. In men with benign prostatic hyperplasia, these drugs can be used to relax the bladder neck muscles to allow urine to flow more easily.

Angiotensin-converting enzyme (ACE) inhibitors decrease detrusor overactivity and urethral sphincter tone, leading to reduced urge incontinence and increased stress incontinence. A dry cough can occur with the use of an ACE inhibitor, provoking stress incontinence.

Diuretics increase urinary frequency and may cause urinary urgency and incontinence through overwhelming the bladder's capacity.

Antidepressants result in urinary retention and eventually overflow incontinence.

Antipsychotics can cause urinary incontinence through complex pathways that may not occur for weeks after initiation.

Sedative-hypnotics may cause sedation and immobility, leading to functional incontinence.

Anti-Parkinson medications

Estrogen (oral and transdermal)

Antihistamines relax the bladder, causing it to retain urine and cause overflow incontinence.

(Data from https://www.uspharmacist.com/article/druginduced-urinary-incontinence)

Impact on Rehabilitation

UI and LUTS negatively impact rehabilitation outcomes across all levels of care. Patients who have UI and any other orthopedic or neurologic diagnosis in inpatient rehabilitation have lower Functional Independence Measure scores.[7] The presence of UI/LUTS is a negative predictor of functional improvement in home health care.[24] Urinary incontinence predicts disability, rehospitalization, and institutionalization.[32,33] Importantly, the most relevant admission factor related to posthospital physical function at 3, 6, 9, and 12 months was UI.[34]

Falls

The compelling evidence of a positive relationship between UI/LUTS and falls should alert physical therapists to the need for screening and intervention in both institutionalized and community-dwelling adults.[2,23] The relationship between UI and falls may be explained by the fact that people experiencing urinary urgency and urge urinary incontinence feel the need to rush to the toilet/commode.[35] If mobility is impaired, as indicated by slower Timed Up and Go (TUG) scores[36] (or other standardized measures), then the risk of falls increases. Concern about not being able to get to the toilet in time combined with the cognitive demands of multitasking to get to the toilet quickly may negatively affect balance in older people.[37,38] For example, an elder may report having no sense of urge to urinate while sitting, but when he or she stands up, he or she is overwhelmed by the urge to urinate. Multiple tasks must be executed successfully to avoid leaking, including walking to the bathroom, concentrating on not allowing urine flow to start, negotiating household obstacles, undressing before initiating urination, and negotiating the transfer to the commode. As a result, elders commonly fall in the bathroom.[39] Both moderate to severe overactive bladder (OAB) and mild OAB were associated with any falls in a large ($n = 2505$) cross-sectional study of male adults.[40] Overactive bladder symptoms were found to have a greater impact on falls than mobility problems and depressive symptoms. Additionally, two or more incidents of nocturia increased risk of falls and fractures.[41,42] Nocturia in men was consistently shown to be associated with increased risk of any fall in a 2016 systematic review.[43]

AGING OF THE GENITOURINARY SYSTEM

The LUT and genitourinary system undergo predictable changes with aging in both men and women.[44] Decreased circulating estrogen and decreased arterial blood flow associated with menopause are directly responsible for age-related changes in the LUT in women. As a result, thinning of the vaginal mucosa and vaginal wall increases the potential for perineal skin breakdown and contributes to weakening of the connective tissue structures supporting the bladder neck. Decreased bladder neck support may contribute to its hypermobility and result in stress incontinence. Decreased arterial blood flow to the submucosal vasculature and a decrease in the number of striated muscle fibers results in decreased mucosal coaptation of the urethra and a decrease in urethral closure pressure, which may allow the escape of urine, resulting in leakage. Decreased urethral closure pressure may also allow bacteria to enter the urethra. Retrograde movement of bacteria may then be a cause of increased urinary tract infections (UTIs) in aging women.[45]

All older adults experience age-related changes that may impact bladder control. The pelvic floor muscles are subject to sarcopenia and thus muscle weakness.[46] Bladder sensation diminishes significantly with age, so that an older adult may better manage LUTS by urinating at a scheduled time rather than waiting to feel the urge to urinate. Bladder capacity does not change as a result of aging; however, the strength and effectiveness of the detrusor muscle contraction decline with age, and the rate of urine flow may be diminished. The clinical significance of postvoid residual volume and whether it is expected to change with age is not clear.[47]

The circadian rhythm impacting the sleep cycle changes with age. Secretion of the diuretic hormone vasopressin decreases, leading to an increase in nighttime urine production. For this reason, some consider waking up two times per night to be an age-related change and within normal limits,[42] whereas others question whether any amount of nocturia, or waking to urinate, is normal.[48] Though common, nocturia should not be considered normal as two or more episodes of nocturia followed by sleep are associated with poor sleep quality, daytime dizziness, drowsiness, decreased function,[49] and cardiovascular events in addition to falls as mentioned earlier.[42]

In middle-aged men the prostate gland may begin to enlarge, a condition called benign prostatic hyperplasia (BPH).[50] Around half of men over the age of 65 report symptoms related to BPH, in which growth of prostatic tissue begins to encroach on the prostatic urethra. Typical symptoms include increased urgency and frequency of urination and difficulty emptying the bladder or initiating urine flow. BPH can lead to the development of a wide range of LUTS[51]; however, not all LUTS in aging men are a result of BPH.[52]

Lower Urinary Tract Symptoms and Bladder Control Problems

The most common LUTS in older adults are urinary incontinence, urgency and frequency, nocturia, and feeling of incomplete emptying.[1] Urinary urgency is the complaint of a sudden, compelling desire to pass urine that is difficult to defer and often leads to a frequency of urination of more than eight times in a day. Urinary urgency may be caused by an OAB, expressed by the complaint that the bladder does not feel empty after micturition. A patient with this complaint may require a referral for measurement for postvoid residual (PVR). The symptom of

TABLE 22.2 Types of Urinary Incontinence, Definition, and Cause

Type of Urinary Incontinence (UI)	International Continence Society Definition[62]	Cause: Storage Versus Emptying?
Urgency UI	Complaint of involuntary loss of urine associated with urgency	Storage problem due to overactivity of the bladder detrusor muscle contracting
Stress UI	Complaint of involuntary loss of urine on effort or physical exertion (e.g., sporting activities) or on sneezing or coughing	Storage problem due to decreased outlet resistance such as decreased activation, atrophy, or functional impairment of pelvic floor muscles and/or decreased closure of urinary sphincters
Mixed UI	Complaint of involuntary loss of urine associated with both stress and urgency UI	Storage problem (see Urgency UI and Stress UI)
Postural UI	Complaint of involuntary loss of urine associated with change in body position, e.g., rising from a seated or lying position	Storage problem due to decreased outlet resistance during postural change
UI associated with chronic retention of urine	Complaint of involuntary loss of urine, which occurs in conditions where the bladder does not empty completely (formerly known by the term *overflow UI*)	Emptying problem
Functional UI	Complaint of involuntary loss of urine that results from an inability to reach the toilet due to cognitive, functional, or mobility impairments in the presence of an intact lower urinary tract system	Storage problem
Insensible incontinence	Complaint of urinary incontinence where the person has been unaware of how it occurred	Further investigation is warranted

incomplete emptying may or may not be indicative of an elevated PVR volume or other pathology.[53] The basics of screening for medical causes of UI/LUTS listed in Box 22.3 are discussed in a later section. Table 22.2 describes the types of UI and their causes and are further explored next.

Stress Urinary Incontinence. Stress UI can also be referred to as activity-related incontinence. A small amount of urine leaks during an increase in intra-abdominal pressure. As mentioned earlier, a history of having a vaginal delivery is one factor that predisposes women to stress UI.[54] Although the exact relationship between pregnancy/childbirth and stress UI is unclear, it is typically attributed to pudendal nerve injury, stretching/tearing of the pelvic ligaments and/or levator ani muscles, or damage to the urethra.[55] Trauma caused by the passage of the fetal head and body through the vaginal canal may lead to a loss of anatomic support (levator ani muscles, endopelvic fascia, and pelvic ligaments) to the proximal urethra. This loss of anatomic support is one mechanism of female stress UI. Without support, the bladder neck and/or urethra descend and decompress during increases in intra-abdominal pressure. The urethra then cannot be sufficiently compressed or closed, abdominal pressure exceeds urethral pressure, and leakage of urine occurs.[56] After the age of 60 years, other stress UI risk factors and/or age-related physiological changes in muscle and connective tissue, such as the changes in the quality of collagen and loss of elasticity, play a greater role in the development of stress UI in older women.[10] Reported risk factors for female stress UI include age, estrogen loss, Caucasian race, family history of stress UI, obesity, smoking, chronic cough/respiratory disease, pelvic surgery, chronic constipation, and neurologic disorders.[57]

Men with prostate cancer who undergo radical prostatectomy (RP) are at great risk of developing some form of UI. At least 50% of men experience UI immediately following this procedure.[58] Following RP, the proximal urethral sphincter, consisting of the bladder neck, prostate, and prostatic (proximal) urethra, is removed. Consequently, continence depends on the integrity of the rhabdosphincter, the distal urethral sphincter. Stress UI following RP is largely attributed to incompetence of the rhabdosphincter. Surgery-related scar tissue, pudendal nerve injury, reduced sphincter mobility secondary to scar tissues, an underdeveloped/weak distal sphincter, and/or weak PFMs are considered possible causes of rhabdosphincter incompetence following RP. Although the incidence of UI decreases over time, those men who remain incontinent report a negative impact on their quality of life.[51]

Urge Urinary Incontinence. An estimated one-third of persons with OAB,[59] characterized by feelings of urinary urgency and frequency of urination, also suffer from urge UI. OAB is defined as urgency, with or without urge UI, usually with frequency and nocturia. People with OAB experience a sudden strong urge to urinate and may leak a moderate to large volume of urine before reaching the toilet. Overactive bladder symptoms can be caused by low bladder compliance (a high rise in bladder pressure during bladder filling) and/or detrusor overactivity (the presence of involuntary bladder contractions during the filling phase). The exact cause of urge UI in many cases is unknown.[60] Detrusor overactivity can occur owing to idiopathic, neurogenic (associated with a neurologic condition, such as stroke, Parkinson disease, multiple sclerosis, brain injury or tumor, spinal cord injury or tumor, or diabetes mellitus), or nonneurogenic (bladder infection, bladder outlet obstruction, bladder tumors, bladder stones, and aging) causes. In women with a history of stress UI, chronic decompression of the proximal urethra may lead to a decrease in detrusor muscle inhibition and urge UI, resulting in "mixed UI"—a combination of stress and urge UI symptoms. Urethral obstruction secondary to POP may lead to detrusor muscle changes and subsequently detrusor overactivity. Other factors associated with female OAB and/or urge UI include advancing age, hysterectomy, caffeine intake >400 mg/day (about 2.5 cups),[61] consumption of carbonated drinks, obesity, arthritis, and impaired mobility and/or impaired activities of daily living.[62] In men, obstruction caused by benign or malignant prostatic enlargement can result in OAB by altering bladder physiology or neural regulation, restricting bladder emptying, and/or affecting PFM strength. Following surgical removal of the obstruction (as in RP), the bladder may continue to be overactive, potentially causing postsurgical urge UI.[63]

URINARY TRACT INFECTIONS AND URINARY RETENTION

UTIs are a common medical condition in the older adult population affecting 20% in the community and over 50% of institutionalized elders.[64] They are more common in women because the female urethra is shorter and bacteria from the vagina and rectum may contaminate the distal third of the urethra. A simple preventative measure is to wipe from front to back and then drop the toilet paper after urination to avoid contamination of the urethra. Another contributing factor to UTIs is urinary retention allowing residual urine to colonize bacteria. During intercourse, bacteria are introduced into the urethra and bladder. Additionally, changes in the vaginal flora secondary to estrogen depletion lead to bacterial colonization of the urethra and bladder. Younger women may experience acute UTI symptoms of dysuria (painful urination), urinary urgency and frequency, suprapubic pain, and hematuria (red blood cells in the urine). However, UTIs in older adults may present atypically with symptoms such as confusion, delirium, and falls.[65] They may not experience the discomfort of a UTI common to younger women. Therefore, UTI in an older woman should be suspected with any

TABLE 22.3 Clinical Presentation and Severity of Urinary Tract Infection (UTI)[67]

Clinical Features	Type of UTI
No urinary symptoms in the presence of bacteria	Asymptomatic bacteriuria
Dysuria, urinary urgency, urinary frequency, nocturia, suprapubic pain	Acute UTI
Flank pain, unilateral costovertebral tenderness, ipsilateral shoulder pain, fever and chills, skin hypersensitivity (hyperesthesia of dermatomes)	Acute pyelonephritis

sudden change in cognition or urinary frequency. Clinical features of UTIs are listed in Table 22.3. The onset of a UTI may be more difficult to recognize in a patient who already has other LUTS, such as urinary urgency and frequency, because UTIs share similar symptoms.[1] Questions that should raise suspicion of a UTI requiring referral to a physician are listed in Table 22.4.

Older women are at increased risk for recurrent UTIs, defined as three or more episodes of UTI in 12 months. Medical management of UTIs is complex and controversial because UTIs are often misdiagnosed and medically mistreated.[66] Asymptomatic bacteriuria is common on older women and may not always need to be treated with antibiotics.[65] Symptomatic UTIs are diagnosed with urine dipstick testing for nitrites and leukocytes, and by urine culture to isolate the causative organism. Recurrent UTIs may need to be treated with prophylactic antibiotics.

TABLE 22.4 Red Flag Questions for Medical Screening for Urinary Incontinence *(Positive response indicates the need for physician referral)*

Questions	Possible Medical Concern
Was there a sudden onset of incontinence?	Infection
Did leaking occur after surgery or with a medication change?	Incontinence as unexpected side effect of surgery or medication
Is there burning/blood with urine/stool?	Infection
Is there a change in vaginal discharge? Odor?	Infection, atrophic vaginitis
Is there difficulty initiating the stream?	Acute urinary retention
Are there moderate/large amounts of incontinence without warning?	Diabetes, heart failure, venous insufficiency, hypercalcemia, hyperglycemia
Is there an acute change in mental status?	Infection

Intravaginal estrogen may be prescribed for women with recurrent UTIs to decrease vaginal pH and reverse microbiological changes in the vagina following menopause.[67]

Urinary retention is the inability to empty the bladder completely and can be acute or chronic. Acute urinary retention happens suddenly. People with acute urinary retention cannot urinate at all, even though they have a full bladder. Acute urinary retention can cause great discomfort or severe suprapubic pain and is a potentially life-threatening medical condition requiring immediate emergency treatment. Urinary retention is diagnosed by bladder ultrasound or catheterization to determine the postvoid residual volume left in the bladder after an attempt to urinate.

Incomplete bladder emptying can be caused by a chronic condition. Remarkably, a postvoid residual volume of urine of up to 100 to 200 mL in older adults may be considered normal.[14] Often people are not even aware they have this condition until they develop another problem, such as UI or a UTI.

IDENTIFICATION, SCREENING, AND ASSESSMENT OF BLADDER CONTROL PROBLEMS

Screening

In health care and rehabilitation settings, screening for UI/LUTS in older adults should be a routine component of every physical therapy evaluation. In the absence of a verbal patient history, a variety of indicators of bladder control problems are often readily identifiable in the course of routine review of the patient's medical record and history. Patients may have a documented preexisting diagnosis of urinary incontinence. The patient may be taking medications for UI/LUTS (see http://emedicine.medscape.com/article/452289-medication#showall for more information). The observant clinician may also be able to detect that a patient is experiencing bladder control problems by noticing environmental and contextual cues. For example, the person may choose to wear dark polyester pants to hide wet spots and stains. The physical therapist may notice pads or garment products in the person's home or room, and the therapist may notice that he or she is wearing a garment or pad. Sometimes, there may be an odor about a person who is experiencing incontinence.

Patient Interview and History Taking

When evaluating a patient for UI/LUTS, a thorough medical history should be taken from the patient and/or primary caregiver. The history should review medical conditions that influence bladder function directly and conditions and/or lifestyle factors that precipitate UI (see Box 22.3). Surgical history, including urethral, bladder, bowel, rectal, obstetric and gynecological (female), and prostate (males), should be obtained. Conditions that may limit physical activity, such as arthritis or pain, should be discussed, as impaired mobility and activities of daily living are risk factors for UI.

Medications should be reviewed, including those that alter cognition, fluid balance, and bladder and/or sphincter function. Through various mechanisms, medications can directly affect urinary function. For example, antihypertensive medication, neuroleptics, and benzodiazepines can reduce urethral pressure. Diuretics are known to increase the production of urine. Anticholinergic medications and β-blockers may affect one's ability to empty the bladder completely. Other medications can affect urinary function indirectly via their side effects. Constipation, a risk factor for stress UI, is a side effect associated with narcotic analgesic and iron use. Another risk factor for stress UI, a dry cough, is a side effect of angiotensin-converting enzyme (ACE) inhibitors.[68]

A bladder symptom history identifies onset, type, frequency, and severity of symptoms; precipitating factors; and need for further medical evaluation. Key questions of a bladder symptom history are found in Table 22.5. The International Consultation on Incontinence Modular Questionnaire-Urinary Incontinence Short Form (ICIQ-UI SF) found in Fig. 22.3 is a 4-item questionnaire that can be used to identify, quantify, and characterize UI/LUTS. Further information about the ICIQ-UI SF is shared in the section on Outcome Measures later in this chapter. Red flag conditions described in Table 22.4 should also be obtained. Patients should be asked whether or not they experience regular constipation, as it is a known risk factor for stress UI.[57] Double incontinence, when a person experiences both UI and fecal incontinence at least once a month, has been reported to occur in about 8% of women and 5% of men with UI.[69]

Patients should be asked about their daily fluid intake. Adults should drink at least six to eight 8-oz drinks per day, or half an ounce of fluids per pound of body weight.[70] A bladder diary can be used to quantify bladder function, including voiding frequency, volume of each void, number of UI episodes per day, sensations such as the intensity of urgency leading to leakage or to voiding, the size or severity of each UI episode, and daily pad usage.[53] A 3-day bladder diary has been shown to be superior to 7-day recording.[71] For someone with UI/LUTS, drinking enough water to make up half of the daily fluid intake may serve to dilute and reduce irritability of other fluids, such as coffee. Restricting fluids is a common coping strategy used by elders with UI/LUTS to reduce urinary frequency, urgency, and incontinence. Yet, reducing fluids may lead to dehydration, increased concentration of bladder irritants in the bladder, and/or constipation or urinary tract infection, and paradoxically make symptoms worse. Conversely, a patient may report excessive fluid intake, which may increase urinary urgency, frequency, and UI. Patient and caregiver education is critical to optimize fluid management for continence and bladder health. A patient education sheet about bladder health prepared by the author for general use that describes

TABLE 22.5 Key Questions to Include in the Initial Assessment of UI/LUTS[53]

Circumstances Surrounding UI/LUTS Symptoms	Implications
*Never—urine does not leak	No incontinence; consider asking about other LUTS
Leaks before you can get to the toilet? Feel an urge to urinate that is so sudden and strong that you don't make it to the bathroom in time?	Urgency UI, increased risk for falls
Leaks when you cough or sneeze?	Stress UI
Leaks when you are asleep?	Enuresis—bladder contracts during sleep
Urge to urinate wakes you up from sleep to urinate during the night? If yes, how many times?	OAB, increased fall risk for waking more than one time per night
Leaks when you are physically active/exercising?	Stress UI
Leaks when you have finished urinating and are dressed?	Stress UI or urge UI
Leaks for no obvious reason?	Needs further investigation
Leaks all the time?	Needs further investigation
Are you wearing pads or garments? How many do you use in a day?	Severity of leakage, risk for UTI and skin breakdown
What type of fluids do you drink? How much? Do you drink any water?	Lifestyle factors contributing to symptoms, risk for dehydration
Pain with urination?	Possible UTI
Need to strain to empty?	Possible urethral obstruction, incomplete emptying, or urinary retention
(Female) Feeling of bulging in the vagina?	Possible pelvic organ prolapse

LUTS, lower urinary tract symptoms; *OAB*, overactive bladder; *UI*, urinary incontinence; *UTI*, urinary tract infection. (Copyright Cynthia E. Neville)

the kind of information valuable to the patient and caregiver is located in Box 22.4.

Taking a Bladder History. Discussing the sensitive topic of bladder control problems can be uncomfortable for physical therapists not accustomed to the types of questions inherent in a bladder history. Incorporating routine questions, asked in a sensitive manner of every older adult, will quickly develop confidence and comfort in formally screening patients for the presence of UI/LUTS. Patients often do not disclose their LUT symptoms without being specifically asked because UI/LUTS are associated with embarrassment. By phrasing questions in ways that avoid embarrassment and preserve the patient's dignity, the physical therapist may more effectively gain important information. For example, the word *incontinent* may be frightening or offensive to the patient. He or she may think that incontinence means a complete lack of bowel and bladder control. Instead of asking if a person is incontinent, the therapist might ask, "Do you ever leak urine when you cough or sneeze or during exercise?" Leakage is a very common symptom and the patient may be more likely to answer yes and engage in further discussion about symptoms. Key questions and their possible implications to include in the initial assessment of UI/LUTS are listed in Table 22.5.

Although it is true that symptoms alone cannot be used to make a definitive medical diagnosis of specific lower urinary tract condition, internationally agreed-upon guidelines support the fact that conservative therapies may be started for urgency, stress, and mixed incontinence[53] and for bothersome LUTS such as urinary frequency without a formal diagnosis. Physical therapists can and should confidently develop an assessment of the type and severity of bladder control problem. Further medical testing for definitive diagnosis is not necessary or required to begin basic treatments, unless there is a suspicion of a UTI.

Physical Examination

Box 22.5 summarizes the components of the physical therapist examination of persons with UI/LUTS and suspected pelvic floor muscle dysfunction. All licensed physical therapists can perform external examination procedures to evaluate pelvic floor and abdominal muscle function. This includes external observation of pelvic floor muscle contraction and external palpation of pelvic floor muscle contraction (Fig. 22.4). However, not all physical therapists have undergone specific training in the internal examination and evaluation of pelvic floor muscle function and dysfunction. Internal (vaginal and rectal) examination of the pelvic floor is consistent with description of physical therapist practice in all 50 states in the United States but is generally regarded as an advanced practitioner skill and is not taught in entry-level education programs. It is strongly recommended that physical therapists undergo specific training in the internal vaginal and anorectal examination of the pelvic floor prior to performing these examinations on patients/clients. For clients with pelvic pain and/or additional musculoskeletal complaints or conditions, a comprehensive examination of the spine, pelvis, and hips is warranted.

Pelvic Floor Muscle Palpation and Testing

The purpose of pelvic floor muscle palpation is to assess the ability of the patient to contract and relax the PFMs correctly, to assess other elements of PFMs such as tone and pain, and to measure both the power of the contraction and the elevation of the pelvic floor muscles. Two

ICIQ-UI Short Form

Initial number

CONFIDENTIAL

DAY MONTH YEAR
Today's date

Many people leak urine some of the time. We are trying to find out how many people leak urine, and how much this bothers them. We would be grateful if you could answer the following questions, thinking about how you have been, on average, over the PAST FOUR WEEKS.

1 Please write in your date of birth: DAY MONTH YEAR

2 Are you *(tick one)*: Female ☐ Male ☐

3 How often do you leak urine? *(Tick one box)*

never	☐	0
about once a week or less often	☐	1
two or three times a week	☐	2
about once a day	☐	3
several times a day	☐	4
all the time	☐	5

4 We would like to know how much urine <u>you think</u> leaks.
How much urine do you <u>usually</u> leak (whether you wear protection or not)?
(Tick one box)

none	☐	0
a small amount	☐	2
a moderate amount	☐	4
a large amount	☐	6

5 Overall, how much does leaking urine interfere with your everyday life?
Please ring a number between 0 (not at all) and 10 (a great deal)

0 1 2 3 4 5 6 7 8 9 **10**
not at all a great deal

ICIQ score: sum scores 3+4+5 ☐☐

6 When does urine leak? *(Please tick all that apply to you)*

- never – urine does not leak ☐
- leaks before you can get to the toilet ☐
- leaks when you cough or sneeze ☐
- leaks when you are asleep ☐
- leaks when you are physically active/exercising ☐
- leaks when you have finished urinating and are dressed ☐
- leaks for no obvious reason ☐
- leaks all the time ☐

Thank you very much for answering these questions.

FIG. 22.3 International Consultation on Incontinence Modular Questionnaire-Urinary Incontinence Short Form (ICIQ-UI SF). Diagnostic questions of the ICIQ-UI SF Question #4: When does urine leak?

scales, the Brink scale[72] and Modified Oxford Grading Scale,[73] have been described for grading PFM function through digital palpation. The Brink scale is based on three muscle contraction variables: intensity of the "squeeze" generated by the muscle contraction, vertical displacement of the examiner's two fingers as the muscles lateral to the vagina contract, and muscle contraction duration. Each variable is rated separately on a 4-point categorical scale. The three subscale scores are summed to obtain a composite score. The Brink scale does not discriminate between right and left pelvic floor muscle contraction. The Modified Oxford Scale uses a 6-point numerical scale to grade PFM contraction. Vaginal or rectal digital palpation is performed and muscle strength is graded on the right and the left using this scale. The Modified Oxford Grading Scale may be applied to digital rectal PFM examination; however, this scale has not been validated when performed via the anorectum. Studies reporting

BOX 22.4 **Patient and Caregiver Information About Bladder Health**

What Is Considered Normal?

- The bladder's job is to fill with urine, store it, and then empty on a regular basis.
- The normal range of voiding urine is six to eight times during a 24-hour period. As we get older, we may need to pass urine more frequently but usually not more than every 2 hours.
- The average bladder can hold about 2 cups of urine before it needs to be emptied.
- Urine should flow easily without discomfort in a good, steady stream until the bladder is fully or almost completely empty.
- No pushing or straining is necessary to empty the bladder.
- An "urge" is a signal that you feel as the bladder stretches to fill with urine. Urges can be felt even if the bladder is not full. Urges are NOT commands to go to the toilet. An urge is merely a signal and can be controlled.

What Are Good Bladder Habits?

- Take your time when emptying your bladder. Don't strain or push to empty your bladder.
- Allow your bladder to empty completely each time you urinate. Do not rush the process or stop before emptying is finished. (Note: It is normal for many people to have some urine left in the bladder after urination.)
- Try not to ignore your bladder. Do not wait for more than 4 hours between toileting during the day.
- Try not to urinate too frequently. Avoid going to the toilet more often than every 2 hours and avoid going "just in case." Try to go only when your bladder is full.
- It is usually not necessary to go when you feel the first urge to urinate. Urgency and frequency of urination can be improved by retraining the bladder and spacing your fluid intake throughout the day.
- After urinating, women should wipe from front to back and then drop the tissue in the toilet to decrease the chance of getting a urinary tract infection.
- Maintain good bladder habits, and don't let your bladder control your life!

Tips to Maintain Good Bladder Habits

- Stay hydrated and maintain a good fluid intake starting early in the day. Depending on your body size and environment, drink 4 to 8 cups (8 oz each) of fluid per day unless otherwise advised by your doctor. Half of the fluids that you drink should be water or water-like. Not drinking enough fluid concentrates urine, making it more irritating, and may create a foul odor and dark color of the urine.
- Limit the amount of caffeine (coffee, cola, chocolate, or tea) and citrus fruit juices and fruits that you consume as these drinks and foods can irritate the bladder and be associated with increased sensation of urinary urgency and frequency.
- Limit the amount of alcohol you drink. Alcohol increases urine production and also makes it difficult for the brain to coordinate bladder control.
- Stop drinking 2 to 3 hours before going to sleep to decrease the chance that bladder urges will wake you up and disrupt your sleep.
- Avoid constipation by maintaining a balanced diet of dietary fiber, drinking enough water, and getting regular cardiovascular exercise.

BOX 22.5 **Components of a Basic Physical Examination for Persons with Urinary Incontinence**

General Examination

- Observation for lower extremity edema
- Lower extremity functional strength and joint mobility
- Lower extremity neurological screening examination: reflexes, myotome and dermatome testing
- Functional mobility

Specific Examination of Female Clients

Perineal Observation

- Perineal skin for inflammation, excessive vaginal discharge, lesions, scars
- Demonstration of pelvic floor muscle voluntary and involuntary contraction and relaxation

External Examination

- Sensation around the perineum
- Palpation to identify painful tissues
- Sacral reflexes: anal wink, bulbocavernosal reflex

Internal Examination (After Medical Clearance Postsurgery)

- Sensation within the vagina
- Palpation to identify painful tissues
- Pelvic floor muscle bulk right and left
- Pelvic floor muscle contraction right and left
- Pelvic floor muscle function testing
- Pelvic floor muscle manual muscle test or Brink score
- Examine rectally if no contraction palpable vaginally
- Presence and quantification of pelvic organ prolapse

Specific Examination of Male Clients

Genital Observation

- Irritation of skin or skin breakdown on penis from urine exposure, genital lesions
- Demonstration of pelvic floor muscle voluntary and involuntary contraction and relaxation contraction

External Examination

- Perineal and perianal sensation
- Sacral reflexes: anal wink, bulbocavernosal reflex

Rectal Examination (After Medical Clearance Postsurgery)

- Pelvic floor muscle contraction right and left
- Pelvic floor muscle function testing
- Pelvic floor muscle manual muscle test

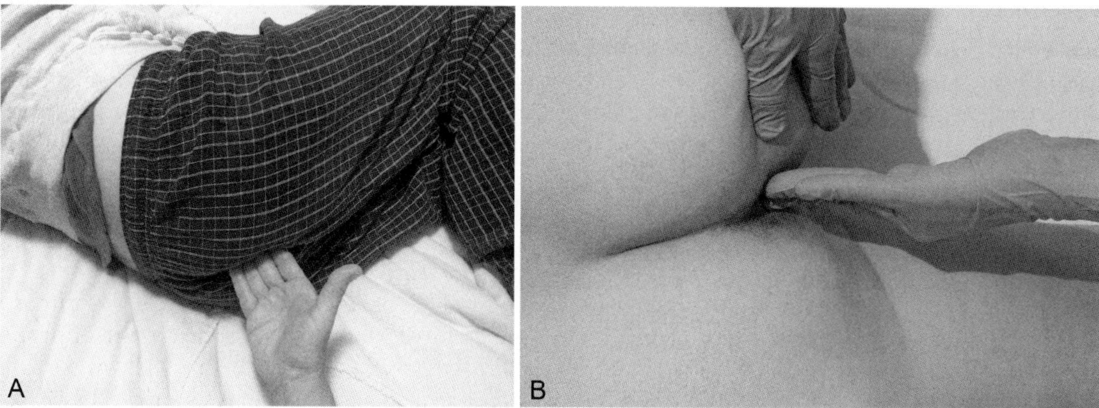

FIG. 22.4 External palpation of the pelvic floor muscle (PFM): Palpation of the levator ani externally placing fingertips between the external anal sphincter and ischial tuberosity (ischiorectal fossa). During levator ani muscle contraction the muscle elevates and pushes fingertips out of the ischiorectal fossa space. **A,** Palpation through clothing. **B,** External perineal palpation. © *Cynthia E. Neville.*

inter- and intrarater reliability for the Modified Oxford Grading Scale for vaginal palpation are conflicting[74] and therefore this method may not be robust enough to be used for scientific purposes to measure muscle strength. However, this method is recommended as a good technique for physical therapists to understand, teach, and give feedback to patients about their ability to perform PFM contraction correctly.

Outcome Measures

LUTS and health-related quality of life (HRQOL) can be measured with condition-specific standardized assessment tools. These tools can also be used to measure change in symptoms and quality of life before and after intervention and to demonstrate the outcome or efficacy of the physical therapy interventions for UI/LUTS. Therefore, they are optimally administered pre- and postintervention. A review of studies using outcome measures after surgery for incontinence found over 42 different measures used, indicating a lack of uniformity in outcome reporting in the research.[75] The validated tools described to follow are clinically useful and are commonly used in PT practice.

The *International Consultation on Incontinence Modular Questionnaire-Urinary Incontinence Short Form (ICIQ-UI SF)* is a 4-item self-report measure used to assess the impact of UI symptoms on quality of life as well as symptom severity. This measure assesses frequency of UI, amount of leakage, and overall impact of UI. The fourth question of the ICIQ-UI SF provides a specific symptoms checklist, which can be of use to the evaluating clinician to develop an understanding of the circumstances surrounding bladder symptoms (Fig. 22.3). The total score of the ICIQ-UI SF ranges from 0 to 21, with greater scores indicative of increased symptom severity and impact.[76] The ICIQ-UI SF demonstrates good construct validity and reliability.[77] The minimum clinical important difference (MCID) for a population of adult women with stress incontinence is a decrease of 2.52 points at 4 months,[77] a decrease of 5 points at 12 months, and a decrease of 4 points at 24 months.[78]

The Pelvic Floor Distress Inventory (PFDI) measures urinary, colorectal (bowel), and pelvic organ prolapse symptoms.[79] Its companion measure, the Pelvic Floor Impact Questionnaire (PFIQ), measures the impact of these symptoms on HRQOL. Both the PFDI and PFIQ were found to be internally consistent, reliable, and valid and to demonstrate responsiveness in women undergoing surgery for a variety of pelvic floor disorders.[79] As the PFDI and PFIQ are quite lengthy, shorter versions (PFDI-20 and PFIQ-7) were developed and also found to have good reliability, validity, and responsiveness.[80] In addition, based on global ratings of improvement defined as at least "a little better" after surgery for pelvic floor disorders, a change of 45 points on the PFDI-20 summary score (summary of the three scale scores) and a change of 36 points on the PFIQ-7 summary score were found to be clinically important.[81]

The American Urological Association Symptom Index (AUA-SI) is a 7-item self-report measure used to assess urinary urgency, frequency, and voiding symptoms.[82,83] The total score of 0 to 35 is used to assess symptom severity, where <8 indicates mild symptoms, 8 to 19 indicates moderate symptoms, and 19+ indicates severe symptoms. There is no established MCID.

INTERVENTIONS

Physical therapists can initiate conservative therapies immediately for urgency incontinence, stress incontinence, mixed incontinence,[53] and bothersome LUTS such as nocturia and urinary frequency, even in the absence of a definitive medical diagnosis or specific referral to physical therapy for treatment of symptoms as mentioned earlier. Interventions can be initiated based on patient report of LUTS and/or assessment of pelvic floor muscle impairments of an inability to contract and relax, endurance, and coordination. Interventions should be initiated immediately if there is a suspicion that UI/LUTS and/or pelvic floor dysfunction are causing or contributing to fall risk or other neuromusculoskeletal impairments. Medical testing for definitive diagnosis of UI/LUTS such as urodynamic evaluation by a urologist or urogynecologist is not necessary or required to begin basic treatment interventions for UI/LUTS.

The role of regular physical activity cannot be emphasized enough, for general health and well-being as well as for pelvic floor health. The recommendations of a minimum of 150 minutes/week of moderate-intense aerobic activity and resistive exercises that allow 8 to 13 repetitions to volitional fatigue on 2 or more days per week are widely accepted. Because skeletal muscle requires an adequate supply of oxygen, adenosine triphosphate (ATP), and nutrients for contractile function, it stands to reason that general fitness will enhance pelvic floor health and have a positive effect on stress UI.[16] Core muscle training such as Pilates or yoga are encouraged to enhance PFM health and optimal function.[16]

The primary physical therapy interventions for UI/LUTS aimed toward improving PFM function include PFM training, biofeedback, and electrical stimulation. Those interventions aimed toward improving behaviors affecting the bladder include education, fluid management, bladder management, and nocturnal management.[74] Each is discussed next.

Pelvic Floor Muscle Training

Poor pelvic floor strength is associated with pelvic organ prolapse and urinary or fecal incontinence. Therefore, pelvic floor muscle training (PFMT) is the first-line intervention for stress and mixed UI.[84,85] PFMT is a program of repeated PFM contraction focusing on the repetitive, selective, voluntary contraction and relaxation of the PFMs.[16] The aim of PFMT is to change the morphology of the PFMs by achieving exercise-induced hypertrophy of the levator ani muscle group, to improve the tone of the PFMs, and to increase motor unit recruitment and activation during PFM contraction.[74] Increasing the PFMs' thickness and responsiveness is thought to improve urethral pressure and structural support of the pelvic organs, thus preventing urethral descent during abrupt rises in intra-abdominal pressure.[86] Patients can also be taught to purposefully contract the PFMs prior to abrupt increases in intra-abdominal pressure as an effective strategy to stop leakage.[87] All trials in one systematic review reported that women who performed PFMT were statistically significantly more likely to report symptom improvement or cure.[88]

PFMT is believed to reduce stress UI by improving urethral closure and pelvic organ support. A properly timed PFM contraction can stop stress UI by compressing the urethra against the symphysis pubis. PFMT is thought to reduce urge UI in the short term by compressing the urethra, which in turn neurologically inhibits the detrusor (bladder) muscle contraction[89] and, in the long term, stabilizes the inhibitory neurogenic activity with changes in muscle morphology.

As with any other skeletal muscle, correct performance of PFM contraction and relaxation requires precise training with appropriate monitoring and feedback.[90] However, many people do not know how to contract and relax the PFM for effective exercise training and functional use. Specific verbal cueing to "squeeze and lift your muscles as if stopping both gas and/or urine" may be the most effective verbal cue for instructing a person to perform a PFM contraction.[17] Many elders are unable to perform a proper PFM contraction with verbal instructions alone. Patients benefit from education regarding the anatomy of the PFMs,[91] specific instructions, demonstration, and palpation when appropriate to learn the correct contraction. General instructions for how to contract PFMs are included in Box 22.6.

For specificity and motor learning, PFM contractions can be initially integrated into other movements and exercises often prescribed by physical therapists, such as the bridge exercise performed when a patient is lying supine with hips and knees flexed and then lifts the pelvis and the hips off of the floor. Activation of both the pelvic floor muscles and hip rotator muscles[92] or the PFM and gluteals[93] has a faciliatory effect to PFM exercises.

BOX 22.6 General Instructions for How to Contract Pelvic Floor Muscles

- The pelvic floor muscles attach from the pubic bone in the front of the pelvis to the tailbone or coccyx and to the side walls of the pelvis at the hip joints.
- The pelvic floor muscles are those that you would use to stop the flow of urine and to prevent the passage of stool or gas from the rectum. You should feel a tightening around the urethra, where urine passes; the vagina (for females); and the anus, where gas and stool passes.
- The muscle contraction should combine both a squeeze around the openings and a lift of the muscles upward toward your head.
- Squeeze and lift the muscles and hold the contraction for 3 to 5 seconds and repeat at least 8 to 10 times. Practice these exercises 2 to 3 times per day.
- Once this becomes easy to do, try to hold the contraction for 8 to 10 seconds and repeat 8 to 10 times, 2 to 3 times per day.
- Never hold your breath when you are doing these exercises. Try counting out loud to avoid breath holding.
- Never strain or bear down, like you are trying to produce a bowel movement.
- Always fully relax these muscles after each contraction for at least 5 seconds.
- Try to relax your abdominal, buttocks, and thigh muscles during exercise. Concentrate on the pelvic floor muscles only.

Coactivation of these muscles stimulates PFM activation even when they are too weak to contract effectively and/or independently. Rehabilitation should progressively be targeted at training the patient to perform relatively isolated contractions of the PFMs, with minimal to no co-contraction of the abdominals, gluteals, adductors, or hip rotators. This specificity will then allow for the performance of intense maximum contractions of the PFMs. Isolated PFM contractions satisfy the American College of Sports Medicine (ACSM) "overload" principle requirement, because rarely do people perform maximal contractions of the PFMs during daily functional activity. PFMT should be performed for a duration of 8 weeks minimum.[74] In geriatric rehabilitation, this may be best accomplished by incorporating PFMT into therapeutic exercise routines and regular physical activity. Hypertrophy of the PFMs will take at least 6 weeks and may not be fully achieved for up to 4 to 6 months, so even after a rehabilitation intervention is completed, a patient should be encouraged to continue the PFM training program.

The physical therapist who does not perform an internal palpation exam of the PFMs can estimate the capacity of the PFMs to perform and sustain a quality contraction. Progression of PFMT begins with attention to training both slow-twitch and fast-twitch PFM fibers. In general, most elders can start with a 3-second contraction followed by a 6- to 10-second relaxation. Physical therapists should verbally emphasize the feeling of the muscle "squeezing and lifting." The imagery of an elevator going up and down can be effective. The levator ani's name is indicative of this elevator-like action. "Squeeze" means the elevator doors are closing (sphincters close) and "lift" means the PFMs elevate toward the head. "Hold" is staying on the top floor, then the elevator "drops" or descends, and the "doors open" when the sphincters relax. Establishing the coordination of PFM contraction and relaxation is a key initial component of PFMT.

PFMT has been extensively studied and is well supported in the literature.[85] Protocols in the literature vary widely; however, a meta-analysis of PFMT supports the prescription of 24 daily contractions.[94] This translates into two sessions of 12 repetitions or three sessions of 8 repetitions of both sustained and fast-twitch contractions on a daily basis. Muscle training exercises should be performed at least 2 days per week, with 5 days/week the most prescribed.[95] Contraction intensity should be both maximal and submaximal with both sustained and rapid types (1 to 20 seconds).[95] Rest periods between sets can be 1 to 20 seconds and the number of sets from 2 to 40.[95] Training positions have been described most often as supine followed by standing, seated, and in the lateral decubitus position.[95] Duration was 12 weeks in most studies.[95]

Effective muscle training requires several exercise principles that are applicable to PFMT.[16] The principle of exercise specificity enhances effectiveness. Appropriate cueing to target the desired type of contraction is described later. A good knowledge of the anatomy of the pelvic floor is necessary to prescribe the correct movements and exercises. The techniques of motor learning to facilitate neural recruitment and control are also necessary. Motor learning techniques include relevance (aligned with specific patient goals), repetition to fatigue, and random practice. Random practice can include PFMT in different situations and positions. Feedback (described later) is an additional element of motor learning. External feedback may be required initially, during the early training period, but should be gradually withdrawn to enhance the patient's internal feedback mechanism. The principle of overload is critical to achieve gains in muscle strength and hypertrophy in any skeletal muscle, and the pelvic floor is no different.[16] Overload can be achieved by using a rate of perceived effort (RPE) of 6 to 8 on a 10-point scale to fatigue (a 10% drop in force, which generally occurs in approximately 10.5 seconds).[16] However, some authors postulate that fatigue is a reason pelvic floor muscles fail and therefore hypothesize that failure during a training program is probably contraindicated.[16] A 60% effort is necessary to achieve sufficient overload to promote changes in muscle morphology. Finally, progression of the program should be included. Progression includes exercises in different settings and positions, harder contractions, and the use of quick contractions (power). The principle of reversibility means that any gains achieved with a training program will be lost if the program is terminated. Therefore, the patient should be educated that when symptoms are under control, the program can be reduced to a maintenance level but not terminated.

Expected results of PFMT include decreasing episodes of incontinence and symptoms of urgency and frequency, which can be tracked using a bladder diary. Symptoms of nocturia are decreased as well, thus improving sleep, including all the benefits associated with improved sleep. By decreasing UI and LUTS, PFMT decreases the risk of adverse events such as falls and infections. Ultimately, both the outcomes of rehabilitation and the patient's quality of life are improved.

Pelvic floor muscle training should continue for at least 6 weeks and up to 4 to 6 months to achieve hypertrophy and optimum results. Once a person knows how to perform PFM exercise, the exercises can be done anytime and anywhere. Patients should be encouraged to incorporate PFMT into routine activities, such as while sitting and before rising after a meal. After 4 to 6 months, a patient may continue with a maintenance program. The minimum number of contractions required to maintain normal PFM function has not been determined; however, there is some evidence that as few as 10 repetitions per week are enough to maintain PFM function and reduced symptoms of UI.[74]

Feedback and Biofeedback

Gaining skill in correct performance of PFM contraction and relaxation is often difficult for people with pelvic floor disorders. Individuals often report that they cannot feel the muscle contracting and relaxing. Visualization might be advantageous, but obviously individuals cannot easily observe pelvic floor muscle contraction and relaxation. Therefore, perineal biofeedback may be an effective component to promote awareness of pelvic floor muscle activation, coordination, and motor learning. Women who received biofeedback during PFMT were significantly more likely to report that their incontinence was improved compared to women who received PFMT alone.[96] Some systematic reviews provide support for PFMT and biofeedback for pelvic floor rehabilitation in women with UI,[97] people with fecal incontinence,[98] and men with UI following RP (limited support).[99]

Simple feedback can be provided by physical therapists who palpate the levator ani muscles externally (Fig. 22.4) or intravaginally or intrarectally and provide verbal and manual kinesthetic feedback and cueing for contraction and relaxation of the muscles. Asking the patient to sit on a small, inflated ball is a technique to assist patients in obtaining kinesthetic awareness and feedback of the PFMs contraction and relaxation. The patient will feel the ball between the ischial tuberosities where the PFMs reside. As the patient contracts the PFMs, he or she can feel the muscles lift off of the ball, and as he or she relaxes, the PFMs move back down onto the ball. This type of feedback can also be accomplished by having the patient sit on a folded or rolled-up towel placed between the ischial tuberosities.

Pressure biofeedback uses devices that are placed inside the vagina or anus to detect squeeze pressure. When the person contracts the muscles, the device measures the amount of pressure produced by the squeeze component of the contraction and provides information and feedback to the patient about the amount of pressure generated. The feedback information may be as simple as a pressure gauge reading or a sound when a certain pressure is achieved. The feedback may be in the form of both an auditory cue and a visual display on a cell phone application. There are a variety of relatively low-cost pressure feedback devices available for patients to purchase and use at home. The drawback of pressure feedback devices is that they cannot distinguish whether the patient is generating squeeze pressure with facilitation using the abdominal or gluteal muscles or if he or she is able to generate squeeze pressure by contracting the PFMs independently.

Surface electromyography (sEMG) perineal biofeedback (Fig. 22.5) is the gold standard for biofeedback during PFMT. sEMG can be recorded from internal vaginal or rectal sensors or from surface electrodes placed externally near the anus. The abdominal, adductor, and gluteal muscles can also be monitored to determine if the patient is correctly isolating the PFMs. Patients with bladder control problems, especially symptoms of urgency and frequency, may initially benefit from sEMG feedback to learn how to relax the PFMs prior to initiating strengthening exercises. sEMG is an effective tool to increase patients' understanding of both the contraction and the relaxation activity of their PFMs. Advanced training is required for physical therapists to become competent in the performance and analysis of sEMG perineal biofeedback for the treatment of pelvic floor disorders.

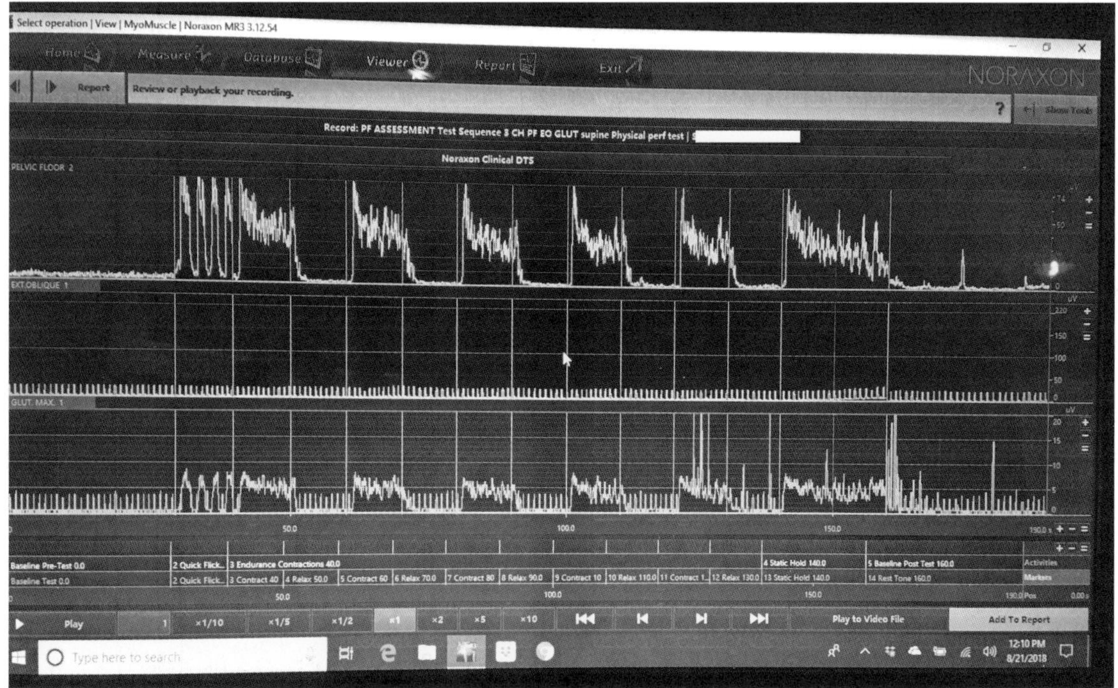

FIG. 22.5 Surface electromyography (sEMG) biofeedback. Channel 1 top graph: pelvic floor muscle (PFM) performance. Channel 2 middle graph: abdominal muscles; note heartbeat artifact. Channel 3 bottom graph: gluteal muscles; note gluteal muscle co-contraction during PFM contraction. © *Cynthia E. Neville.*

Electrical Stimulation

Electrical stimulation (ES) for the treatment of bladder control problems is a noninvasive low-cost treatment well tolerated by most individuals. Compelling, but limited, evidence supports the use of ES for bladder control in pelvic floor muscle rehabilitation as an intervention for symptoms of urinary urgency and overactive bladder[100,101] as well as for facilitating pelvic floor and urinary sphincter muscle contraction.[102] Sacral nerve, tibial nerve,[101] and intravaginal stimulation have effectiveness in treating urge urinary incontinence in some studies.[100,101] Intravaginal ES can improve quality of life, urine leakage, pelvic floor muscle strength, and the squeeze pressure of a PFM contraction.[103] Electric stimulation improved incontinence symptoms and enhanced the quality of life in patients with urinary incontinence following stroke.[104] Improved urethral closure and improved neuromotor function of the PFMs have been repeatedly demonstrated with electrical stimulation with nonimplanted surface or internal electrodes.[103,105,106] However, a recent systematic review indicates that it is currently not known if ES is as effective as, or more effective than, PFMT for the treatment of incontinence.[107]

Electric stimulation should be performed as a component of multimodal physical therapy intervention for pelvic floor disorders and not as a stand-alone treatment. The objectives of ES treatment include neuromodulation of pelvic nerves to regulate the diverse population of nerves related to bladder control and pelvic floor muscle function, to facilitate sensory awareness of pelvic floor muscles, to inhibit reflex bladder contractions and decrease urinary urgency, and to facilitate the contraction of the PFM. Theoretically, neuromodulation by ES reflexively influences the neural activity to the pelvic parasympathetic nerve and the hypogastric sympathetic nerves of the bladder, as well as the sensory and motor inputs to the pelvic floor.

A variety of ES electrode placement options are available (Fig. 22.6). Two or four electrodes placed over the sacrum at the levels of S2–4 nerve roots, two electrodes placed suprapubically over the bladder 2 to 3 inches apart, or two electrodes placed on either side of the anus on the perineum in the S2–3 dermatome provide neuromodulation to the pudendal nerve S2–4. Surface electrodes placed above the medial malleolus and at the medial aspect of the calcaneus stimulate the distal tibial nerve, which shares the S3 nerve to the bladder and pelvic floor.

Physical therapists trained in pelvic floor rehabilitation may also recommend internal vaginal or internal rectal electrodes for appropriate patients; however, internal electrodes are not necessary to provide ES treatment for improving bladder and pelvic floor muscle control. For example, a systematic review indicates that transcutaneous tibial nerve stimulation for adults with OAB was effective.[108] Table 22.6 provides suggested parameters for ES treatment.

Education

Community-dwelling elders have poor knowledge of normal bladder function and UI.[109] It is doubtful that education alone can improve symptoms of incontinence and improve bladder control[110]; however, some research shows that education and training including Internet-based education[111] can result in improvements in symptoms when included in a pelvic floor training program. Education about normal bladder control should include the topics listed in Box 22.7.

Fluid Management Strategies

Individuals with UI will often self-initiate fluid restriction to better manage their urinary symptoms.[112] However, there are conflicting results in the effects of decreasing fluid intake on incontinence[113] and overactive bladder,[114] with concerns that dehydration must be avoided. Fluid intake over 2,400 mL (80 oz) or under 1,500 mL (50 oz) can contribute to UI.[115] Thus, leeway exists in making recommendations for changes in fluid intake, which may be to either increase fluids or decrease fluids depending on the patient's fluid intake behaviors.

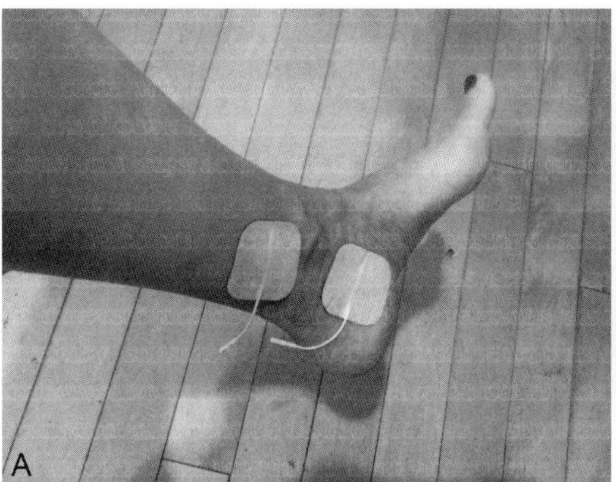

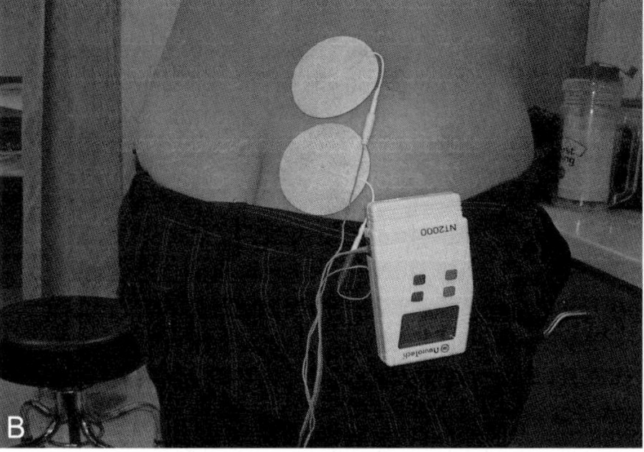

FIG. 22.6 Surface transcutaneous electric nerve stimulation (TENS)/neuromuscular electrical nerve stimulation (NMES) electrode placement for stimulation and neuromodulation. **A,** Tibial nerve. **B,** S2–4 sacral 3 nerve root. © *Cynthia E. Neville.*

TABLE 22.6 Parameters for TENS/NMES for Bladder Control

	Typical Protocol for Urinary Urgency and Urge Urinary Incontinence, Overactive Bladder, Nocturia	Typical Protocol for Stress Urinary Incontinence and Underactive Pelvic Floor	Possible Parameters
Electrode placement	Two electrodes: options • Medial ankle over distal tibial nerve • Suprapubic over bladder 2 inches apart • Over S2–4 nerve roots on sacrum	Two electrodes next to the anal sphincter, perform active PFM contraction during stimulation "on" time	Internal vaginal or internal rectal electrodes for appropriate patients provided by trained PT can also be used for either protocol
Frequency	10–30 Hz	35–50 Hz	5–50 Hz (underactive PFM) 5–20 Hz (urgency) 100–200 Hz (pain)
Pulse duration (width)	100–350 μsec	100–350 μsec	100–1000 μsec Note: Wider pulse duration requires less amplitude to depolarize nerves and so is more comfortable
Waveform	Asymmetrical biphasic	Asymmetrical biphasic	Symmetrical or asymmetrical biphasic
Amplitude (intensity)	To patient tolerance	To patient tolerance or anal wink	To patient tolerance or anal wink
Duty cycle	5–10 seconds on 5–10 seconds off	Correlate with PFM training program Start: 5 seconds on, 10 seconds off Progress to: 10 seconds on, 4 seconds off	Equal rest Double rest If combining with active PFM training, then work up to less than half of on time as rest time
Duration	10–20 minutes	10–20 minutes	5–30 minutes
Frequency of prescription	1 to 7 ×/week BID if possible	BID to 3 ×/week	BID to 1 ×/week
Length of prescription	8–12 weeks May decrease to 1 ×/week for long term	8–16 weeks	Once to ongoing
Comments	Can be done in sitting or lying position Consider treatment before bedtime if patient has nocturia	Progress to a standing position, performing active contractions with stimulation	Both protocols can be used for a patient who has mixed urinary incontinence or who has both PFM weakness and urinary urgency

BID, two times per day; *NMES*, neuromuscular electrical nerve stimulation; *PFM*, pelvic floor muscle; *PT*, physical therapist; *TENS*, transcutaneous electric nerve stimulation.

BOX 22.7 Education About Normal Bladder Function

Education about normal bladder function should include:

Role of the normal bladder and its function:

- Bladder typically fills at a fairly constant rate
- Bladder stores urine 2 to 4 hours during the day and longer, 6 to 8 hours, at night
- Bladder empties but not always completely: Normal postvoid residual may be 100 to 200 mL (3 to 7 oz)

Definition of incontinence: what it means, signs, symptoms, risk factors, self-care, and prevention

Relationship between fluid intake and bladder function and symptoms

Relationship between bladder muscle and pelvic floor muscles

- Role of pelvic floor muscles in controlling urine flow
- How to perform pelvic floor muscle exercises
- Pelvic floor muscle contractions can inhibit bladder urgency

Avoid urinating when there is not an urge to do so (except when on a schedule for voiding)

Frequently emptying bladder to avoid leaking contributes to urinary urgency and frequency and decreased perceived bladder capacity

Normally we can override the urge to urinate. We may need to retrain the brain and bladder, and re-learn bladder control:

- "Mind over bladder"

The physical therapist and patient/caregiver can assess fluid intake behaviors and formulate fluid management strategies by discussing fluid intake habits or by evaluating a bladder diary. The goal of fluid management is symptom reduction, not deprivation or forced fluid intake. Changes in fluid intake can initially be made in small increments of 2 to 8 oz at a time and gradually progress over 2 to 4 weeks. The physical therapist can often identify bladder irritants on the bladder diary or hypothesize which fluids in the patient's diet may be contributing to symptoms. Common bladder irritants often contain caffeine and include coffee, tea, soda, and alcohol.[116] Other bladder irritants include some medications and chocolate.[61] Daily consumption of >204 g (2 to 3 cups) of caffeine per day was significantly associated with any UI.[117,118] Awareness of the effects of certain fluids on UI/LUTS may lead to behavior that will reduce or eliminate the problematic fluid. A person may not want to give up coffee but may be willing to decrease the amount of coffee intake, or can be aware of impending symptoms when he or she drinks coffee so that he or she can manage those symptoms.

The gradual normalization of water and fluid intake to recommended guidelines to maintain hydration and to minimize the negative effects of bladder irritants on LUTS is a key goal. The patient can be advised how to dilute bladder irritants with water. For example, drinking an ounce or two of water before or after drinking coffee may minimize the effects of the coffee. Optimally, fluids should be evenly spaced throughout the day, with most hydration coming in the morning and afternoon hours. Thirst and fluid intake are often impaired, even in the healthy older individual,[119,120] so the individual may need to initiate adequate fluid intake rather than waiting until feeling thirsty. The total fluid intake should be about six to eight 8-oz glasses/day or 48 to 64 oz total. The U.S. Food Science Board–recommended guidelines for older adults are half an ounce of fluids per pound of body weight.[70]

Bladder Training

Bladder training is a behavioral exercise used to improve bladder control in all treatment settings. Bladder training is also called timed voiding, habit training, or promoted voiding. A key component of bladder training is education about the function of the bladder to fill, store, and empty. Timed voiding is a program of mandatory scheduled voiding, whether there is an urge to urinate or not, with progressive increases or decreases in the intervals between voiding.[121] Habit training is a program of identifying the patient's typical voiding habits and then scheduling voiding based on those habits, whether there is an urge to urinate or not.[121] Prompted voiding is used with cognitively impaired patients. The caregiver is responsible for verbally cueing the patient to identify the need to urinate and identify if leakage has occurred and then offer the patient the opportunity to urinate in the bathroom.[122] Bladder management has conflicting evidence as to its effectiveness, owing in part to the variability of individuals' abilities and type of bladder control problems included in studies.[123,124]

Strategies for Deferral and Inhibition of Urinary Urgency and Nocturia

The urge to urinate resulting in urinary urgency and urinary leakage can be deferred or inhibited with a number of different strategies. PFM contractions, mental distraction, and calf muscle exercises may inhibit or decrease the feeling of the strong urge to urinate so that the urge will dissipate. A reciprocal inhibition relationship exists between the bladder detrusor muscle and the pelvic floor muscles. When the bladder muscle contracts to empty, the pelvic floor muscles must be relaxed. Conversely, when the pelvic floor muscles contract, the bladder muscle is reflexively inhibited. Performing 8 to 12 strong quick pelvic floor muscle contractions can work to inhibit detrusor/bladder contractions and decrease associated feelings of urgency. The PFM contractions inhibit the bladder by closing the external urinary sphincter, elevating the bladder neck and thus closing the internal urinary sphincter, and activating a detrusor inhibition reflex.[125] Another technique shown to reduce bladder contractions is to perform heel raises, or "self-induced plantar flexion."[126] Active plantar flexion movements and heel raises can be done in the sitting, lying, or standing position for 10 to 20 repetitions to decrease the sensation of urgency. Diaphragmatic breathing to decrease sympathetic output may be effective. Mental distraction techniques including meditation, visualization of a calming scene, concentration on a poem or song, and keeping the mind busy with a task (such as counting in another language) are all strategies that may be effective. Sitting down and putting pressure on the perineum between the legs, such as sitting on the arm of a couch, can also decrease the urge and inhibit the bladder.

Nocturia Management

Waking from sleep with the urge to urinate (nocturia) is a common scenario leading to falls in older people. The more a person drinks in the evening, the more likely he or she is to have to get up to urinate. Fluid management strategies, as described previously, are recommended for nocturia management. Stopping fluids 2 to 3 hours before sleep and avoiding drinking fluids in the evening and during the night are recommended for patients with nocturia. When a person does wake with the need to void, he or she can use urgency inhibition strategies as described earlier. Physical therapists can advise patients to perform PFM contractions while lying in bed, while sitting on the edge of the bed, or before standing up to reduce urinary urgency. Pelvic floor muscle contractions potentially inhibit urgency and concurrent bladder contractions and reduce the risk of leaking urine on the way to the bathroom. This may potentially prevent a fall on the way to the bathroom. For men, providing a urinal near the bed may be a reasonable management strategy for nighttime voiding. For both men and women, a bedside commode may be beneficial to reduce the risk of falling while trying to ambulate to a bathroom. Finally, if a person has lower extremity swelling, it may be helpful to elevate the feet 2 to 3 hours before sleep to encourage processing of fluids before going to bed to reduce nocturia.

Bladder Emptying

Older adults may report that they feel as if they are not emptying the bladder completely. Physical therapists should provide education that there can be a normal postvoid residual volume of urine left in the bladder after emptying. For the bladder to initiate emptying, and to empty efficiently, the pelvic floor muscles must be relaxed. Physical therapists can teach the patient to contract and relax the PFMs and to feel the difference between the contraction and the relaxation. The patient should then be more aware of the tone of the PFMs and actively relax the PFMs when initiating urination.

Position and posture during urination may impact the ability to empty the bladder. Sitting in what is referred to as the "potty posture" or the "defecation posture"[127] (Fig. 22.7) with the hips flexed to >100 degrees facilitates relaxation of the PFMs and may also improve emptying of the bowels. This posture should be used every time a person urinates or defecates. For some, sitting on a public toilet seat is not acceptable. Some women may hover over the toilet seat. This position may lead to contraction of the hip and pelvic floor muscles and make it more difficult to initiate urination and to fully empty. The PFMs also must be relaxed in males to initiate urination in the standing position.

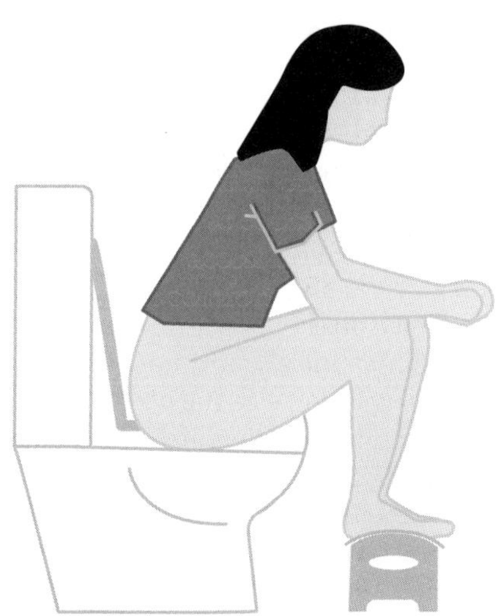

FIG. 22.7 Squatting or defecation posture for bladder and bowel evacuation.

The Frail Elder and Cognitively Impaired

Multiple integrating risk factors such as age-related changes in physiology, cognitive changes, polypharmacy, and comorbidities may lead to UI/LUTS in the elder with frailty.[1] A comprehensive, multicomponent, and multidisciplinary approach is optimal because of this multifactorial nature of UI. A lack of clinical trials to guide practice in the treatment of UI in this population makes clinical decision making a challenge.[1] The most common strategy for management of UI in the frail elder is the use of pads and garments; however, they may be misused and potentially increase the risk of developing UI and associated conditions such as UTIs. Conservative interventions may be effective so that pad usage can possibly be decreased or potentially eliminated. The health care team's assessment, choice of interventions, and timing of interventions for incontinence must take into consideration the patient's multisystem involvement and the service delivery processes that are involved in the care of the patient or resident in his or her environment. Rehabilitation providers typically focus on promoting strength, safety, mobility, and dexterity relating to toileting. Physical therapists should also actively collaborate with nursing care providers to promote regular or scheduled voiding intervals. Elders with cognitive impairments or sensory impairments may not recognize the need to urinate, so therapists can reinforce and promote scheduled voiding as a strategy for the elder to regularly empty the bladder, even during therapy sessions. One study successfully used PFMT for older women with mild cognitive impairment or Alzheimer disease (mean Mini-Mental State Examination score = 23) and UI. The intervention group received six sessions of training for 12 weeks. The primary outcome was change in UI episodes measured with a frequency volume chart. After 12 weeks of training, the mean number of UI episodes per 24 hours decreased from 3.3 to 1.7 in the intervention group and by 0.5 in the control group.[128] The International Continence Society Committee on Incontinence in the Frail Elderly provides evidence-based recommendations for practice in caring for frail elders with incontinence, listed in Box 22.8. Health care providers are more likely to succeed in supporting bladder control in frail elder people when the health care team is knowledgeable about conservative evidence-based interventions, and members collaborate to support each other to provide all interventions as much as possible.

SUMMARY

Bladder control problems such as urinary incontinence negatively impact rehabilitation outcomes and patient quality of life. Health professionals caring for elders must identify and assess incontinence and other LUTS, even while other conditions and diagnoses take precedence in the plan of care. Bladder control problems should be identified during the initial patient assessment. Baseline

BOX 22.8 Summary of International Continence Society Recommendations for Practice for Frail Elders with Incontinence

Environmental cues—toilet visibility, signs, color differentiation, images, arrows, and directions should be used to compensate for visual-perceptual deficits in frail older adults with urinary incontinence (UI).

Each component of the toileting process requires skill dexterity and physical strength. Individual strength and dexterity impairments relating to toileting should be identified and treatment provided in frail individuals and those with cognitive impairments

Day-to-day continence care processes (such as scheduled voiding) in health care settings should be promoted by awareness-raising activities for the patient, family and caregivers, and clinical staff.

Planning for services for frail elders should ensure that time, resources, knowledge, and skill required to conduct an assessment are provided to health care providers, including active, effective, conservative management of UI episodes and promotion of bladder control.

Gaps in health care practitioner knowledge about preventing, managing, and treating incontinence should be continually addressed with training and education.

Evidence-based guidelines for the use of continence aids, such as pads and garments, should be implemented to promote an active approach to diagnosis, treatment, and prevention of UI.

Fonda D, DuBeau CE, Harari D, et al. Incontinence in the Frail Elderly. In P. Abrams, L. Cardozo, S. Khoury, & A. Wein (Eds.), *Incontinence: Proceedings of the Fourth International Consultation on Incontinence*, July 5–8, 2008, 1165–1240. Health Publications Limited Paris. https://www.ics.org/Publications/ICI3/v2.pdf/chap18.pdf.

measurement of the severity of symptoms, types of symptoms, and impact of UI/LUTS on quality of life can be obtained early in the rehabilitation episode of care using standardized validated outcome measures such as the ICIQ-UI SF. Therapists should consider the potential negative impact of symptoms on achievement of rehabilitation-related goals, such as reducing fall risk and preventing rehospitalization. Improvement in bladder control and reduction of UI/LUTS should be stated goals of rehabilitation.

If a patient is leaking urine, it can be inferred that he or she likely has a pelvic floor disorder. The patient ideally should complete a 3-day bladder diary to further assess symptoms and behaviors relating to symptoms; however, the therapist can obtain valuable information about a patient's fluid intake and voiding habits simply by asking questions and engaging in a conversation about them. Even in elder patients with multiple impairments and comorbidities, basic interventions to improve bladder control can be initiated immediately and are best reinforced by all members of the rehabilitation and nursing care team. External examination of pelvic floor muscle contraction can be performed, and patients can begin to perform pelvic floor muscle exercises to improve the function of this critical muscle group. Bladder training and timed voiding are simple and effective enough strategies to influence and improve bladder storage and emptying patterns. Small and/or gradual changes in fluid intake volumes, timing of fluid intake, and identification of bladder irritants can lead to symptom improvement in a short period of time. Techniques to defer urinary urgency, such as heel raises and fast-twitch pelvic floor muscle contractions, are often easy to incorporate into a daily schedule and are often immediately effective. Being able to control urgency may not only return some feeling of control to the patient with symptoms of urinary urgency, frequency, and UI but also ultimately reduce the risk of a fall occurring while rushing to the bathroom. Electrical stimulation applied externally to the distal ankle or sacral spine can be effective at reducing urgency and urgency incontinence, with little to no side effects. Every therapist should be proficient in teaching PFMT because of its effectiveness for bladder control problems. If an individual has UI/LUTS, then PFMT should be incorporated into the therapeutic exercise prescription. Many elders require additional strengthening of the hip and gluteal muscles, and PFM contractions can be performed at the same time as these exercises to promote improved PFM function and strength. Conservative interventions are all well tolerated and may yield satisfying results in the form of symptom reduction, improved patient satisfaction and self-efficacy, reduced fall risk, and improved overall outcomes of rehabilitation.

Although UI/LUTS are highly prevalent in the aging population, prevention of PFM disorders leading to UI/LUTS is being intensively investigated.[129] Prevention of incontinence is not yet an integral part of the present health care paradigm but may be achievable in the future. Physical therapists can identify bladder control problems in the evaluation of patients and during any episode of care. Physical therapists can provide basic interventions described in this chapter, which may improve health and rehabilitation outcomes. When basic interventions are not effective, physical therapists can refer to a physical therapist with advanced training in pelvic health rehabilitation. Elders with UI/LUTS are at risk for poor rehabilitation outcomes. Physical therapists should identify and coordinate management, just as they would do for osteoporosis, hypertension, or diabetes. Because pelvic floor rehabilitation is strongly supported in the literature, physical therapists should confidently incorporate PFMT and rehabilitation of the PFMs into clinical care.

REFERENCES

1. Wagg A, Gibson W, Ostaszkiewicz J, et al. Urinary incontinence in frail elderly persons: report from the 5th International Consultation on Incontinence. *Neurourol Urodyn.* 2015;34(5):398–406. https://doi.org/10.1002/nau.22602.
2. Foley AL, Loharuka S, Barrett JA, et al. Association between the geriatric giants of urinary incontinence and falls in older people using data from the Leicestershire MRC Incontinence Study. *Age Ageing.* 2012;41(1):35–40. https://doi.org/10.1093/ageing/afr125.

3. Holroyd-Leduc JM, Straus SE. Management of urinary incontinence in women: scientific review. *JAMA*. 2004;291(8): 986–995. https://doi.org/10.1001/jama.291.8.986.
4. Coyne KS, Sexton CC, Irwin DE, Kopp ZS, Kelleher CJ, Milsom I. The impact of overactive bladder, incontinence and other lower urinary tract symptoms on quality of life, work productivity, sexuality and emotional well-being in men and women: results from the EPIC study. *BJU Int*. 2008;101:1388–1395. https://doi.org/10.1111/j.1464-410X.2008.07601.x.
5. Ramage-Morin PL, Gilmour H. Urinary incontinence and loneliness in Canadian seniors. *Health Rep* 2013;24:3–10.
6. Coyne KS, Sexton CC, Thompson CL, et al. Impact of overactive bladder on work productivity. *Urology*. 2012;80:97–103. https://doi.org/10.1016/j.urology.2012.03.039.
7. Mallinson T, Fitzgerald CM, Neville CE, et al. Impact of urinary incontinence on medical rehabilitation inpatients. *Neurourol Urodyn* 2017;36(1):176–183. https://doi.org/10.1002/nau.22908.
8. Powell LC, Szabo SM, Walker D, Gooch K. The economic burden of overactive bladder in the United States: a systematic literature review. *Neurourol Urodyn* 2018;37:1241–1249. https://doi.org/10.1002/nau.23477.
9. Milsom I, Altman D, Lapitan MC, et al. Epidemiology of urinary (UI) and faecal (FI) incontinence and pelvic organ prolapse (POP). In: Abrams P, Cardozo L, Khoury S, Wein A, eds. *Incontinence: Proceedings of the Fourth International Consultation on Incontinence*. Health Publications Limited Paris; July 5–8, 2008:1165–1240. https://www.ics.org/Publications/ICI_4/files-book/comite-1.pdf.
10. Landi F, Cesari M, Russo A, Onder G, Lattanzio F, Bernabei R. Potentially reversible risk factors and urinary incontinence in frail older people living in community. *Age Ageing* 2003;32: 194–199. https://doi.org/10.1093/ageing/32.2.194.
11. Xu D, Kane RL. Effect of urinary incontinence on older nursing home residents' self-reported quality of life. *J Am Geriatr Soc*. 2013;61(9):1473–1481. https://doi.org/10.1111/jgs.12408.
12. Lukacz ES, Sampselle C, Gray M, et al. A healthy bladder: a consensus statement. *Int J Clin Pract*. 2011;65:1026–1036. https://doi.org/10.1111/j.1742-1241.2011.02763.x.
13. Livingston BP. Anatomy and neural control of the lower urinary tract and pelvic floor. *Top Geriatr Rehabil*. 2016;32(4):280–294. https://doi.org/10.1097/TGR.0000000000000123.
14. Park J, Lavelle JP, Palmer MH. Voiding dysfunction in older women with overactive bladder symptoms: a comparison of urodynamic parameters between women with normal and elevated post-void residual urine. *Neurourol Urodyn*. 2016;35(1):95–99. https://doi.org/10.1002/nau.22689.
15. Eickmeyer SM. Anatomy and physiology of the pelvic floor. *Phys Med Rehabil Clin N Am*. 2017;28:455–460. https://doi.org/10.1016/j.pmr.2017.03.003.
16. Marques A, Stothers L, Macnab A. The status of pelvic floor muscle training for women. *Can Urol Assoc J*. 2010;4: 419–424. https://www.ncbi.nlm.nih.gov/pmc/articles/PMC2997838/.
17. Crotty K, Bartram CI, Pitkin J, et al. Investigation of optimal cues to instruction for pelvic floor muscle contraction: a pilot study using 2D ultrasound imaging in pre-menopausal, nulliparous, continent women. *Neurourol Urodyn*. 2011;30:1620–1626. https://doi.org/10.1002/nau.21083.
18. Bø K, Lilleås F, Talseth T, Hedland H. Dynamic MRI of the pelvic floor muscles in an upright sitting position. *Neurourol Urodyn*. 2001;20:167–174. https://onlinelibrary.wiley.com/doi/abs/10.1002/1520-6777%282001%2920%3A2%3C167%3A%3AAID-NAU19%3E3.CO%3B2-4.
19. Dietz HP. Pelvic floor ultrasound: a review. *Clin Obstet Gynecol*. 2017;60:58–81. https://doi.org/10.1097/GRF.0000000000000264.
20. Sapsford RR, Hodges PW, Richardson CA, Cooper DH, Markwell SJ, Jull GA. Co-activation of the abdominal and pelvic floor muscles during voluntary exercises. *Neurourol Urodyn*. 2001;20:31–42. https://doi.org/10.1002/1520-6777(2001)20:1<31::AID-NAU5>3.0.CO;2-P.
21. Junginger B, Baessler K, Sapsford R, et al. Effect of abdominal and pelvic floor tasks on muscle activity, abdominal pressure and bladder neck. *Int Urogynecol J*. 2010;21:69. https://doi.org/10.1007/s00192-009-0981-z.
22. Smith EM, Shah AA. Screening for geriatric syndromes. *Clin Geriatr Med*. 2018;34(1):55–67. https://doi.org/10.1016/j.cger.2017.08.002.
23. Hasegawa J, Kuzuya M, Iguchi A. Urinary incontinence and behavioral symptoms are independent risk factors for recurrent and injurious falls, respectively, among residents in long-term care facilities. *Arch Gerontol Geriatr*. 2010;50(1): 77–81.
24. Fusco D, Bochicchio GB, Onder G, Barillaro C, Bernabei R, Landi F. Predictors of rehabilitation outcome among frail elderly patients living in the community. *J Am Med Dir Assoc*. 2009;20:335–341. https://www.jamda.com/article/S1525-8610(09)00082-6/fulltext.
25. Frick AC, Huang AJ, Van den Eeden SK, et al. Mixed urinary incontinence: greater impact on quality of life. *J Urol*. 2009;182(2):596–600. https://doi.org/10.1016/j.juro.2009.04.005.
26. Alappattu M, Neville C, Beneciuk J, Bishop M. Urinary incontinence symptoms and impact on quality of life in patients seeking outpatient physical therapy services. *Physiother Theory Pract* 2016;32(2):107–112. https://doi.org/10.3109/09593985.2015.1116648.
27. Tadic SD, Zdaniuk B, Griffiths D, Rosenberg L, Schäfer W, Resnick NM. Effect of biofeedback on psychological burden and symptoms in older women with urge urinary incontinence. *J Am Geriatr Soc*. 2007;55:2010–2015. https://doi.org/10.1111/j.1532-5415.2007.01461.x.
28. Jenkins KR, Fultz NH. Functional impairment as a risk factor for urinary incontinence among older Americans. *Neurourol Urodyn*. 2005;24:51–55. https://doi.org/10.1002/nau.20089.
29. Tannenbaum C, Johnell K. Managing therapeutic competition in patients with heart failure, lower urinary tract symptoms and incontinence. *Drugs Aging*. 2014;31:93–101. https://doi.org/10.1007/s40266-013-0145-1.
30. Tamanini JTN, Santos JLF, Lebrao ML, Duarte YAO, Laurenti R. Association between urinary incontinence in elderly patients and caregiver burden in the city of Sao Paulo/Brazil: Health, Wellbeing, and Ageing Study. *Neurourol Urodyn*. 2011;30:1281–1285. https://doi.org/10.1002/nau.21040.
31. Doughty D, Junkin J, Kurz P, et al. Incontinence-associated dermatitis: consensus statements, evidence-based guidelines for prevention and treatment, and current challenges. *J Wound Ostomy Continence Nurs*. 2012;39:303–315. https://doi.org/10.1097/WON.0b013e3182549118.
32. Kolominsky-Rabas PL, Hilz MJ, Neundoerfer B, Heuschmann PU. Impact of urinary incontinence after stroke: results from a prospective population-based stroke register. *Neurourol Urodyn*. 2003;22:322–327. https://doi.org/10.1002/nau.10114.
33. Meijer R, Ihnenfeldt DS, de Groot IJM, van Limbeek J, Vermeulen M, de Haan RJ. Prognostic factors for ambulation and activities of daily living in the subacute phase after stroke. A systematic review of the literature. 2003;17:119–129. https://doi.org/10.1191/0269215503cr585oa.
34. Lee J, Rantz M. Correlates of post-hospital physical function at 1 year in skilled nursing facility residents. *J Adv Nurs*. 2008;62: 479–486. https://doi.org/10.1111/j.1365-2648.2008. 04612.x.
35. Chiarelli P, Weatherall M. The link between chronic conditions and urinary incontinence. *Aust New Zeal Cont J*. 2010;

16:7–14. https://www.continencexchange.org.au/journals.php/2/anzcj-vol-16-no-1-pp7-14.pdf.
36. Hunter KF, Voaklander D, Hsu ZY, Moore KN. Lower urinary tract symptoms and falls risk among older women receiving home support: a prospective cohort study. *BMC Geriatr.* 2013;13:46. https://doi.org/10.1186/1471-2318-13-46.
37. Chiarelli PE, Mackenzie LA, Osmotherly PG. Urinary incontinence is associated with an increase in falls: a systematic review. *Aust J Physiother.* 2009;55(2):89–95.
38. Wolf SL, Riolo L, Ouslander JG. Urge incontinence and the risk of falling in older women. *J Am Geriatr Soc.* 2000; 48(7):847–848. https://doi.org/10.1111/j.1532-5415.2000.tb04765.x.
39. Aminzadeha F. Utilization of bathroom safety devices, patterns of bathing and toileting, and bathroom falls in a sample of community living older adults. *Technol Disabil.* 2000;13: 95–103.
40. Kurita N, Yamazaki S, Fukumori N, et al. Overactive bladder symptom severity is associated with falls in community-dwelling adults: LOHAS study. *BMJ Open.* 2013;3: e002413. https://doi.org/10.1136/bmjopen-2012-002413.
41. Teo JSH, Briffa NK, Devine A, Dhaliwal SS, Prince RL. Do sleep problems or urinary incontinence predict falls in elderly women? *Aust J Physiother.* 2006;52:19–24. https://doi.org/10.1016/S0004-9514(06)70058-7.
42. Cornu J-N, Abrams P, Chapple CR, et al. A contemporary assessment of nocturia: definition, epidemiology, pathophysiology, and management—a systematic review and meta-analysis. *Eur Urol.* 2012;62:877–890. https://doi.org/10.1016/j.eururo.2012.07.004.
43. Noguchi N, Chan L, Cumming RG, Blyth FM, Naganathan V. A systematic review of the association between lower urinary tract symptoms and falls, injuries, and fractures in community-dwelling older men. *Aging Male.* 2016;19(3):168–174. https://doi.org/10.3109/13685538. 2016.1169399.
44. Vahabi B, Wagg AS, Rosier PFWM, et al. Can we define and characterize the aging lower urinary tract?—ICI-RS 2015. *Neurourol Urodyn.* 2017;36:854–858. https://doi.org/10.1002/nau.23035.
45. Birder LA, Ruggieri M, Takeda M, et al. How does the urothelium affect bladder function in health and disease? ICI-RS 2011. *Neurourol Urodyn.* 2012;31:293–299. https://doi.org/10.1002/nau.22195.
46. Walston JD. Sarcopenia in older adults. *Curr Opin Rheumatol.* 2012;24(6):623–627. https://doi.org/10.1097/BOR.0b013e328358d59b.
47. Huang AJ, Brown JS, Boyko EJ, et al. Clinical significance of postvoid residual volume in older ambulatory women. *J Am Geriatr Soc.* 2011;59:1452–1458. https://doi.org/10.1111/j.1532-5415.2011.03511.x.
48. Bosch JLHR, Everaert K, Weiss JP, et al. Would a new definition and classification of nocturia and nocturnal polyuria improve our management of patients? ICI-RS 2014. *Neurourol Urodyn.* 2016;35:283–287. https://doi.org/10.1002/nau.22772.
49. Asplund R. Nocturia in relation to sleep, health, and medical treatment in the elderly. *BJU Int.* 2005;96 Suppl 1:15–21. https://doi.org/10.1111/j.1464-410X.2005.05653.x.
50. Schulman C, Lunenfeld B. The ageing male. *World J Urol.* 2002;20(1):4–10. https://doi.org/10.1007/s00345-002-0258-3.
51. Parsons JK. Benign prostatic hyperplasia and male lower urinary tract symptoms: epidemiology and risk factors. *Curr Bladder Dysfunct Rep.* 2010;5:212–218. https://doi.org/10.1007/s11884-010-0067-2.
52. Abdelmoteleb H, Jefferies ER, Drake MJ. Assessment and management of male lower urinary tract symptoms (LUTS). *Int J Surg.* 2016;25:164–171. https://doi.org/10.1016/j.ijsu.2015.11.043.
53. Staskin D, Kelleher C, Avery K, et al. Initial assessment of urinary and faecal incontinence in adult male and female patients. In: Abrams P, Cardozo L, Khoury S, Wein A, eds. *Incontinence: Proceedings of the Fourth International Consultation on Incontinence.* Health Publications Limited Paris; July 5–8, 2008:331–412. https://www.ics.org/Publications/ICI-3/v1.pdf/chap9.pdf.
54. Memon HU, Handa VL. Vaginal childbirth and pelvic floor disorders. *Women's Health.* 2013;9:265–277. https://doi.org/10.2217/whe.13.17.
55. Dietz HP, Lanzarone V. Levator trauma after vaginal delivery. *Obstet Gynecol.* 2005;106:707–712. https://doi.org/10.1097/01.AOG. 0000178779.62181.01.
56. Wyndaele M, Hashim H. Pathophysiology of urinary incontinence. *Surgery (United Kingdom).* 2017;35:287–292. https://doi.org/10.1016/j.mpsur.2017.03.002.
57. Luber KM. The definition, prevalence, and risk factors for stress urinary incontinence. *Rev Urol.* 2004;6 Suppl 3:S3–S9.
58. Shamliyan TA, Wyman JF, Ping R, Wilt TJ, Kane RL. Male urinary incontinence: prevalence, risk factors, and preventive interventions. *Rev Urol.* 2009;11:145–165. https://www.ncbi.nlm.nih.gov/pmc/articles/PMC2777032/.
59. Banakhar MA, Al-Shaiji TF, Hassouna MM. Pathophysiology of overactive bladder. *Int Urogynecol J.* 2012;23:975–982. https://doi.org/10.1007/s00192-012-1682-6.
60. Nygaard I. Idiopathic urgency urinary incontinence. *N Engl J Med.* 2010;363:1156–1162. https://doi.org/10.1056/NEJMcp1003849.
61. Gleason JL, Richter HE, Redden DT, Goode PS, Burgio KL, Markland AD. Caffeine and urinary incontinence in US women. *Int Urogynecol J.* 2013;24:295–302. https://doi.org/10.1007/s00192-012-1829-5.
62. Wein AJ. Re: An International Urogynecological Association (IUGA)/International Continence Society (ICS) Joint Report on the Terminology for the Conservative and Nonpharmacological Management of Female Pelvic Floor Dysfunction. *J Urol.* 2017;198(3):488–489. https://doi.org/10.1016/j.juro.2017.06.050.
63. Yu Ko WF, Sawatzky JAV. Understanding urinary incontinence after radical prostatectomy: a nursing framework. *Clin J Oncol Nurs.* 2008;12:647–654. https://doi.org/10.1188/08.CJON.647-654.
64. Saliba W, Fediai A, Edelstein H, Markel A, Raz R. Trends in the burden of infectious disease hospitalizations among the elderly in the last decade. *Eur J Intern Med.* 2013;24: 536–540. https://doi.org/10.1016/j.ejim.2013.06.002.
65. Robinson D, Giarenis I, Cardozo L. The management of urinary tract infections in octogenarian women. *Maturitas.* 2015;81(3):343–347. https://doi.org/10.1016/j.maturitas.2015.04.014.
66. Schulz L, Hoffman RJ, Pothof J, Fox B. Top ten myths regarding the diagnosis and treatment of urinary tract infections. *J Emerg Med.* 2016;51(1):25–30. https://doi.org/10.1016/j.jemermed.2016.02.009.
67. Smelov V, Naber K, Bjerklund Johansen TE. Improved classification of urinary tract infection: future considerations. *Eur Urol Suppl.* 2016;15(4):71–80. https://doi.org/10.1016/j.eursup. 2016.04.002.
68. Goode PS, Burgio KL, Richter HE, Markland AD. Incontinence in older women. *JAMA.* 2010;303:2172–2181. https://doi.org/10.1001/jama.2010.749.
69. Markland AD, Goode PS, Burgio KL, et al. Correlates of urinary, fecal, and dual incontinence in older African-American and white men and women. *J Am Geriatr Soc.* 2008;56:285–290. https://doi.org/10.1111/j.1532-5415.2007.01509.x.

70. *Dietary Reference Intakes for Water, Potassium, Sodium, Chloride, and Sulfate.* Washington, DC: National Academies Press; 2005.
71. Dmochowski RR, Sanders SW, Appell RA, Nitti VW, Davila GW. Bladder-health diaries: an assessment of 3-day vs 7-day entries. *BJU Int.* 2005;96:1049–1054. https://doi.org/10.1111/j.1464-410X.2005.05785.x.
72. FitzGerald MP, Burgio KL, Borello-France DF, et al. Pelvic-floor strength in women with incontinence as assessed by the Brink scale. *Phys Ther.* 2007;87:1316–1324. https://doi.org/10.2522/ptj.20060073.
73. Ferreira CHJ, Barbosa PB, Souza F de O, Antônio FI, Franco MM, Bø K. Inter-rater reliability study of the Modified Oxford Grading Scale and the Peritron manometer. *Physiotherapy.* 2011;97:132–138. https://doi.org/10.1016/j.physio.2010. 06.007.
74. Bo K, Berghmans B, Morkved S, Van Kampen M. *Evidence-Based Physical Therapy for the Pelvic Floor.* St Louis: Churchill Livingstone; 2014; https://doi.org/10.1016/B978-0-443-10146-5.X5001-1.
75. Finsterbusch C, Carmel M, Zimmern P. Outcome measures most commonly used in the literature to assess stress incontinence surgery in women over the past 5 years : can we come to some agreement to improve our reporting? ICS 2016;S19 ePoster 2:Abstract 326 https://www.ics.org/2016/abstract/326.
76. Avery K, Donovan J, Peters TJ, Shaw C, Gotoh M, Abrams P. ICIQ: a brief and robust measure for evaluating the symptoms and impact of urinary incontinence. *Neurourol Urodyn.* 2004;23:322–330. https://doi.org/10.1002/nau.20041.
77. Nyström E, Sjöström M, Stenlund H, Samuelsson E. ICIQ symptom and quality of life instruments measure clinically relevant improvements in women with stress urinary incontinence. *Neurourol Urodyn.* 2015;34:747–751. https://doi.org/10.1002/nau.22657.
78. Sirls LT, Tennstedt S, Brubaker L, et al. The minimum important difference for the International Consultation on Incontinence Questionnaire-Urinary Incontinence Short Form in women with stress urinary incontinence. *Neurourol Urodyn.* 2015;34:183–187. https://doi.org/10.1002/nau.22533.
79. Barber MD, Kuchibhatla MN, Pieper CF, Bump RC. Psychometric evaluation of 2 comprehensive condition-specific quality of life instruments for women with pelvic floor disorders. *Am J Obstet Gynecol.* 2001;185:1388–1395. https://doi.org/10.1067/mob.2001.118659.
80. Barber MD, Walters MD, Bump RC. Short forms of two condition-specific quality-of-life questionnaires for women with pelvic floor disorders (PFDI-20 and PFIQ-7). *Am J Obstet Gynecol.* 2005;193:103–113. https://doi.org/10.1016/j.ajog.2004.12.025.
81. Rogers RG, Kammerer-Doak D, Villarreal A, Coates K, Qualls C. A new instrument to measure sexual function in women with urinary incontinence or pelvic organ prolapse. *Am J Obstet Gynecol.* 2001;184:552–558. https://doi.org/10.1067/mob.2001.111100.
82. Barry MJ, Fowler FJ, O'Leary MP, et al. The American Urological Association symptom index for benign prostatic hyperplasia. The Measurement Committee of the American Urological Association. *J Urol.* 1992;148(5):1549–1557. discussion 1564. http://www.ncbi.nlm.nih.gov/pubmed/1279218. Accessed August 19, 2018.
83. Barry MJ, Avins AL, Meleth S. Complementary and Alternative Medicine for Urological Symptoms Study Group. Performance of the American Urological Association Symptom Index with and without an additional urge incontinence item. *Urology.* 2011;78(3):550–554. https://doi.org/10.1016/j.urology.2011.04.017. Epub 2011 Jul 8. PubMed PMID: 21741692; PubMed Central PMCID: PMC3166397.
84. Qaseem A, Dallas P, Forciea MA, Starkey M, Denberg TD, Shekelle P. Nonsurgical management of urinary incontinence in women: a clinical practice guideline from the American College of Physicians. *Ann Intern Med.* 2014;161:429–440. https://doi.org/10.7326/M13-2410.
85. Dumoulin C, Hay-Smith EC, Mac Habée-Séguin G. Pelvic floor muscle training versus no treatment, or inactive control treatments, for urinary incontinence in women. *Cochrane Database Syst Rev.* 2014;5:CD005654.
86. Price N, Dawood R, Jackson SR. Pelvic floor exercise for urinary incontinence: a systematic literature review. *Maturitas.* 2010;67:309–315. https://doi.org/10.1016/j.maturitas.2010.08.004.
87. Miller JM, Sampselle C, Ashton-Miller J, Hong GRS, DeLancey JOL. Clarification and confirmation of the Knack maneuver: the effect of volitional pelvic floor muscle contraction to preempt expected stress incontinence. *Int Urogynecol J.* 2008;19:773–782. https://doi.org/10.1007/s00192-007-0525-3.
88. Angelini K. Pelvic floor muscle training to manage overactive bladder and urinary incontinence. *Nurs Womens Health.* 2017;21(1):51–57.
89. Shafik A, Shafik IA. Overactive bladder inhibition in response to pelvic floor muscle exercises. *World J Urol.* 2003;20:374–377. https://doi.org/10.1007/s00345-002-0309-9.
90. Bø K. Pelvic floor muscle training in treatment of female stress urinary incontinence, pelvic organ prolapse and sexual dysfunction. *World J Urol.* 2012;30:437–443. https://doi.org/10.1007/s00345-011-0779-8.
91. Jácomo RH, Alves AT, Dos Santos Bontempo AP, Botelho TL, Teixeira FA, De Sousa JB. Effect of increasing awareness of genital anatomy on pelvic floor muscle strength in postmenopausal women: a randomized controlled trial. *Top Geriatr Rehabil.* 2016;32(4):274–279. https://doi.org/10.1097/TGR.0000000000000122.
92. Tuttle LJ, DeLozier ER, Harter KA, Johnson SA, Plotts CN, Swartz JL. The role of the obturator internus muscle in pelvic floor function. *J Women's Heal Phys Ther.* 2016;40(1):15–19. https://doi.org/10.1097/JWH.0000000000000043.
93. Asavasopon S, Rana M, Kirages DJ, et al. Cortical activation associated with muscle synergies of the human male pelvic floor. *J Neurosci.* 2014;34:13811–13818. https://doi.org/10.1523/JNEUROSCI.2073-14.2014.
94. Choi H, Palmer MH, Park J. Meta-analysis of pelvic floor muscle training: randomized controlled trials in incontinent women. *Nurs Res.* 2007;56:226–234. https://doi.org/10.1097/01.NNR.0000280610.93373.e1.
95. Oliveira M, Ferreira M, Azevedo MJ, Firmino-Machado J, Santos PC. Pelvic floor muscle training protocol for stress urinary incontinence in women: a systematic review. *Rev Assoc Med Bras (1992)* 2017;63(7):642–650.
96. Herderschee R, Ejc H, Gp H, et al. Feedback or biofeedback to augment pelvic floor muscle training for urinary incontinence in women. 2011;7. https://doi.org/10.1002/14651858.CD009252.Copyright.
97. Fitz FF, Resende APM, Stüpp L, Sartori MGF, Girão MJBC, Castro RA. Biofeedback for the treatment of female pelvic floor muscle dysfunction: a systematic review and meta-analysis. *Int Urogynecol J.* 2012;23:1495–1515. https://doi.org/10.1007/s00192-012-1707-1.
98. Norton C, Cody JD. Biofeedback and/or sphincter exercises for the treatment of faecal incontinence in adults. *Cochrane Database Syst Rev.* 2012;11(7):CD002111. https://doi.org/10.1002/14651858.CD002111.pub3.
99. Anderson CA, Omar MI, Campbell SE, Hunter KF, Cody JD, Glazener CM. Conservative management for postprostatectomy urinary incontinence. *Cochrane Database Syst Rev* 2015;1:CD001843. https://doi.org/10.1002/14651858.CD001843.pub5.

100. Schreiner L, Santos TG Dos, Souza ABA De, Nygaard CC, Silva Filho IG Da. Electrical stimulation for urinary incontinence in women: a systematic review. *Int Braz J Urol* 2013;39:454–464. https://doi.org/10.1590/S1677-5538.IBJU.2013.04.02.
101. Slovak M, Chapple CR, Barker AT. Non-invasive transcutaneous electrical stimulation in the treatment of overactive bladder. *Asian J Urol.* 2015;2:92–102. https://doi.org/10.1016/j.ajur.2015.04.013.
102. Correia GN, Pereira VS, Hirakawa HS, Driusso P. Effects of surface and intravaginal electrical stimulation in the treatment of women with stress urinary incontinence: randomized controlled trial. *Eur J Obstet Gynecol Reprod Biol.* 2014;173:113–118. https://doi.org/10.1016/j.ejogrb.2013.11.023.
103. Sung MS, Hong JY, Choi YH, Baik SH, Yoon H. FES-biofeedback versus intensive pelvic floor muscle exercise for the prevention and treatment of genuine stress incontinence. *J Korean Med Sci.* 2000;15:303–308. https://doi.org/10.3346/jkms.2000.15.3.303.
104. Guo ZF, Liu Y, Hu GH, Liu H, Xu YF. Transcutaneous electrical nerve stimulation in the treatment of patients with poststroke urinary incontinence. *Clin Interv Aging.* 2014;9:851–856.
105. Yamanishi T, Yasuda K, Sakakibara R, Hattori T, Suda S. Randomized, double-blind study of electrical stimulation for urinary incontinence due to detrusor overactivity. *Urology.* 2000;55:353–357. https://doi.org/10.1016/s0090-4295(99)00476-8.
106. Berghmans B, Hendriks E, Bernards A, de Bie R, Omar MI. Electrical stimulation with non-implanted electrodes for urinary incontinence in men. *Cochrane Database Syst Rev.* 2013;(6):CD001202. https://doi.org/10.1002/14651858.CD001202.pub5.
107. Stewart F, Berghmans B, Bø K, Glazener CM. Electrical stimulation with non-implanted devices for stress urinary incontinence in women. *Cochrane Database Syst Rev.* 2017;12.
108. Booth J, Connelly L, Dickson S, Duncan F, Lawrence M. The effectiveness of transcutaneous tibial nerve stimulation (TTNS) for adults with overactive bladder syndrome: a systematic review. *Neurourol Urodyn.* 2018;37(2):528–541.
109. Day MR, Patricia L-W, Loughran S, O'Sullivan E. Community-dwelling women's knowledge of urinary incontinence. *Br J Community Nurs.* 2014;19:534–538. https://doi.org/10.12968/bjcn.2014.19.11.534.
110. Novick BJ, Angie M, Walker E, et al. The effect of intensive education on urinary incontinence following radical prostatectomy: a randomized control trial. *Urol Nurs.* 2014;34:246–251. https://doi.org/10.7257/1053-816X.2014.34.5.246.
111. Sjöström M, Umefjord G, Stenlund H, Carlbring P, Andersson G, Samuelsson E. Internet-based treatment of stress urinary incontinence: a randomised controlled study with focus on pelvic floor muscle training. *BJU Int.* 2013;112:362–372. https://doi.org/10.1111/j.1464-410X.2012.11713.x.
112. Anger JT, Nissim HA, Le TX, et al. Women's experience with severe overactive bladder symptoms and treatment: insight revealed from patient focus groups. *Neurourol Urodyn.* 2011;30(7):1295–1299. https://doi.org/10.1002/nau.21004.
113. Imamura M, Williams K, Wells M, Mcgrother C. Lifestyle interventions for the treatment of urinary incontinence in adults. *Cochrane Database Syst Rev.* 2015;(12):CD003505. https://doi.org/10.1002/14651858.CD003505.pub5.
114. Corcos J, Przydacz M, Campeau L, et al. CUA guideline on adult overactive bladder. *Can Urol Assoc J.* 2017;11(5):E142–E173. https://doi.org/10.5489/cuaj.4586.
115. Swithinbank L, Hashim H, Abrams P. The effect of fluid intake on urinary symptoms in women. *J Urol.* 2005;174:187–189. https://doi.org/10.1097/01.ju.0000162020.10447.31.
116. Jura YH, Townsend MK, Curhan GC, Resnick NM, Grodstein F. Caffeine intake, and the risk of stress, urgency and mixed urinary incontinence. *J Urol.* 2011;185:1775–1780. https://doi.org/10.1016/j.juro.2011.01.003.
117. Segal S, Saks EK, Arya LA. Self-assessment of fluid intake behavior in women with urinary incontinence. *J Women's Health.* 2011;20:1917–1921. https://doi.org/10.1089/jwh.2010.2642.
118. Gleason JL, Richter HE, Redden DT, Goode PS, Burgio KL, Markland AD. Caffeine and urinary incontinence in US women. *Int Urogynecol J.* 2013;24(2):295–302. https://doi.org/10.1007/s00192-012-1829-5.
119. Hooper L, Bunn D, Jimoh FO, Fairweather-Tait SJ. Water-loss dehydration and aging. *Mech Ageing Dev.* 2014;136–137:50–58. https://doi.org/10.1016/j.mad.2013.11.009.
120. Begg DP. Disturbances of thirst and fluid balance associated with aging. *Physiol Behav.* 2017;178:28–34. https://www.sciencedirect.com/science/article/abs/pii/Soo31938416307235?via%3Dihub.
121. Ostaszkiewicz J, Johnston L, Roe B. Timed voiding for the management of urinary incontinence in adults. *Cochrane Database Syst Rev.* 2004;(1):CD002802. Review. https://doi.org/10.1002/14651858.CD002802.pub2.
122. Engberg S, Sereika SM, McDowell BJ, et al. Effectiveness of prompted voiding in treating urinary incontinence in cognitively impaired homebound older adults. *J Wound Ostomy Continence Nurs.* 2002;29(5):252–265.
123. Milne JL. Behavioral therapies at the primary care level: the current state of knowledge. *J Wound Ostomy Continence Nurs.* 2004;31:367–372.
124. Health Quality Ontario. Behavioural interventions for urinary incontinence in community-dwelling seniors: an evidence-based analysis. *Ont Health Technol Assess Series.* 2008;8(3):1–52.
125. Danziger ZC, Grill WM. Sensory and circuit mechanisms mediating lower urinary tract reflexes. *Auton Neurosci Basic Clin.* 2016;200:21–28. https://doi.org/10.1016/j.autneu.2015.06.004.
126. Stav K, Leibovici D, Yoram SI, Ronny O, Zisman A. Self-induced plantar-flexion objectively reduces wave amplitude of detrusor overactivity and subjectively improve urinary urgency: a pilot study. *Neurourol Urodyn.* 2014;33:1247–1250. https://doi.org/10.1002/nau.22493.
127. Takano S, Sands DR. Influence of body posture on defecation: a prospective study of "The Thinker" position. *Tech Coloproctol.* 2016;20:117–121. https://doi.org/10.1007/s10151-015-1402-6.
128. Lee BA, Kim SJ, Choi DK, Kwon O, Na HR, Cho ST. Effects of pelvic floor muscle exercise on urinary incontinence in elderly women with cognitive impairment. *Int Neurourol J.* 2017;21(4):295–301. https://doi.org/10.5213/inj. 1734956.478.
129. Bazi T, Takahashi S, Ismail S, et al. Prevention of pelvic floor disorders: international urogynecological association research and development committee opinion. *Int Urogynecol J.* 2016;27:1785–1795. https://doi.org/10.1007/s00192-016-2993-9.

CHAPTER 23

Wellness in the Older Adult

David M. Morris, Rita A. Wong

OUTLINE

INTRODUCTION

The World Health Organization (WHO) defines health as "a state of complete physical, mental, and social well-being and not merely the absence of disease or infirmity."[1] The National Wellness Institute defines wellness as "an active process through which people become more aware of, and make choices toward, a more successful existence."[2] Wellness is often described in terms of three interconnected domains of well-being: physical, psychological (mental), and social. Wellness is considered both a process and an outcome achieved through health promotion and disease prevention efforts. Wellness programs give participants skills and tools that promote optimal health and maximize personal potential.

Two related terms, *health promotion* and *disease prevention*, are often used in conjunction with the term *wellness*. The WHO defines health promotion as "the process of enabling people to increase control over, and to improve, their health."[3] It moves beyond a focus on individual behavior toward a wide range of social and environmental interventions. *The Guide to Physical Therapist Practice (The Guide)*[4] describes prevention services provided by physical therapists (PTs) as a mechanism to "forestall or prevent functional decline and the need for more intensive care." Prevention is divided into three categories: (1) primary prevention: identifying risk factors and implementing services to individuals and populations before health effects occur; (2) secondary prevention: preventing or slowing progression of functional decline and disability from an identified condition; and (3) tertiary prevention: reducing or slowing the progression of disability and deterioration from an ongoing health condition to optimize activity and participation.

Health promotion and disease prevention programs typically focus on enhancing wellness across one or more of the three broad domains of physical, psychological, and social health, as well as one or more of the six interconnected dimensions of personal wellness: physical, emotional, spiritual, social, occupational/vocational, and intellectual (Table 23.1 and Fig. 23.1).[2] Although these dimensions are frequently described in the wellness literature, there is little scientific evidence to confirm or reject these dimensions as the primary underlying factors making up the broad construct of "wellness." Despite the lack of a clear understanding of the various components of the construct of wellness, wellness is generally accepted as a multidimensional entity that includes factors associated with physical, psychological, and social health. Wellness becomes a philosophy of life that utilizes health promotion and disease prevention strategies to achieve the goal of optimal aging. Optimal aging implies maximizing one's ability to function across physical, psychological, and social domains to one's satisfaction and despite one's medical conditions.[5]

Wellness is a critical component of contemporary physical therapy practice.[6–8] In a 2009 two-part review,[6,7] Dean made a compelling argument for physical therapist clinical competencies in promoting healthy lifestyle behaviors concerning physical activity, dietary habits, weight management, stress management, smoking, and

TABLE 23.1 Wellness Domains

Health Domain	Wellness Dimension	Description
Physical	Physical	Physical functioning to the degree that allows one to perform roles in family and society
Mental	Emotional	Sense of well-being and the ability to cope effectively with life's "ups and downs"
	Spiritual	Aspect of life that provides meaning and direction that connects to something greater than one's self
	Intellectual	Ability to learn and use information effectively and to reason and use self-efficacy in wellness endeavors
Social	Social	Meaningful relationships and presence of a social support structure
	Occupational/ vocational	Purpose in life, a reason to get up in the morning

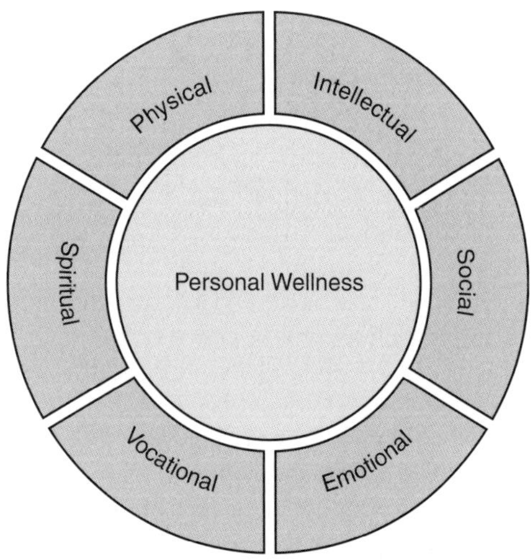

FIG. 23.1 Six dimensions of wellness. *(Courtesy of Lifetime Wellness, Ltd., Longview. Texas.)*

sleep.[6,7] She emphasized the relationship of lifestyle behaviors to mortality and morbidity from such common health conditions as ischemic heart disease, smoking-related conditions, hypertension and stroke, obesity, diabetes, and cancer. She described physical therapists as particularly well positioned for this role because of their educational background and their relatively lengthy contact with patients that often leads to a close and trusting relationship, an important component of behavior change intervention. The American Physical Therapy Association (APTA)[9] position statement "Physical Therapists' Role in Prevention, Wellness, Fitness, Health Promotion and Management of Disease and Disability" (Box 23.1) describes the PT as uniquely qualified to promote wellness in clinical practice, research, advocacy, and collaborative consultation as well as serving as a dynamic link between health promotion and health services delivery. The APTA position statement on "Health Priorities for Population and Individuals"[10] includes critical statements about the importance of PTs in promoting active living in individual older adults and within older adult populations. Injury prevention in the areas of falls, workplace injury, and community-based injury is specifically identified in the position statement. Educational, patient advocacy, and referral opportunities, applicable across age groups, are also highlighted in the position statement and listed Box 23.2.

In 2017, Lein and colleagues published a consensus-driven and validated Health-Focused Physical Therapy (HFPT) model as a framework for PT educators to integrate prevention, wellness, and health promotion content

BOX 23.1 Physical Therapists' Role in Prevention, Wellness, Fitness, Health Promotion, and Management of Disease and Disability[9]

For their role as a dynamic link between health and health services delivery, physical therapists:

1. apply their expertise in exercise and physical activity to adapt health recommendations for individuals and populations, from clinical settings to the home and community;
2. function as a member of an interprofessional team of health providers, wellness and fitness providers, community health workers, public health providers, and other diverse professionals to help individuals and populations reduce their disease risk and improve their health and quality of life; and
3. communicate and collaborate with relevant health professionals to help individuals and populations receive appropriate health services.

Excerpt from APTA position statement: *Physical Therapists' Role in Prevention, Wellness, Fitness, Health Promotion, and Management of Disease and Disability*. HOD P06-16-05 [Initial: HOD P06-15-23-15] [Position].[9]
APTA, American Physical Therapy Association.

BOX 23.2 Health Priorities for Populations and Individuals

Physical therapists provide education, behavioral strategies, patient advocacy, referral opportunities, and identification of supportive resources after screening for the following additional U.S. NPS health priorities:

- Stress management
- Smoking cessation
- Sleep health
- Nutrition optimization
- Weight management
- Alcohol moderation/substance-free living
- Violence-free living
- Adherence to health care recommendations

Excerpt from APTA position statement: "Health Priorities for Populations and Individuals", HOD P06-15-20-11 [Position].[10]
APTA, American Physical Therapy Association; *NPS*, National Prevention Strategy.

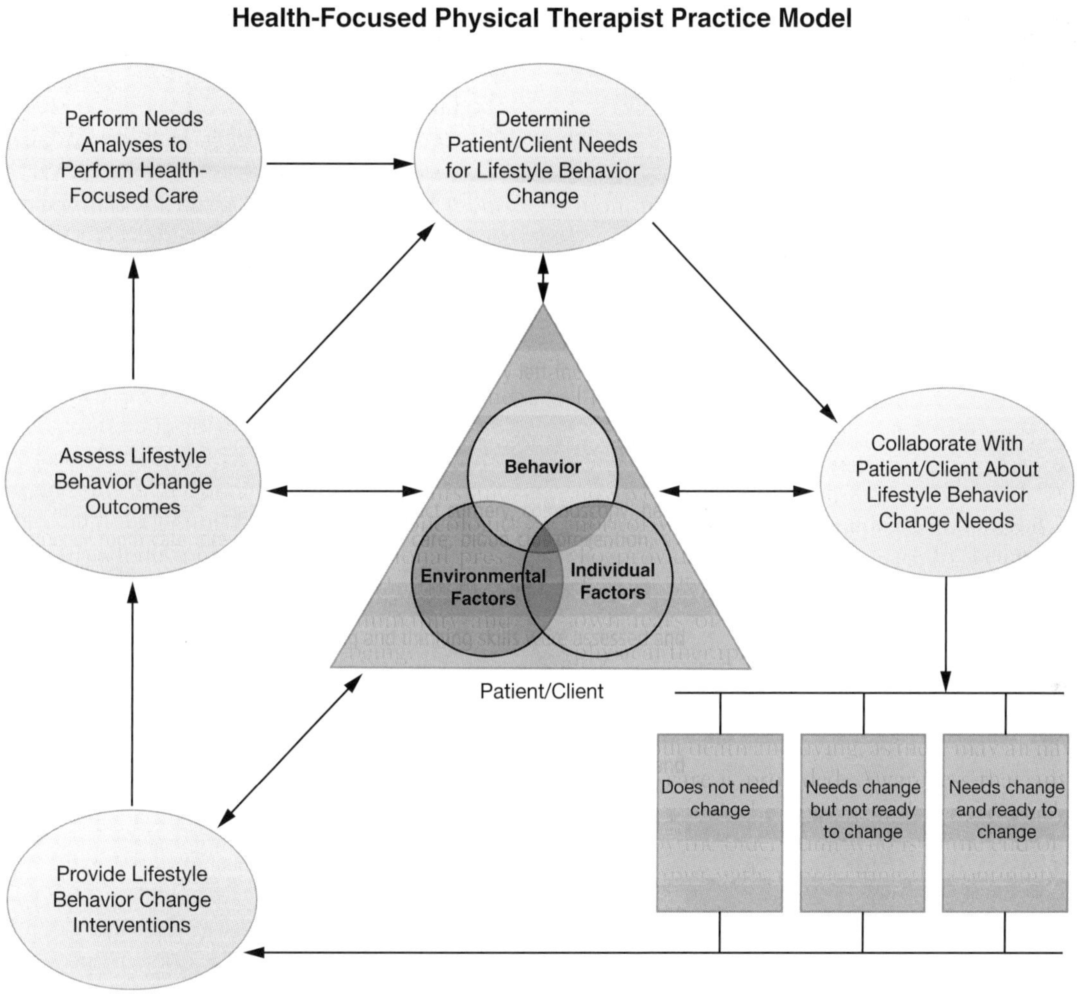

Health-Focused Physical Therapist Practice Model

FIG. 23.2 Health-Focused Physical Therapy (HFPT) model. *(From Lein DH, Clark D, Graham C, Perez P, Morris DM. A model to integrate health promotion and wellness in physical therapist practice: development and validation. Phys Ther. 2017;97:1169–1181.)*

into customary PT clinical care coursework.[11] This model, displayed in Fig. 23.2, includes screening and management of lifestyle behaviors framed to be consistent with and integrated into the APTA's *Guide to Physical Therapist Practice*. The model describes wellness-oriented activities as well as emphasizing use of health data surveillance systems to assess the anticipated needs of your patient/client population, developing wellness-oriented consultancy networks, gathering wellness-oriented patient education materials, and using effective communication strategies (e.g., motivational interviewing) to assist patients/clients to adopt healthier lifestyles.

In this chapter, each of the three dimensions of wellness will be explored, with emphasis placed on important considerations for providing PT services for older adults. All health care practitioners have a role in promoting wellness to their older adult patients/clients. The PT practitioner is particularly well suited/positioned to address the physical health domain of adopting/maintaining an active lifestyle.[6–8] As such, promoting physical activity will be explored in greater depth, including examples of successful programs/strategies for achieving active lifestyles in older patients/clients. Finally, resources and tools for further study about wellness, older adults, and PT will be provided.

A comprehensive approach to wellness considers all three health dimensions and the overlapping lifestyle issues most commonly identified as contributing to poor health and mortality: physical inactivity, poor dietary habits, obesity, uncontrolled and chronic stress, smoking, and insufficient/ineffective sleep.[6–8] The physical dimension of health will focus on the lifestyle considerations of physical activity, healthy eating, weight management, smoking cessation, and sleep health. The psychological dimension will address stress management. The social dimension will focus on the impact of social connectedness and social networks on physical and emotional well-being.

PHYSICAL WELLNESS

The physical dimension of wellness is primarily influenced by physical activity, nutrition, weight management, sleep, and tobacco use plus the early detection and treatment of diseases and medical conditions and avoidance of iatrogenic complications. Physical fitness involves cardiorespiratory endurance (aerobic power), skeletal muscle endurance, skeletal muscle strength, skeletal muscle power, flexibility, balance, speed of movement, reaction time, and body composition.[12] An individual's fitness and health goals dictate the fitness dimensions of most importance to achieving those goals.

Physical Activity. Exercise is the single most important health-promoting activity for older adults.[12] Current recommendations for physical activity to achieve health benefits are a minimum of 150 minutes per week of *moderate to intense* aerobic activity and strengthening of the major muscle groups 2 or more days per week (Table 23.2).[12] However, the Centers for Disease Control and Prevention (CDC) reports that only 17% of individuals aged 65 and older achieve these aerobic plus muscle-strengthening guidelines.[13] Physical therapists are uniquely qualified to guide older adults to improve physical wellness through individualized fitness and physical activity programs.[6–8] Physical therapists, as movement specialists, can provide information, guidance, and help that is particularly relevant to older adults striving to optimize their aging—by maintaining and enhancing function, and adapting physical activity and exercise programs to accommodate pain or other disability that challenges movement ability. Communicating and marketing the value of having a physical therapist engaged in wellness programs (e.g., directly or as a consultant) are key to promoting the functional abilities and wellness of aging adults. The important role of PTs in promoting physical activity is addressed in greater detail later in this chapter.

TABLE 23.2 2018 Physical Activity Guidelines for Older Adults
Move more and sit less throughout the day—some physical activity is better than none
At least 150 minutes to 300 minutes a week at moderate intensity, or 75 minutes to 150 minutes a week at vigorous intensity, or an equivalent combination; preferable to spread these activity bouts throughout the week
Additional benefits are gained by engaging in physical activity beyond 300 minutes at moderate intensity
Muscle strengthening—at moderate or greater intensity 2 or more days/week that work all major muscle groups
Multicomponent physical activity that includes balance training as well as aerobic and muscle strengthening
Should determine their level of physical activity relative to their fitness level
Older adults with chronic conditions should understand whether and how their conditions affect their ability to do regular physical activity safely
When unable to do 150 minutes of moderate activity a week because of chronic conditions, should be as physically active as their abilities and conditions allow

Healthful Eating and Weight Management. Poor nutrition can lead to either excessive weight loss or excessive weight gain (obesity). Both are associated with mortality, frailty, and lower quality of life. In 2015, <42% of U.S. adults reported eating fruit on a daily basis and <22% reported eating vegetables each day.[13] For adults aged 65 and older, 34.3% and 21.4%, respectively, consumed fruit and vegetables on a daily basis. As reported by the CDC in 2016, 28% of individuals aged 65 years and older adults are obese and 39% are overweight.[13] Maintaining a healthy body weight promotes optimal aging. There is strong evidence that a body mass index (BMI) over 20 to 21 is associated with the risk of developing a wide range of chronic health conditions including type 2 diabetes, heart disease, and hypertension.[14] Weight loss in obese individuals is associated with improved functional status and amelioration of frailty in older adults.[15] Dietary interventions may decrease the risk or progression of macular degeneration, stroke, heart attacks, lipid abnormalities, osteoarthritis and osteoporosis, and a number of cancers.[16–19] There is growing evidence that older adults can benefit from regular use of a daily multivitamin containing age-appropriate recommended amounts of folic acid and vitamins B_6, B_{12}, D, and E, as older adults are often deficient through dietary intake. Suboptimal vitamin D levels (serum 25-hydroxyvitamin D) have been associated with poor balance, weakness, and increased risk of hip fracture.[20] Table 23.3 provides a summary of the key nutritional considerations outlined in the U.S. Department of Agriculture MYPLATE nutritional guidelines for older adults, advocated by many gerontologists.[21]

The taste buds for salt and sweet decline with increasing age. By 60 years of age, most people have lost approximately half of their taste buds, a change that further accelerates after age 70.[22] These factors often result in increased use of salt and sweetner in food to achieve the comparable taste intensity experienced as a younger adult. Increased use of salt and sugar can pose problems for

TABLE 23.3 Recommendations from the U.S. Department of Agriculture's MYPLATE for Older Adults

1. Add flavor to foods with spices and herbs instead of salt, and look for low-sodium packaged foods.
2. Add sliced fruits and vegetables to your meals and snacks. Look for presliced fruits and vegetables on sale if slicing and chopping is a challenge.
3. Ask your doctor to suggest other options if the medications you take affect your appetite or change your desire to eat.
4. Drink 3 cups of fat-free or low-fat milk throughout the day. If you cannot tolerate milk try small amounts of yogurt, buttermilk, hard cheese, or lactose-free foods. Drink water instead of sugary drinks.
5. Consume foods fortified with vitamin B_{12}, such as fortified cereals.

older individuals with hypertension or diabetes. Other age-related changes that impact taste and enjoyment of food include decreased saliva flow and changes in oral secretions, increased incidence of gum and tooth disease, smoking and chronic diseases such as diabetes, and interventions used in cancer management (medications, radiation, and surgery), which may each contribute to the decline of taste sensitivity and overall food enjoyment. Increasing the color, aroma, and texture of food by supplementing with spices, herbs, and flavor extracts, as well as use of sugar and salt substitutes, can greatly enhance taste and flavor without compromising health conditions.

Physical therapists should be ready to advise older adults on basic nutrition principles to manage weight or accommodate high levels of physical activity.[6–8] The APTA position statement titled *The Role of the Physical Therapist in Diet and Nutrition*[23] states that diet and nutrition are key components of primary, secondary, and tertiary prevention of many conditions managed by physical therapists. Physical therapists have a role in screening for and providing information about diet and nutritional issues to patients, clients, and the community within the scope of PT practice. A variety of screening tools can assist the PT to identify poor eating. This includes appropriate referrals to nutrition and dietary health professionals when the required advice and education lies outside the education level of the PT.[24] The PT will also work with nutrition specialists who can provide individualized assessment of nutritional needs and recommendations for nutritional modifications in managing special diets (e.g., control of diabetes or morbid obesity).

When assessing eating patterns and weight management, the PT should look for overeating and undernourishment as well as obesity and underweight status. Some helpful assessment tools for examining eating patterns include Rate your Plate[25]; Rapid Eating Assessment for Patients Scale (REAPS)[26]; Common Measures, Better Outcomes (COMBO) questionnaire[27]; the Mini Nutritional Assessment (MNA)[28]; and the DETERMINE Your Nutritional Health Questionnaire.[29] The DETERMINE is particularly helpful for detecting undernourishment as the name is an acronym for common reasons for undernourishment (i.e., Disease, Eating poorly, Tooth loss/mouth pain, Economic hardship, Reduced social contact, Multiple medicines, Involuntary weight loss/gain, Needs assistance in self-care, Elder years above age 80). Common assessments for overweight and obesity include BMI calculations, waist circumference calculations, and skinfold caliper assessments.[30]

PT management of poor eating habits is mostly directed at patient education, ensuring that the patient understands good nutritional practices. It may be helpful to share one of the many consumer-focused educational resources identified in Box 23.3 with your patients needing nutritional guidance. It is important to avoid sharing "fad diet" information and resources that include unproven advice.[21,31–33] When the patient's/client's nutritional needs exceed the PT's scope of practice, the most common referral resource is a registered dietitian nutritionist (RDN). An RDN has completed an accredited educational program on dietetics, has completed a supervised practicum, and has passed a national examination administered by the Commission on Dietetic Registration. You can find RDNs in your area by going to the "find an expert" section of Eatright.org.[33]

BOX 23.3 Sources of Consumer-Focused Nutritional Recommendations for Older Adults

Name of Initiative	Sponsor	Web Link
ChooseMyPlate.gov[21]	U.S. Department of Agriculture	https://www.choosemyplate.gov/
Eat Healthy	President's Council on Fitness, Sports and Nutrition, the National Center on Health; US Department of Health and Human Services.[30]	https://www.hhs.gov/fitness/eat-healthy/index.html
Nutrition	National Center on Health, Physical Activity, and Disability (NCHPAD)[31]	https://www.nchpad.org/Articles/12/Nutrition
Eatright	Academy of Nutrition and Dietetics[33]	https://www.eatright.org/

Sleep Health. Proper sleep is an important factor in maintaining a healthy body and mind. In general, although older adults spend less time asleep than younger adults,[34] experts recommend that older adults get 7 to 8 hours of quality sleep each night.[34] Certain types of sleep disorders are particularly problematic with older adults.[35–37] For example, older adults are more likely to experience sleep architecture problems (e.g., they spend more time in the lighter stages of sleep and decreased time in the deep, more restorative stage of sleep). This altered sleep pattern results in low-quality, ineffective sleep. Older adults with sleep insufficiency are less likely to report their symptoms and seek a solution than younger adults, often thinking it is a normal part of aging. Even worse, when the concern is finally mentioned, the complaint may be disregarded and considered a normal part of aging by the health care provider. Although there are changes in sleep patterns with aging, poor sleep is not an inevitable consequence of aging. The prevalence of poor sleep among older adults is higher in individuals with multiple physical and psychiatric conditions.

Sleep is a behavior. As such, it is subject to learning and can be influenced by intentional, motivational, and habit-related factors, discussed later in this chapter. Spielman and colleagues[38] describe a 3P model for describing the underlying causes of sleep insufficiency: (1) predisposing factors—risk factors that increase the likelihood that the older adult will experience poor sleep (e.g., physical and mental health problems, family history of sleep insufficiency, low socioeconomic status, genetic factors); (2) precipitating factors—events that acutely disrupt sleep (e.g., depressive episodes, hospitalization, loss of a loved one, changing place of residence); and (3) perpetuating factors—behavioral, psychological, environmental, and physiological factors that maintain poor sleep (e.g., drinking alcohol close to bedtime, physical inactivity, certain medications). The predisposing and precipitating factors lead to the development of poor sleep, and the perpetuating factors contribute to the ongoing continuation of poor sleep. Medical conditions may also be the source of poor sleep. The top most common sleep disorders are insomnia, sleep apnea, and restless leg syndrome.

Questions about sleep health can and should be incorporated into the PT examination of older adults. Bezner recommends questions like "Do you get 7-8 hours of sleep each night?; Are you tired in the morning?; Do you fall asleep quickly?; Are you sleepy during the day?; and Do you wake up at night?"[8] If further assessment is warranted, screening tools are available to assess common sleep disorders. For example, the Insomnia Severity Index[39] and the STOP-Bang questionnaire[40] are helpful for identifying chronic insomnia and obstructive sleep apnea, respectively. More detailed questionnaires are also available including the Pittsburgh Sleep Quality Index[41] and Epworth Sleepiness Scale.[42] The formal assessment strategies can be particularly helpful for identifying the need for a referral to a sleep professional.

Patients/clients with more serious sleep issues that fall outside the PT's scope of practice should be referred to another professional for a more extensive sleep evaluation.[43] A general medical practitioner can often identify and manage many sleep issues (e.g., identifying a medication interaction or a need to treat depression symptoms). However, a certified sleep physician may be required for a thorough sleep examination of a persistent sleep issue.

PT management of poor sleep is typically focused around educating about sleep hygiene, promoting exercise, advising on proper positioning in bed to decrease pain or discomfort affecting sleep quality, and referring patients/clients to other professionals.[43] Sleep hygiene is defined as behaviors/routines that help to promote good sleep. Patient/client education about better sleep hygiene practices can be easily integrated into usual PT services. Some of the more common sleep hygiene recommendations are listed in Table 23.4.[44–46] If the PT has limited time to discuss these sleep hygiene principles, they can be shared on handouts and/or on the clinic's website. Box 23.4 provides a listing of websites and organizations that provide credible and informative consumer-focused resources about principles of sleep hygiene.

Exercise can positively influence many health issues, including poor sleep.[43] Studies suggest that acute and chronic exercise has a moderately positive benefit on sleep duration and quality. The exact mechanism by which exercise improves sleep is unknown, however. Although exercise is beneficial, most individuals should avoid exercising in the evening because an increase in body temperature is believed to interfere with natural sleep mechanisms. Relaxation or meditative exercise can also be helpful (e.g., tai chi, yoga, deep breathing, progressive relaxation).

TABLE 23.4 Commonly Accepted Sleep Hygiene Tips

Commonly Accepted Sleep Hygiene Tips
Go to bed and get up at the same time every day.
Drink caffeinated drinks only in the mornings.
Avoid alcohol.
Avoid smoking, especially in the evenings.
Lose weight if overweight.
Exercise regularly, but not before bedtime.
Use your bed only for sleep and sex.
Avoid looking at a screen before bedtime.
Get out of bed if you cannot get to sleep in 20 minutes and return when sleepy.
Create a comfortable, quiet, and cool environment in your bedroom.
Avoid daytime napping.

BOX 23.4 Resources for Consumer Educational Materials on Principles of Sleep Hygiene

National Sleep Foundation[44]
American Academy of Sleep Medicine[45]
Centers for Disease Control and Prevention
U.S. Department of Health and Human Services
National Institute for Neurological Disorders and Stroke[46]

Pain is a common complaint associated with poor sleep.[43] As such, the PT can be helpful for assessing sleep positioning issues and making recommendations for comfort. This might include identifying optimal positions (e.g., side-lying or supine), use of pillows to support body parts, and bed mobility skill training. In 2017, Siengsukon and colleagues published a seminal article in *Physical Therapy* that addressed the role of the PT in sleep health promotion.[43] This article is highly recommended for PTs wishing to learn more.

Many interventions outside the scope of PT practice may be helpful for improving sleep with older adults. For example, sleeping medications may help improve sleep, especially when used along with better sleep habits. It is recommended that sleeping pills be used for only short time periods. Common medications for poor sleep include antidepressants, benzodiazepines, doxepin, eszopiclone, ramelteon, suvorexant, zaleplon, zolpidem, and over-the-counter sleep aids. Side effects include daytime sedation, drowsiness, dizziness, lightheadedness, cognitive impairment, incoordination, dependence, respiratory suppression, and rebound insomnia. Older adults taking sleep medications should be monitored closely for fall risks.

Cognitive-behavioral therapy (CBT) includes strategies that correct cognitive distortions about insomnia, improve sleep hygiene, address maladaptive behaviors, reduce stimuli that promote wakefulness, and incorporate relaxation training and/or biofeedback.[47] Patients can receive CBT from a trained therapist or through self-guided modules. CBT has been found to be superior to medication use in short- and long-term management of insomnia in older adults to improve sleep efficiency, reduce sleep latency, and decrease time awake at night.

Used for sleep apnea, continuous positive airway pressure (CPAP) is a form of positive airway pressure that applies mild air pressure to keep the airways continuously open. When used properly, the therapy has been shown to reduce the number of respiratory events during sleep, decrease daytime sleepiness, and improve overall quality of life of older adults.[48,49] Adherence to CPAP is related to the severity of the symptoms. Individuals with severe symptoms tend to have the highest adherence at about 89%, but this decreases to around 55% for those with low severity.[50] Proper fit of the mask is essential to adherence and effectiveness. Also, newer devices are smaller, quieter, and more portable.

Smoking Cessation. Cigarette smoking is a major public health concern. In 2016, 15.5% of U.S. adults reported that they smoke.[51] Though down from 20.9% reported in 2005, smoking is still the leading cause of preventable death in the United States. Billions of U.S. dollars are spent annually on smoking-related health issues. Nearly 9 of every 100 (8.8%) adults aged 65 years or older identify as smokers. Individual with disabilities report higher rates of smoking (20.5%) than those without disabilities. Smoking harms nearly every organ in the body, can impede recovery from disease or injury (e.g., slows wound and fracture healing), and is strongly linked to cancer, heart disease, stroke, lung disease, diabetes, and chronic obstructive pulmonary disease. It also increases risk for tuberculosis, certain eye diseases, and problems of the immune system.[51] It is important to note that significant health benefits can be realized by quitting smoking regardless of age or length of time smoking. Quitting smoking can be difficult, however, with an average of nine attempts reported before a smoker quits smoking for good. The barriers and challenges to quitting include withdrawal symptoms (e.g., feeling nervous and anxious), fear of failure, weight gain, lack of support from friends/family, and depression.[52] Although critically important for comprehensive health care for smokers, a survey of PTs reported that few PTs engage in smoking cessation counseling with their patients/clients who smoke.[53] PTs report multiple barriers to smoking cessation counseling including low confidence and feeling unprepared to do so.[53]

As part of the PT examination, older adult patients/clients should routinely be asked if they smoke cigarettes. Further, if they answer yes, they should be advised on strategies for quitting.[8] When asking about sensitive issues like smoking, it is helpful to use a structured approach. Some examples of such an approach are the National Institute on Drug Abuse Quick Screen,[54] Tobacco Questions for Survey from the Global Tobacco Surveillance System,[55] and the Fagerstrom Nicotine Dependence Test.[56] The Fagerstrom is unique in that it gives the practitioner an idea of the degree of the patient's/client's nicotine dependency.

The primary PT management strategy for smokers is to educate and advise them. Physical activity is known to assist with smoking cessation by decreasing stress/anxiety and reducing weight gains commonly experienced. To educate and advise effectively, the PT must gain an in-depth knowledge of smoking cessation. A great resource for doing this is the Treating Tobacco Use and Dependence website created by the U.S. Agency for Healthcare Research and Quality (AHRQ).[57] This resource highlights the AHRQ's clinical guidelines and recommendations for health care practitioners. It also directs the health care provider to educational resources for patients/clients and to state-based quit phone lines where they can access advice and resources from trained counselors. PTs should also know about medications that aid in smoking cessation so that they can advise and encourage their patients/clients to explore these with their physicians. Finally, several excellent resources for smoking cessation are tailored for older adults. These include a National Institute on Aging website titled Quitting Smoking for Older Adult[58] and another one specifically tailored for patients/clients titled Smokefree60+.[59]

PSYCHOLOGICAL WELLNESS

Psychological wellness includes the emotional, cognitive, and spiritual dimensions of wellness. Emotional wellness involves the control of stress and effective coping with life situations. High stress levels combined with poor coping mechanisms can lead to negative physiological (e.g., cardiovascular, musculoskeletal), emotional (e.g., depression, anxiety, anger), and behavioral (e.g., inability to work, inefficiency) responses.[60] Cognitive wellness occurs when you are confident that you have the skills needed to accomplish a task or achieve a goal (self-efficacy) and you are interested in actively engaging in the world.

Spiritual health includes the values, morals, and ethics that guide an individual's search for a state of harmony and inner balance. Spirituality is about a person's existence and relationships with self, others, and the universe. Spirituality does not necessarily connote religiosity.[60] The spirituality dimension may increase with age, perhaps because of increased time to reflect about one's role in the universe and the meaning of life.[61]

Ryff and Keyes,[61] in a confirmatory factor analysis of a large group of adults across a wide age range, identified six distinct dimensions associated with psychological wellness that integrate elements from several theorists such as Erikson, Maslow, and Rogers. They labeled these six dimensions: (1) positive self-regard, (2) mastery of the surrounding environment, (3) continued growth and development, (4) the belief that life is purposeful and meaningful, (5) quality relationships with other people, and (6) capacity for self-determination. A healthy psychological outlook can reduce the intensity and duration of illnesses, creating the so-called mind–body interaction. Although the absence of mental distress or illness does not equate to psychological well-being, attention to these six domains can promote a sense of well-being and hope that encompasses psychological health.

The classic definition of stress is a condition or feeling experienced when a person perceives that demands exceed the personal and social resources the individual is able to mobilize.[62] However, it is difficult to quantify what constitutes "excessive stress" because contributors to stress are very broad and reactions to the stressors are very subjective. Stress is associated with a family of related experiences, pathways, responses, and outcomes. Stress is extremely subjective (i.e., something that is stressful to one individual may not be to another) and can be caused by a range of different events or circumstances.[62] In actuality, stress is a part of daily life for most everyone. It is not necessarily a "bad" thing. A certain level of stress can be motivating, beneficial, and even enjoyable. Stress becomes negative when it is chronic, defeating, and/or humiliating. The "fight or flight" phenomenon is commonly used to describe the physiologic effects of stress. This response occurs when a person perceives a threat. In this situation, hormones are released that influence physiologic systems that help to make the person faster and stronger (e.g., heart rate and blood pressure increase). This response can also make a person overexcitable, anxious, jumpy, and irritable, reducing the effectiveness of his or her response. A more contemporary view of the harmful effects of stress involves allostasis and allostatic load. Allostasis is an adaptive process that maintains homeostasis through the production of mediators such as adrenalin, cortisol, and other chemical messengers.[63,64] It occurs when the fight or flight response is induced repeatedly. When induced chronically, it can result in an imbalance of primary mediators of homeostatic responses (some excessive and some inadequate). Eventually, this "ramped up" state leads to wear and tear on the body's systems, a state referred to as "allostatic overload." The negative effect of allostatic overload can include poor brain function (e.g., impaired sleep, impaired memory, neuron atrophy), cardiovascular stress (e.g., hypertension, atherosclerotic plaques), impaired immune system response (e.g., suppressed immunity), and metabolic dysfunction (e.g., insulin resistance, reduced glucose uptake). When experienced, physical symptoms commonly reported include irritability, fatigue, muscle aches, headaches, gastrointestinal distress, and insomnia. Associated medical conditions include hypertension, angina, gastrointestinal ulcers, obesity, myalgia, and arthralgia. In a 2012 survey, the American Psychological Association reported that 77% of U.S. respondents reported regularly experiencing physical symptoms caused by stress and 33% believed that they were living with extreme stress.[62] Common causes of stress reported (from worst to least) were job pressure, money, health, relationships, poor nutrition, media overload, and sleep deprivation.

PTs can screen patients for stress using the Psychological Stress Measure (PSM-9)[65] and the Patient Stress Questionnaire.[66] The General Anxiety Disorder-7 (GAD-7)[67] and the Zung Self-Rating Anxiety Scale[68] can also be helpful for distinguishing general stress from more severe mental health conditions needing a referral to a mental health professional.

PTs can assist their patients with stress management in a variety of ways including stress management education, promoting physical activity and a healthy diet, and promoting relaxation strategies, meditation, and mindfulness. Table 23.5 provides some helpful tips to share with patients as common stress management strategies, and Box 23.5 provides examples of available resources for stress management.[69–72]

A variety of stress-reducing techniques, falling under the categories of relaxation, meditation, and mindfulness, can be taught to and encouraged with patients. These three categories are different yet share some common elements. Progressive muscle relaxation (PMR) exercises induce stress reduction by sequentially tightening or tensing one muscle group at a time followed by a deliberate relaxation phase or release of tension. First described by Jacobson in the 1930s, these techniques are easy to learn

TABLE 23.5 Commonly Accepted Stress Management Tips

To change stress you can: • Set boundaries—learn to say "no." • Spend time with people you enjoy—limit time with those who "stress you out." • Change your environment. • Express your feeling (assertively, respectfully, prepared to negotiate).
When the situation cannot be changed, change your response: • Try to reframe the situation. • Take the long view. • Avoid the trap of perfectionism. • Recognize what is beyond your control—focus on the things you can influence and "let go" of that you cannot control. • Learn to forgive—"let go" of anger and resentment.
Healthy habits that help: • Talk things over with those you trust. • Make time for yourself. • Keep a sense of humor. • Eat right, sleep enough, exercise, and avoid alcohol and drugs as an escape.

BOX 23.5 Examples of Publicly Available Patient Education Materials and Resources for Stress Management

National Institutes of Mental Health[69]	https://www.nimh.nih.gov/index.shtml
Mental Health America[71]	http://www.mentalhealthamerica.net/
U.S. Department of Health and Human Services	https://www.hhs.gov/
American Psychological Association	https://www.apa.org/

and require only short periods of time to execute (e.g., 10 to 20 minutes each day).

Whereas the focus of PMR is the individual muscles, the focus of meditation is to develop a focused and tranquil mind state.[73] During meditation, patient/clients are encouraged to focus their attention and eliminate the excessive stream of thoughts that may be crowding their minds and causing stress. A wide array of meditation forms are available including guided meditation, mantra meditation, mindfulness meditation, and transcendental meditation. Qui gong, tai chi, and some forms of yoga are also considered to have meditation-oriented qualities. Mindfulness can be defined as an awareness that arises through intentionally attending in an open, accepting, and discerning way to whatever is arising in the present moment.[74] Mindfulness can be cultivated, at least in part, using strategies like meditation.

SOCIAL WELLNESS

Social wellness includes the social and occupational dimensions of wellness. In general, social well-being involves the ability to develop and maintain healthy relationships with others, to feel connected to a community or group, to interact well with other people, and to have a support structure to call on during difficult times. Social supports significantly influence the ability to cope with life's stressors. Social networks also help to protect older people against harm and promote emotional and physical well-being. For older adults, social connectedness is often a priority need and helps people find a balance between quality of life and compromised health. People considered socially well are usually involved with others, rather than isolated, and they report satisfactory levels of perceived social support.

Five major factors make up the construct of social wellness.[75] These five factors are:

1. Social integration ("I feel close to other people in my community")
2. Social contribution ("My daily activities are worthwhile to my community")
3. Social coherence ("I can make sense of what's going on in the world")
4. Social actualization ("Society is improving for people like me")
5. Social acceptance ("People care about the social issues that are important to me")

In a large-scale set of two studies that included adult subjects between 18 and 74 years of age, Keyes found that social well-being increased with age (although more slowly with increasing age) in all categories except for social coherence, which decreased with increasing age.

Social supports and caregiving can be both formal and informal. Formal caregiving involves paid services, usually from agencies and organizations that address basic needs of individuals such as personal care, meals, and transportation. Informal (unpaid) caregiving, typically provided by family, friends, and significant others, often is the main source of emotional and psychosocial support for the older adult. A healthy social network provides a safety net for older adults. Older adults who lack adequate social supports are more vulnerable to safety risks such as abuse and substance misuse and are at risk for depression, impaired decision making, isolation, loneliness, poor health, and decreased life expectancy.[68]

Occupational/vocational wellness is closely linked to social wellness. A basic tenet of occupational/vocational wellness is a balance between work, home, and leisure activities, with the opportunity to engage in meaningful activity.[76] Occupational wellness refers to one's attitude about one's work and to having an occupational or vocational interest in life. An occupationally well person is one who is involved in paid and nonpaid activities that are personally rewarding and make a contribution to the well-being of the community at large. As older individuals leave paid work, purposeful employment (occupation) can be replaced with purposeful and meaningful activity such as volunteer activities (vocation). Vocational wellness occurs through matching core values with interests, hobbies, employment, and volunteer work. Retirement can bring opportunities for vocational wellness. Employment or vocational endeavors can provide a sense of purpose, enrichment-enhanced mental health indices, and overall wellness in older adults.[77]

The dimensions of wellness described earlier demonstrate the capacity of older adults to live optimally throughout their days. Wellness is a concept to strive for regardless of health conditions. Although PTs deal primarily with the domain of physical wellness, familiarity with the other domains of wellness will enhance the PT's ability to promote optimal aging.

PHYSICAL ACTIVITY AND EXERCISE–FOCUSED WELLNESS PROGRAMS

In the past two decades, the efficacy of physical activity for facilitating wellness of older adults, whether through community-, clinic-, or home-based programs, is well established. Fundamental and meaningful change in strength, balance, flexibility, function, and community participation is possible with exercise regardless of age.[78,79] Therefore, the inclusion of activity promotion, purposeful physical engagement, and/or exercise should be a goal of any wellness program for all older adults.

PHYSICAL THERAPISTS' SCOPE OF PRACTICE

Providing health promotion and wellness services in the area of physical fitness and patient education in healthy lifestyle principles is considered a practice expectation of physical therapists.[9,10] However, when licensed health professionals such as physical therapists deliver wellness services, they must function within the scope of practice allowed by their state licensing laws. Each state has its own laws regarding the practice of physical therapists. Many states now allow full and direct access to patients; some states require a physician referral for any access to a patient. Most states allow physical therapists to evaluate and screen individuals without physician referral but then have varying provisions regulating the implementation of an intervention. For several states, the language of the state physical therapy practice act makes a clear statement allowing physical therapists to provide wellness and fitness programs without physician referral when the purpose is for prevention of illness or improved functional ability (in the absence of an acute illness or injury). However, other state practice acts do not provide this option. Thus, physical therapists must be familiar with the licensing regulations in their state and organize wellness services to comply with these regulations.

The ability to legally evaluate and provide wellness services to older adults is a separate consideration from the ability to be reimbursed by health care insurers. Frequently, patients' rehabilitative needs far exceed their Medicare benefits. For example, older individuals with fractured hips frequently show continued improvement with extended exercise rehabilitation programs offered beyond the regular rehabilitation period.[80] Other clients with chronic conditions may be ineligible for traditional physical therapy because they require "maintenance," an area that many insurance providers do not cover. In recent years, however, some insurers have directed benefits toward supporting physical activity in older adults. For example, some Medicare supplemental plans will support selected evidence-based exercise programs and gym memberships (e.g., SilverSneakers). General deconditioning (e.g., following treatment for cancer or even severe flu), neurologic disease such as Parkinson disease, and dizziness are examples of chronic conditions that fall into the cracks of our health care system. These patient groups are examples of older adult clients who may benefit substantively from follow-up care or wellness for which the expertise of a physical therapist could be particularly useful.

Screening for Physical Activity and Wellness Programs

Screening is an essential part of a physical activity/exercise-focused wellness program to determine the appropriateness of individuals to participate and may help to stratify individuals to the appropriate program or level within a program. Screening is a precursor to baseline and outcomes assessment.

The Physical Activity Readiness Questionnaire (Par-Q), validated for adults between 18 and 69 years of age, is a popular screening tool to identify readiness to exercise. The freely available Par-Q tool consists of seven questions that address possible contraindications to exercise.[81] A positive answer on any of these seven risk items indicates a need to further investigate the individual's readiness for more intense physical activity. However, a concern expressed by users of the Par-Q is that the tool's emphasis on identifying potential contraindications to increasing physical activity has been an unnecessary barrier in many instances to encouraging self-initiated and safe exercise participation. The original Par-Q has been modified over time to add a MED PAR-X form that can be used to communicate with the client's medical team as well as a Par-Q+ and a Physical Activity Readiness Medical Examination Online (ePARmed-X+).[82] The newer forms are intended to enhance risk stratification by including follow-up questions about the medical conditions identified (Par-Q+). If concerns are identified in the Par-Q+, the person is encouraged to complete the ePARmed-X+, with more in-depth guidance through an online screening and exercise recommendation.

In response to the limitations of the Par-Q, the Exercise Assessment and Screening for You (EASY) tool was developed.[83] This six-question online screening tool (Table 23.6) identifies potential health problems that require health care provider clearance before exercising, provides education about each problem and the value of exercise, and helps older adults choose appropriate exercises that may not first require a physician's approval. The EASY tool emphasizes the benefits of exercise and physical activity for all individuals while educating the older adult about how to exercise within the individual's limitations. The EASY tool provides instant recommendations

TABLE 23.6 Exercise and Screening for You (EASY)

1. Do you have pains, tightness, or pressure in your chest during physical activity (walking, climbing stairs, household chores, similar activities)?
2. Do you currently experience dizziness or lightheadedness?
3. Have you ever been told you have high blood pressure?
4. Do you have pain, stiffness, or swelling that limits or prevents you from doing what you want or need to do?
5. Do you fall, feel unsteady, or use assistive device while standing or walking?
6. Is there a health reason not mentioned why you would be concerned about starting an exercise program?

(Adapted from Exercise and Screening for You. http://www.easyforyou.info/index.asp. Accessed January 5, 2019.)

regarding the safety of exercise or the need for the client to see a physician before exercising.

Finally, in 2015, the Canadian Society for Exercise Physiology (CSEP) created the Get Active Questionnaire. The new screening tool is recommended as it was developed by consensus, grounded in evidence, includes individuals older than 69 years of age, is user friendly, and is believed to encourage and "screen in" older adults to engage in regular physical activity. The Get Active Questionnaire is self-administered on the CSEP website created for that purpose.[84]

Regardless of which screening tool is used, additional questions about the presence of osteoporosis and falls history are helpful with older clientele. Certain movements such as excessive thoracic flexion, common in the presence of osteoporosis, have been linked to thoracic fractures,[85] and fractures result more easily with falls.[86] In addition, fear of falling may be more acute in individuals who know they have a heightened risk of fracture.[87] The physical therapist can provide valuable information and exercise cueing to avoid potential problems if awareness of osteoporosis is present. Table 23.7 describes screening questions for osteoporosis. Although no one tool exists as a criterion standard of fall risk,[88] a recent systematic review identified five medical screening questions, two self-report measures, and five performance-based tools that each contribute to the determination of fall risk and provide supporting evidence.[89] A summary of the scores and level of support of each tool is provided as Fig. 7.2 in Chapter 7.[89]

Baseline and Outcomes Assessment

Baseline measures for physical activity/exercise-focused wellness programs can help establish program goals and identify specific areas to target, such as flexibility, strength, and aerobic fitness. Baseline measures can also be used to stratify clients to an appropriate exertional and skill level. Ideally, baseline information should be gathered that determines health issues, prior exercise history, functional deficits, impairments such as poor cardiovascular endurance, strength deficits, and balance issues. In addition, clients' adherence and self-efficacy can improve when regular feedback is given about their progress.[90]

TABLE 23.7 Screening for Osteoporosis
The physical therapist can ask for:
The results of previous dual-energy x-ray (DEXA), heel scan indicating (T-score of −2.5 or more)
Family history of osteoporosis (mother, sisters, grandmother)
Low body mass index
History of vertebral or wrist fractures[190]
Observe presence of kyphosis[191]
Loss of height of >4 cm[192]

Many objective and responsive tools are available to measure different aspects of physical ability, and many of these tools have age-based normative data. The specific measurements or assessments used depend on the amount of time available, the condition of the client, and the focus of the program.

The Senior Fitness Test (SFT) is a readily available physical performance tool to assess general older adult fitness. The test was developed by Rikli and Jones to assess fitness and physical parameters associated with functional ability in those over 60 years of age. It is a reliable and valid test in community-dwelling older individuals and those with dementia.[22,91,92] The test is responsive to change in high-intensity and functional exercise programs.[93] The SFT can identify whether an older adult may be at risk for loss of functional ability, making it also suitable as a screening tool in the community setting.[94] The SFT has six functional tasks in the domains of strength, endurance, balance, agility, and flexibility, which are scored separately. Each item has percentile norms for men and women aged 60 to 94-plus based on a national study of more than 7000 Americans, making it possible to compare one's performance against similarly aged individuals. Additionally, the SFT provides threshold values on each test item that help to identify if an older adult is at risk for mobility loss.[95] More recently, the authors developed valid and reliable criterion-referenced standards to indicate thresholds to preserve mobility and independence in later years (Table 23.8).[96]

Directions for test administration are freely available on the web (https://www.interactivehealthpartner.com/pdf/fft_overview.pdf). The test takes approximately 30 minutes to complete and is suitable for a community wellness environment. The normative values for the SFT [94–95] have been broadly reproduced in many online resources as a component of directions for interpretation of the test. Threshold criteria from Rikli and Jones are listed in Table 23-9.[95]

The normative values for the SFT[94–95] have been broadly reproduced in many online resources as a component of directions for interpretation of the test. The test takes approximately 30 minutes to complete and is suitable for a community wellness environment.

For example, if a walking program is the focus of the wellness activity, then the assessment may be heart rate response to walking in a 6-minute walk test, gait speed, 1-mile walk, or a 24-hour pedometer reading. If the intended outcome is improved balance, then baseline measures of balance capacity should be used. A wide range of functional assessment tools are described in Chapter 7, including data on the validity and reliability of each tool as well as normative data across various age groups.

Knowledge of the clients' physical activity history can provide valuable baseline information if a goal is to improve physical activity. Knowledge of clients' physical activity history can help determine a starting point for the physical activity/exercise class. A detailed history of prior training is likely important if preparing older adults for an

TABLE 23.8 Criterion-Referenced Fitness Standards for Maintaining Physical Independence in Older Adults

Task	Age Groups							% of Decline Reflected over 30 Years
	60–64	65–69	70–74	75–79	80–84	85–89	90–94	
Lower body strength (no. of chair stands in 30 seconds)								
Men	15	15	14	13	12	11	9	40.0
Women	17	16	15	14	13	11	9	47.1
Upper body strength (no. of arm curls in 30 seconds)								
Men	17	17	16	15	14	13	11	35.3
Women	19	18	17	16	15	13	11	42.1
Aerobic endurance (no. of yards walked in 6 minutes)								
Men	625	605	580	550	510	400	400	36.0
Women	680	650	620	580	530	400	400	41.2
Alternate aerobic endurance (no. of steps in 2 minutes)								
Men	97	93	89	84	78	60	60	38.1
Women	106	101	95	88	80	60	60	43.4
Agility/dynamic balance (8-foot Up and Go, seconds)								
Men	5.0	5.3	5.6	6.0	6.5	7.1	8.0	37.5
Women	4.8	5.1	5.5	5.9	6.4	7.1	8.0	40.0
Mean decline = 40.1								

From Rikli RE, Jones CJ. Development and validation of criterion-referenced clinically relevant fitness standards for maintaining physical independence in later years. *Gerontologist* 2013;53(2).262.

intense exercise activity such as a competitive senior Olympic sport. If working with a group of frail seniors in an assisted living facility, the only question that may be needed is, "Have you ever been active?"

Outcome measures for program evaluation can be used to provide individual feedback on progress, to evaluate and determine whether the class has met its purpose, and to provide data on the program's effectiveness. Individual client feedback focused on the clients' wellness goals can be provided at the end of the program. Consideration should be made for the time it takes to realize a change in the desired outcome. For example, 12 months or more may be needed to achieve weight loss goals, to increase physical activity to recommended wellness levels, or to realize quality-of-life changes.[97,98] However, specific strength and endurance gains may occur in as little as 12 to 15 weeks.[99] Recognizing that several months may be required to achieve functionally important physical changes, it is important to provide feedback that highlights the short-term successes the patient is achieving along the longer-term path to more functionally visible outcomes—for example, sticking with a commitment for regular attendance and participation in physical activity, lower perceived exertion with the same workload, and additional repetitions of exercises or distance walked without a rest. Early success in physical activity endeavors positively reinforces commitment to pursuit of long-term physical activity goals. Individual results can be provided in terms of age-based norms for additional value to the client.

Program evaluation can also be determined by factors such as class attendance, clients' adherence, and satisfaction with the various components of the program, such as self-perception of health and lifestyle changes. Summary scores of performance-based outcome tools can provide an indication of general strength gains, weight loss, and balance improvement in the group. Program evaluation outcomes should relate to the purpose and focus of the program.

Types of Physical Activity and Exercise Programs

There are literally hundreds of opportunities for physical therapists to promote wellness for the older adult client. Fortunately, there are resources available, some in book or monograph form, many on the Internet, and numerous video-based protocols that may be used to assist in the design of an activity program. Several types of programs are presented here. Utilizing existing resources is encouraged when a specialty wellness activity program is chosen. Physical activity/exercise-focused wellness programs can be developed in any venue such as health clubs, outpatient offices, older adult residences, senior centers, health-related clinics, nursing homes, rehab hospital gyms, religious facilities, or individually. Wellness programs can also take the form of consultant-type services. The following section provides an overview of physical activity programs. Chapter 8 provides a more detailed discussion of many of these programs.

Balance and Fall Prevention Programs. Many older adults are justifiably afraid of falling as their balance is beginning to decline and reaction times are slower than they were in younger years. Balance programs are quite varied, particularly if they capitalize on popular programs such as tai chi. Tai chi is known to be effective in improving balance and reducing fall risk, and its movements and principles can be incorporated into any balance activity.[100] Tai chi was also shown to reduce symptoms of knee osteoarthritis[101] and reduce blood pressure.[102]

Tai chi is one of many approaches to enhancing balance in older adults. Literature has demonstrated that balance will improve if multimodal programs are used.[103,104] The programs should include challenge to static and dynamic balance provided two to three times a week for at least 8 weeks, environmental assessment and remediation, visual assessment and remediation (if needed), vestibular assessment, and promotion of strength, particularly of the lower extremity muscles.[105,106] In 2015, the CDC published a compendium of specific interventions for which there is evidence for reducing falls in community-dwelling older adults.[107] The CDC also provides a comprehensive set of materials that address falls prevention through the Stopping Elderly Accidents, Deaths, and Injuries (STEADI) initiative. This CDC website provides a wide range of information for consumers, health professions, and caregivers as well as training and educational materials.

Strength Training. The efficacy of strength training for older adults has been demonstrated by numerous investigators. From the seminal article by Fiatarone et al.[108] in 1990 to more contemporary issues of power versus velocity versus traditional weights, a multitude of evidence overwhelmingly supports the inclusion of strength training for all older adults, including those who are frail, have multiple comorbidities, and have never done any type of resistance activity.[109–112]

Strength training can be done in myriad ways, including traditional free weights, isotonic-type machines, elastic bands, functional activities (e.g., weighted chair stands, stair climbing), and incorporating high-velocity training into, and emphasizing power-based training in, class-type activity or individual exercises. Unless medically contraindicated, resistance training should be incorporated into all activity programs for older adults.[113–115] Chapter 8 provides dose-specific recommendations to increase strength.

Exercise for Frail Older Adults. The number of 80-plus-year-old individuals is increasing rapidly in the United States, and these individuals are at greatest risk for loss of independence.[116] A large proportion of this population is deconditioned, with poor muscular and cardiovascular endurance as well as muscle weakness, associated with sedentary lifestyle and periodic bouts of bed rest from illnesses and hospitalizations. More than 50% of individuals older than age 80 years are physically inactive; at least 60% have difficulty with functional activities such as stooping, crouching, kneeling, lifting or carrying 10 pounds, and standing from an armless chair; and 30% have difficulty with very basic activities of daily living such as dressing and bathing.[117] Individuals who have low physical activity levels, need help with daily activities, fatigue easily, are weak, and have slow motor performance and balance abnormalities are likely to be classified as frail.[118]

Wellness classes are greatly needed for frail and near-frail older adults. However, this is the most challenging group to tackle given preexisting medical conditions, lack of endurance, low physical activity levels, and generalized weakness.[118] Nonetheless, developing and implementing programs for the frail is interesting, gratifying, and wonderfully challenging. Exercise focused on remediating frailty and improving function in frail older adults can be task specific, as research has shown that task-specific exercise is equivalent to resistance training.[119,120] Task-specific exercise has the advantage of being relevant to the frail older adult, which may promote participation.

General conditioning exercises are extremely effective for prefrail older adults and can be done in groups.[121–123] These classes should focus on strengthening activities, particularly the lower extremities, dynamic balance (in standing position), and functional activities such as getting up and down from the floor, stair climbing, and walking distances of 0.25 to 1 mile. An advantage of group classes is the socialization they provide that may promote exercise adherence.

Exercise to Enhance Bone Quality/Quantity. One of every two women older than age 50 years is on a trajectory to develop osteoporosis if she does not have it already.[124] Consequently, wellness programs that emphasize bone loading are important and highly pertinent. Key components to all of the approaches to enhance bone health are core strengthening exercises for abdominals and back extensors, possible use of a weighted vest (if there is no kyphosis), strengthening exercises for the scapular retractors and upward rotators, and lower extremity loading.[125] Physical activity recommendations for enhancing bone quality include progressive resistive training, walking activities, high-impact weight-bearing activities, and whole-body vibration.[126]

Aerobic Training. The vast majority of older adults have cardiovascular deconditioning, most of which is the consequence of a sedentary lifestyle.[127] The presence of cardiovascular disease does not preclude aerobic training; to the contrary, the presence of disease makes aerobic training even more important.[128,129] There is no evidence indicating a worsening of cardiovascular disease with exercise. In fact, exercise actually improves the disease state (e.g., congestive heart failure, post–myocardial infarction) and raises the level of conditioning. The only time exercise is contraindicated for heart disease is if a client is in the midst of an acute crisis.[113] In the presence of substantial deconditioning, nearly all exercise constitutes an aerobic challenge. Thus, it is often not necessary to consider aerobic exercise within the narrow framework of running, cycling, Nordic track, elliptical trainer, or stair stepper. Dance, tai chi, brisk walking, and resistive strengthening functional activities are often of sufficient intensity to achieve an aerobic training effect in deconditioned individuals.

Enhancing Physical Activity and Mobility. Mobility-challenged older adults are often one fall or illness away from admission to assisted care or a nursing home. Mobility programs for sedentary and frail older adults that are chair based have very limited mobility benefit. Wellness activities for this population should heavily incorporate daily functional mobility skills, such as handling pots and pans, carrying items, sweeping and vacuuming, putting clothes away, and stooping to pick up items from the floor. Gait activities are also important and should include changing direction suddenly, walking backward, changing gait speed quickly in response to a command, walking under time pressure the distance required to cross a street with the light, and stepping up and down from a curb. Obstacle courses and circuit training activities can be fun, meaningful, and effective for individuals struggling to stay independent.[130]

Walking Programs. Walking programs are very easy to set up, require little supervision, and can provide numerous benefits such as socialization, sense of well-being, self-efficacy, and health benefits such as decreased pain (in the presence of knee osteoarthritis) and improved glycemic control.[131] Pedometers are effective in tracking steps and can promote physical activity more so than encouragement alone to be more physically active. Recommendations of 10,000 steps/day (5 miles) are associated with health benefits.[132] The Walk with Ease program, a program of the Arthritis Foundation,[133] is acknowledged by the CDC as a community-based program with demonstrated benefit in the management of arthritis symptoms and mobility limitations.

SUMMARY

Given the burgeoning older adult population, an increasing life span, and the greater risk of frailty and loss of independence for people over 80 years of age, wellness programs and self-management of chronic health conditions are increasingly important. Because increased physical activity and exercise is most important for health and physical and cognitive well-being, every physical therapist should be involved in promoting physical activity and exercise programs. Physical therapists have the skills required to prevent the spiraling decline in independence among the aging and aged population. The efficacy of physical activity and exercise programs has been demonstrated. Elements of endurance as in walking, strengthening, and balance should be incorporated. All that is required is willingness to begin and an appropriate assessment of resources.

REFERENCES

1. World Health Organization. Constitution of the World Health Organization. *Chronicle World Health Organ.* 1947;1:29–43.
2. National Wellness Institute. *Definition of wellness.* https://www.nationalwellness.org/page/Six_Dimensions; 2019. Accessed 27 December 2019.
3. World Health Organization. Health promotion. https://www.who.int/healthpromotion/fact-sheet/en/. Accessed March 18, 2019.
4. American Physical Therapy Association. *Guide to Physical Therapist Practice.* http://guidetoptpractice.apta.org/. Last updated November 27, 2016.
5. Brummel-Smith K. Optimal aging. Part II: evidence-based practical steps to achieve it. *Ann Long Term Care.* 2007;15(12):32–40.
6. Dean E. Physical therapy in the 21st century (part I): toward practice informed by epidemiology and the crisis of lifestyle conditions. *Physiother Theory Pract.* 2009;25(5–6):330–353.
7. Dean E. Physical therapy in the 21st century (part II): evidence-based practice within the context of evidence-informed practice. *Physiother Theory Pract.* 2009;25(5 6):354–368.
8. Bezner JR. Promoting health and wellness: implications for physical therapist practice. *Phys Ther.* 2015;95:1433–1444.
9. American Physical Therapy Association. Physical Therapist's Role in Prevention, Fitness, Health Promotion, and Management of Disease and Disability. http://www.apta.org/uploadedFiles/APTAorg/About_Us/Policies/Practice/PTRoleAdvocacy.pdf. Last updated September 2, 2016.
10. American Physical Therapy Association. Health Priorities for Populations and Individuals. http://www.apta.org/uploadedFiles/APTAorg/About_Us/Policies/Practice/HealthPrioritiesPopulationsIndividuals.pdf. Last updated June 3, 2015.
11. Lein DH, Clark D, Graham C, Perez P, Morris DM. A model to integrate health promotion and wellness in physical therapist practice: development and validation. *Phys Ther.* 2017;97:1169–1181.
12. U.S. Health and Human Services, Office of Disease Prevention and Health Promotion. Physical Activity Guidelines for Americans, 2nd edition. https://health.gov/paguidelines/second-edition/pdf/Physical_Activity_Guidelines_2nd_edition.pdf
13. Centers for Disease Control and Prevention. Nutrition, Physical Activity, and Obesity: Data Trends and Maps. https://www.cdc.gov/nccdphp/dnpao/data-trends-maps/index.html. Accessed January 1, 2019.
14. Fontana L, Hu FB. Optimal body weight for health and longevity: bridging basic, clinical, and population research. *Aging Cell.* 2014;13(3):391–400.
15. Villareal DT, Banks M, Sinacore DR, et al. Effect of weight loss and exercise on frailty in obese older adults. *Arch Intern Med.* 2006;166(8):860–866.
16. Wu J, Cho E, Willett WC, Sastry SM, Schaumberg DA. Intakes of lutein, zeaxanthin, and other carotenoids and age-related macular degeneration during 2 decades of prospective follow-up. *JAMA Ophthalmol.* 2015;133(12):1415–1424.

17. Van Horn L, Carson JA, Appel LJ, et al. Recommended dietary pattern to achieve adherence to the American Heart Association/American College of Cardiology (AHA/ACC) guidelines: a scientific statement from the American Heart Association. *Circulation.* 2016;134:e505–e529.
18. Agarwal P, Wang Y, Buchman AS, Bennett DA, Morris MC. Dietary patterns and self-reported incident disability in elderly. *J Gerontol A Biol Sci Med Sci.* 2019;74(8):1331–1337.
19. Maggini S, Pierre A, Calder PC. Immune function and micronutrient requirements change over the life course. *Nutrients.* 2018;10(10):1531. https://doi.org/10.3390/nu10101531.
20. Lv QB, Gao X, Liu X, et al. The serum 25-hydroxyvitamin D levels and hip fracture risk: a meta-analysis of prospective cohort studies. *Oncotarget.* 2017;8(24):39849–39858.
21. U.S. Department of Agriculture. ChooseMyPlate.gov. https://www.choosemyplate.gov/. Accessed January 2, 2019.
22. Hesseberg K, Bentzen H, Bergland A. Reliability of the Senior Fitness Test in community-dwelling older people with cognitive impairment. *Physiother Res Int.* 2015;20(1):37–44. https://doi.org/10.1002/pri.1594.
23. American Physical Therapy Association. The Role of the Physical Therapist in Diet and Nutrition. http://www.apta.org/uploadedFiles/APTAorg/About_Us/Policies/Practice/RolePTDietNutrition.pdf; 2019. Accessed 11 March 2019.
24. Morris DM, Kitchin EM, Clark DE. The physical therapist as an important member of the nutrition management team. *Physio Theory Practice.* 2009;25:408–423.
25. Brown University Institute for Community Health. Rate Your Plate. https://www.brown.edu/academics/public-health/research/health-equity/sites/brown.edu.academics.public-health.research.health-equity/files/uploads/RYPALL%20Revised.pdf; 2019. Accessed 2 January 2019.
26. Brown University Institute for Community Health. Rapid Eating Assessment for Patients (REAP). https://txpeds.org/sites/txpeds.org/files/documents/reap.pdf; 2019. Accessed 2 January 2019.
27. Fernald DH, Froshaug DB, Dickinson M, et al. Common measures, better outcomes (COMBO): a field test of brief health behavior measures in primary care. *Am J Prev Med.* 2008;35(5S):S414–S422.
28. Kaiser MJ, Bauer JM, Ramsch C, et al. Validation of the Mini Nutritional Assessment Short-Form: a practical tool for identification of nutritional status. *J Nutr Health Aging.* 2009;13:782–788.
29. Nutritional Screening Initiative. DETERMINE Your Nutritional Health. https://nutritionandaging.org/wp-content/uploads/2017/01/DetermineNutritionChecklist.pdf; 2019. Accessed 2 January 2019.
30. Racette SB, Deusinger SS, Deusinger RH. Obesity: overview of prevalence, etiology, and treatment. *Phys Ther.* 2003;83(3):276–288.
31. U.S. Department of Health and Human Services. President's Council on Sports, Fitness and Nutrition. https://www.hhs.gov/fitness/index.html; 2019. Accessed 2 January 2019.
32. National Center on Health. Physical Activity, and Disability (NCHPAD). Building Healthy Inclusive Communities. https://www.nchpad.org/; 2019. Accessed 2 January 2019.
33. Academy of Nutrition and Dietetics. Eatright. https://www.eatright.org/; 2019. Accessed 2 January 2019.
34. Hirshkowitz M, Whiton K, Albert SM, et al. The National Sleep Foundation's sleep time duration recommendations: methodology and results summary. *Sleep Health.* 2015;1(1):40–43.
35. Gooneratne NS, Vitiello MV. Sleep in older adults: normative changes, sleep disorders, and treatment options. *Clin Geriatr Med.* 2014;30(3):591–627.
36. Suzuki K, Miyamoto M, Hirata K. Sleep disorders in the elderly: diagnosis and management. *J Gen Fam Med.* 2017;18:61–71.
37. Rodriguez JC, Dzierzewski JM, Alessi CA. Sleep problems in the elderly. *Med Clin North Am.* 2015;99:431–439.
38. Spielman AJ, Caruso LS, Glovinsky PB. A behavioral perspective on insomnia treatment. *Psychiatr Clin North Am.* 1987;10(4):541–553.
39. Bastien CH, Vallieres A, Morin CM. Validation of the Insomnia Severity Index as an outcome measure for insomnia research. *Sleep Med.* 2001;2:297–307.
40. Nagappa M, Wong J, Sign M, Wong DT, Chung F. An update on the various practical applications of the STOP-Bang questionnaire in anesthesia, surgery, and perioperative medicine. *Curr Opin Anaesthesiol.* 2017;30:118–125.
41. Backhaus J, Junghanns K, Broocks A, Riemann D, Hohagen F. Test-retest reliability and validity of the Pittsburgh Sleep Quality Index in primary insomnia. *J Psychom Res.* 2002;53:737–740.
42. Johns MW. A new measure for measuring daytime sleepiness: the Epworth Sleepiness Scale. *Sleep.* 1991;14(6):540–545.
43. Siengsukon CF, Aldughmi M, Stevens S. Sleep health promotion: practical information for physical therapists. *Phys Ther.* 2017;97(8):826–836.
44. National Sleep Foundation. Sleep.org. https://www.sleepfoundation.org/. Accessed January 2, 2019.
45. American Academy of Sleep Medicine. https://aasm.org/; 2019. Accessed 2 January 2019.
46. National Institute for Neurological Disorders and Stroke. Brain basics: understanding sleep. https://www.ninds.nih.gov/Disorders/Patient-Caregiver-Education/Understanding-Sleep; 2019. Accessed 2 January 2019.
47. Bloom HG, Ahmed I, Alessi CA, et al. Evidence-based recommendations for the assessment and management of sleep disorders in older persons. *J Am Geriatr Soc.* 2009;57(5):761–789.
48. Yan B, Jin Y, Hu Y, Li S. Effects of continuous positive airway pressure on elderly patients with obstructive sleep apnea: a meta-analysis. *Med Sci (Paris).* 2018;34:66–73.
49. Serrano Merino J, Torres LP, Bardwell W, et al. Impact of positive pressure treatment of the airway on health-related quality of life in elderly patients with obstructive sleep apnea. *Biol Res Nurs.* 2018;20(4):452–461.
50. Jacobsen AR, Eriksen F, Hansen RW, et al. Determinants for adherence to continuous positive airway pressure therapy in obstructive sleep apnea. *PLoS One.* 2017;12(12):e0189614.
51. Centers for Disease Control and Prevention. Current Cigarette Smoking Among Adults in the United States. https://www.cdc.gov/tobacco/data_statistics/fact_sheets/adult_data/cig_smoking/index.htm; 2019. Accessed 18 March 2019.
52. Pignataro RM, Ohtake PJ, Swisher A, Dino G. The role of physical therapists in smoking cessation: opportunities for improving treatment outcomes. *Phys Ther.* 2012;92(5):757–766.
53. Bodner ME, Miller WC, Rhodes RE, Dean E. Smoking cessation and counseling: knowledge and views of Canadian physical therapists. *Phys Ther.* 2011;91:1051–1062.
54. National Institute on Drug Abuse. The NIDA Quick Screen. https://www.drugabuse.gov/publications/resource-guide-screening-drug-use-in-general-medical-settings/nida-quick-screen; 2019. Accessed 4 January 2019.
55. Centers for Disease Control and Prevention and the World Health Organization. Tobacco Questions for Surveys: A Subset of Key Questions from the Global Tobacco Survey (GATS). https://www.who.int/tobacco/publications/surveillance/en_tfi_tqs.pdf; 2019. Accessed 4 January 2019.
56. Heatherson TF, Kozlowski LT, Frecker RC, Fagerstrom K. The Fagerstrom Test for nicotine dependence: a revision of the Fagerstrom Tolerance Questionnaire. *Br J Addict.* 1991;86(9):1119–1127.

57. U.S. Department of Health and Human Services, Agency for Healthcare Research and Quality. Treating Tobacco Use and Dependence: 2008 Update. https://www.ahrq.gov/professionals/clinicians-providers/guidelines-recommendations/tobacco/index.html. Accessed January 5, 2019.
58. U.S. Department of Health and Human Services, National Institute on Aging. Quitting Smoking for Older Adults. https://www.nia.nih.gov/health/topics/smoking. Accessed January 5, 2019.
59. U.S. Department of Health and Human Services. National Institute on Aging, National Cancer Institute. Smoke free 60+. https://60plus.smokefree.gov/; 2019. Accessed 5 January 2019.
60. Atchley RC. *Spirituality and Aging*. Baltimore: Johns Hopkins Press; 2009.
61. Ryff CD, Keyes CL. The structure of psychological well-being revisited. *J Pers Soc Psychol*. 1995;69(4):719–727.
62. American Psychological Association. Stress in America: The State of Our Nation. https://www.apa.org/news/press/releases/stress/2017/state-nation.pdf; 2017. Accessed 5 January 2019.
63. McEwen BS. Stressed or stressed out: what is the difference? *J Psychiatry Neurosci*. 2005;30(5):315–318.
64. Ramsay DS, Woods SC. Clarifying the roles of homeostasis and allostasis in physiological regulation. *Psychol Rev*. 2014;121(2):225–247.
65. Lemyre L, Lalande-Markon MP. Psychological Stress Measure (PSM-9): integration of an evidence-based approach to assessment, monitoring, and evaluation of stress in physical therapy practice. *Physiother Theory Pract*. 2009;25(5–6):453–462.
66. Levenstein S, Prantera C, Varvo V, et al. Development of the perceived stress questionnaire: a new tool for psychosomatic research. *J Psychosomatic Res*. 1993;37(1):19–31.
67. Integrated Behavioral Health Partners. Generalized Anxiety Disorder (GAD)-7 Scale. http://www.ibhpartners.org/wp-content/uploads/2016/04/TheGeneralizedAnxietyDisrorder.pdf; 2019. Accessed 9 January 2019.
68. Zung WW. A rating instrument for anxiety disorders. *Psychosomatics*. 1971;12(6):371–379.
69. National Institute of Mental Health. 5 Things You Should Know About Stress. https://www.nimh.nih.gov/health/publications/stress/5thingsshldknowaboutstress-508-03132017_142898.pdf; 2019. Accessed 9 January 2019.
70. Anxiety and Depression Association of America. Understand the Facts. https://adaa.org/understanding-anxiety; 2019. Accessed 5 January 2019.
71. Mental Health America. http://www.mentalhealthamerica.net/; 2019. Accessed 5 January 2019.
72. U.S. Department of Health and Human Services. Stress Management. https://healthfinder.gov/FindServices/SearchContext.aspx?topic=825; 2019. Accessed 9 January 2019.
73. McManus CA. *Group Wellness Programs for Chronic Pain and Disease Management*. Butterworth-Heinemann: Oxford; 2003.
74. Shapiro SL, Carlson LE. *The Art and Science of Mindfulness: Integration Mindfulness into Psychology and the Helping Professions*. Washington, DC: American Psychological Association; 2017.
75. Keyes CB. Social well-being. *Soc Psychol Q*. 1998;61:121–140.
76. Thompson CR. *Prevention Practice and Health Promotion: A Health Care Professional's Guide to Health, Fitness, and Wellness*. Thorofare, NJ: Slack; 2015.
77. Mandal B, Roe B. Job loss, retirement and the mental health of older Americans. *J Ment Health Policy Econ*. 2008;11(4):167–176.
78. Taylor D. Physical activity is medicine for older adults. *Postgrad Med J*. 2014;90:26–32.
79. Gries KJ, Raue U, Perkins RK, et al. Cardiovascular and skeletal muscle health with lifelong exercise. *J Appl Physiol*. 2018;125(8):1636–1645.
80. Auais MA, Eilayyan O, Mayo NE. Extended exercise rehabilitation after hip fracture improves patients' physical function: a systematic review and meta-analysis. *Phys Ther*. 2012;92(11):1437–1451.
81. American College of Sports Medicine. Physical Activity Readiness Questionnaire (PAR-Q) and You. http://uwfitness.uwaterloo.ca/PDF/par-q.pdf; 2019. Accessed 5 January 2019.
82. Par-Q+ Collaboration. The New Par-Q+ and eParmed-X+: Official Website. http://eparmedx.com/; 2019. Accessed 6 January 2019.
83. Resnick B, Ory MG, Hora K, et al. A proposal for a new screening paradigm and tool called Exercise Assessment and Screening for You (EASY). *J Aging Phys Act*. 2008;16(2):215–233.
84. Canadian Society for Exercise Physiology. Get Active Questionnaire-Reference Document. http://www.csep.ca/CMFiles/publications/GAQ_ReferenceDoc_2pages.pdf. Accessed January 6, 2019. Alternative – Get Active Questionnaire.
85. Wong CC, McGirt MJ. Vertebral compression fractures: a review of current management and multimodal therapy. *J Multidiscip Healthc*. 2013;6:205–214.
86. Sambrook PN, Cameron ID, Chen JS, et al. Influence of fall related factors and bone strength on fracture risk in the frail elderly. *Osteoporos Int*. 2007;18(5):603–610.
87. Arnold CM, Busch AJ, Schachter CL, et al. The relationship of intrinsic fall risk factors to a recent history of falling in older women with osteoporosis. *J Orthop Sports Phys Ther*. 2005;35(7):452–460.
88. Gates S, Smith LA, Fisher JD, Lamb SE. Systematic review of accuracy of screening instruments for predicting fall risk among independently living older adults. *J Rehabil Res Dev*. 2008;45(8):1105–1116.
89. Lusardi MM, Fritz S, Middleton A, et al. Determining risk of falls in community dwelling older adults: a systematic review and meta-analysis using posttest probability. *J Geriatr Phys Ther*. 2017;40(1):1–36.
90. Cress ME, Buchner DM, Prohaska T, et al. Best practices for physical activity programs and behavior counseling in older adult populations. *J Aging Phys Act*. 2005;13(1):61–74.
91. Rikli RE, Jones CJ. Development and validation of a functional fitness test for community-residing older adults. *J Aging Phys Act*. 1999;7(2):129–161.
92. Jones CJ, Rikli RE, Beam WC. A 30-s chair-stand test as a measure of lower body strength in community-residing older adults. *Res Q Exerc Sport*. 1999;70(2):113–119. https://doi.org/10.1080/02701367.1999.10608028.
93. Todde F, Melis F, Mura R, et al. A 12-week vigorous exercise protocol in a healthy group of persons over 65: study of physical function by means of the Senior Fitness Test. *Biomed Res Int*. 2016;2016:1–6. https://doi.org/10.1155/2016/7639842.
94. Jones CJ, Rikli RE. Measuring functional fitness in older adults. *J Act Aging*. 2002;(March–April):24–30.
95. Rikli RE, Jones CJ. *Senior Fitness Test Manual*. Champaign, IL: Human Kinetics; 2001.
96. Rikli RE, Jones CJ. Development and validation of criterion-referenced clinically relevant fitness standards for maintaining physical independence in later years. *Gerontologist*. 2013;53(2):255–267. https://doi.org/10.1093/geront/gns071.
97. Madureira MM, Bonfa E, Takayama L, Pereira RM. A 12-month randomized controlled trial of balance training in elderly women with osteoporosis: improvement of quality of life. *Maturitas*. 2010;66(2):206–211.

98. Kahn EB, Ramsey LT, Brownson RC, et al. The effectiveness of interventions to increase physical activity. A systematic review. *Am J Prev Med.* 2002;22(4):73–107 Suppl.
99. Macera CA, Cavanaugh A, Bellettiere J. State of the art review: physical activity and older adults. *Am J Lifestyle Med.* 2017;11 (1):42–57.
100. Low S, Ang LW, Goh KS, Chew SK. A systematic review of the effectiveness of tai chi on fall reduction among the elderly. *Arch Gerontol Geriatr.* 2009;48(3):325–331.
101. Wang C, Schmid CH, Hibberd PL, et al. Tai chi is effective in treating knee osteoarthritis: a randomized controlled trial. *Arthritis Rheum.* 2009;61(11):1545–1553.
102. Wolf SL, O'Grady M, Easley KA, et al. The influence of intense tai chi training on physical performance and hemodynamic outcomes in transitionally frail, older adults. *J Gerontol A Biol Sci Med Sci.* 2006;61(2):184–189.
103. Sherrington C, Whitney JC, Lord SR, et al. Effective exercise for the prevention of falls: a systematic review and meta-analysis. *J Am Geriatr Soc.* 2008;56(12):2234–2243.
104. Shumway-Cook A, Silver IF, Lemier M, et al. Effectiveness of a community-based multifactorial intervention on falls and fall risk factors in community-living older adults: a randomized, controlled trial. *J Gerontol A Biol Sci Med Sci.* 2007;62 (12):1420–1427.
105. Karinkanta S, Piirtola M, Sievanen H, et al. Physical therapy approaches to reduce fall and fracture risk among older adults. *Nat Rev Endocrinol.* 2010;6(7):396–407.
106. Silsupadol P, Lugade V, Shumway-Cook A, et al. Training-related changes in dual-task walking performance of elderly persons with balance impairment: a double-blind, randomized controlled trial. *Gait Posture.* 2009;29 (4):634–639.
107. Stevens JA, Burns E. A CDC Compendium of Effective Fall Interventions: What Works for Community-Dwelling Older Adults. https://www.cdc.gov/homeandrecreationalsafety/pdf/falls/CDC_Falls_Compendium-2015-a.pdf#nameddest=intro; 2019. Accessed 6 January 2019.
108. Fiatarone M, Marks E, Ryan N, et al. High-intensity strength training in nonagenarians. *JAMA.* 1990;263(22): 3029–3034.
109. Orr R, Raymond J, Fiatarone Singh M. Efficacy of progressive resistance training on balance performance in older adults: a systematic review of randomized controlled trials. *Sports Med.* 2008;38(4):317–343.
110. Campbell AJ, Robertson MC, Gardner MM, et al. Falls prevention over 2 years: a randomized controlled trial in women 80 years and older. *Age Ageing.* 1999;28:513–518.
111. Buchner DM, Cress ME, de Lateur BJ, et al. The effect of strength and endurance training on gait, balance, fall risk, and health services use in community-living older adults. *J Gerontol A Biol Sci Med Sci.* 1997;52(4): M218–M224.
112. Guizelini P, de Aguiar R, Denadai B, Caputo F, Greco C. Effect of resistance training on muscle strength and rate of force development in healthy older adults: a systematic review and meta-analysis. *Exper Gerontol.* 2018;102:51–58.
113. American College of Sports Medicine. *ACSM's Guidelines for Exercise Testing and Prescription.* 10th ed. Baltimore, MD: American College of Sports Medicine; 2018.
114. Peterson MJ, Giuliani C, Morey MC, et al. Physical activity as a preventative factor for frailty: the health, aging, and body composition study. *J Gerontol A Biol Sci Med Sci.* 2009;64 (1):61–68.
115. Avers D, Brown M. White paper: strength training for the older adult. *J Geriatr Phys Ther.* 2009;32(4):148–152.
116. Seeman TE, Merkin SS, Crimmins EM, Karlamangla AS. Disability trends among older Americans: National Health and Nutrition Examination Surveys, 1988-1994 and 1999-2004. *Am J Public Health.* 2010;100(1):100–107.
117. Fried LP, Ferrucci L, Darer J, et al. Untangling the concepts of disability, frailty, and comorbidity: implications for improved targeting and care. *J Gerontol A Biol Sci Med Sci.* 2004;59 (3):255–263.
118. Bandeen-Roche K, Xue Q, Ferrucci L, et al. Phenotype of frailty: characterization in the women's health and aging studies. *J Gerontol A Biol Sci Med Sci.* 2006;61(3):262–266.
119. Henwood TR, Riek S, Taaffe DR. Strength versus muscle power-specific resistance training in community-dwelling older adults. *J Gerontol A Biol Sci Med Sci.* 2008;63(1):83–91.
120. Manini T, Marko M, VanArnam T, et al. Efficacy of resistance and task-specific exercise in older adults who modify tasks of everyday life. *J Gerontol A Biol Sci Med Sci.* 2007; 62(6):616–623.
121. de Vreede PL, van Meeteren NL, Samson MM, et al. The effect of functional tasks exercise and resistance exercise on health-related quality of life and physical activity. A randomised controlled trial. *Gerontology.* 2007;53(1):12–20.
122. Silva RB, Aldoradin-Cabesa H, Eslick GD, et al. The effect of physical exercise on frail older persons: a systematic review. *J Frailty Aging.* 2017;6(2):91–96.
123. Cadore EL, Rodriquez-Manas L, Sinclair A, Izquierdo M. Effects of different exercise interventions on risk of falls, gait ability, and balance in physical frail older adults: a systematic review. *Rejuvenation Res.* 2013;16(2). 1050114.
124. Berry SD, Kiel DP, Donaldson MG, et al. Application of the National Osteoporosis Foundation guidelines to postmenopausal women and men: the Framingham Osteoporosis Study. *Osteoporos Int.* 2010;21(1):53–60.
125. Sinaki M, Itoi E, Wahner HW, et al. Stronger back muscles reduce the incidence of vertebral fractures: a prospective 10 year follow-up of postmenopausal women. *Bone.* 2002;30(6):836–841.
126. McMillan LB, Zengin A, Ebeling PR, Scott D. Prescribing physical activity for the prevention and treatment of osteoporosis in older adults. *Healthcare.* 2017;5(4):85–100.
127. Owen N, Healy GN, Matthews CE, Dunstan DW. Too much sitting: the population health science of sedentary behavior. *Exerc Sport Sci Rev.* 2010;38(3):105–113.
128. Ades PA, Keteyian SJ, Balady GJ, et al. Cardiac rehabilitation exercise and self-care for chronic heart failure. *JACC Heart Fail.* 2013;1(6):540–547.
129. Taylor RS, Sagar VA, Davies EJ, et al. Exercise-based rehabilitation for heart failure. *Cochrane Database Syst Rev.* 2014;2014(4):CD003331. Published 2014 Apr 27. https://doi.org/10.1002/14651858.CD003331.pub4.
130. Chtara M, Chaouachi A, Levin GT, et al. Effect of concurrent endurance and circuit resistance training sequence on muscular strength and power development. *J Strength Cond Res.* 2008;22(4):1037–1045.
131. Fletcher GF, Balady G, Blair SN, et al. Statement on exercise: benefits and recommendations for physical activity programs for all Americans. A statement for health professionals by the Committee on Exercise and Cardiac Rehabilitation of the Council on Clinical Cardiology, American Heart Association. *Circulation.* 1996;94(4):857–862.
132. Yates T, Davies M, Gorely T, et al. Effectiveness of a pragmatic education program designed to promote walking activity in individuals with impaired glucose tolerance: a randomized controlled trial. *Diabetes Care.* 2009;32 (8):1404–1410.
133. Callahan LF, Shreffler J, Altpeter M, et al. Evaluation of group and self-directed formats of the Arthritis Foundation's Walk with Ease Program. *Arthritis Care Res.* 2011;63 (8):1098–1107 PMID: 21560255.

CHAPTER 24

Acute Care Management of the Older Adult

Chris L. Wells, Jenny Forrester

OUTLINE

INTRODUCTION

The population of the United States is aging, with a projected estimate of 83.7 million adults over 65 years of age living in the United States by 2050.[1] The U.S. Census Bureau projects that by 2050, older adults 85 years and older will have a life expectancy of an additional 7.0 to 8.5 years, and of 19.2 to 23.5 additional years for those 65 years and older,[2] leading to another, larger group of old-old adults. The 85-year-old age group is expected to grow faster than the working-age population. This economic problem is compounded with the advances in medical management and surgical procedures that are making it possible for older adults to live longer with multiple comorbidities and to survive acute hospitalization.[3] This current model is leading to a growing crisis in health care. The U.S. government pays 65% of the medical expenses for older adults, which is five times the average annual cost per person for health care when compared to children and three times that of the working-age group. It has been reported that the United States spends $25,000 annually on medical expenses for the 85-and-older adult population.[1]

The American Hospital Association reported that there were over 35 million hospital admissions in 2016, of which more than 40% were for adults over the age of 65 years, which accounts for more than half of the $991.5 million spent on hospital care.[4] According to the Centers for Disease Control and Prevention (CDC), in 2010 those aged 65 and over were hospitalized at a rate five times the rate of those younger than 65 years old, which speaks to the increase in comorbidities and frailty.[5] The cost continues to climb despite a decrease in the number of admissions and the decrease in length of stay from 7.7 to 5.5 days.[6]

ISSUES WITH HOSPITALIZATION OF THE OLDER ADULT

What makes the care of the older adult more complex is the normal effects of aging compounded with the presence of multiple comorbidities, which leads to frailty and a decline in physiological reserve.[7] Table 24.1 describes age-related changes and possible complications.[8–11] Chronic conditions such as cardiovascular disease including arrhythmias, coronary and valvular disease and heart failure, infections (pneumonia and septicemia), management of chronic obstructive pulmonary disease (COPD), diabetes, and problems with medications are the leading admitting diagnoses.[12] In 2012 surgical stays accounted

TABLE 24.1 Age-Related Changes and Possible Complications[8–11]

System	Normal Aging	Complications
Neurological	↓ Sensory information (hearing, vision, taste, sensation) ↓ Cognitive process	↑ Risk of delirium ↑ Balance and fall risk ↑ Pressure injuries
Cardiovascular	↓ ANS (SNS) response ↓ CO and reserve	↑ Risk of not meeting metabolic demand ↑ Risk of orthostatic hypotension ↑ Risk of arrhythmias
Pulmonary	↓ Airway clearance ↓ Chest wall compliance ↑ Lung compliance ↓ Muscle strength	↑ Risk of pneumonia ↑ Work of breathing/ fatigue ↑ Atelectasis ↑ Aspiration
Musculoskeletal	Sarcopenia ↓ Joint ROM and flexibility ↓ Bone density	↑ Fatigue ↑ Risk of falls/ fractures ↑ Caloric demand for a given activity
Integumentary	↓ Elasticity ↓ Vascularity	↑ Risk of pressure injuries and tears ↓ Wound healing
Visceral function	↓ Renal filtration ↓ Liver clearance ↓ GI motility ↓ Sphincter control	↑ Risk of edema Poor drug clearance Electrolyte imbalances ↓ Cognitive and motor function

ANS, autonomic nervous system; *CO*, cardiac output; *GI*, gastrointestinal; *ROM*, range of motion; *SNS*, sympathetic nervous system.

for 15.2% of hospital stays for adults aged 85 and over, and medical stays made up the other 84.8%.[13]

A unique challenge of managing the older adult in the acute care setting is that those aged 85 and older are particularly more likely to be hospitalized with an injury or medical condition that requires postdischarge institutional care when compared to the younger older adult (65 to 74 years of age). In fact, 56% of adults over age 85 years require discharge to other medical/rehabilitation institutions for further care.[5,13] This creates a large challenge to the acute care facility to find postacute beds for all of these patients, which can lead to a decrease in throughput, a term that refers to the ability of a hospital to admit, medically stabilize, and discharge patients to free the bed for the next medically needy individual.

The older adult appears to be more vulnerable to the hospital environment. Table 24.2 lists the iatrogenic effects associated with hospitalization, and Table 24.3 lists the environmental barriers that contribute to these effects. Recent literature reviews show that functional decline is one of the most common negative outcomes of hospitalization, with up to 60% of older adults losing the ability to complete at least one activity of daily living (ADL), 40% reporting losses in instrumental ADLs, and only 30% obtaining full recovery 1 year after admission.[14,15] The unfamiliarity with their hospital room and the disruption of their sleep and wake cycle cause older patients to get easily disoriented and even suffer delirium within a few days of admission.

TABLE 24.2 Iatrogenic Effects Associated with Hospitalization[22,23]

Delirium	Pressure injuries
Pneumonia	Muscle weakness
Infections	Functional mobility declines
Dehydration	Anxiety, depression, posttraumatic stress disorder
Loss of control, helplessness	Malnutrition

TABLE 24.3 Hospital Barriers to Maintaining and Restoring Function

Poor pain management	Sedation
Tethering with lines and tubes	Unfamiliar and unfriendly environment
Hospital furniture	Sleep disturbance
Social and cognitive isolation	Polypharmacy
Access to and use of glasses, hearing aids, and dentures	Inconsistent staff and schedules

Modified from Resnick B, Wells CL, Brotemarkle BA, Payne AK. Exposure to therapy of older people with trauma and factors that influence provision of therapy. *Phys Ther.* 2014;94:40–51; Fisher SR, Galloway RV, Kuo YF, et al. Pilot study examining the association between ambulatory activity and falls among hospitalized older adults. *Arch Phys Med Rehabil.* 2011;92(12):2090–2092. doi:10.1016/j.apmr.2011.06.022; and Boltz M, Resnick B, Capezuti E, Shuluk J, et al. Functional decline in hospitalized older adults: can nursing make a difference? *Geriatr Nurs.* 2012;33:272–279.

Delirium

Delirium is an acute change in mental state that has four characteristics: altered mental state, inattentiveness, altered level of consciousness, and disorganized thinking. Delirium is a serious condition that is associated with prolonged mechanical ventilator use, longer length of stays, and higher hospital and 1-year mortality rates.[16–19] Further discussion of delirium and its management can be found in Chapter 19. Another adverse environmental condition is that hospitals have policies and procedures in place to provide a safe environment and reduce falls, but these procedures along with the older patient being tethered by lines, tubes, and medical monitoring devices lead to severe restrictions in patient's mobility, increasing the fear of falling which can lead to self-limited mobilization and contribute to hospital acquired deconditioning.

Falls in the Hospital

Patients attempting to get out of bed alone or ambulate to/from the bathroom account for approximately 30% falls in the acute setting.[20] A fall alone can cause decreased willingness and confidence to ambulate once medically stable, and if the fall resulted in injury, it could increase the length of hospitalization, affect discharge, and increase mortality. Patients' beliefs and thoughts about their ability to safely move, known as falls efficacy, is directly correlated with fall risk. Fifty percent of community-dwelling older adults report a fear of falling, and this number only increases when they are in an unfamiliar setting and acutely ill.[21] Other factors that are associated with loss of function for the older adult include isolation and patients not having access to such items as their eyeglasses, hearing aids, dentures, and shoes.[22] Isolation and the fear of loss of independence can lead to depression and anxiety, which can lead to a lack of motivation to participate in therapy and mobility programs that can minimize the loss of function and facilitate institutional discharge.[23]

Vulnerability to Medical Deterioration

Another effect of hospitalization is older adults' vulnerability to critical illness. Think about a three-sided assault that occurs when the older adult faces a critical illness. First, many adults have personal risk factors besides age that are associated with higher morbidity rates, including decline in cognitive function and decreased physical function, malnutrition, and sarcopenia. Second, there are the iatrogenic effects of the hospital environment like restricted movement, cognitive isolation and depression, polypharmacology, and underprescribed rehabilitation.[14] The third assault is the physiological stress of a critical illness that typically occurs from a cardiac or pulmonary dysfunction or failure, or sepsis from postoperative complications. Of all critical care days in 2005, 36.5% were Medicare receipients.[24]

Critical illness is commonly associated with a systemic inflammatory process that can lead to a catabolic state. The reader should refer to Chapter 14, Management of the Acutely Ill Older Patient, for an update on cachexia. The result can be persistent skeletal muscle weakness that can leave up to 60% of survivors with at least one additional limitation in an ADL and prolonged mechanical ventilation.[14] Once again, the older adult has a higher burden for personal risk factors, such as comorbidities, underlying dementia, and poor hearing and eyesight, that are associated with the development of delirium.[25,26] Finally, there is a higher level of psychiatric impairments like anxiety and depression and further cognitive dysfunction associated with surviving a critical illness.[16,27]

The iatrogenic effects of critical illness and hospitalization leave the older adult more vulnerable to these potentially long-term physical, emotional, and cognitive impairments. This complicates the clinician's job in trying to mitigate these adverse effects and maintain or restore function for a successful discharge, and burdens the health care system by delaying discharges, requiring more postacute rehabilitation beds, and increasing the financial and physical burden on families and the communities at large.

PREVENTATIVE INITIATIVES AND PROGRAMS

Various organizations including the Society of Critical Care Medicine (SCCM) and the American Association of Critical Care Nurses (AACN) have developed national initiatives to decrease the adverse effects associated with the ICU. The SCCM developed the ICU Liberation initiative, which focuses on controlling pain and decreasing agitation and delirium (PAD guidelines).[28]

The AACN proposed an interdisciplinary evidence-based practice bundle referred to as the ABCDEF Bundle (Table 24.4),[29] which encourages nursing, respiratory, and physical therapy providers and others to address early waking, daily assessment to promote early weaning from the ventilator, team communication, delirium assessment and management, early exercise and mobilization, and family engagement. The physical therapist should be involved with any ICU and acute care unit's initiatives to assist in reducing the complications associated with hospitalization. The E within the Bundle should include some type of nursing screening to assess the patient's basic functional ability (Fig. 24.1). The physical therapist can utilize the results of such nursing screening to determine patients' rehabilitation needs. The collaboration between nursing and physical therapy is vital to maintaining and progressing functional recovery and preparing for discharge. The physical therapist can play a critical role throughout the hospitalization in contributing to the reduction of pain, delirium, and agitation with early rehabilitation, reorientation, and basic cognitive stimulation. Therapy can assist in positioning and airway clearance to aid in ventilator liberation, and physical therapists can lead the initiative in patient and family engagement.

The Acute Care for the Elderly (ACE) program reduces costs, decreases length of stay (LOS), improves functional abilities, decreases fall rates, decreases delirium and use of urinary catheters, reduces readmissions, improves home discharge, and prevents adverse events.[30–32] These programs target the typical adverse events from hospitalization such as functional decline or delirium. The multidisciplinary team, made up of a hospitalist in geriatric medicine or a geriatrician, a pharmacist, a social worker, a physical therapist, and a nurse, performs a comprehensive geriatric assessment (CGA) on an at-risk elder, identifying risk factors and specific needs and then implementing a comprehensive

TABLE 24.4 ABCDEF Bundle and Role of Physical Therapy[42]

	Definition and Purpose	Rehab Role
A	Spontaneous Awakening Trials (SATs): lighten sedation to determine medical stability to stay awake and interact within the environment	Coordinate assessment and intervention during awakening trials to engage the patient
B	Spontaneous Breathing Trials (SBTs): If patient is on mechanical ventilation, this step is to determine if the patient is ready to be extubated or weaned off of the ventilator	Prior to SBTs, position patient to maximize breathing pattern, complete airway clearance techniques, and teach breath control techniques; if extubation is questionable, assess pulmonary tolerance during functional training and exercise
C	Communication and Coordination within the medical team to advance the patient's recovery process	Work with the team to maximize the patient's progression with functional restoration; provide team with questions and concerns that are a barrier to recovery
D	Delirium assessment and management	Assess for delirium and engage the patient in functional mobility and functional cognitive activities to restore cognitive function
E	Early exercise and mobilization	Collaborate with RN with basic activities so the therapist can provide more advanced rehabilitation services to promote recovery
F	Family engagement	Engage the family in exercises and functional activities and keep family informed regarding rehabilitation findings and recommendations

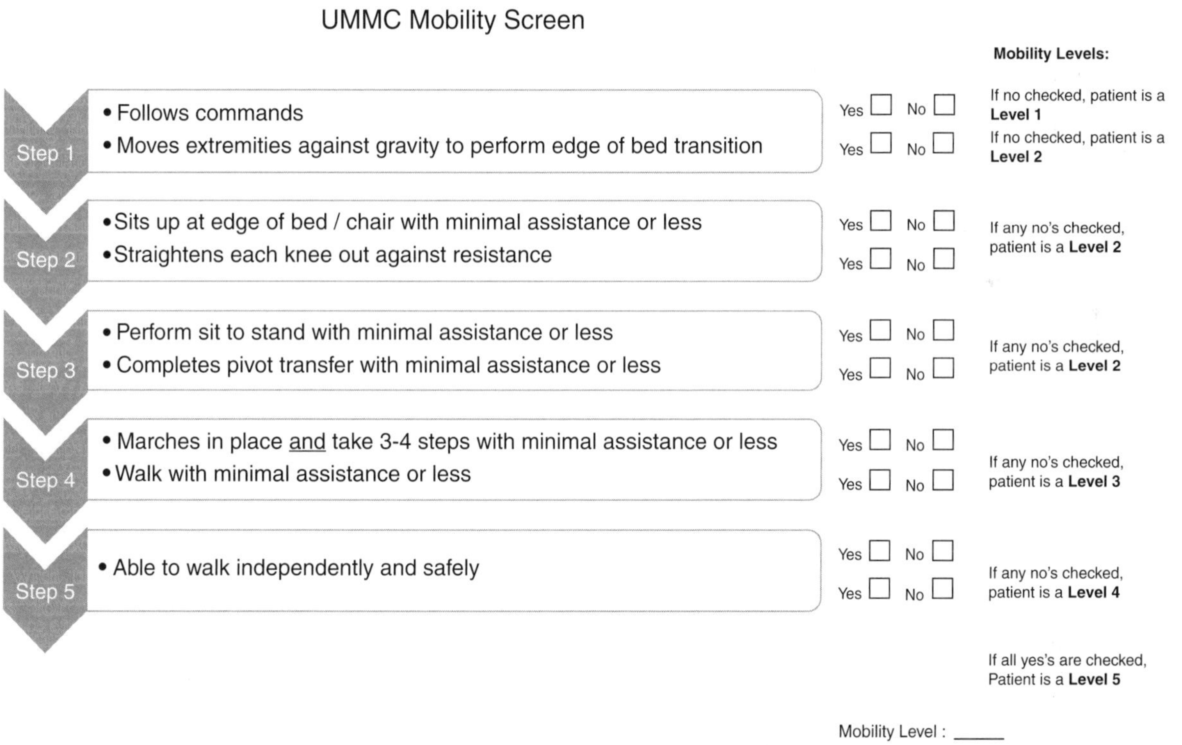

UMMC Mobility Screen

			Mobility Levels:
Step 1	• Follows commands	Yes ☐ No ☐	If no checked, patient is a **Level 1**
	• Moves extremities against gravity to perform edge of bed transition	Yes ☐ No ☐	If no checked, patient is a **Level 2**
Step 2	• Sits up at edge of bed / chair with minimal assistance or less	Yes ☐ No ☐	If any no's checked, patient is a **Level 2**
	• Straightens each knee out against resistance	Yes ☐ No ☐	
Step 3	• Perform sit to stand with minimal assistance or less	Yes ☐ No ☐	If any no's checked, patient is a **Level 2**
	• Completes pivot transfer with minimal assistance or less	Yes ☐ No ☐	
Step 4	• Marches in place and take 3-4 steps with minimal assistance or less	Yes ☐ No ☐	If any no's checked, patient is a **Level 3**
	• Walk with minimal assistance or less	Yes ☐ No ☐	
Step 5	• Able to walk independently and safely	Yes ☐ No ☐	If any no's checked, patient is a **Level 4**
		Yes ☐ No ☐	
			If all yes's are checked, Patient is a **Level 5**

Mobility Level : _____

FIG. 24.1 University of Maryland Medical Center Mobility Screen. *(From Wells CL, Pittas J, Roman C, Lighty K, with collaboration from the University of Maryland Rehabilitation Network and the Rise & Shine Committee at the University of Maryland Medical Center. Property of UMMC. Not to be duplicated without express permission of the author.)*

treatment plan. Mobility is a key aspect, thus emphasizing the need and benefit of having a physical therapist on the team. In one unique model, health profession students (medical, physical therapy, and nursing students) assisted patients with mobility throughout the day.

Two programs implemented because of the Affordable Care Act have significance to older adults. The Hospital-Acquired Condition Reduction Program (HACRP) was implemented in 2015 and the Hospital Readmission Reduction Program (HRRP) was implemented in 2012.

These programs have mandated hospitals to focus their care on quality with the goal to prevent circumstances that increase costs. The emphasis on reduction in hospital-acquired complications and decreased readmissions should lead to efforts to change hospital policies, procedures, and cultures for the betterment of patients' health.

The HACRP financially penalizes hospitals 1% of reimbursed costs when their performance on certain reportable outcomes is in the lower 25% of hospitals with similar case mixes. Conditions under the HACRP include unacceptable levels of central line–associated bloodstream infections (CLABSIs), catheter-associated urinary tract infections (CAUTIs), reported surgical site infections (SSIs), methicillin-resistant *Staphylococcus aureus* (MRSA) bacteremia, and *Clostridium difficile* infections (CDIs). Patient safety issues and adverse events can also affect reimbursement penalties. These events are referred to as the Patient Safety and Adverse Events Composite, known as PSI 90, and include such medical complications as deep vein thrombus (DVT), pressure injuries, fall-related hip fractures, postoperative kidney injury, postoperative respiratory failure, postoperative sepsis, and abdominal surgical complications like an unexpected laceration or puncture.[33] One successful team-based program to assist in reducing readmissions of older adults is the Hospital Elder Life Program (HELP) focused on preventing delirium and described in Chapter 19, Cognitive Issues in the Older Adult.[34] Physical therapists need to be intimately involved in hospital policies and procedures related to the reduction of infections, fall prevention initiatives, and early mobilization and rehabilitation programs to reduce the risk of DVTs when interacting with older adults.

The HRRP also financially penalizes hospitals for any patient who is unexpectedly readmitted within 30 days of their initial discharge. This program targets the following admitting diagnoses: acute myocardial infarction, heart failure, pneumonia, exacerbation of COPD, coronary artery bypass surgery, and total hip and knee arthroplasties.[35] The HRRP makes everyone in the acute setting focus on two large areas: workload and capacity (Box 24.1).[36] These financial penalties have forced hospitals to fully prepare the patient for discharge (Box 24.1). Hospitals have created discharge and transitional care coordinators and teams that remain in contact with patients after discharge to ensure they are able to follow their care plan and have access to their medications and outpatient medical services.[37] Some transitional care programs work within the community, some in the hospitals. Some programs have shown to be useful in reducing readmissions, as well as saving thousands of dollars over a year, but at this time they are not individually reimbursable.[38] The acute care physical therapist can also play a substantial role in hospital initiatives by providing proper and effective education; making appropriate discharge recommendations; delivering effective rehabilitation sessions to improve functional mobility and activity tolerance, particularly for those patients who are anticipated to be discharged home; constantly screening for any signs and symptoms suggestive of medical complications; screening for any apparent gaps in the discharge plan; and being an active member of the health care team so any concerns can be voiced and addressed.

BOX 24.1 Workload and Capacity

	Description	Examples
Workload	All the work of being a patient and includes efforts to understand and plan for care, to enroll the support of others, and to access and use health care services	Case management Patient education Caregiver training Telemonitoring Home visits Self-management support
Capacity	Quality and availability of resources to enable the patient to accomplish required self-care tasks	Physical and mental health Collaboration with social and community services Transitional care (acute and community) Financial resources Environmental assets Establishing follow-up plans

Leppin AL, Giofriddo MR, Montori VM. Preventing 30-day hospital readmissions: a systematic review and meta-analysis of randomized trials. *JAMA Intern Med*. 2014;174(7):1095–1107.

CARE COORDINATION AND COMMUNICATION

Effective communication among an inclusive health care team is at the foundation of successful programs to improve workload and capacity and reduce adverse outcomes in the acute care setting. Each professional has a unique set of skills and there are many areas of professional overlap. It is imperative that the health care team decide the primary and supportive roles for each professional. The physical therapist's primary role may be assessment for discharge recommendations and restoration of function for those patients who are likely to be discharged home, but the physical therapist should not be limited to this important role. For example, the therapist has other areas in which to contribute to patient care and support other members of the health care team such as airway clearance, pain management, prevention of pressure injuries with positioning, splint selection and fitting, and cognitive retraining, just to name a few.

The health care team's effectiveness is through effective communication. The team's communication may occur in patient care or discharge planning rounds, transfer and handoff communications, and process improvement meetings. Many of these meetings address the daily plan for the patient. These rounds should ensure that the patient is proceeding to the expected discharge date, and if not, there should be a decision about the barriers and what the plan is to address the issues. These communications commonly occur in person and the therapist may struggle to attend these rounds and still maintain productivity requirements. The therapist has to determine how best to interface with the other team members and still meet patients' needs. Process improvement meetings are important to attend because these meetings usually examine practices and identify shortcomings; the therapist will want to participate in establishing common practice and the culture in which health care is delivered.

ROLE OF THE PHYSICAL THERAPIST IN THE ACUTE CARE ENVIRONMENT

A physical therapist who focuses his or her practice on treating the critically ill is in a unique, demanding, and rewarding area of practice. In addition to competence in traditional patient management, the acute care therapist must manage mechanical support of the patient (e.g., ventilation and hemodialysis), effects of inappropriate medication dosing and polypharmacy, and physiological system effects of medical interventions. Table 24.5 lists various medical equipment and the rehabilitation implications that need to be part of the management of the patient. To effectively pull these disparate knowledge and skill bases together, the therapist needs to have sound critical reasoning and communication skills. The therapist needs to assimilate an enormous amount of medical and surgical information; determine the impact to medical stability, function, and activity tolerance prior to starting the session; and determine when the patient has achieved a positive physiological response to the activities, all the while monitoring closely enough to look for signs of intolerance. The therapist needs to be adaptive in how to anticipate and respond to a patient who is decompensating during the therapy session. Effective communication with the nursing staff, the various medical service teams, and family members is critical. Providing early rehabilitation to critically ill patients requires the therapist to know the roles of the other members of the health care team, how to utilize them to help during the therapy session, and how to command the environment to achieve safe functional training.

Throughput

Another area of mastery required of the acute care therapist is systems knowledge of how hospitals work from a reimbursement and regulation perspective. For example, in today's acute care environment, the primary role of the physical therapist is to facilitate throughput. Throughput is the term used to describe the flow of patients through the hospital system. Throughput is extremely important to serve the needs of the community in getting the sickest patients into the right medical location for care; it is also important for the financial health of the hospital.

The physical therapist affects throughput in several ways (Box 24.2). The most obvious role physical therapists play is in the evaluation of patients to determine functional status, social and environmental situation, and prior level of function to make a discharge recommendation. Once the discharge recommendation is made, the case manager and the other members of the medical team can begin preparing for that discharge. The therapist will frequently be asked to update assessments to confirm or amend recommendations based on any changes in the patient's status. The discharge recommendation process can be a very complex process owing to the medical complexity and frailty of the older patient's health, social and environmental circumstances, prognostic indicators for recovery, and the patient's wishes.

The need to keep physically active while in the hospital is a key factor to returning home for any older adult, which aids in expediated discharge and improves throughput. There are multiple studies that show maintaining the activity level of the older adult leads to less pain, less delirium, improved cognitive function, maintained mental health, and fewer iatrogenic effects like infections and DVTs.[39] Maintaining the functional mobility of the older adult also leads to lower readmission rates.

Objective Assessment

Besides making discharge recommendations, the physical therapist is critical in collaborating with nursing to maintain and progress the functional mobility and physical activity of the older adult. The physical therapist's assessment of the patient's functional deficits leads to a treatment plan that guides the nursing staff and rehabilitation services to promote functional mobility and address limitations. Several outcome measures have been identified to be useful to determine a care plan to address the needs that make older adults more vulnerable. One of the most predictive outcome measures for identifying 1-month readmissions is the ability of the adult to rise from a standard chair without the use of the upper extremities. Gait speed <0.6 m/sec and a score of 5 or less on the Cumulative Ambulation Score, which examines the patient's ability to get out of bed, stand up from a chair, and walk a short distance, are also strong outcomes that can be used to identify patients at risk and direct resources to address needs. Handgrip strength is a good indicator of physical reserve and screening for sarcopenia with cutoff at <16 kg for females and <26 kg for males, but not a strong predictor of readmissions.[15]

Nursing Mobility Programs

Many health care institutions have implemented a nursing-driven mobility program that is directed at assessing the patient's current physical abilities (Box 24.3) and developing an activity plan for the day. These mobility programs can be used to promote safe mobility of the patient and maximize utilization of rehabilitation services. A successful nursing-directed mobility program includes five components (Box 24.3).[3,40] The rehabilitation staff

TABLE 24.5 UMMC General Information Regarding Acute Care Medical Equipment and Rehabilitation Implications for Patient Care Management

Gastrointestinal, Genitourinary, and Renal Systems

		General Information	Rehab Implications
Arterial lines		• Pressurized line used to continuously monitor blood pressure and to obtain arterial blood • Inserted into the arterial system (most commonly radial or femoral artery)	• Transducer must be level with the right atrium of the heart (fourth intercostal space, midpoint between the anterior and posterior chest wall) to ensure accurate reading • If dislodged, place the patient in a safe position, call for the RN immediately, and apply strong direct pressure (will bleed excessively); if disconnection occurs along the tubing, clamp line and call for the RN
Venous lines	Infusion pump	• Machine used to deliver medication(s) to the patient at a set rate	• May be unplugged from wall for mobility • Should only be reset by the RN • May be paused/disconnected depending on the type of fluid or medication
	Peripheral intravenous line (IV)	• Used to deliver medications, fluids, and blood transfusions; obtain venous blood • Inserted into any peripheral vein	• Avoid ROM that interferes with the infusion, causes pain, or jeopardizes the IV site • Ensure adequate slack of IV tubing prior to ROM/mobility • If dislodged, place the patient in a safe position, call for the RN, and apply direct pressure
	Central venous catheter (central line)	• Used to deliver medications, fluids, blood transfusions, and TPN; obtain venous blood; monitor central venous pressure • Inserted into a central vein (most commonly femoral, subclavian, jugular) and terminates in the superior vena cava	• See Rehab Implications for Peripheral IV • Ensure integrity of dressing prior to mobility owing to increased infection risk • Monitor for signs of DVT
	Tunneled central venous catheter (Hickman, Permacath)	• Used (often in the community setting) to deliver long-term fluids/medications (TPN, chemotherapy) or for hemodialysis • Inserted into the jugular vein and terminates in the superior vena cava; has a portion that is tunneled in the subcutaneous tissue and exits the skin from the anterior chest wall	• See Rehab Implications for Peripheral IV
	Peripherally inserted central catheter (PICC)	• Used (often in the community setting) to deliver long-term fluids/medications (antibiotics, TPN) • Inserted into the brachial vein and travels through the axillary vein to terminate in the superior vena cava	• See Rehab Implications for Peripheral IV • Axillary crutch use may be contraindicated • Avoid manual blood pressure on involved extremity
	Vascular access port (Mediport, Port-A-Cath)	• Used (often in the community setting) to deliver long-term fluids/medications (TPN, chemotherapy) • Inserted into the subclavian or jugular vein and terminates in the superior vena cava; has a tunneled portion attached to a port that is implanted in a subcutaneous pocket in the anterior chest wall • Needle is used to access the port	• When needle is in place, see Rehab Implications for Peripheral IV • Otherwise, no rehab implications noted

	Quinton catheter	• Central line used for short-term dialysis access • Most commonly seen for CRRT, but can also be used for intermittent hemodialysis	• See Rehab Implications for Central Venous Catheter
	Sheath introducer (Cordis)	• Large-bore single-lumen central line • Can be used alone for rapid/heavy fluid resuscitation or as an introducer for placement of a PA catheter, transvenous pacer, or central line	• If being used for fluid resuscitation, see Rehab Implications for Central Venous Catheter • If being used as introducer, see Rehab Implications for the line being introduced
	Patient-controlled analgesia (PCA)	• Used to deliver pain medication via a patient-controlled pump • Inserted via peripheral IV (PCA), but can also be placed as an epidural catheter (PCEA)	• See Rehab Implications for Peripheral IV • Avoid disconnecting as patient will not receive pain meds during this time • With PCEAs, patients may have decreased strength/sensation in lower extremities; complete a lower quarter screen (notify LIP of any positive findings) and monitor for orthostatic hypotension
Gastrointestinal, Genitourinary, and Renal Systems		**General Information**	**Rehab Implications**
Urinary/ rectal drainage devices	Indwelling/Foley catheter	• Inserted into the bladder for drainage of urine • A balloon holds the catheter in place	• Maintain collection bag below the level of the bladder to prevent backflow/infection • Tubing should be secured to patient (via an attached clip and/or adhesive on the leg) prior to mobility
	Suprapubic catheter	• Surgically inserted into the bladder to drain urine by bypassing the lower urinary tract	• See Rehab Implications for Foley Catheter • Be aware of exit point to avoid compromise of the catheter when using a gait belt
	Condom/Texas catheter	• Used to drain urine in males only • A condom-like catheter is placed over the penis and collects urine into a collection bag	• Ensure catheter is secured prior to mobility • Easily dislodged during mobility
	Purewick	• Used to drain urine in females only • An external sponge-like wick absorbs urine and is connected to a low-pressure suction source	• Can be removed prior to mobility • Postsession, either replace Purewick or notify RN of need to replace (depending on therapist comfort/discretion)
	Fecal collection devices (rectal tube, Flexiseal)	• Used to drain stool via a tube inserted inside the rectum • May have an internal balloon to hold the device in place	• Easily dislodged during mobility • Alert RN if dislodged/leaking to prevent skin compromise
	Ostomy	• Surgical procedure to divert urine or stool through the abdominal wall • Collection bag is attached over the stoma for collection of contents	• May be helpful to have the RN empty the ostomy bag of its contents prior to mobility • Be aware of positioning of gait belt to avoid pressure over ostomy

Continued

TABLE 24.5 UMMC General Information Regarding Acute Care Medical Equipment and Rehabilitation Implications for Patient Care Management—cont'd

Gastrointestinal, Genitourinary, and Renal Systems		General Information	Rehab Implications
Feeding tubes	Nasogastric/orogastric tubes	• Used to provide nutrition/medications or to drain stomach contents • If being utilized for feeding, tube will be connected to tube feeds • If being utilized for drainage, tube may be placed to gravity (via a collection device) or to suction	• If dislodged, pause tube feeds, hold tube in place, do not attempt to replace, alert RN, place patient in side-lying/upright position to prevent aspiration • If being utilized for feeding: tube feeds may be disconnected for mobility (if patient is not on insulin) and should be paused before placing head of bed below 30 degrees (to prevent aspiration) • If being utilized for drainage: maintain collection device below the level of insertion; if connected to wall suction, may only disconnect with LIP clearance
	Percutaneous endoscopic gastrostomy/jejunostomy (PEG/PEJ)	• See General Information for Nasogastric/Orogastric Tubes • Inserted surgically/endoscopically through the abdominal wall for long-term nutrition • A PEG is prepyloric (enters the stomach); a PEJ is postpyloric (enters the jejunum) and decreases the risk of aspiration	• See Rehab Implications for Nasogastric/Orogastric Tubes • Note that risk of aspiration does not apply for PEJ tubes
Dialysis	Intermittent hemodialysis	• Used to filtrate the blood for patients in chronic renal failure; typically scheduled several times per week and runs 2–4 hours • Delivered via a fistula (surgically created arteriovenous anastomosis) or a central catheter	• Patients can participate in therapy without restriction, though must ensure patency of the line during activity • Monitor vital signs and access site closely • Dialysis technician will be present to manage machine
	Peritoneal hemodialysis	• Used to filtrate the blood for patients in chronic renal failure; typically performed in the home several times a week and can run between 45 minutes and 9 hours • Delivered via an indwelling catheter in the abdomen	• Consult with RN/LIP to best determine timing of therapy around exchanges
	Continuous renal replacement therapy (CRRT)	• Used to filtrate the blood continuously for critically ill patients who cannot tolerate intermittent hemodialysis • Delivered via a central catheter • Can run multiple modalities of dialysis, including slow continuous ultra-filtration (SCUF)	• Patients can participate in therapy without restriction, though must ensure patency of the line during activity • Monitor vital signs and access site closely
	Aquadex	• Used to provide ultrafiltration for the removal of salt and water in patients with fluid overload • Delivered via a central catheter or a peripheral IV	• Easily portable for ease of mobility • Monitor vital signs and access site closely
	Molecular adsorbent recirculating system (MARS)	• Used to filtrate the blood and detoxify the liver continuously for patients in severe acute liver failure as a bridge to liver transplantation • Delivered via a central catheter	• Patients can participate in therapy without restriction, though must be aware that these patients are very critical • Consider utility of therapy during this time as machine is typically only used in short duration

Respiratory System		General Information	Rehab Implications
Low-flow systems	Nasal cannula	• Placed in the nares to provide supplemental oxygen to the spontaneously breathing patient	• Oxygen is considered to be a medication and should not be adjusted without RN/LIP clearance • Ensure adequate slack of tubing prior to ROM/mobility • Can deliver up to 44% FiO_2
	Simple face mask/ face tent	• Placed over the face to provide supplemental oxygen to the spontaneously breathing patient • Face tent may be used for patients with facial trauma, large jaw, or discomfort	• See Rehab Implications for Nasal Cannula • Can deliver up to 55% FiO_2 (for simple face mask) or 40% (for face tent)
	Trach collar	• Placed over a tracheostomy to provide supplemental oxygen to the spontaneously breathing patient after patient has been weaned from the ventilator	• See Rehab Implications for Nasal Cannula • See Rehab Implications for Tracheostomy • Can deliver up to 70% FiO_2
	Partial rebreather	• Placed over the face to provide supplemental oxygen to the spontaneously breathing patient • Has a reservoir bag that acts as another source of oxygen by collecting both FiO_2 AND a percentage of expired air that is rebreathed • The remaining amount of expired air is vented through holes on the mask	• See Rehab Implications for Nasal Cannula • Can deliver up to 85% FiO_2
	Nonrebreather (NRB)	• Placed over the face to provide supplemental oxygen to the spontaneously breathing patient • Has a reservoir bag that acts as another source of oxygen by collecting 100% FiO_2 • All of the expired air is vented through holes on the mask	• See Rehab Implications for Nasal Cannula • Can deliver up to 100% FiO_2
High-flow systems	Venturi system	• Used to deliver an exact amount of FiO_2, at a set oxygen inflow rate, to the spontaneously breathing patient • The number of liters of O_2 required to achieve desired FiO_2 is listed on colored diluter jets	• Used to make trach collar portable during mobility • Select the colored diluter jet that corresponds to the amount of FiO_2 the patient is prescribed • Can deliver up to 50% FiO_2
	Vapotherm/Optiflow	• Used to deliver high-flow, humidified, thermal-controlled, supplemental oxygen to the spontaneously breathing patient • Can deliver aerosol pulmonary medications	• Must consult with RT to determine how to best meet patient's O_2 needs when planning for mobility out of the room (only certain Vapotherm machines can run on battery); sometimes an NRB may be used as an alternative means of oxygenation • RT will need to be present to manage the portable Vapotherm/Optiflow machine and/or to assess patient tolerance to alternative means of oxygenation • Can deliver up to 100% FiO_2
	Manual resuscitation bag (MRB)	• Used to provide respirations in emergent situations; facilitate larger tidal volume/cough; provide respiratory support while off of mechanical vent; provide preoxygenation prior to suctioning • Can be used for patients with natural airways (via facemask) or artificial airways (via an adaptor that connects to a tracheostomy/endotracheal tube) • Can be used to support respiration during ambulation	• Should be available in room and connected to a flow meter during treatment of any ICU patient and during airway clearance procedures • PEEP valve should be set to 5 (for spontaneously breathing patients) or matched to the PEEP setting prescribed on the ventilator (for mechanically ventilated patients)

Continued

TABLE 24.5 UMMC General Information Regarding Acute Care Medical Equipment and Rehabilitation Implications for Patient Care Management—cont'd

Respiratory System		General Information	Rehab Implications
	NIOV (noninvasive open ventilation) Life 2000®	• Lightweight, wearable, noninvasive, ventilator used (often in the community setting) for patients with chronic lung disease • Nasal pillows are placed in the nares and are connected to a portable ventilator with an oxygen source	• Has three activity settings: low (resting), medium (moderate activity), and high (exercise) • During mobility out of the room, must use the "Auxiliary" setting on the portable oxygen tank
	Noninvasive CPAP (continuous positive airway pressure)	• Used to decrease the work of breathing in the spontaneously breathing patient by providing positive end-expiratory pressure • Most commonly used for OSA	• Mask needs to have a good seal against the face to provide effective delivery of pressure • Equipment may be noisy and communication can be difficult
	Noninvasive BiPAP (bilevel positive airway pressure)	• Used to decrease the work of breathing in the spontaneously breathing patient by providing positive inspiratory and positive end-expiratory pressure • Most commonly used to decrease CO_2 retention	• See Rehab Implications for Noninvasive CPAP
Artificial airways	Endotracheal tube (ETT) and nasotracheal tube	• Short-term artificial airway that acts as an interface between the patient and a mechanical ventilator • Inserted into the trachea via the mouth (endotracheal tube) or nose (nasotracheal tube) to preserve the patient's airway	• Ensure that the Hollister is secure prior to mobility • Ventilator tubing should always be supported during mobility • If there is a loss of the endotracheal/nasotracheal tube, monitor vitals, provide ventilation using the MRB via face mask (if indicated), and call for assistance immediately
	Tracheostomy	• Used for patients who require long-term ventilation, or who have face/neck dysfunction/injury • Inserted directly into the trachea via a surgical incision; usually sutured in place and secured with ties around the neck • Tracheostomy cuff may be found inflated or deflated: patients who are on the ventilator must have their cuff inflated; patients who are on trach collar may have their cuff inflated to limit the risk of aspiration or deflated to decrease the work of breathing and to allow for placement of a Passy-Muir speaking valve	• Ensure that trach ties are secure prior to mobility • Ventilator tubing should always be supported during mobility • If there is a loss of the tracheostomy tube, monitor vitals, seal off the stoma with your hand via multiple gauze pads, provide ventilation using the MRB via face mask (if indicated), and call for assistance immediately • Cuff must be fully deflated prior to placement of a Passy-Muir speaking valve (as valve only allows for one-way passage of air and would otherwise result in patient suffocation)
Secretion clearance modalities	Intrapulmonary percussive ventilation (IPV)	• Machine used to loosen and mobilize secretions by providing percussive bursts of gas throughout the entire respiratory cycle • Typically utilized for the mechanically ventilated patient, but can also be used for the spontaneously breathing patient (via a mouthpiece or mask interface)	• May be useful to time therapy with RT to assist with airway clearance pre- or postsession
	Cough assist	• Machine used to stimulate a productive cough by gradually providing positive pressure during inspiration and rapidly shifting to negative pressure	• See Rehab Implications for Intrapulmonary Percussive Ventilation
	Airway clearance vest	• Machine used to loosen and mobilize secretions by generating compressions via a noninvasive vest wrapped around the chest	• See Rehab Implications for Intrapulmonary Percussive Ventilation

Cardiopulmonary System	General Information	Rehab Implications
Chest tube	• Used to remove air, fluid, or blood from the thoracic cavity • Indications include pneumothorax, hemothorax, pleural effusion, empyema, or for drainage following thoracic/cardiac procedures • Inserted into an intercostal space and threaded into the pleural or mediastinal space • Pigtail chest tubes consist of smaller-bore tubing and are typically used for drainage over a longer period of time	• Maintain collection chamber below level of insertion site and avoid tipping of chamber • Tubing should not be kinked or occluded at any time • Ensure integrity of exit site dressing prior to mobility • Requires LIP clearance to disconnect from suction for mobility • If dislodged, cover with gauze, apply pressure, sit the patient upright, monitor vitals, and notify the RN immediately • If the chest tube is disconnected from the collection chamber, kink/fold the tubing still attached to patient and notify the RN immediately
Heimlich/ Pneumostat	• Used (often in the community setting) to replace traditional chest tube drainage systems for uncomplicated pneumothoraces/hemothoraces or chronic effusions • One-way valve allows air to flow out of chest with exhalation; distal end may be connected to a traditional chest tube collection chamber or a built-in collection chamber	• Typically placed just prior to discharge • Secure to clothing during mobility
Temporary pacemaker and wires	• Used to help control abnormal heart rates/rhythms • Three types: transvenous, transcutaneous, and transthoracic	• Transvenous: LIP order is needed for mobility • Transcutaneous: typically mobility is held until another form of pacer has been established but can discuss with LIP if mobility is feasible • Transthoracic: patients can be easily mobilized; avoid tension on wires during mobility and ensure pacer wires are connected to leads and pacer box; patient will be on bed rest for 1 hour following wire removal
Diaphragm pacer	• Consists of surgically implanted wires that stimulate the phrenic nerve to contract the diaphragm • Allows patients (who would otherwise be ventilator dependent) to liberate partially/fully from mechanical ventilation	• Ensure integrity of wires and exit site dressing prior to mobility • Avoid tension on wires
Pulmonary artery (PA) catheter (Swan-Ganz catheter)	• Used to measure a variety of pressures and volumes (central venous pressure, pulmonary arterial pressure, pulmonary capillary wedge pressure, cardiac output, cardiac index, SvO_2, fluid balance) • Inserted into the subclavian or internal jugular vein; the line is then threaded through the right atrium/ventricle and into the pulmonary artery	• Make sure that the PA catheter is not in wedge position • Monitor waveform and presence of PVCs prior to and during treatment session • Depending on unit, RN may need to be present during mobility for line management (refer to service line orientation for further details)
Vigileo/ Vigilance	• Used to continuously measure cardiac output, stroke volume, and SvO_2 • Attaches to a central venous catheter, an arterial line, or a PA catheter	• See Rehab Implications for Arterial Lines • See Rehab Implications for PA Catheters
Intra-aortic balloon pump	• Used to improve myocardial perfusion and decrease the work of the left ventricle • Inserted into the femoral, brachial, or axillary artery; balloon catheter is then advanced until it sits above the renal arteries and below the subclavian artery	• Patients are typically on bed rest when placed via femoral artery; patients may be mobilized if placed via brachial or axillary artery • May be seen for bed-level therapy if line will remain in place for a prolonged period of time; do not flex hip beyond 30 degrees on leg on which femoral access is obtained, monitor for signs of vascular insufficiency

Continued

TABLE 24.5 UMMC General Information Regarding Acute Care Medical Equipment and Rehabilitation Implications for Patient Care Management—cont'd

	General Information	Rehab Implications
Cardiopulmonary System		
Extracorporeal membrane oxygenation (ECMO)	• Used to oxygenate the blood and remove CO_2 outside of the body to maintain the body's pH • Provides prolonged cardiac and respiratory support to patients whose heart and lungs are unable to provide an adequate amount of gas exchange for perfusion	• Perfusionist or ECMO specialist must be present for mobility and for MBS transport • Ensure cannulas are secure and assess integrity of cannula sites prior to and following mobility • See ECMO education materials for more information
Ventricular assist device (VAD)	• Used to assist the function of the right, left, or both ventricles in circulating blood • Classified based on duration (temporary or long-term) and pulsatility (pulsatile or nonpulsatile)	• Must be VAD competent to treat VAD patients, otherwise RN must be present • Vital signs are not typical for this population; obtain MAP for reference • Ensure that drive line is anchored and dressing is secure • Do not perform CPR • See VAD education materials for more information
Neurological System	**General Information**	**Rehab Implications**
Lumbar drain	• Used to drain cerebrospinal fluid • Inserted through a lumbar puncture	• If being continuously drained, patients are typically on bed rest with head of bed flat • If being intermittently drained, patients can be mobilized only after the RN clamps the drain
Subdural drain	• Used to drain blood or cerebrospinal fluid from the subdural space • Inserted directly through the skull via a burr hole	• Patients are typically on bed rest with HOB flat
External ventricular drains (EVDs)	• Used to measure intracranial pressure (when clamped) and drain cerebrospinal fluid/blood (when open) • Inserted directly through the skull via a burr hole	• The EVD transducer must be level with the foramen of Monro to ensure accurate ICP reading (only accurate when EVD is clamped) • The zero point of the EVD must be level with foramen of Monro to ensure accurate rate of drainage (therefore must never move bed or patient while EVD is open) • Once the EVD is clamped by the RN the patient can be mobilized without restriction; the EVD must be releveled by the RN postmobility
Camino Bolt	• Used to measure intracranial pressure • Inserted into the subarachnoid space or the parenchyma via a burr hole	• Adapter needs to be anchored during mobility to prevent increased traction on the bolt
Licox	• Used to measure interstitial brain tissue oxygenation ($PbtO_2$) and brain temperature • Inserted below the dura into the white matter of the brain via a burr hole	• Adapter needs to be anchored during mobility to prevent increased traction on the bolt

General Surgical Drains

	General Information	Rehab Implications
Hemovac	• Used to drain localized fluid/blood from a surgical site • May be placed to either gravity or to suction	• Secure to clothing during mobility • If found open and has lost suction, confirm with RN if drain should be to gravity or to suction prior to reapplying suction
Jackson-Pratt (JP) drain	• Used to drain localized fluid/blood from a surgical site • May be placed to either gravity or to suction	• Secure to clothing during mobility • If found open and has lost suction, confirm with RN if drain should be to gravity or to suction prior to reapplying suction
PleurX	• Used for management of malignant ascites and recurrent pleural effusions (often in the community setting, to limit the need for hospitalization for repeat paracentesis/thoracentesis) • Includes an indwelling catheter and vacuum bottle	• Secure to clothing during mobility • Ensure integrity of exit site dressing prior to mobility
Biliary, nephrostomy, and abdominal drains	• Used to drain fluid from the applicable organ or region • May be placed to either gravity (via a collection bag) or to suction	• Secure collection bag during mobility • Keep collection bag below insertion site if draining to gravity
Vacuum-assisted closure (Wound VAC)	• Used to provide an optimal wound-healing environment via a negative pressure system • Indicated for deep extensive wounds, soft tissue infections, grafts/flaps, or while awaiting definitive closure of surgical incisions	• Suction must be maintained at all times • Notify the RN if the VAC dressing appears loose or if the vacuum unit is alarming • May be unplugged from power cord during mobility
Penrose drain	• Soft, flexible, straw-like tube • Can be placed directly into a surgical site to drain localized fluid/blood, or can be looped into and out of the surgical site to prevent premature wound closure and facilitate continued drainage	• Care must be taken to prevent dislodgment as drain is delicate

CPR, cardiopulmonary resuscitation; *DVT*, deep vein thrombosis; *HOB*, head of bed; *ICU*, intensive care unit; *LIP*, licensed independent practitioner; *MAP*, mean arterial pressure; *OSA*, obstructive sleep apnea; *PA*, pulmonary artery; *PCEA*, patient-controlled epidural analgesia; *PEEP*, positive end-expiratory pressure; *PVC*, premature ventricular contraction; *RN*, registered nurse; *ROM*, range of motion; *RT*, respiratory therapist; *TPN*, total parenteral nutrition.

(From Wells CL, Pittas J, Heyman K, Barron K, in collaboration with the Department of Rehabilitation Services Clinical Practice Committee at the University of Maryland Medical Center. Property of UMMC.)

BOX 24.2 Role of Physical Therapist in Acute Care

1. Make discharge recommendation based on determination of functional abilities, social and environmental circumstances, patient wishes and prognosis
2. Promote and facilitate safe physical activity while in hospital
3. Collaborate with health care team in developing care plan
4. Provide acute rehabilitation (management of critical lines, etc.)
5. Assess functional abilities through objective tests and measures

BOX 24.3 Successful Nursing-Directed Mobility Program

1. Physiological assessment to determine readiness for mobilization and exercise
2. Objective mobility screen to assess patient's physical ability
3. Collaboration with formal rehabilitation services to focus on developing mobility process to mitigate hospital-acquired deconditioning and restore functional mobility
4. Become nurse unit–based early mobility champions
5. Utilize nursing tools to promote treatment plans to assist patients with exercises, self-care, functional mobility

is vital in training and assisting the nursing team in basic safe patient handling, like how to help transfer a patient to a chair and walk to the bathroom, and basic functional mobility and exercises to promote follow-through of the treatment plan.

A successful nursing mobility program permits the physical therapist to focus on the rehabilitation process and aid in throughput with the patient being discharged to a higher level of care. Physical therapists can provide directed functional activities and exercises for the nurse to complete with the patient, leaving therapists to be able to focus on higher faciliatory skills within their session to progress the patient's status. With the collaboration between therapy and nursing, the families are more likely to be engaged in receiving similar information regarding the functional status and mobility plan for the day.[41] Finally, a well-supported nursing-driven mobility program allows therapy services to be directed to the right patient at the right time, which should allow for improved utilization of therapy services.

Beyond the discharge recommendation role and directed therapy to facilitate effective discharge home, acute care physical therapists also provide acute rehabilitation services to patients. Patient care can include optimizing discharge placement or preparing patients for additional medical or surgical procedures. Physical therapists also collaborate with the intensive care team to liberate patients from prolonged mechanical ventilation and the ICU setting. Physical therapists have become key members of the ICU team in addressing functional retraining, increasing activity tolerance, and problem-solving ways to overcome the barriers of many ICU devices with the goal to promote mobility[42,43] and contribute to less ventilator-supported days and shorter ICU lengths of stay.[44–46]

An effective therapist is routinely obtaining and providing information to progress the patient care plan. The critical care therapist must be familiar with, and able to manipulate, critical lines such as a Camino bolt, lumbar drain, endotracheal tube, swan, left ventricular assist device, and/or extracorporeal membrane oxygenation to successfully and safely mobilize patients. Every device, line, and tube should be identified and their function known. Precautions should be implemented to care for them while mobilizing the patient. The therapist needs to be prepared to respond in case a line becomes displaced or dislodged.

HOSPITAL-ACQUIRED DECONDITIONING AND POST-ICU SYNDROME

Hospital-acquired deconditioning and post-ICU syndrome (PICS) are receiving increased attention as conditions that can be prevented. For example, during an acute hospitalization, older adults spend approximately 83% of their hospital stay in bed and 12% of their time in a chair,[47] contributing to the well-known adverse effects of bed rest. Up to 60% of older adults admitted to the hospital report posthospital decline in completing ADLs, and more than 40% were unable to complete their prior instrumental ADLs. Only about 30% of older adults ever achieve their prior level of function at 1 year.[14,15] Physical therapists have a critical role in mitigating loss of muscle, strength, and functional limitations. Mehlhorn et al. found that patients who received physical therapy immediately upon ICU admission had better functional outcomes at ICU discharge as well as hospital discharge.[48] Patients who lose less muscle and functional mobility are able to return home after discharge versus needing a postacute rehabilitation stay.

Physical therapists can assess strength and report loss of strength using the ICU-acquired weakness (ICU-AW) score that assesses six muscle groups and document functional levels using various outcome measures such as the ICU Mobility Scale, the Functional Status Score for the ICU (FSS-ICU), or the Activity Measure for Post Acute Care (AM-PAC) "6 clicks" form. Strength and function are associated with outcomes of decreased ventilator days, ICU length of stay, and mortality. Wieske et al.[49] found that an ICU-AW is independently associated with post-ICU mortality and clinically relevant lower physical function in those who survive their critical illness. Additionally, Herman and colleagues found increased 1-year mortality in patients diagnosed with ICU-AW.[50a]

Falvey and colleagues suggest that traditional exercise prescription for older adults at risk for hospital-acquired deconditioning (HAD) be reassessed for appropriate intensity and functional mobility training to reverse the loss of functional reserve and physical performance.[50]

These authors advocate for a similar approach to that used to treat frailty (described in Chapter 13, The Older Adult Who Is Frail). This approach emphasizes high-intensity resistance training as a foundation for mobility training and aerobic training. Because no adverse effects from a high-intensity approach are reported, therapists should use this evidence-based approach to HAD while carefully monitoring the patient's physiological response and perceived effort to activity.

PHYSICAL THERAPY CONTRIBUTION TO FALL PREVENTION

Falls in the acute care setting are a grave concern for all involved. Fall prevention takes center stage within the hospital setting because it leads to direct patient care costs, longer hospital stays, and financial burden from litigation. Fall rates range from 3.3 to 11.5 falls per 1000 patient-days. Twenty-five percent of falls lead to injuries and 2% result in fractures, leading to an average of 6 to 12 days longer in length of stay.[51] Falls occur more on medicine nursing units when compared to ICUs or surgical units. Older adults fall more often perhaps owing to age-related changes, preexisting disabilities and comorbidities, increased risk of delirium and dementia, fear of falling, depression, polypharmacy, and dependency on unavailable eyeglasses. Hospital policies tend to focus on fall prevention through the use of alarms, restraints, and sitters. However, these methods are not supported by peer-reviewed evidence. Rather, a focus on an environment of mobility and prevention of functional loss, while more labor intensive, has better outcomes.[52–55]

Physical therapists have a key role to play in fall reduction within the acute care setting. Collaborating with nursing to establish accurate functional levels for each patient's needs can quickly identify a plan to promote safe patient activities. Therapists should make equipment and functional mobility recommendations, provide exercises to improve strength and balance, screen for or instruct in safe compensatory strategies to encourage mobility, and work with nursing to establish safer environments. Finally, therapists can lead hospital initiatives and committee work to promote functional mobility and walking programs, and rule out medical issues such as orthostatic hypotension, arrhythmias, and improper-fitting splints or braces that may contribute to falls.

PHYSICAL THERAPIST ROLE IN THE ICU

The physical therapist who treats patients in the ICU is required to have not only knowledge of the patient, lines and tubes, and common medications, but also knowledge and understanding of multiple diagnoses in their most critical forms and the possible complications and rehabilitation implications. Most larger hospitals separate their ICUs by population (i.e., surgical, medical, neurological, etc.), so a therapist may have the opportunity to become familiar with certain critical diagnoses related to the population he or she treats most frequently. Regardless of specific population, knowledge of human pathology in critical care is necessary for the physical therapist treating in the ICU (e.g. understanding hemodynamics and the volume shifts that can occur with changes in position, understanding the effect of one system in crisis and how it can affect other body systems).

Working in the ICU requires a closer relationship with nursing staff and intensivists, ICU doctors. Discussing with nursing how the patient tolerated daily care activities, such as rolling to change sheets, can give the physical therapist information regarding how the patient may tolerate exercise and mobility. Another benefit of working more closely with nursing is that the physical therapist can discuss medications and the potential for more, if needed, and push the patient a little more perhaps than if the nurse was not able to titrate drips to assist the patient in recovery, if the session is poorly tolerated. Working in closer proximity to the critical care physicians and providers is a unique benefit of critical care physical therapy. The ability to discuss, in real time, a patient's (in)tolerance for activity and address any concerns one may have allows the physical therapist to provide the best care. Sometimes a decision needs to be made mid–treatment session regarding ventilatory or pharmaceutical support to optimize the treatment; having a doctor or provider on the unit allows for a quick discussion and decreases missed therapy time compared to having to page a physician and wait for a call back.

Though there are some general principles to critical care physical therapy, each ICU and population has specifics of which the therapist assigned to that unit needs to have intimate knowledge. An understanding of each common diagnosis and the general paths taken as the patient progresses toward recovery, as well as regresses, is necessary to properly treat these ICU patients. This allows the physical therapist to be a member of the critical care team with pertinent information to offer based on treatment sessions. Specific patient populations will be discussed next.

Cardiac Surgery and ICU

One-third of all surgeries involving patients 65 years or older are cardiac or colorectal in nature.[56] Over half a million individuals undergo some type of open heart procedure, with more than 50% involving the older adult,[57] including coronary artery bypass, valvular repair or replacement, combined procedures, and aortic repairs owing to aneurysm or dissections.

Surgeons are operating more frequently on individuals over the age of 70 with survival rates close to 90% at 1 year and 62% at 5 years.[58,59] More recently attention has been focused on preoperative characteristics of the individual to determine potential predictors of postoperative outcomes and the quality of recovery after open heart surgery.

Frailty is a better predictor of mortality than chronological age in studies on the association between surgical outcomes and frailty.[60] Frailty has also been associated with longer dependence on mechanical ventilation.[61] Robinson et al. reported that the presence of frailty was associated with postoperative complications and the severity of frailty was associated with more than one postoperative complication after coronary artery bypass grafting (CABG), valve surgery, or a combined procedure.[56] Therefore, assessing for the presence of frailty preoperatively, if possible, can provide important information to the surgical team. Postoperatively, the presence of frailty may inform prognosis and discharge planning. The reader is encouraged to read Chapter 13, The Older Adult Who Is Frail, for a comprehensive discussion of the implications of frailty.

Other risk factors for poor outcomes for older adults included being age 85 years or older, having a body mass index (BMI) of <25, and having atrial fibrillation, renal failure, or a history of depression, gastrointestinal (GI) bleeds, cerebrovascular accident (CVA), or cancer. Certain outcome measures were also associated with higher mortality rates, including gait speeds slower than 0.54 m/sec, five times sit to stand in over 60 seconds, handgrip of <20 kg, balance deficits, and existing ADL impairments.[62] Interestingly, gait speed, sit-to-stand time, and grip strength are components of frailty.

Depending on the type of open heart surgery that is performed and the individual risk factors, potential complications that need to be discussed with the older adult include stroke, delirium, renal and pulmonary dysfunction, and arrest, to mention a few common ones (Table 24.6). Diagnosis and management of heart failure are important components of postoperative care because heart failure is the most common complication after open heart surgery. Heart failure is associated with longer mechanical ventilation time and longer ICU and hospital lengths of stay. Patients also tend to present with a higher incidence of depression and decreased social and activity engagement.[63] The physical therapist can be a key member of the health care team to monitor for plateaus or declines in function so that the medical team can make prompt changes to optimize the medical management plan to decrease avoidable delays. The therapist should provide education regarding the expected course of functional recovery and continued assessment to make the most appropriate discharge recommendation.

Hospitals are returning to the utilization of postoperative clinical pathways to standardize routine care and improve efficiency. These clinical pathways reduce variability between health care services, improve interdisciplinary collaboration and communication, and allow the team to quickly identify when a patient is not meeting expected goals. Adoption of such pathways can lead to reduction in mechanical ventilation time, improved feeding, and reduced ICU and hospital LOSs, as well as promote early mobilization.[64] The team can be tasked to assess the cause of the deviation from expected outcomes and take corrective measures to address the cause with the goal to return the patient to the pathway or determine a new plan of care.

Physical therapy is a key component of open heart procedure clinical pathways. From the initial evaluation on postoperative day 0 or 1 therapists assess functional ability and stability of vital signs, begin to instruct the patient and family on sternal precautions if appropriate, and make discharge recommendations. Over recent years it has been shown that patients can safely use their upper extremities to perform functional activities such as transfers out of bed and to rise from a seated position. These patients should be encouraged to restore the range of motion of their shoulders over the next several postoperative days. Use of the upper extremities for transfers and ADLs should be completed with the upper extremities positioned to approximate the sternum and decrease the length of the pectoralis muscles to reduce the stress to the skin and sternum. Literature is now available to report that the patient can lift 10 to 20 pounds safely when the weight is held close to the body, and patients should be able to resume prior activities after 6 weeks, as pain permits, unless there is concern regarding healing.[65,66] Physical therapy should also be collaborating with nursing to progress walking tolerance with the goal for patients to ambulate at least three times a day for at least 30 total

TABLE 24.6 Common Postoperative Complications

Postoperative Complication	Physical Therapy Role
Wound infection or dehiscence	Wound protection by teaching alternative functional mobility strategies to minimize incisional stress Wound management
Arrhythmias	Monitor for changes in electrocardiogram, determine associated signs and symptoms
Insufficient airway clearance or pneumonia	Airway clearance techniques, exercises and functional activities progression
Renal insufficiency or failure	Edema management, techniques and equipment to reduce pressure injuries
Pressure injuries	Repositioning strategies, mobility, recommendations for specialty bed surfaces and splints
Stroke	Neuromuscular examination and intervention
Delirium	Reorientation and cognitive retraining
Infection (urinary tract infection, line infection)	Monitor for signs and symptoms of infection and increase mobility to facilitate decrease in Foley catheters

minutes, increase airway clearance to normalize ventilation, and instruct in splinting and cough strategies.

Another source of postoperative complications is the use of cardiopulmonary bypass during open heart surgery. Browndyke et al. found that postoperative cognitive changes were associated with changes documented by magnetic resonance imaging (MRI) in the regions of the posterior cingulate cortex and right superior frontal gyrus. These structures are involved in self-awareness, internally driven cognition, focused attention, and global cerebral communication processes. Clinically, these patients showed deficits in such cognitive testing as the Trail A, Stroop Color and Word, and Rey Auditory Learning tests.[67] The therapist should screen for cognitive and attentional deficits during the initial evaluation and follow-up sessions and alert the surgical team if there are concerns because delirium is negatively associated with LOS and functional outcomes, as mentioned earlier. The therapist may consider recommending an occupational therapy or speech consult to the team for their further assessment of deficits and recommendations.

Pulmonary complications after open heart surgery are the leading cause of mortality, ranging as high as 76% depending on type of complication, type of surgery, and individual risk factors. Pulmonary complications are associated with complete heart block and altered chest wall mechanics from the sternotomy or thoracotomy surgical approach, which may lead to insufficient ventilation, systemic inflammatory response syndrome, phrenic nerve injury, alveolar edema due to insufficient left ventricular function, increased pulmonary vascular pressures, atelectasis, and pneumonia.[68] Besides functional progression, addressing pulmonary dysfunction is a substantial part of the care a physical therapist should provide to a patient after an open heart procedure. This may include but not be limited to airway clearance techniques, breath control exercises, mobility, positioning to normalize breathing patterns, and strengthening of the respiratory muscles.

Preoperative education and preparation are becoming part of routine surgical management of patients undergoing open heart procedures to improve outcomes and decrease LOS. Individualized patient-centered education has been found to reduce anxiety and depression and improve self-care after open heart surgery.[69] It is important for the surgical team to provide education across various media including written, video, and face to face to meet the learning styles and needs of patients. The reader is referred to Chapter 11, Patient Education, within this text.

It is also important to address physical limitations and behaviors that contribute to postoperative complications in the preoperative period, when possible. Having patients participate in physical therapy to address functional impairments, teach postoperative functional mobility modification, and increase activity tolerance has contributed to LOS reduction and improved quality of life. Smoking cessation, use of inspiratory muscle trainers, and teaching breath control exercises also have postoperative benefits.[70] These preoperative education and therapy interventions also need to be provided to the patients who are admitted to the hospital prior to surgery to avoid preoperative hospital-acquired deconditioning, which can lead to a decrease in functional recovery, delays in discharge, and increased risk of acquiring a hospital-associated complication like pneumonia, urinary tract infection, or pressure injury.[71]

A part of the physical therapist's management of patients after open heart surgery is the consistent assessment of functional progression, pulmonary function, and vital signs. Therapists should monitor vitals during functional training including monitoring electrocardiography changes. Atrial fibrillation is one of the most common arrhythmias for older adults after open heart procedures and is one of the leading causes of readmission. Determining that the patient experiences a normal heart rate and rhythm, blood pressure, and saturation response to exercise and functional training is very important to inform progression and contribute to a successful discharge. Another area where physical therapists can contribute to the care of these patients is in educating the patient in how to move and exercise safely while the soft tissue and sternum heal. Education should also include the signs and symptoms of wound infections, which are also a common cause for readmission.[72]

Finally, the physical therapist should work closely with case management and social work on developing a discharge plan. The patient will need continued support for 4 to 8 weeks after hospital discharge. Patients typically need assistance with ADLs such as bathing, housework, and driving for 1 to 2 months after surgery.[73] This time may be longer for those patients who demonstrate ADL deficits prior to surgery, who have multiple comorbidities, or who experienced delirium during the hospital stay.[73]

Cardiac Surgical Procedures

The most common procedures that are included in open heart surgery are CABG and valvular repairs or replacements. CABG remains the gold-standard surgical management for coronary artery disease. CABG, for either isolated left anterior disease or multivessel disease, is associated with lower mortality and lower incidences of future cardiovascular events like myocardial infarctions and strokes when compared to less radical surgical options such as minimally invasive direct coronary artery bypass (MIDCAB) and angioplasty with arterial stenting.[74] MIDCAB tends to show longer LOSs but is also associated with fewer future cardiovascular events and need for additional revascularization when compared to angioplasty.[75] For the older adult who has a high surgical risk secondary to multiple comorbidities, MIDCAB for isolated disease or MIDCAB with angioplasty with stenting may be the best option. Surgeons can complete many of these surgical procedures off cardiopulmonary bypass with reduced rates of stroke than traditional on-pump procedures.

Off-pump procedures may reduce mortality and morbidity for high-risk elderly patients.[76]

Aortic Valve Stenosis. is the most frequent valvular disease that impairs ejection from the left ventricle and is associated with other comorbidities like carotid artery stenosis, stroke, peripheral arterial disease, and chronic renal failure. Sixty-three percent of patients with aortic stenosis also have clinically significant coronary arterial disease. Langanay et al. reported favorable outcomes for the older adult over 80 years of age using a surgical approach with a late median survival of 7.1 years.[59] More recently older adults who were considered high risk for an aortic valve replacement or not considered surgical candidates at all have undergone transcatheter aortic replacement as opposed to an open heart procedure. The mortality and morbidity outcomes for patients undergoing transcatheter aortic valve replacement are lower than with the surgical approach, but the literature is not definitive on the selection criteria for a surgical versus transcatheter approach owing to study design, sample size, and selection.[62,77]

Mitral Valve Repair. Moderate to severe mitral value disease affects 5 million individuals and can be classified as primary or secondary disease. Primary disease is related to intrinsic abnormalities of the valve such as a congenital deformity of the leaflets of the valve. Secondary disease is related to left ventricular failure with the most common cause from ischemic coronary artery disease that leads to mitral regurgitation owing to either papillary muscle ischemia, rupture, or left ventricular remodeling.[78]

It is commonplace for a patient to undergo mitral valve repair or replacement and a CABG for coronary disease at the same time. These patients may experience longer times on cardiopulmonary bypass during surgery, longer time on mechanical ventilators, and longer LOSs, but the outcomes are favorable. By improving myocardial perfusion and correcting the dysfunctional mitral valve, the left ventricle can remodel and blood can flow forward through the heart and out to the systemic circulation, and patients show improvement in physical capacity.[78]

The outcomes between mitral valve repair versus replacement are variable. It appears that there is more consistent left ventricular remodeling with less recurrent regurgitation when the mitral valve is replaced. Other surgeons have reported that if there is no recurrent regurgitation at 2 years postoperation for a mitral valve repair, then the ventricle remodeling is actually better with the natural valve.[77,78]

Minimally invasive mitral valve surgery (MIMVS) has become an effective alternative approach, and this type of surgical approach has expanded to include partial sternotomy and anterior thoracotomy. The types of repair can be customized to fit the valvular dysfunction and can include the replacement of a ruptured chordae tendinea and repair of the valvular ring or leaflet. More recently transcatheter appropriate to repairs are also being performed via a femoral vein approach. There appears to be no difference in mortality from MIMVS when compared to conventional sternotomy mitral valve replacement, although there is an increased risk for future surgical intervention owing to recurrent regurgitation.[79]

Neurological ICU

In the neurological ICU common diagnoses are CVAs, subarachnoid hemorrhages (SAHs), and intracerebral hemorrhages (ICHs). There are specific best-practice recommendations for physicians based on patient presentation and wishes, but there are also similarities in treatment of these conditions that are more relevant to rehabilitation and treatment in the ICU.

Blood pressure (BP) management is critically important to prevent further bleeding and neurological insult. BP is variable and affected by activity; one patient may tolerate getting out of bed and into a chair without exceeding his or her BP goal, whereas another patient with the same diagnosis may only tolerate bed mobility. It is important that a physical therapist be aware of the specific BP goal for individual patients and modify treatment to adhere to these parameters. For example, patients with recent neurological insult will have a target blood pressure goal. This may include permissive hypertension, allowing a systolic blood pressure (SBP) up to 220 mmHg, in the case of an ischemic CVA to try to reperfuse the area of ischemia, or maintaining SBP <140 mmHg for ICH and SAH conditions to prevent rebleeding.[80]

Another common event seen in the neurocritical care population is vasospasm. This is the sudden narrowing of vessels, leading to further ischemia. Patients experiencing vasospasm will display symptoms of new focal deficits and/or decreased level of consciousness.[81] If a patient begins to show symptoms of vasospasm during physical therapy treatment, it is important that the physical therapist recognize these symptoms and respond appropriately. It may be that the patient is hypovolemic and simply needs IV fluids, or it may be that the patient requires endovascular treatment; either way, the physical therapist should know the symptoms and recognize that treatment should be terminated and notify the critical care team of the new symptoms.

As with other critically ill patients, patients in the neurological ICU can experience setbacks. Whether related to something relatively simple such as hemodynamics or electrolyte imbalance or to something more critical such as blood pressure management or rebleeding, patients can appear ready to progress to an intermediate care (IMC) or floor unit one day and later that same day be deemed too unstable for transfer. These patients can present differently from one treatment to another. It is the job of the critical care physical therapist to work within the limitations and most current presentation, provided the patient is medically stable for therapy, to functionally progress these patients until they are able to go to a rehabilitation center. Frequent assessments (i.e., strength, alertness, coordination, etc.), even if similar to ones documented by the critical care team, can provide the therapist and team with pertinent information regarding patients' tolerance to treatment, progress, and readiness for transfer out of the ICU to a stepdown unit.

Medical ICU

In the medical ICU a therapist will be exposed to a variety of diagnoses. Commonly, patients with worsening respiratory distress or renal failure and those experiencing side effects and effects of cancer are transferred to a medical ICU for a higher level of care. Like other ICUs, a patient can be stable and appropriate for therapy and still begin to decompensate during a treatment; therefore, it is important to know the signs and symptoms and appropriate courses of action.

Ventilation in the ICU. Patients who experience respiratory distress in an ICU are usually going to require intubation for ventilation. Knowledge and understanding of mechanical ventilation and the ventilator itself are necessary to progress patients in therapy. Treatment and duration of ventilation may vary depending on the diagnosis. Common diagnoses requiring ventilation include pneumonia, COPD, and asthma. Familiarity with the ventilator will allow the therapist to confidently manage tubing for optimal positioning for mobility. As mentioned earlier, recognition of various alarms and how/when to respond is important for optimal patient management. Understanding ventilator settings and modes will give the therapist knowledge of how hard the patient is working and whether he or she is breathing with assistance or initiating each breath independently. Some modes of ventilation are known to be weaning modes (pressure or volume support) and may be an indicator that the patient is nearing extubation. The physical therapist can assist and treat patients while weaning from ventilation, even if the patient isn't able to tolerate mobility or ambulation at that time. A physical therapist can assist in positioning for optimal breathing as well as educate patients on deep breathing techniques and secretion clearance to make the weaning process successful. Though it varies by facility, it is common practice to mobilize and ambulate patients while they are still intubated. Maintaining strength, endurance, and functional mobility is paramount when recovering from respiratory distress/failure. It is important to note that although a patient may be comfortable at rest on a weaning mode, he or she may require more ventilatory support to participate in therapy, especially for ambulation and endurance training. Discussing the possibility of changing the mode of ventilation for participation in therapy can be done with the critical care team prior to treating the patient.

Hemodialysis in the ICU. It is not uncommon to encounter a patient with renal failure in the medical ICU, either as the primary reason for admission or as a secondary problem caused by critical illness. Whether acute or chronic renal failure, treatment in critical care will have similarities, and familiarity with the diagnosis and treatment will aid the physical therapist in functional progression. Five to six percent of patients admitted to the ICU will have acute renal failure. Of those patients, 75% will be treated with continuous renal replacement therapy (CRRT).[100] According to research, approximately 4% to 5% of all critically ill patients require renal replacement therapy.[101] CRRT is a gentler form of hemodialysis (HD) that removes fluid and solutes at a slower rate over a longer period of time. Because the therapy is stretched over 16 to 24 hours (versus 3 to 5 hours for intermittent HD), patients who are hemodynamically unstable can better tolerate this treatment without becoming severely hypotensive. These patients can better tolerate, and participate in, physical therapy. Although slower, prolonged fluid removal appears better for the kidneys, it can present a challenge for the physical therapist who wishes to mobilize the patient with renal failure. The catheter needs to be monitored closely and may be very sensitive to joint position, which can disrupt filtration. The actual machines are also typically difficult to maneuver during the mobilization activity. Though it is generally accepted that early mobility in critical care is advantageous to the patient, many providers and nurses are hesitant to extend this to patients receiving CRRT. CRRT is delivered via a double-lumen central line catheter, usually located in the internal jugular, subclavian, or femoral areas. Though many studies[102–106] have demonstrated the safety and feasibility of mobilizing patients with catheters, especially femoral, many people are uncomfortable because of the renal replacement therapy itself. The CRRT machine and supplies do have a significant cost associated with them, and the circuit itself is vulnerable to clotting if not managed by a skilled professional. However, Wang and associates noted in their prospective study of patients on CRRT, with all of the aforementioned catheter sites, that mobilization was associated with prolonged filter life for the machine itself and was associated with no adverse events for the patients or the circuits, and in fact may prolong the life of the filter in some cases.[100] Even with a treatment team that is comfortable with mobilizing patients on CRRT, the physical therapist is limited to in-room activities because the CRRT machine is not battery operated. Some facilities will allow the patient to be removed from CRRT (once the blood has been returned to the patient) for a short period of time to allow for ambulation. This needs to be coordinated with the bedside nurse, because the circuit can only be "paused" for a short period of time before the circuit cannot be reconnected. Alternatively, some physicians will run the CRRT only at night, allowing the patient more freedom to mobilize throughout the day.

TRAUMA MANAGEMENT

Older adults with trauma requiring hospitalization account for more ICU days, longer hospital LOSs, higher utilization of hospital services, and higher admission rates to skilled nursing facilities.[82] Hospital LOS is positively correlated with patients' age owing to the likelihood of comorbidities including arrythmia, hypertension, coronary artery disease, diabetes mellitus, drug abuse, liver dysfunction, hemophilia, coagulopathy, peripheral vascular disease, and electrolyte imbalance.[83]

Trauma is the seventh leading cause of death in older adults with a higher 30-day mortality for those individuals unable to be discharged home. There is an association between death and cardiac and pulmonary disease, psychiatric disorders, hematological disorders, cognitive impairments, stroke, and diabetes.[8,83] Older adults have poorer outcomes when compared to younger adults despite a lower severity index, which may be associated with comorbidities, frailty, and a decrease in physical reserve.[83]

The older adult will respond differently to the stress of trauma. Factors such as decreases in cellular function, a decline in physical reserve, and the possible presence of sarcopenia can lead to medical complications and higher morbidity and mortality rates.[82–84] There is an increase in physiological burden after a traumatic event. This places additional stress on the myocardium, which may already be compromised owing to chronic disease. The natural decline in cellular organ function with aging compounded by chronic diseases can lead to organ dysfunction, such as respiratory failure due to pneumonia, renal failure, and infections that further complicate medical recovery and hamper the rehabilitation and recovery process.[83,84] The use of anticoagulation owing to increased incidence of atrial fibrillation in the older adult also increases the risk of bleeding.[83]

The presence of sarcopenia at the time of the traumatic event directly relates to the prediction of functional recovery. Every centimeter increase in the size of the psoas muscles measured from the abdomen and pelvis computed tomography scan, which is a very common diagnostic tool related to trauma admission, is correlated with a 20% increase in the likelihood of achieving independent living.[85] Possibly, the consideration of the stage of sarcopenia may shed even more light on the clinical value for intervention and discharge recommendations.

The acute inflammatory response that is triggered by a significant traumatic event or critical illness such as sepsis, emergency surgery, respiratory failure, and traumatic injury amplifies the catabolic process of skeletal muscle that is associated with sarcopenia. The older adult can quickly experience profound muscle wasting and functional dependence owing to the development of a catabolic state, leading to mitochondrial dysfunction and a decrease in muscle protein synthesis.[84] Muscle atrophy and loss of strength and function can occur within the first 5 days of a critical illness, and by 10 days there may be profound dysfunction of the sarcomere of the skeletal muscle.[86,87] Within the first week of hospitalization 50% to 80% of patients will experience further muscle weakness,[88,89] and 100% will experience muscle weakness in the presence of sepsis.

Clinical management can be further compromised by malnutrition despite BMI. In this stressed physiological state glycogen stores are significantly utilized within the first 24 hours and then the body turns to the amino acids of skeletal muscle to make energy, leading to proteolysis, which appears to affect type 2 muscle fibers more than type 1 fibers. Along with a decrease in physical activity, there is a reduction in oxidative enzymes to make sufficient energy, leading to further mitochondrial dysfunction and muscle function impairments.[84]

The treatment approach to address traumatic injuries in the older adult is to first start with prevention. Keeping the older adult active and engaged is critical in sustaining the physiological reserve and the ability of the body to more likely overcome the stress of a traumatic event. Optimizing medication management and examining drug interactions is a key part of geriatric medical care. Routine examinations and management of chronic diseases may also improve outcomes after hospitalization.

Once hospitalization has occurred, the staff should implement a screening process to identify individuals at risk for poor outcomes. The Identification of Seniors at Risk (ISAR) questionnaire is an easy screening tool that considers the following risk factors: premorbid and acute changes in function, recent hospitalizations, memory deficits, impaired vision, and polypharmacy. An individual who scores a 2 or greater is at risk for poor outcomes. The CGA is typically performed by a geriatrician and assesses several domains of an older adult's function. Patients who show deficits in both the ISAR and the CGA were at the highest risk for poor functional outcomes after a traumatic event.[90] Another tool that can be helpful is the Vulnerable Elderly Survey (VES-13), which assigns points, 0 to 4 (0 = no disability), in four domains: physical function, ADLs, self-health status, and age. For physical function the person is asked if he or she can complete the following tasks independently or with difficulty requiring assistance or is unable to complete the following activities: physical tasks like stooping or kneeling, walking .25 miles, lifting 10 pounds, reaching overhead, writing, and completing heavy housework. The survey also asks about one's ability to walk and to complete ADLs such as shopping, managing money, doing light housework, and bathing. The individual is also asked to rank his or her health compared to others of similar age, and finally his or her age. A VES-13 score of >2 along with an Injury Severity Score of 16 or higher was associated with hospital complications and poor outcomes.[91]

Hospitals should implement a collaborative model between rehabilitation services and nursing to promote early mobilization and rehabilitation to maintain functional mobility and cognitive engagement as soon as possible.[41] Facilities need to adopt policies to reduce the level of sedation and use of restraints, encourage family engagement, minimize sensory isolation, and make the environment mobility friendly for the older adult.[31,92] Rehabilitation services need to examine how patients are prioritized and use screening tools to treat patients at risk for severe functional declines; this may include making patients suffering from trauma such as hip fractures and chest wall trauma high priorities to aggressively promote mobility to prevent the age-related and iatrogenic effects of hospitalization with the goal to obtain the highest level of function and placement.[9]

Falls-Related Trauma

Falls are the number one cause of trauma in the older adult, with older males having a higher in-hospital death rate.[93,94] Risk factors related to falls are listed in Table 24.7. Annually, approximately 35% of community-dwelling older adults over the age of 65 will experience a fall, with 20% to 30% sustaining moderate to severe injuries. Adults over the age of 85 years are four to five times more likely to suffer severe injuries related to a fall and are more prone to polytrauma.[95,96] Trauma-related admissions for older adults account for 25% of all trauma admissions and are projected to increase to 40% by 2050.[8]

Falls in the elderly are associated with a certain type of injuries. There is an increase in a traumatic brain injury as an individual ages, particularly when the individual is over 75 years.[94] Traumatic brain injuries (TBIs) resulting from a fall can be the result of a subdural bleed, contusion injury, or intracerebral hematomas, which are more common than in the young adult. TBIs are common following a fall on the head because of the increase in subdural space associated with a reduction in brain volume. This increased space leads to increased movement of the brain when the head is struck. Additionally, a decrease in vascular compliance can lead to a risk of bleeding after a fall, especially in the presence of anticoagulant use in older adults.[95,97,98] It is important that the physical therapist be aware that the 20% to 30% of older adults who have sustained a TBI related to a fall may deteriorate over 48 hours of the initial injury. This delay may be related to a slow bleed and decreased tolerance to cerebral ischemia. The therapist should obtain objective measures to assess and monitor neurological changes over the acute phase of recovery.[97]

Older adults frequently have asymptomatic degenerative cervical disease, but with a fall there is an increased risk for cervical injuries, including spinal cord injury. Required and necessary immobilization can lead to increased muscle weakness, which is associated with impaired cough and gag abilities, predisposing the patient to a risk for pneumonia. Additionally, atelectasis may occur and thus require mechanical ventilator support. Given the decrease in lung and chest wall compliance and risk of malnutrition, the therapist needs to be constantly assessing and providing airway clearance to reduce the risk of pneumonia.[8,95]

Hip fractures lead to 30% 1-year mortality owing to frailty and a decrease in physical reserve. Males over the age of 80, delay in surgical repair, comorbidities of cardiac and renal disease, and anticoagulation use increase the risk of postoperative complications and death associated with hip fractures.[9] Thirty-five percent of older adults who suffer a hip fracture will experience delirium. The physical therapist and other members of the health care team should complete risk screens for all older adults prior to and following surgery with the goal to decrease the incidence and duration of delirium. Risk factors for delirium in the presence of hip fracture, in addition to previously described risk factors, include low hemoglobin, blood transfusion, dementia, frailty, preoperative functional limitations, and institutionalization.[99]

TABLE 24.7 Risk Factors Associated with Falls

Infections	Immobility
Visual impairment	Arrhythmias
Delirium	Dehydration
Polypharmacy	Cardiovascular disease
Comorbidities: diabetes, stroke (sensory deficits)	Anemia
Age	Decrease in functional mobility
Preadmission cognitive deficits	History of falls
Incontinence	Arthritis
Sarcopenia	Orthostatic hypotension

(Modified from Ambrose, AF, Paul Geet, Hausdorff, JM. Risk factors for falls among older adults: a review of the literature. *Maturitas*. 2013;75:51–61.)

ONCOLOGY CONSIDERATIONS

Whether identified pretreatment or not, many older adults diagnosed with cancer will have one or more geriatric syndromes than can be exacerbated by treatment, including radiation or chemotherapy, as well as a prolonged hospital admission to administer these treatments. All of the previously mentioned effects of being in the hospital—prolonged bed rest, increased fall risk, delirium, and so forth—are potential complications for the geriatric oncology patient, in addition to the effects of being treated for cancer.

Chemotherapy and radiation are common treatments for a number of cancers and are known to cause nausea, vomiting, fatigue, and neuropathy. Any one of these effects alone, even more so in combination, can make it difficult for a patient to want to, or be able to, participate in physical therapy treatment. Decreased platelet count (thrombocytopenia) is also a possible side effect of chemotherapy that can limit ability to participate in therapy.[107]

Strenuous exercise performed by a older patient with thrombocytopenia could lead to hemorrhage of the skin, muscles, or even brain. It is important for the physical therapist to look at recent lab values and plan treatment accordingly based on accepted recommendations. Chapter 14, Management of the Acutely Ill Older Adult Patient, provides more information. Patients experiencing excessive pain and/or nausea secondary to a cancer diagnosis or treatment are at times additionally treated with steroids. Though steroids can alleviate these symptoms, prolonged use can cause other problems, including increased susceptibility to infection and/or psychosis. Steroid psychosis can present as mania and depression, and up to 75% of the time as delirium and psychosis. Given that older adults face a high risk for delirium with prolonged hospitalization and with use of certain medications, distinguishing delirium due to steroid psychosis can be difficult and can delay appropriate treatment.

Fatigue is the most commonly reported symptom of those being treated for cancer.[107] There are many potential causes of this fatigue, including the treatment itself, thrombocytopenia, lack of proper nutrition, decreased physical activity, lack of sleep, and emotional stress. One study[108] compared patients older than 60 with those 18 to 50 years old and found that though fatigue status and type were not significantly different, the impact of fatigue on daily activities was significantly higher in the older age group. This may make a patient less willing to participate in therapy or cause decreased tolerance for activity. The physical therapist treating this patient population will need to be aware of the effects of cancer as well as the treatments and plan therapy sessions accordingly. Knowing that patient tolerance may change day to day, the therapist should have multiple treatment options of varying difficulties to choose from to allow the patient to be successful in therapy. It should also be noted that there will be days when the patient does not feel up to the task of therapy; though it is the job of the physical therapist to motivate patients to do their very best, it is also imperative to know when to allow patients to rest and recover. This is even more true with the oncology population.

One area where physical therapy can especially benefit this patient population is in positioning in bed and chairs. Patients being treated for cancer are known to be frail, potentially malnourished, and weak; this, in addition to increased time in bed and prolonged hospitalization, leaves a patient at risk for skin breakdown and pressure ulcers. With decreased muscle mass and adipose tissue, patients are at a higher risk for pressure-related injuries over protruding bony prominences, which may happen quickly. Already immunocompromised from cancer treatment, elderly patients with skin tears take a long time to heal. Physical therapists are trained to position patients in a manner that will minimize excess pressure on bony prominences and to recognize signs of pressure when mobilizing patients. Patients and families can be educated on proper positioning and pressure relief schedules. Physical therapists can coordinate with nursing to ensure proper positioning is reproduced when patients are mobilized.

DIFFERENTIATING "SIMPLE" FROM "COMPLEX" MANAGEMENT CONSIDERATIONS

Before beginning an examination on a patient, a physical therapist should complete a review of systems, the process that allows a therapist to gain as much knowledge as possible about a patient from the medical record and by speaking to the nurse, patient, and other caregivers. Patients will have varying degrees of complexity, even within units devoted to complexity such as the ICU and IMC unit. Reading the medical chart, including the history and physical, trending vital signs, and recent progress notes, will give insight into how stable the patient has been over the past few hours. Chapter 14, Management of the Acutely Ill Older Patient, describes the art of chart review and history taking. The physical therapist should be able to take available information from the chart, team meetings, and rounds, and determine appropriate courses of action including the need for further clarification.

The acute care therapist needs to rapidly obtain and synthesize pertinent information from multiple sources. The therapist then selects and executes appropriate tests and measures to determine prognosis for recovery and recommend accurate discharge recommendations to facilitate hospital throughput. The overarching skill that is necessary to be an effective acute care therapist is clinical reasoning. A therapist who demonstrates clinical reasoning can effectively and efficiently complete a review of systems that may come from various sources in a systematic end-focused manner to lead the therapist to a planned direction for the examination. For a patient with a health medical history who was admitted for a common procedure like a debridement of the knee owing to osteoarthritis, the therapist may only really need to attend to gait, including stairs, balance, and coordination to use an assistive device and a home exercise program to restore knee function and control edema. This case is quite simple with little need for integrative clinical reasoning. Let us consider this same hospital procedure but now the individual has significant comorbid burdens including diabetes with severe peripheral neuropathy, and retinopathy with limited vision and poor depth perception, and a history of a CVA with residual hemiparesis. For this patient the therapist has a complex situation that will take more clinical reasoning to produce a successful outcome. In this case the therapist needs to generate a working priority framework about what might be anticipated as barriers to functional recovery and discharge, generate questions to return to further information gathering, and redevelop a plan for the examination or systems review. The therapist may anticipate that this patient will have difficulty using an assistive device and significant safety concerns regarding functioning in unfamiliar surroundings. This patient may have a history of falls that would warrant further examination of probable causes and further understanding of the home environment and social support. The therapist will also need to consider that this patient may be more prone to abnormal vitals response, poor healing, and perception of pain that may lead to a high risk for readmissions. During the examination and future interventions, the therapist will need to be constantly reassessing and determining the impact the acute situation and past medical history have on progress and discharge planning. This simple surgical intervention becomes a complex scenario for the therapist to manage to ensure proper throughput.

Simple and complex management may also refer to the length of time a patient is hospitalized. A simple case may be a patient who is expected to have a short length of stay with few to no complications. In this situation when evaluating a simple patient case in the acute care setting, the hospital course for the procedure, management, and discharge is predictable. The goal for the therapist is usually clearance for a safe discharge from the hospital. The physical therapist will focus on restoring safe functional independence with basic mobility like bed mobility, transfers, gait, and stair negotiation. The physical therapist will need to complete an in-depth subjective interview to say with authority that the patient can safely discharge home and that he or she has the necessary physical assistance and supervision available. On the other hand, a complex management may involve a patient who is not following the expected hospital course owing to complications that will lead to progressive weakness and functional limitations. The acute care therapist will need to implement a more complex plan of care that may include interventions that are commonly used in rehabilitation centers and outpatient clinics like manual skills, neuromuscular facilitation, splinting, and airway clearance. Care of the complex patient extends beyond making a recommendation of disposition and in many cases requires providing frequent rehabilitation services to assist in weaning from the mechanical ventilator and addressing progression of basic mobility tasks and activity tolerance to ensure the patient is stable enough with exertion to be discharged to another institutional setting. With these complex cases clinical reasoning becomes critical because the patient's medical status can change frequently, and the therapist will need to continue to assess and reassess addressing the most pressing issues during each session with the goal to achieve functional mobility and activity tolerance sufficient for discharge.

Medication Considerations

Beyond the direct interaction with the patient, the therapist must be familiar with the common medications and their effects on exercise and activity tolerance. The therapist also needs to be comfortable with the common medications that are administered within a specific population. By screening the medication list as well as the dosages, the therapist can obtain a better understanding of the medical complexity of the patient that should guide the clinical decision to intervene with the patient and, if so, how to proceed. This is extremely important in the ICU setting because the types of medications the patient is being administered will help the therapist to determine the level of critical illness and medical stability, the appropriateness to see the patient, and how to plan the treatment session. For example, consider that you have two patients who are on Levophed for hypotension. Patient A is on a low dosage, but patient B's dosage is at maximal administration parameters. The therapist's clinical reasoning may lead to the conclusion that patient A may be more appropriate to evaluate and slowly progress functional activities, whereas the more appropriate intervention for patient B would be to address skin care needs and positioning, and defer mobility assessment until the patient is more stable. The therapist is in a perfect position to also examine the effects of medication on functional mobility and activity tolerance. For example, a patient could be progressing poorly with therapy and constantly reporting excessive fatigue. If the therapist recognizes that the patient is on a nonselective β-blocker like propranolol and determines that the patient has little heart rate and blood pressure response during exertion and is reporting dyspnea, the therapist needs to share his or her findings with the provider, who may change the type of medication, the dosage, or the time of administration, which will likely improve activity tolerance and may positively impact discharge.

POSTSURGICAL ACUTE MANAGEMENT OF COMMON ORTHOPEDIC SURGERIES

Given the estimated increase in the number of older adults over the next few decades, there will likely be an increase in number of surgeries performed, both elective and nonelective. With age, multiple comorbidities, and potential frailty, considerations must be taken before, during, and after surgical intervention. Complications in this population can lead to prolonged hospitalizations, or even death, more so than with younger persons.

Irrespective of type of surgery, the main goal postoperatively is early mobility and preventing complications. This cannot be accomplished without appropriate and adequate pain management. There are multiple considerations a physician must take when prescribing pain control after surgery; when possible a baseline pain assessment, including pain history and any narcotic use, will be beneficial in postoperative management. The risk for delirium and drug interactions can occur rapidly as a result of inappropriate dosing. The results of medication side effects can adversely affect the patient's ability and desire to participate in mobilization efforts and can predispose the patient to falls. Additionally, overmedication can affect the respiratory and/or cardiac systems, necessitating a higher level of care and prolonged hospitalization.

For these reasons, and more, research shows that older patients, especially those undergoing surgery for a hip fracture, tend to be undermedicated.[109] Insufficient pain control limits patient progress and functional outcomes. Uncontrolled pain following lower extremity orthopedic surgery has been associated with increased lengths of stay, increased complications, delayed start to ambulation, impaired functional recovery, and increased suffering by the elderly patient.[110] In addition, patients without sufficient pain control were less likely to be ambulating by 3 days after surgery and showed less mobility at 6-month follow-ups.[109] Pain can be a major limiting factor to mobility and ambulation, more so when a patient is unable to verbalize his or her pain. One study found that among nursing home residents, those with decreased cognition were prescribed, and administered, significantly fewer analgesics than their cognitively intact peers.[109] It is important to look for nonverbal indicators of pain such as restlessness, agitation, guarding, splinting, rapid blinking, or facial expression, or to look for physiological changes such as tachycardia, hypertension, or tachypnea to assess how a patient is handling his or her pain. In the acute setting, pain control should be a priority of the therapist prior to mobilization.

Depending on the facility, there may be a service team dedicated to pain management that can be consulted to help appropriately treat the surgical patient. Multimodal pain management has been shown to be helpful in patients after a total joint arthroplasty.[111] The goal of multimodal management is less reliance on opioids and finding a combination of available options to appropriately treat the acute pain associated with surgery. Use of cryotherapy, nerve blocks, epidural analgesics, nonsteroidal anti-inflammatory drugs (NSAIDs) like acetaminophen, or nonopioid narcotics like tramadol, managed appropriately, can control pain enough to allow the patient to participate in therapy. Appropriate pain control has been associated with decreased lengths of hospitalization, decreased readmissions for pain, and overall reduction in cost of care.

Older age may be an independent risk factor for postoperative development of pneumonia.[112] Pneumonia and other pulmonary complications such as pneumothorax can increase the risk of mortality after a surgery. In addition to early and frequent mobilization, there are other strategies available to prevent pulmonary complications. Encouraging deep breathing, coughing, and use of respiratory tools such as the incentive spirometer can keep the lungs open and free of secretions pressuring the alveoli. Screen patients for safe swallowing and maintain an upright head of bed during meals and drinking to prevent aspiration. Recognition of signs and symptoms of dysphagia, coughing with meals, hoarse voice, desaturation, and engaging a speech-language pathologist in a timely manner can prevent further aspiration that could lead to pneumonia.

Early and frequent mobility is important and necessary in this older postoperative population, and although getting up to the chair frequently is encouraged, it is equally important that patients are performing pressure relief. Most pressure ulcers occur in the hospital, and usually in the first 2 weeks. Given the risk factors associated with older age and the time associated with surgery alone, usually multiple hours, a patient can potentially already have the beginnings of a pressure ulcer before the initial evaluation. There are multiple validated scales that can, and should, be used to assess patients' risk for skin breakdown and ulceration. Use of cushions designed to allow offloading with small movements while sitting in the chair and specialty mattresses that allow increased airflow while the patient is lying in bed are effective interventions. Educating patients and nursing staff on the importance of unweighting when sitting upright for a prolonged time can assist in prevention even after the evaluation is completed.

Awareness of practice guidelines to prevent potential complications described earlier, such as delirium, falls, skin breakdown, and pneumonia, is essential when managing an older adult in the acute care setting, regardless of diagnoses. The physical therapist has an important role in what should be a multidisciplinary team with the goal of safely and appropriately treating postoperative older adults. Coordinating with the team; encouraging early mobility to aid in prevention of delirium, pulmonary complications, and functional decline; and helping to address acute pain limitations to assist in safe and timely discharge from the acute care setting are considered optimal management.

ROLE OF THE PHYSICAL THERAPIST IN EMERGENCY DEPARTMENT

Older adults' utilization of emergency department (ED) services is on the rise. In 2013, 12% to 14% of ED admissions were of individuals over the age of 65, and this percentage increases as age increases.[113] In the fast pace of the ED where triaging and directing necessary medical care is the mission, many EDs are not equipped to address the complex needs of the older adult.[114] Often, in the presence of a medical emergency, the impact of functional limitation and altered cognition is not recognized or addressed in the ED. For example, cognitive deficits are present in 15% to 40% of older adults who present to the ED but only recognized 50% of the time by the ED staff.[113] Older adults who present to the ED but who are not admitted have an increased risk of needing future medical care. These individuals have a 20% rate of readmission within the first month, 19% to 24% within 3 months, and 40% within 6 months.[113] Those readmitted to the ED tend to have higher rates of comorbidities and will require more home health services to return to the community.

Recognizing the unique needs of older adults and the known and expected future medical burden to care for the growing older adult population, EDs are developing different management plans to attempt to meet patient needs, minimize cost, and still sustain throughput. Some hospitals are adopting such programs as the Geriatric ED Innovation in Care Through Workforce, Informatics, and Structural Enhancement (GEDI WISE), which is a comprehensive approach from a geriatric-focused team that assesses and treats the older adult. This program manages how medical information is integrated across various medical settings, altering the ED environment to promote mobility, and improving noise and lighting.[115] Acute care facilities are beginning to explore the benefit of staffing physical therapists in EDs or including physical therapists as a consult service in the ED to facilitate the assessment and intervention of musculoskeletal injuries, expediate discharge planning, reduce the length of stay in the ED, and address the needs of the older adult. Some EDs have nurses perform a mobility screen or the Timed Up and Go (TUG) to determine which patients would benefit from a physical therapist's assessment.[116] Although Mesa et al. reported results that included all adults, their pilot work is appropriate to include here for readers' consideration. They allotted a physical therapist to be stationed for 4 hours a day during the week in a busy urban ED. They were able to reduce the length of stay in the ED by almost 20 hours, increase the number of patients discharged home by 15%, and expedite the discharge of patients classified in an observation status by 72 hours.[117]

Other EDs are implementing CGA protocols. The CGA includes medical, psychosocial, and functional assessment to determine level of frailty and community needs to provide support for the older adult in his or her community. The physical therapist can contribute to the CGA by completing a functional assessment and implementing outcome measures to determine the effectiveness of care. EDs that have implemented CGA have reported the identification of new issues that needed to be addressed. This process has led to a reduction in ED readmissions and mitigation of further functional declines.[113,118]

The current literature is clearly showing the special needs of older adults and the future health care crisis to deal with these needs. These findings are pushing hospitals to develop new approaches to improve health care delivery and ensure throughput to meet community needs in the ED. Primarily, work is showing that there needs to be a screening process completed by the nurse or ED team to identify frailty that leads to increased risk for further physical decompensation and readmissions.[116,119] Furthermore, it appears promising to consider physical therapists as key members of the ED health care team to address functional limitations and musculoskeletal deficits of older adults to promote comprehensive and cost-effective health care.

SUMMARY

The role of the physical therapist is rewarding and ever changing in the acute care setting. Therapists are key members of the health care team in the diagnosis and management of mobility disability while improving the hospital environment to mitigate the adverse effects of illness and hospitalization. Therapists are also critical in contributing to patient throughput throughout the system, which impacts the availability of hospital beds for new admissions, directs patients to optimal services upon discharge, and adds to cost containment for the institution.

The acute care therapist must have a broad range of knowledge and skills unique to the acute care setting to effectively manage the hospitalized patient and communicate with the health care team. Knowledge of tubes, lines, ventilation, and hemodialysis systems as well as medications and implications of dosing and interactions is used every day with a variety of patients. Additionally, therapists need to be acutely aware of the effects of immobilization and develop innovative strategies to mitigate these effects in complex situations.

The hospitalized older adult is vulnerable to many adverse situations and functional decline; therefore, the acute care therapist must process multiple compounding factors like the decline in multisystem physiological reserve, impact of multiple comorbidities, presentation of acute dysfunction, and prognosis for recovery when evaluating patients, developing a treatment plan, and making discharge recommendations. The physical therapist who is progressive and aggressively promotes the safe functional recovery within the challenges of the acute care environment will have a profound impact on the recovery and quality of life of the older adult.

REFERENCES

1. DeNardi M, French E, Jones J, et al. Medical Spending of the US Elderly. National Bureau of Economic Research Working Paper. 2015. http://journalistresource.org/studies/government/health-care/elderly-medical-spneding-medicare. Updated February 22, 2015. Accessed April 30, 2018.
2. Ortman J, Velkoff V. An Aging Nation: The Older Population in the United States Population Estimates and Projections Current Population Reports. https://www.census.gov/prod/2014pubs/p25-1140.pdf; May 2014.
3. Nelson JE, Cox CE, Hope AA, Carson SS. Chronic critical illness. *Am J Respir Crit Care Med.* 2010;182:446–454.
4. American Hospital Association. Fast facts on U.S. hospitals, 2019. http://www.aha.org/statistics/fact-facts-us-hospitals. Updated January 2019. Accessed August 2, 2019.
5. Levant S, Chiar K, DeFrances CJ. https://www.cdc.gov/nchs/data/databriefs/db182.htm; January 2015. Accessed 15 April 2018.
6. Weiss AJ, Elixhauser A. H-CUP Statistical Brief # 180. Overview of hospital stays in the US, 2012, published in October 2012. https://www.hcup-us.ahrq.gov/reports/statbriefs/sb180-Hospitalizations-United-States-2012.pdf. Accessed August 7, 2019.

7. Mattison M. Hospital management of older adults. http://uptodate.com/contents/hospital-management-of-older-adults; March 2018. Accessed 30 April 2018.
8. Cutugno C. The "graying" of trauma care: addressing traumatic injury in older adults. *Am J Nurs.* 2011;111(11):40–48.
9. Joyce M, Gupta A, Azocar R. Acute trauma and multiple injuries in the elderly population. *Curr Opin Anaesthesiol.* 2015;28(2):145–150. https://doi.org/10.1097/aco.0000000000000173.
10. Bianchi L, Abete P, Bellelli G, et al. Prevalence and clinical correlates of sarcopenia, identified according to the EWGSOP definition and diagnostic algorithm, in hospitalized older people: the GLISTEN Study. *J Gerontol A.* 2017;72(11):1575–1581. https://doi.org/10.1093/gerona/glw343.
11. Guyton AC, Hall JE. *Guyton and Hall Textbook of Medical Physiology.* 13th ed. St Louis: Elsevier; 2016:1095.
12. Foltz-Gray D. Most common causes of hospital admissions for older adults. AARP. https://www.aarp.org/health/doctors-hospitals/info-03-2012/hospital-admissions-older-adults.html. Accessed August 3, 2019.
13. Weiss AJ, Elixhause A. Overview of Hospital Stays in the United States, 2012. Healthcare Cost and Utilization Project, AHRQ. https://www.hcup-us.ahrq.gov/reports/statbriefs/sb180-Hospitalizations-United-States-2012.pdf. Accessed April 15, 2018.
14. Admi H, Shadmi E, Baruch H, Zisberg A. From research to reality: minimizing the effects of hospitalization on older adults. *Rambam Maimonides Med J.* 2016;6(2):e0017.
15. Bodilsen AC, Klasen HH, Petersen J, et al. Prediction of mobility limitations after hospitalization in older medical patients by simple measures of physical performance obtained at admission to the emergency department. *PLoS One.* 2016;11(5):e0154350.
16. Mikkelson ME, Christie JD, Lanken PN, et al. The adult respiratory distress syndrome cognitive outcomes study. *Am J Crit Care Med.* 2012;185(12):1307–1315.
17. Pisani MA, Kong SY, Kasl SV, et al. Days of delirium are associated with 1-year mortality in an older intensive care unit population. *Am J Respir Crit Care Med.* 2009;180(11):1092–1097.
18. Ely EW, Margolin R, Francis J, et al. Evaluation of delirium in critically ill patients: validation of the Confusion Assessment Method for the Intensive Care Unit (CAM-ICU). *Crit Care Med.* 2001;29(7):1370–1379.
19. Ely EW, Shintani A, Truman B, et al. Delirium as a predictor of mortality in mechanically ventilated patients in the intensive care unit. *JAMA.* 2004;291(14):1753–1762.
20. Tzeng HM. Understanding the prevalence of inpatient falls associated with toileting in adult acute care settings. *J Nurs Care Qual.* 2010;25(1):22–30.
21. Resnick B, Wells CL, Brotemarkle BA, Payne AK. Exposure to therapy of older people with trauma and factors that influence provision of therapy. *Phys Ther.* 2014;94:40–51.
22. Fisher SR, Galloway RV, Kuo YF, et al. Pilot study examining the association between ambulatory activity and falls among hospitalized older adults. *Arch Phys Med Rehabil.* 2011;92(12):2090–2092. https://doi.org/10.1016/j.apmr.2011.06.022.
23. Boltz M, Resnick B, Capezuti E, et al. Functional decline in hospitalized older adults: can nursing make a difference? *Geriatr Nurs.* 2012;33:272–279.
24. Halpern NA, Pastores SM. Critical care medicine in the United States 2000-2005: an analysis of bed numbers, occupancy rates, payer mix, and costs. *Crit Care Med.* 2010;38(1):65–71. https://doi.org/10.1097/CCM.0b013e3181b090d0.
25. Teale E, Young J. Multicomponent delirium prevention: not as effective as NICE suggest? *Age Ageing.* 2015;44:915–917.
26. Tabet N, Howard R. Pharmacological treatment for the prevention of delirium: review of current evidence. *Int J Geriatr Psychiatry.* 2009;24:1037–1044.
27. Pandharipande PP, Girard TD, Jackson JC, et al. Long-term cognitive impairment after critical illness. *N Engl J Med.* 2013;369:1306–1316.
28. Society of Critical Care Medicine. ICU Liberation. https://www.sccm.org/ICULiberation/About. Accessed August 3, 2019.
29. Critical econnections. June 19, 2014. http://www.enews.SCCM.me/benfits-ofothe-ABCDE-bundle-in-icu-patients Accessed February 2017.
30. Hung WW, Ross JS, Farber J, Siu AL. Evaluation of the Mobile Acute Care of the Elderly (MACE) service. *JAMA Intern Med.* 2013;173(11):990–996.
31. Flood KL, MacLennan PA, McGrew D, Green D, Dodd C, Brown CJ. Effects of an acute care for elders unit on costs and 30-day readmissions. *JAMA Intern Med.* 2013;173(11):981–987.
32. Abdalla A, Adhaduk M, Haddad RA, Alnimer Y, Ríos-Bedoya CF, Bachuwa G. Does acute care for the elderly (ACE) unit decrease the incidence of falls? *Geriatr Nurs.* 2018;39(3):292–295.
33. Hospital-Acquired Condition Reduction Program (HACRP). https://www.cms.gov/Medicare/Medicare-Fee-for-Service-Payment/AcuteInpatientPPS/HAC-Reduction-Program.html. Accessed 14 May 2018.
34. Rubin FH, Bellon J, Bilderback A, et al. Effects of the hospitalized elder life program on risk of 30-day admission. *J Am Geriatr Soc.* 2017;66(1):45–149.
35. Centers for Medicare & Medicaid Services. Hospital Readmissions Reduction Program (HRRP). https://www.cms.gov/medicare/medicare-fee-for-service-payment/acuteinpatientpps/readmissions-reduction-program.html. Accessed August 3, 2019.
36. Leppin AL, Giofriddo MR, Kessler M, et al. Preventing 30-day hospital readmissions: a systematic review and meta-analysis of randomized trials. *JAMA Intern Med.* 2014;174(7):1095–1107.
37. Leppin AL, Gionfriddo MR, Kessler M, Brito JP. MBBS preventing 30-day hospital readmissions: a systematic review and meta-analysis of randomized trials. *JAMA Intern Med.* 2014;174(7):1095–1107.
38. Naylor M, Keating S. Transitional care: moving patients from one care setting to another. *Am J Nurs.* 2008;108(9):58–63. https://doi.org/10.1097/01.NAJ.0000336420.34946.3a.
39. Boltz M, Resnick B, Capezuti E, et al. Functional decline in hospitalized older adults: can nursing make a difference? *Geriatr Nurs.* 2012;33(4):272–279.
40. Booth K, Rivet J, Flici R, et al. Progressive mobility protocol reduced venous thromboembolim rate in trauma intensive care patients: a quality improvement project. *J Trauma Nurs.* 2016;23(5):284–289.
41. Balas M, Buckingham R, Braley T. Extending the ABCDE Bundle to the post-intensive care unit setting. *J Gerontol Nurs.* 2013;39(8):39–51. https://doi.org/10.3928/00989134-20130530-06.
42. Garzon-Serrano J, Ryan C, Waak K, et al. Early mobility in critically ill patients: patients' mobilization level depends on health care provider's profession. *J Phys Med Rehabil.* 2011;3:307–313.
43. Jolley SE, Regan-Baggs J, Dickson R, et al. Medical intensive care unit clinician attitudes and perceived barriers towards early mobility of critically ill patients: a cross-sectional survey study. *Biomed Anesthesiol.* 2014;14:84–93.
44. Needham DM, Korupolu R, Zanni JM, et al. Early physical medicine and rehabilitation for patients with acute respiratory failure: a quality improvement project. *Arch Phys Med Rehabil.* 2010;91:536–542.

45. Morris PE, Goad A, Thompson C, et al. Early intensive care unit mobility therapy in the treatment of acute respiratory failure. *Crit Care Med*. 2008;36(8):2238–2243.
46. Damluji A, Zanni JM, Mantheiy E, et al. Safety and feasibility of femoral catheters during physical rehabilitation in the intensive care unit. *J Crit Care*. 2013;28(4):535. e9–e15.
47. Brown CJ, Redden DT, Flood KL, Allman RM. The underrecognized epidemic of low mobility during hospitalization of older adults. *J Am Geriatr Soc*. 2009;57 (9):1660–1665.
48. Mehlhorn J, Freytag A, Schmidt K, et al. Rehabilitation interventions for postintensive care syndrome: a systematic review. *Crit Care Med*. 2014;42(5):1263–1271. https://doi.org/10.1097/ccm.0000000000000148.
49. Wieske L, Dettling-Ihnenfeldt DS, Verhamme C, et al. Impact of ICU acquired weakness on post ICU physical functioning: a follow up study. *Crit Care*. 2015;19:196–204.
50. Falvey JR, Manione KK, Stevens-Lapsly JE. Rethinking hospital-associated deconditioning: proposed paradigm shift. *Phys Ther*. 2015;95(9):1307–1315.
50a. Ali NA, O'Brien JM, Hoffmann SP, et al. Acquired weakness, handgrip strength and mortality in critically ill patients. *Am J Respire Crit Care Med* 2008;178:261–268.
51. Bouldin ED, Andresen EM, Dunton NE, et al. Fall among adult patients hospitalized in the United States: prevalence and trends. *J Patient Saf*. 2013;9(1):13–17.
52. Resnick B, Galik E, Enders H, et al. Functional and physical activity of older adults in acute care settings: where we are and where we need to go. *J Nurs Care Qual*. 2011;26(2): 169–177.
53. Resnick B, Wells C, Galik E, et al. Feasibility and efficacy of function focused care for orthopedic trauma patients. *J Trauma Nurs*. 2016;23(3):144–155.
54. Boltz MRB, Capezuti E, Shuluk J, et al. Functional decline in hospitalized older adults: can nursing make a difference? *Geriatr Nurs*. 2012;33(4):272–279.
55. So C, Pierluissi E. Attitudes and expectations regarding exercise in the hospital of hospitalized older adults: a qualitative study. *J Am Geriatr Soc*. 2012;60:713–718.
56. Robinson T, Wu D, Pointer L, et al. Simple frailty score predicts postoperative complications across surgical specialties. *Am J Surg*. 2013;206:544–550.
57. Kim D, Kim C, Placide S, Lipsitz L, Marcantonio E. Preoperative frailty assessment and outcomes at 6 months or later in older adults undergoing cardiac surgical procedures: a systematic review. *Ann Intern Med*. 2016;165(9):650–660. https://doi.org/10.7326/m16-0652.
58. Govers A, Buurman B, Jue P, De Mol BAJM, Dongelmans D, Rooij S. Functional decline of older patients 1 year after cardiothoracic surgery followed by intensive care admission: a prospective longitudinal cohort study. *Age Ageing*. 2014;43(4):575–580. https://doi.org/10.1093/ageing/afu058.
59. Langanay T, Rouze S, Tomasi J, et al. Conventional aortic valve replacement in 2005 elderly patients: a 32-year experience. *Eur J Cardio-Thorac Surg*. 2018;54:446–452. https://doi.org/10.1093/ejcts/ezy072.
60. Song X, Mitnitski A, Rockwood K. Prevalence and 10-year outcomes of frailty in older adults in relation to deficit accumulation. *J Am Geriatr Soc*. 2010;58(4):681–687. https://doi.org/10.1111/j.1532-5415.2010.02764.x.
61. Kovacs J, Moraru L, Antal K, Cioc A, Voidazan S, Szabo A. Are frailty scales better than anesthesia or surgical scales to determine risk in cardiac surgery? *Korean J Anesthesiol*. 2017;70 (2):157–162. https://doi.org/10.4097/kjae.2017.70.2.157.
62. Afilalo J, Lauck S, Kim D, et al. Frailty in older adults undergoing aortic valve replacement. *J Am Coll Cardiol*. 2017;70(6):689–700.
63. Ogawa M, Izawa KP, Satomi-Kobayashi S, et al. Impact of delirium on postoperative frailty and long term cardiovascular events after cardiac surgery. *Plos One*. 2017;12(12):e0190359. https://doi.org/10.1371/journal.pone.0190359.
64. Kebapcı A, Kanan N. Effects of nurse-led clinical pathway in coronary artery bypass graft surgery: a quasi-experimental study. *J Clin Nurs*. 2018;27:980–988. https://doi.org/10.1111/jocn.14069.
65. Katijjahbe MA, Denehy L, Granger CL, et al. The Sternal Management Accelerated Recovery Trial (S.M.A.R.T) – standard restrictive versus an intervention of modified sternal precautions following cardiac surgery via median sternotomy: study protocol for a randomised controlled trial. *Trials*. 2017;18(1):290. https://doi.org/10.1186/s13063-017-1974-8.
66. Adams J, Lotshaw A, Exum E, et al. An alternative approach to prescribing sternal precautions after median sternotomy, "keep your move in the tube". *Baylor Univ Med Center Proc*. 2016;29(1):97–100. https://doi.org/10.1080/08998280.2016.11929379.
67. Browndyke J, Berger M, Harshbarger TB, et al. Resting-state functional connectivity and cognition after major cardiac surgery in older adults without preoperative cognitive impairment: preliminary findings. *J Am Geriatr Soc*. 2017;65:E6–E12.
68. Naveed A, Azam H, Murtaza HG, et al. Incidence and risk factors of pulmonary complications after cardiopulmonary bypass. *Pakistan J Med Sci*. 2017;33(4):1–4.
69. Rushton M, Howarth M, Grant M, Astin F. Person-centred discharge education following coronary artery bypass graft: a critical review. *J Clin Nurs*. 2017;26(23–24):5206–5215. https://doi.org/10.1111/jocn.14071.
70. Perelló-Díez M, Paz-Lourido B. Prevention of postoperative pulmonary complications through preoperative physiotherapy interventions in patients undergoing coronary artery bypass graft: literature review. *J Phys Ther Sci*. 2018;30 (8):1034–1038. https://doi.org/10.1589/jpts.30.1034.
71. Falvey JR, Mangionne KK, Stevens-Lapsley JE. Rethinking hospital associated deconditioning: proposed paradigm shift. *Phys Ther J*. 2015;95(9):1307–1315.
72. Feng TR, White RS, Gaber-Baylis LK, et al. Coronary artery bypass graft readmission rates and risk factors - a retrospective cohort study. *Int J Surg*. 2018;54:7–17.
73. Min L, Mazzurco L, Gure TR, et al. Longitudinal functional recovery geriatric cardiac surgery. *J Surg Res*. 2015;194:25–33.
74. Lee C, Ahn J, Cavalcante R, et al. Coronary artery bypass surgery versus drug-eluting stent implantation for left main or multivessel coronary artery disease. *JACC Cardiovasc Interv*. 2016;9:2481–2489.
75. Patel A, Yates M, Soppa G. What is the optimal revascularization technique for isolated disease of the left anterior descending artery: minimally invasive direct coronary artery bypass or percutaneous coronary intervention? *Interact Cardiovasc Thorac Surg*. 2014;19 (1):144–148. https://doi.org/10.1093/icvts/ivu076.
76. Kowalewski M, Pawliszak W, Malvindi PG, et al. Off-pump coronary artery bypass grafting improves short-term outcomes in high-risk patients compared with on-pump coronary artery bypass grafting: meta-analysis. *J Thorac Cardiovasc Surg*. 2016;151(1):60–77. e58.
77. Mamane S, Mullie L, Piazza N, et al. Psoas muscle area and all-cause mortality after transcatheter aortic valve replacement: the Montreal-Munich Study. *Can J Cardiol*. 2016;32:177–182. https://doi.org/10.1016/j.cjca.2015.12.002.
78. Sandoval Y, Sirahha P, Harris K. Contemporary management of ischemic mitral regurgitation: a review. *Am J Med*. 2018;131(8):456–465.

79. Algarni K, Suri R, Schaff H. Minimally invasive mitral valve surgery: does it make a difference? *Trends Cardiovasc Med*. 2015;25(5):456–465. https://doi.org/10.1016/j.tcm.2014.12.007.
80. Casaubon LK, Boulanger J-M, Blacquiere D, et al. Canadian stroke best practice recommendations: hyperacute stroke care guidelines, update 2015. *Int J Stroke*. 2015;10(6):924–940. https://doi.org/10.1111/ijs.12551.
81. Frontera J, Fernandez A, Schmidt JM, et al. Defining vasospasm after subarachnoid hemorrhage: what is the most clinically relevant definition? *Stroke*. 2009;40(6):1963–1968.
82. Charles E. Outcomes after falls continue to worsen despite trauma and geriatric care advancements. *Am Surgeon*. 2018;84(3):392–397.
83. Calvo RY. *The Association of Chronic Conditions with Clinical Outcomes Following Traumatic Injury in Older Adults (Unpublished doctoral dissertation)*. San Diego: University of California; 2015.
84. Hanna JS. Sarcopenia and critical illness: a deadly combination in the elderly. *J Parenteral Enteral Nutr*. 2015;39(3):273–281. https://doi.org/10.1177/0148607114567710.
85. Fairchild B, Webb TP, Xiang Q, Tarima S, Brasel KJ. Sarcopenia and frailty in elderly trauma patients. *World J Surg*. 2015;39(2):373–379. https://doi.org/10.1007/s00268-014-2785-7.
86. Apostolaskis E, Papakonstantinou NA, Baikoussis NG, Papadopoulos G. Intensive care unit-related generalized neuromuscular weakness due to critical illness polyneuropathy/myopathy in critical ill patients. *J Anesth*. 2015;29:112–121.
87. Wollersheim T, Woehlecke J, Krebs M, et al. Dynamics of myosin degradation in intensive care unit-acquired weakness during severe critical illness. *Intensive Care Med*. 2014;40(4):528–538.
88. Schorl M, Valerisu-Kukula SJ, Kemmer TP. Critical illness polyneuropathy as sequelae of sever neurological illness: incidence and impact on ventilator therapy and rehabilitation. *Neurorehabilitation*. 2013;32:149–156.
89. Kress JP, Hall JB. ICU acquired weakness and recovery from critical illness. *N Engl J Med*. 2014;370:1626–1635.
90. Gronewold J, Dahlmann C, Jäger M, Hermann DM. Identification of hospitalized elderly patients at risk for adverse in-hospital outcomes in a university orthopedics and trauma surgery environment. *Plos One*. 2017;12(11):e0187801. https://doi.org/10.1371/journal.pone.0187801.
91. Min L, Ubhayakar N, Saliba D, et al. The Vulnerable Elders Survey-13 predicts hospital complications and mortality in older adults with traumatic injury: a pilot study. *J Am Geriatr Soc*. 2011;59(8):1471–1476. https://doi.org/10.1111/j.1532-5415.2011.03493.x.
92. Resnick B, Wells CL, Brotemarkle BA, Payne AK. Exposure to therapy of older patients with trauma and factors that influence provision of therapy. *Phys Ther*. 2014;94(1):40–51. https://doi.org/10.2522/ptj.20130087.
93. Axmon A, Sandberg M, Ahlström G, Midlöv P. Fall-risk-increasing drugs and falls requiring health care among older people with intellectual disability in comparison with the general population: a register study. *Plos One*. 2018;13(6):e0199218. https://doi.org/10.1371/journal.pone.0199218.
94. Fu W, Fu T, Jing R, Mcfaull S, Cusimano M. Predictors of falls and mortality among elderly adults with traumatic brain injury: a nationwide, population-based study. *Plos One*. 2017;12(4):e0175868. https://doi.org/10.1371/journal.pone.0175868.
95. Grimm D, Mion L. Falls resulting in traumatic injury among older adults. *AACN Adv Crit Care*. 2011;22(2):161–168. https://doi.org/10.1097/nci.0b013e3182157cb3.
96. Devries RD, Reininga IH, Pieske O, Lefering R, Moumni ME, Wendt K. Injury mechanisms, patterns and outcomes of older polytrauma patients—an analysis of the Dutch Trauma Registry. *Plos One*. 2018;13(1):e0190587. https://doi.org/10.1371/journal.pone.0190587.
97. Karibe H, Hayashi T, Narisawa A, Kameyama M, Nakagawa A, Tominaga T. Clinical characteristics and outcome in elderly patients with traumatic brain injury: for establishment of management strategy. *Neurol Med Chir*. 2017;57(8):418–425. https://doi.org/10.2176/nmc.st.2017-0058.
98. Krishnamoorthy V, Distelhorst J, Vavilala M, Thompson H. Traumatic brain injury in the elderly. *J Trauma Nurs*. 2015;22(4):204–E4. https://doi.org/10.1097/jtn.0000000000000145.
99. Mosk C, Mus M, Vroemen J, et al. Dementia and delirium, the outcomes in elderly hip fracture patients. *Clin Interv Aging*. 2017;12:421–430.
100. Wang Y, Haines TP, Ritchie P, et al. Early mobilization on continuous renal replacement therapy is safe and may improve filter life. *Criti Care*. 2014;18:1–10.
101. Srisawat N, Lawsin L, Uchino S, Bellomo R, Kellum JA. Cost of acute renal replacement therapy in the intensive care unit: results from the Beginning and Ending Supportive Therapy for the Kidney (BEST Kidney) Study. *Crit Care*. 2010;14(2):R46. https://doi.org/10.1186/cc8933.
102. Fields C, Trotsky A, Fernandez N, Smith BA. Mobility and ambulation for patients with pulmonary artery catheters: a retrospective description study. *J Acute Care Phys Ther*. 2015;6(2):64–70.
103. McGarrigle L, Caunt J. Physical therapist–led ambulatory rehabilitation for patients receiving CentriMag short term ventricular assist device support: respective case series. *Phys Ther J*. 2016;96(10):1–11.
104. Perme C, Lettivin C, Throckmorton T, Mitchell K, Masud F. Early mobility and walking for patients with femoral arterial catheters in intensive care unit: a case series. *J Acute Care Phys Ther*. 2011;2(1):32–36.
105. Lima NP, Silva GM, Park M, Pires-Neto RC. Mobility therapy and central or peripheral catheter related adverse events in an ICU in Brazil. *J Bras Pneumol*. 2015;41(3):225–230.
106. Wells CL, Forrester J, Vogel J, et al. Safety and feasibility of early physical therapy for patients on extracorporeal membrane oxygenation: University of Maryland Medical Center Experience. *Crit Care Med*. 2018;46(1):53–59.
107. Ching W, Luhmann M. Neuro-oncologic physical therapy for the older person. *Top Geriatr Rehabil*. 2011;27(3):184–192. https://doi.org/10.1097/tgr.0b013e3182198f25.
108. Eyigor S, Eyigor C, Uslu R. Assessment of pain, fatigue, sleep and quality of life (QoL) in elderly hospitalized cancer patients. *Arch Gerontol Geriatr*. 2010;51(3):e57–e61. https://doi.org/10.1016/j.archger.2009.11.018.
109. Egol KA, Strauss EJ. Perioperative considerations in geriatric patients with hip fracture: what is the evidence? *J Orthop Trauma*. 2009;23(6):386–394.
110. Morrison RS, Flanagan S, Fischberg D. A novel interdisciplinary analgesic program reduces pain and improves function in older adults after orthopedic surgery. *J Am Geriatr Soc*. 2009;57(1):1–10. https://doi.org/10.1111/j.1532-5415.2008.02063.x.
111. Parvizi J, Miller AG, Gandhi K. Multimodal pain management after total joint arthroplasty. *J Bone Joint Surg*. 2011;93-A(11):1075–1084.
112. Mohanty S, Rosenthal RA, Russell MM, et al. Optimal perioperative management of the geriatric patient: a best practices guideline from the American College of Surgeons NSQIP and the American Geriatrics Society. *J Am Coll Surg*. 2016;222(5):930–947.
113. Deschodt M, Devriendt E, Sabbe M, et al. Characteristics of older adults admitted to the emergency department (ED)

and their risk factors for ED readmission based on comprehensive geriatric assessment: a prospective cohort study. *BMC Geriatr*. 2015;15(1):54. https://doi.org/10.1186/s12877-015-0055-7.

114. Latham L, Ackroyd-Stolarz S. Emergency department utilization by older adults: a descriptive study. *Can Geriatr J*. 2014;17(4):118–125. https://doi.org/10.5770/cgj.17.108.

115. Hwang U, Dresden S, Rosenberg M, et al. Geriatric emergency department innovations: transitional care nurses and hospital use. *J Am Geriatr Soc*. 2018;66(3):459–466.

116. Tousignant-Laflamme Y, Beaudoin A, Renaud A, et al. Adding physical therapy services in the emergency department to prevent immobilization syndrome – a feasibility study in a university hospital. *BMC Emerg Med*. 2015;15(1):35. doi:10.1186/s12873-015-0062-1

117. Mesa G, Swoboda M, Wilson F, Ayres A, Johnson D. *Outpatient Physical Therapy in the Emergency Department: A Descriptive and Prospective Analysis*. New Orleans, Louisiana: Poster presented at American Physical Therapy Combined Section Meeting; 2018.

118. Southerland LT, Vargas AJ, Nagaraj L, Gure TR, Caterino JM. An emergency department observation unit is a feasible setting for multidisciplinary geriatric assessments in compliance with the geriatric emergency department guidelines. *Acad Emerg Med*. 2017;25(1):76–82. https://doi.org/10.1111/acem.13328.

119. Huded J, Dresden S, Gravenor S, Rowe T, Lindquist L. Screening for fall risks in the emergency department: a novel nursing-driven program. *West J Emerg Med*. 2015;16(7):1043–1046. https://doi.org/10.5811/westjem.2015.10.26097.

CHAPTER 25

Postacute Care Management of the Older Adult

Greg W. Hartley, Rosanna Gelaz

OUTLINE

INTRODUCTION

Postacute care of geriatric patients has undergone massive change over the past 20 years. According to the United States Department of Health and Human Services, Agency for Healthcare Research and Quality, approximately 7.96 million inpatient stays were discharged to postacute care settings, accounting for 22.3% of all hospital discharges in 2013.[1] New payment methodologies such as prospective payment systems (PPSs) have significantly altered patterns of patient placement upon discharge from acute care settings.[1] These changes have forced physical therapists working in postacute environments to broaden the rehabilitation services offered and to expand upon traditional roles, especially skilled nursing facilities (SNFs). This chapter focuses on several, but not all, inpatient postacute care settings. Rehabilitation hospitals are discussed briefly because regulatory changes in this environment have subsequently impacted the patient population of other postacute care environments.[2] The bulk of the chapter focuses on the nursing home environment, both short-term skilled (subacute) care and long-term care (LTC). Specifically, this chapter addresses how physical therapy practice has evolved to keep pace with the changing population in these settings. In the United States, Medicare is the predominant payor in all of these settings, and because Medicare is the predominant payor for geriatric patients, a discussion of Centers for Medicare & Medicaid Services (CMS) regulations that impact the provision of physical therapy services in these settings is provided where applicable.

INPATIENT REHABILITATION FACILITIES

Profile of an Inpatient Rehabilitation Facility and Its Patients

Rehabilitation hospitals, or inpatient rehabilitation facilities (IRFs), are either free-standing hospitals or units within an acute care hospital whose purpose it is to provide multidisciplinary, team-oriented services to patients with intense rehabilitation needs. For the purposes of Medicare (and most other payors), for a patient to be admitted to an IRF, patients must meet specific criteria, including reasonable and necessary care and a significant rehabilitation potential. Patients must also require the coordinated care of at least two therapy disciplines, including physical therapy, occupational therapy, and speech–language pathology. One of the two disciplines must be either physical therapy or occupational therapy. Patients are also required to participate in a minimum of 3 hours of therapy per day, at least 5 days a week at the time of admission. Therefore, IRFs must be reasonably assured that patients require these services and can fully participate at the time of admission. Trial admissions are not permitted. Care must be coordinated and team oriented, with an emphasis on discharging patients to the community.

For geriatric patients in a rehabilitation hospital, Medicare is most often the payor. Since 2002, CMS has reimbursed IRFs prospectively, a system referred to as the PPS.[3] Because of the level of care that is required in IRFs, CMS's payments are typically higher than other settings. Because payment is at a higher tier, CMS requires IRFs to meet specific criteria to be paid under the PPS. Chief among these criteria is a requirement that at least 60% of all patients have a diagnosis that qualifies for the setting.[3] There are currently 13 diagnoses, or diagnostic categories, that qualify. These diagnostic categories are collectively called the CMS-13. The qualifying diagnoses in the CMS-13 are listed in Box 25.1. The remaining 40% of patients admitted to IRFs may have any diagnosis; however, the patients must still meet all of the requirements, including admission requirements, a need for multidisciplinary rehabilitation, and intensity of service (3 hours/day).[3]

CMS regulations for IRFs have undergone significant change since PPS became the means of reimbursement for IRFs in 2002. One of the most significant changes occurred in 2004 with the elimination of unilateral total joint replacements from the CMS-13 list of qualifying diagnoses. After analysis by CMS, it was determined that these patients could achieve similar outcomes in a less expensive setting (skilled nursing facility [SNF], home health, outpatient). Some patients may continue to qualify for the rehabilitation hospital setting (in the other 40%) if they meet requirements for IRF admission, including requiring more than one discipline (e.g., physical therapy and occupational therapy as well as a coordinated team approach that cannot be provided in a less "intense" environment). But in general, patients with uncomplicated unilateral total joint replacements no longer qualify for an inpatient rehabilitation hospital level of care. When possible, these patients go directly home from acute care, where they typically receive home health care or outpatient therapy. However, in many cases, patients are not able to go directly home after acute care.[4] Whereas patients in this category are frequently discharged from acute care to SNFs, they might have been sent to a rehabilitation hospital several years ago. The effects of the changes in CMS policy have contributed to a change in SNF patient populations over the past several years, particularly in urban areas, where IRFs are more abundant.[5] As a result, the total population of patients with major joint replacement in IRFs has decreased as the numbers of these patients in SNFs has been increasing.[4] Subsequently, many SNFs

BOX 25.1 CMS-13: Qualifying Diagnoses for Inpatient Rehabilitative Facility Reimbursement

The following list includes the medical conditions that require intensive rehabilitative services (i.e., qualify for inpatient rehabilitation hospital) under revised Title 42 CFR 412.23(b)(2)(iii).

Stroke.

Spinal cord injury.

Congenital deformity.

Amputation.

Major multiple trauma.

Fracture of femur (hip fracture).

Brain injury.

Neurological disorders, including multiple sclerosis, motor neuron diseases, polyneuropathy, muscular dystrophy, and Parkinson disease.

Burns.

Active, polyarticular rheumatoid arthritis, psoriatic arthritis, and seronegative arthropathies resulting in significant functional impairment of ambulation and other activities of daily living that have not improved after an appropriate, aggressive, and sustained course of outpatient therapy services or services in other less intensive rehabilitation settings immediately preceding the inpatient rehabilitation admission or that result from a systemic disease activation immediately before admission, but have the potential to improve with more intensive rehabilitation.

Systemic vascularities with joint inflammation, resulting in significant functional impairment of ambulation and other activities of daily living that have not improved after an appropriate, aggressive, and sustained course of outpatient therapy services or services in other less intensive rehabilitation settings immediately preceding the inpatient rehabilitation admission or that result from a systemic disease activation immediately before admission, but have the potential to improve with more intensive rehabilitation.

Severe or advanced osteoarthritis (osteoarthrosis or degenerative joint disease) involving two or more major weight bearing joints (elbow, shoulders, hips, or knees, but not counting a joint with a prosthesis) with joint deformity and substantial loss of range of motion, atrophy of muscles surrounding the joint, significant functional impairment of ambulation and other activities of daily living that have not improved after the patient has participated in an appropriate, aggressive, and sustained course of outpatient therapy services or services in other less intensive rehabilitation settings immediately preceding the inpatient rehabilitation admission, but have the potential to improve with more intensive rehabilitation. (A joint replaced by a prosthesis no longer is considered to have osteoarthritis, or other arthritis, even though this condition was the reason for the joint replacement.)

Knee or hip joint replacement, or both, during an acute hospitalization immediately preceding the inpatient rehabilitation stay and also meet one or more of the following specific criteria:

- The patient underwent bilateral knee or bilateral hip joint replacement surgery during the acute hospital admission immediately preceding the IRF admission.
- The patient is extremely obese with a body mass index of at least 50 at the time of admission to the IRF.
- The patient is age 85 or older at the time of admission to the IRF.

CMS, Centers for Medicare & Medicaid Services; *IRF,* inpatient rehabilitative facility.

Data from Centers for Medicare & Medicaid Services. *Inpatient Rehabilitation Facility PPS.* 2018. https://www.cms.gov/Medicare/Medicare-Fee-for-Service-Payment/InpatientRehabFacPPS/index.html.

have reconfigured themselves to better care for this type of patient (i.e., subacute rehabilitation).

Although rehabilitation hospitals play a large role in postacute rehabilitation, the vast majority of Americans needing postacute rehabilitation receive this care in an SNF. Although this is partly related to the IRF criteria described earlier, it is more likely related to accessibility issues.[6,7] Many communities simply do not have access to an IRF. Accordingly, the remainder of this chapter will focus on patients and residents in short-term (skilled and subacute) and LTC facilities.

SKILLED NURSING AND LONG-TERM CARE FACILITIES

Profile of a Skilled Nursing Facility, Long-Term Care Facility, and Their Patients (Residents)

An SNF is a nursing home that has been certified by CMS to provide Medicare-reimbursable short-term skilled nursing or therapy services (or both). Among SNF residents, the most common diagnoses are joint replacements, heart failure, pneumonia, septicemia, hip fracture, and kidney or urinary tract infections.[1] Because the participation and payment rules for SNFs were created as a "subset" of nursing home rules and regulations, CMS refers to clients in an SNF as "residents" (a product of LTC language).[8] Historically, patients treated in SNFs were those with lower functional levels and required longer courses of treatment (nursing or rehabilitation) to return to the community. If a return to the community was not possible, patients could potentially stay as LTC residents. In the past, SNFs also had a greater variety of diagnoses than rehabilitation facilities (there is no "60% rule" in SNFs), with more individuals having lower functional levels.[7] Although SNFs have continued to care for the complex, lower functional-level patients who may (at least initially) require less intense rehabilitation services and longer lengths of stay, SNFs also care for a myriad of patients with advanced rehabilitation needs who require relatively short stays, who have the potential to return home or to the community quickly, and who tolerate intense levels of rehabilitation services. In fact, in the calendar year 2015, the average length of stay for patients with Medicare in SNFs nationwide was 26.78 days.[9] The regulatory changes in other settings have meant more patients in SNFs have elective joint replacements, "acute" rehabilitation needs, and the potential to make rapid, substantial progress with an expected discharge to the community.[4] The growth in this group of patients has led to greater use of the term *subacute* to describe this cohort more effectively. In addition, the growth of Medicare Advantage (MA) programs has also affected rehabilitation utilization in SNFs. More and more, patients enrolled in MA programs are referred to SNFs instead of other, higher cost settings such as IRFs.[10]

After skilled care has been completed, in some cases, residents stay in a nursing home as an LTC patient after the SNF benefit is exhausted or when they no longer require ongoing skilled services. The leading reasons for LTC admission are decreased cognition, incontinence, and falls leading to a decrease in functional status.[11] About 1.4 million residents of all ages lived in 15,600 nursing facilities in 2014. Of them, 85% were age 65 years or older.[12] In 2010, only 3.1% of people older than age 65 years lived in nursing facilities, a decline from 7.5% in 1982.[13,14] It is unknown exactly why the percentage decreased so much during this time. It could be due to economic reasons because the cost of care has risen drastically. Alternatively, it might be related to improved social support systems, accessibility, or a greater focus on health promotion and wellness over the past several years. However, the percentage is likely to increase again in future years because the numbers of individuals surviving into their 8th, 9th, and 10th decades of life will represent the fastest growing segment of the population.[14] Disability rates are strongly related to age; about 50% of the population ages 85 years and older has a disability compared with only 10% of the population ages 65 to 74 years.

By definition, long-term *institutional* care is custodial. Of course, LTC can be interpreted to include much more than institutional care. The broader definition of LTC would include assisted living (where less supervision is provided, but typically some supervised services are offered), adult day care (per day or daytime-supervised care), home care or sitter services (nonskilled home care under the Medicare Part A benefit), and many other local or community-based services, whether paid or unpaid. As the population of aging adults who require these services increases, the availability and variety of these alternative LTC settings and services will also expand. However, for the purposes of this chapter, the focus will remain on institutional LTC.

In the LTC setting, no *regular, skilled* intervention is provided under the LTC benefit. The staff administer medications and provide ongoing restorative, recreational, and social activities for residents. Because LTC is, in fact, nonskilled, Medicare does not cover this cost. LTC is paid out of pocket, by private insurance, or by Medicaid for residents who qualify based on their income.[15] Medicaid is the primary payor for most nursing facility residents. Almost two-thirds (62.9%) of LTC residents had Medicaid as the primary payor in 2013. The remaining nursing facility residents had other sources of payment such as private LTC insurance or paid out of pocket.[12] *Institutionalization* is a term that unfortunately conjures up images of an older person being abandoned forever at the door of some dark building. However, admission to LTC institutions is not permanent in many cases. In fact, it has been reported that between 22% and 25% of all LTC residents are discharged to the community because they have either stabilized or recovered.[16]

Risk factors for permanent residency in LTC include hospitalization, advanced age, dementia, female gender, and discharge from the hospital to an SNF. Additionally, frailty and prefrailty have been found to be significant predictors for nursing home placement among community-dwelling older adults who have not had a previous stay in an SNF.[17,18]

If permanent residence is required, a wide variety of services are available to residents to ensure a high quality of life. In long-term settings, staff perform periodic screens for the need for skilled rehabilitation services. When the need for skilled therapy is identified, residents are treated under the Medicare Part B (outpatient) benefit, assuming Medicare is their payor, or a similar benefit if the individual has an MA product or private insurance. The same rules that apply to regular outpatient (Part B) also apply in the LTC setting. A study commissioned by CMS indicates that in 2008, 32.3% of all Part B therapy claims were billed from an SNF or LTC setting, more than private practice settings (28.8%) or hospitals (16.7%).[19] From these data, one can hypothesize that many of the residents who reside in LTC have the potential to benefit from physical therapy.

PHYSICAL THERAPY PATIENT MANAGEMENT IN THE SKILLED NURSING FACILITY AND LONG-TERM CARE SETTINGS

The remainder of the chapter focuses on clinical management of SNF patients as well as the LTC residents who are not receiving the "skilled" benefit (i.e., not in SNF). Long-term residents are different from patients who are in a nursing home for short stays receiving skilled services. As discussed previously, in today's health care environment, SNF residents present clinically as "subacute" patients. On the other hand, long-term residents are those patients who, for whatever reason, reside in the nursing home for extended periods of time, often for the remainder of their lives. There are a wide variety of functional abilities among these patients. Although many individuals in LTC are frail, not all fit this description. Of the settings discussed in this chapter, long-term residents show the most variability in functional abilities, ranging from being independent ambulators to being totally bed bound.

The SNF patient typically arrives from the acute care setting after hospitalization with the aim of discharging the patient to her or his previous residence or for possible transition into LTC if indicated. In the LTC setting, the goal is often to return the resident to a prior level of function or higher. The prior level of function, though, may be lower than that of a patient in a rehabilitation hospital or even SNF. For example, the prior level of function may be ambulation of short distances with a rolling walker, or perhaps it is simply the ability to sit independently. However, therapists should not underestimate residents' ability to make significant improvements, sometimes beyond the prior level of function. Residents whose status commonly declined by virtue of disuse can, with physical activity along with physical therapy, reasonably expect the achievement of a higher functional level. This variability of patient function coupled with altered mental status (in some cases) and complex regulations can make for challenges as well as opportunities in the LTC setting. These opportunities create a perfect environment for autonomy in decision making and interprofessional collaboration with other health professionals, especially nurses and physicians. In the LTC setting, the therapist must function as a team member who will delegate tasks and follow through with other team members. Collaboration between team members is vital to the success of any LTC therapeutic program and can be one of the greatest challenges of this setting. Next we will highlight important differences and nuances in the physical therapy assessment and management of residents in the SNF and LTC settings.

EXAMINATION AND EVALUATION

History

When performing a chart review for an SNF patient, the skilled clinician needs to do more than simply scan for a medical diagnosis. See Box 25.2 for a list of the components of a thorough chart review. It is the responsibility of the therapist to confirm with the patient and/or family or caregiver that the information obtained from the chart review is in fact accurate and complete, note if there are discrepancies, and communicate such information with the medical or rehabilitation team as needed. When the patient is a poor historian, the examining clinician should make an attempt to contact the patient's next of kin or authorized representative to obtain further details, including prior level of function and type of residence as well as bathroom set-up, assistance available in the home environment, and what medical equipment the patient owns.

BOX 25.2 Components of Chart Review

- Reason for admission and admitting diagnosis
- Recent and relevant physician orders
- Weight-bearing status and other precautions (if applicable)
- Current medications and allergies
- Imaging reports and findings
- Laboratory values (trends)
- Surgical and procedure reports (if applicable)
- Diet, dietary restrictions, and swallowing precautions
- Past medical and surgical history
- Cognitive status
- Social history, living situation, educational level, and primary language
- Funding source
- Recent clinical notes from nursing and physicians
- Rehabilitation notes from acute care, if available

Although information provided in the chart of an LTC resident, such as history of condition, minimum data set (MDS) scores on activities of daily living (ADLs), nutritional status, and laboratory values, is important when determining the plan of care and setting goals; history taking should not be limited to the medical chart. Interviewing the resident and staff most involved with the resident is key. Certified nursing assistants, restorative nursing staff, nutritionists, and any other staff who have regular interaction with the resident can provide information, such as how much assistance the resident needs and whether the resident's ability to perform ADLs has changed recently. The individuals in regular contact with the resident may be the first ones to recognize a resident's change in functional status and behavior.

Any history of falls and mitigating circumstances for the falls should be noted, both for SNF and LTC residents. Some facilities may have fall assessment teams, often directed by a physical therapist, in which the team analyzes the reasons for a particular fall or looks for patterns that may be contributing to falls, and then discusses and plans ways to intervene.

Approximately half of nursing home residents in the United States fall annually, and about 30% of those who fall will fall two or more times in a year.[20] This high incidence of falls is caused both by the nature of persons living in institutions and by more accurate reporting of falls in institutions. Falls are a major determinant of functional decline, increased risk of death, and restricted activity.[20] Unsafe behaviors, cognitive status, chronic disease, deconditioning from inactivity, medication side effects, and unsafe equipment have been identified as risk factors contributing to falls among nursing home residents.[20] All of these factors are linked to falling, and determining the cause of the fall through an extensive history can be fundamental in establishing an appropriate intervention and prevention. Box 25.3 lists the common causes of falls in nursing home residents.[21]

Physical therapists are often the ones identifying residents at risk for falls resulting from medications, including their adverse effects and polypharmacy concerns, and this information should be shared with the nursing and medical staff. Sometimes falls may be reduced by just decreasing or reducing a medication. Studies conducted with nursing home residents have found that the use of multiple medications and the prescription of psychotropic drugs have been associated with increased fall risk, and antipsychotics and antidepressants are linked to an almost threefold increase in fall incidence.[22,23] This increase in fall risk was observed for both prescriptions on scheduled dosage as well as those on an as-needed basis.[22] Other studies targeting the reduced use of psychotropic, cardiovascular, and analgesic drugs have also reported success in decreasing the rate or risk of falls in older people.[24–26] The role of the physical therapist in identifying these risk factors by taking a thorough history cannot be underestimated. For example, adverse drug reactions such as orthostatic hypotension and dizziness are common, and medications should be reviewed carefully for their contribution to the cause of falls. These characteristics can help the therapist consider the contribution of orthostasis to falls and fall risk.

BOX 25.3 Risk Factors for Falls in Nursing Homes

- Gait, mobility, or balance disorder
- Sedentary behavior and weakness
- Psychological status (e.g., fear of falling)
- Environmental hazards (e.g., poor lighting, wet floors, incorrect bed height, inadequate wheelchair size and maintenance)
- Certain types of medications (e.g., benzodiazepines, psychotropics, class 1a antiarrhythmics, digoxin, diuretics, and other sedatives)
- Medication changes (types and doses)
- Impaired cognition
- Visual impairments
- Nutritional deficiencies including low body mass index and vitamin D deficiency
- Dizziness or vertigo
- Improper foot care or ill-fitting footwear
- Improper use or inadequate maintenance of walking aids or other durable medical equipment

Data from Todd C, Skelton D. *What Are the Main Risk Factors for Falls Among Older People and What Are the Most Effective Interventions to Prevent These Falls?* Copenhagen: WHO Regional Office for Europe; 2004. http://www.euro.who.int/document/E82552.pdf.

Systems Review

The senses of hearing and vision are expected to decline as a normal part of aging, and losses are common findings in most nursing home residents. Hearing loss is the most prevalent of all sensory losses, affecting an estimated 75% of individuals older than 70 years of age, with fewer than 30% of individuals who could benefit from use of a hearing aid actually having used one in the past.[27] Vision losses from cataract, glaucoma, diabetic retinopathy, and macular degeneration have all been shown to decrease quality of life.[28] Population-based studies have reported the prevalence of moderate to severe visual impairment or blindness to be 81% among individuals aged 50 years and older.[29] Hearing and vision impairments have been linked to dependence in ADLs, depressive symptoms, and early death in community-dwelling older adults.[30]

Residents often wear corrective lenses. However, in a study looking at the need for an eye examination in 371 nursing home residents, although 32% of the participants were already using corrective lenses, 15% were recommended glasses, but 36% required further examination by an ophthalmologist.[31] Information about residents' hearing and vision is important when the therapist is determining the best way to teach and cue a patient and should be noted in the initial evaluation and the plan of care. Specific visual pathologies such as cataracts, macular degeneration, and glaucoma have different presentations and visual effects that can impede physical therapy interventions. Awareness of visual pathology presentations will help the therapist provide the most effective education and cueing. Therapists need to be cautious to differentiate poor cognition from poor hearing and lack of interest from poor vision.

Control of bowel and bladder functioning also should be noted. Approximately 31.8% of residents in LTC are incontinent of urine.[32] Incontinence is reported to be highly associated with impairment in ADL, cognitive impairments, depression, chronic obstructive pulmonary disease, and malnutrition.[32] For many residents, incontinence or bowel or bladder accidents may likely be caused by impairments in ADLs.

Residents may have chronic conditions affecting the heart and lungs, and many have mobility constraints, which may affect skin condition. Therefore, the cardiac, pulmonary, and integumentary systems require special attention. Aerobic capacity and endurance tests include vital signs at rest and after activity, autonomic responses to positional change, and functional tests of endurance.

Tests and Measures

Strength. Muscle strength is a predictor of function in older adults, and because most LTC residents have difficulty with ADLs, it can be safely presumed that most LTC residents have severe strength deficits.[33] For example, to stand from a normal chair without the use of arms requires leg strength of nearly half of the body weight.[34] If a resident cannot walk without weight bearing on his or her arms secondary to leg weakness, it can be presumed the resident has lost 75% of his or her reserve strength.[35] Therefore, strength assessment is vital to the physical therapy examination. However, the traditional manual muscle testing (MMT) has inherent limitations, especially in the LTC setting. MMT is not a quantitative assessment method for strength and has been shown to lack accuracy when used as a screening test.[36] Bohannon and Corrigan have shown that MMT has severe ceiling effects for grades higher than 5 of 5 in the lower extremity with a range from 85.4 to 650.0 Newtons.[37] MMT may not be easily performed in some patients with cognitive impairments or, range of motion (ROM) or mobility limitations. Therefore, MMT will not correlate with functional tasks on certain patients. Therapists may over- or underrate strength by observing function. For example, Bohannon found that if a patient is able to stand up from a chair without the use of his or her arms, it is safe to assume that strength on the quadriceps is at least 4+ of 5.[34] The therapist may determine the resident has "normal" strength and not incorporate appropriate strength training. Besides strength deficits, the resident may also exhibit poor balance or be afraid of falling, affecting task performance. The resident may have difficulty understanding instructions or simply not want to perform the task, issues insensitive to MMT. For these reasons, we advocate a functional testing perspective.

Functional Assessment. Functional assessment plays a vital role in demonstrating and documenting the outcomes of rehabilitation and should be an assumed standard of practice for all geriatric practitioners.[38,39] Many assessment tools that measure and analyze gait and balance require some level of resident comprehension and willingness to participate. Considering the number of residents with dementia and depression in LTC settings, the use of some of these standard tests may be challenging for the patient to complete and the therapist to administer.[40,41] However, many standardized tests and measures are appropriate and clinically meaningful in the LTC setting. We have listed some functional tools we find most valuable for residents of LTC settings in Table 25.1.[42]

The data obtained from the tests and measures are used to make a clinical judgment (evaluation), to establish a diagnosis and prognosis, and to determine an appropriate plan of care. These functional outcome measures can be used not only to determine a baseline of performance but also to help guide treatment interventions and when establishing objective and meaningful goals for both SNF and LTC patients by comparing the results with established clinometric properties when available. A clinician is able to reflect skilled care by careful test selection that accurately gauges a patient's level of impairment without over- or underchallenging the patient, provides as little patient distress as possible, and is administered faithfully as per testing instructions and conditions, and through observation and assessment of the patient's physical performance and physiological responses. In the LTC setting, the physical therapist has great autonomy and will determine the dosage of interventions and when to discharge from skilled therapy. It is imperative to constantly reassess the individual to determine when to begin a maintenance program or refer to restorative nursing.

Screening in Long-Term Care

The continuous-care nature of LTC requires ongoing and regular screening of the functional status of each resident. Although there is no regulation that designates a specific discipline to conduct screens, physical therapists are aptly qualified to perform them. Screenings are not meant to replace an evaluation and should be used to determine a change in status, for better or worse. Important information on residents' status can be obtained from the MDS, but the therapist should obtain information beyond the MDS. A more comprehensive picture of any change is usually obtained from nursing staff, nutritionists, and residents themselves. The therapist performing the screening should then visually inspect or observe the resident. Changes in ability to transfer or ambulate; any new onset of pain; worsening or development of contractures; new difficulty in eating, swallowing, or speaking; and difficulty propelling a wheelchair should be noted. Inspection of the prosthesis, braces, wheelchair, or splints can identify problems that may impair mobility or comfort and safety. Periodic

TABLE 25.1 Selected Standardized Assessments Useful for Long-Term Care Patients[a]

Functional Test	Rationale
Timed Up and Go (TUG)	General test of mobility and fall risk; may be done as dual task as well; cut score for fall risk; validated in multiple groups, including older adults with dementia
Gait speed	Used to determine rehabilitation potential, prognostication, and pre- and postmeasure; considered the "sixth vital sign"; validated in subacute care
6-Minute Walk	Gold standard test of functional endurance; measure of aerobic function and general mobility; pre- and postmeasure (2-minute version also available); validated In multiple populations. including those with Alzheimer disease
Four Square Step Test	Quantifies dynamic balance in four directions; includes a cognitive skill; valid and reliable in population of interest
Modified Clinical Test for Sensory Interaction of Balance (m-CTSIB)	Measures the way the balance triad (vision, vestibular, somatosensory) interacts to maintain balance; useful in diagnosing impairments and directing interventions appropriately; modified version is appropriate for population of interest
Berg Balance Scale	Measures static and dynamic balance and falls risk; assessment of patient performance on each of its components helps identify impairments and guides intervention; clinimetrics are sound for population of interest; a shortened version is available
30 Second Sit to Stand	Assesses lower extremity strength and ability to rise from a chair; functional marker
5 Time Sit to Stand	Assesses lower extremity strength and ability to rise from chair; functional marker (use 30-sec sit to stand if patient is unable to complete at least five repetitions)
Sitting Balance Scale	Quantifies sitting balance for frail older adults who are primarily nonambulatory; clinimetrically sound in population of interest
Foot Posture Index	Easy quantification of standing foot posture (a contributor to fall risk); sound clinimetrics in the population of interest
Chair Sit and Reach Test[b]	Objectively assesses general hamstring flexibility; highly relevant in population of interest; gender-specific norms available up to age 94 yr (*not appropriate for all patients, e.g., those with severe osteoporosis, confirmed or suspected vertebral fractures*)
Back scratch test[b]	Objectively assesses general shoulder flexibility; highly functional and relevant in population of interest; gender-specific norms available up to age 94 yr
Tandem stance	Measures balance, fall risk; tests for cerebellar or vestibular involvement
Single-leg stance, one-legged stance test	Measures static postural control and fall risk; clinimetrically sound in frail older adults

[a]Not an exhaustive list
[b]Flexibility norms differ for women and men, with women having higher flexibility norms than men.

assessment of the fit of the prosthesis or orthosis is necessary because the resident may experience muscle atrophy and weight loss over time. When function is measured over time, a snapshot of the resident's ability to maintain basic self-care activities is obtained and indicates if there has been a decline, improvement, or stabilization of a condition. After recognizing the resident's change in functional status, physical therapists working in an LTC setting may determine that skilled intervention is required, or they may refer the resident to a restorative nursing program. Therapists should attempt to make this decision process as objective as possible. Therefore, it is of paramount importance for the physical therapist to understand payor definitions of skilled therapy.

Medicare sets forth its definition of skilled physical therapy services in §220 and §230 of Chapter 15 of the Medicare Benefit Policy Manual.[43] The CMS definition of skilled therapy is presented in Box 25.4. It is incumbent upon the physical therapist to understand the requirements of each specific payor; however, many payors follow CMS's lead.

Active ROM or passive ROM provided to maintain the range does not require the skills of a physical therapist and can be performed in a restorative nursing program. However, exercise to improve ROM or to maintain range in a complex circumstance, such as in a joint near an unstable fracture, should be performed by a physical therapist or physical therapist assistant. It is important to understand that goal setting and plans of care in an LTC setting will be different compared with goals and plans of care provided in a rehabilitation hospital, where patients tend to quickly improve in function. LTC residents may not require treatment for mobility deficits at all. The potential for skin breakdown alone may warrant admission to skilled services for positioning, education, devices, contracture management, and prevention. As with all patients, a thorough history and chart review are the first two steps to determine the need for skilled therapy.

BOX 25.4 Medicare Coverage for Skilled Therapy in Long-Term Care (Part B)

- Service must be of a level of complexity and sophistication, or the condition of the patient must be of a nature that requires the judgment, knowledge, and skill of a qualified therapist. This means that the services can only be performed by a qualified therapist. If a CNA, family member or other caregiver can perform the treatment, then it probably does not meet this criterion. Document tests and measures, functional assessments, special techniques and specialized teaching that only you can provide as part of your scope of practice.
- Positive Expectation for Improvement: The condition of the patient is expected to improve materially in a reasonable and generally predictable period of time or services must be necessary for the establishment of a safe and effective maintenance program. Ask yourself what you see in the patient's environment and behavior that suggests intervention would be beneficial (i.e., social support, prior level of function, motivation and attention, ability to follow directions).
- The services must be considered under accepted standards of medical practice to be a specific and effective treatment for the patient's condition. This requires knowledge of the research. Know the tests and techniques that have been found to be effective within our scope of practice.
- The service must be reasonable and necessary for the treatment of the patient's condition including amount, frequency and duration of services. Documentation of a change of condition, ongoing problems and risk factors can add support to the necessity of your treatment. Documentation of the patient's complications and safety issues related to his or her impairments and functional deficits is important to meet this criterion.

From *Medicare Benefit Policy Manual*. Chapter 15: Covered medical and other health services. https://www.cms.gov/Regulations-and-Guidance/Guidance/Manuals/Downloads/bp102c15.pdf.

INTERVENTIONS

Exercise

As in most physical therapy settings, exercise is one of the cornerstones in the rehabilitation of a patient in an SNF or LTC. As dictated by their impairments and activity limitations, these patients benefit from properly dosed skilled strength training, aerobic conditioning, endurance training, ROM and flexibility activities, and power training, and have the potential to make significant improvements at discharge to the community. It is the responsibility of the clinician to take into consideration prior level of function, comorbidities, precautions and contraindications to exercise, current functional status, activity tolerance, cognitive status, and patient's goals and motivating factors to effectively prescribe and dose exercises for optimal and efficient recovery. It is the ethical and legal duty of the therapist to demonstrate clinical judgment, reasoning, and decision making when both prescribing and documenting skilled interventions for all patients as a reflection of our specialized knowledge base, formal education, and clinical training. This includes monitoring and interpreting vital signs at initiation and as a response to exercise with use of the Borg rate of perceived exertion (RPE) as appropriate, careful consideration of cardiopulmonary status for effective conditioning, awareness of the impacts of cognition, taking current medications and their side effects into consideration, and tailoring exercise selection for each patient. Probably the most crucial type of training in LTC is active participation in meaningful activities. Residents may not understand why they are asked to perform certain exercises and may not see the potential benefit of exercise performance.[44] Patients must see the connection between their resistance training improvements and the performance of ADLs. The connection can be enhanced by relating the activity to the patient-stated goal.

One of the strongest motivators affecting exercise adherence in older adults is self-efficacy, the confidence in one's ability to carry out a planned behavior.[45] When an exercise directly improves ADLs, it may then generate exercise adherence. A second motivator is outcome expectation, which is the belief that desirable outcomes will result from specific personal actions.[45] Self-efficacy has been shown to be a predictor of stair-climbing ability, balance, and general functional decline in older adults.[46] Self-efficacy beliefs have also been found to play a significant role as predictors of exercise behaviors in community-dwelling older adults, and exercise interventions that serve to improve the self-perception of exercise self-efficacy can instill confidence and help begin and maintain physical activity.[47,48]

Age is not an appropriate characteristic to determine application of specific interventions. Too often, in the authors' opinion, physical therapy practice in SNFs and especially LTC reflects low expectations by the therapist and often by the resident. Frequently, LTC residents are viewed by therapist as too frail or too cognitively impaired to benefit from best practices such as high-intensity strengthening, motor learning principles, electromodalities, and task-specific training. Unfortunately, there is a tendency to be too conservative when prescribing exercises to older patients even though studies have long shown that older adults can gain as much benefit from intense strength training as younger individuals.[51] The principles of intensity and specificity need to be used in a conscientious manner for strength gains to occur, with constant monitoring of sufficient overload and proper form to assure the patient is being challenged and progressed in a safe manner that avoids injury and pain, as well as monitoring vital signs and rate of perceived effort and providing adequate warm-up and cool-down periods. Prescribing exercise that is intense enough to provoke a strength-training effect of at least 60% of a 1 repetition maximum (RM; or 15 RM) for 1 set or 75% of 1 RM (or 10 RM) will achieve functional gains and can be motivating as well.[52] To obtain greatest strength improvements, 10 repetitions, or 80% of 1 RM, with form deterioration during the last one or two repetitions is most effective, even in frail populations.[52] Exercises that are meaningful to the older adult not only improve exercise adherence but also provide gains in functional capacities. It has been documented that older adults can adapt physiologically to exercise training similarly to younger adults, if specificity is incorporated.[49] Kato and coworkers studied the effects of a 12-week exercise program on ADL performance and functional mobility in frail older adults.[50] Participants (age 79.6 ± 7.7 years) completed low- to moderate-intensity training consisting of marching in place and chair rise, with gradual increase in speed of movements to address power training as training progressed. The 20-minute sessions were completed 7 days per week. Significant improvements were noted in those who received the intervention for the Barthel Index, mean power during chair rise, and 10-m walk test. These data suggest an important role of task specificity when designing exercise programs to improve physical function in lower functioning older adults.

It is well known that frail older adults can achieve improvements in strength, mobility, fall prevention, body composition, balance, functional ability, and endurance with training at any age, as well as experience a positive effect on cognition and psychological health.[53,54] Some studies suggest that exercise may help to prevent or delay the onset of frailty in older adults, which can improve quality of life.[53] Ferreira and coworkers studied a group of 37 frail, institutionalized older adult participants (mean age, 76 years) randomly assigned to a control group or an exercise group.[55] The physical training program focused on improving mobility, flexibility, strength, and aerobic resistance, with exercises prescribed individually to participants after an initial assessment. The exercises were performed up to moderate intensities according to each individual's perception of effort (between 5 and 7 according to an adapted OMNI Scale of Perceived Exertion), three times per week for 40 minutes for 12 weeks. Outcome measures included anthropometrics, clinical history, biochemical indices, inflammatory markers, and functional performance. Participants who completed the exercise training demonstrated improved functional performance, including strength, speed, and agility, as well as biochemical markers such as glucose insulin, triglycerides, total cholesterol, and C-reactive protein. Research also indicated a decrease or reversal in frailty as measured by the number of criteria for frailty syndrome. Based on evidence, we advocate and strongly encourage the prescription of moderate to vigorous exercises centered on a program established according to the patient's 1 RM for patients and residents in LTC. If high-intensity exercise is not appropriate, however, older adults with frailty can still make gains that may be more related to improved motor learning and movement efficiency than actual strength gains with a low- to moderate-intensity program.

In the frail population, lower intensities of 30% to 70% 1 RM produce some strengthening effects of significance. A recent systematic review of resistance training in physically frail aging adults concluded that a training volume of 1 to 3 sets of 6 to 15 repetitions and intensity of 30% to 70% 1 RM promoted significant enhancement on muscle strength, muscle power, and functional outcomes (which included Timed Up and Go [TUG] score and gait speed among others).[56] Another study compared high-intensity resistance training (70% 1 RM), low-intensity resistance training (40% 1 RM), and no training in a group of 48 aging adults in LTC. High-intensity training produced better results on the Short Physical Performance Test, but both the high- and low-intensity groups improved on other measures of ADLs (Barthel Index), depression (Geriatric Depression Scale), and quality of life (World Health Organization Quality of Life Instrument–Older Adults Module). Of important significance, the control group (no exercise) got worse on all measures.[57]

The intensity principle should be applied to aerobic conditioning as well, using a percentage of heart rate reserve and aerobic exercise tests such as the 2-Minute Walk Test, 6-Minute Walk Test, or 2-Minute Step Test to determine cardiovascular endurance and effectively gauge progression with therapy. Cardiorespiratory capacity is positively associated with muscle power and strength, so aerobic endurance interventions in frail adults should be included within a multicomponent exercise program. Endurance training of sufficient intensity induces improvements on VO_{2max} and submaximal endurance capacity in frail older adults. Evidence suggests endurance training should be performed at moderate to high intensity (i.e., 60%–85% of VO_{2max}), and moderate volume (i.e., 25–40 minutes).[58] Forms of skilled endurance training found to be effective in improving cardiovascular and functional performance in older adults with frailty should include treadmill walking, walking with changes in pace and direction, stair climbing, step-ups, and stationary cycling; these exercises may start at 5 to 10 minutes during initial training then progress to 15 to 30 minutes for the remainder of the program, with an intensity of 12 to 14 on the Borg scale as a suitable alternative to resistance training.[59] It is important to remember what constitutes skilled treatment in the context of aerobic capacity. Although aerobic training can (and arguably should) be provided concurrent with strength or power training, it is often documented as a stand-alone intervention ("endurance training") and lends itself to scrutiny by third party reviewers. Why is it scrutinized so closely? In the author's opinion, it is because there is often a lack of clinical judgment or reasoning evident in the documentation. Therapists must document heart rate, blood pressure, and pulse oximetry before, during, and after exercise. In addition to assessing pre- and postexercise cardiovascular response, dosage adjustments must be made based on the patient's individual response. Knowledge of the patient's target heart rate, maintenance of heart rate within the target zone, or use of an exertion scale (e.g., Borg RPE, Omni RPE) to determine exercise intensity is required. Failure to demonstrate this basic level of clinical judgment when prescribing and providing exercise designed to address aerobic capacity does not meet the definition of skilled care. Thus, having a patient perform "endurance training" on a recumbent bike, upper body ergometer, or restorator without evidence of measuring and monitoring heart rate, oximetry, blood pressure, or exertion levels and subsequently using this information to adjust exercise intensity is not considered skilled care.

Another form of training that is often overlooked in older adults in the postacute setting is power training. Muscle power decreases earlier than muscle strength with advancing age, and evidence suggests it is more strongly associated with function than strength.[60] Research indicates that muscle power is more important than muscle strength in maintaining physical function in older adults, and high-velocity resistance training has been accepted as a practical, successful, and safe intervention to improve lower extremity muscle power in older adults with frailty.[61] In the postacute setting, power training can be geared toward meaningful functional tasks, such as standing from a bed or chair, step training, or stair training. A controlled trial performed on 24 institutionalized frail nonagenarians (mean age, 91.9 years) investigated the effect of a multicomponent intervention, including power, balance, and gait training on muscle power, muscle mass, and functional outcomes.[60] Power training for the upper and lower body was performed at 40% to 60% of 1 RM for 8 to 10 repetitions twice a week for 12 weeks. Training sessions lasted about 40 minutes, with 10 minutes of balance and gait training and 20 minutes of resistance training. Results showed improvements in TUG with single and dual tasks, balance performance, ability to rise from a chair, muscle power and strength, muscle mass, and reduced incidence of falls. Izquierdo and Cadore state, "Routine multicomponent interventions that include muscle power training should be prescribed to institutionalized oldest old because such interventions improve the overall physical status of frail elderly individuals and prevent disability and other adverse outcomes. This result is especially important in frail subjects, who urgently need to improve their functional capacities to prevent adverse outcomes such as falls, hospitalizations, disability, or even death."[62] It is therefore beneficial to not only prescribe multicomponent exercise interventions to nonagenarians but to also include challenging interventions that are not traditionally associated with aging adults, such as power training, to maximize functional outcomes in this population.

It is important to remember that older adults themselves may have misconceptions and lack knowledge about strength training and therefore be skeptical or even resistant to an intense exercise regimen. In a study by Manini and coworkers, 129 older adults (77.5 ± 8.6 years) responded to questions about their opinions, experiences, and knowledge of strength training recommendations.[63] Forty-eight percent of older adults believed that strength training would not increase muscle mass, 45% said that increasing weight is not more important than number of repetitions for building strength, and 37% responded that walking is more effective than lifting weights at building strength. Clearly, physical therapists have an important role in educating older adults on the benefits and appropriateness of strength training as well as providing the reassurance and motivation often needed to overcome fear or apprehension.

Gait Training

Older adults often recognize changes in their gait patterns and speed, and believe that they cannot walk "the way they used to." Gait speed has been shown to be a predictor of functional decline, nursing home placement, and mortality.[64–67] Gait speed declines with age and reductions in activity levels and has been referred to as the "sixth vital sign."[68] Potter and coworkers reported that older adults in a geriatric unit who had a gait speed of less than 0.25 m/s were more likely to be dependent in ADLs.[69] Gait speeds of 0.5 m/s or less are common in LTC settings and indicate the severe loss of strength that is associated with frailty and sedentary behavior.[70] Multicomponent exercise programs that include endurance, lower extremity strength, and balance training have been shown to be the most effective strategy for improving gait, strength, and balance as well as decreasing rate of falls in aging adults; when systematic resistance training is performed, either alone or as part of multicomponent exercise programs, greater strength improvements have been observed in frail adults or those with severe functional declines.[59] We advocate the measurement of gait speed over a 4-m walkway for every resident. Usual and fast gait speed should be measured with an expectation of a difference between the two, to indicate the reserve available. Although a difference of 0.33 m/s is usual for well-functioning community-dwelling older adults, 0.22 m/s is seen in women with difficulty in two or more ADLs.[71] It is hypothesized that the smaller the reserve, the poorer the potential of being able to tolerate and gain from skilled physical therapy sessions.

Gait training in the institutionalized older adult should be no different than in other settings in which the therapist analyzes stance and swing phases, observes step length and symmetry, notes compensations, and generates hypotheses as to the causes of the limitations (impairments). Therapists should realize that causes of gait dysfunction in institutionalized older adults may be of a chronic nature and that some of the impairments may not be reversible. However, any impairment noted should not be assumed to be attributable to "geriatric gait" but rather an indication of an underlying gait impairment that may be corrected or modified. The therapist should use different feedback strategies to improve the patient's awareness of gait impairments and attempt self-correction as well as carryover. Although the impairment may not be reversible, the functional limitations may improve if treatment is directed at balance, speed, and compensatory strategies. Improving gait to decrease the risk of falls is of extreme importance in most LTC settings. Slowed gait speed in the older adult population has been related to an increased risk for falls, which in turn often leads to a loss of independent living and to institutionalization.[72,73]

Gait training and ambulation are clear differentiators of a skilled service and a nonskilled service. Gait training provided by a physical therapist or physical therapist assistant is considered skilled care under CMS criteria under three conditions: (1) when a therapist needs to give specific instructions, verbally or manually, to a resident to improve the gait pattern; (2) a gait assessment needs to be made to determine the impairments causing any abnormalities; or (3) recommendations need to be made for assistive devices. When a therapist determines that no improvement can be made in the gait pattern but a resident should continue walking to maintain the functional status or simply improve distance ambulation for endurance, it can be performed in a restorative nursing program and does not require the skill of a therapist. It is also important to differentiate between manual cues and physical assistance. A resident can be in a restorative nursing program even when physical assistance is required to ambulate as long as the referring therapist believes it is safe and the person assisting is providing support to the resident when no significant functional improvement is expected.

Skilled gait training should focus on adequately challenging the patient while taking the overload principle into consideration to improve performance. This can include multidirectional stepping activities; start–stop exercises; use of compliant surfaces; over obstacles; curb, stair, or ramp training; using a less restrictive assistive device; in outdoor parking areas; using different footwear; and use of an elastic band to resist lateral or forward movement. Dual-task training with gait activities, including use of a cognitive task such as reacting to signs for changing directions, task management, and simulating daily situations while negotiating a crowded environment and reacting to signs, has been found to improve walking performance under single- and dual-task conditions in aging adults with and without concern about falling.[74] Dual-task training, including task-managing strategies such as task prioritization or task switching, when combined with coordination and balance tasks, was found to have greater benefits on gait performance and reduced fear of falling than strength and resistance training.[75] Recording and monitoring vital signs and the patient's physiological response will provide information about the level of intensity and challenge being provided in a gait training session.

Balance Training

Balance training has been shown to be effective in improving static and dynamic balance, proactive, and reactive balance as well as performance in balance test batteries in older adults, with recommendations made for three training sessions per week for total duration of 91 to 120 minutes of balance training per week to improve overall balance.[76] Balance training for frail older adults should include varied exercise stimuli, such as multidirectional weight lifts, tandem stance, line walking, heel–toe walking, single-limb stance, stepping practice, and weight shifting between lower extremities.[59] Free-weight resistance training, in the form of squats, lunges, and bridging exercises, performed on unstable surfaces such as wobble boards, inflatable discs, and BOSU balls was found to be as effective as machine-based stable resistance training and machine-based unstable surface training in increasing lower extremity power, strength, and balance in older adults with notably lower training loads.[77] Balance training should include specific strategies to address the identified balance impairments and should be directed at the system(s) contributing to the balance condition (somatosensory, vestibular, and visual) while facilitating compensation or challenge to the appropriate system. Therapists must also have knowledge of the neuromuscular (strength, power) and biomechanical (arthrokinematics, ROM) contributors to being upright. Skilled balance training includes an awareness that normal walking is a series of balance recoveries and preventing the loss of balance, as opposed to preventing a fall, is actually detrimental because a patient must learn how to recover his or her balance. Balance training is progressive in nature, meaning the activities included are progressively challenging to the three systems of balance control. Static activities may progress from standing on a level surface with the eyes open to standing with the eyes closed, to standing on a compliant surface with eyes open then closed. The base of support can be narrowed to make static activities more challenging. Dynamic activities can be challenged by incorporating head or eye movements, and progressing these activities to compliant surfaces, with and without visual input. Dynamic activities may include changing gait speed or direction, avoiding obstacles, stepping tasks, tandem walking, reverse walking, gait over varied surfaces, obstacle course negotiation, and using varying level of support. Variety is important and activities should not be repetitive in nature because normal balance requires individuals to maintain an upright position (not fall) in novel situations.

When describing balance in patients, terms such as "poor," "fair," or "good" are not helpful. These terms are vague, not standardized, and ultimately meaningless. For example, "fair" standing or sitting balance is not defined and may mean different things depending on context. How would another clinician know when "fair" balance has improved to "good" balance, for example? A description of balance (in sitting or standing) should be based on standardized quantifiable measurements that demonstrate adequate clinimetric properties (e.g., validity, reliability, responsiveness). There are a number of balance tools that are appropriate for patients in SNF and LTC settings (see Table 25.1). These tools may be used to describe balance at any point in the episode of care and often serve as a component of a comprehensive fall risk assessment.

Transfer Training

Transfer training is a frequent intervention provided to patients in postacute settings because relearning how to move from one surface to another is a fundamental activity required for increased independence and participation. The provision of transfer training as a therapeutic activity is skilled when the therapist or therapist assistant uses evidence, critical thinking, and clinical reasoning to design, implement, and progress the activity. Skilled transfer training should incorporate the concepts and theories surrounding motor learning and adult learning. For example, a patient may perform a transfer activity repeatedly until performance deteriorates, indicating motor fatigue. Varying the surface or the side of the bed or mat as well as eliminating the use of handrail or bed rail also introduces novelty and promotes motor learning. Skilled transfer training also should include the concepts of overload and specificity. Removing upper extremity assistance or adding resistance (holding weight or a ball, for example) accomplish overload during the training. Interventions should address identified impairments. So, if performance is impaired by poor lower extremity strength, for example, the height of the surface could be altered until strength or power gains are accomplished and similarly can be lowered or made compliant to adequately challenge the patient as progress is made.

Although cueing is important, transfer training that overemphasizes cueing for safety or hand placement without a documented knowledge or performance deficit in safety awareness does not constitute skilled therapy. The intervention should be directed at an identified impairment. Repetition is important; therefore, multiple repetitions are necessary for the intervention to be therapeutic and for learning to occur. Simply performing a transfer for the sake of moving from one surface to another does not constitute skilled transfer training. Furthermore, the fact that a patient requires assistance with transfers does not make provision of assistance during a transfer a skilled activity. An awareness of impairments, linked to the performance of the activity, along with accepted theories of motor and adult learning are required elements of skilled transfer training.

UNIQUE CHALLENGES IN THE LONG-TERM CARE SETTING

Fall Risk Reduction

Falls prevention is an important component of caring for aging adults. Although what constitutes successful fall intervention in nursing homes has not been determined, some program characteristics are promising. For example, Vlaeyen and coworkers studied the characteristics and effectiveness of fall prevention programs in nursing homes.[78] This systematic review included 22,915 nursing home residents and examined number of falls, fallers, and recurrent falls. Fall prevention interventions, whether single, multiple, or multifactorial intervention components, were found to significantly reduce the number of recurrent falls by 21%. Multifactorial interventions were also found to significantly decrease falls and the number of recurrent fallers as opposed to single or multiple interventions. According to the Academy of Geriatric Physical Therapy's Clinical Guidance Statement on fall risk in community-dwelling older adults, treatment interventions indicated to have the greatest effect on fall prevention are those in which balance training focuses on standing balance, upper extremity support is minimized, intervention are progressed appropriately, and the minimum training dosage is 50 hours.[79] Although this guidance statement is directed at community-dwelling older adults, therapists working with residents in LTC settings should be aware of the extended time that may be required to engage in effective fall reduction activities. Low-dose, short-term interventions may not be effective. Furthermore, some of these residents may go home where treatment should continue. For patients in nursing homes, multidisciplinary interventions delivered by a multidisciplinary team have been found to be the most successful interventions. Where more medically complex patients are concerned, examining and managing medical risk factors along with physical therapy may be an effective way to decrease fall risk. These results suggest that high rates of falls can be lowered through interdisciplinary approaches in LTC settings. Physical therapists should be active members of the falls reduction teams present in most facilities.

Clinical reasoning and decision making must be clearly evident (i.e., documented) for a falls risk assessment to be a skilled activity. The therapist must choose evidence-based fall risk assessment tools appropriate for the patient and for the setting. The therapist must interpret the results of these tests accurately, having a clear understanding of the test administration protocol as well as the test clinimetrics (e.g., validity, reliability, responsiveness). Pre- and postintervention measures should be compared to ensure a clinically meaningful change has occurred that has exceeded any measurement error ('noise") in the test itself. Skilled risk assessment also includes a process of prioritizing risk factors, addressing those that can be addressed by a physical therapist, and referring to other providers when the treatment is outside the scope of physical therapy. When a plan of care is created to address physical impairments and activity limitations contributing to fall risks, skill rests in demonstrating judgment and clinical reasoning for the interventions chosen. For further information on skilled interventions used to decrease fall risk, please refer to the chapter of this book that pertains to balance.

Restraint Reduction

The Omnibus Reconciliation Act of 1987 specified that residents have the right to be free from restraints; therefore, restraints are used only when all other alternatives to prevent injuries have failed.[80] Most institutions have programs in place to reduce the use of restraints. In the LTC setting, physical therapists are often consultants and assume leadership roles in finding alternatives for the use of restraints. Some of the alternatives for the use of restraints include engaging residents in physical activities, increasing participation in leisure activities, and increased supervision from staff, which can be difficult and sometimes overwhelming. Commonly used alternatives to restraints are low beds, mattresses on the floor to prevent injury in case of a fall out of bed, wheelchair or bed alarms, and beds with no railings. Some facilities have adopted the use of hip protectors to reduce the likelihood of fracture if a fall were to occur; however, the evidence on hip protectors is equivocal.[81]

There are many reasons why residents prefer having a bed rail, including the sense of security it seems to offer and the bed rail's ability to enable rolling. Bed rails are common in LTC but are considered a restraint if the resident is unable to lower the rail independently. And although the rail may seem to prevent injury and falls, the opposite is actually the case. Evidence indicates that use of physical restraints is not associated with a reduction in falls nor fall-related injuries.[82] In addition, the use of restraints has led to reduced mobility, decreased psychosocial wellbeing, entrapment, and strangulation.[82] Physical therapists should consider these facts when assessing functional independence in the LTC setting.

Contracture management and risk reduction of contractures are a common consequence of prolonged physical immobility among nursing home residents and further reduce mobility, social participation, and ADL performance, as well as increase the risk of other ill effects of decreased mobility, such as pressure ulcers.[83] Almost two-thirds of the LTC residents in a study performed by Wagner and coworkers had at least one contracture, with the most common locations being the shoulder and knee.[84] In this study, the greatest predictors of contractures were pain, physical restraints, and urinary incontinence. Recent systematic reviews considering both passive and active interventions (stretching and positioning) for the treatment of disability caused by acquired joint contractures is conflicting. Some studies show improvement with more active intervention, but results are still based on weak evidence.[85,86] Researchers suggest that in addition to functional issues, activities and social participation should also be studied as outcomes.

When contracture is already present, the therapist should not only take the accurate ROM measurement but also assess the nature of the contracture by differentiating fixed contractures (with no give in ROM by passive stretch) from a nonfixed restriction (with a gain in ROM with stretch), and rigidity from spasticity (neurologic) to establish the best intervention. The therapist must also be certain that any intervention is a skilled physical therapy service. When clinical judgment and reasoning are required, and when adjustments and changes are made based on demonstrable clinical characteristics, one could deem contracture management skilled. However, the routine donning and doffing of splints or positioning devices would not necessarily be skilled therapy and in some facilities may be delegated to the restorative care team.

Pressure Ulcer Management and Risk Reduction

Physical therapists are often the first ones to observe redness or tender points in nursing home residents, frequently in bed-bound, nonverbal patients. Careful skin inspection should be part of the physical therapist's assessment, including to all aspects of the feet and toenails. Routine screening should also include sensory examination to note whether sensation is absent or diminished with particular attention paid to areas prone to skin break down, especially for patients with a history of diabetes, neuropathy, or other neurologic condition such as a stroke. Sharing the findings with nursing staff and providing alternatives for positioning is a primary task of the physical therapist in this scenario.

The prevalence of pressure ulcers varies from 2% to 28% among nursing home residents, with stage 2 pressure ulcers being the most common, accounting for about 50% of all pressure ulcers in 2004.[87] However, according to the CMS, the percentage of nursing home residents in the United States with pressure ulcers has decreased from 5.9% to 5.1% from 2011 to 2014.[88] Risk factors for pressure ulcers include immobility or restricted mobility, loss of bowel and bladder control, polypharmacy, and recent weight loss.[87] Preventive interventions, such as frequent repositioning, tissue load management, and ensuring adequate nutrition, have been shown to help prevent pressure ulcer formation among patients at risk.[89]

The most practical method for reducing pressure is to turn and position the patient frequently. Although repositioning is a widely used and integral component of pressure ulcer prevention and treatment, there is a lack of high-quality evidence on the effect of repositioning frequency and position for pressure ulcer prevention and healing rates.[90,91] Because of the limitations and cost of turning patients frequently, a number of devices have been developed for preventing pressure injury. A recent systematic review indicates that those at high risk of developing pressure ulcers should use higher specification foam mattresses rather than standard hospital foam mattresses.[92] Although the relative advantage of alternating- and constant low-pressure devices are unclear, alternating-pressure mattresses are possibly more cost effective than alternating-pressure overlays.[92] Malnutrition has been linked to an increase in the risk of skin ulcers and to delayed healing.[93] During periodic screenings, therapists should speak with dieticians and certified nursing assistants involved in feeding to identify residents who are malnourished or at high risk for malnourishment, thereby attempting to indirectly reduce the risk of pressure sores. Some useful questions that can be asked are the following:

- Has there been any weight loss?
- If the resident wears dentures, do they fit appropriately, and are they being used?
- Does the resident eat independently or with assistance?
- If the resident requires assistance with eating, has there been a recent change in the level of assistance required?

In summary, the list below highlights the role of the physical therapist in managing and preventing pressure sores in institutionalized older adults:

- Educate nursing staff whenever needed on proper transfers and lifting techniques to avoid skin injury from friction or shear.
- Recommend a turning and repositioning schedule for residents who are at risk.
- Leave residents with pillows or other devices to keep bony prominences from direct contact with each other.
- Teach residents to perform small and regular weight shifts.
- Recommend proper pressure-reducing devices for the wheelchair and bed, and be familiar with current products available.
- Keep residents as active as possible; promote mobilization by referring to restorative programs and encouraging participation in social events.

Readers are referred to the chapter on the integument for more information of the assessment and management of pressure ulcers.

RESTORATIVE PROGRAMS

When it is determined by the therapist's evaluation that a resident is not appropriate for skilled services, physical therapists also have an active role in teaching nursing staff the most appropriate transfer techniques, aids for proper positioning, donning and doffing braces and splints, guarding techniques during ambulation, and development of a restorative nursing program to maintain current status and prevent risk of functional decline. Physical therapists often refer patients to these restorative nursing programs upon discharge from skilled physical therapy as a type of "step-down" program for the residents or if the therapist determined that the resident does not require the skills of a physical therapist. Restorative programs may include turning and positioning programs, wheelchair mobility and endurance programs, ambulation, ADL programs, active ROM programs, and restorative dining programs, among others. Programs that encourage walking as part of the resident's daily routine (e.g., walking to the dining room) have been reported to increase overall ambulatory endurance, decrease fall rates, decrease incidences of incontinence, and inhibit functional decline.[94,95] A 6-month walking program has also been found to improve ADL performance, increase endurance, and delay cognitive decline in nursing home residents with Alzheimer disease.[96]

Trained restorative aides generally carry out restorative nursing programs. These programs can be quite effective if both nursing and rehabilitation staff are committed to their success. Communication between the therapist referring the resident to a restorative program and the clinician running it is fundamental. Some facilities keep a log with descriptors of their residents' participation and restorative goals that have or have not been achieved. This may be a quick and effective way to supervise a resident's performance. A good time to interview the staff member responsible for the restorative program is during a periodic screen. The physical therapist should ask about residents' participation in the program and whether they are achieving the desired results. It is common for residents to improve slowly, over time, while on a restorative program. Do not confuse this with skilled therapy, in which significant functional gains are expected in a reasonable time frame.[43] Any major changes in performance, for better or worse, should warrant a complete physical therapy evaluation.

It is important to consider the difference between restorative care and skilled maintenance. Skilled maintenance is a covered service under Medicare.[97] However, for skilled maintenance to be considered billable, the services must require the skills of a physical therapist or physical therapist assistant. This means that the services are of a complexity that they cannot be performed by a restorative aide, nursing assistant, nurse, or family member. Documentation of skill is paramount for patients being seen under a maintenance plan of care. For a full explanation of skilled maintenance, see the Medicare Benefit Policy Manual (MBPM), Chapter 15, Section 220 (Part B) and MBPM Chapter 8, Section 30.2.2.1 (Part A).

DEALING WITH DEMENTIA AND DEPRESSION

Dementia is one of the most common reasons for placement of older adults in nursing facilities.[98] Depression affects a median of 10% of patients in LTC settings with a median of 29% demonstrating depressive symptoms and is associated with significant morbidity, mortality, disability, and suffering for patients and their families.[37,99,100] The presence of dementia or depression may pose challenges for physical therapists that require creativity in engaging the resident. A resident who is depressed may be more inclined to participate in activities that were enjoyed before the onset of depression. For example, if the resident enjoyed dancing, it could be incorporated into treatment by having the resident move according to the music to improve balance or move according to the beat during gait training. Ball toss or kicking as well as competitive tasks or obstacle courses could be incorporated into treatment sessions for residents who enjoy sports. Consideration of how to build self-efficacy as described earlier can be included. Residents who are cognitively impaired may not understand exercising for the sake of exercising, or in severe cases, not even understand the instructions given. Therapists often struggle with this challenge and unfortunately may exclude these residents from skilled therapy, claiming that they are unable to participate. However, therapists should attempt to include confused residents in activities that are meaningful, practical, or functional. For example, a resident who was a housewife for her whole life may be able to fold towels and sheets. The therapist can use this activity to work on balance, standing tolerance, or upper extremity motion. A resident who refuses to stand up from a chair when asked to may automatically stand up to answer the phone or the door and may agree to "go for a walk" to look for something or someone. It is in the authors' experience that although they may experience difficulty completing rote therapeutic exercises, these patients often benefit from massed practice functional training to help tap into motor memory and improve safety and carryover with functional tasks.

Evidence suggests that cognitively impaired older adults who participate in exercise rehabilitation programs have similar strength and endurance training outcomes as age- and gender-matched cognitively intact older participants.[37] Research also indicates that exercise interventions can improve not only physical fitness and functional performance but also cognitive function in persons with dementia.[101] These findings are consistent with those of Littbrand and coworkers.[102] The results of this study suggest that a high-intensity functional weight-bearing exercise program is applicable for use, regardless of cognitive function, among older people who are dependent in ADLs, living in residential care facilities, and have a Mini-Mental State Examination (MMSE) score of 10 or higher. Cadore and coworkers studied the effects of an exercise program involving gait training, balance and resistance training, and cognitive exercises in frail adult patients with dementia after long-term physical restraint.[103] They found that the 8-week program improved muscle strength, balance, and gait ability, and reduced the incidence of falls. Clearly, cognitively impaired individuals should not be excluded from rehabilitation programs. For further information and resources, please refer to the chapter on cognition in this textbook.

Blumenthal and coworkers assessed whether patients receiving aerobic training achieved reduction in depression compared with standard antidepressant medication (sertraline HCl) and a greater reduction in depression compared with placebo control participants.[100] Their findings indicate that the efficacy of exercise in patients seems generally comparable with patients receiving antidepressant medication and both tend to be better than the placebo. Clearly, given these results, physical therapists need to be engaged in the discussion and treatment of patients with depression in LTC and other settings.

FUTURE TRENDS IN POSTACUTE CARE

Health care delivery and systems in the United States are changing rapidly. Any initiatives from states and the federal government to ensure the solvency of Medicare and Medicaid programs are likely to affect postacute care settings in great measure. In coming years, there may be massive changes in health care payment methodology, systems of delivery, and continuity of care. Postacute care settings, including IRF, SNF, and LTC, will undoubtedly see widespread change. It is clear that our current system will need to change to keep up with the large numbers of aging adults who have (and will) create the biggest demand on the Medicare system the program has experienced since its inception. Physical therapists will continue to have an important role in the delivery of care in postacute care settings. Knowledge of evidence-based interventions, which are both clinically effective and fiscally efficient, will be especially important. Health promotion and wellness efforts should become standard practice for geriatric physical therapists as our society shifts toward a more preventive model of health care delivery. The postacute care environments, especially LTC, offer many opportunities for physical therapists to make substantive contributions to changes in how aging adults regain function and are able to have a meaningful, productive quality of life.

REFERENCES

1. Tian W. (AHQR). *An All-Payer View of Hospital Discharge to Postacute Care*, 2013. HCUP Statistical Brief #205; May 2016. Rockville, MD; 2016.
2. Kaplan SJ. Growth and payment adequacy of medicare postacute care rehabilitation. *Arch Phys Med Rehabil.* 2007;88(11):1494–1499.
3. Centers for Medicare & Medicaid Services. *Inpatient Rehabilitation Facility PPS*. https://www.cms.gov/Medicare/Medicare-Fee-for-Service-Payment/InpatientRehabFacPPS/index.html; *2018*.
4. Haghverdian BA, Wright DJ, Schwarzkopf R. Length of stay in skilled nursing facilities following total joint arthroplasty. *J Arthroplasty.* 2017;32(2):367–374.
5. Buntin MB, Garten AD, Paddock S, Saliba D, Totten M, Escarce JJ. How much is postacute care use affected by its availability? *Health Serv Res.* 2005;40(2):413–434.
6. Buntin MB. Access to postacute rehabilitation. *Arch Phys Med Rehabil.* 2007;88(11):1488–1493.
7. Buntin MB, Colla CH, Escarce JJ. Effects of payment changes on trends in post-acute care. *Health Serv Res.* 2009;44(4):1188–1210.
8. Centers for Medicare & Medicaid Services. *Skilled Nursing Facility PPS*. https://www.cms.gov/Medicare/Medicare-Fee-for-Service-Payment/SNFPPS/index.html; 2018.
9. Centers for Medicare & Medicaid Services. *Skilled Nursing Facilities Data*. 2018. https://www.cms.gov/Research-Statistics-Data-and-Systems/Statistics-Trends-and-Reports/Medicare-Provider-Charge-Data/SNF2015.html; *2015*.
10. Picariello G, Hanson C, Futterman R, Hill J, Anselm E. Impact of a geriatric case management program on health plan costs. *Popul Health Manag.* 2008;11(4):209–215.

11. Johnson RW, Toohey D, Wiener JM. *Meeting the Long-Term Care Needs of the Baby Boomers.* Washington, DC: *How Changing Families Will Affect Paid Helpers and Institutions*; 2007.
12. Centers for Disease Control and Prevention. *FastStats—Nursing Home Care.* https://www.cdc.gov/nchs/fastats/nursing-home-care.htm; 2017.
13. Manton KG, Gu X, Lamb VL. Change in chronic disability from 1982 to 2004/2005 as measured by long-term changes in function and health in the U.S. elderly population. *Proc Natl Acad Sci U S A.* 2006;103(48):18374–18379.
14. West LA, Cole S, Goodkind D, He W. *65+ in the United States: 2010 Special Studies Current Population Reports.* Washington, DC: U.S. Census Bureau; 2014:23–212.
15. Medicaid.gov. https://www.medicaid.gov/index.html.
16. Holup AA, Gassoumis ZD, Wilber KH, Hyer K. Community discharge of nursing home residents: the role of facility characteristics. *Health Serv Res.* 2016;51(2):645–666.
17. Goodwin JS, Howrey B, Zhang DD, Kuo Y-F. Risk of continued institutionalization after hospitalization in older adults. *J Gerontol A Biol Sci Med Sci.* 2011;66(12):1321–1327.
18. Kojima G. Frailty as a predictor of nursing home placement among community-dwelling older adults: a systematic review and meta-analysis. *J Geriatr Phys Ther.* 2018;41(1):42–48.
19. Ciolek DE, Hwang W. *Short Term Alternatives for Therapy Services (STATS) Task Order: Final report on short term alternatives. Report prepared for the* Centers for Medicare & Medicaid Services (CMS). Baltimore, MD: Computer Sciences Corporation; 2010.
20. Agency for Healthcare Research and Quality. *Chapter 1. Introduction and program overview. Falls Manag Progr A Qual Improv Initiat Nurs Facil.* https://www.ahrq.gov/professionals/systems/long-term-care/resources/injuries/fallspx/fallspxman1.html; 2017.
21. Todd C, Skelton D. *What Are the Main Risk Factors for Falls amongst Older People and What Are the Most Effective Interventions to Prevent These Falls?* Copenhagen: World Health Organization Regional Office for Europe; 2004.
22. Cox CA, van Jaarsveld HJ, Houterman S, et al. Psychotropic drug prescription and the risk of falls in nursing home residents. *J Am Med Dir Assoc.* 2016;17(12):1089–1093.
23. Sterke CS, Verhagen AP, van Beeck EF, van der Cammen TJM. The influence of drug use on fall incidents among nursing home residents: a systematic review. *Int Psychogeriatrics.* 2008;20(05):890–910.
24. Gillespie LD, Robertson MC, Gillespie WJ, et al. Interventions for preventing falls in older people living in the community. *Cochrane Database Syst Rev.* 2012;9:CD007146.
25. Okada K, Okada M, Kamada N, et al. Reduction of diuretics and analysis of water and muscle volumes to prevent falls and fall-related fractures in older adults. *Geriatr Gerontol Int.* 2017;17(2):262–269.
26. Rolita L, Spegman A, Tang X, Cronstein BN. Greater number of narcotic analgesic prescriptions for osteoarthritis is associated with falls and fractures in elderly adults. *J Am Geriatr Soc.* 2013;61(3):335–340.
27. Rooth MA. The prevalence and impact of vision and hearing loss in the elderly. *N C Med J.* 2017;78(2):118–120.
28. Thapa R, Bajimaya S, Paudyal G, et al. Prevalence and causes of low vision and blindness in an elderly population in Nepal: the Bhaktapur retina study. *BMC Ophthalmol.* 2018;18(1):42.
29. Bourne RRA, Flaxman SR, Braithwaite T, et al. Magnitude, temporal trends, and projections of the global prevalence of blindness and distance and near vision impairment: a systematic review and meta-analysis. *Lancet Glob Heal.* 2017;5(9):e888–e897.
30. Michikawa T. Prevalence, adverse health, and risk factors in association with sensory impairments: data from a prospective cohort study of older Japanese. *Environ Health Prev Med.* 2016;21(6):403–409.
31. Jensen H, Tubæk G. Elderly people need an eye examination before entering nursing homes. *Dan Med J.* 2017;64(2):A5325.
32. Saga S, Vinsnes AG, Mørkved S, Norton C, Seim A. What characteristics predispose to continence in nursing home residents? A population-based cross-sectional study. *Neurourol Urodyn.* 2015;34(4):362–367.
33. Cadore EL, Izquierdo M. How to simultaneously optimize muscle strength, power, functional capacity, and cardiovascular gains in the elderly: an update. *Age (Dordr).* 2013;35(6):2329–2344.
34. Bohannon RW. Body weight-normalized knee extension strength explains sit-to-stand independence: a validation study. *J Strength Cond Res.* 2009;23(1):309–311.
35. Bassey EJ, Fiatarone MA, O'Neill EF, Kelly M, Evans WJ, Lipsitz LA. Leg extensor power and functional performance in very old men and women. *Clin Sci.* 1992;82(3):321–327.
36. Bohannon RW. Manual muscle testing: does it meet the standards of an adequate screening test? *Clin Rehabil.* 2005;19(6):662–667.
37. Bohannon RW, Corrigan D. A broad range of forces is encompassed by the maximum manual muscle test grade of five. *Percept Mot Ski.* 2000;90:747–750.
38. Pardasaney PK, Latham NK, Jette AM, et al. Sensitivity to change and responsiveness of four balance measures for community-dwelling older adults. *Phys Ther.* 2012;92(3):388–397.
39. Wrisley DM, Kumar NA. Functional gait assessment: concurrent, discriminative, and predictive validity in community-dwelling older adults. *Phys Ther.* 2010;90(5):761–773.
40. Harris Y. Depression as a risk factor for nursing home admission among older individuals. *J Am Med Dir Assoc.* 2007;8(1):14–20.
41. Heyn P, Johnson K, Kramer A. Endurance and strength training outcomes on cognitively impaired and cognitively intact older adults: a meta-analysis. *J Nutr Health Aging.* 2008;12(6): 401–409.
42. Avers D, VanBeveren P. *Course Notes, SUNY Upstate Medical University;* 2009.
43. US Center for Medicare and Medicaid Services. *Medicare Benefit Policy Manual, Chapter 15: Covered Medical and Other Health Services.* Washington DC: Government Printing Office; 2018.
44. Martin Ginis KA, Latimer AE, Brawley LR, et al. Weight training to activities of daily living: helping older adults make a connection. *Med Sci Sport Exerc.* 2006;38(1):116–121.
45. Neupert SD, Lachman ME, Whitbourne SB. Exercise self-efficacy and control beliefs: effects on exercise behavior after an exercise intervention for older adults. *J Aging Phys Act.* 2009;17(1):1–16.
46. Paterson D, Jones G, Rice C. Ageing and physical activity: evidence to develop exercise recommendations for older adults. *Can J Public Heal.* 2007;98(suppl 2):S69–S108.
47. Kroll T, Kratz A, Kehn M, et al. Perceived exercise self-efficacy as a predictor of exercise behavior in individuals aging with spinal cord injury. *Am J Phys Med Rehabil.* 2012;91(8):640–651.
48. Lee L-L, Arthur A, Avis M. Using self-efficacy theory to develop interventions that help older people overcome psychological barriers to physical activity: a discussion paper. *Int J Nurs Stud.* 2008;45(11):1690–1699.
49. Manini T, Marko M, VanArnam T, et al. Efficacy of resistance and task-specific exercise in older adults who modify tasks of everyday life. *J Gerontol A Biol Sci Med Sci.* 2007;62(6):616–623.
50. Kato Y, Islam MM, Koizumi D, Rogers ME, Takeshima N. Effects of a 12-week marching in place and chair rise daily exercise intervention on ADL and functional mobility in frail older adults. *J Phys Ther Sci.* 2018;30(4):549–554.

51. Frontera W, Meredith C, O'Reilly K, Knuttgen H, Evans W. Strength conditioning in older men: skeletal muscle hypertrophy and improved function. *J Appl Physiol.* 1988;64(3):1038–1044.
52. Avers D, Brown M. White paper: strength training for the older adult. *J Geriatr Phys Ther.* 2009;32(4):148–152.
53. Silva RB, Aldoradin-Cabeza H, Eslick GD, Phu S, Duque G. The effect of physical exercise on frail older persons: a systematic review. *J Frailty Aging.* 2017;6(2):91–96.
54. de Labra C, Guimaraes-Pinheiro C, Maseda A, Lorenzo T, Millán-Calenti JC. Effects of physical exercise interventions in frail older adults: a systematic review of randomized controlled trials. *BMC Geriatr.* 2015;15(1):154.
55. Ferreira CB, Teixeira P dos S, Alves dos Santos G, et al. Effects of a 12-week exercise training program on physical function in institutionalized frail elderly. *J Aging Res.* 2018;2018:1–8.
56. Lopez P, Pinto RS, Radaelli R, et al. Benefits of resistance training in physically frail elderly: a systematic review. *Aging Clin Exp Res.* 2018;30(8):889–899.
57. Sahin UK, Kirdi N, Bozoglu E, et al. Effect of low-intensity versus high-intensity resistance training on the functioning of the institutionalized frail elderly. *Int J Rehabil Res.* 2018;41 (3): 211–217.
58. Cadore EL, Pinto RS, Bottaro M, Izquierdo M. Strength and endurance training prescription in healthy and frail elderly. *Aging Dis.* 2014;5(3):183–195.
59. Cadore EL, Rodríguez-Mañas L, Sinclair A, Izquierdo M. Effects of different exercise interventions on risk of falls, gait ability, and balance in physically frail older adults: a systematic review. *Rejuvenation Res.* 2013;16(2):105–114.
60. Cadore EL, Casas-Herrero A, Zambom-Ferraresi F, et al. Multicomponent exercises including muscle power training enhance muscle mass, power output, and functional outcomes in institutionalized frail nonagenarians. *Age (Omaha).* 2014;36(2):773–785.
61. Reid KF, Martin KI, Doros G, et al. Comparative effects of light or heavy resistance power training for improving lower extremity power and physical performance in mobility-limited older adults. *J Gerontol Ser A Biol Sci Med Sci.* 2015;70 (3):374–380.
62. Izquierdo M, Cadore EL. Muscle power training in the institutionalized frail: a new approach to counteracting functional declines and very late-life disability. *Curr Med Res Opin.* 2014;30(7):1385–1390.
63. Manini TM, Druger M, Ploutz-Snyder L. Misconceptions about strength exercise among older adults. *J Aging Phys Act.* 2005;13(4):422–433.
64. Spirduso WW, Cronin DL. Exercise dose-response effects on quality of life and independent living in older adults. *Med Sci Sports Exerc.* 2001;33(6):S598–S608.
65. Guralnik JM, Ferrucci L, Simonsick EM, Salive ME, Wallace RB. Lower-extremity function in persons over the age of 70 years as a predictor of subsequent disability. *N Engl J Med.* 1995;332(9):556–562.
66. Gill TM, Williams CS, Tinetti ME. Assessing risk for the onset of functional dependence among older adults: the role of physical performance. *J Am Geriatr Soc.* 1995;43(6):603–609.
67. Brach JS, VanSwearingen JM, Newman AB, Kriska AM. Identifying early decline of physical function in community-dwelling older women: performance-based and self-report measures. *Phys Ther.* 2002;82(4):320–328.
68. Fritz S, Lusardi M. White paper: "walking speed: the sixth vital sign". *J Geriatr Phys Ther.* 2009;32(2):2–5.
69. Potter JM, Evans AL, Duncan G. Gait speed and activities of daily living function in geriatric patients. *Arch Phys Med Rehabil.* 1995;76(11):997–999.
70. Kuys SS, Peel NM, Klein K, Slater A, Hubbard RE. Gait speed in ambulant older people in long term care: a systematic review and meta-analysis. *J Am Med Dir Assoc.* 2014;15:194–200.
71. Onder G, Penninx BWJH, Lapuerta P, et al. Change in physical performance over time in older women: the Women's Health and Aging Study. *J Gerontol A Biol Sci Med Sci.* 2002;57 (5):M289–M293.
72. Rubenstein LZ, Powers CM, MacLean CH. Quality indicators for the management and prevention of falls and mobility problems in vulnerable elders. *Ann Intern Med.* 2001;135 (8 part 2):686.
73. Rogers ME, Rogers NL, Takeshima N, Islam MM. Methods to assess and improve the physical parameters associated with fall risk in older adults. *Prev Med.* 2003;36(3):255–264.
74. Wollesen B, Schulz S, Seydell L, Delbaere K. Does dual task training improve walking performance of older adults with concern of falling? *BMC Geriatr.* 2017;17(1):213.
75. Wollesen B, Mattes K, Schulz S, et al. Effects of dual-task management and resistance training on gait performance in older individuals: a randomized controlled trial. *Front Aging Neurosci.* 2017;9:415.
76. Lesinski M, Hortobágyi T, Muehlbauer T, Gollhofer A, Granacher U. Effects of balance training on balance performance in healthy older adults: a systematic review and meta-analysis. *Sport Med.* 2015;45(12):1721–1738.
77. Eckardt N. Lower-extremity resistance training on unstable surfaces improves proxies of muscle strength, power and balance in healthy older adults: a randomised control trial. *BMC Geriatr.* 2016;16(1):191.
78. Vlaeyen E, Coussement J, Leysens G, et al. Characteristics and effectiveness of fall prevention programs in nursing homes: a systematic review and meta-analysis of randomized controlled trials. *J Am Geriatr Soc.* 2015;63(2):211–221.
79. Avin KG, Hanke TA, Kirk-Sanchez N, et al. Management of falls in community-dwelling older adults: clinical guidance statement from the academy of geriatric physical therapy of the American Physical Therapy Association. *Phys Ther.* 2015;95(6):815–834.
80. Center for Medicaid and State Operations/Survey and Certification Group. *Freedom from Unnecessary Physical Restraints: Two Decades of National Progress in Nursing Home Care.* Vol S&C-09-11. Baltimore, MD: US Government Printing Office; 2008.
81. Hartley Greg, Kirk-Sanchez N. Fall risk in community-dwelling elders. *PT Now*; 2017. https://www.ptnow.org/clinical-summaries-detail/fall-risk-in-communitydwelling-elders#Examination.
82. Möhler R, Meyer G. Development methods of guidelines and documents with recommendations on physical restraint reduction in nursing homes: a systematic review. *BMC Geriatr.* 2015;15(1):152.
83. Bartoszek G, Fischer U, Grill E, Müller M, Nadolny S, Meyer G. Impact of joint contracture on older persons in a geriatric setting. *Z Gerontol Geriatr.* 2015;48(7):625–632.
84. Wagner LM, Capezuti E, Brush BL, Clevenger C, Boltz M, Renz S. Contractures in frail nursing home residents. *Geriatr Nurs.* 2008;29(4):259–266.
85. Saal S, Beutner K, Bogunski J, et al. Interventions for the prevention and treatment of disability due to acquired joint contractures in older people: a systematic review. *Age Ageing.* 2017;46(3):373–382.
86. Prabhu RK, Swaminathan N, Harvey LA. Passive movements for the treatment and prevention of contractures. *Cochrane Database Syst Rev.* 2013;12:CD009331.
87. Park-Lee Eunice, Caffrey C. *Pressure ulcers among nursing home residents: United States, 2004. NCHS Data Br No 14.* https://www.cdc.gov/nchs/products/databriefs/db14.htm; 2009.
88. Centers for Medicare and Medicaid Services. *Nursing Home Data Compendium.* 2015 Edition. Washington, DC: Department of Health & Human Services; 2015. https://www.cms.gov/Medicare/Provider.../nursinghomedatacompendium_508-2015.pdf.

89. Jaul E. Assessment and management of pressure ulcers in the elderly: current strategies. *Drugs Aging.* 2010;27(4): 311–325.
90. Gillespie BM, Chaboyer WP, McInnes E, Kent B, Whitty JA, Thalib L. Repositioning for pressure ulcer prevention in adults. *Cochrane Database Syst Rev.* 2014;4:CD009958.
91. Moore ZE, Cowman S. Repositioning for treating pressure ulcers. *Cochrane Database Syst Rev.* 2015;(1): CD006898.
92. McInnes E, Jammali-Blasi A, Bell-Syer SE, Dumville JC, Middleton V, Cullum N. Support surfaces for pressure ulcer prevention. *Cochrane Database Syst Rev.* 2015;9: CD001735.
93. Posthauer ME, Banks M, Dorner B, Schols JMGA. The role of nutrition for pressure ulcer management. *Adv Skin Wound Care.* 2015;28(4):175–188.
94. MacRae PG, Asplund LA, Schnelle JF, et al. A walking program for nursing home residents: effects on walk endurance, physical activity, mobility, and quality of life. *J Am Geriatr Soc.* 1996;44(2):175–180.
95. Koroknay VJ, Werner P, Cohen-Mansfield J, Braun JV. Maintaining ambulation in the frail nursing home resident: a nursing administered walking program. *J Gerontol Nurs.* 1995;21(11):18–24.
96. Venturelli M, Scarsini R, Schena F. Six-month walking program changes cognitive and ADL performance in patients with Alzheimer. *Am J Alzheimer's Dis Other Dementias.* 2011; 26(5):381–388.
97. Centers for Medicare & Medicaid Services. *MLN Matters®. Number: MM8458 Related Change Request Number: 8458*; U.S. Government Printing Office; 2014.
98. Buhr GT, Kuchibhatla M, Clipp EC. Caregivers' reasons for nursing home placement: clues for improving discussions with families prior to the transition. *Gerontologist.* 2006;46(1): 52–61.
99. Seitz D, Purandare N, Conn D. Prevalence of psychiatric disorders among older adults in long-term care homes: a systematic review. *Int Psychogeriatrics.* 2010;22(07):1025–1039.
100. Blumenthal JA, Babyak MA, Doraiswamy PM, et al. Exercise and pharmacotherapy in the treatment of major depressive disorder. *Psychosom Med.* 2007;69(7):587–596.
101. Heyn P, Abreu BC, Ottenbacher KJ. The effects of exercise training on elderly persons with cognitive impairment and dementia: a meta-analysis. *Arch Phys Med Rehabil.* 2004;85 (10):1694–1704.
102. Littbrand H, Rosendahl E, Lindelöf N, Lundin-Olsson L, Gustafson Y, Nyberg L. A high-intensity functional weight-bearing exercise program for older people dependent in activities of daily living and living in residential care facilities: evaluation of the applicability with focus on cognitive function. *Phys Ther.* 2006;86(4):489–498.
103. Cadore EL, Moneo ABB, Mensat MM, et al. Positive effects of resistance training in frail elderly patients with dementia after long-term physical restraint. *Age (Omaha).* 2014;36(2): 801–811.

CHAPTER

26

Home Health Management of the Older Adult

Christine E. Fordyce

OUTLINE

INTRODUCTION

Providing care in the home is a unique way to deliver geriatric rehabilitation to older adults who are homebound. On any given day, the home care clinician may be the only health care professional to see the patient. Although home care offers a great deal of autonomy, the home care clinician must be able to coordinate the patient's care with other members of the team, work in collaboration with other health care providers, and teach available caregivers. Home care has several advantages. The clinician spends one-on-one time with the patient in average durations of 45 to 60 minutes, with a relatively low full-time caseload of about five or six patients a day. Most home health agencies and patients allow the therapist to set the time of the visit, often accommodating the therapist's schedule. The therapist can work with the family caregiver, or both, within the patient's actual setting to provide care that is relevant to the patient's environment and needs. Home care also presents unique challenges for the physical therapist. Although the home care setting has inherent autonomy, it also presents situational isolation from other health professionals, documentation requirements, variability, and unanticipated circumstances, and requires efficient time management.

Nearly all older adults prefer to age in their homes and communities as opposed to an institutional facility. An unsafe environment and inaccessibility to the home can pose challenging obstacles to aging in place. Therefore, clinicians caring for older adults need to be prepared to make best-practice decisions regarding the reality of honoring the patient's goal of aging in place. This chapter discusses the unique features, as well as federally mandated characteristics, of the home care provision benefit under Medicare Part A, and the sequence and scope of an episode of care.

DEFINITION OF HOMEBOUND

To receive coverage under the Medicare benefit, patients must be "homebound" or "confined to the home."[1] An individual is considered confined to home if the following criteria are met:

Criteria One

- "the patient must either, because of an injury or illness, need the aid of support devices (such as crutches, canes, wheelchairs and walkers; the use of special transportation; or the assistance of another person to leave the home)"

- "OR have a condition that leaving the home is medically contraindicated."

If the patient meets one of the above conditions, then the patient must also meet two additional requirements, referred to as Criterion Two:

Criterion Two
- "there must exist a normal inability to leave home
- "AND leaving the home must require a considerable and taxing effort."[1]

However, "considerable and taxing effort" is not defined and therefore is left to the interpretation of the therapist, agency, and intermediary. See Box 26.1 for examples of how to document considerable and taxing effort.

Thus, as part of the initial home health visit and on all subsequent visits, the clinician must identify the functional criteria that support the patient's homebound status. Medicare provides for the patient to leave the home under certain conditions and still be homebound if the absences from the home are infrequent or for periods of relatively short duration or are attributable to the need to receive health care treatment. Examples of home bound criteria defined by Centers for Medicare & Medicaid Services (CMS) are listed in Box 26.2. Therapy services can also be provided to patients in their homes under the Medicare Outpatient Part B benefit. For this benefit, patients do not need to be considered homebound, but the travel time to the patient's home is not reimbursable.

BOX 26.1 Examples of Statements That Can Justify Home Care

- After returning home from an outing, the patient requires 2 hours of rest as a result of exhaustion from the trip.
- The patient scored >15 seconds on the Four Square Step Test, indicating the need for assistance of one person to safely exit the home as a result of fall risk.
- The patient reports a Borg score of >12 while ambulating inside the home and is therefore homebound as a result of the taxing effort ambulation requires.
- Decreased cognition as evidenced by the Mini Mental Status score indicates the patient requires the assistance of one person to exit the home safely.
- The patient lives in an apartment building and is unable to safely negotiate stairs as a result of partial weight-bearing status after total hip arthroplasty to exit home.
- The patient reports a Borg RPE of >12 after descending and ascending 14 stairs required to enter his or her home and is therefore homebound as a result of the taxing effort required to leave the home.
- The patient is unable to ambulate >1000 feet and has a gait speed of <0.8 m/s and a reported Borg RPE of ≥11 and is therefore homebound because the patient is unable to safely ambulate community distances at a gait speed required for community ambulators.

RPE, rate of perceived exertion.

BOX 26.2 Centers for Medicare & Medicaid Services Definition of Homebound Status

If the patient does in fact leave the home, the patient may nevertheless be considered homebound if the absences attributable to the need to receive health care treatment include, but are not limited to:
- Attendance at adult day centers to receive medical care;
- Ongoing receipt of outpatient kidney dialysis; or
- The receipt of outpatient chemotherapy or radiation therapy.

Examples of allowed visits so long as they are infrequent and of short duration include:
- health care treatment.
- an occasional trip to the barber,
- a walk around the block or a drive,
- attendance at a family reunion, funeral, graduation, or
- other infrequent or unique event

Some examples of homebound patients that illustrate the factors used to determine whether a homebound condition exists are listed below.
- A patient paralyzed from a stroke who is confined to a wheelchair or requires the aid of crutches in order to walk.
- A patient who is blind or senile and requires the assistance of another person in leaving their place of residence.
- A patient who has lost the use of their upper extremities and, therefore, is unable to open doors, use handrails on stairways, etc., and requires the assistance of another individual to leave their place of residence.
- A patient in the late stages of ALS or neurodegenerative disabilities. In determining whether the patient has the general inability to leave the home and leaves the home only infrequently or for periods of short duration, it is necessary (as is the case in determining whether skilled nursing services are intermittent) to look at the patient's condition over a period of time rather than for short periods within the home health stay. For example, a patient may leave the home (meeting both criteria listed above) more frequently during a short period when the patient has multiple appointments with health care professionals and medical tests in 1 week. So long as the patient's overall condition and experience is such that he or she meets these qualifications, he or she should be considered confined to the home.
- A patient who has just returned from a hospital stay involving surgery, who may be suffering from resultant weakness and pain because of the surgery and; therefore, their actions may be restricted by their physician to certain specified and limited activities (such as getting out of bed only for a specified period of time, walking stairs only once a day, etc.).
- A patient with arteriosclerotic heart disease of such severity that they must avoid all stress and physical activity.
- A patient with a psychiatric illness that is manifested in part by a refusal to leave home or is of such a nature that it would not be considered safe for the patient to leave home unattended, even if they have no physical limitations.

The aged person who does not often travel from home because of feebleness and insecurity brought on by advanced age would not be considered confined to the home for purposes of receiving home health services unless they meet one of the above conditions. Although a patient must be confined to the home to be eligible for covered home health services, some services cannot be provided at the patient's residence because equipment is required that cannot

Continued

BOX 26.2 Centers for Medicare & Medicaid Services Definition of Homebound Status—cont'd

be made available there. If the services required by an individual involve the use of such equipment, the HHA may make arrangements with a hospital, SNF, or a rehabilitation center to provide these services on an outpatient basis. (See §50.6.) However, even in these situations, for the services to be covered as home health services the patient must be considered confined to home and meet both criteria listed above.

If a question is raised as to whether a patient is confined to the home, the HHA will be requested to furnish the Medicare contractor with the information necessary to establish that the patient is homebound as defined above.

From Medicare benefit policy manual, Chapter 7, Home health services; 2017. http://www.cms.hhs.gov/manuals/Downloads/bp102c07.pdf. Accessed April14, 2018.

ROLE OF THE PHYSICAL THERAPIST IN HOME HEALTH

The fundamental roles of the older adult–oriented home care physical therapist is to promote independence in essential activities of daily living (ADLs), promote reintegration of the patient into the community, and minimize the risk for recurrent acute care hospitalizations and/or nursing home admission. According to a 2015 study of 1248 participants conducted by the National Alliance for Caregiving (NAC) and the AARP Public Policy Institute, caregivers spend 24.4 hours a week on average providing care to their loved ones.[2] Sixty percent of caregivers report helping their loved ones with at least one ADL, and most commonly report helping with bed and chair transfers.[2] Thus, home care therapists play a key role in teaching caregivers a variety of safety techniques, including proper patient positioning for transfers and fall prevention. The patient's home environment provides a rich context for the therapist to gain insight into the patient's functional abilities, particularly the performance of essential ADLs such as bathing, dressing, walking inside the house, and transferring from a chair. Frequently, hospitalization or inactivity leads to the development of restriction of essential ADLs. Furthermore, individuals who lose their ability to perform valued functional and social activities are more likely to become dissatisfied with their quality of life and are likely to experience depression, increasing the likelihood of being homebound.[3] The effect of decreased physical activity and functioning promotes further decline on the slippery slope of aging[4] and increases the risk for physical frailty, recurrent disability, multiple hospitalizations, and eventual nursing home admission.[5] The home care physical therapist has a critical role to play in this transitional setting between a higher level of function and institutionalization.

Rehospitalization

The process by which patients move from hospitals to other care settings is increasingly problematic as hospitals shorten lengths of stay and care becomes more fragmented. Within 30 days of discharge, there was a 17.5% rate of hospital readmissions in 2015 for targeted conditions of myocardial infarction, heart failure, and pneumonia.[6] Patients between the ages of 75 and 84 years accounted for the highest number of 30-day hospital readmissions and 35.6% of hospital readmissions in 2015.[7] Eleven percent of hospital readmissions are directly related to nonadherence to medication recommendations.[7] Medicare's cost for these unplanned readmissions is estimated to be nearly $40 billion.[8] The most frequent reasons for unplanned readmissions were acute myocardial infarction, heart failure, pneumonia, sepsis, dehydration, postoperative infection, and gastrointestinal bleeding.[8] Unplanned rehospitalizations are almost always medical emergencies and often signal failure of the transition from the hospital to another source of care.

Avoidable admissions and readmissions can be related to a lack of care coordination and poor discharge planning. However, environmental, community, and patient-level factors, including sociodemographic factors, can also affect the risk of readmission. The complexity of what causes avoidable admissions and readmissions means that providers across the health care continuum, including hospitals, skilled nursing facilities, and clinicians in the community, must work together to ensure high-quality care transitions by improving care coordination across providers and engaging patients and their families.[8]

The three main drivers of unplanned rehospitalizations are (1) the patient and family not being engaged in the health care process, (2) gaps in processes within a provider or provider group (e.g., not having a focused plan of care for patients with congestive heart failure or not having a uniform discharge transfer tool), and (3) no existing process to communicate information between providers at discharge such as the next care provider and the primary care physician (PCP). The evidence of national and individual home health agency's success is demonstrated with publicly reported comparative measures (Box 26.3).

Rosati and coworkers[9] identified several risk factors for medical adverse events (listed in Box 26.4) among home health care recipients and found that home health agencies that focused on these risk factors were more likely to improve the effectiveness and efficiency of their efforts to prevent rehospitalization of their patients.[9] Home health physical therapists who address a patient's fall risk and physical functioning decline can play a key role in the prevention of unplanned hospital readmissions. A continued focus on reducing the factors contributing to rehospitalization to promote cost containment will continue in the foreseeable future, with physical therapists continuing to play a significant role.

BOX 26.3 Publicly Reported Comparative Measures for Home Health Agencies (Star Ratings)

List of Quality Measures

Process of Care Measures

Process of care measures show how often home health agencies gave recommended care or treatments that research shows get the best results for most patients. The list of process measures includes:

Process Measures	As Listed on Home Health Compare	Data Source
Timely initiation of care	How often the home health team began their patients' care in a timely manner.	OASIS
Influenza immunization received for current flu season	How often the home health team made sure that their patients have received a flu shot for the current flu season.	OASIS
Pneumococcal polysaccharide vaccine ever received	How often the home health team made sure that their patients have received a pneumococcal vaccine (pneumonia shot).	OASIS
Diabetic foot care and patient education implemented	For patients with diabetes, how often the home health team got doctor's orders, gave foot care, and taught patients about foot care.	OASIS
Depression assessment conducted	How often the home health team checked patients for depression.	OASIS
Drug education on all medications provided to patient/caregiver	How often the home health team taught patients (or their family caregivers) about their drugs.	OASIS
Multifactor fall risk assessment conducted for all patients who can ambulate	How often the home health team checked patients' risk of falling.	OASIS

Process of Care Measures

Outcome of Care Measures

Outcome of care measures show the results of care given by the home health agency. There are 2 types of outcome measures reported on Home Health Compare:

- Improvement measures
- Health care utilization measures

Improvement measures fall into 3 categories: those describing a patient's ability to get around, those describing a patient's ability to perform activities of daily living, and those describing their general health status.

Health care utilization measures describe how often patients access other health care resources either while home health care is in progress or after home health care is completed.

The list of outcome measures includes:

Outcome Measures	As Listed on Home Health Compare	Data Source
Improvement in ambulation	How often patients got better at walking or moving around.	OASIS
Improvement in bed transfer	How often patients got better at getting in and out of bed.	OASIS
Improvement in pain interfering with activity	How often patients had less pain when moving around.	OASIS
Improvement in bathing	How often patients got better at bathing.	OASIS
Improvement in management of oral medications	How often patients got better at taking their drugs correctly by mouth.	OASIS
Improvement in dyspnea	How often patients' breathing improved.	OASIS
Improvement in status of surgical wounds	How often patients' wounds improved or healed after an operation.	OASIS
Acute care hospitalizations	How often home health patients had to be admitted to the hospital.	Medicare Claims
Emergency department use without hospitalization	How often patients receiving home health care needed any urgent, unplanned care in the hospital emergency room—without being admitted to the hospital.	Medicare Claims
Rehospitalization during the first 30 days of home health	How often home health patients, who have had a recent hospital stay, had to be readmitted to the hospital.	Medicare Claims
Emergency department use without hospital readmission during the first 30 days of home health	How often home health patients, who have had a recent hospital stay, received care in the hospital emergency room without being readmitted to the hospital.	Medicare Claims

From Medicare—the official U.S. Government site for people with Medicare. Home health compare. https://www.medicare.gov/HomeHealthCompare/Data/List-Quality-Measures.html. http://www.medicare.gov/HHCompare/Home.asp?dest=NAV|Home|DataDetails#TabTop. Accessed April 29, 2010.

BOX 26.4 Risk Factors for Medical Adverse Events

- Pattern of one or more hospitalizations or emergency room visits in the past 12 months
- History of falls
- Chronic conditions such as congestive heart failure, skin ulcers, or congestive obstructive pulmonary disease
- Social and cognitive factors such as inadequate support network, low literacy level, dementia, needing help with managing medications, or low socioeconomic status

Modified from Rosati RJ, Huang L, Navaie-Waliser M, Feldman PH. Risk factors for repeated hospitalizations among home healthcare recipients. *J Healthc Qual.* 2003;25(2):4–10.

In 2012, CMS introduced the Hospital Readmissions Reduction Program. CMS measures excess hospital readmissions by a ratio determined by adding up a hospital's predicted 30-day readmissions for the penalty diagnosis (heart attack, heart failure, pneumonia, chronic obstructive pulmonary disease, hip and knee replacement, and coronary artery bypass graft surgery) divided by the number that would be expected based on average hospital readmission with similar patients.[10] Since the introduction of this program, many home health agencies have introduced performance improvement plans targeted on decreasing patient hospital readmissions, specifically targeting those cases with the penalty diagnoses. Rehospitalization percentages are publicly reported for consumers on Home Health Compare (see Box 26.3).

Variability of the Home Environment

In addition to the medical management of the patient, providing physical therapy care in the patient's home presents unique personal challenges. Whether or not the home is one of cramped conditions or a well-maintained residence with lots of space, the therapist is literally a guest in someone's home and must be able to project a sincere attitude of caring while conveying respect for the desire of the older adult to remain at home. The clinician has to be sensitive to and respectful of any boundaries the patient sets with respect to the home environment and aspects of care provided. The home health clinician may encounter a wide variety of socioeconomic, ethnic, and cultural situations. Sensitivity to patient beliefs and background is needed to help gain trust and establish rapport with the home health patient. Clinicians in the home setting are likely to encounter a variety of cultural dynamics. Depending on the patient's culture, self-care may not be an important personal goal, and therefore it may be inappropriate to insist that an older adult patient provide self-care, especially when family members or paid caregivers are available and willing to provide care.

In some cultures, older adults are considered to be "entitled" to rest and to be cared for at home. In fact, the majority of cultures do not consider self-care to be an important goal of aging, including Asian, Hispanic, African, and almost all other cultures other than Anglo American. These cultures value family interdependence over independence and therefore may believe it is inappropriate for an older adult to insist on self-care when family members are available to provide care. Moreover, younger caregivers may be quite willing to attend to older loved ones as a natural and normal family dynamic. However, although there is great diversity in American culture, American health care providers typically promote continued self-reliance and the maintenance of independence with age. Whereas independence in traditional American culture is not only the expectation but also a source of self-esteem, dependence can be a source of significant emotional and psychological distress.

Some clients or patients may prefer to have family members present during physical therapy sessions and, depending on the degree of family involvement, there may be the need for additional teaching and explanations. By contrast, the physical therapist may be able to work more effectively with the patient when there are no family "observers" because the patient may be reluctant to demonstrate functional independence in front of family caregivers. Sensitivity to cultural differences, such as acceptability of being touched, in particular by someone of the opposite gender; verbal and nonverbal expressions of pain; and patient-specific goal setting, allows clinicians to adapt care in a manner that is congruent with their patients' cultural expectations.

Lastly, providing care in the home involves having to adapt to a variety of structural barriers, sensitivity to the homeowner who may not be the patient, and lifestyle preferences of the patient and caregivers. Patients typically have daily routines, routines that when disrupted can be sources of stress and conflict. Home health therapists have to take these concerns into account when scheduling treatment times. In addition, homes can range widely from being very tidy to being cluttered, presenting fall risk hazards. All of these variables can make it challenging to prescribe an effective exercise program, and a substantial degree of creativity is needed to make the best of a particular situation. Box 26.5 lists universal recommendations and resources for improving knowledge about different cultures and ethnicities.

DOCUMENTATION

The Medicare Payment Advisory Commission (MedPAC) classifies Home Health as a postacute setting,[11] and payment is administered under the Medicare Part A program. MedPAC advises CMS on setting payment rates for all Medicare providers. Similar to other settings, Medicare sets payment rates based on the patient's medical complexity and expected resource use. In 2015, Medicare spent $18.1 billion on home health services for about 3.5 million Medicare beneficiaries.[11] From 2002 to 2015, home health utilization has increased significantly with a noted 60% increase in the number of episodes of care.[11]

BOX 26.5 Universal Recommendations for Improving Cultural and Ethnicity Knowledge

1. Learn from patients.
   - Respectfully ask patients about their health beliefs and customs. For example: "Is there anything I should know about your culture, beliefs, religious practices, or preferences that would help me take better care of you."
   - Avoid stereotyping based on religious or cultural background. Recognize each person as an individual who may or may not adhere to certain cultural beliefs or practices common to his or her culture.
2. Learn from other sources.
   - Think Cultural Health offers several options for free continuing education credit. https://www.thinkculturalhealth.hhs.gov/education
   - EthnoMED contains information about cultural beliefs, medical issues, and related topics pertinent to the health care of immigrants and refugees. This site also has patient information in a variety of languages. http://ethnomed.org/
   - Race/Ethnicity culture, language and health literacy resources provides resources about several races and ethnicities, including African Americans, Asian Americans, Native Hawaiians and other Pacific Islanders, Native American, Hispanics and Latinos, and special populations such as farm and migrant workers; homeless populations; and lesbian, gay, bisexual, and transgender populations. https://www.hrsa.gov/cultural-competence/race.html
   - Community organizations such as religious institutions and cultural organizations (e.g., invite a member of a relevant cultural group to address a staff meeting)
   - Use interpreters as cultural brokers who can educate regarding specific meanings and cultural differences.

Adapted from: "Tool 10. Consider Culture, Customs, and Beliefs." Health Literacy Universal Precautions Toolkit (2e). Agency for Healthcare Research and Quality; Rockville, MD. February 2015. http://www.ahrq.gov/professionals/quality-patient-safety/quality-resources/tools/literacy-toolkit/healthlittoolkit2-tool10.html.

The Outcome and Assessment Information Set (OASIS) instrument, in use since July 1999, is used by the Home Health Agency (HHA) nurse or therapist to assess the patient's condition. The OASIS instrument has been revised several times since then, with the latest version at the time of this writing called the OASIS-C2. Physical therapy is one of the three qualifying disciplines authorized to collect the initial OASIS data as part of the patient's comprehensive assessment at the start of care. Skilled nursing and speech–language pathology are the other two qualifying disciplines authorized to collect OASIS data at the start of care. This initial visit serves to assess if the patient meets home health coverage criteria; the patient's condition; and the patient's likely needs for skilled nursing care, therapy, medical social services, and home health aide services.

Home Health Documentation Requirements

The Medicare Conditions of Participation for Home Health mandate an initial comprehensive, individual, and specific assessment of each patient. Whether the therapist is documenting on paper-based forms or electronically, the initial home health visit can average 90 minutes to complete the initial comprehensive assessment. In addition to the OASIS instrument, therapists may also have to document the patient's medication profile that includes all of the prescription and over-the-counter medication, including herbs and supplements. When a home health case is "therapy only," the physical therapist may spend a great deal of time at the initial visit on resolving medication discrepancies between the hospital discharge medication list and the patient's actual medications in the home. Follow-up with the primary care physicians and specialists to resolve discrepancies or to obtain a referral for a nurse is often necessary. Until the therapist becomes familiar with the OASIS instrument and more practiced in completing medication profiles, the initial home health visit with an OASIS assessment can take as much as 2 hours. Most importantly, the primary focus for a physical therapist conducting a home health admission is to ensure that the patient is safe at home and to refer to other disciplines or services when appropriate. An explanation of the services covered by Medicare for Home Health is presented in Box 26.6.

OASIS rules and conventions are described in detail in the OASIS Guidance Manual and are periodically updated with information available at the CMS website.[12] In 2017, CMS issued a final rule on the Conditions of Participation for Home Health Agencies that became effective in January of 2018 representing a comprehensive update for home health agencies to adopt into practice.[13] Competence in assessment of all areas of the OASIS may require additional knowledge and practice skills in differential diagnosis, pharmacology, skin assessment, depression screening, and home safety assessment. Given the uniqueness of the home health admission, the therapist new to the home care setting can benefit greatly from a guided practical orientation with a peer mentor. The mentor can role model how to efficiently conduct the sequence of interview questions that correspond with OASIS data items.

Specific observations of the patient's functional abilities such as transfers, dressing, and walking are also necessary for accurate responses to OASIS items and serve as the basis for planning the teaching that a therapist would provide the patient. The length of time a patient, family, or caregiver may require for education interventions should be determined by assessing each patient's individual condition and other pertinent factors such as the skill required to teach the activity and the unique abilities of the patient. It is important to know that teaching activities must be related to the patient's functional loss, illness, or injury. When a patient or caregiver is incapable of learning, more visits to provide patient and caregiver education are subject to Medicare payment denials. Medicare's home health benefit is not intended to provide training and education to patients, families, or caregivers for an infinite period of time.

BOX 26.6 Skilled Services for Home Health Covered by Medicare Part A

Skilled Nursing (SN)
- Observation and assessment of the patient's condition
- Medication management, assessment, and teaching
- Tube feedings
- Nasopharyngeal and tracheotomy aspiration
- Catheters, wound care, heat treatments, medical gases, rehabilitation nursing, venipuncture, psychiatric evaluation, therapy, and teaching

Speech–Language Pathology (SLP)
- A change in functional speech or motivation
- Clearing of confusion
- The remission of some other medical condition that previously contraindicated SLP services

Occupational Therapy (OT)
- Selecting and teaching task-oriented therapeutic activities designed to restore physical function
- Planning, implementing, and supervising therapeutic tasks and activities designed to restore sensory-integrative function (vision and cognition)
- Planning, implementing, and supervising individualized therapeutic activity programs as part of an overall "active treatment" program with a patient diagnosed with psychiatric illness
- Teaching compensatory techniques to improve the level of independence in the activities of daily living
- Designing, fabricating, and fitting of orthotic and self-help devices
- Vocational and prevocational assessment and training
- Patient must have a continued need for OT when: the services meet the definition of OT and the patient's eligibility has been established by virtue of a prior need for skilled nursing care, SLP, or PT in the current or prior certification period

Medical Social Services (MSW)
- Assessment of the social and emotional factors related to the patient's illness, need for care, response to treatment, and adjustment to care
- Assessment of the relationship of the patient's medical and nursing requirements to the patient's home situation, financial resources, and availability of community resources
- Appropriate action to obtain available community resources to assist in resolving the patient's problem
- Medicare does not cover the services of MSWs to complete application for Medicaid
- Counseling services that are required by the patient
- Services of MSWs are covered if they are necessary to resolve social or emotional problems that are or expected to be an impediment to the effective treatment of the patient's medical condition *and* the plan of care indicates how the services necessitate the skills of a qualified MSW to be performed safely and effectively
- Covered on a short-term basis and agency must demonstrate that a brief MSW intervention is necessary to remove a clear and direct impediment to the effective treatment of the patient's medical condition or to the patient's rate of recovery

Home Health Aide (HHA)
- Patient care
- Simple dressing changes that do not require the skills of a licensed nurse
- Assistance with medications which are ordinarily self-administered and do not require the skills of a licensed nurse to be provided safely and effectively
- Assistance with activities that are directly supportive of skilled therapy services but do not require the skills of a licensed nurse to be provided safely and effectively
- Assistance with activities that are directly supportive of skilled therapy services but do not require the skills of a therapist to be safely and effectively performed, such as routine maintenance exercises and repetitive practice of functional communication skills to support SLP services
- Provision of services incidental to personal care services; however, the purpose of an HHA visit may not be only to provide incidental services (light cleaning, preparation of a meal, taking out the trash, shopping, and so on)
- Must be intermittent and patient is being case managed by an SN, PT, OT, or SLP

From Centers for Medicare & Medicaid Services: Medicare benefit policy manual. http://www.cms.hhs.gov/manuals/Downloads/bp102c07.pdf. Accessed August 24, 2018.

THE INITIAL VISIT

This section describes the features of best practices for the first visit for a home care patient under Medicare Part A. The author suggests contacting the patient before the initial visit to arrange a time that is convenient and to request the patient have a Medicare card and all medications (including over-the-counter medications) available and ready for review. Also, the patient may prefer to have a family member or friend present. Calling ahead is useful because Medicare does not require a patient to be home 24/7 to be considered homebound. Asking the patient or family member to have the Medicare card and medications ready will help to make the time spent in the patient's home more efficient. Items recommended to have available on the first and subsequent visits are listed in Box 26.7. It is valuable to carry everything in a clinical travel bag. In addition to the bag, home health therapists should always carry a cell phone and keep car keys on their person at all times in case of an emergency.

The Comprehensive Start of Care OASIS and Consent (Full Disclosure)

Opening a Case. Arguably, the primary focus of opening a case is to complete the OASIS, assure the patient is safe to be in his or her home, and refer to other skilled services when appropriate. As mentioned previously, opening a case for an experienced clinician typically takes 1 to 2 hours depending on the complexity of the patient and home situation. The OASIS document serves as a guideline for the clinician to ensure a comprehensive assessment.

BOX 26.7 Items for the Clinical Bag

The Clinical Bag—Essential Items to Pack for the Trip

Blood pressure cuff
Cardiopulmonary resuscitation mask
Disinfectant wipes for equipment
Gait belt
Girth measurement tape
Goniometer
Hand soap
Paper towels
Personal protective equipment (gloves, mask, gowns)
Reflex hammer
Sterile wound care supplies
Stethoscope
Stopwatch
Tape measure
Thermometer

Additional Useful Items

1000 feet or more measuring wheel
Balance pad
Elastic tube/bands
Masking tape
Pedal ergometer
Pulse oximeter
Weighted vest

Tip: Assessment of Urinary and Bowel Incontinence

The OASIS assessment requires the physical therapist to assess for urinary and bowel incontinence. When interviewing the patient, he or she may deny this condition especially in the presence of family members or friends. The clinician may need to do some "detective work" (or sense of smell) to answer this question correctly. During the assessment of activities of daily living and instrumental activities of daily living section of the OASIS when the patient is up and moving around the house, look for adult diapers in the bathroom or next to the patient's bed.

The results of the OASIS will help the clinician determine if there are issues in an area beyond the scope of physical therapy. The clinician is ethically obligated to refer to the appropriate service for additional assessment and intervention. For example, if the patient is having difficulty in the OASIS area of Living Arrangements, Supportive Assistance, and Emotional/Behavioral status, the physical therapist may consider a referral to social work services. If the patient is having difficulties in the areas of sensation, cognition, vision, ADLs, or instrumental activities of daily living (IADLs), the clinician may consider a referral for speech–language pathology or occupational therapy. An occupational therapist can also assist the patient with equipment needs and management. If the patient is having difficulties in the areas of integumentary, respiratory, cardiovascular, urinary, gastrointestinal, or medication management, the clinician may consider a referral to a skilled nurse. The need for a home health aide should also be assessed at the start of care. A patient who is receiving home health services under the Medicare Part A benefit is entitled to receive all the skilled health care provider services needed under the Medicare benefit. See Box 26.6 for a detailed explanation of skilled services covered by Medicare Part A in Home Health. After the systems review has been completed using the OASIS as a guide, a medication reconciliation is required.

The Medication Reconciliation

Pharmacology in physical therapy has been defined by the American Physical Therapy Association (APTA).[14] These competencies state that the physical therapist should, at a minimum, integrate an understanding of a patient's prescription and nonprescription medication regimen with consideration of its impact on health, function, and disability for the patient. Importantly, it is not within a physical therapist's scope of practice to provide instructions about how to take drugs or assess for possible drug interactions. However, the physical therapist should be aware of adverse drug reactions for the patient's safety and recognize when it is necessary to contact the patient's physician to obtain an order for a skilled nursing assessment.

Physical therapists should then perform a reconciliation of the medication list. This reconciliation includes assessment of whether the medications correlate with past medical history or current diagnosis. For this skill, the physical therapist needs to have knowledge of medications, indications, and common side effects. The therapist should reconcile the patient's symptoms with possible adverse drug reactions. For example, if a patient complains of dizziness and is taking multiple medications to lower blood pressure, the patient may be experiencing an adverse drug event. Finally, the therapist should assess whether there are medication implications for the therapy plan of care. In the previous example, if the patient is experiencing dizziness from hypotension, a clinical hypothesis regarding decreased exercise tolerance should be explored.

When reviewing medications with the patient, the home care physical therapist should consider if a skilled nursing assessment is warranted. It should be noted that there are differing state regulations for physical therapists on medication reviews and providing patient education about high-risk medications by physical therapists.[14] For example, as a result of the implementation of OASIS-C, in January 2010, the New York State Department of Health ruled that a physical therapist may complete the comprehensive assessment only if the home health agency has implemented a policy and procedure that requires collaboration between the physical therapist and other agency staff.[15] It is important for home health therapists to be aware of their state regulations regarding medication review.

Older adults are at a higher risk for adverse drug reactions than younger individuals. The increased risk occurs for several reasons discussed elsewhere in this text. Physical therapists need to be aware that adverse events most often occur during the first 30 days after hospital discharge or when the patient fails to adhere to medical advice about medication use.[16] If the patient or family member is unable to tell the clinician what medications the patient is taking or the usage and purpose of the medication, it is likely that the patient is at risk for an adverse drug event.

Several red flags pertinent to the physical therapist may become apparent during the medication reconciliation. For example, polypharmacy (three or more drugs) and certain drug types can increase fall risk.[17] The Beers criteria for potentially inappropriate medication (updated nearly annually) can be used to screen the medication profile for inappropriate or problematic drugs and predict the likelihood of the patient experiencing an adverse drug reaction.[18,19] The Screening Tool of Older Persons' Potentially Inappropriate Prescriptions (STOPP) published in 2008 is another valuable reference for home care physical therapists.[20] The STOPP criteria focus on avoiding use of medications potentially inappropriate in older adults, similar to the Beers list. The author recommends that the home health therapist have current copies of both the Beers' list and STOPP when in the home to use as a quick reference tool during medication reconciliation.

Apart from a medication review, the therapist should determine if the patient or caregiver has difficulty with managing the medication regimen such as being able to visually recognize each drug, describe the purpose, verbalize when to take each medication, and determine if the patient uses any type of medication-organizing system. The therapist should be aware of the strain on caregivers when the burden of managing and administering the patient's medication regimen falls to the caregiver. This strain is more pronounced in caregivers of patients with moderate cognitive impairment as opposed to those patients with normal or very low cognitive functioning.[21] When a home health therapist recognizes caregiver strain, it may be appropriate to refer to skilled nursing or a medical social worker to help the patient and caregivers cope with these types of issues. Thus, physical therapists, as frontline professionals, have an important role to play in the home health setting by evaluating the extent to which the patient or caregiver are competent in the management of the patient's medication regimen. Some elements of an interdisciplinary medication assessment are listed in Box 26.8.

BOX 26.8 Elements of an Effective Interdisciplinary Approach to Medication Management in the Home

- Assessment of the medication regimen, which includes the patient's understanding of degree of adherence to the prescribed regimen
- Evaluation of the complexity of the regimen for patient and caregivers, which includes consistency of correct administration
- Monitor responses to drug actions, interactions, and side effects
- Provide education

Fall-Risk Screening

An important area to assess at the first visit is fall risk. Reducing fall risk and fall-related injuries can prevent significant declines in function and independence, allowing older adults to be active in the community and age in their home. Risk factors for falling are diverse and many of them, such as balance impairment, muscle weakness, polypharmacy, and environmental hazards, are common but potentially modifiable in the homebound patient. Frail older adults are more likely to fall indoors and most commonly on level surfaces during walking.[22,23] Falls are the leading cause of injuries that result in hospitalization for older adults.[24] After hospital discharge, fall rates are higher as compared with community-dwelling older adults.[25] Multifactor falls risk assessments and individually tailored follow-up interventions that include appropriate exercise intensity and specificity are recommended in the evidence-based literature and are discussed elsewhere in this text. Home health therapists are in an ideal position to address many fall-related factors within the home, a functional and relevant environment.

The home health assessment of potential fall risk begins with a history of a prior fall or a fear of falling. A prior fall predicts a decline in function, hospitalization, and adverse events among older adults and remains independently predictive of a likelihood of future hospitalization as well as a future fall.[26] Those who sustain ground-level falls and are admitted to hospital inpatient are subsequently readmitted within a year in 44% of cases and 33% have a 1 year mortality rate.[27] In addition, falls occurring indoors and an inability to get up after a fall are positive predictors of falls in older adults.[28] Therefore, the physical therapist should routinely assess the homebound older adult's ability to rise from the floor, both as a potential predictor of fall risk and as a safety issue if the person falls. If the person cannot safely rise unassisted, a Lifeline or similar device may be recommended and strategies for how to get up off the floor implemented. The ability to get up off the floor is also an important goal for patients who are home bound.

Fear of falling is also a predictor of fall risk. Many older individuals limit their mobility and become increasingly sedentary and homebound because of their awareness of declining balance, near falls, or fear of falling. Interviewing a patient about his or her fear of falling, including the completion of a fear of falling index such as the Falls Efficacy Scale or the Activities Balance Confidence Scale (ABC), may provide useful information that will inform goals and intervention strategies.

Home health therapists need to be aware of the possible underreporting of falls and near falls. Older adults may believe that reporting a fall might result in nursing home placement or notification of the fall incident to other family members who might arrange for relocation. Therefore, it is likely that an older adult may deny or minimize a fall history or a fall injury. Because only 20% of older adults who fall seek medical attention, the health care provider may not know about a fall.[28] Our recommendation is to assume fall risk and create a safe environment for the homebound patient to report a fear of falling and near and actual falls, and to implement appropriate strategies to improve the patient's balance.

Home Safety Assessment

Home assessment should be carried out at the first visit. Safety and mobility barriers are the prime focus of the home assessment. Because the majority of all falls and fall-related injuries in older adults occur inside the home,[29] it is imperative that the therapist address any potential hazards.

Within the home, the majority of falls, injurious or not, occur on level surfaces. Regardless of whether the fall resulted in an injury or not, most indoor falls happened in the living room (25%) and bedroom (23%).[23] Another five occur on the stairs or from a height with 14% resulting in an injury.[23,30] More injurious falls (17%) occurred in the bathroom compared with 8% of noninjurious falls.[23] The majority of falls resulting in injury resulted from slipping, tripping, or stumbling.[30]

The fundamental goals of home safety assessments and interventions are to improve and maintain the older adult's ability to function safely at home in all seasons. For example, an antislip shoe device reduced the rate of falls in icy conditions.[31] A home safety assessment is especially effective in people with severe visual impairment and in those at higher risk of falling. The most common home modifications are extra handrails or grab bars, wide doors and hallways, accessibility features in the bathroom, and ramps.[30] Although the evidence is not clear on the effectiveness of home modifications to reduce falls and improve safety in the home,[32] it seems prudent to advise the home health patient and caregiver about significant potential hazards and is one of the recommendations of the American Geriatrics Society/British Geriatrics Society Clinical Practice Guidelines for the Prevention of Falls in Older Persons.[33]

Interestingly, although many older households could make modifications that could potentially reduce falls, most do not.[30] The home health therapist may be familiar with the resistance of many older adults to changing their home environments on the recommendation of a therapist. Resistance to recommendations may be because the patient does not believe the hazard will cause a fall, the patient may be resistant to change and the associated costs of the change, or the patient may resist the perceived lack of control in incorporating a change to his or her home. Strategies that may be effective in overcoming resistance include sensitive communication with the patient and family member or friend about why the changes are necessary, and the implications associated with falls and health status in older adults and providing the patient with a list of community resources. These types of resources may be found at senior centers, rehabilitation centers, physician offices, and on the Internet. Some states may provide financial assistance for home modifications. In addition, all recommendations should be presented in a way that allows the older adult to remain in control of his or her home environment. Presenting recommendations in terms of choices, such as grab handles or a slip-proof stair covering, may allow the older adult to feel more in control.

Home safety checklists should address three basic areas: the presence of environmental hazards, problem areas, and lack of supportive or safety features. Checklists are commonly available to help organize the home safety assessment. For example, the Centers for Disease Control and Injury Prevention publishes a "Home Fall Prevention Checklist for Older Adults" that is available in English and several other languages.[34]

In addition to the home safety assessment, the home health therapist also has a role in recommending modifications to improve mobility. These recommendations may be to remove or modify potential hazards to mobility, such as adapting stairs with a ramp, or recommend an assistive device. Examples of adaptive or structural changes are listed in Table 26.1.

Functional Assessment Testing

Functional assessment testing can provide valuable information in any setting but is particularly relevant in the home health setting because of its specificity to home care activities. Functional assessment is an effective way to objectively document a patient's functional status, progress through the episode of care, and justify homebound status. Functional assessment testing can also justify discharge from physical therapy services. The functional tests of gait speed, timed chair rise, 6-minute walk test, floor rise, timed stair climb, and balance tests described in elsewhere in this text are particularly relevant for homebound patients

TABLE 26.1 Common Home Safety Interventions
Nonslip mats under loose rugs
Night lights and other indirect lighting in bathroom, hallways, and stairs
Move or tape down electrical cords or cover with rug that will not slip
Install railings on both sides of stairs
Use adaptive equipment such as tub transfer bench or shower chair, elevated toilet seat
Use cane or walker at top of stairs
Use bedside commode
Install grab bars in bathroom and at floor- or stair-height transitions
Hospital bed
Wheelchair

transitioning to the community. Gait speed is the single best predictor of functional decline and disability and therefore should always be assessed in the home setting. The home health therapist should be familiar with normative scores and make appropriate clinical decisions based on published data described elsewhere in this text.

Emergency Situations

Being prepared for emergency situations in the home is considered best practice in home health. Because of the autonomous nature of the home care practice, the therapist is often alone with the patient and needs to be adaptable to creating a safe and clear space for treatment as well as remain cognizant of the patient's and therapist's personal safety. The author recommends that the home health therapist always use a gait belt when working with patients in the home and to keep a cell phone on one's person at all times in case of an emergency when the patient cannot be left.

It is assumed that home health therapists are aware of their limitations and know when to call for help. Options include 911, the patient's physician, or a clinical manager of the home health agency. Basic clinical assessment skills such as taking baseline vital signs and assessing the patient's perceived rate of exertion during exercise are standard requirements for most home health agencies. Moreover, current certification in Basic Life Support for Healthcare Providers is the minimum requirement for patient safety. A cardiopulmonary resuscitation mask should be included in the therapist's tool bag.

The potential for a situation that requires activation of emergency medical services (EMS) always exists. An advance directive is an official document. When completed correctly, this form allows a patient with a life-threatening illness or injury to forgo specific resuscitative measures that may keep the individual alive. Home health providers are trained to inquire at the start of care if the patient has an advance directive form and to identify where the document is kept. The document serves to express the patient's wishes when the patient cannot speak for himself or herself. The patient should be instructed to keep the advance directive notice easily visible—mounted by a magnet on the refrigerator door is recommended by state medical associations. The location of the advance directive form should be ascertained at the first visit and made more visible if necessary. Home health clinicians are usually advised by their clinical managers to begin life-saving measures until EMS personnel arrive on the scene if there is any doubt about the patient and family's wishes.

The most recent CMS Conditions of Participation update requires agencies to comply with all applicable federal, state, and local emergency preparedness requirements.[13] The emergency preparedness plan must be comprehensive and collaborative with local, state, regional, and federal officials to maintain an integrated response during a disaster or emergency situation (Box 26.9).

Tip: Storing Medical Information

Medical information can be stored in the refrigerator in an empty vial or pill bottle designated with a sticker that would alert emergency responders such as paramedics or firefighters to its contents.

BOX 26.9 Centers for Medicare & Medicaid Services Requirements for Emergency Preparedness

The Home Health Agency (HHA) must comply with all applicable Federal, State, and local emergency preparedness requirements. The HHA must establish and maintain an emergency preparedness program that meets the requirements of this section. The emergency preparedness program must include, but not be limited to, the following elements:

(a) *Emergency plan.* The HHA must develop and maintain an emergency preparedness plan that must be reviewed, and updated at least annually. The plan must do all of the following:
  (1) Be based on and include a documented, facility-based and community-based risk assessment, utilizing an all-hazards approach.
  (2) Include strategies for addressing emergency events identified by the risk assessment.
  (3) Address patient population, including, but not limited to, the type of services the HHA has the ability to provide in an emergency; and continuity of operations, including delegations of authority and succession plans.
  (4) Include a process for cooperation and collaboration with local, tribal, regional, state, and federal emergency preparedness officials' efforts to maintain an integrated response during a disaster or emergency situation, including documentation of the HHA's efforts to contact such officials and, when applicable, of its participation in collaborative and cooperative planning efforts.

(b) *Policies and procedures.* The HHA must develop and implement emergency preparedness policies and procedures, based on the emergency plan set forth in paragraph (a) of this section, risk assessment at paragraph (a)(1) of this section, and the communication plan at paragraph (c) of this section. The policies and procedures must be reviewed and updated at least annually. At a minimum, the policies and procedures must address the following:
  (1) The plans for the HHA's patients during a natural or man-made disaster. Individual plans for each patient must be included as part of the comprehensive patient assessment, which must be conducted according to the provisions at § 484.55.
  (2) The procedures to inform state and local emergency preparedness officials about HHA patients in need of evacuation from their residences at any time due to an emergency situation based on the patient's medical and psychiatric condition and home environment.
  (3) The procedures to follow up with on-duty staff and patients to determine services that are needed, in the event that there is an interruption in services during or due to an emergency. The HHA must inform state and local officials of any on-duty staff or patients that they are unable to contact.

BOX 26.9 Centers for Medicare & Medicaid Services Requirements for Emergency Preparedness—cont'd

(4) A system of medical documentation that preserves patient information, protects confidentiality of patient information, and secures and maintains the availability of records.

(5) The use of volunteers in an emergency or other emergency staffing strategies, including the process and role for integration of state or federally designated health care professionals to address surge needs during an emergency.

(c) *Communication plan.* The HHA must develop and maintain an emergency preparedness communication plan that complies with federal, state, and local laws and must be reviewed and updated at least annually. The communication plan must include all of the following:

(1) Names and contact information for the following:
- (i) Staff.
- (ii) Entities providing services under arrangement.
- (iii) Patients' physicians.
- (iv) Volunteers.

(2) Contact information for the following:
- (i) Federal, state, tribal, regional, or local emergency preparedness staff.
- (ii) Other sources of assistance.

(3) Primary and alternate means for communicating with the HHA's staff, federal, state, tribal, regional, and local emergency management agencies.

(4) A method for sharing information and medical documentation for patients under the HHA's care, as necessary, with other health care providers to maintain the continuity of care.

(5) A means of providing information about the general condition and location of patients under the facility's care as permitted under 45 CFR 164.510(b)(4).

(6) A means of providing information about the HHA's needs, and its ability to provide assistance, to the authority having jurisdiction, the Incident Command Center, or designee.

(d) *Training and testing.* The HHA must develop and maintain an emergency preparedness training and testing program that is based on the emergency plan set forth in paragraph (a) of this section, risk assessment at paragraph (a)(1) of this section, policies and procedures at paragraph (b) of this section, and the communication plan at paragraph (c) of this section. The training and testing program must be reviewed and updated at least annually.

(1) *Training program.* The HHA must do all of the following:
- (i) Initial training in emergency preparedness policies and procedures to all new and existing staff, individuals providing services under arrangement, and volunteers, consistent with their expected roles.
- (ii) Provide emergency preparedness training at least annually.
- (iii) Maintain documentation of the training.
- (iv) Demonstrate staff knowledge of emergency procedures.

(2) *Testing.* The HHA must conduct exercises to test the emergency plan at least annually. The HHA must do the following:
- (i) Participate in a full-scale exercise that is community-based or when a community-based exercise is not accessible, an individual, facility-based exercise. If the HHA experiences an actual natural or man-made emergency that requires activation of the emergency plan, the HHA is exempt from engaging in a community-based or individual, facility-based full-scale exercise for 1 year following the onset of the actual event.
- (ii) Conduct an additional exercise that may include, but is not limited to the following:
  - (A) A second full-scale exercise that is community-based or individual, facility-based.
  - (B) A tabletop exercise that includes a group discussion led by a facilitator, using a narrated, clinically-relevant emergency scenario, and a set of problem statements, directed messages, or prepared questions designed to challenge an emergency plan.
- (iii) Analyze the HHA's response to and maintain documentation of all drills, tabletop exercises, and emergency events, and revise the HHA's emergency plan, as needed.

(e) *Integrated healthcare systems.* If a HHA is part of a healthcare system consisting of multiple separately certified healthcare facilities that elects to have a unified and integrated emergency preparedness program, the HHA may choose to participate in the healthcare system's coordinated emergency preparedness program. If elected, the unified and integrated emergency preparedness program must do all of the following:

(1) Demonstrate that each separately certified facility within the system actively participated in the development of the unified and integrated emergency preparedness program.

(2) Be developed and maintained in a manner that takes into account each separately certified facility's unique circumstances, patient populations, and services offered.

(3) Demonstrate that each separately certified facility is capable of actively using the unified and integrated emergency preparedness program and is in compliance with the program.

(4) Include a unified and integrated emergency plan that meets the requirements of paragraphs (a)(2), (3), and (4) of this section. The unified and integrated emergency plan must also be based on and include all of the following:
- (i) A documented community-based risk assessment, utilizing an all-hazards approach.
- (ii) A documented individual facility-based risk assessment for each separately certified facility within the health system, utilizing an all-hazards approach.

(5) Include integrated policies and procedures that meet the requirements set forth in paragraph (b) of this section, a coordinated communication plan and training and testing programs that meet the requirements of paragraphs (c) and (d) of this section, respectively.

From Centers for Medicare & Medicaid Services. Medicare and Medicaid Programs; Emergency Preparedness Requirements for Medicare and Medicaid Participating Providers and Suppliers. https://www.federalregister.gov/documents/2016/09/16/2016-21404/medicare-and-medicaid-programs-emergency-preparedness-requirements-for-medicare-and-medicaid#p-amd-27. Accessed August 25, 2018.

Personal Safety

As the home care environment grows, so does the potential for encountering occupational hazards in the home. For example, in 2007, 27,400 recorded injuries occurred among more than 896,800 home health care workers.[35] Home health care workers are frequently exposed to a variety of potentially serious or even life-threatening hazards. These dangers include overexertion, stress, guns and other weapons, illegal drugs, verbal abuse and other forms of violence in the home or community, bloodborne pathogens, needlesticks, latex sensitivity, temperature extremes, and unhygienic conditions (including lack of water, unclean or hostile animals, and animal waste).[35] For these reasons, cell phones and other mobile communication devices are considered essential for home health care workers. The author strongly believes that employee safety is fundamental to being able to provide patient care, and policies that promote a culture of safety for employees as an organizational priority are essential. Although incidents of violence in the home health environment are rare, situations do occur. When risk factors for violence are suspected, prescreening of the patient's home using a security escort or supervisory visits by a home health agency clinical manager may be necessary. Patients may be discharged from home health services after the physician is contacted in situations when the clinician is in imminent danger in the patient's home environment.

GOAL SETTING

There is some evidence that when the therapist and patient work together to establish meaningful goals for the patient, the patient has improved enthusiasm, buy-in, and outcomes.[36] Many home health patients have the potential and desire to become community-dwelling ambulators, returning to their prior or higher level of function. Others may be more limited or not desire to be integrated back into the community. Therefore, it may be advisable and necessary to involve the patient's chosen representative in the goal-setting process. Patient representatives and caregivers can help with information on prior level of function that is useful in setting realistic goals. For example, the patient may indicate a desire to return to full community integration, including driving. However, when discussing this goal with the family, the therapist may discover the patient has had several near-accidents and is often confused about the actual location when out in the community. This information may require a refocusing of the patient on shorter term goals with the expectations that the individual may come to a realization of limitations.

In setting goals to reintegrate a patient into the community, it may be useful to refer to Shumway-Cook and coworkers' required tasks of community-dwelling older adults.[37] These authors observed older adults for a 1-week period to identify required tasks in community-dwelling older adults for the purpose of helping home health therapists set goals. They found that older adults routinely:

- Walked a minimum of 300 m per errand (often making two or three separate trips at a time)
- Carried packages averaging 6.7 lb while walking,
- Frequently encountered stairs, curbs, and slopes
- Engaged in frequent postural transitions (changes in direction, reaching up, looking up, moving backward, and so on)

A systemic review about the speed and distance requirements for community ambulation investigated literature from three countries, the United States, Australia, and Singapore. Three sites with the largest mean distances were club warehouses (677 m), superstores (183–607 m), and hardware stores (566 m). The average speed to cross the street in the time of a walk signal varied from 0.44 to 1.32 m/s.[38]

Ideally, the goals set for patients who desire to return to the community should reflect these community standards. Box 26.10 lists some examples of evidence-based goals useful for a home health physical therapist.

There may be cases in which a patient may well intend to be a community ambulator and home health care is used as part of the continuum of care to transition the patient to outpatient care. An example is a patient who is discharged to home from the hospital a few days after total hip arthroplasty (THA). The patient may have a goal of getting to outpatient therapy as soon as possible, so goal setting would include increasing ambulation distance, stairs, and car transfers in order to transition to the outpatient setting.

It is the opinion of the author that often patients are discharged far too early from home health services. Criteria for community mobility have been clearly established and

BOX 26.10 Examples of Evidence-Based Goals for Home Health Patients Who Have the Potential to Become Community Ambulators Upon Discharge

- The patient will score <12 sec on the Timed Up and Go without an assistive device without loss of balance.
- The patient will score ≥50/56 on the Berg Balance Test to transition from floor to standing, and safely transfer from a variety of surfaces.
- The patient will score <12 sec on the 4 Square Step Test without loss of balance to demonstrate dynamic stability while changing directions.
- The patient will score >85% on the Activity-specific Balance Confidence Scale demonstrating confidence in common mobility tasks.
- The patient will ambulate >1000 ft (300m) without an assistive device with a gait speed >0.8 m/s with a reported Borg RPE of 10 or less to meet community standards for mobility.
- The patient will score <10 s on the 5 Repetition Sit to Stand to demonstrate adequate reserve in performing multiple transitions from chair to standing.

RPE, rate of perceived exertion.

should be used as goals for the patient desiring to be reintegrated into the community.[37,38] In addition, objective fall risk should be considered when preparing for discharge. When a person demonstrates substantial fall risk per an objective tool designed to identify fall risk, the person may benefit from further therapy to decrease fall risk and improve balance.

Unfortunately, the author has seen arbitrary standards for justification of discharge that have no basis in Medicare guidelines. For example, one therapist may discharge a patient from home health services simply because the patient went out to get a haircut. Another therapist may discharge a patient because the patient can ambulate 200 feet or can drive. However, under Medicare guidelines, a homebound patient is allowed to occasionally and infrequently leave the home to get a haircut, attend physician appointments, and participate in religious services. They are also permitted to leave their homes for special occasions such as holidays or visiting relatives as long as the trip away from home is physically taxing (see Box 26.1). It is important to note that no Medicare guideline establishes a prescribed ambulation distance to determine homebound status. Box 26.2 lists some examples of statements that may justify continued homebound care.

Home health physical therapists have a professional obligation to provide the needed patient services while complying with CMS guidelines and regulations. Objective documentation and thorough examination of the patient will help drive an appropriate plan of care. Each subsequent visit note must stand alone to justify medical necessity. The purpose of this section was to assist the home health therapist to think critically about patient-centered goals and justify the provision of in-home therapy services under Medicare guidelines.

EPISODE OF CARE

Projecting Number of Physical Therapy Visits and Episode Timing

Currently, a 60-day certification period applies to home health patients admitted for home health services under the Medicare Part A benefit. A detailed description of what Medicare considers skilled physical therapy services is available on the CMS website.[1] Briefly, the skilled services should be appropriate, reasonable, necessary, and safe for the patient. Skilled physical therapy will be covered throughout the 60-day certification period under the condition that supporting documentation justifies the need for skilled services. The documentation needs to include homebound status at the time of start of care and on every subsequent visit note.

The individual with frailty poses a challenge with respect to predicting the frequency and duration of services because frailty is linked with a poor prognosis.[39] Frailty is a biological condition characterized by three or more of the following characteristics: unexplained weight loss of 10 lb or more in the past year, self-reported exhaustion, weakness (as measured by grip strength), slow walking speed, and low physical activity.[40] A patient who is frail requires more visits on average, spread out throughout the certification period to move her or him to a higher functional level. However, if the person is so frail that the individual is almost bedbound and cannot participate in the kind of exercise program that will allow the patient to make meaningful functional gains, fewer therapy visits will be needed to educate the patient and family on safe mobility and a home exercise program.

Application of clinical decision making is imperative when determining frequency and duration of physical therapy services. Appropriate exercise for older adults—including intensity, overload, and specificity—is needed to effect change. Use of these principles will help the home health physical therapist determine the frequency and duration for the home health episode of care and avoid a premature discharge. In all cases, the home health therapist is responsible for ordering the number of therapy visits that are medically necessary. The patient's needs must remain the therapist's foremost concern when determining the number of therapy visits, regardless of reimbursement models or pressures. Considering that all therapy visits must be medically necessary, each visit note must justify the visit.

Initial Patient Education Interventions

Skilled home health therapy includes patient education interventions *and* the patient's, as well as caregivers', response to education. Patient education at the start of care may be the primary intervention and include information about the patient bill of rights, the agency's complaint process, the agency's emergency disaster plan, home safety interventions, pain management interventions, home exercise program, orthopedic precautions, fall prevention strategies, and the plan of care. Any patient education provided must be documented at the initial and subsequent visits. Suggestions for documentation of patient education are explained further in the subsequent visit section of this chapter.

The volume of information to be shared and taught may necessitate several educational sessions. Effective patient education is considered a skilled intervention as teaching must be tailored to meet the older adult's physical, cognitive, and psychosocial functioning level. Clinicians who take the time to assess their patients' individual abilities, learning preferences, and motivational differences will find teaching to be more rewarding and meaningful for the patient.

Start of Care Case Conference and Physician Communication

Discharge Planning at the Start of Care. As in all settings, discharge planning in home health begins at the start of care. The patient is required to sign a consent form at the first visit that includes the agreed upon frequency and duration of home physical therapy. Rarely can an older adult afford the luxury of being sedentary; thus, some plan for continued physical activity and exercise should be discussed with the patient within the first few visits. The patient may be discharged to outpatient services, self-care, or a home program with assistance from a family or friend. The home health physical therapist is expected to coordinate the discharge plan with the physician, the patient, and anyone else who may be involved in the patient's care. In many cases, a patient who is expected to reintegrate into the community could benefit from additional outpatient physical therapy services to help move the person to as high a level of function as possible. This will help prevent future functional decline by building up functional reserve and protecting the person against future hospitalizations.

Subsequent Visits

Documentation. Documentation for each home health visit may differ from other clinical settings. Issues need to be documented each visit as appropriate, such as complete vital sign assessment, objective pain assessment, documentation of subjective and objective assessment, and the reassessment of the physical therapy plan. The therapist may also document the observance of universal precautions or the use of "clean bag" technique to reduce the risk of using contaminated equipment between patients. Documentation of discharge planning and homebound status should be noted throughout the episode of care.

Documentation of skilled teaching and progress toward goals should also be included on every visit. For example, the home health therapist may document the provision of patient education regarding THA precautions knowing that the patient will require further teaching. The teaching intervention may be documented in the following way: "The patient was provided with education on THA precautions; further teaching is required because the patient was only able to verbalize two of three hip precautions." This example includes what the patient was taught and the patient's response to teaching. This example requires follow-up documentation on subsequent visit notes because "further teaching is required" was documented. When full understanding of THA precautions is demonstrated by the patient, the home health therapist may document the following: "The patient verbalized understanding of THA precautions." If understanding the THA precautions was a goal for the patient, the therapist would also document that goal was met on that date in the progress toward goals section on the note.

Coordination of Patient Care

Although the home health visit may occur in isolation from other health care team members, communication about the case occurs frequently between clinicians and clinical managers in the office. This communication is so important that it is termed *care coordination* and is required for each patient under CMS Conditions of Participation. Care coordination is characterized by communication among all members of the interdisciplinary team. Specific documentation of patient notification of care provided, the disciplines involved, the frequency of proposed visits, notification 48 hours before planned discharge, and any changes to the plan of care is required. The Conditions of Participation also require the agency to notify the physician of changes in the patient's condition that may necessitate a change in the treatment plan that was established on the first visit. For example, if the physical therapist determines 2 weeks after the start of care that the patient is exhibiting a change in cognition or having signs of skin breakdown, a referral for a skilled nursing assessment is warranted because of the change in the patient's medical condition. An interim order from the physician is required for the newly required skilled nursing assessment. Also, if a patient is not progressing as anticipated or not participating with therapy, the physician must be notified that skilled services may no longer be necessary and thus need to end before what was originally planned. In such an example, the home health therapist may work with the physician and possibly the agency's social worker to coordinate options for a different level of care for those individuals who are not safe in the home and yet not progressing sufficiently with rehabilitative efforts.

Coordination of care also requires communication between disciplines and typically with the agency's clinical manager; however, these requirements are agency specific. Care coordination needs to take place at the start of care, resumption of care, recertification of care, and at discharge. There are other cases when documentation of communication between the interdisciplinary team and the clinical case manager are warranted, such as when reporting patient complaints or infections and incidents, lack of progress toward goals, and when providing supervision of other associates (home health aide, physical therapist assistant [PTA], and licensed practical nurse).

In the home health setting, the case manager is responsible for overseeing the care plan and coordination of that care with all disciplines. The physical therapist, registered nurse, speech–language pathologist, or occupational therapist is allowed under Medicare guidelines to be the patient's case manager. If nursing is involved in a patient's care, the nurse is considered the patient's case manager by default. When physical therapy but not nursing is involved, the physical therapist is the case manager regardless of what other disciplines are involved on the case.

The interdisciplinary team is expected to work together to set goals with the patient to ensure a cohesive plan of care. Physical and occupational therapists work particularly closely with each other when both are involved in the same episode of care because of the similarity in goals and focus. Both professionals collaborate on the duration and frequency of the plan of care and specific intervention focus. Care coordination is also important when scheduling visits with patients to ensure that the services are not overlapping. If two individuals are needed to provide a service, two visits may be covered by CMS.[1] An example given by CMS is when an occupational therapist is at a patient's home supervising the certified occupational therapist assistant. In this instance, only one visit is billable to Medicare. CMS reimburses for joint visits (e.g., physical therapy and occupational therapy) only in special circumstances.[1]

Care coordination with all disciplines at the time of discharge is necessary. Skilled services of various disciplines of the interdisciplinary team may be discharged at different times during the episode of care. The last discipline on the case will be responsible for completion of the OASIS discharge assessment, with the exception of home health aides. Disciplines that discharge before the OASIS discharge are responsible for completing less labor-intensive documentation in accordance with CMS, state, and agency guidelines.

A home health physical therapist may help facilitate the patient's discharge from home health and any transition to outpatient physical therapy by communication with the physician and outpatient clinic of the patient's choice. If the patient does not go to outpatient physical therapy at the time of discharge, it is recommended that the physical therapist ensure that the patient and the family or caregivers understand the home exercise program instructions. The Home Health Section of the APTA provides additional information on discharge planning and documentation requirements for home health (Box 26.11).

BOX 26.11 Documentation Requirements for Home Health Care

Guideline

The physical therapist and physical therapist assistant complete timely documentation for each visit performed, providing clear justification for services rendered that is consistent with the essential requirements specified by APTA, state and federal regulations, home health agency policy, and payer sources.

Criteria

1. Physical therapists and physical therapist assistants follow general principles of documentation, which include but are not limited to:
   a. Abbreviations—minimal use, "do not use," per home health agency policy
   b. Addendums/errors—documentation errors must be corrected by drawing a single line through the error and initialing and dating the error or through the appropriate mechanism for electronic documentation
   c. Functional progress—document status regularly
   d. Skilled care—includes problem solving, clinical decision making, objectively measuring patient response, and standardized testing
   e. Timeliness—documentation should be completed the same day as the encounter/visit
   f. Terms/phrases to avoid—Avoid generalized statements such as "tolerated treatment well," "continue POC," and "as above"
2. Documentation required for all visits
   a. Name of patient
   b. Visit date and start/end times
   c. Objective tests and measures
   d. Vital signs
   e. Homebound status, if applicable
   f. Medication review (eg, changes, side effects, new medications)
   g. Physical therapist intervention(s), including:
      i. Rationale/explanation for intervention(s)
      ii. Education/cueing (eg, mobility training, body mechanics, safety, home exercise program, medication effects on exercise and physical activity)
      iii. Detailed description of treatment(s)
      iv. Objective measure of patient response (eg, Borg scale, vital signs)
      v. Assistance required
   h. Comparative statement(s) to identify patient progress or lack thereof
      i. Current visit vs prior visit
      ii. Current visit vs goals
      iii. Existing impairments/functional limitations vs prior level of function
   i. Identification of barriers to progress, if applicable
   j. Plan for next visit, to include specific modifications/progression of interventions for unmet goals
   k. Modification/update of discharge plan as needed
   l. Applicable physician/interdisciplinary communication
   m. Appropriate signature(s) that include:
      i. Legible physical therapist/physical therapist assistant signature, with full name and designation
      ii. If required by home health agency policy, signature of patient or caregiver/power of attorney

BOX 26.11 Documentation Requirements for Home Health Care—cont'd

3. Additional documentation pertaining to evaluation visits
   a. Start of care/admission visits include:
      i. Signed consent forms
      ii. Explanation of services
      iii. Outcome Assessment Information Set (OASIS)
      iv. Acuity/priority status
      v. Education regarding advance directives and privacy rights (HIPAA)
   b. Initial evaluation/examination visits include:
      i. Medical history
      ii. Current medical status and diagnoses (eg, medical, rehab)
      iii. Medication review/allergies
      iv. Prior vs current level of function
      v. Impairments and functional limitations
      vi. Activity limitations/participation restrictions
      vii. Environment/equipment and personal factors
      viii. Interventions provided
      ix. Patient-centered goals with expected time frame for achievement
      x. Rehab potential to achieve plan-of-care goals
      xi. Planned interventions and frequency/duration of visits
      xii. Discharge plan
   c. Reassessment
      i. Reassessments performed by PTs in association with the following visits:
         1. Resumption of care (ROC)
         2. Follow-up due to change of patient condition
         3. Recertification
         4. Functional reassessment required by state/federal regulations
      ii. Reassessment documentation should include:
         1. Standardized testing with explanation of relevance to goals
         2. Summary of progress toward goals, or lack thereof
         3. Summary of barriers to progress toward goals
         4. Justification for why patient requires continued treatment
         5. Rationale for any plan of care modifications, including updated goals and visit frequency changes
   d. Discharge visits should include the following components:
      i. OASIS assessment when needed
      ii. Current level of function with objective measures
      iii. Interventions received
      iv. Discharge disposition
      v. Discharge instructions/discharge notice provided per regulatory requirement
      vi. Medication reconciliation
      vii. Goals met
      viii. Explanation for any unmet goals
      ix. Communication with physician regarding recommendations for any ongoing care
4. Nonvisit documentation
   a. Supervision
      i. PTA supervision may be done with or without a visit per state requirements
      ii. Documentation of onsite observation of PTA visit, or review and follow-up of PT plan of care of PTA notes
      iii. Ongoing PT and PTA communication regarding patient care and any medical issues that come up during visits made by PTA
   b. Care coordination
      i. Conferencing to include communication with physician, interdisciplinary team, and equipment companies
      ii. Missed visit/refusal, including date, time, reason, and physician notification
      iii. Patient visit scheduling
   c. Nonvisit OASIS
      i. Transfer to inpatient facility
      ii. Nonvisit discharge

APTA, American Physical Therapy Association.

From American Physical Therapy Association. Home Health Section—Guidelines for the provision of physical therapy in the home. https://www.homehealthsection.org/global_engine/download.aspx?fileid=9BAAE903-74A0-4560-BF9F-AA801056CEAA&ext=pdf. Accessed August 25, 2018.

CMS uses the Start of Care OASIS and Discharge OASIS scores as a way to determine the effectiveness of the services provided by the home health agency. The results for all agencies are available for public reviewing at "Home Health Compare" on Medicare's website.[41] Box 26.3 lists the quality measures for home health agencies. Written notification and signature of the patient is required 48 hours *before* discharge from home health services. The purpose of this is to make sure that the patient is aware that the discharge planned by the home health agency may be disputed by contacting Medicare. A copy of the information is left with the patient and kept in the clinician record. The patient has a right to appeal the agency discharge by contacting Medicare.

PHYSICAL THERAPY INTERVENTION IN THE HOME

Exercise is one of the most often used interventions in the home health setting because it has been shown to be effective in improving functional abilities given appropriate intensity and specificity. The lack of formal exercise equipment can make the provision of evidence-based exercise challenging, requiring creativity to achieve the necessary parameters of an effective exercise program. Box 26.12 provides some suggestions for exercises and activities easily done in the home. Box 26.7 lists a few items that are useful and feasible to carry with the therapist when prescribing exercise in the home. The drive spent between patients can often be used to develop creative exercises that are functional and of interest to the patient.

BOX 26.12 Examples of Exercises for Home Health

Examples of Practical Exercises in and Outside the Home

Car transfers
Dynamic balance activities
Floor transfer training
Heel raises, progressing to unilateral heel raises
Quick toe tapping
Repeated sit to stand, progressing to one-leg sit to stand
Stair climbing
Step ups
Walking on uneven surfaces outside

Examples of Task-Specific Activities

Repeatedly getting in and out of bed
Repeatedly performing dressing tasks
Reaching up into cupboards lifting cans of food, dishes, or weights
Carrying items (e.g., dishes pots) across room from kitchen to dining area
Putting in and removing items from refrigerator or stove
Repeatedly opening and closing refrigerator or exterior door of home
Transferring up and down from commode repeatedly
Bending over to pick up pet's food or water dishes from floor
Stand at bedside and put shirts onto hanger and then hang shirts in closet
Vacuuming or sweeping
Transferring clothes from washer to dryer

Home Exercise Programs

Home health patients are typically seen two to three times a week initially during the episode of care; therefore, exercise performance between sessions may be necessary depending on the goals of treatment. If strengthening is a goal and the patient is seen three times a week, it would be best practice to prescribe endurance or flexibility exercises between sessions (assuming appropriate intensity is performed to require recovery). A home program could consist of a physical activity prescription such as a daily walking program with alternating days working on speed or strength. The home health therapist may also choose to have the patient work on task-specific activities on the nontherapy days (see Box 26.12). The home exercise program should be updated as the treatment progresses. The literature shows that it is best practice to give a patient only two to three exercises for the home exercise program to ensure correct form and perhaps compliance.[42] Written exercise prescriptions with pictures may be useful for patients. The exercises should be reviewed regularly with the patient to ensure that technique is safe and correct. In some cases, the most effective way to prescribe a home exercise program is to involve family members, especially in cases when the patient has an existing cognitive or visual deficit.

Physical Therapist Assistant Utilization

Under CMS guidelines, the PTA can provide therapy without onsite supervision of the physical therapist, another unique aspect of the home care setting. However, physical therapist supervision and utilization must be in accordance with CMS and state regulations. The Home Health Section of the APTA provides information on the role of the PTA in the home as well as the necessary qualifications.

Individual states can also regulate how the PTA is used in the home care setting. For example, in New York State, the physical therapist and the PTA must make the initial joint visit together, with the physical therapist performing a follow-up visit every sixth occasion or 30 days (whichever comes first). This example demonstrates how each physical therapist should be aware of his or her state's requirements regarding supervision of PTAs in the home care setting.

CARE TRANSITIONS AND PATIENT SELF-MANAGEMENT: A VISION FOR HOME HEALTH

According to the American Geriatrics Society (AGS) position statement "Improving the Quality of Transitional Care for Persons with Complex Care Needs," practitioners across health care settings often operate independently, which interferes with the ability to have seamless transitions of the patient among care settings.[43] During transitions, patients are at risk for medical errors, service failures, and ultimately poor clinical outcomes. Intervention strategies to improve care transitions involve a timely transfer of health care information from the acute care setting to post–acute care health care providers and vice versa. Organizational tools such as care transition coaches who support patients and teach self-management skills will enhance health information exchange across care settings. When patients and their caregivers are able to easily track key medical information, health care concerns, medications from all prescribers, and their history of provider contacts, patients' competence in self-management and likelihood to remain independent at home increase. Thus, the author believes that if tools become widely used to promote seamless transitions, home health becomes the only truly scalable infrastructure to deliver transitional, postacute, and primary care and chronic care management for older adults.

SUMMARY

Although Medicare may limit the definition of home health to short-term, intermittent, treatment-focused medical care for homebound patients, these restrictions historically came from when home care was initially designed to be *incident* to acute care. Moreover, rehabilitation programs for older adults were considered possible only if delivered in facilities with therapy gyms and an array of therapeutic equipment. Home health is now recognized as a transition in the continuum of care that provides a window of opportunity to affect the functional abilities of older adults. There are many functional assessment tests and interventions that are extraordinarily adaptable to being performed in the patient's home. The provision of evidence-based exercise in the home allows for comparisons of outcomes across settings and overall sound clinical decisions about the patient's readiness to progress to self-management. All physical therapists should advocate for their patients to reintegrate into the community and progress to outpatient care or community-based exercise programs. The challenges in the home health setting present opportunities for physical therapists to demonstrate their expert clinical decision making while practicing in the most functional environment for their patients.

REFERENCES

1. Centers for Medicare & Medicaid Services. Medicare benefit policy manual, Chapter 7, Home health services. http://www.cms.hhs.gov/manuals/Downloads/bp102c07.pdf. Accessed April 14, 2018.
2. Caregiving in the US. AARP Public Policy Institute; 1995. https://www.caregiving.org/wp-content/uploads/2015/05/2015_CaregivingintheUS_Executive-Summary-June-4_WEB.pdf. Accessed August 23, 2018.
3. Katula JA, Rejeski WJ, Wickley KL, Berry MJ. Perceived difficulty, importance, and satisfaction with physical function in COPD patients. *Health Qual Life Outcomes*. 2004;2:18.
4. Schwartz RS. Sarcopenia and physical performance in old age: introduction. *Muscle Nerve Suppl*. 1997;5:S10–S12.
5. Gill TM, Allore HG, Holford TR, Guo Z. Hospitalization, restricted activity, and the development of disability among older persons. *JAMA*. 2004;292(17):2115–2124.
6. Zuckerman R, Sheingold S, Orav E, et al. Readmissions, observation, and the hospital readmissions reduction program. *N Engl J Med*. 2016;374(16):1543–1551.
7. Walker B. Insights on patient engagement and behavior change. In: *Hospital Readmission Statistics You Need to Know*; 2017. http://insights.patientbond.com/blog/hospital-readmission-statistics-you-need-to-know. Accessed August 23, 2018.
8. All-cause Admissions and Readmission 2015–2017 Technical Report. National Quality Forum. All-cause Admissions and Readmission 2015–2017; 2017. Washington, DC: National Quality Forum. http://www.qualityforum.org/Publications/2017/04/All-Cause_Admissions_and_Readmissions_2015-2017_Technical_Report.aspx. Accessed August 23, 2018.
9. Rosati RJ, Huang L, Navaie-Waliser M, Feldman PH. Risk factors for repeated hospitalizations among home healthcare recipients. *J Healthc Qual*. 2003;25(2):4–10. quiz 10–11.
10. Centers for Medicare & Medicaid Services. Readmissions Reduction Program (HRRP)2018. https://www.cms.gov/medicare/medicare-fee-for-service-payment/acuteinpatientpps/readmissions-reduction-program.html. Accessed August 23, 2018.
11. MedPAC. Home health care services payment system; 2017. http://www.medpac.gov/docs/default-source/payment-basics/medpac_payment_basics_17_hha_final37a311adfa9c665e80adff00009edf9c.pdf?sfvrsn=0. Accessed July 27, 2018.
12. Centers for Medicare & Medicaid Services. OASIS User Manuals. https://www.cms.gov/Medicare/Quality-Initiatives-Patient-Assessment-Instruments/HomeHealthQualityInits/HHQIOASISUserManual.html; 2018. Accessed August 24, 2018.
13. Medicare and Medicaid Programs. Conditions of Participation for Home Health Agencies; 2017. https://www.federalregister.gov/documents/2017/01/13/2017-00283/medicare-and-medicaid-program-conditions-of-participation-for-home-health-agencies. Accessed August 24, 2018.
14. American Physical Therapy Association. *Medication management and physical therapists*; 2013. http://www.homehealthquality.org/getattachment/UP/UP-Event-Archives/PTs_and_Medication_State_Law_and_Regs_4-13_(2).pdf.aspx. Accessed August 24, 2018.
15. New York State Department of Health; 2010. http://www.op.nysed.gov/prof/pt/HCBS10-01MedicationReviewsByPTs.pdf. Accessed August 24, 2018.
16. Field TS, Mazor KM, Briesacher B, et al. Adverse drug events resulting from patient errors in older adults. *J Am Geriatr Soc*. 2007;55(2):271–276.
17. de Jong M, Van der Elst M, Hartholt K. Drug-related falls in older patients: implicated drugs, consequences, and possible prevention strategies. *Ther Adv Drug Saf*. 2013;4(4):147–154.
18. American Geriatrics Society. American Geriatrics Society 2015 updated Beers criteria for potentially inappropriate medication use in older adults; 2015. https://www.guidelinecentral.com/summaries/american-geriatrics-society-2015-updated-beers-criteria-for-potentially-inappropriate-medication-use-in-older-adults/#section-420. Accessed August 24, 2018.
19. Chang CM, Liu PY, Yang YH, et al. Use of the Beers criteria to predict adverse drug reactions among first-visit elderly outpatients. *Pharmacotherapy*. 2005;25(6):831–838.
20. Gallagher P, O'Mahony D. STOPP (Screening Tool of Older Persons' Potentially Inappropriate Prescriptions): application

to acutely ill elderly patients and comparison with Beers' criteria. *Age Ageing*. 2008;37(6):673–679.
21. Travis SS, McAuley WJ, Dmochowski J, et al. Factors associated with medication hassles experienced by family caregivers of older adults. *Patient Educ Couns*. 2007;66(1):51–57.
22. Timsina LR, Willetts JL, Brennan MJ, et al. Circumstances of fall related injuries by age and gender among communitydwelling adults in the United States. *PLoS One*. 2017;12(5):e0176561. http://journals.plos.org/plosone/article?id=10.1371/journal.pone.0176561. Accessed August 24, 2018
23. Stevens JA, Mahoney JE, Ehrenreich H. Circumstances and outcomes of falls among high risk community-dwelling older adults. *Inj Epidemiol*. 2014;1:5. https://www.ncbi.nlm.nih.gov/pmc/articles/PMC4700929/pdf/40621_2013_Article_5.pdf. Accessed August 24, 2018.
24. Centers for Disease Control and Prevention. Falls are the leading cause of injury and death in older Americans. https://www.cdc.gov/media/releases/2016/p0922-older-adult-falls.html; 2016. Accessed August 24, 2018.
25. Hill AM, Hoffmann, T, McPhail, S et al. Evaluation of the sustained effect of inpatient falls prevention education and predictors of falls after hospital discharge—follow up to a randomized controlled trial. *J Gerontol A Bio Sci Med Sci*. 20111;66(9):1001–112.
26. Laird RD, Studenski S, Perera S, Wallace D. Fall history is an independent predictor of adverse health outcomes and utilization in the elderly. *Am J Manag Care*. 2001;7(12):1133–1138.
27. Ayoung-Chee P, McIntyre L, Ebel BE, Mack CD, McCormick W, Maier RV. Long-term outcomes of ground-level falls in the elderly. *J Trauma Acute Care Surg*. 2014;76(2):498–503.
28. Close JC, Hooper R, Glucksman E, et al. Predictors of falls in a high risk population: results from the prevention of falls in the elderly trial (PROFET). *Emerg Med J*. 2003;20(5):421–425.
29. Runyan CW, Perkis D, Marshall SW, et al. Unintentional injuries in the home in the United States, part II: morbidity. *Am J Prev Med*. 2005;28(1):80–87.
30. Kochera A. Falls among older persons and the role of the home: an analysis of cost, incidence, and potential savings from home modification. https://assets.aarp.org/rgcenter/il/ib56_falls.pdf. Accessed August 24, 2018.
31. Gillespie LD, Robertson M, Gillespie WJ, et al. Interventions for preventing falls in older people living in the community. *Cochrane Database Syst Rev*. 2012;12(9):CD007146.
32. Tse T. The environment and falls prevention: do environmental modifications make a difference? *Aust Occup Ther J*. 2005;52:271–281.
33. Panel on Prevention of Falls in Older Persons, American Geriatrics Society and British Geriatrics Society. Summary of the Updated American Geriatrics Society/British Geriatrics Society clinical practice guideline for prevention of falls in older persons. *J Am Geriatr Soc*. 2011;59(1):148–157.
34. Centers for Disease Control and Prevention. Check for safety: a home fall prevention checklist for older adults. http://www.cdc.gov/ncipc/pubres/toolkit/Falls_ToolKit/DesktopPDF/English/booklet_Eng_desktop.pdf. Accessed August 24, 2018.
35. Centers for Disease Control and Prevention. NIOSH Hazard Review. Occupational Hazards in Home Healthcare; 2010. https://www.cdc.gov/niosh/docs/2010-125/default.html. Accessed August 24, 2018.
36. Tripicchio B, Bykerk K, Wegner C, Wegner J. Increasing patient participation: the effects of training physical and occupational therapists to involve geriatric patients in the concerns-clarification and goal-setting processes. *J Phys Ther Educ*. 2009;23(1):53–63.
37. Shumway-Cook A, Patla AE, Stewart A, et al. Environmental demands associated with community mobility in older adults with and without mobility disabilities. *Phys Ther*. 2002;82(7):670–681.
38. Salbach NM, O'Brien K, Brooks D, et al. Speed and distance requirements for community ambulation: a systematic review. *Arch Phys Med Rehabil*. 2014;95(1):117–128.
39. Hatheway OL, Mitnitski A, Rockwood K. Frailty affects the initial treatment response and time to recovery of mobility in acutely ill older adults admitted to hospital. *Age Ageing*. 2017;46(6):920–925.
40. Fried LP, Tangen CM, Walston J, et al. Frailty in older adults: evidence for a phenotype. *J Gerontol A Biol Sci Med Sci*. 2001;56A(3):M146–M156.
41. Medicare—The official U.S. government site for people with Medicare. Home health compare. http://www.medicare.gov/HHCompare/Home.asp?destNAV|Home|DataDetails#TabTop. Accessed August 24, 2018.
42. Henry KD, Rosemond C, Eckert LB. Effect of number of home exercises on compliance and performance in adults over 65 years of age. *Phys Ther*. 1998;79(3):270–277.
43. Coleman EA, Boult C. American Geriatrics Society Health Care Systems Committee. Improving the quality of transitional care for persons with complex care needs. *J Am Geriatr Soc*. 2003;51(4):556–557, 2003.

CHAPTER 27

Hospice and End of Life

Karen Mueller, Christopher Wilson, Richard Briggs

OUTLINE

INTRODUCTION

The Concept of a "Good Death"

Health care outcomes, regardless of one's discipline, are generally focused on the enhancement of patient quality of life. For each person, quality of life is a subjective, broad, and multifaceted construct, which includes all elements that provide life satisfaction. Physical therapists have a critical role in optimizing quality of life through the application of skills related to the evaluation and treatment of conditions affecting movement and function from the moment of birth until the moment of death.

Nevertheless, because the typical expectation of physical therapy intervention is related to the attainment of improved function, the benefits of our services to those facing end of life are often not considered. To that end, patients in a hospice setting may be told that "nothing more can be done" by health professionals who are unaware of the value of physical therapy in maintaining safe and comfortable function in the presence of physical decline. Unfortunately, such lack of awareness may prevent the optimization of quality of life in persons for whom death may be imminent yet whose life is still potent with opportunities for rich interactions.

It does not have to be this way. The indignities of a lonely, painful, and helpless death are among the greatest fears of Americans.[1] Fortunately, in the past few decades, these fears have forced a reexamination of end-of-life care, resulting in the development of the compassionate, patient-centered approach that defines hospice and palliative care.

Central to the hospice approach is the construct of a "good death," the inevitable outcome to which all effective end-of-life care is directed. This construct is the obvious antithesis of our worst fears. Simply put, a good death is one where the dying person is free of discomfort, in the presence of those they love, and in the environment of their choosing.

This patient-centered approach is certainly not a foreign concept in other areas of health care. For example, just as expectant mothers can orchestrate the manner in which their labor and delivery proceed, dying patients can be given similar options for the ways in which they affect their end of life. One of the most important contributions of hospice and palliative care is to assist patients in making and carrying out these choices.

Physical therapists have an important role in supporting a good death through a host of interventions to reduce pain, optimize the patient's remaining function, and enhance the quality of life for whatever time is left. In end-of-life care, physical therapy outcomes may not be solely functional but can include improved sleep quality, decreased physiological and psychological stress, improved respiratory function, and a decreased need for analgesic medication. More importantly, skilled physical therapy intervention can help the patient and family to maintain safe, energy-efficient mobility in the presence of declining systemic function, a process that can best be described as "rehabilitation in reverse."

A primary goal of this chapter is to examine the current structure and process of hospice and palliative care, a growing health setting for all Americans, particularly those in their later years. In addition, the roles, benefits, and outcomes of physical therapy intervention in the realms of hospice and end-of-life care will be explored. Most importantly, the information presented here should enable the reader to advocate for the ongoing involvement of physical therapists in this important area of care. Accordingly, because hospice and palliative care is a newer area of physical therapist practice, rich opportunities exist for engagement in outcome studies to support the value of these services. Finally, we should remember that participation in hospice and palliative care is an elegant reflection of the American Physical Therapy Association's Vision Statement, which directs us to "Transform society by optimizing movement to *improve the human experience* for all people of all ages."[2] Given that the overall outcome of interventions in hospice and palliative care relates to a death with dignity, it is important to understand the physiological elements of the dying process. This knowledge is critical in providing compassionate support to patients and families as they navigate the poignant experience of this natural process.

AN OVERVIEW OF HOSPICE AND PALLIATIVE CARE

Hospice Versus Palliative Care

In the realm of end-of-life care, two related terms, *hospice* and *palliative care*, are often used. Both terms pertain to the optimization of comfort and quality of life of patients with life-threatening conditions. Although hospice programs have delivered palliative care for more than 30 years, palliative care is also used in many other settings that focus on the treatment of the chronically, but not terminally, ill. As discussed later in this chapter, hospice is a specific set of services that is covered by the Medicare hospice benefit. Patients admitted to hospice must meet certain requirements, including a physician-determined prognosis of less than 6 months to live and the acknowledgment that they are no longer seeking curative measures. In contrast, payment for palliative care services is not tied to a specific health care initiative such as Medicare; instead, services are reimbursed through the patient's regular health insurance. Thus, payment for services must be in line with the range of covered benefits within each insurer's plan. Regardless of the payment system or stage of the patient's illness, a central theme in the management of serious disease is palliative-based interventions. For some patients, disease progression may result in admission to hospice. For others, effective palliative care may result in significant improvements, including cure. Accordingly, although all patients in hospice receive palliative care, not every patient who receives palliative care will do so in a hospice setting.

The World Health Organization defines palliative care as "an approach that improves the quality of life of patients and their families facing the problem associated with life-threatening illness, through the prevention and relief of suffering by means of early identification and impeccable assessment and treatment of pain and other problems, physical, psychosocial and spiritual."[3] Palliative care programs also help patients to coordinate their care, to understand their condition, and to cope with related physical, emotional, and psychological distress. Payment for services rendered is the same as that for any other health-related treatment.

In reality, the philosophy of palliative care is nothing new to physical therapists as it relates to preserving human dignity and maintaining an optimal quality of life whatever the circumstances. The profession's long history of compassionately enhancing the quality of life for all patients is only one of the ways in which we are well positioned for important contributions in palliative care.

In many communities, hospice and palliative care services are offered through the same facility. Reimbursement for palliative care services is administered through the patient's primary medical insurance, enabling patients in palliative care to receive coverage for monthly visits from the hospice/palliative care nursing staff. Patients may remain on palliative services for months or years while seeking curative or supportive measures for their condition.

The Evolution of Palliative Care and Hospice in the 21st Century

Over the last several years the health care system has undergone a dramatic shift toward better health care management for individuals with chronic, life-threatening, or terminal illnesses specifically with the growth and proliferation of palliative care programs. Fig. 27.1 illustrates the rapid growth of such programs since 2000.

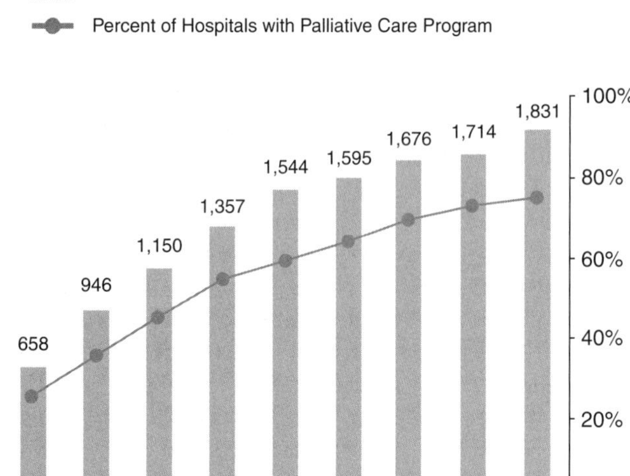

FIG. 27.1 The proliferation of palliative care programs in U.S. hospitals (with 50 or more beds) from 2000 to 2016. *(From Center to Advance Palliative Care. Growth of Palliative Care in U.S. Hospitals 2016 Snapshot. Reprinted with permission.)*

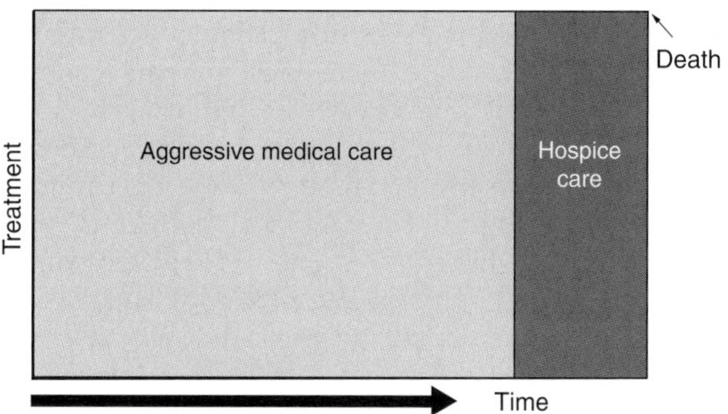

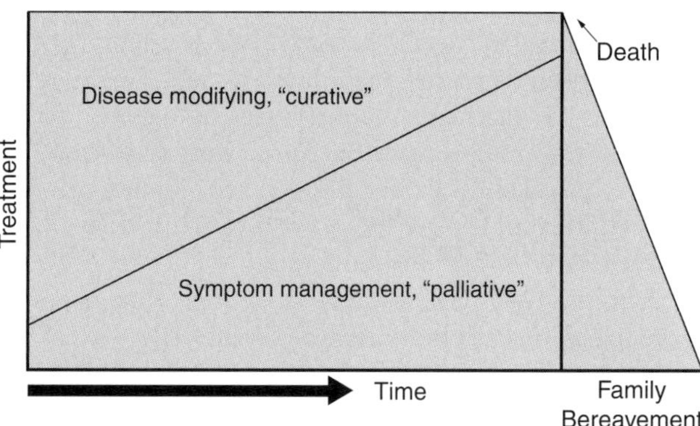

FIG. 27.2 The older "transition" model of care versus a "trajectory" model of palliative and hospice. *(From Lynn J, Adamson DM. Living Well at the End of Life. White Paper. Santa Monica, CA: Rand Corporation; 2003. Reprinted with permission.)*

Palliative care is often perceived as a transition from active "curative" care to hospice care, but palliative care also includes patients with life-threatening illness who are not imminently dying but in physical decline who need holistic, patient-centered multidisciplinary support services.[4] The Center to Advance Palliative Care describes palliative care as "specialized medical care for people with serious illness. It focuses on providing patients with relief from the symptoms, pain and stress of a serious illness - whatever the diagnosis."[5] According to the Institute of Medicine, 60% of all health care costs in the United States were attributed to only 5% of patients—those with serious illness.[6] Of this small but costly group of patients, 11% were in the last year of their life, and 89% will remain alive for longer than a year.[6] This highlights the need for comprehensive, focused care for those with serious illness to help contain health care costs and optimize remaining quality of life (QOL). Within this health care paradigm, physical therapists can demonstrate their value by keeping these individuals safe at home and in their community by optimizing health, preventing falls, providing for safe discharge, and reducing unwarranted hospital readmissions. Fig. 27.2 illustrates the change in models of palliative care to hospice toward a trajectory model.

Providing physical therapy care to patients who are not expected to demonstrate functional recovery is a recent phenomenon in the United States, perhaps owing to insurance regulations requiring documented gains—commonly termed the "improvement standard." In 2013, a number of seriously ill individuals initiated a class action lawsuit to challenge standards of access to medical services including physical therapy in the United States. The *Jimmo v. Sebelius* settlement in the U.S. federal court establishes that the Centers for Medicare and Medicaid Services (CMS) must reimburse for skilled services (including physical therapy) if the services are medically necessary to maintain or slow the decline of function during a serious or life-threatening illness even if there is not the expectation of physical or functional improvement.[7] This settlement does not differentiate between different payment methodologies for Medicare and would include both Medicare part A and Medicare part B payment services for physical therapy. Once a patient with a life-threatening illness enrolls in the Medicare hospice benefit, the payment structure does shift toward a per diem model where a hospice organization receives a certain dollar amount per day for all services. In this hospice payment model, physical therapy availability may be more restricted owing to financial limitations and the patient's advanced disease process. Although the *Jimmo v. Sebelius* settlement agreement pertains to the United States' CMS, it is an important factor for other private insurances or agencies to consider when determining which services to cover or provide during the care of the individual with a life-threatening illness.

Clinical Scenario. Elaine was a 54-year-old woman with a 2-year history of cervical cancer. During this time, Elaine had received three courses of chemotherapy with good results. Elaine sought palliative care services through her local hospital system for the purpose of expert pain management. She received monthly visits from the palliative care nurse, who assisted Elaine in determining appropriate pharmacologic measures for pain control. Elaine's medications were covered by her primary insurance. In the meantime, Elaine underwent an additional course of chemotherapy, and this episode left her considerably weaker than prior courses. As a result, Elaine was unable to engage in her aerobics classes at her local gym. A physical therapy consult was requested to assist Elaine in developing an exercise and wellness prescription. During the consult, the physical therapist worked with Elaine to develop a slowly progressive walking program, using a pedometer to measure her progress. Elaine remained on palliative services for an additional 8 months, whereupon her physician determined that further curative measures were unlikely to be successful. Elaine transferred to hospice and received services for another 2 months before her death.

The Physical Therapist's Role in Hospice and Palliative Care

In the United States and globally, there remains inconsistent access to hospice and palliative care (HPC) services, with more traditional underserved regions or areas such as rural or low-income areas having decreased access to consistent HPC services. In these areas limited HPC services may be compounded with inconsistent access to physical therapy (PT) services within HPC.[8] Other health professionals may be unaware of the value of physical therapy in maintaining safe and comfortable function in the presence of physical decline. This lack of access to physical therapy may prevent the optimization of the remaining part of life and its rich interactions. The American Physical Therapy Association's (APTA) House of Delegates has endorsed and clarified the physical therapist's role in HPC through a motion passed in 2011 (RC 17-11)[9] that included concepts related to continuity of care, appropriate and adequate access to PT services, the importance of an interdisciplinary approach, and education of PTs, physical therapist assistants (PTAs), and students in HPC, as well as pursuing appropriate and comparable coverage and payment.

Fig. 27.3 depicts a conceptual framework that represents the roles of physical therapy in various aspects of hospice and palliative care. The conceptual framework was developed after qualitative interviews with experienced

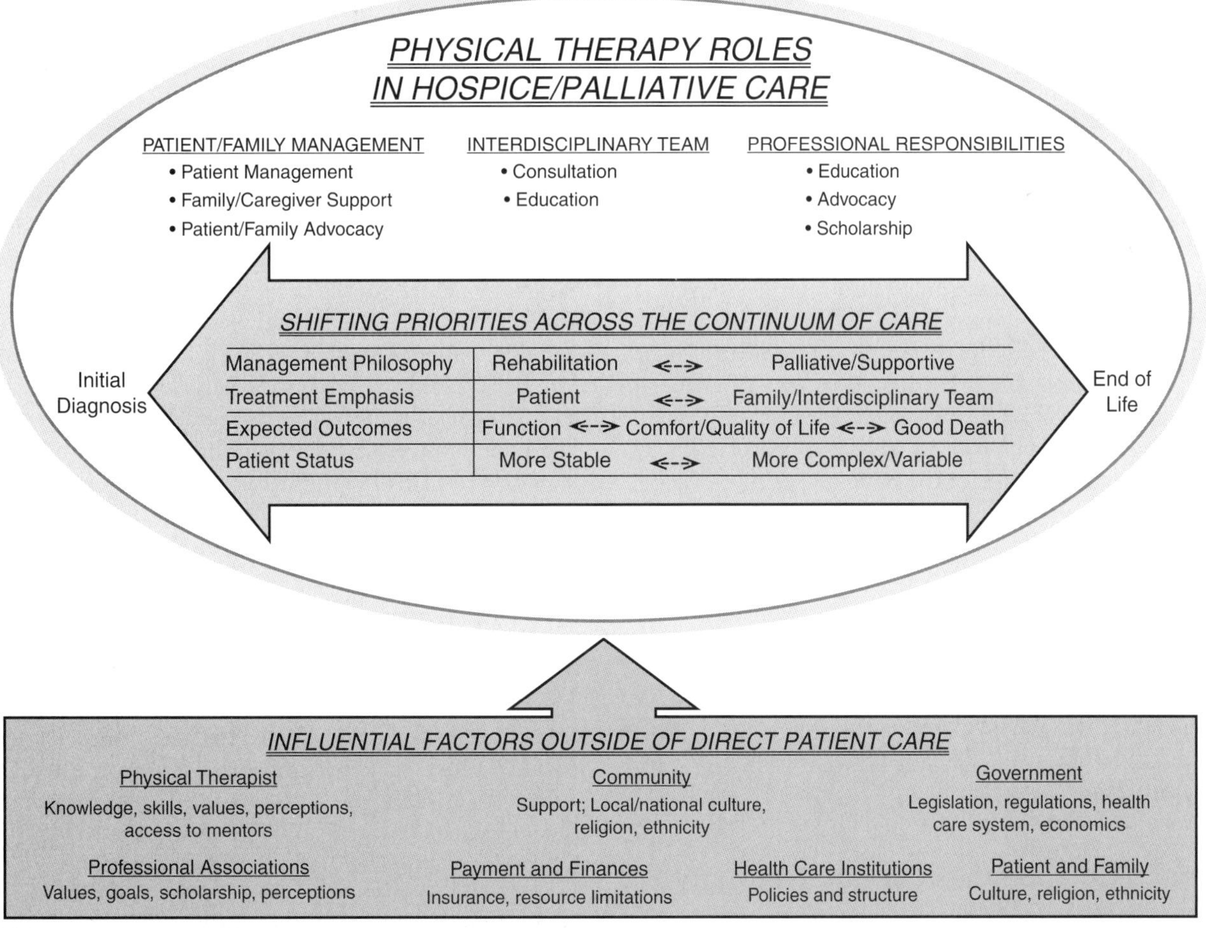

FIG. 27.3 Conceptual framework for physical therapist involvement in hospice and palliative care. *(From Wilson CM, Stiller CH, Doherty DJ, Thompson KA. The role of physical therapists within hospice and palliative care in the United States and Canada. Am J Hospice Palliative Med. 2017 Feb;34[1]:34–41. Reprinted with permission.)*

HPC physical therapists in the United States and Canada.[10] Within the large oval is the physical therapist's role as it relates to hospice and palliative care. At the top of the oval are the PT's roles within hospice and palliative care that are present at all times in the management of a patient with a late-stage chronic disease or life-limiting illness (patient and family management, the PT's role as an interdisciplinary team member, and professional responsibilities).

The large bidirectional arrow represents care concepts related to shifting patient care priorities across the continuum as the patient advances through his or her disease trajectory from initial diagnosis through death. These shifting priorities may include the PT's patient management philosophy, the shift in emphasis in treatment and expected outcomes, and anticipating shifting patient status from more stable to more complex and variable. For example, a patient with a degenerative condition such as multiple sclerosis may have frequent and dramatic fluctuations in function between periods of stability with associated varying needs for physical therapy. The small double-sided dashed arrows represent shifting priorities—double-sided because individuals/therapists can go back and forth between the two extremes and dashed because there may be some cases where therapy is interrupted because of medical issues, patient and family preference, financial issues, or other external factors.

Below the oval that outlined the PT's role in HPC is a large rectangle that describes factors that influence the physical therapist's HPC management beyond direct patient care. Factors include influences inherent to an individual physical therapist including his or her comfort level with end-of-life care, patient access, and knowledge of HPC care philosophy. Additional factors are the community and government, payment and finances, physical therapists' professional association, and perceptions and infrastructure of individual health care institutions. Finally, the patient and family circumstances were influential factors on physical therapy outside of direct patient care, including willingness and ability to participate in rehabilitation, acceptance of the patient's current disease state and trajectory, and the emotional resources of the patient and family to participate in rehabilitation during this difficult time. For example, several physical therapists noted that financial barriers, governmental regulations, or institutional structure was not always conducive to performing their role within hospice or palliative care, and physical therapists need to advocate for their services or establish strategic alliances to integrate physical therapy services into currently existing or newly developing hospice or palliative care programs.[10]

Determining and Documenting Necessity of PT Services in HPC

As noted earlier, the *Jimmo v. Sebelius* settlement further clarified that a patient or client is still eligible to receive skilled services even if there is no clear potential for physical or functional improvement. The patient/client would also be eligible when skilled physical therapy services are required to maintain the patient's current status or slow the decline of the patient's condition. It is anticipated that additional insurance payers may consider adopting this payment methodology. A key concept of this methodology is that these services must require the skills of a licensed PT or PTA and the provider's clinical documentation must reflect the need for the services and why these services cannot be safely or appropriately performed by a different provider (such as nursing, massage therapist, etc.) or by volunteers or family caregivers. Fig. 27.4 outlines key clinical decision-making points to assist therapists to determine if their individual patient situation would be appropriate for skilled physical therapist services.

If the clinical documentation does not clearly establish these key tenets on a regular basis, the physical therapy services are at a higher risk of rejection for payment or additional audits by insurance companies. As most rehabilitation professionals focus their clinical documentation on demonstrating progress with impairments or improvements in functional limitations, this patient population may demonstrate some confounding factors to conventional clinical documentation. If a therapist only reports objective measures such as range of motion, strength, or functional mobility status and these measures do not demonstrate improvement, it may increase the likelihood of insurance nonpayment or audit. Therefore, it is imperative that HPC PTs and PTAs also quantify contextual factors as well as patient-reported QOL. Even if a patient's range of motion, strength, or gait distance worsens, if the therapist is able to demonstrate that the skilled services have improved or maintained QOL, even in the presence of an advancing disease process, then payment denials are less likely. There are a number of widely utilized, valid, reliable patient-reported QOL outcome measures that can be accessed at www.facit.org including the Functional Assessment of Cancer Therapy—General (FACT-G) and the Functional Assessment of Chronic Illness Therapy—Fatigue (FACIT-F). Table 27.1 provides some clinical documentation examples to justify physical therapy services for a variety of palliative or hospice scenarios.

Acute Care Palliative Care

Within palliative care, there are two main locales where programs are generally being developed: hospital-based acute care and postacute care. Postacute care may include locations such as home care services, skilled nursing facilities, transitional care units, long-term acute care hospitals, inpatient rehabilitation units, and some outpatient facilities.[11] In addition to patient-centered outcome measures including improvement in QOL, maintenance of high level of functioning (as able), and optimal symptom management, key outcomes for these organizations include reducing unwarranted readmissions into the hospital, falls

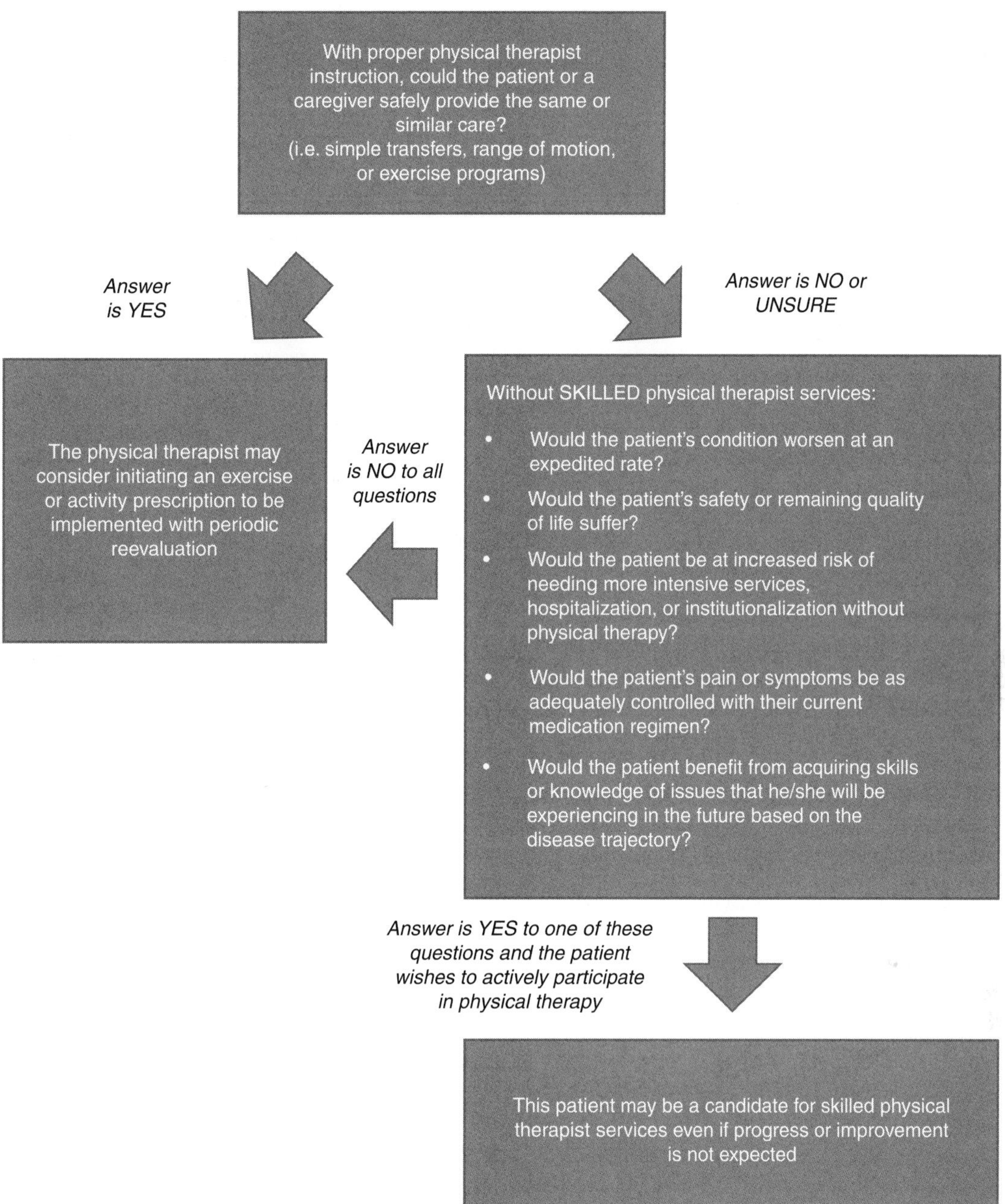

With proper physical therapist instruction, could the patient or a caregiver safely provide the same or similar care?
(i.e. simple transfers, range of motion, or exercise programs)
Answer is YES
Answer is NO or UNSURE
The physical therapist may consider initiating an exercise or activity prescription to be implemented with periodic reevaluation
Answer is NO to all questions
Without SKILLED physical therapist services:
Would the patient's condition worsen at an expedited rate?
Would the patient's safety or remaining quality of life suffer?
Would the patient be at increased risk of needing more intensive services, hospitalization, or institutionalization without physical therapy?
Would the patient's pain or symptoms be as adequately controlled with their current medication regimen?
Would the patient benefit from acquiring skills or knowledge of issues that he/she will be experiencing in the future based on the disease trajectory?
Answer is YES to one of these questions and the patient wishes to actively participate in physical therapy
This patient may be a candidate for skilled physical therapist services even if progress or improvement is not expected

FIG. 27.4 Considerations for determining medical necessity for physical therapy. *(From Wilson CM, Boright L. Documenting medical necessity for palliative care and degenerative or chronic conditions. Rehabil Oncol. 2017 Jul 1;35[3]:153–156. Reprinted with permission.)*

(especially injurious falls), and avoiding unwarranted diagnostic testing or surgical procedures that do not improve the patient's quality of remaining life or disease trajectory. A key component of this transition from acute to postacute care is clear handoff communication and integrated services between acute care and the postacute setting—all services that acute care physical therapists are equipped to assist with. A study by Wilson and Roy[12] examined the overlap between acute care palliative consultations and physical therapy consultations and demonstrated that for 963 palliative care consultations, physical therapists were consulted 83% of the time during that hospital admission, indicating that there is a significant role for physical therapists with the acute palliative population. In addition, it was noted that physical therapy was ordered before palliative care 70% of the time, which may indicate that attending physicians may be utilizing physical therapy as a part of the decision-making process as to whether to initiate palliative care services or not. For example, if a patient is participating in PT during a hospitalization and is not demonstrating improvement, it provides further evidence that palliative care may be necessary.

In the hospital setting, many health care systems have begun to hire palliative care midlevel providers such as specialty-trained nurse practitioners or physician assistants. Key roles for these midlevel providers, working under the

TABLE 27.1 Examples of Documentation That Justify Need for Physical Therapist Services in Hospice and Palliative Care

Clinical Scenario/ *Patient Description*	Interventions Performed or Objective Findings	Assessment or Evaluation	Expected Outcomes or Goal Setting
Maintenance of a status that is anticipated to decline without skilled PT *47 y.o. female with progressive multiple sclerosis*	The patient was able to perform her lower extremity exercises at the same resistance and dosage despite documented disease progression.	Without PT services, it is expected that the patient's lower extremity strength status would worsen over the next 2 to 3 weeks.	The patient's bilateral quadriceps strength will remain 4/5 as opposed to declining to 3+/5 as would be expected without skilled PT intervention.
Ensuring safety via skilled PT services *74 y.o. male with stage 4 lung CA with bone metastasis to femurs*	Patient requires continuous monitoring and manual or verbal cueing from PTA during gait training with standard walker to maintain non–weight bearing due to femoral bone metastases.	Patient requires continued skilled physical therapy services to maintain safety with functional transfers/mobility in preparation for home discharge on hospice.	The patient will be able to ambulate with standard walker with caregiver or therapist assistance to protect the restricted weight-bearing status.
Anticipating future decline *63 y.o. male with amyotrophic lateral sclerosis*	Patient was able to tolerate gait training with standby assistance with standard cane for 100 feet. The patient was instructed in the use of two-wheeled walker in anticipation of functional status declining as a result of disease trajectory.	In addition to interventions to address current clinical deficits, the patient would benefit from preparatory training in use of rolling walker and wheelchair, to promote continued safe home mobility through anticipated progressive decline in lower extremity strength (functional endurance) expected as a result of chronic disease process.	The patient will demonstrate the ability to transfer and ambulate safely with the two-wheeled walker to safely perform functional activities as the disease process progresses.
Slower progress or decreased tolerance anticipated *79 y.o. female with COPD*	X, Y, and Z interventions had planned to be implemented but were modified (or held) on this date owing to decreased endurance and tolerance.	Patient does require continued skilled physical therapy services but will likely need frequent rest breaks and decreased intensity of interventions to optimize comfort and physical outcomes.	Patient's Timed Up and Go test time will only increase by 5 seconds as opposed to improving by 10 or more seconds as would be expected without the patient's COPD.
Emphasizing quality of life *89 y.o. female with Alzheimer dementia and Parkinson disease*	Although subacute rehab was recommended after discharge by care team, patient and family prefer to d/c home. Caregiver training was completed for safe home mobility in anticipation of home discharge.	As the patient's functional status and strength are declining, the PT will focus on optimizing remaining quality of life and safe, comfortable, active participation in life events as quantified by FACT-G questionnaire.	The patient's FACT-G QoL score will increase to 65 even though objective physical measures are expected to decline.
Nonopioid pain management *64 y.o. male with stage IV lung CA with spinal metastasis*	Patient's pain reports remained less than 4/10 on visual analog scale throughout exercise session with a reported decreased need for prescription pain medications prior to therapy.	Patient demonstrates ability to effectively manage pain through positioning and exercise techniques.	Patient will be independent in home pain management techniques as evidenced by decreased need for oral opioid use.

CA, cancer; *COPD*, chronic obstructive pulmonary disorder; *d/c*, discharge; *FACT-G*, Functional Assessment of Cancer Treatment: General (www.facit.org); *PT*, physical therapist; *PTA*, physical therapist assistant; *QoL*, quality of life; *y.o.*, year old.
(From Wilson CM, Boright L. Documenting medical necessity for palliative care and degenerative or chronic conditions. *Rehabil Oncol*. 2017 Jul 1;35[3]:153–156. Reprinted with permission.)

supervision of a physician leader trained in palliative care, are to discuss the patient's goals of care, advance directives, and transition to next level of care. Hospitals have begun to convene formal or informal palliative care interdisciplinary rounds within the hospital. These are often attended by physicians, palliative care midlevel providers, social workers, chaplains/pastoral care professionals, rehabilitation professionals (such as physical therapists), and representatives from postacute care settings. Within these interdisciplinary team meetings, physical therapists should report on the patient's current or anticipated functional capabilities and deficits, provide input on safe discharge planning and fall prevention, and assist with procurement of durable medical equipment that the patient may need as their functional status changes.[13] It may not be feasible for every physical therapist within the hospital setting who works with a palliative care patient to attend these rounds. Best practice may be if one key physical therapist attends and serves as the conduit for communicating information to and from the rest of the care team with his or her physical therapist colleagues. An example of best-practice interdisciplinary communication would be if a treating physical therapist noted that the patient's functional status was declining despite continued participation in physical therapy. This information would be important to communicate to the palliative care team. The treating physical therapist would communicate this information to the PT who attends palliative care rounds to convey to the rest of the interdisciplinary team. After the meeting was completed, the PT who attended the rounds updates the treating physical therapist as to the status of the patient, and the outcome and recommendations from the interdisciplinary care team. Because a goal of interdisciplinary hospice and palliative care rounds is to improve the communication and continuity of care, there may be opportunities for post-acute physical therapists to either attend via telecommunications or convey information to their representative who attends the rounds regarding steps that may be taken to avoid unwarranted readmission to keep the patient safe and active in his or her home.[14]

PLANNING FOR DEATH WITH DIGNITY: ADVANCED DIRECTIVES

Advanced Care Planning

As autonomous human beings, we desire the ability to identify, plan, and execute important elements of our lives. Planning is a central process by which we direct our lives in concert with our values and preferences. The vast majority of human activities, particularly those involving health care interactions, require the cooperation of others. Thus, the ability to communicate values and preferences surrounding health care choices is central in patient satisfaction and quality of life. The end of life is no exception. Planning for the type of care we want at this juncture can help ensure a death with dignity and comfort in the setting of our choice. More importantly, in situations where we are no longer able to convey our preferences, a clear plan for the type of health care we desire assures our family and loved ones that they are supporting us in concert with our wishes. Advanced care planning (ACP) involves making decisions, identifying strategies, and enlisting the support of family members and health professionals to ensure medical care that is congruent with personal values and preferences.[15]

Health care preferences at end of life are typically conveyed through a document known as an *advanced directive*. An advanced directive enables a person to identify a trusted individual to convey the individual's preferences for medical care in the event that the individual is no longer able to do so. This document also enables a person to select options for life-sustaining care. Ideally, an advanced directive is completed before circumstances require it.

The absence of an advanced directive can have a devastating impact for family members, particularly if they disagree about the best course of action. Such disagreement was illustrated in the 2005 case of Terri Schiavo, a young woman living in a persistent vegetative state for 15 years following a cardiac arrest.[16] Schiavo was incapable of purposeful interaction and required a feeding tube to sustain her nutrition; however, she was able to breathe independently. She had been in a persistent vegetative state for 8 years when her husband petitioned the Sixth Circuit Court of Florida to remove her feeding tube, stating that Schiavo would have never wanted to live in her current condition. However, her parents, both devout Catholics, disagreed, stating that removal of the feeding tube was tantamount to murder. Unfortunately, Schiavo had not completed an advanced directive and her family members were unable to agree on a course of action. A nationally prominent court battle ensued over the next 7 years before the feeding tube was removed. Schiavo died on March 31, 2005.[16]

In spite of the publicity around the Schiavo case, the use of advanced directives remains limited. In one study, only half of persons aged 60 or older reported the completion of these documents.[17] Even in the case of serious illness, the issue of advanced directives may be ignored. Another study found that only 27% of patients with advanced cancer had discussed advanced directives with their oncologist and only 13% had discussed palliative care with any physician.[18] Even when advanced directives are in place, health care professionals may not have access to these, resulting in the use of unwanted interventions.

As a result of these missteps, ACP has gained increased recognition as a health care intervention intended to reduce unwanted care at the end of life. As of January 1, 2016, the CMS has reimbursed physicians and other health professionals for ACP conversations with patients as part of the annual wellness visit.[19] The outcomes of these discussions will be documented in the patient's medical record so that all providers are informed of the patient's end-of-life preferences. Evidence supports the value of ACP in promoting better patient outcomes at end of life, including decreased use of inappropriate care, lower health care costs, and better physician adherence to patient wishes.[20]

Physical therapists should be prepared to engage in ACP discussions, many of which may arise in the context of discharge planning, identifying equipment needs in the face of decline, or referring a patient for a palliative care consult.[21] When addressing ACP during a clinical encounter, a broad, open-ended question will invite the patient to explore a wide range of possibilities that can be further explored. For example, when working with a patient who is declining rapidly from amyotrophic lateral sclerosis (ALS), the physical therapist might inquire, "What future support might you need to have the best quality of life with your disease?" A follow-up question such as "How have you conveyed these desires?" can lead to a discussion on the value of ACP in ensuring that such needs are met. Any elements of an ACP-related discussion should be documented to facilitate communication between other providers.

Elements of the Advanced Directive

Advanced care plan (ACP) documents allow individuals to identify their preferences for care in the event that they are no longer able to speak for themselves. There are two types of ACP documents, each with a distinct purpose and intended audience, explained in detail next. Healthy individuals over the age of 18 are encouraged to complete a DPAHC and living will as a general indication of their preferences for future care. In contrast, a DNR or MOLST is typically completed when an individual is terminally ill and facing the possibility of imminent death. Accordingly, the MOLST enables a terminally ill person to explicitly identify the extent and nature of life-sustaining interventions, which range from comfort care only to hospitalization and full resuscitation. Although a DNR and/or MOLST are not required as a condition for admission to hospice and palliative care programs, patients are encouraged to complete these to prevent unwanted aggressive treatment such as cardiac resuscitation.

Durable power of attorney is the appointment of a trusted individual aged 18 years or older (typically a family member or close friend) to make decisions on one's behalf (act as a surrogate) when a person is no longer able to do so him- or herself. A DPAHC can be granted for decisions related to financial matters, mental health care, and general health care. The DPAHC is a written document, which, depending on the person's state of residence, becomes a legal document when signed by the patient (also known as "grantor") in the presence of a witness. Notarization is required in some states.

The extent of DPAHC responsibilities typically involve coordinating care with health care providers and family members to ensure that the grantor's preferences are honored. Many of the challenges around end-of-life care involve the execution of patient desires involving the refusal, initiation, or withdrawal of life-sustaining treatments such as ventilators, enteral feeding ("feeding tubes"), and cardiac resuscitation. Refusal or withdrawal of such measures inevitably leads to death, and some health care providers may be reluctant to execute these measures. Thus, patients should engage family members and health care team members in the process of ACP. These discussions support the patient as well as the providers who carry out the patient's requests.

A living will identifies the patient's specific requests for the type of health care desired in the event of a serious illness. The living will can even be broadened to include special provisions for pregnant women to determine the extent of life-saving measures for their unborn offspring. Some living wills are integrated into the DPAHC document, and others are stand-alone documents. In either case, family members and health care providers should all receive copies of these documents and their contents should be thoroughly discussed with family and health care providers. Documentation of the patient's advanced directive should also be noted in the medical record.

A DNR is a document that clearly specifies the patient's refusal for cardiac resuscitation in the event of a life-threatening event. Most persons do not complete a DNR as part of their advanced directive until a serious terminal illness raises QOL issues. Although a DNR is not required as a condition of hospice admission, the topic typically arises in patient discussions about care options. For patients receiving in-home hospice care, the DNR is typically printed on orange paper and prominently placed in clear sight (often on the kitchen refrigerator door). Enacting a DNR can be a difficult decision for family members or health providers who are present when a person shows clear signs of imminent death, however, hospice personnel are highly skilled in providing support and other interventions to allow a peaceful and comfortable death. Moreover, patients who cannot provide evidence of their enacted DNR may receive unwanted resuscitation with potentially devastating consequences such as brain anoxia or chest/rib trauma. DNR orders are not typically signed by the patient's physician, which may contribute to inconsistent follow-through if the patient is admitted to a hospital. The reasons for this are varied and include a lack of visible DNR documentation and disagreements between family members that result in a 911 call. In such cases, the medical response team is required to institute aggressive life support measures that include CPR or electrocardioversion.

For persons with serious, life-limiting medical conditions or advanced frailty, there are 2 advanced care documents which fall under the category *of medical orders*. The first is the Do Not Resuscitate (DNR) order which addresses the use of cardiac resuscitation. The other document is the POLST (physician orders for life sustaining treatment,) or MOLST (medical orders for life sustaining treatment). The purpose of these documents is to direct emergency personnel to provide specific interventions (such as cardiac resuscitation as well as medically assisted nutrition, hydration or ventilation) in a medical emergency. These documents are medical orders which are signed by the appropriate health professional after a conversation with the patient in which treatment options are agreed upon. Although signature requirements for a valid POLST form vary by state, these health professionals typically include physicians, advanced practice registered nurses and physician assistant. Completion of the

TABLE 27.2 Comparison of Advanced Directives and Physician Orders for Life-Sustaining Treatment (POLST) Documents

	POLST Paradigm Form	Advance Directive
Type of document	Medical order	Legal document
Who completes the document	Health care professional (which health care professional can sign varies by state)	All competent adults
What document communicates	Specific medical orders	General treatment wishes
Can this document appoint a surrogate decision maker?	No	Yes
Surrogate decision maker role	Can engage in discussion and update or void form if patient lacks capacity	Cannot complete
Can emergency personnel follow this document?	Yes	No
Ease in locating/portability	Patient has original and a copy is in patient's medical record; a copy may be in a state registry (if state has one)	No set location; individuals must make sure surrogates have most recent version
Periodic review	Health care professional responsible for reviewing with patient or surrogate	Patient is responsible for periodically reviewing

(Comparison of Advanced Directives and POLST Documents. Used with permission from the National POLST Paradigm. Available at http://www.POLST.org.)

POLST form is strictly voluntary. The National Hospice and Palliative Care Organization provides information about ACP on its website and also provides access to state-specific forms.[24]

Advanced directives and POLST documents are similar in that they are both intended to allow individuals to identify their individual preferences for care in the event of incapacitation due to serious illness or injury. However, they have distinct differences as shown in Table 27.2.

5 Wishes: A User-Friendly Advanced Directive

In 1996, attorney Jim Towey founded Aging with Dignity after his experiences at Mother Teresa's homes for the dying inspired him to promote better care for people facing the end of life. He developed a user-friendly advanced directive known as 5 Wishes, which uses simple language and an interactive written format to facilitate the appointment of a DPAHC, the type of care desired, and the type of emotional, physical, and spiritual support desired.[25] The 5 Wishes program is used in all 50 states and meets the requirements for a legal advanced directive in 42 states (in the other states, 5 Wishes can be made legal through the process of notarization). Thus far, 5 Wishes has become one of the most popular forms of advanced directive, with 25 million persons having used this document.[25]

Death with Dignity: Physician-Assisted Death

Physician-assisted death allows mentally competent patients with a terminally ill condition to request and receive a prescription medication to hasten their imminent and inevitable death. As of 2018, seven states (California, Colorado, District of Columbia, Hawaii, Oregon, Vermont, and Washington) have enacted death with dignity laws, which permit physician-assisted death.[26] Although the intent of physician-assisted dying is to ensure complete patient autonomy in the decision to die with peace and comfort at the time and place of their choosing, the practice has raised ethical concerns that patients may choose this instead of seeking appropriate palliative care. Accordingly, a recent position paper from International Association for Hospice and Palliative Care has asserted that no country or state should consider the legalization of physician-assisted death until it ensures universal access to palliative care services and to appropriate medications, including opioids for pain and dyspnea. The position paper further states that palliative care units should not be responsible for involvement in these practices.[27]

HOSPICE CARE: SUPPORTING DEATH WITH DIGNITY AND COMFORT

The Medicare Hospice Benefit

The Medicare hospice benefit was enacted by Congress in 1982 and since that time has been the major source of payment for U.S. hospice services. In 2016, Medicare provided services for 48% of all patients served.[28] To qualify for hospice, both the hospice physician and the patient's primary care provider must certify the presence of a terminal condition with a prognosis of <6 months. In addition, patients must certify that they are willing to accept comfort-based care and are no longer seeking curative measures for their condition. Finally, patients must be entitled to Medicare Part A services (inpatient). Patients who elect the Medicare hospice benefit begin with two initial 90-day periods, which can then be followed by unlimited 60-day periods as long as documentation shows the continued need and appropriateness for services. Patients may revoke their hospice benefit if they decide to pursue curative measures.[29] Medicare requires that all core services (nursing, physician, psychological, and spiritual support) be available on a 24-hour basis to ensure support and comfort whenever needed. The levels of service and types of care covered under the Medicare hospice benefit are illustrated in Boxes 27.1 and 27.2.

History of Hospice Care

The term *hospice* derives from the Latin term *hospitum*, which originally described a place of shelter for sick and weary travelers. Nirmal Hriday (Pure Heart), one of the first known homes for the dying, was established in 1952 by Mother Teresa in Calcutta, India.[29,30] Working in the most destitute slums of Calcutta, she and her sister nuns took indigents who were dying off the streets to nurse them at this home, enabling "persons who lived like animals to die like angels, loved and wanted."[30] This noble work continues today in more than 500 worldwide centers.

Dame Cicely Saunders, MD (1918–2005), is recognized as the founder of the modern hospice movement. As a nurse working at an English cancer hospital after World War II, she was disturbed by the pain and isolation she witnessed among dying patients. These observations compelled her to enter St. Thomas's Medical School in 1951 at the age of 33, qualifying as a physician in 1957. Following the completion of her medical studies, Saunders sought additional training in pharmacology, when she explored the effective use of analgesic medications for the treatment of pain at end of life. In an environment where medication underutilization was common because of fears of addiction, she challenged rationales that were grounded mainly in conjecture. Accordingly, instead of requiring patients to wait until their pain medications wore off before requesting another dose, Saunders advocated medicating at a level to produce continual analgesia and wrote several papers that described and provided support for her approach. Furthermore, instead of the sterile and lonely hospital rooms where she had worked as a young nurse, Saunders proposed treating dying patients in a warm and comfortable setting with a home-like atmosphere. In 1967, Saunders opened St. Christopher's Hospice in London where she put her vision into action.[31] Saunders served as the medical director of St. Christopher's until 1985, and was awarded England's Order of Merit in 1989. By the time she died in 2005, at the same hospice she established, there were more than 8,000 hospices worldwide.

The U.S. hospice movement began in 1974 upon the opening of the Connecticut Hospice in Branford. Many of Cicely Saunders' original ideals have been successfully integrated into current hospice practice, contributing to the hospice movement's significant growth and making it the preferred approach to end-of-life care.

BOX 27.1 Specific Services Covered by Medicare Hospice Benefit

- Physician services*
- Nursing care*
- Medical equipment (like wheelchairs or walkers)
- Medical supplies (like bandages and catheters)
- Prescription drugs
- Hospice aide and homemaker services
- Physical and occupational therapy
- Speech–language pathology services
- Social worker services*
- Dietary counseling*
- Grief and loss counseling for patient and family*
- Short-term inpatient care (for pain and symptom management)
- Short-term respite care
- Any other Medicare-covered services needed to manage the terminal illness and related conditions, as recommended by the hospice team

* Denotes core service required for Medicare reimbursement.

BOX 27.2 Levels of Care Provided by Hospice Benefit

Home-Based Care

1. Routine home care: Patient receives hospice care at the place he or she resides.
2. Continuous home care: Patient receives hospice care consisting predominantly of nursing care on a continuous basis at home. Continuous home care is only furnished during brief periods of crisis and only as necessary to maintain the terminally ill patient at home.

Inpatient Care

1. General inpatient care: Patient receives general inpatient care in an inpatient facility for pain control or acute or chronic symptom management that cannot be managed in other settings.
2. Inpatient respite care: Patient receives care in an approved facility on a short-term basis to provide respite for the caregiver.

Growth of Programs and Services

Since the inception of hospice in 1974, the number of Medicare-certified American hospices has steadily grown, numbering 4,382 in 2017.[27] Hospice services are delivered through a variety of facilities that include the patient's residence, freestanding facilities, hospice programs in home health agencies, units attached to hospitals, and nursing homes. In 2016, 1.43 million Americans received at least one day of hospice services.[28] The National Hospice and Palliative Care Organization reported that of the 2.7 million U.S. deaths occurring in

2016, 1.04 million (38.8%) occurred while enrolled in hospice care. Nearly 45% occurred in the patient's residence.[28] Interestingly, 235,200 patients (16.8%) were discharged from hospice, either because of an extended prognosis or because of a desire to pursue curative measures.[28] This is a noteworthy statistic, which dispels the misperception that hospice is an irrevocable or predictably ominous choice for patients with terminal illness.

Profile of Hospice Patients

According to 2017 outcome data from the National Hospice and Palliative Care Organization, 58.6% of all hospice patients were female. The vast majority (84%) of these hospice patients were age 65 years or older.[28] Thus, hospice is and will continue to be primarily a geriatric treatment setting, with numbers increasing significantly with the aging of the baby boomer generation.

Currently, hospice patients are predominately Caucasian (48.9%). The existence of racial and ethnic disparities in end-of-life care has been confirmed in several studies.[32,33] A systematic review of 13 retrospective cohort studies found statistically significantly lower hospice utilization rates among African Americans compared to Caucasians.[32] Another retrospective study examined Medicare hospice database records of 40,960 Caucasian, Hispanic, African American, and Asian beneficiaries who received services for end-stage cancer between 1992 and 2001.[33] The results of the study showed that Caucasians had the highest hospice utilization rate (49%) followed by African Americans (36%), Hispanics (37%), and Asians (32%) (Table 27.3).

The study also found that nonwhite groups had higher numbers of hospitalizations for longer periods of time as well as a higher likelihood of an intensive care unit admission in their last month of life. Finally, members of these nonwhite racial groups were also more likely to die in the hospital.[33] The reasons for these ethnic and racial disparities are not yet clear, and further research is needed to explore the impact of cultural differences, belief systems, and patient preference on selections related to end-of-life care. As the American population becomes increasingly diverse, health care professionals may need to explore culturally sensitive approaches for educating patients of different racial and ethnic backgrounds about the value of hospice care.

Diagnoses

The major diagnostic categories of the patients seen in U. S. hospices in 2016 are shown in Table 27.4.

A notable trend with respect to these diagnostic categories is the increasing number of patients with Alzheimer dementia and debilitation. Currently it is estimated that 5.7 million Americans are living with Alzheimer disease, and projections are as high as 16 million by 2050.[34] Patients with this disease may survive and deteriorate for a period of years while their family members struggle to provide care.

As patients with Alzheimer disease become more debilitated, they may ultimately develop a host of conditions that are considered indications of the end stage of the disease. To be considered for hospice coverage, Medicare guidelines require patients with Alzheimer disease to exhibit at least one of the following signs in the previous 12 months: muscle wasting and malnutrition (inanition) with a 10% decrease in body weight, septicemia, decubitus ulcer, aspiration pneumonia, recurrent fever, or urinary tract infection.[35] Unfortunately, by the time patients qualify for hospice care under the current guidelines, many patients with end-stage Alzheimer disease are completely dependent and show significant cognitive impairments. The extent of these impairments can challenge caregivers, especially in the realm of determining patient needs for pain medications and other comfort measures. As patients with end-stage dementia enter the hospice system in increasing numbers, further guidelines are needed to determine appropriate indications for pain control and comfort as patients approach end of life. As the burden of caregiving can be considerable in such cases, hospice staff can also provide assistance to family members so that patients can remain in their homes during this process.

TABLE 27.3 Hospice Deaths by Race in 2017

Race	Percentage
Caucasian	48.9%
African American	35.6%
Hispanic	37.4%
Asian	31.7%
Other	36.2%
Native American	32.9%
Unknown	34.3%

(Source: National Hospice and Palliative Care Organization. Facts and Figures, 2017 Edition. https://www.nhpco.org/sites/default/files/public/Statistics_Research/2017_Facts_Figures.pdf.)

TABLE 27.4 Diagnostic Categories of Hospice Deaths

Principal Diagnosis Causing Terminal Prognosis	
Cancer	27.2%
Cardiac and circulatory	18.7%
Dementia	18.0%
Respiratory	11.0%
Stroke	9.5%
Other	15.6%

(Source: National Hospice and Palliative Care Organization. Facts and Figures, 2017 Edition. https://www.nhpco.org/sites/default/files/public/Statistics_Research/2017_Facts_Figures.pdf.)

Length of Stay

The average length of stay for patients in hospice in 2016 was 71 days, with 74.9% of all patients receiving care for <90 days.[28] However, 16.8% of beneficiaries were discharged from hospice during that year, with 6.4% being patient-initiated discharges (revocation of benefits), presumably to pursue curative measures. An additional 6.6% were hospice-initiated discharges for patients who were no longer considered terminally ill. These statistics indicate that patient survival is possible even when initially qualifying with the Medicare requirement of an expected prognosis of 6 months or less. Furthermore, this data indicates that a majority of patients and families receive services long enough to benefit from hospice's compassionate and expert approach to comfort measures.

It can be emotionally difficult for family members when admission to hospice is delayed in spite of a compelling need. This can occur when lack of health care provider awareness precludes a timely referral, or when the disease process becomes so acute that the patient dies in the hospital. In an illustrative case, Cheryl, an 83-year-old woman with ovarian cancer, was admitted to the hospital with severe pain. Her attending physician, perhaps fearing the possibility of an overdose, refused to prescribe opioid medications at the level needed for analgesia. When Cheryl's son arrived from another state 2 days later, he arranged for Cheryl's immediate transfer to a hospice residence where she died only hours later, still without adequate pain control. Cheryl's case raises troubling questions. How can health care providers be better educated about the value of hospice services? How can candidates for hospice services be identified in a timelier manner? What are sources of barriers to effective pain control at end of life, and how can they be mitigated? As the discussions related to U.S. health care reform continue, it will be important to identify any additional barriers to timely hospice admission.

Hospice Outcomes

Data on hospice outcomes are slowly emerging and showing promising results. One of the most encouraging outcomes, from a study of 4,493 patients, indicates that admission to hospice prolongs life by a mean of 29 days.[36] The authors of this study suggested that the reason for this finding was the administration of adequate pain control and its favorable impact on enhancing comfort and quality of life.

Another promising trend is that hospice care is a cost-efficient approach to reducing Medicare expenditures, 25% of which have been reported to occur in the last year of life.[37] A study from Duke University reported that the use of hospice services reduced Medicare expenditures by $2,309 during this same period.[38]

A major quality outcome of hospice care involves the discussion of advanced directives and DNR, the implantation of which is associated with greater patient satisfaction.[39] A 2011 study of 591 US hospice facilities indicates that these discussions occur at an average rate of 82% (range=77%–89%). This study also found that 87% of these hospice facilities assess patient pain at regular intervals.

Areas of physical therapy intervention in hospice have been described in a growing number of studies, and considerable agreement among them suggests that pain control, relaxation, respiratory care, and mobility are the major areas of focus.[41–48] These interventions are discussed in forthcoming sections.

The Hospice Interdisciplinary Model of Care

Today, hospice care involves an interdisciplinary medical, psychological, and spiritual approach to the promotion of comfort and quality of life in patients with a terminal illness and a life expectancy of 6 months or less. Medicare-certified hospice facilities require the involvement of several distinct health professionals who compose the interdisciplinary team (IDT). These professionals represent four domains of care: (1) *physical* (physician and nurse), (2) *functional* (consulting therapists, nurses, and nurses' aides), (3) *interpersonal* (social workers, psychologists, and counselors), and (4) *spiritual* (chaplain, psychologists, and social workers).[49] Coverage for core services, medications, and equipment is provided to Medicare-certified hospices through a specified daily, or per diem, rate. A 2014 provision in the Affordable Care Act links the extent of payment to compliance with Medicare quality data reporting requirements. For the 2018 fiscal year, Medicare reimbursed hospices who submitted the required quality data at a daily rate of $193.03 for each patient receiving routine home care, $976.80 for continuous home care, and $743.55 for inpatient hospice care.[50] Volunteers, who complete a comprehensive training course on the philosophy of hospice, are an important element of each domain of hospice care. Accordingly, volunteers assist with light housework or meal preparation. They can also provide supportive companionship for patients and family members.

Physical therapists are not a required "core service" on the hospice IDT, meaning that Medicare does not require their services to be provided for all patients. Rather, physical therapists are part of a group of professionals (including occupational therapists and speech–language pathologists) who must be made available to any patient on an "as needed" or "consultative basis." Thus, the Medicare hospice benefit includes coverage for physical therapy provided in a hospice setting on a consultative basis. This policy is supported by the 2008 Medicare Conditions of Participation for hospice (section 418.72), which was revised to include the following language: "Physical therapy, occupational therapy, and speech–language pathology must be—

1. Available, and when provided, offered in a manner consistent with accepted standards of practice; and
2. Furnished by personnel who meet the qualifications specified in part 484 of this chapter (individuals who are licensed in the relevant disciplines)."[51]

Although this mandate suggests that physical therapy is an important component of the IDT, individual hospice programs must develop their own guidelines for our inclusion. Research is currently underway to help determine these guidelines as well as to support the cost-effectiveness of physical therapist inclusion as a core service on the IDT. Fig. 27.5 illustrates the disciplines that make up the IDT.

Interdisciplinary Team Meetings

The *Medicare Conditions of Participation*[51] mandates that each patient in a Medicare-certified hospice receive an interdisciplinary plan of care at the time of admission, which must be updated by the team at least every 2 weeks. Thus, most hospices hold weekly IDT meetings, which facilitate the coordination of care for both new and existing patients. The reports of each core discipline provide a comprehensive picture of the status of each patient and his or her support system. The patient and his or her family members may also request the option to attend the IDT.

The IDT model of hospice care prevents many of the communication pitfalls that can impede quality of care and create patient dissatisfaction. By the thoughtful coordination of every aspect of care, patients and their families can have every element of their quality of life addressed at a time when it is most needed. Because physical therapists are not considered a core member of the IDT, they may not feel that their presence at the weekly meetings is appropriate or necessary. However, it has been the experience of these authors that a consistent presence at weekly IDT meetings is invaluable for educating team members about the value of our services. In addition, we can identify patients who could benefit from a physical therapist examination and intervention.

Case Scenario. Alicia was an 86-year-old woman who was admitted to hospice after a series of several strokes that resulted in failure to thrive. Alicia had a long prior history of back pain that had recently exacerbated. At the IDT meeting, a long discussion ensued about appropriate options for pain control, as Alicia wanted to avoid sedation as much as possible. At that point, the physical therapist suggested a trial of transcutaneous electrical nerve stimulation (TENS), describing the use and benefits of this modality in the treatment of back pain. The team agreed that a trial of TENS might provide Alicia with a nonsedating approach to pain control. A physical therapy consult was initiated and TENS turned out to be a successful pain control option for Alicia.

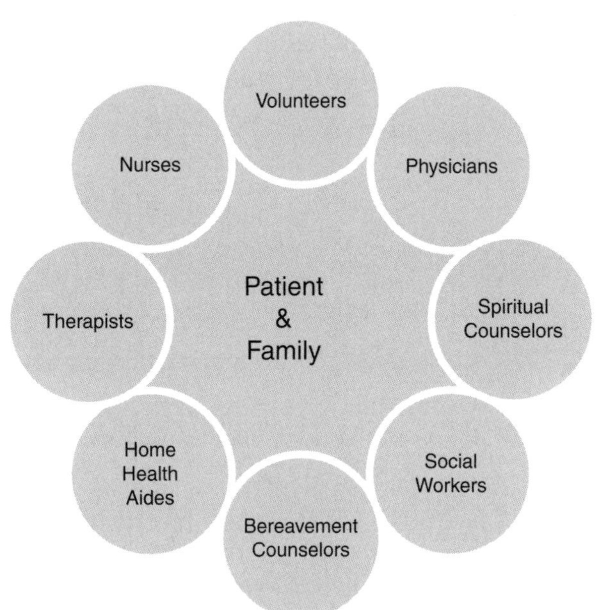

FIG. 27.5 Hospice interdisciplinary team.

MODELS OF PHYSICAL THERAPY PRACTICE IN HOSPICE AND PALLIATIVE CARE

Advanced and progressive disease requires a different orientation to goal setting and treatment than care to regain a premorbid level of function. Dietz identified palliative care strategies in patients with cancer, recognizing the need to address ongoing problems and minimizing complications.[52,53,53a] Briggs[52] further defined models of care in the palliative spectrum by integrating the framework from the *Guide to Physical Therapist Practice*[54] in response to a variety of reimbursement structures. Briggs' models include rehabilitation light, rehabilitation in reverse, case management, skilled maintenance, and supportive care. As the models are described, keep in mind that they are not necessarily exclusive of one another and may be used together or in succession as a framework to support important interventions of end-of-life physical therapy practice.[53]

Rehabilitation Light

Some patients are admitted to hospice or palliative care after a long course of disease and uncontrolled symptoms, or when experiencing the adverse effects of treatment interventions such as chemotherapy, surgery, or radiation treatment. Likely their pain management has been poor.

Initial nursing care may improve symptom control so that for the first time in many weeks or months, the person may feel like he or she might be able to make some headway toward a stronger and more functional state. Physical therapy at a traditional frequency of two to three times each week might be more than the person can tolerate and is often considered cost-prohibitive in the per diem reimbursement model of a hospice benefit program. An alternative model is a slowly progressive modified "rehabilitation light" program that provides exercise and functional training during each weekly or biweekly visit. Activities can include targeted strengthening exercises that minimize the number of exercises and functional activities such as a timed sitting program or other ambulation activity that provides both increased strength and endurance as well as improved quality of life. Home exercise program follow-through is an essential part of this approach. Progress toward goals may be extremely slow, though measurable, over a few weeks or even several months. The rehabilitation light approach uses the skilled care of the therapist in providing timely and appropriate exercise instruction and functional training, and it works within the hospice framework emphasizing quality of life despite a terminal diagnosis. Close contact and communication with the interdisciplinary team is vital to ensure all team members recognize and concur with this approach to care, as it may initially appear to conflict with the hospice goal of acceptance of a natural death. The following case scenario illustrates the use of the rehabilitation light approach.

Case Scenario. Thelma, age 78 years, was discharged from the hospital with end-stage renal disease and begrudgingly chose hospice because the only alternative offered was to begin dialysis three times a week. She faced multiple other conditions, including chronic obstructive pulmonary disease, diabetes, obesity, an indwelling catheter, osteoporosis, and a fractured metatarsal, but maintained a lifelong outlook that she would overcome these conditions. She accepted hospice care but did not plan on dying. Initially bed-bound and on a pressure-relieving mattress because of her inability to reposition herself, she tolerated minimal exercise but wanted to know what she could do to work toward the goal of getting out of bed to the commode. Beginning with a sitting program in the semielectric bed, within a month she was able to sit at bedside. Each day she worked on her own on a few basic exercises with the support of her granddaughters. At each weekly physical therapist visit she was able to do more, such as come to stand and then transfer with less assistance as her foot pain subsided to allow more weight bearing. By the end of the second month, transfers with family assist to the commode or wheelchair were happening almost daily, though actual sitting tolerance was less than an hour. After continued work in standing for strength, balance, and self-support with weight shifting, Thelma took several steps with a front-wheeled walker by month 3 and declared, "I want to be able to walk out to the kitchen so I can enjoy a cigarette." Slowly, progressive gait training ensued, followed by instruction of caregivers to assist with limited ambulation, with a wheelchair following. By 6 months, she had achieved her goal as well as transfers with a tub transfer bench and wheelchair negotiation of a ramp to the yard. Thelma's physical therapy goals had been met with Thelma reaching her maximum potential, and she was shortly discharged from hospice, to live another 2 years. This case demonstrates how physical therapy intervention can help achieve a person's desired outcome by using restorative therapy principles within the palliative care model in the hospice care environment.

Rehabilitation in Reverse

Traditional rehabilitation progresses a person from a lower to higher level of functional ability. Rehabilitation in reverse is the utilization of skilled patient training and instruction to caregivers as a person moves through the transitions from an independently mobile level to a more dependent one as the disease progresses and as strength and balance wane. Transfers may also become increasingly difficult, necessitating the use of equipment (wheelchair, bedside commode, shower bench) and the assistance of another person. Eventually, bed mobility may require assistance for positioning and comfort, and determination of the proper bed surface for skin pressure management. Throughout this course, the physical therapist can use his or her skill and knowledge of optimal ways to move and assist, allowing the patient and family to negotiate this transition toward the end of life. By being able to problem-solve functional dilemmas and anticipate the loss of activities, the physical therapist can enhance the family's ability to adjust along an unpredictable course of decline and prevent unsafe conditions resulting in falls or caregiver injuries. At each new functional level, the therapist might consider what the short-term goals are for the visit in light of the long-term hospice goal of a safe and comfortable patient-directed death at home. Frequency for such care may be quite variable, and the use of PRN (as needed) visits can be appropriate. Regular communication with the patient, family, and other hospice IDT staff may help identify when visits are needed. The following case scenario illustrates rehabilitation in reverse.

Case Scenario. Frank, age 84 years, developed back and abdominal pain while traveling in a recreational vehicle one summer and eventually was diagnosed with advanced adenocarcinoma. Frank and his family decided not to pursue treatment but rather to try to enjoy the remaining time they had together, at home. When Frank was admitted to home-based hospice, nursing was able to manage his pain while social work fostered family support, with daughters traveling for respite and help when needed. Frank had been losing weight but had been active doing household and garden chores. Some unsteadiness in the yard one day made the IDT and family concerned about the possibility of falling and a physical therapy referral was made. Frank's lower extremity strength was decreased, with significant muscle atrophy visible, although his gait appeared symmetrical. However, any challenge or advanced balance activity revealed unsteadiness. He was willing to accept a standard cane after a trial and instruction in several alternative assistive devices. A therapy visit frequency of two to four times a month was established to follow his adaptations. Within a week he requested a quad cane, which was properly fitted. He was instructed in use of the quad cane within his home, on the steps to the driveway, and about his shop. Frank declined any exercises, stating his preference was to spend his time and energy doing what he loved most. By the end of a month, it was evident that bilateral support was needed as he walked about with the cane in one hand while constantly reaching for support on the nearest wall or furniture. A trial of a front-wheeled walker was offered, providing new freedom, despite some difficulty in navigating about his favorite spots.

His wife and daughters watched over him with concern as they could see his continued weight loss and declining energy level. Within the second month, a second near fall occurred, making it apparent that the options of having a family member provide contact assist or use of a wheelchair would become necessary. This transition required more instruction and significant discussion of his physical course. Soon Frank was spending almost all of his time sitting, and the wheelchair became his more ready companion. Moving from sitting to standing was becoming more difficult, so instruction was provided to Frank and his family on his wheelchair setup and body positioning for a transfer, as well as assistance techniques. His reluctance to use a bedside commode required an increasing number of transfers throughout the day and night—a strain on all involved. Frank was preparing to let go, as his sense of meaningful participation in life was ebbing. A sudden change in level of awareness and physical status required family training on bed positioning and turning for pressure relief. After 3 days of intermittent consciousness, Frank died in his own bed, with his wife and two daughters nearby.

This case illustrates the type of effective care a physical therapist can provide in the face of a terminal diagnosis and declining mobility, rather than the traditional care of expecting participation in progressive-resistive exercise to achieve goals of enhanced mobility. Interestingly, the patient and family's acceptance of Frank's impending death made this approach feasible and appropriate.

Case Management

Case management is a frequently used model of care for nursing and physical therapy in many specialty clinics to provide long-term, ongoing care for challenging and changing conditions such as amyotrophic lateral sclerosis, spinal cord injury, amputation, and diabetes. In home health, case management is used to provide similar follow-up, care, and instruction for people with complicated care, multiple comorbidities, and unskilled or multiple caregivers.[55] This model is useful in palliative and hospice care as well. With a person who is relatively stable though gradually declining over weeks or months, periodic reevaluation can identify physical and functional changes that need to be addressed to prevent complications. Interventions can include instructing the caregivers in providing optimal assistance, updating the home exercise program, and outlining problems that might be anticipated. Monthly or bimonthly visits with appropriate instruction and follow-up intervention can accomplish this end. The case of Evelyn illustrates case management.

Case Scenario. At 94 years, Evelyn retained a regal demeanor, sitting in her chair holding court with four generations of offspring attending to her, although she did not allow much to be done for her. With end-stage heart disease as an admitting diagnosis, along with osteoarthritis, cataracts, and hearing loss, life had become a challenge. She insisted on doing almost everything herself, despite exerting high levels of energy. An initial physical therapy visit offered recommendations to make the environment safer and easier to move around and adjust her equipment for improved comfort and efficiency. Monthly visits were scheduled to reassess her safety and mobility and to instruct various caregivers in different ways to assist as Evelyn's condition became more fragile. Begrudgingly she allowed more help with bathing, dressing, and other tasks.

Because sitting was her primary position of comfort both day and night, skin integrity and pressure relief concerns were addressed. Adapting her chair to an optimal height with the fabrication of a platform underneath the entire chair elevated the seat height while maintaining the other comfort features and eliminated the instability of multiple cushions. She enjoyed doing some exercises while she sat, if someone did them along with her, and the family was more than willing to comply. Her family's concerns about potential falls were discussed repeatedly and at length in the context of physical limitations, Evelyn's variable willingness to have assistance or use devices, and her right to self-determination. Evelyn was under hospice care for 8 months, long enough to celebrate her 95th birthday. Just a week later, her daughter found her in her chair one morning, having expired peacefully during the night.

Traditional physical therapy might have been offered on a very short-term basis to achieve a specific short-term goal and then the patient would have been discharged as she did not have rehabilitation potential. However, under hospice, supportive, palliative care can be provided, easing the transition to dependency and facilitating a safe and comfortable patient-directed death.

Skilled Maintenance

When a patient must perform an activity that is medically necessary, skilled maintenance has been identified for use under Medicare home health guidelines.[55] In traditional home health situations, care that might, under usual circumstances, be taught to a caregiver may require skilled physical therapist intervention because of specific complexity. An example might be the performance of range of motion to a joint proximate to an unstable fracture. In hospice, skilled maintenance is used to perform an important functional activity, which the patient is no longer able to perform alone or with a family caregiver yet can complete with the assistance of the physical therapist. For example, because of extensive weakness, tone or balance deficits, or caregiver limitations, a therapist may be needed to provide help with ambulation or bed transfers. Under hospice rules, when these activities provide for significant quality of life, they are considered skilled care. Consultation with the IDT is important to establish a care plan that provides for the frequency needed, as well as patient and family support through the process of letting go of activities during the course of care.

Case Scenario. Roger, age 74 years, was a retired rancher and businessman. His life was changed with the diagnosis of an astrocytoma and the resultant physical trauma of brain surgery to resect the tumor, radiation treatments, and the array of medications to control seizures, swelling, and other adverse effects. He was eventually admitted to hospice, and a physical therapy consult was initiated because the patient's wife was having difficulty helping him transfer because of the dense left-sided paresis and spasticity he experienced. The primary focus of physical therapy was problem-solving environmental challenges and transfer techniques to allow his petite spouse to assist with the patient's transfers to every surface.

In conversation, it became clear that Roger's sense of self had been dramatically affected by confinement to a chair. What he missed more than anything was being able to walk about his home and gaze through the windows at "his spread." A trial of gait with a hemi-cane, a plastic ankle–foot orthosis, and a gait belt on the next visit revealed Roger's ability to walk up to 50 feet with help to maintain balance, weight shift, and control the advance of his left leg during swing phase. He was elated at this recovered ability, and his physical therapist decided with the patient that it could become a part of a weekly physical therapy visit. Other issues arose, including travel plans to a national rodeo and training other family caregivers.

As the disease progressed, Roger lost the ability to walk, even with assistance, but was able to stand at the counter with support to look out over land he loved. The opportunity to continue being mobile until it was no longer possible, even with assistance, gave meaning to his existence.

Supportive Care

Supportive care is often provided throughout the course of care and is composed of the psychosocial support associated with end-of-life process, as well as physical measures. The frequency of supportive care measures is variable. Physical measures may include range of motion and massage. Physical therapy pain management techniques should coincide with the frequent use of a medication regimen by nursing. Some mechanical pain that is not treatable with even high levels of opiates can be diminished using a physical therapist's knowledge of biomechanics and positioning.

Pressure relief becomes an issue with progressive weakness, decreased mobility, insufficient nutrition, and fragile skin. Both seating and bed surfaces should be considered to manage a failing body's integumentary system. A more complete discussion of these clinical supportive care measures follows in the next section.

CLINICAL ISSUES—CONSIDERATIONS FOR CARE

As with the models for practice in hospice and palliative care, the circumstances of declining function and often very limited performance status demand the attention of the physical therapist to reexamine elements of clinical practice in this light. Subtle changes in the way knowledge is used and clinical skills are applied can result in substantially improved short-term outcomes for those individuals in the last stage of life.

The Role of Exercise

Exercise plays a critical role in maintaining strength to allow adequate functional mobility for quality of life. When determining the appropriateness of exercise for a body that is failing at the end of life, the cause of the weakness should be considered to determine if increased strength is possible and/or realistic. Weakness that can be reversed may be caused from chemotherapy or radiation therapy,[56] prolonged hospitalization,[57] or a period of immobility or forced bed rest.[58]

The client's prior exercise and fitness history is also significant.[59] A person with substantial prior participation in some strength and endurance activities will respond in a different way than someone who has never participated in exercise as a lifestyle behavior. Ability to differentiate effort, fatigue, and workload from soreness or pain will play a role in performance and success as well. Some patients will decline an exercise program as part of their end-of-life care, choosing only to participate in activities that provide quality of life—a decision that must be respected by the therapist.

The limited physical capacity that may be present in a chronically debilitated person can guide us toward the use of "rehabilitation light" as previously discussed. Focusing the exercise program on maximum strength outcomes with a limited number of exercises can enhance success. Recent evidence indicates that a home exercise program for people older than age 65 years with two exercises results in a better performance outcome than with eight exercises.[59]

All exercise should address functional goals[59] and thus be directly seen by patients as a means to an end, rather than something to keep them occupied. Positively reinforcing experiences gives feedback that will provide the best outcome. If the patient feels overwhelmed or experiences significant delayed-onset soreness following activity, it is likely that the decreased quality-of-life satisfaction will inhibit further participation.[60]

Even patients with severe chronic obstructive pulmonary disease have been found to benefit from a biweekly supervised home exercise program over a 4-month period, with a 3% gain as opposed to 28% deterioration in the nonexercising control. These results are not overwhelming evidence of the effectiveness of exercise training, but the patients in this study belong to a severely disabled population with a progressive disease and a grim outlook.[61]

Measuring resting heart rate (RHR) and activity-related heart rate is useful in determining physical performance status, when related to the predicted maximum heart rate (age-adjusted maximum heart rate) (using 220 - age, or less, or 220 - RHR × exercise level). With a failing body, resting heart rate may be much higher than 100 beats per minute. A 75-year-old man with a predicted maximum heart rate (PMHR) of 145 and an RHR of 120 is already performing at more than 80% of maximum (82%). After walking 30 feet to the bathroom using a wheeled walker, he nearly collapses with a heart rate of 144, more than 99% of PMHR. This adverse event represents not only a significant fall risk from collapse but also an effort comparable to that of a sprint performance on a running track. An explanation of this relative maximum aerobic effort is often affirming to the patient and reassuring to the family. Similarly, patients with progressive weakness and muscle atrophy will experience difficulty moving from sitting to standing, especially from their favorite chair. Physical therapists have a critical opportunity to educate patients, their families, and their caregivers regarding maximal physical capacity for anaerobic muscle contraction and the work that is done just to move from one position to another. Sharing these examples with both patient and family can lead to an affirmation that perceived exertion is extremely high while in the process of decline and also some recognition of the effort it takes to accomplish even the smallest of tasks.

In conclusion, it is important that the physical therapist offer the option of specific exercises and activities that are both accomplishable and meaningful to the patient's life condition, along with education that puts exercise and physical performance in the perspective of physical changes toward the end of life. If such a program is well integrated into a daily routine, the optimal understanding and outcomes will be achieved.

Equipment and the Environment

The ability to move from sitting to standing may require greater effort or assistance with increased weakness. Adapting a favorite recliner chair to an optimal height can be achieved by instruction to the family in fabrication of a platform underneath the entire chair, often of 4 to 6 inches. This elevates the seat height, maintains the other comfort features, and eliminates the instability of multiple cushions. Some families may choose to purchase an electric lift recliner as another option. Other equipment in the home such as a bedside commode or shower bench might need to be elevated accordingly.

Energy conservation can be of great significance, as patients are often performing at near-maximal energy output levels and fatigue rapidly as noted earlier. Standard measurement for walker heights allows for significant elbow flexion. In younger populations and people with adequate strength, the energy costs of this upper extremity use may be easily within their ability. In tests of upper extremity forces with variable walker heights while maintaining a stressful lower extremity non–weight-bearing status, evidence shows that more complete elbow extension can reduce elbow force moments.[58] With the older adult in terminal decline, adjusting a walker height to allow almost complete elbow extension can provide energy savings that will allow safer and easier ambulation for an extended time during their illness.

Comfort Care Measures

Comfort care of the terminally ill has risen to the forefront with increased awareness of the physical and psychosocial variables that affect and accompany the process.[62] One of the primary goals of end-of-life care through hospice is pain relief and comfort. Physical therapy has much to offer through appropriate direct interventions and the education and training of family caregivers.

Edema is a frequent symptom as the body fails, whether from adverse effects of treatment (surgery and radiation), decreased mobility and stasis of position,[63] or failure of body systems as disease progresses. Swollen limbs can become extremely uncomfortable from the internal pressure on sensory receptors. Manual lymphatic drainage and other massage techniques can provide temporary and longer-term relief in many such situations. Positioning and wrapping with short stretch bandages also may be helpful to reduce limb size and allow easier functional mobility with unweighted limbs.[64] By demonstrating these techniques effectively and teaching the caregivers to follow a modified program that is not overly taxing on the family, caregivers can be taught by a physical therapist to provide a successfully satisfying activity with their loved one. It is understood and should be explained that in some cases the efforts to control edema may fail because of the body's system failure, and this is not a failure of the caregivers. Despite this eventual outcome, comfort from the touch of massage may still be enjoyed.

End-of-life experiences may include a sense of "needing to go," as the person undergoes transitional changes and separation. Younger and more able-bodied patients can become very restless and walk or pace endlessly. This phenomenon becomes a more challenging management problem if the terminal restlessness occurs in someone unable to get up from bed safely.[65] Therapeutic techniques such as holding and rocking (in bed or at the bedside) may be used and also taught to caregivers as a way to provide the physical and vestibular sensation of movement and the "going" that is so keenly desired.[66] This is an excellent adjunct to the medications frequently offered by the hospice team to control this symptom.

Range of motion is another intervention that must be considered from a different perspective. Range of motion may be provided to maintain enough range to allow for personal care or limiting finger flexion to prevent palm injury. If movement is painful, range of motion should be limited to this practical standard. Some people may very much enjoy the stimulus of having their otherwise immobile and understimulated limbs moved for comfort. With proper instruction, caregivers or other volunteers may be able to do passive or assistive range of motion regularly. Another application of range of motion in end-of-life care is to provide the gentle stimulus of passive, assistive, or active movements of the lower extremities, along with the verbally guided visualization images of a favorite walk that the person might have enjoyed (e.g., to a park, the ocean, or community locations). This "walking together" can provide the patient and caregivers with a sense of doing something purposeful and pleasurable as they reflect on their memories and life closure issues together.

Perspectives on Falls at End of Life

Falls are always a consideration for physical therapists and require special considerations during the end-of-life course.[67] The questions one must ask are, "Is it possible for a person to transition from active and functional to a premorbid state without increased risks of falling?" and "What should we do about that?" Much research has been done to assess and limit falls with appropriate intervention. The wide range of patient abilities in palliative care and hospice practice necessitate targeting assessment tools to the abilities of the person such as the Timed Up and Go or even just observation. Interventions also must be carefully considered as well, with the variable and often progressive nature of the disease or condition. Zero risk and zero falls cannot be the goal with any kind of quality of life. Risk management at an acceptable level with quality-of-life considerations as determined by patient desires for independence and family concerns should be the outcome. Falls will happen in the course of decline, and for some a fall may even be the natural way out of this world.

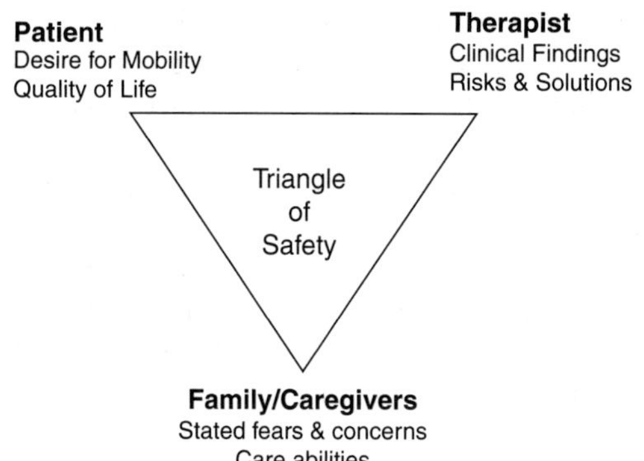

FIG. 27.6 Briggs' Triangle of Safety when considering addressing falls and safety risks. *(From Briggs 2018.)*

The Joint Commission supports having a program in place that is consistent with the provider organization, the clients served, and the environment of care.[68] A reasoned approach in the hospice environment is to use a concept such as the Triangle of Safety, identified by Briggs in Fig. 27.6.

The Triangle of Safety involves the three main parties involved in care decisions: the patient, the family/caregivers, and the clinician. Communication and sharing of concerns and experiences are essential. This alliance[69] empowers the patient to decide what is agreeable, the family caregivers to voice their concerns, and the therapist to identify clinical findings and solution options to consider.[69] Together an acceptable level of support and intervention can be found, which may include environmental changes, equipment use, assistance, or other changes. People who perceive that they are being "called by others" or "going to the light" may even try to get up though no longer physically able, which is beyond anyone's control.[70]

The therapist's role evolves in the hospice environment from directly being a care provider when fall training and interventions no longer are beneficial or accepted to that of a risk and solution identifier. Our role is to support the decline and dying process and trust that those in our care will make the most informed decisions in line with their understanding of the outcomes. Two case examples follow.

Case Scenarios. Tony was in his 40s and had lived with HIV/AIDS for nearly 18 years. Now on hospice and living alone, he recently fell while answering the phone, which led him to reluctantly agree to a physical therapy referral. His father met the therapist outside and demanded that we make his son be safe. Muscle wasting, lethargy, and massive edema were the primary conditions affecting Tony's gait and balance. Multiple devices were offered and tried: a straight cane, quad canes, pick-up and front wheeled walkers. Considerations were discussed including weight, stability, and even appearance. Tony went back and forth but eventually chose the front-wheeled walker, which made him more stable and reassured his family. This choice allowed him to live his last days without further falls.

Martha was 93 years old and had graduated from hospice admissions for cardiac failure twice and was now referred by neurology to palliative care home health for gait training and balance. She was quite determined and able to make some gains in both strength and balance using a walker or cane with constant assistance. As discharge was nearing, a moment of inattention by her live-in attendant allowed a fall, which resulted in compression fractures of the spine. With significant pain, now suddenly bedfast, and having difficulty with air exchange, Martha was again open to hospice. As her daughters gathered and accepted Martha's preparing to let go this time, she lived just 2 more weeks. Through a fall, Martha had found her way "home."

PAIN AND SYMPTOM MANAGEMENT

Defining Pain at End of Life

A painful death is among the greatest fears surrounding the end-of-life process; accordingly, one of the most important goals in the management of terminally ill persons is timely and effective pain management.[48] The hospice approach to pain supports this goal, specifically in terms of reducing the level of related distress to a tolerable level within 48 hours of admission.

Although pain can be academically defined as "an unpleasant sensory experience associated with actual or potential tissue damage,"[70] the definition used in hospice is "whatever the patient says it is."[71] Thus, any patient report of pain is acknowledged and addressed in a compassionate and efficacious manner.

In the hospice setting, pain assessment is considered the "fifth vital sign,"[1] an important indication of the patient's physiological homeostasis and well-being. In addition, pain is viewed as an impediment to the patient's spiritual, psychological, and emotional processes of life review and meaningful closure with loved ones. Hospice nurses are experts in the area of pharmacologic approaches to pain management. Working with the patient and family, they can quickly identify strategies to reduce, and in many cases eliminate, discomfort. Physical therapists can also provide the nonpharmacologic interventions described in the previous section on comfort measures, which may enhance the effectiveness of medications. In many cases, physical therapy interventions such as massage, guided breathing for relaxation, TENS, and gentle movement can even reduce the need for pharmacologic agents.

In cases where the patient is unresponsive, delirious, or aphasic, potential causes of pain are identified and addressed. For example, an unresponsive patient with a severe urinary tract infection would most likely be treated for pain. In addition, if a patient has previously reported a consistent pattern of pain during periods of consciousness, it will probably be assumed that this discomfort remains even when the patient is no longer able to verify this.

Prevalence of Pain at End of Life

Although the prevalence of pain at end of life will vary depending on the nature of the terminal disease process, research indicates that two–thirds of patients with advanced cancer experience pain.[72] Pain and discomfort are multidimensional constructs. One assessment known as the Memorial Symptom Assessment Scale-Short Form (MSAS-SF)[73] is a patient self-report of the spectrum of cancer-related sources of physical and psychological distress (Fig. 27.7).

The MSAS-SF also enables patients to rate the extent to which particular symptoms affect them, using a 5-point continuum between *not at all* (0) and *very much* (4).

The two most common forms of discomfort in 299 patients with advanced cancer completing the MSAS-SF included pain (72%) and lack of energy (70%).[73] Furthermore, more than 50% of these patients rated these symptoms as affecting them "quite a bit" or "very much." Finally, between 35% and 39% of these patients reported occasional psychological distress such as worrying, feeling irritable, and feeling sad. Clearly, the physical and psychological effects of advanced cancer frequently affect most patients.

The multidimensional element of pain, particularly at end of life, was first recognized by Cicely Saunders, who defined pain as "not just an event, or a series of events, but rather a situation in which the patient is held captive."[74] Saunders defined the collective impact of these discomforting "events" as "Total Pain," which is illustrated in Fig. 27.8.

In developing the interdisciplinary model of hospice care, Saunders considered that each professional member had a role in helping ease the various contributions to a patient's total pain. For example, a hospice chaplain could address spiritual pain, whereas a social worker might mitigate the issues of bureaucratic pain (i.e., the frustration of filling out the endless and tedious forms required for insurance claims). By addressing the many contributions to distress, patients' energy resources can then be marshaled for meaningful and comforting activities, thus enhancing their quality of life. In the context of total pain, Saunders' approach to management was to employ both pharmacologic and nonpharmacologic measures proactively rather than reactively.

Without a doubt, effective pain management is one of the most important of Saunders' many contributions to the development of a standardized approach to compassionate end-of-life care. She was among the first to demonstrate that inadequate pain management at the end of life hastens death by increasing physiologic stress, myocardial oxygen demand, and the work of breathing.[74]

Patient's Name ______________________ Date ___/___/___ ID # ______________

MEMORIAL SYMPTOM ASSESSMENT SCALE – SHORT FORM [MSAS-SF]

I. INSTRUCTIONS: Below is a list of symptoms. If you had the symptom **DURING THE PAST WEEK,** please check YES. If you did have the symptom, please check the box that tells us how much the symptom DISTRESSED or BOTHERED you.

Check *all* the symptoms you have had during the PAST WEEK.	**IF YES:** How much did it DISTRESS or BOTHER you? Yes (√)	Not at all (0)	A little bit (1)	Some-what (2)	Quite a bit (3)	Very much (4)
Difficulty concentrating						
Pain						
Lack of energy						
Cough						
Changes in skin						
Dry mouth						
Nausea						
Feeling drowsy						
Numbness/tingling in hands and feet						
Difficulty sleeping						
Feeling bloated						
Problems with urination						
Vomiting						
Shortness of breath						
Diarrhea						
Sweats						
Mouth sores						
Problems with sexual interest or activity						
Itching						
Lack of appetite						
Dizziness						
Difficulty swallowing						
Change in the way food tastes						
Weight loss						
Hair loss						
Constipation						
Swelling of arms or legs						
"I don't look like myself"						
If you had any other symptoms during the PAST WEEK, please list them below, and indicate how much the symptom DISTRESSED or BOTHERED you.						
1						
2						

II. Below are other commonly listed symptoms. Please indicate if you have had the symptom **DURING THE PAST WEEK,** and if so, how **OFTEN** it occurred.

Check *all* the symptoms you have had during the PAST WEEK.	**IF YES:** How **OFTEN** did it occur? Yes (√)	Rarely (1)	Occasionally (2)	Frequently (3)	Almost constantly (4)
Feeling sad					
Worrying					
Feeling irritable					
Feeling nervous					

FIG. 27.7 Memorial Symptom Assessment Scale-Short Form (MSAS-SF).

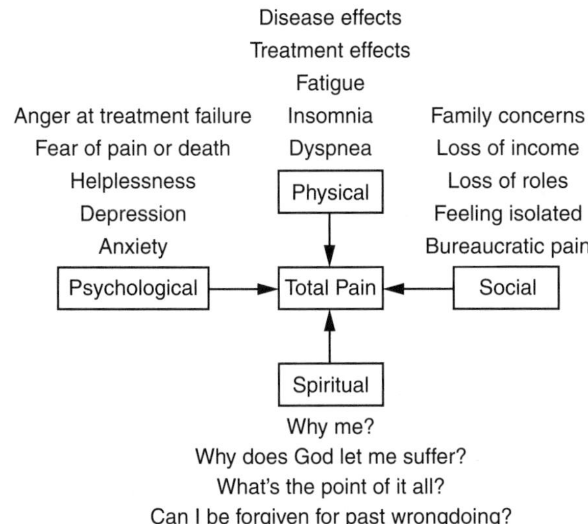

FIG. 27.8 Saunders' model of total pain.

BOX 27.3 Definitions of Terms Related to Addiction

Addiction: a primary, neurobiological, social, and environmentally based disease characterized by behaviors that include one or more of the following: impaired control over drug use, continued use despite harm, and craving

Physical dependence: a normal state of adaptation manifested by a drug class–specific withdrawal syndrome that can be provoked by abrupt cessation, rapid dose reduction, decreasing blood levels of the drug, or administration of an antagonist

Tolerance: a state of adaptation in which exposure to a drug induces changes that result in a diminution of one or more of the drug's effects over time

Pseudoaddiction: the false assumption of addiction in a person seeking relief from pain

Pseudotolerance: the false assumption that the need for increasing doses of a medication is the result of tolerance rather than disease progression or other factors[77]

Furthermore, inadequate pain relief increases the burden of total pain, causing significant anguish for both the patient and family. Accordingly, given the prevalence and intensity of physical pain among terminally ill patients, Saunders advocated the use of opioid medications in sufficient doses to maintain a consistent level of relief. Her well-known maxim in this regard was "constant pain needs constant control."[74] Nevertheless, despite considerable evidence for their use, barriers exist within society and the medical system that can prevent adequate dosing of the highly effective opioid medications. Because of their potential for abuse and addiction as well as opioids' popularity as street drugs, many states have restrictive laws that can limit their availability in both rural and inner-city pharmacies.[1] Accordingly, it is critical for health professionals working in pain management to understand the true nature of addiction as well as physical dependence, tolerance, pseudo-tolerance, and pseudo-addiction to avoid perpetuating existing barriers to appropriate pain management at end of life. In reality, both past and recent studies have found addiction rates of anywhere between 0% and 7% in patients receiving opioids for end-stage cancer pain.[75,76] In end-of-life care, concern for patient comfort is first and foremost. Moreover, nurses and other health professionals working in a hospice setting may need to educate and advocate for their patients to ensure their access to appropriate medications and need for optimal comfort.

To educate health professionals, the American Academy of Pain Medicine generated a consensus document in 2001 defining the terms *addiction*, *physical dependency*, and *tolerance*.[77] These definitions are defined in Box 27.3.

Types of Physical Pain

To achieve the outcome of consistent analgesia, it is important to understand the physiological sources that contribute to pain. For example, physical pain can derive from organs, neural tissue, or musculoskeletal components, each of which produces a distinct type of discomfort and requires a specific class of pharmacologic agents. *Nociceptive* pain (from disease or damage to skin, muscles, bones, or connective tissue) and *neuropathic* pain (from disease or damage to neurons involved in pain signaling) are the two most common pain syndromes at end of life. Another form of discomfort is known as *breakthrough pain*, which is a sudden increase in pain intensity lasting up to an hour or more despite the use of continuous opioid medication. An understanding of pain's sources and behavior promotes the physical therapist's effective advocacy and pain management. In the presence of advanced disease (particularly with cancer), it is not uncommon for patients to experience brief intermittent episodes of severe pain lasting from several seconds to several minutes. In most cases, this "breakthrough pain" occurs in the presence of overall effective baseline analgesia. Although these episodes can occur without apparent provocation, they may also correlate with changes in activity. Breakthrough pain can be effectively managed, usually by providing a fast-acting medication in a specific percentage of the patient's overall daily dose. It can be helpful for patients to maintain a pain diary, which allows them to record the impact of activities and other factors on their pain levels. The American Cancer Society has developed a pain diary found on their website.[78] The pain diary includes useful questions that can help physical therapists in the assessment of pain such as location, nature (e.g., stabbing, throbbing, shooting), pain rating, and provoking factors.

Decisions related to appropriate medications for pain control are based on patient or caregiver reports. It is important for health professionals to recognize that patients, especially older ones, may be reluctant to report the true nature, extent, and severity of their pain. Barriers to accurate reports are numerous, including cultural differences, fear of being seen as complaining, lack of knowledge about pain control, and fears of medication adverse effects, tolerance, or addiction.[1]

Pharmacologic Measures for Pain Control

There are several effective medications that can be used for pain control in patients facing the end of life. This section will provide a brief overview of the unique aspects of pain medications in chronic, palliative, and hospice situations. For a more detailed description of these medications, the reader is referred to Chapter 6 on pharmacology.

The selection of the appropriate class of medications is determined by the source of the pain as well as its severity. The World Health Organization (WHO) has developed a pain ladder that can also be used to determine the appropriate medications in end-stage cancer (Fig. 27.9).

Nonopioid Analgesics. This class of medications includes acetaminophen (Tylenol) and nonsteroidal anti-inflammatory drugs (NSAIDs). The WHO pain ladder recommends nonopioid analgesics for mild pain, which is <3 on a 1 to 10 numerical scale, where 0 is *no pain* and 10 is the *worst imaginable* pain.[48] Specific medications, indications, side effects, and mechanisms of action are described in Chapter 6, Pharmacology.

Opioid Analgesics. Opioid analgesics are considered the most effective medications for the management of moderate to severe pain and morphine is a staple in end-of-life situations. Accordingly, the WHO pain ladder recommends these as the preferred medication in such instances.[79]

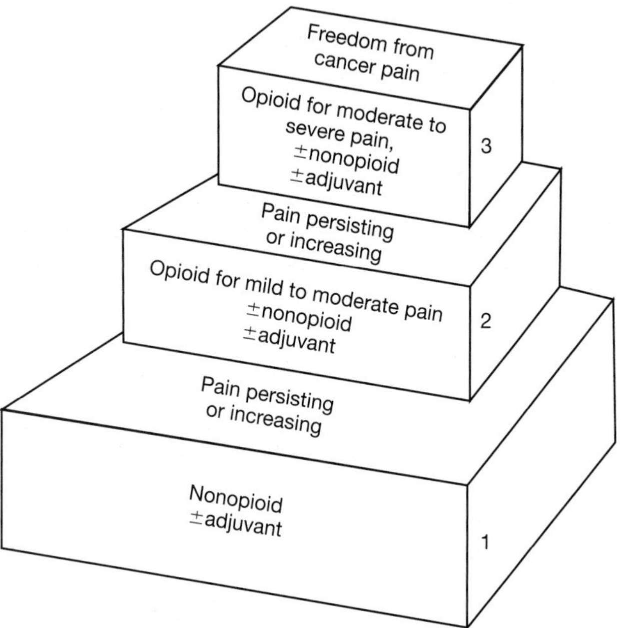

FIG. 27.9 World Health Organization's pain ladder. *(Accessible at http://www.who.int/cancer/palliative/painladder/en/. Reprinted with permission.)*

Moderate pain is defined as between 4 and 6 on a 0 to 10 numerical scale, where 0 is *no pain* and 10 is the *worst imaginable pain*. Severe pain is defined as between 7 and 10 on the same numerical scale.[48] These medications bind to opioid receptors in the brain, blocking the release of neurotransmitters involved in processing pain perception. In addition to their pain-relieving effect, opioid medications are also useful in treatment of dyspnea at end of life.

In end-of-life care, optimal pain control is the ultimate goal of pharmacologic treatment; thus, dosing is determined by the level required to attain this outcome. Fortunately, many of the opioid medications can be delivered in either extended- or immediate-release formulations, allowing for a more consistent level of control. Often, both types of medications are used.

Opioid Adverse Effects. Fortunately, allergic reactions to opioid medications are extremely rare, and the only contraindication to their use at end of life is a history of a hypersensitivity reaction such as rash or wheezing. One of the more common opioid adverse effects is constipation, and it is thus recommended that a prophylactic bowel regimen be started immediately upon the initiation of these medications. In addition to stimulant laxatives and the encouragement of adequate fluid intake when possible, interventions such as abdominal massage, range of motion, and upright mobility training can also assist bowel evacuation.

Sedation is another common adverse effect of opioid use, particularly with the initial doses, and it is important to recognize that although many patients may view sedation as a barrier to quality waking time with family and loved ones, others may consider it a welcome opportunity for rest, particularly if insomnia has been problematic.

One of the most feared (yet relatively rare) complications of opioid use is respiratory suppression. Fortunately, this adverse event is usually preceded by sedation, which provides an opportunity for symptom reversal through the use of an opioid antagonist such as naloxone. Indications for reversal generally include lack of arousability and a drop in oxygen saturation. The highest risk for respiratory depression occurs with the first doses of opioids in patients without a prior history of their use (opioid naïve). Opioid-tolerant patients who have achieved good pain control generally do not develop this complication.

The Opioid Crisis and Physical Therapy. Over the past several years, the United States has experienced an increased use and abuse of opioid medications. In 2016, the White House and the Centers for Disease Control and Prevention declared an opioid epidemic and announced initiatives to address these issues. These initiatives included modernizing regulations, prescription practices, and production of opioids. Although these initiatives are warranted and important in light of the number of deaths due to opioid misuse, there remains concerns about the potential inadvertent consequences on the management of those at end of life. As this patient population often requires opioids for management of symptoms, a reduction in availability or increased social stigma of using opioids could reduce their comfort and quality of life.

Physical therapists are experts in nonopioid management of pain. As the role of the PT in HPC is increasing, therapists should look for opportunities to assist with providing symptom control without excessive opioid use. The therapist should be cognizant that although a goal is to reduce the overutilization of opioids, in the HPC population, opioids are a necessary and beneficial medication for symptom control and to ensure death with dignity and comfort.[80]

Adjuvant Analgesics. This class of medications includes an array of agents that produce analgesic effects. These include antidepressants, anticonvulsants, corticosteroids, local anesthetics, and calcium channel blockers. Although these medications can be effective for milder pain when used in isolation, they are most typically used in conjunction with opioids. They can be particularly effective in the presence of severe neuropathic or bone pain.

Routes of Administration. Analgesic medications can be administered through a variety of methods. Although many patients with advanced disease are able to take medications orally (either in pill or liquid form), others may require alternative forms of delivery. Thus, medications can be administered through a variety of routes, including mucosal, transdermal, rectal, or topical approaches. One of the most common routes for patients without oral function is through rectal or vaginal suppositories. Medications also can be delivered through intravenous or intrathecal methods; however, whenever possible, the least invasive approach is used.

Intramuscular injections are generally not used in end-of-life care because they are painful in themselves, and because rates of vascular drug absorption are highly variable when using this approach. In selecting the preferred route of delivery for pain medications, the hospice nurse will work closely with the patient and family to determine the most effective, consistent, and efficient approach.

Medical Marijuana. Over the last decade there has been increased acceptance of the use of medical marijuana for a number of conditions, including advanced cancer, chronic disease, and end-of-life situations.[81] With the recent legislative changes and associated media coverage, individuals with a life-limiting condition may be employing marijuana or its derivative products to assist with symptom control. There are two active cannabinoid compounds most commonly used, delta-9-tetrahydrocannabinol (THC) and cannabidiol (CBD). The THC compound is commonly associated with psychoactive effects, whereas CBD is associated with nonpsychoactive effects such as controlling pain and spasticity. Medical marijuana and cannabinoids have been used for treatment of pain including cancer-related pain, neuropathic pain, and spasticity. Medical marijuana has also been used to treat chemotherapy-induced nausea and vomiting, as an appetite stimulant, and for psychological or neurological conditions such as anxiety or spasticity. Dronabinol (Marinol, Syndros) is a THC-based capsule or solution taken by mouth and is approved by the Food and Drug Administration for treatment of nausea and vomiting when symptoms are not controlled using other conventional methods.[82] Because this medication contains THC, psychotropic effects may be encountered with individuals using dronabinol.

Because there remains a potential social stigma to this medical marijuana or its derivatives, some patients may not be forthright with disclosing its use; therefore, clinicians may need to specifically ask about this use in patients with a life-limiting condition.[81] Finally, physical therapists who encounter terminally ill patients with symptoms not managed with traditional medication regimens may consider a discussion with physician colleagues to assess if marijuana products may be beneficial.

PALLIATIVE SEDATION

For some individuals, the end-of-life process may involve levels of pain that are intractable even with aggressive pain management efforts. In such cases, the only remaining approach is to induce sedation to alleviate conscious awareness of pain. Palliative sedation (PS) is defined as "the monitored use of medications (sedatives, barbiturates, neuroleptics, hypnotics, benzodiazepines or anesthetic medication) to relieve refractory and unendurable physical, spiritual, and/or psychosocial distress for patients with a terminal diagnosis, by inducing varied degrees of unconsciousness."[83]

The American Academy of Hospice and Palliative Medicine describes mild and deep levels of PS, which vary in terms of the level of consciousness preserved.[84] With mild sedation, smaller doses of short-acting medications such as midazolam at an infusion rate of 0.5 mg/hour are used, promoting enough alertness to allow the patient to engage in conversation. Should mild sedation not be sufficient, a deeper level may be required, and in this case, higher doses of midazolam may be used in addition to longer-acting medications such as benzodiazepines and morphine sulfate.[84] In having two progressive levels of PS available, patients and their families can maintain a level of choice, which enables them to fully direct their care with the assistance of the hospice team.

Ethical Framework for Palliative Sedation

The intent of palliative sedation is to provide comfort when all appropriate methods of pain control are inadequate. Patients and families must clearly understand that the overall intent of PS is to provide relief from unendurable suffering, but not to hasten death. Nevertheless, the end result for many patients undergoing PS will be the eventual cessation of respiration followed by death. Although death is an expected outcome from the disease process itself, the addition of PS cannot be definitively excluded as a contributory factor. Thus, the ethical framework in which PS is grounded is that of "double effect," which suggests that the beneficent intention of reducing suffering may produce the unintentional effect of death. In addition, the principle of proportionality suggests that the selection of PS should be proportionate to the extent of patient suffering, treatment alternatives, expected benefits, and possible harm.[84] A 1997 ruling of the U.S. Supreme Court declared that there is no constitutional right to physician-assisted suicide.[85] Terminal sedation is intended for symptom relief and is appropriate in the aggressive practice of palliative care.[85]

Initiating Palliative Sedation

The decision to initiate PS is based on the assessment of patient symptoms and, often, the patient's stated desire to be free of his or her discomfort. Once it is clear that PS is the only remaining treatment option, the patient or health care surrogate (the individual appointed to make medical decisions on the patient's behalf) must be clearly instructed in the goals and expected outcomes of treatment. Informed consent is typically required. Members of the hospice team are also available to provide any support that may be needed by the patient or family.

In most cases, PS is initiated at the onset of terminal restlessness, an indication that death is imminent within days or hours. Although the most common indication for PS is agitated delirium, others include pain, seizures, and dyspnea and severe anxiety. Many patients have more than one symptom, which greatly compounds their distress. One patient of the authors described the feelings of terminal restlessness as "a horrible sense of doom and fear, like a weight crushing down on me."

There are many different medications that can be used for PS. They include central nervous system depressants such as midazolam, benzodiazepines, lorazepam, and pentobarbital. Most of these medications are administered intravenously. Another common formulation known as a hospice suppository contains metoclopramide to prevent gastrointestinal distress, diphenhydramine to dry up secretions, morphine sulfate for pain, lorazepam for anxiety, and haloperidol for delirium. These suppositories are inserted rectally every 3 to 8 hours as needed and are often a preferred method for home use.

A recent study exploring trends in the use of palliative sedation in one European country indicated that the frequency with which PS is used at end of life decreased from 14.5% in 2007 to 12.0% in 2013.[86] A retrospective study of 374 patients receiving tertiary care for terminal cancer indicated that 203 (54.2%) received PS. Interestingly, the patients who received PS had a significantly longer survival period than patients who were not sedated (33 days vs. 16 days, respectively).[87] However, other studies comparing survival length between patients receiving PS with those who did not showed no significant differences.[88,89]

When a patient is undergoing PS, family members should be encouraged to talk to them and touch them. Gentle massage can be helpful in assisting the letting-go process, and patients may respond with a change in breathing that suggests relaxation. Sometimes, patients may respond in other poignant and life-changing ways.

THE PHYSIOLOGICAL PROCESS OF DYING

It has been stated that "we die of old age because we have been worn and torn and programmed to cave in. The very old do not succumb to disease, they implode their way to eternity."[90] As this quote suggests, advances in medicine have prolonged our lives so that the typical American death is most likely to occur in the old and very old from a chronic condition involving a period of physiological decline. Accordingly, the Centers for Disease Control and Prevention reported that of the 2,744,248 U.S. deaths that occurred in 2016, the five leading causes were heart disease (24.1%), cancer (22.7%), chronic lower respiratory tract disease (5.9%), unintentional injuries (5.6%), and stroke (5.3%).[91] In fact, 75% of all American deaths occur from these or other chronic conditions. Although a slow and progressive deterioration can be disheartening for the patient to experience and challenging for the family to observe, a centered presence in the face of impending death optimizes opportunities for meaningful closure. Accordingly, patients can rally when least expected, often to fulfill one last important goal. For example, in the days before his death, Bill, a 70-year-old man with end-stage brain cancer, decided that he would leave his bed to have one last meal at the table with his family. Physical therapy services were requested and provided to help Bill carry out this goal. In other cases, patients may also linger in an unresponsive state for a period of time, dying shortly after a long-awaited loved one finally arrives. Joseph, a 72-year-old man with liver cancer, died the day after his six adult children finally arrived from their locations around the country.

The end-of-life process is unique for every individual. There are many different ways in which the journey to the end of life begins so that each person dies in his or her own unique way, and in his or her own time.[5] Supporting this individual process is the purpose and focus of hospice care. In the context of hospice care, approaching death is viewed as a physical, psychological, and spiritual event. Patients and their families require information and compassionate support to ensure that their collective needs are honored during this critical time. The interdisciplinary hospice approach involves considerable involvement of the patient's nurse, who will administer medications for comfort. The hospice chaplain may be involved for spiritual support at the request of the individual or family, especially when impending death provokes questions by the dying person or family members related to the presence of, or the prospect of, life after death. Trained hospice volunteers may provide caregiver respite or provide a reassuring presence at the bedside. The hospice social worker may assist the family in a number of practical ways, such as addressing financial concerns. Physical therapy interventions such as edema reduction, breathing exercises for relaxation, positioning, and gentle massage or stretching may be performed in the days or even hours before death. In one study exploring the feasibility of physical therapy interventions among 528 terminally ill patients, 90% of these patients received a variety of effective interventions that included physical activity (50%), relaxation training (22%), breathing training (10%), and lymphedema management (6%).[48] A recent study examined the impact of physical therapy intervention among patients in a community hospice. The most prevalent symptoms included weakness, pain, edema, and breathlessness.[45] The results of this study indicated that physical therapy intervention improved several elements of these patients' function and symptoms. The most commonly reported benefit was a significant reduction in musculoskeletal pain, followed by improvements in performance of activities of daily living and mobility. Other reported benefits included improvements in endurance, mood, and energy. The most common assessment tool was the visual analog scale for pain, followed by varying measures of functional mobility, balance, and patient-reported quality of life. Common forms of intervention included functional skills training, breathing exercises, and manual therapy such as lymphedema massage.

The following section includes a description of common physiological changes that accompany the death process, but it is important to note that these will vary among persons.

The Dying Process

Physiological Changes Associated with Death. The dying process involves the decline and ultimate failure of all major organ systems. Depending on the nature of the contributory disease, this process may take anywhere from several months to several hours. Box 27.4 depicts the broader progressive changes that occur in the final months of life.

As a patient declines in function, physical therapy intervention can be helpful in providing education, adaptive devices, or alternative movement strategies to optimize safe function. These interventions are fully described in the section on models of physical therapy practice in hospice and palliative care earlier in this chapter.

Of equal importance to providing appropriate interventions is working closely with the hospice team to ensure that all forms of pain and discomfort are minimized. This is important not only for the patient but also for family members who, whenever possible, must be freed of the burden inherent in watching a loved one suffer. In the weeks or days before death, multisystem decline results in a host of signs, which are illustrated in Table 27.5 and further described in this chapter.

It is very common for patients to sleep most of the time in the days before death. They may no longer be interested in food or fluid, and family members must be assured that for the dying person, the process of digestion can be uncomfortable or even painful. Furthermore, as death approaches, patients may have increased difficulty swallowing. Even in the absence of discomfort, dying patients do not need, nor can their bodies assimilate, the energy provided from food. When patients refuse food and fluids, or in cases where they are withdrawn in accordance with an advance directive, family members need assurance that the patient will not experience hunger or any sense of deprivation. In such instances, the hospice nurse will work with the patient and family to provide medications and other interventions to ensure optimal comfort. The ethical and legal aspects of intentional food and fluid withdrawal will be further discussed later in this chapter.

"Terminal restlessness" is a specific form of delirium and agitation that occurs in the final weeks, days, or hours of life. It is very common, although the degree may vary greatly, affecting up to 85% of terminally ill patients, and includes signs such as restlessness, agitation, confusion, hallucinations, or nightmares.[92] The experience of terminal restlessness can be highly upsetting for families and patients alike. One patient of the authors described his terminal restlessness as a feeling of "just wanting to crawl out of my skin." Terminal restlessness is thought to be the result of failing metabolic processes occurring as death approaches. In addition, terminal restlessness may be exacerbated by physical distress from severe constipation, decreased oxygen exchange, or changes in body temperature. Thus, terminal restlessness could be described as a condition involving considerable physiological and psychological pain, occurring at all levels of consciousness. Unresponsive patients may demonstrate terminal restlessness by pulling

BOX 27.4 Progressive Changes in the Terminal Phase

Month 6	Generally, patient is ambulatory, coherent, some adverse effects from curative measures/medications, initial stages of grief, anger, denial
Month 5	Some weight loss, weakness, symptoms manifested (i.e., pain, dyspnea, organic dysfunction), showing signs of stress, growing acceptance of terminal state, fear, depression
Month 4	Continuing weight loss, decreasing appetite, physical manifestations, symptoms more pronounced; grief work, planning, resolving
Month 3	Physical deterioration apparent, symptomatology and pain increase, beginning of withdrawal, acceptance of terminal disease
Month 2	Progressive physical deterioration, symptoms increase, pain management primary, may be bedridden, increasing withdrawal, resolution, and closure
Final month	End stage: pronounced withdrawal, requires total care, intensive management of symptoms and pain, no appetite

(Adapted from National Hospice and Palliative Care Organization [NHPCO]. Time line phases of terminal care. 1996. Reprinted with permission.)

TABLE 27.5 Multisystem Physiologic Signs of Approaching Death

System	Sign or Symptom	Contributing Factors
Central nervous system	Confusion, delirium Disorientation Increased time spent sleeping (from a few hours a day to most of the day) Decreased levels of responsiveness, eventual coma Anxiety and restlessness, hallucinations or reports of seeing things, hearing voices	Hypoxemia from disease process or decreased function, metabolic imbalances such as acidosis, toxicity from renal or liver failure, pain, adverse effects of opioid medication (this may be reversible)
Musculoskeletal	Weakness, loss of function, fatigue	Progression of disease process, prolonged inactivity
Cardiopulmonary	Drop in blood pressure Heart rate variability and irregularity Breathing rate may be very rapid, alternating with periods of apnea, or very slow gurgling in chest	Disease process, organ failure, adverse effect from chemotherapy (not reversible) Respiratory failure may result in fluid accumulation in lungs
Integumentary	Cool and clammy skin, distal extremities may be bluish Edema	Loss of cardiovascular perfusion Pump failure Loss of muscle tone
Gastrointestinal	Loss of interest in food and fluid Constipation or diarrhea Incontinence, decreasing urine output as death approaches	Adverse effects of medications (opioid medications are constipating)

at their bed clothes, making random movements, or attempting to remove their medical appliances. Patients who are more wakeful may repeatedly ask to get up or attempt to do so without help. They may talk about seeing and speaking with deceased friends or family members (e.g., a patient may sit up in bed and tell family members, "They're coming!"). Understandably, the behaviors of terminal restlessness can be disconcerting for patients and families. Reassurance, support, and skilled pharmacologic intervention, often involving the use of sedating medications, are important measures that can reduce the duration and severity of these symptoms.

"Active death" typically occurs in the final days or hours and involves observable signs of systemic failure.[93] Terminal restlessness may increase. Respirations may become extremely irregular and include periods of very rapid breathing, followed by several seconds of apnea (Cheyne–Stokes breathing). Other types of irregular breathing patterns may occur as well, along with "death rattles" from congested and fluid-congested lungs. Urine output decreases significantly, and the urine may be dark. Blood pressure will often drop 20 to 30 points below the patient's normal blood pressure range, with systolic pressure as low as 70 mmHg and diastolic readings as low as 50 mmHg. This lack of perfusion may result in extremities that are very cold, blue, or purple. Patients may also complain of numbness in their distal extremities.

The patient may be unresponsive, or even comatose. Family members need to be assured that the patient hears them as hearing is one of the last senses to fail[94] and thus should be encouraged to talk to their loved one even if they do not receive a response. In contrast, other patients may be relatively wakeful and able to converse with family members almost to the moment of death.

As stated previously, dying is not only a physical event, many patients experience significant psychological and social signs as well. Table 27.6 illustrates the spectrum of these, along with their possible causes and helpful interventions.

One of the many benefits of hospice involvement is the preparation of the patient and his or her family about the signs and symptoms related to the death process. Such preparation dispels inaccuracies (i.e., death is painful), reducing fear, regret, and guilt over not doing enough for their loved one. Most of all, skillful management of death-related discomfort allows the patient and family to be comfortably and lovingly present to each other throughout the process. Finally, when a loved one dies peacefully in the manner of a "good death," family members can focus their grief on mourning their loss and finding comfort in their memories.

Nearing Death Awareness. A variety of altered mental states may be experienced as the end of life approaches. The "out of body" experience has been reported after brushes with death, such as an accident.[93] Others have reported incidents of knowledge of things that they attribute to awareness of another dimension.[94] All of this work recognizes the mystery that surrounds the dying process, which exceeds the physical indicators that medical professionals can use to quantify the ceasing of life in the body.

Callahan and Kelley[70] recommend from their years of working with individuals during end-of-life experiences that clinical caregivers as well as family members learn from close listening and observation of the person in their care. Caregivers who do not have an understanding of this communication may experience more anxiety.

The dying person may speak in metaphoric language. For example, imagine this dialogue between a mother

TABLE 27.6 Psychosocial and Spiritual Signs, Symptoms, and Interventions of the Actively Dying

Signs and Symptoms	Cause/Etiology	Interventions
Fear of the dying process. Fear of the dying process may be greater than the fear of death.	Cause of fear will be specific to the individual. Fear of the unknown: how the person will die, what will happen during the dying process. Fear of painful death and suffering such as breathlessness, physical pain, loss of mental competence and decision-making ability, loss of control, loss of ability to maintain spiritual belief systems and faith. Fear of judgment, punishment related to guilt, and subsequent pain and suffering during the dying process.	Explore fears and cause/etiology of fears, including physical, psychosocial, and spiritual. Educate patient and family on physical, psychosocial, and spiritual signs and symptoms of dying process. Ask patient/family how they would like the dying process to happen. Normalize feelings. Provide reassurance that patient will be kept as comfortable as possible. Provide presence and increase as needed.
Fear of abandonment. Most patients do not want to die alone. May present as patient anxiety, pressing call button frequently, or calling out for help at home. Family members may continuously stay at bedside to honor patient wish to not be left alone.	Fear of being alone. Fear of who will care for the person when he or she is unable to care for him- or herself.	Provide reassurance that everything will be done to have someone with the patient. Provide presence. Explore options for increasing presence around the clock, including health care professionals (nurse, social worker, nurse's aide) and family, friends, volunteers, church members, etc. For family member doing bedside vigil, encourage frequent breaks; offer respite. Family members may also be anxious and need permission from nurse to care for themselves.
Fear of the unknown.	Fear of what will happen after the person dies: afterlife or cultural/faith system beliefs in relation to death. Fear that belief systems regarding afterlife will be different than perceived and/or lived.	Assist in exploration of fear. Provide companionship, presence. Offer pastoral care or patient's clergy for exploration of life, afterlife, faith system beliefs. Support cultural and faith system beliefs.
Nearing death awareness. Patients state they have spoken to those who have already died or have seen places not presently accessible or visible to family and/or nurse. May describe spiritual beings, bright lights, "another world." Statements may seem out of character, gesture or request. Patients may tell family members, significant others when they will die.	Attempt by the dying to describe what they are experiencing, the dying process, and death. Transitioning from this life. Attempting to describe something they need to do/accomplish before they die, such as permission from family to die, reconciliation, see someone, reassurance that survivor will be okay without them.	Do not contradict, explain away, belittle, humor, or argue with the patient about these experiences. Attentively and sensitively listen to the patient, affirm the experience, and attempt to determine if there is any unfinished business, patient needs. Encourage family/significant others to say goodbye, give permission for patient to die as appropriate. Support family and other caregivers. Educate about the difference between nearing death awareness and confusion, education to family, and other caregivers.
Withdrawal from family, friends, the nurse, and other health care professionals: decreased interest in environment and relationships; family may feel they have upset or offended patient.	Transition from this life, patient "letting go" of this life.	Normalize withdrawal by educating family about transition. Provide presence, gentle touch. Family members may need to be educated, encouraged to give permission to patient to die. Family may need to be encouraged to say goodbyes.

(From The Hospice of the Florida Suncoast, 1999. Reprinted with permission.)

and daughter. "I need to go home," states the older patient. "Mom, you are home. This is your house. See the family photos on the mantle above the fireplace, and there is your favorite chair," replies her daughter in frustration after several repetitions. Could there be another sense of *home* to which she is referring, perhaps even a spiritual resting place consistent with her lifelong beliefs?

Another example of misinterpreting metaphorical speech would be this hypothetical conversation between a father and son. "The door is locked," declares Mr. Thompson emphatically as he arouses from a lethargic state. His family is glad to hear him communicate. Son Robert steps from the bedside to the sliding glass door across the room. "No, Dad. Look, the door is open," he responds as he demonstrates the sliding door out to the patio moving freely. Perhaps there is some unfinished business Mr. Thompson needs to address, or it is his way of indicating that he does not believe he is ready to die.

Patients will commonly report seeing things that are not visible to others. Insects, reptiles, or other animals may be reported as hallucinations related to the introduction or dosing changes of opioid medications, but the visualization of people is worth exploring. Often these may be recognizable to the dying individual as previously deceased friends or family members, who are perceived as calling and communicating in some way with the dying person. Understanding this as a relatively common but often unacknowledged experience, perhaps because of a societal reluctance to grapple with complex metaphysical issues, may provide recognition that this is a normal end-of-life process occurring and afford some individuals comfort that the dying loved one will not be alone after passing away as may be consistent with their personal beliefs.

Other patients may voice their beliefs about the timing of their deaths in ways that may not seem to coincide with apparent physical parameters. The insights offered by those in our care offer us an opportunity to support their caregivers and loved ones in helping meet the desire to have a peaceful death. By listening carefully, then recognizing such communication, physical therapists can educate family members, allowing them to become more intimately involved in this experience of accompanying their dying loved one and preparing for their own time of bereavement.

CULTURAL ISSUES WITH ACCEPTANCE OF DEATH

A consideration in the acceptance of the dying process is the diverse cultural backgrounds of patients and families. It is incumbent that the therapist is sensitive and aware of the cultural norms and desires of the clients being served.[95] Expressions of pain vary significantly across races and ethnic groups.[96] Concurrently, the social roles during illness can have a significant impact on goal setting, intervention, and the desire or expression of success or independence.[97] Attitudes about the language that health care providers use in discussing the condition and possible outcomes, the use of metaphors, and considerations of death are other topics that should be understood.[98] Historically, the hospice philosophy evolved in nations such as England and France; subsequently, HPC has proliferated to regions that had historical or colonial ties to these nations.[99] Patients and families that are more familiar with the HPC care philosophy may be more willing to consider and accept HPC care tenets; however, individual or family preferences still have a strong influence.

Making death a clinical, medical matter often does not keep with many cultural or religious traditions.[100] Relatives may request traditional healers to try to elicit a cure or relatives may explore facilitating death at home or a sacred location as well as visitation by extended family and friends. Examples of good practice before death include providing privacy for prayer, respect and care for sacred texts or icons, and gender-sensitive patient care providers for selected procedures.[99] Even the concept of a "good death," though generally accepted in Western nations, varies significantly in other continents or nations, including the belief of the causes of death and illness.[49] Behaviors and expectations may be influenced by customs and traditional healers as opposed to Western medical care. These differences in practices present barriers but also opportunities for alliances between HPC practitioners, physical therapists, and traditional healers.

As the history and evolution of HPC concepts has followed the proliferation of a Western-hemispheric, Christian growth pattern, there is value in exploring how all religions and cultures approach this concept.[101] Gatrad and Sheikh[100] highlighted challenges when discussing any large heterogeneous group, such as those who follow Islam. They noted that the more rooted an individual was within the local culture or religion, the more it was felt that the family should be the ones to look after the ill, but those individuals who had exposure, had schooling, or lived in a Western culture were more open to having external assistance caring for the terminally ill. Many families do not wish their dying relative to be informed of the prognosis as the family may be concerned about a "loss of hope." These may create challenging ethical conflicts between a well-intentioned health care provider who may feel this was a violation of an individual's right to autonomy and the relatives' rights to care for their loved one in a culturally and traditionally appropriate fashion. Culture, religion, and spirituality tend to play an increased influence on provision of HPC care (including physical therapy) in end-of-life situations and physical therapists must anticipate these issues and work closely with the patient, family, and interdisciplinary team to best provide for patient-centered, culturally sensitive care to optimize remaining quality of life and a good death.[9]

CONFRONTING THE REALITY OF DEATH

Being comfortable with dying is a challenge for many therapists and individuals because of the limited exposure during our training and clinical practice, and the nature of modern culture. The process of understanding the meaning and nature of death, then being able to speak of living and dying with comfort and ease, takes time and practice through repeated exposure and experience. This development can occur through reading, conversations with professional peers, and eventually during work with people approaching the end of life. This section will introduce conversation topics that arise in clinical settings and promote adjustment to the dying process.

Decline, if not reversible, will lead to death. Fully understanding the universality of death as more than an abstract concept can make us open to the possibility of improvement, maintaining a functional level, or further decline and death during the course of clinical care. Death is not failure by the patient or the therapist, but the natural course of life. The ability to give voice to this natural event as it occurs during the process of care can provide a sense of understanding that will support the coping of patients and family members.

Death is an experience fraught with an array of emotion. Patients often have limited experiences with death during their lifetimes and may find themselves struggling with unfamiliar circumstances and feelings as their conditions progress. How health professionals address the events that occur at the end of life can offer support and understanding to allow the completion of this process with less distress and better understanding. Patients and family members have identified geriatric and oncologic medical care that includes physical and intentional presence, developing an understanding of their individualized experience, and maintaining the patient's humanity and dignity, as essential to their spiritual well-being.[102]

Reframing Physical Loss and Dying

Loss and suffering are a natural, albeit unpleasant, part of the dying process. Often there is a component of significant physical loss such as the inability to walk, stand, or even get out of bed during this experience. The physical therapist can use clinical observations made during initial examination or ongoing assessments to affirm the person's maximal efforts at mobility and function in light of a progressive or deteriorating condition. Understanding these losses can change the aspects of suffering that are then experienced and one can discover a meaning to life by the attitude taken toward this unavoidable suffering.[103]

Spiritual Awareness

In the past century, perhaps because of the advances of medicine, emphasis has been on the physical changes that occur as the body deteriorates in the process of dying rather than on the spiritual changes with dying, as in past centuries. Previously, societies have examined death as a spiritual event and created treatises such as the Christian *Ars Moriendi* or "Art of Dying"[104] and the Buddhist *Tibetan Book of the Dead*.[105] Evidence of spiritual well-being is found to improve coping with terminal illness.[106,107] It is important that members of the IDT meet the spiritual needs of patients and families receiving hospice care, even if their spiritual/religious tradition or beliefs differ from one's own.[108]

Dealing with Death and Dying

In physical therapy practice of aging adults, it is common to provide care to individuals who are facing death either imminently or in the not-so-distant future. Many physical therapists' first experience of death is with an older patient with whom they have grown close through the therapeutic relationship. When confronted with the inevitability of the patient's death, a physical therapist may feel anxiety or feel incapable of coping with such a situation.[108] A common and natural emotional reaction is fear that can be perceived by the patient from the therapist's body language and facial expression as pity.[109] The therapist's recognition that death is inevitable and naturally occurring can bring about a freedom from the fear and a recognition that everyone has choices in how one's days can be lived. Listening to the patient with empathy and unconditional positive regard is a way of communicating compassion[109] without using nonsensical statements such as "I know how you feel" (you don't) or "It will be all right" (it may not) or worse, "You shouldn't feel that way" (why not?). To provide compassionate care by being present to the dying individual, health professionals must face their own fears of loss, suffering, and death. To be effective, physical therapists need to recognize their own as well as the aging adult's feelings, have a sense of their strengths and weaknesses, and be aware of their thoughts and feelings about death and dying, as these may all have an impact on how care is provided. Awareness that any discomfort the therapist feels is a personal reaction and may not be shared by the older adult who is at the end of life can help the therapist with appreciating the continuity of life.

Unfinished Business

Often, the older patient may be comfortable with death, even anticipating it as a means of meeting a spouse or other loved one who predeceased him or her. However, the patient's family may still be resisting the finality of death and may express discomfort as wanting more therapy, pushing the patient to do more, to not give up, and so forth. This lack of acceptance of the loved one's death may be a result of unfinished business. Clinically this can be addressed through using the various practice patterns identified earlier in this chapter to sustain a sense of hope rather than the abandonment that may be felt from a discharge from having "failed" therapy. The personal issues of unfinished business can be addressed as well.

Unfinished business has been identified by Elizabeth Kubler Ross[110] and others[111] as tasks and relationships that need completion or resolution before the end of life, or to get through any difficult situation. Byock[112] has outlined four communication tasks of the dying and their families: "Please forgive me," "I forgive you," "Thank you," and "I love you." Offering these words of goodbye may help families find closure. Being in the presence of those close to the end of life and struggling with their own issues of pending loss will in many cases bring to the level of awareness of the family and/or practitioner feelings and emotions related to their own past or anticipated life losses.

Being able to process and resolve one's own personal issues of unfinished business is a healthy and life-affirming process that is recognized as anticipatory grief for patients and families. Patients can be teachers to therapists as well. Those at the end of life may report increased comfort and peace as this occurs. They may report a clarity and meaning in life that was not evident previously. For the health and well-being of physical therapists as end-of-life caregivers, reflection around such issues can promote more effective listening ability and long-term work satisfaction. Most hospice workers have a spiritual belief system, which may not be connected to an organized religion or be well defined, but consist of some belief in something beyond the self, some way of making meaning of the world and life.[113] Patients and families can be guided to access their own religious or spiritual support system, or that of the hospice program, to cope with the realities and unknown of death.

SUMMARY

End-of-life care is a challenge for both the new and experienced physical therapist. Clinical expertise is developed through an ongoing practice of reflection and mindfulness.[114] Knowledge of aging and disease processes, pain and symptom management, and the different patterns of care used to support a palliative care approach is essential. Understanding the physical therapy role within the hospice interdisciplinary team approach is important for successful practice integration. Personal exploration of one's own feelings and issues with loss, grief, and death is necessary to maintain personal health while providing the best intervention and support to individuals as they die.

REFERENCES

1. American Association of Colleges of Nursing and City of Hope National Medical Center. *End-of-Life Nursing Education Consortium (ELNEC) Module 1: Nursing care at the end of life*. Duarte, CA.
2. American Physical Therapy Association. *Vision Statement for the Physical Therapy Profession*. http://www.apta.org/Vision/. Accessed February 14, 2018.
3. World Health Organization. WHO definition of palliative care. http://www.who.int/cancer/palliative/definition/en/. Accessed March 6, 2018.
4. Lynn J, Adamson DM. *Living Well at the End of Life. White Paper*. Santa Monica, CA: Rand Corporation; 2003.
5. Center to Advance Palliative Care. Improving Care for People with Serious Illness Through Innovative Payer-Provider Partnerships, 2014. A Palliative Care Toolkit and Reference Guide. National Business Group on Health. https://www.capc.org/payers/palliative-care-payer-provider-toolkit/. Accessed April 10, 2018.
6. Institute of Medicine of the National Academies. Policies and payment systems to support high-quality end-of-life care. In: *Dying in America: Improving Quality and Honoring Individual Preferences Near the End of Life*. Washington, DC: National Academies Press; 2015.
7. Center for Medicare and Medicaid Services. *Jimmo v. Sebelius Settlement Agreement Fact Sheet*. http://www.cms.gov/Medicare/Medicare-Fee-for-Service-Payment/SNFPPS/Downloads/Jimmo-FactSheet.pdf. Published January 23, 2013. Accessed August 27, 2015.
8. Drouin JS, Martin K, Onowu N, Berg A, Zuellig L. Physical therapy utilization in hospice and palliative care settings in Michigan: a descriptive study. *Rehabil Oncol*. 2009;27:3–8.
9. American Physical Therapy Association. The Role of Physical Therapy in Hospice and Palliative Care HOD P06-11-14-11. [Position]. http://www.apta.org/uploadedFiles/APTAorg/About_Us/Policies/Health_Social_Environment/RoleHospicePalliativeCare.pdf. Published August 1, 2012. Accessed May 6, 2018.
10. Wilson CM, Stiller CH, Doherty DJ, Thompson KA. The role of physical therapists within hospice and palliative care in the United States and Canada. *Am J Hospice Palliative Med*. 2017;34(1):34–41.
11. Hanson LC, Ersek M. Meeting palliative care needs in post–acute care settings: "to help them live until they die" *JAMA*. 2006;295(6):681–686.
12. Wilson C, Roy D. Relationship between physical therapy, occupational therapy, palliative care consultations, and hospital length of stay. *J Acute Care Phys Ther*. 2017;8(3):106–112.
13. Kumar SP, Jim A. Physical therapy in palliative care: from symptom control to quality of life: a critical review. *Ind J Palliative Care*. 2010;16(3):138.
14. Mitchell G, Del Mar C, O'Rourke P, Clavarino A. Do case conferences between general practitioners and specialist palliative care services improve quality of life? A randomised controlled trial (ISRCTN 52269003). *Palliative Med*. 2008;22:904–912.
15. Centers for Disease Control and Prevention. Give peace of mind: advanced care planning. http://www.cdc.gov/aging/advancecareplanning/index.htm. Published March 3, 2014. Accessed April 6, 2018.
16. Neporent L. Terri Schiavo: 10 years after her death, "end of life" debate rages on. ABC News. http://abcnews.go.com/Health/terri-schiavo-10-years-death-end-life-debate/story?id=30013571. Published March 31, 2015.
17. Downey L, Au DH, Curtis JR, et al. Life-sustaining treatment preferences: matches and mismatches between patients' preferences and clinicians' perceptions. *J Pain Symptom Manage*. 2013;46(1):9–19.
18. Mack JW, Cronin A, Taback N, et al. End-of-life discussions among patients with advanced cancer: a cohort study. *Ann Intern Med*. 2012;156(3):204–210.
19. Department of Health and Human Services Medical Learning Network. Advanced Care Planning. Center for Medicare and Medicaid Services. https://www.cms.gov/Outreach-and-Education/Medicare-Learning-Network-MLN/MLNProducts/Downloads/AdvanceCarePlanning.pdf. Accessed April 10, 2018.
20. Nguyen KH, Sellars M, Agar M, Kurrle S, Kelly A, Comans T. An economic model of advanced care planning is Australia: a cost-effective way to respect patient choice. *BMC Health Serv Res*. 2017;17(1):797.
21. Wilson C. Advanced directives, advanced care planning and the physical therapists' role in these challenging conversations. *Rehab Oncol*. 2016;34(2):72–74.
22. Deleted in Proof.
23. Deleted in Proof.
24. National Hospice and Palliative Care Organization. *Advance Care Planning*. https://www.nhpco.org/advance-care-planning. Accessed April 10, 2018.
25. Aging with Dignity. *5 Wishes*. https://agingwithdignity.org/five-wishes. Accessed April 10, 2018.
26. Death with Dignity National Center. *About us*. https://www.deathwithdignity.org/about/. Accessed April 10, 2018.

27. De Lima L, Woodruff R, Pettus K, et al. International Association for Hospice and Palliative Care position statement: euthanasia and physician-assisted suicide. *J Palliative Med.* 2017;20(1):8–14.
28. National Hospice and Palliative Care Organization. *NHPCO Facts and Figures: Hospice Care in America.* 2017 Edition, https://www.nhpco.org/sites/default/files/public/Statistics_Research/2017_Facts_Figures.pdf. Accessed April 10, 2018.
29. Centers for Medicare and Medicaid Services. *Medicare Hospice Benefits.* https://www.medicare.gov/Pubs/pdf/02154-Medicare-Hospice-Benefits.PDF. Accessed April 10, 2018.
30. Mother Teresa Center. *Mother Teresa of Calcutta Important Dates.* http://www.motherteresa.org/important-dates.html. Accessed April 10, 2018.
31. Obituary. Dame Cicely Saunders, founder of the modern hospice movement. *BMJ.* 2005;331. https://doi.org/10.1136/bmj.331.7510.238. Accessed April 10, 2018.
32. Johnson KS. Racial disparities in palliative care. *J Palliat Med.* 2013;16(1):1329–1334.
33. Smith AK, Craig EC, McCarthy EP. Racial and ethnic differences in end of life care in fee for service Medicare beneficiaries with advanced cancer. *J Am Geriatr Soc.* 2009;57(1):153–158.
34. Alzheimer's Association. 2018 Alzheimer's Disease Facts and Figures. *Alzheimers Dement.* 2018;14(3):367–429. https://www.alz.org/documents_custom/2018-facts-and-figures.pdf. Accessed 10 April 2018.
35. National Hospice and Palliative Care Organization. Medicare Hospice Criteria. http://www.nhhpco.org/scontent/uploads/files/HospiceCriteriaCard.pdf. Accessed April 6, 2018.
36. Conner SR, Pyenson B, Fitch K, et al. Comparing hospice and nonhospice patient survival among patients who die within a three year window. *J Pain Symptom Manage.* 2007;33(3):238–246.
37. Shugarman LR, Decker SL, Bercovitz A. Demographic and social characteristics and spending at the end of life. *J Pain Symptom Manage.* 2009;38(1):15–26.
38. Taylor DH, Ostermann J, VanHoutven CH, et al. What length of hospice use maximizes reduction in medical expenditures near death in the US Medicare Program? *Soc Sci Med.* 2007;65(7):1466–1478.
39. Carlson MD, Barry C, Schlesinger M, et al. Quality of palliative care at US hospices: results of a national survey. *Med Care.* 2011;49(9):803–809. https://doi.org/10.1097/MLR.0b013e31822395b2.
40. Deleted in Proof.
41. Wilson C, Mueller K, Briggs R. Physical therapists' contribution to the hospice and palliative care interdisciplinary team: a clinical summary. *J Hospice Palliative Nurs.* 2017;19(60):588–596.
42. Mueller K, Hamilton G, Rodden B, et al. Functional assessment and intervention by nursing assistants in hospice and palliative care inpatient care settings: a quality improvement pilot study. *Am J Hosp Palliat Care.* 2016;33(2):136–143.
43. Jensen W, Bialy L, Ketels G, Baumann FT, Bokemeyer C, Oechsle K. Physical exercise and therapy in terminally ill cancer patients: a retrospective feasibility analysis. *Support Care Cancer.* 2014;22(5):1261–1268.
44. Dal Bello-Haas V. A framework for rehabilitation of neurodegenerative diseases: planning care and maximizing quality of life. *Neurol Rep.* 2002;26(3):115–129.
45. Mueller K, Decker I. Impact of physical therapy intervention on function and quality of life in a community hospice. *Top Geriatr Rehabil.* 2011;27(1):2–9.
46. Frost M. The role of physical, occupational, and speech therapy in hospice: patient empowerment. *Am J Hosp Palliat Care.* 2001;18(6):397–402.
47. Mackey KM, Sparling JW. Experiences of older women with cancer receiving hospice care: significance for physical therapy. *Phys Ther.* 2000;80:459–468.
48. Putt K, Faville KA, Lewis D, McAllister K, Pietro M, Radwan A. Role of physical therapy intervention in patients with life-threatening illnesses: a systematic review. *Am J Hospice Palliative Med.* 2017;34(2):186–196.
49. Ferrell BR, Coyle N, Paice J, eds. *Oxford Textbook of Palliative Nursing.* 4th ed. New York: Oxford University Press; 2014:1311–1314.
50. Center for Medicare and Medicaid Services. *Annual Change in Hospice Rates.* https://www.medicaid.gov/medicaid/benefits/downloads/medicaid-hospice-rates-ffy-2018.pdf. Accessed April 10, 2018.
51. National Hospice and Palliative Care Organization. *Medical Hospice Conditions of Participation, Allied Therapists.* www.nhpco.org/sites/default/files/public/regulatory/Allied_therapist_tip_sheet.pdf. Accessed April 8, 2018.
52. Briggs R. Physical therapy in hospice care. *Rehabil Oncol.* 1997;15(3):16–17.
53. Briggs R. Models for physical therapy practice in palliative medicine. *Rehabil Oncol.* 2000;18(2):18–19.
53a. Dietz Jr. JH. Rehabilitation of the cancer patient: its role in the scheme of comprehensive care. *Clin Bull.* 1974;4:104–107.
54. American Physical Therapy Association. *Guide to Physical Therapist Practice 3.0.* http://www.apta.org/Guide/. Accessed April 10, 2018.
55. Center for Medicare and Medicaid Services. *Medicare Benefit Policy Manual Chapter 7 - Home Health Services.* https://www.cms.gov/Regulations-and-Guidance/Guidance/Manuals/downloads/bp102c07.pdf. Published February 24, 2017. Accessed April 10, 2018.
56. Squires RW, Shultz AM, Herrmann J. Exercise training and cardiovascular health in cancer patients. *Curr Oncol Rep.* 2018;20(3):27.
57. Barreiro E. Models of disuse muscle atrophy: therapeutic implications in critically ill patients. *Ann Transl Med.* 2018;6(2):29. https://doi.org/10.21037/atm.2017.12.12.
58. Gianoudis J, Bailey CA, Daly RM. Associations between sedentary behaviour and body composition, muscle function and sarcopenia in community-dwelling older adults. *Osteoporos Int.* 2015;26(2):571–579.
59. Pizzi MA, Briggs R. Occupational and physical therapy in hospice: the facilitation of meaning, quality of life, and well-being. *Top Geriatr Rehabil.* 2004;20(2):120–130.
60. Burton E, Farrier K, Lewin G, et al. Motivators and barriers for older people participating in resistance training: a systematic review. *J Aging Phys Act.* 2017;25(2):311–324.
61. Busch AJ, McClements JD. Effects of a supervised home exercise program on patients with severe chronic obstructive pulmonary disease. *Phys Ther.* 1988;68:469–474.
62. Gudas SA. Terminal illness. In: *Psychology in the Physical and Manual Therapies.* New York, NY: Churchill Livingstone; 2004:333–350.
63. Borasio GD, Rogers A, Voltz R. Palliative medicine in non-malignant neurological disorders. In: Doyle D, Hanks G, Cherny N, Calman K, eds. *Oxford Textbook of Palliative Medicine.* 3rd ed. New York, NY: Oxford University Press; 2005.
64. Sterns RH, Emmett M, Forman JP. *Patient education: edema (swelling) (beyond the basics).* UpToDate, https://www.uptodate.com/contents/edema-swelling-beyond-the-basics. Published December 16, 2017.

65. Head B, Faul A. Terminal restlessness as perceived by hospice professionals. *Am J Hosp Palliat Med.* 2005;22(4):277–282.
66. Korner AF, Thoman EB. The relative efficacy of contact and vestibular-proprioceptive stimulation in soothing neonates. *Child Dev.* 1972;43:443–453.
67. Gray J. Protecting hospice patients: a new look at falls prevention. *Am J Hospice Palliative Med.* 2007;24 (3):242–247.
68. The Joint Commission. *National Patient Safety Goals Home Care Accreditation Program.* https://www.jointcommission.org/assets/1/6/2015_NPSG_OME.pdf. Published January 1, 2015. Accessed April 11, 2018.
69. Hall AM, Ferreira PH, Maher CG, et al. The influence of the therapist-patient relationship on treatment outcome in physical rehabilitation: a systematic review. *Phys Ther.* 2010;90:1099–1110.
70. Callahan M, Kelley P. *Final Gifts: Understanding the Special Awareness, Needs, and Communications of the Dying.* New York, NY: Poseidon Press; 2012.
71. International Association for the Study of Pain. IASP Taxonomy. https://www.iasp-pain.org/Taxonomy. Accessed April 8, 2018.
72. McCaffery M, Pasero C. *Pain: Clinical Manual.* 2nd ed. St. Louis, MO: Mosby; 1999.
73. Chang VT, Hwang SS, Feuerman M, et al. The Memorial symptom assessment scale short form. *Cancer.* 2000;89: 1162–1171.
74. Saunders C. Nature and management of terminal pain. In: Shotter EF, ed. *Matters of Life and Death.* London: Dartman, Longman and Todd; 1970.
75. Pinkerton R, Hardy JR. Opioid addiction and misuse in adult and adolescent patients with cancer. *Intern Med J.* 2017;47 (6):632–636.
76. Højsted J, Sjøgren P. Addiction to opioids in chronic pain patients: a literature review. *Eur J Pain.* 2007;11(5):490–518.
77. American Academy of Pain Medicine. *Definitions related to the use of opioids for the treatment of pain.* https://www.asam.org/docs/default-source/public-policy-statements/1opioid-definitions-consensus-2-011.pdf. Published 2001. Accessed April 8, 2018.
78. American Cancer Society. *Daily Pain Diary.* https://www.cancer.org/content/dam/cancer-org/cancer-control/en/worksheets/pain-diary.pdf. Accessed April 8, 2018.
79. World Health Organization. *WHO's cancer pain ladder for adults.* http://www.who.int/cancer/palliative/painladder/en/. Accessed April 8, 2018.
80. Wilson CM, Briggs R. Physical therapy's role in opioid use and management during palliative and hospice care. *Phys Ther.* 2018;98:83–85.
81. Ciccone CD. Medical marijuana: just the beginning of a long, strange trip? *Phys Ther.* 2017;97:239–248.
82. Medline Plus. Dronabinol. U.S. National Library of Medicine. https://medlineplus.gov/druginfo/meds/a607054.html. Updated September 15, 2017. Accessed April 10, 2018.
83. Cherny NI. ESMO clinical practice guidelines for the management of refractory symptoms at the end of life and the use of palliative sedation. *Ann Oncol.* 2014;25(Suppl 3). iii143–152.
84. American Academy of Hospice and Palliative Medicine. *Statement on Palliative Sedation.* http://aahpm.org/positions/palliative-sedation. Published December 5, 2014. Accessed April 8, 2018.
85. Burt RA. The Supreme Court speaks—not assisted suicide but a constitutional right to palliative care. *N Engl J Med.* 1997;337:1234–1236.
86. Robijn L, Cohen J, Deliens L, Chambaere K. Trends in continuous deep sedation until death between 2007 and 2013: a repeated nationwide survey. *PLoS One.* 2016;11(6): e0158188.
87. Prado BL, Bugano DDG, Usón Jr. P, et al. Continuous palliative sedation for patients with advanced cancer at a tertiary care cancer center. *BMC Palliat Care.* 2018;17 (1):13.
88. Beller EM, van Driel ML, McGregor L, et al. Palliative pharmacological sedation for terminally ill adults. *Cochrane Database Syst Rev.* 2015;(1):CD010206.
89. Fainsinger RL, Waller A, Bercovici M, et al. A multicentre international study of sedation for uncontrolled symptoms in terminally ill patients. *Palliat Med.* 2000;14(4):257–265.
90. Nuland SB. *How We Die: Reflections on Life's Final Chapter.* New York, NY: Vintage Books; 1995.
91. Centers for Disease Control National Center for Health Statistics (NCHS). *Data Brief: Mortality in the United States, NCHS Data Brief no. 293, December 2017.* https://www.cdc.gov/nchs/data/databriefs/db293.pdf. Accessed April 10, 2018.
92. Hospice Patients Alliance. *Terminal Agitation.* http://www.hospicepatients.org/terminal-agitation.html. Accessed April 10, 2018.
93. Moody R. *Life After Life.* San Francisco, CA: Harper; 2001.
94. Kubler-Ross E. *Death Is of Vital Importance.* Barrytown, NY: Station Hill Press; 2005.
95. Rothstein JM. Stereotyping or liberating: data on ethnicity and culture. *Phys Ther.* 2004;84(5):406.
96. Murtaugh CM, Beissner KL, Barrón Y, et al. Pain and function in home care: a need for treatment tailoring to reduce disparities? *Clin J Pain.* 2017;33(4):300.
97. Norris M, Allotey P. Culture and physiotherapy. *Diversity Health Social Care.* 2008;5(2):151–159.
98. Altilio T. The power and potential of language. In: Altilio T, Otis-Green S, eds. *Oxford Textbook of Palliative Social Work.* New York, NY: Oxford University Press; 2011.
99. Payne S, Seymour J, Ingleton C. *Palliative Care Nursing: Principles and Evidence for Practice.* Maidenhead: McGraw-Hill/Open University Press; 200839–54.
100. Gatrad AR, Sheikh A. Palliative care for Muslims and issues before death. *Int J Palliative Nurs.* 2002;8(11): 526–531.
101. Bingley A, Clark D. A comparative review of palliative care development in six countries represented by the Middle East Cancer Consortium (MECC). *J Pain Symptom Manage.* 2009;37(3):287–296.
102. Daaelman TP, Usher BM, Williams SW, et al. An exploratory study of spiritual care at the end of life. *Ann Fam Med.* 2008; 6(5):406–411.
103. Gawande A. *Being Mortal: Illness, Medicine and What Matters in the End.* New York, NY: Metropolitan Books; 2014.
104. Atkinson DW. *The English Ars Moriendi.* New York, NY: Peter Lang; 1992.
105. Rinpoche G. Translated by Fremantle F & Trungpa C. *The Tibetan Book of the Dead: The Great Liberation Through Hearing the Bardo.* Boston: Shambhala; 2010.
106. Babler JE. A comparison of spiritual care provided by hospice social workers, nurses, and spiritual care professionals. *Hosp J.* 1997;12(4):15–27.
107. McClain C, Rosenfeld B, Breitbart W. Effect of spiritual well-being on end-of-life despair in terminally-ill cancer patients. *Lancet.* 2003;361(9369):1603–1607.
108. Ogiwara S, Matsubara H. Attitudes of Japanese physiotherapists towards death and terminal illness. *J Phys Ther Sci.* 2007;19(4):227–234.
109. Tulsky JA. Beyond advance directives: importance of communication skills at the end of life. *JAMA.* 2005;294 (3):359–365.

110. Kubler-Ross E. *On Death and Dying*. New York, NY: Macmillan; 1969.
111. Longaker C. *Facing Death and Finding Hope*. New York, NY: Doubleday; 1997.
112. Byock I. *The Four Things That Matter Most*. New York, NY: Simon and Schuster; 2004.
113. Jones SH. A self care plan for hospice workers. *Am J Hospice Palliat Med*. 2005;22(2):125–128.
114. Wainwright SF, Shepard KF, Harman LB, Stephens J. Novice and experienced physical therapy clinicians: a comparison of how reflection is used to inform the clinical decision-making process. *Phys Ther*. 2010;90:75–88.

CHAPTER

28

The Senior Athlete

Jared M. Gollie

OUTLINE

INTRODUCTION

The average life expectancy is increasing globally. According to the World Health Organization's (WHO) *World Report on Ageing and Health*, for the first time in history, most people are expected to live into their 60s.[1] As the older population continues to grow, the concept of healthy aging has become a major focus in an attempt to ensure well-being and quality of life in the later years of life. The WHO defines *healthy aging* as the process of developing and maintaining the functional ability that enables well-being in older age.[1] Figure 28.1 shows a model adapted from the WHO *World Report on Ageing and Health* depicting the hypothetical trajectories of physical capacity in (1) senior athletes, (2) after injury, and (3) in the presence of physical inactivity or disease with aging. Given that senior athletes demonstrate superior functional capabilities compared with their sedentary counterparts, this athletic subgroup of aging adults represents a truly unique example of those who are aging exceptionally well.[2,3] It has been argued that highly trained older athletes provide the most optimal model to understand the physiological processes of human aging.[4] The premise for this argument is based on the absence of physical inactivity as a confounding factor in such individuals; thus, the observed longitudinal decrements in performance are solely the reflection of the aging process.[4] Understanding the reasons behind the inevitable declines in athletic performance nonetheless are essential for effective intervention design to ensure safe and competitive sports participation in senior athletes.

Masters and age-group distance running, cycling, and swimming records are broken at a staggering rate. The masters marathon record for the men's 35-year age group belongs to Haile Gebrselassie of Ethiopia with a time of 2:03:59 set in 2008 at the age of 35 years.[5] Ed Whitlock of Canada owns an astonishing three masters marathon world records with times of 2:54:48, 3:04:54, and 3:15:54 set at the ages of 73, 76, and 80 years for the men's 70-, 75-, and 80-year age groups, respectively.[5] The men's 90-year age group masters marathon world record is held by Ernest Van Leeuwen of the United States with a time of 6:46:34 set at the age of 92 years.[5] The current women's masters marathon world record is held by Irina Mikitenko of Germany set in 2008 at the age of 36 years with a time of 2:19:19.[5] The women's 90-year age group masters marathon world record holder is Mavis Lindgren of the United States with a time of 8:53:08 set in 1997 at the age of 90 years.[5]

Even more impressive has been the emergence of centenarian performances. Tom Lane holds swimming records for the men's 100- to 104-year age group for the 50- and 100-m freestyle and the 50-, 100-, and 200-m backstroke with times of 1:40.46, 4:05.98, 1:50.73, 4:13.84, and 9:04.31, respectively.[6] In the women's 100- to 104-year age group, Anne A. Dunivin holds records for the 50-, 100-, and 200-m freestyle events with times of 2:43.80, 5:42.81, and 12:06.09, respectively.[6] In 2011, at the age of 100 years, Fauji Singh became the first centenarian to complete a marathon, finishing in 8 hours and 11 minutes.[7] Robert Marchand set the 1-hour cycling

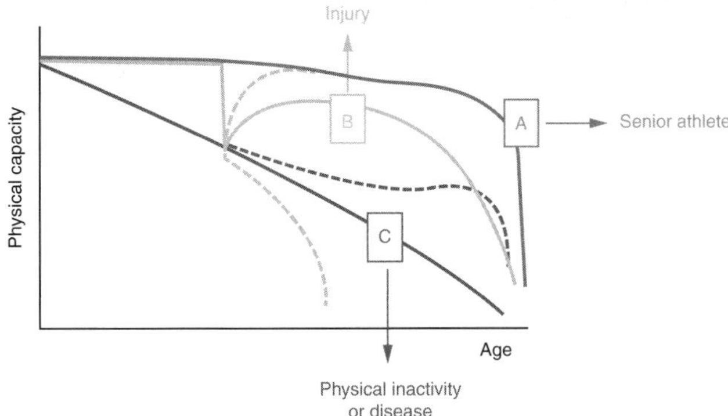

FIG. 28.1 Hypothetical model describing the trajectories of physical capacity in senior athletes (*A*), after injury (*B*), and in the presence of physical inactivity or disease with aging (*C*). *(Adapted from World Health Organization. World Report on Ageing and Health. Geneva: World Health Organization; 2015:31.)*

record for centenarians at the age of 101 years with a performance of 24.25 km and 2 years later broke his own record at the age of 103 years with a performance of 26.92 km.[8] Although there are declines in performance with age, the physical limits of the human body are constantly being challenged by senior athletes of all sports and walks of life. These observations hold significant implications for the potential to improve physiological capacities and functional abilities through rehabilitation and training.

Rehabilitation professionals who expect to treat the older athlete must have experience and a good working knowledge of aging and the potential mechanisms of athletic decline and risk of injury. The ideal professional would have firsthand experience working with older athletes before, during, and after athletic participation and know both the physical and psychological demands of sport. The clinician should be versed in a diversity of areas of human performance, including anatomy, cardiorespiratory and neuromuscular physiology, nutrition, biomechanics and kinesiology, psychology, rehabilitation and exercise sciences, and exercise prescription. Understanding age-related physiological changes and their ramifications relating to physical exercise and rehabilitation is vital to the patient's safe and successful functional return to participation and, in some cases, competition. Knowledge of pathologic changes, comorbidities, and their effects on the ability to participate in athletic activities is critical in the design and implementation of a rehabilitation program for older athletes.

This chapter focuses on individuals who physically challenge themselves by participating at high levels in competitive or recreational sports throughout their adulthood. Descriptions of performance and physiological alterations in senior athletes are described so that rehabilitation professionals have a sound understanding of the unique changes experienced by this population. Information pertaining to the prevalence and location of injury are discussed to highlight common cases that may be encountered by physical therapists. To assist in understanding movement performance of the senior athlete, a conceptual framework based on the interactions of the athlete, task, and environment is reviewed. Last, sport-specific training and programming considerations are detailed with an emphasis placed on neuromuscular and cardiorespiratory systems. The information presented in this chapter will aid rehabilitation professionals' decision-making process for designing safe and effective treatment plans for senior athletes. Additionally, the principles provided in this chapter are applicable to the common older adult looking to become physically active.

DEFINING THE POPULATION: WHO IS THE SENIOR ATHLETE?

There is often confusion about the definition of a senior athlete. The terms "masters athlete," "geriatric athlete," "aging athlete," and "senior athlete" are not synonymous. Masters athletes may not be senior athletes. Masters athletes are competitors in a given sport who exceed a minimum age criterion, which are often in the 20s, 30s, and 40s. For example, in competitive swimming in the United States and Canada, the minimum masters age is 18 years (Table 28.1).[6] For the purpose of this chapter, there are three groups that make up the population described as the senior athlete. Although there may be an overlap, these groups have some apparent differences that influence their need for rehabilitation and training considerations. Each group is dealt with in turn. Table 28.2 provides a description of the level of activity for the wide variety of athletes that may be considered

TABLE 28.1 Masters and Seniors Sport Organizations and Competitions

Sport Organization	Ages (yr)	Age Divisions	Events
World and National Masters Athletics	35–100+	5-yr increments	All stadia (in stadium) and nonstadia track and field events
Masters Running	35+	5-yr increments	Road races
Senior Golf (USGA)	50+	No age divisions	Designated senior golf tournaments
Masters Swimming (USMS)	18–100+	5-yr increments	Designated masters swimming events
Worldwide Senior Tennis Circuit (USTA)	30+	5-yr increments	Designated senior tennis events

Data from www.world-masters-athletics.org, www.seniorjournal.com, www.usga.com, www.usms.org, and www.itftennis.com.

TABLE 28.2 Descriptions of Types of Senior Athletes Using Centers for Disease Control and Prevention (CDC) Guidelines

Descriptors	Sedentary	Recreational	Competitive	Elite
Level and intensity of exercise	CDC recommendation for substantial health benefits	CDC recommendation for substantial health benefits: 150 min/wk of moderate-intensity[a] aerobic activity or 75 min/wk of vigorous-intensity[a] aerobic activity PLUS muscle strengthening 2 or more days/week	CDC recommendation for greater health benefits: 300 min/wk of moderate-intensity[a] aerobic activity or 150 min/wk of vigorous-intensity[a] aerobic activity, *PLUS* muscle strengthening 2 or more days/wk	CDC recommendation for greater health benefits *PLUS* specific and varied intensities of training for high-level competitions in select sports
Typical activities	ADLs and low-level functional tasks only	Home or health club, individual or group exercisers, without competitive participation	Runners, cyclists, tennis players, and golfers who compete in small local events	Registered "senior" or "masters" athletes who train and compete nationally and internationally

ADL, Activity of daily living.
[a]Moderate intensity is equivalent to brisk walking; vigorous intensity is equivalent to jogging or running (http://www.cdc.gov).

senior athletes in relation to the Centers for Disease Control and Prevention (CDC) 2018 Physical Activity Guidelines Advisory Committee Scientific Report[9] and exercise recommendations proposed by the American College of Sports Medicine (ACSM).[10]

The first group consists of former competitive athletes who have continued to exercise recreationally, for example, a football or field hockey team player who is now conditioning on a more individual basis using an activity such as running, swimming, or cycling. Many of these individuals may have sustained a significant injury during their earlier competitive play and therefore may not currently participate in competitions or tournaments; rather, they have adopted independent or group fitness as a part of their way of life. Older recreational athletes encompass lifelong athletes who trained intensively for a period in their lives and currently may or may not be training at a relative intensity that is comparable with their earlier training levels. The physical performances of these noncompetitive athletes are hard to describe and quantify. This group uses a wide variety of sports and training intensities; however, these athletes share the dedication to fitness, healthy living, and regular activity that support this categorization. Virtually all the athletes who played team sports as competitive performers and who are still exercising are training at some other sport or activity, often at the recreational level.

The second group is composed of lifelong athletes. Again, these athletes are involved in a spectrum of activities and training intensities, making their participation rates and physical performances hard to describe and quantify. Most are lifetime "sports people," some of whom are recreationally active and others who compete. They play tennis or golf; they run, cycle, or compete in triathlons. They may even participate in several different activities, but their involvement has been primarily in one sport or group of sports, some at the local level and others at the national or elite level. The definition of a competitive senior athlete for the purposes of this chapter is "one who participates in an organized team or individual sport that requires regular competition against others, places a high premium on excellence and achievement, and requires systematic training."[9] A significant subgroup of athletes in this recreational group are the aging athletes who are considered physically elite. They train and compete at high levels, regionally, nationally, and internationally in events such as the National Senior Games or the Worldwide Senior Tennis Circuit. For these individuals, athletic activity is as much a part of their routine as dressing or eating meals. They are reluctant to stop participating in their chosen activity, even in the face of significant pain or dysfunction.

The final group is made up of nonathletes who began to exercise late in life (arbitrarily, after age 40 years). This is a small but significant group who may be recreationally or competitively active. These individuals present a unique set of problems related directly to beginning physical activity at an older age and indirectly to their reasons for beginning to exercise. In many instances, exercise has been initiated by a health crisis. Common examples of this type of individual may include a patient who has experienced coronary symptoms (or may be a prime candidate for them) that is the direct result of a number of controllable risk factors, including improper diet (obesity) and lack of exercise. In many cases, low-intensity activity such as walking is recommended as a beginning or introduction to exercise and positive health behaviors. Potential differences in an individual's physical capabilities and the demands required in sport underscore the importance of appropriate exercise prescription. Caution should be taken when working with individuals who recently experienced a health crisis to ensure safe participation in sporting activity.

EFFECTS OF AGING ON PERFORMANCE AND PHYSIOLOGICAL CHANGES IN SENIOR ATHLETES

All senior athletes will experience declines in sport performance compared with performances earlier in life because of the aging process. The rate and magnitude of performance decline are influenced by several factors, including genetics, training history, sex, health status, age, and sporting event of interest. Age-related declines in endurance performance are observed across endurance sports such as running, orienteering, rowing, and swimming.[11] Similarly, record performances for masters sporting events for swimming, cycling, triathlon, rowing, and weightlifting all decline with increasing age.[12] Whereas rowing shows the least deterioration, weightlifting performance shows the fastest and greatest reductions with age. Running times in masters athletes become significantly greater as athletes get older with the slope of performance decline gradual from age 50 to 75 years (Fig. 28.2).[2–4,13,14] After 75 years of age, performance decrements become much more dramatic.[2,4,14] In most track and field events, a linear decline in performance is observed up to 70 years of age at which point the rate of performance loss is accelerated.[15] When age-specific world records were compared with current world records, performance was shown to reduce at a rate that approached or exceeded 100% by the 80-year age group for most running events.[16] The evidence provided by the centenarian athletic population supports the continual drop in performance with aging; however, as discussed in later sections of this chapter, the rate and magnitude of decline can be slowed with training and continued sport participation.

Despite reductions in performance with aging, older athletic populations experience greater health and function compared with their nonactive counterparts, which give the rehabilitation specialist some support for including physical activity training for all older adults, not just senior athletes. It is well known that vigorous exercise throughout middle and older ages is associated with reduced disability and increased longevity.[17] For example, runners who were running 60 minutes per week with a mean age of 78 years had strikingly lower disability rates, especially women, and had prolonged survival in a 21-year longitudinal study.[17] Clearly, lifelong athleticism has the potential to slow the functional consequences of aging (Fig. 28.3).[2,3,17,18] Master athletes are capable of maintaining muscle mass and strength, which may suggest that reductions in these factors with aging are associated with physical inactivity in addition to aging.[19] Indicators of functional performance, such as Five Times Sit-to-Stand speed, is shown to be faster in senior athletes compared with norms derived from community-dwelling older adults.[20] Rate of falls has been shown to be considerably lower in senior athletes than their community-dwelling counterparts.[21] Strength-trained masters athletes exhibited greater leg press maximal strength than recreationally active, sedentary, and young adults.[22] In addition, masters athletes' rate of force development was not different from young and higher than recreationally active and sedentary older populations.[22] High-performing octogenarians better maintain neuromuscular stability of the motor unit and mitigate loss of motor units associated with aging well into later decades.[23]

The pattern of sport-specific performance decrements differs between female and male senior athletes. In men,

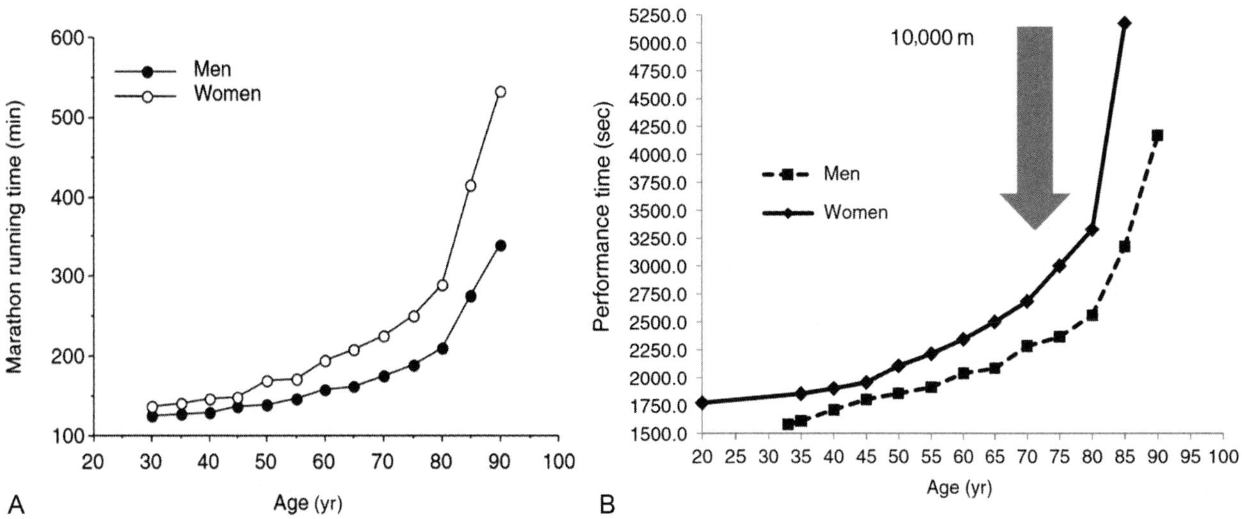

FIG. 28.2 Changes in marathon running times with age (**A**) and world record performances for the 10,000-m track event as of June 2016 for both male and female master athletes (**B**). The data in *B* are from each age category (5-year increments) from age 35 years and include the current world record performances by nonmaster athletes (data from www.world-masters-athletics.org). *Arrow* indicates the accelerated increased in performance times around the eighth decade of life. *(From Tanaka H, Seals DR. Endurance exercise performance in Masters athletes: age-associated changes and underlying physiological mechanisms: endurance performance and Masters athletes. J Physiol. 2008;586(1):56; and Lazarus NR, Harridge SDR. Declining performance of master athletes: silhouettes of the trajectory of healthy human ageing? Ageing and master athletes. Th J Physiol. 2017;595(9):2943.)*

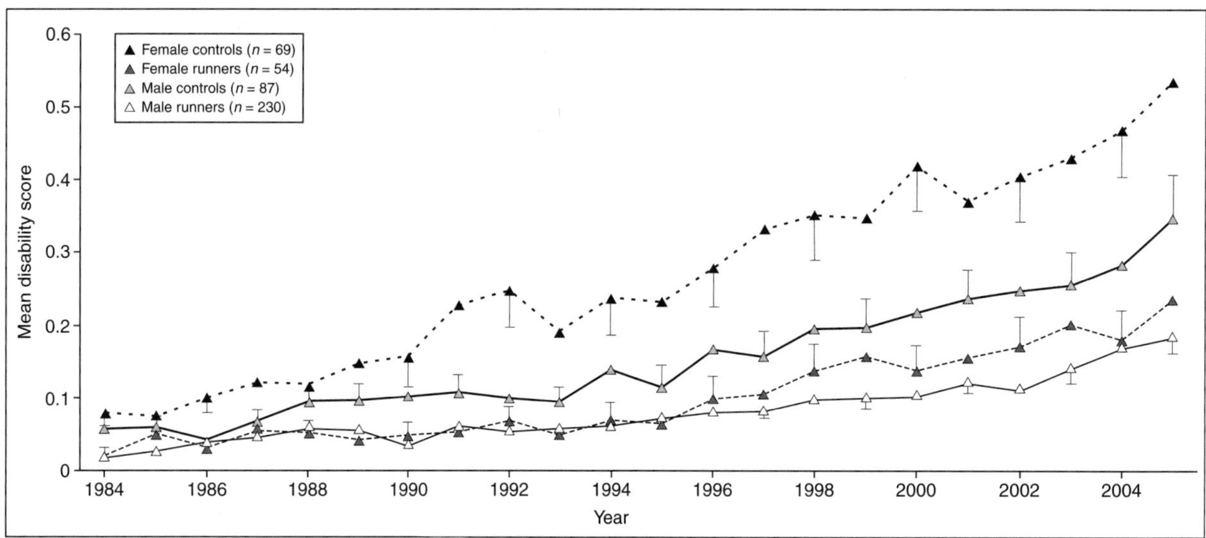

FIG. 28.3 Mean disability levels by year separated by sex. *Solid lines* represent data for runners, and *dashed lines* represent data for control participants who continued participation through 2005. Only participants who completed the 21-year follow-up are included. Errors indicate standard deviation. *(From Chakravarty EF. Reduced disability and mortality among aging runners: a 21-year longitudinal study. Arch Intern Med. 2008;168(15):1642.)*

smaller differences in the rate of performance declines are seen between sprint and endurance running events compared with women.[3,16] In a study of masters athlete world records, the men's world record for the 85-year-old age group was 64.4% slower compared with the currently held world record for the 100-m sprint event at the time of the study, whereas the 10,000-m event was 100.4% slower.[16] Conversely, the women's record for the 85-year-old age group for the 100-m sprint was 100.0% slower, with the 10,000-m world record being 194.7% slower. Fewer data are available regarding gender differences in cycling performances with aging; however, of the reported data, men's world record performance decreased by 9.9% for the 200-m sprint and 6.3% for the 40-km for the 50-year age group. For women, declines of 17.1% and 14.4% for the 200-m and 40-km events, respectively, are observed. These results led to gender differences of 22.2% and 64.3% for the 100- and 10,000-m running events and 17% and 16.6% for the 200-m and 40-km cycling events, respectively. In swimming events, performance has been shown to decline by 76.8% in men and 107% in women for the 100-m event and 99.3% in men and 103.8% in women for the 1500-m event for the 85-year age group.[16] This resulted in gender differences of 34.4% and 12.4% for the 100-and 1500-m events for swimming, respectively.[16] Together, these data demonstrate that women experience greater rates of decline in the running, cycling, and swimming events reported with the largest differences between genders occurring in endurance running events.

Neuromuscular

The neuromuscular system is responsible for the generation of force required for motor performance. The aging process induces numerous structural and functional alterations to the neuromuscular system limiting force generation and power production.[24,25] In the presence of disease and chronic illness, the loss of force-producing characteristics of the neuromuscular system is accelerated. The age-related structural changes include reductions in the number of motor units, muscle fibers, muscle cross-sectional area, satellite cell concentration, and type IIa muscle fibers (Fig. 28.4).[24] The functional consequences of these alterations are seen in decreases in voluntary muscle activation, motor unit discharge rate and recruitment range, contractile velocity, and peak force and power.[24] The ultimate outcome of the combined structural and functional alterations associated with age is decreased motor performance.[24]

Numerous factors contribute to the complex process of age-associated muscle loss, including reductions in anabolic hormones, chronic inflammation, degradation of muscle contractile proteins, loss of regenerative capacity, altered neural activation, and mitochondrial dysfunction.[25] Median values of loss in skeletal muscle mass have been reported to occur at a rate of 0.47% per year in men and 0.37% per year in women when comparing younger (18–45 years) and older (>65 years) adults.[26] After 75 years of age, the loss of skeletal muscle mass is accelerated in both men (0.80%–0.98% per year) and women (0.64–%0.70%).[26] In addition, older adults experience a preferential loss and marked atrophy in type II muscle fibers with relatively preserved type I fiber number and size.[24–26] Women are more vulnerable to loss of function secondary to type IIa muscle atrophy,[27] and women appear to experience greater declines in muscular strength and power (particularly in the upper extremities) than men.[3] Strength is lost at a disproportionate rate compared with skeletal muscle mass with losses in strength experienced at rates two to five times faster than loss of mass, especially in the legs.[26,28] Therefore, mechanisms other than muscle atrophy contribute to the declines in neuromuscular force. Alterations in neural control, increased

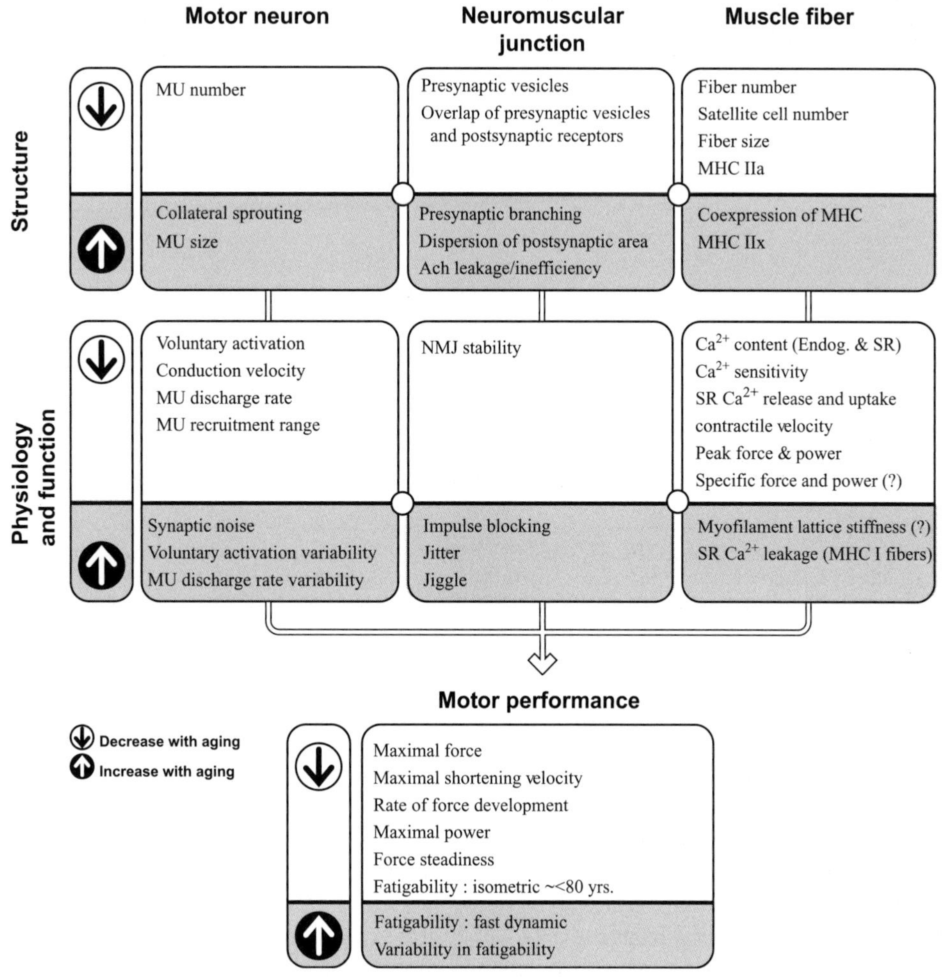

FIG. 28.4 Structural and physiological changes to the aging motor unit and motor performance outcomes. *Arrows (left)* indicate the direction of change that occurs with advanced age. *MHC*, myosin heavy chain; *MU*, motor unit; *NMJ*, neuromuscular junction. *(From Hunter SK, Pereira HM, Keenan KG. The aging neuromuscular system and motor performance. J Appl Physiol. 2016;121(4):984.)*

fat and connective tissue accumulation, and changes in contractile units in addition to muscle atrophy have all been identified as possible mechanisms leading to reductions in neuromuscular force.[24–26]

The combination of muscle atrophy and reductions in voluntary force generation may explain the greater deficits in neuromuscular power observed with aging (Fig. 28.5).[28,29] For example, rate of torque development, an index of neuromuscular power, is shown to be significantly lower in older men than younger men.[30] The age-related decrements in power output are likely to contribute to the observation of greatest rates of performance decline occurring in strength and power dependent events.[31] In masters athletes, the annual rate of loss in power is shown to be 1.25%, with greater declines observed in the upper limbs (1.4% per year) compared with the lower limbs (between 1.1% and 0.6% per year depending on sporting event).[15] However, strength-trained master athletes (mean age, 71 years) have been shown to exhibit greater maximum strength and rate of

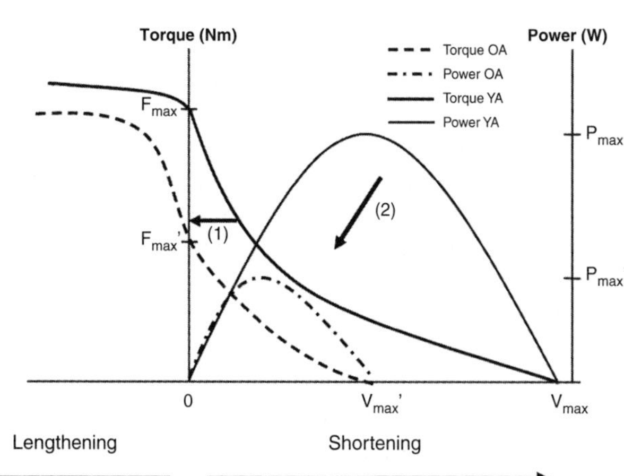

FIG. 28.5 Summary of the changes to the force–velocity and power–velocity relationship with age during shortening and lengthening contractions based on data from studies referenced by Raj and coworkers.[76] *(Modified from Raj IS, Bird SR, Shield AJ. Aging and the force–velocity relationship of muscles. Exp Gerontol. 2010;45(2):85.)*

force development than active older (mean age, 73 years) and moderately active younger adults (mean age, 22 years).[22] These findings were corroborated in a systematic review and meta-analysis demonstrating greater strength in strength and power master athletes compared with age-matched master endurance athletes and untrained individuals and comparable values to young untrained adults.[32] Thus, senior athletes who have specifically trained for strength and power are able to maintain force-generating characteristics similar to younger untrained adults.

Skeletal

Changes common to aging joints include deterioration of joint surfaces, breakdown of collagen fibers, and a decrease in the viscosity of synovial fluid, which can result in loss of flexibility and an increase in joint stiffness. Osteoarthritis (OA) is a common manifestation of these changes and is discussed in a later section of this chapter. Although a decrease in bone mineral density (BMD) is common with advancing age, senior athletes performing higher levels of vigorous *weight-bearing* exercise and resistance training may experience less bone density loss. In fact, the results of a 5-year longitudinal study of male master runners aged 40 to 80 years demonstrated maintenance of BMD despite moderate decreases in training volumes as the runners aged.[33] These runners demonstrated a slower decline from peak bone mass, indicative of bone maintenance, not loss.[33] The influence of sports on skeletal health is determined by the event and the magnitude of skeletal loading. Master cyclists and swimmers who performed little weight-bearing activity showed less bone density than age-matched controls.[34] Runners showed higher BMD in the total hip, intertrochanter and 1/3 distal radius compared with swimmers.[35] When comparing BMD in master sprint (mean age, 71 years; 28 men, 10 women) and endurance athletes (mean age, 70 years; 111 males, 38 women) with control participants, sprint athletes showed the greatest hip and spine BMD.[36] This finding was observed despite a higher number of low and medium impacts experienced by the endurance athletes with no differences in number of high impacts or weekly training hours between sprint and endurance athletes. Therefore, although swimming and cycling offer many other health benefits, such activities do not seem sufficient for maintaining or preventing bone density loss. The forces absorbed by the skeletal system during running activities on the other hand provide a valuable stimulus for maintaining bone integrity. Preventative measures, such as resistance exercise, should be considered when working with lifelong swimming and cycling athletes to promote skeletal health.

Cardiorespiratory

Endurance performance is dependent on the ability of the cardiorespiratory system to deliver and use oxygen at a rate that meets the energetic demands of muscle activity. In community-dwelling adults, the age-associated decreases in maximal aerobic capacity (VO_{2max}) increase progressively from 3% to 6% in the third and fourth decades of life to greater than 20% per decade after age 70 years.[37] In master athletes, reductions in VO_{2max} range from −1% to −4.6% per year for men and −0.5% to 2.4% per year for women beginning in the fourth decade.[38] The relative rate of decline in VO_{2max} is similar between endurance athletes and sedentary adults (Fig. 28.6). However, in absolute terms, athletes experience greater decrements in VO_{2max} compared with sedentary counterparts.[3] The decline in VO_{2max} in athletes is highly dependent on the continued magnitude of the training stimulus (i.e., volume and intensity).[2,7,8,39] The majority of the athletes reduced their training levels over time, resulting in longitudinal reductions in VO_{2max} two to three times as large as those predicted by cross-sectional analyses or longitudinal responses seen in their sedentary peers.[3,39] Despite similar relative and greater absolute reductions in VO_{2max}, masters athletes still possess superior cardiorespiratory fitness levels compared with age-matched nonathletes.

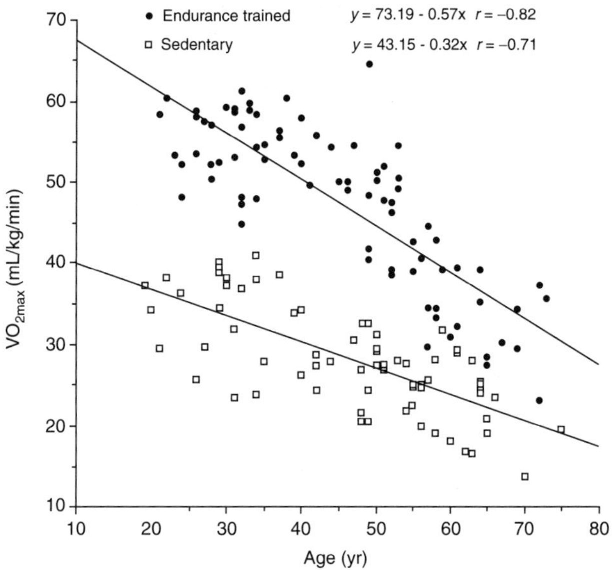

FIG. 28.6 Effects of age on maximal aerobic capacity (VO_{2max}) in endurance trained and sedentary women. Note that even though both trained and sedentary participants show predictable age-related declines, trained participants generally performed better than sedentary participants at all ages. *(From Tanaka H, Seals DR. Invited review: dynamic exercise performance in Masters athletes: insight into the effects of primary human aging on physiological functional capacity. J Appl Physiol. 2003;95(5):2157.)*

The capacity of the cardiorespiratory system to transport and use oxygen depends on both central and peripheral factors (Fig. 28.7).[2,7] Among the central factors contributing to endurance performance, the largest declines with age are seen in cardiac output (stroke volume [SV] × heart rate [HR]) (Table 28.3).[2] SV and HR experience similar responses with about a 10% decline with age when young (28 years) and master (60 years) endurance-trained

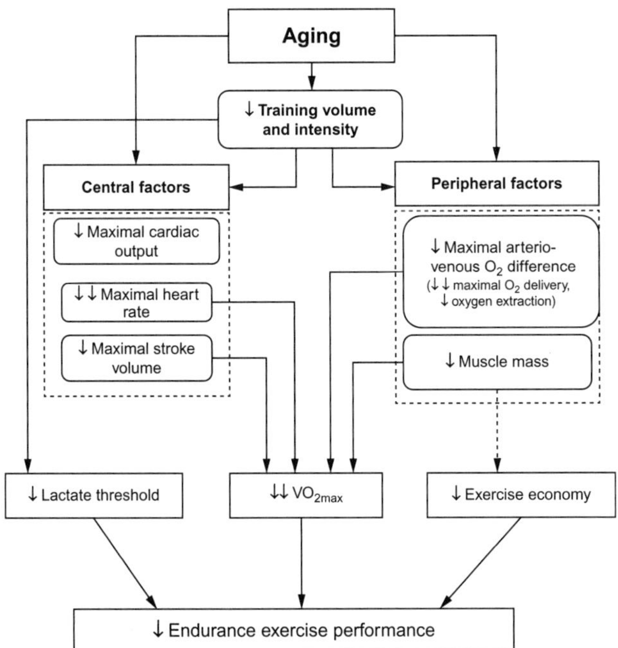

FIG. 28.7 Physiological mechanisms implicated in the age-related decline in endurance exercise performance. *Double arrow* expresses a main influence. *VO_{2max}*, Maximal aerobic capacity. *(From Lepers R, Stapley PJ. Master athletes are extending the limits of human endurance. Front Physiol. 2016;7:5.)*

athletes were compared.[2] Declines in maximal HR (HR_{max}) occur at a rate of an estimated 0.7 beats/min per year beginning during early adulthood.[2] Although HR_{max} is a major contributor to cardiac output, decrements in HR_{max} in master male and female endurance runners was not correlated with change in VO_{2max}.[38] In addition to cardiac output, ventilation also seems to play a key role in the decline in VO_{2max} in aging elite runners.[40] For example, Everman and coworkers[40] demonstrated that decreases in maximal minute ventilation (VE_{max}) was a significant predictor of the decrease in VO_{2max} over a 45-year span.[40]

The reported peripheral factors contributing to reduced VO_{2max} in senior athletes consist of lower arteriovenous oxygen difference (a-vO_2 diff) and loss of muscle mass.[7] The age-related changes associated with peripheral factors are slightly less than those observed for central factors.[2] The peripheral factors determine the muscles' capacity to extract oxygen from the blood to be used for energy synthesis by the mitochondria. The mechanisms of age-related muscle loss have been discussed previously in this section (see the Neuromuscular section). The changes in a-vO_2 diff with age is influenced by oxygen availability (i.e., oxygen delivery), oxidative enzyme concentrations, and mitochondrial and capillary density. For example, in highly active male endurance cyclists (aged 55–79 years), capillarity density and capillary-to-fiber ratio of the vastus lateralis were significantly correlated with VO_{2max}.[41] Thus, interventions that promote peripheral adaptations to maintain or improve muscle oxygen delivery and utilization may be advantageous for delaying declines in aerobic capacity or endurance performance.

Prevalence and Location of Injury

The potential for injury is always present in sports because of the demands of competition, which require the body to function at or near physiological limits. Senior athletes are an understudied population, and therefore information on the prevalence and types of injury is currently lacking. In a 16-year follow-up, Kettunen and associates[42] found that Finnish master athletes (mean age, 55 years) had a greater risk for shoulder region tendinopathy and Achilles tendon rupture after the age of 45 years than age- and gender-matched control participants. However, age-adjusted risk for medically diagnosed OA, hip pain, hip disability, and knee disability was lower in the master athlete group. In a study investigating the injury rates between master runners (≥40 years) and younger runners, the master runners had a significantly greater risk for injury than the younger runners.[43]

The most common locations of injury are the knee and foot. One potential factor leading to an increased risk of injury in senior athletes is inappropriate training load leading to overuse injuries. For example, when comparing master runners who sustained an injury compared with noninjured master runners, a significantly greater number of injured runners ran six or more times per week, but the healthy runners only trained one to three times per week.[43] An analysis of the 2012 European Veteran Athletics Championships (mean age, 53.2 years) revealed that 2.8% of female athletes and 2.2% of male athletes registered an injury.[44] Of the registered injuries, no fractures were experienced, and only one operative treatment was required to repair an Achilles tendon rupture. Lower extremity strength and power events (sprint or middle distance, and jumps) had a significantly higher injury rate

TABLE 28.3 Oxygen Consumption and Its Determinants at Maximal Exercise in Endurance-Trained Men[a]

	Young Men (28 yr)	Older Men (60 yr)	Age-Related Change (%)
Oxygen consumption (mL kg^{-1} min^{-1})	68.2	49.4	28
Cardiac output (L min^{-1})	27.0	21.7	20
Stroke volume (mL $beat^{-1}$)	147	132	10
Heart rate (beats min^{-1})	184	165	10
a-v O_2 difference (mL $[100\ mL]^{-1}$)	16.7	15.2	8

[a]The data were compiled from four studies in which values for all of the variables were reported in younger and older groups.[2]

compared with throws, long-distance, and decathlon and heptathlon events. This was reflected in the anatomical locations for injury with the most injured area being the thigh (22.5%) followed by the Achilles tendon, heel, or lower leg (18.8%) and the knee (11.3%). Thus, soft tissue injuries of the lower extremity seem to be of the greatest concern in senior athletes, especially in sporting events requiring a high degree of neuromuscular force generation. Appropriately managing training load (i.e., volume and intensity) becomes critical for reducing the risk of injury while increasing treatment adherence and promoting health and fitness benefits.

Golf Injuries

In the United States, the occasional golfer is an average of 45 years of age with one-third of all American golfers older than 50 years of age.[45] Golfers aged 50 to 65 years are reported to have a higher prevalence of injury. Golfing is an extremely complex skill and therefore requires many hours of practice positing training volume as a possible risk factor for injury.[45] The golf swing is composed of three main components: the backswing, the downswing, and the follow-through.[45] The majority of injuries occur during the follow-through phase of the swing because this part of the swing is responsible for rapid deceleration of the club. The locations for injuries in amateur golfing athletes occur in the upper extremity with the low back, elbow, wrist and hand, and shoulder being the primary sites (Fig. 28.8).[45] The biomechanics of a golfer's swing seem to contribute to low back pain. Poor posture, overrotation, and decreased abdominal activity during the golf swing have all been identified as risk factors for low back pain.[46] Shoulder injuries are most often the result of overuse and predominantly occur on the lead shoulder (i.e., the left shoulder for a right-handed golfer) as a result of the high eccentric load placed on the shoulder muscles during the transition between the backswing and the downswing).[46] Impingement at the acromioclavicular joint, rotator cuff tendinitis or tear, posterior glenohumeral subluxation, and arthritis are additional factors that may also contribute to shoulder pain.[45] Given the findings on golf-related injuries, many rehabilitation treatment plans focus on addressing deficits in flexibility and strength.

Swimming Injuries

Swimming is another popular sporting activity among older adults. The freestyle stroke is one of the most common swimming strokes performed. This stroke requires the production of propulsive force by adduction and internal rotation with the pectoralis major and latissimus dorsi being the largest muscles involved.[47] The freestyle stroke can be deconstructed into six parts: (1) hand entry, (2) forward reach, (3) pull-through, (4) middle pull-through, (5) hand exit, and (6) middle recovery (Fig. 28.9).[47] Swimming competitively requires performing a high degree of repetitive movements, increasing the risk for overuse injuries, especially at the shoulder. Shoulder pain is often correlated with an increase in training volume and poor technique caused by insufficient or imbalanced strength.[47] Senior athletes participating in swimming activities may be more vulnerable to injury because they have been shown to experience similar rates of shoulder injury compared with collegiate swimmers (master swimmers, 48% vs collegiate swimmers, 47%) despite being exposed to lower training loads.[48] "Swimmer's shoulder" describes a myriad of shoulder pathologies in which the pain is felt in and about the shoulder temporally related to the act of swimming.[49] The potential causes of shoulder pain include subacromial impingement, hyperlaxity, scapular dyskinesis, glenohumeral internal rotation deficit, labral damage, os acromiale, and suprascapular neuropathy.[47] Given the number of possible causes, appropriate screening and examination are critical for accurate diagnosis. Figure 28.10 depicts an algorithm proposed by Matzkin

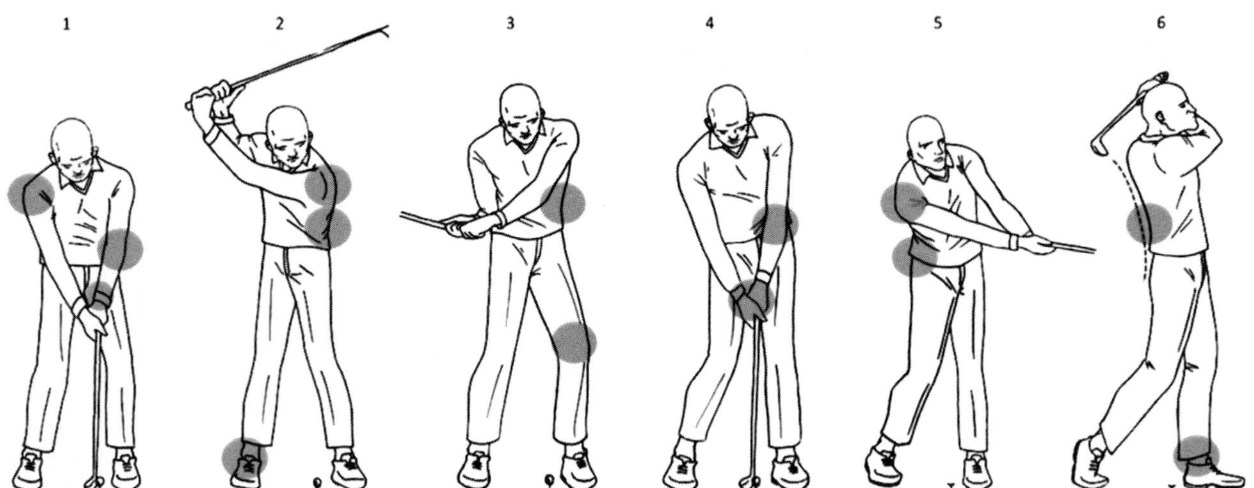

FIG. 28.8 Possible locations of golfing injuries *(shaded areas)* during ball address *(1)*, backswing *(2)*, forward swing *(3)*, ball impact *(4)*, early follow-through *(5)*, and late follow-through *(6)*. *(From Cabri J, Sousa JP, Kots M, Barreiros J. Golf-related injuries: a systematic review. Eur J Sport Sci. 2009;9(6):362.)*

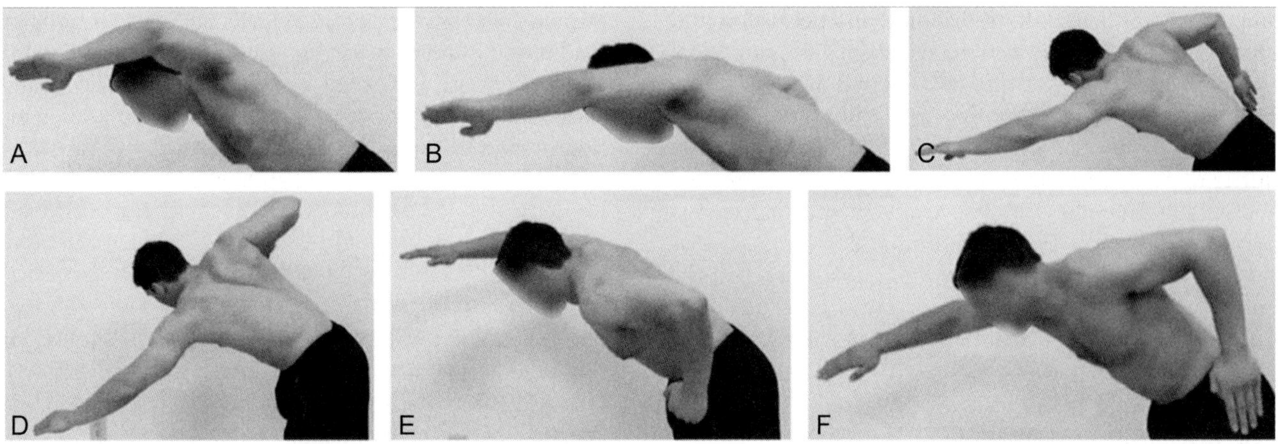

FIG. 28.9 Clinical photographs demonstrating the six parts of the freestyle swim stroke: hand entry (**A**), forward reach (**B**), pull-through (**C**), middle pull-through (**D**), hand exit (**E**), and middle recovery (**F**). *(From Matzkin E, Suslavich K, Wes D. Swimmer's shoulder: painful shoulder in the competitive swimmer. J Am Acad Orthop Surg. 2016;24(8):528.)*

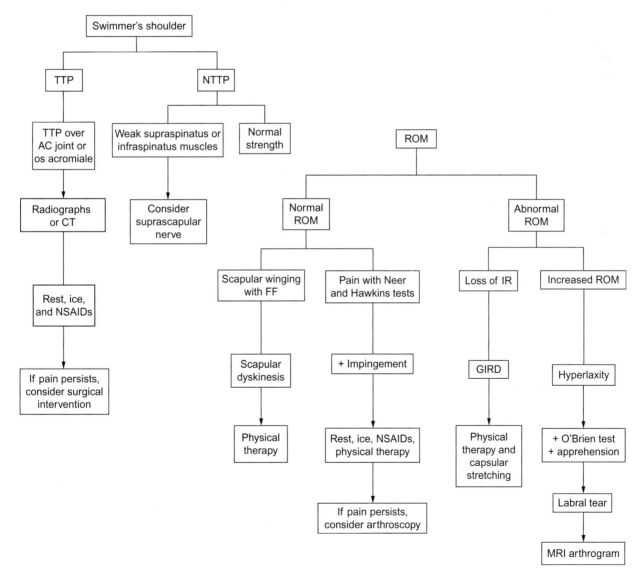

FIG. 28.10 Algorithm depicting diagnosis and treatment pathways for patients presenting with swimmer's shoulder. *AC,* Acromioclavicular joint; *CT,* computed tomography; *FF,* forward flexion; *GIRD,* glenohumeral internal rotation deficit; *IR,* internal rotation; *MRI,* magnetic resonance imaging; *NSAID,* nonsteroidal antiinflammatory drug; *NTTP,* no tenderness to palpation; *ROM,* range of motion; *TTP,* tenderness to palpation. *(From Matzkin E, Suslavich K, Wes D. Swimmer's shoulder: painful shoulder in the competitive swimmer. J Am Acad Orthop Surg. 2016;24(8):531.)*

and coworkers[47] for diagnosing and treating patients presenting with swimmer's shoulder. Stretching and strengthening exercises are often prescribed to maintain or restore complete range of motion (ROM) and muscular balance.[47] Stretching exercises that aggravate the preexisting injury should be avoided and strengthening exercise should be progressed gradually.

Osteoarthritis

Articular degeneration, commonly known as OA, is the most common joint pathology of aging occurring over time. The activity of running is often thought to cause knee OA; however, current evidence suggests that there is no risk of knee OA when running for fitness or recreation.[50] For example, Chakravarty and coworkers[51] examined differences in the progression of knee OA in middle- to older-aged runners and healthy nonrunners (aged 50–72 years) over nearly 2 decades and found that the long-distance runners did not have an increased prevalence of OA compared with nonrunners. Evidence from a narrative review investigating the role of physical activity, recreational and elite sports found that physical activity such as running, cycling, swimming, racquet sports, and weight training did not increase the frequency of self-reported physician-diagnosed hip–knee OA in the absence of a significant joint injury.[52] Magnusson and coworkers[53] examined a prediction model to determine the 40-year risk of knee OA in young men and found that having a body mass index (BMI) of 30 at 18 years of age and a knee injury were primary factors contributing the increased likelihood of having knee OA. These findings suggest that type of sport, training load, BMI, and previous injury are major factors contributing to OA later in life and that running does not increase the risk of knee OA. In middle- and older-aged populations, both resistance and aerobic exercises have been shown to be beneficial for the management of OA.[54] High-quality evidence shows that exercise moderately reduces pain and improves physical function in people with knee OA[55] and slightly reduces pain and improves function in people with hip OA.[56]

MOVEMENT PERFORMANCE IN SENIOR ATHLETES

Compromised foundational movement skills such as kicking, running, and squatting persisting with age is likely to have a negative impact on sport performance and potentially increasing the risk of injury.[57] "Foundational movement skills" reflect a wide variety of skills and are defined as goal-directed movement patterns that directly and indirectly impact an individual's capability to be physically active across the lifespan.[57] Individuals who do not develop sufficient competence in foundational movement skills will have greater difficulty developing and maintaining health-enhancing physical activity habits into old age.[57] Thus, comprehensive approaches to movement performance, which includes a combination of foundational and specialized skills development, may be advantageous for senior athletes to maintain sport participation, improve sport performance, and reduce the risk of sport-related injury. Similar approaches might also be incorporated into treatment planning for all older adults who wish to increase their physical activity, even if their ultimate goal is not competitive participation.

Both physiological and psychological factors contribute to the ability to engage in and successfully perform movement skills. Whereas physiological factors refer to weight status, cardiorespiratory fitness, flexibility, and muscular strength and endurance, psychological factors include perceived competence and self-efficacy.[57] The constraints-led framework to motor control can be used to understand how the numerous physiological and psychological factors interact to influence motor performance.[58,59] Constraints are categorized into organismic (i.e., the person), task, and environment, and are viewed as boundaries or features that limit movement.[59] Organismic constraints refer to constraints residing at the level of the organism. In senior athletes, such constraints may include the neuromuscular or cardiorespiratory changes outlined earlier. Environmental constraints are constraints external to the organism but not task specific (e.g., gravity, natural light). Task constraints relate to the goal of the task, rules specifying or constraining response dynamics, and implements or machines specifying or constraining response dynamics. Examples of task constraints specific to tennis include the size of the tennis racquet, the dimensions of the court, and the height of the net. Thus, movement performance is viewed as the outcome of perception–action coupling influenced by the interactions of constraints to accomplish goal-directed activity (Fig. 28.11).[58,59]

In line with the constraints-led approach, a case study exploring the practical knowledge of an experienced senior tennis athlete determined that the performer perceived the tennis environment in terms of the opportunities afforded by the environment.[60] The performer's practical knowledge centered on performance capabilities and strategic planning that revealed opponent limitations. The knowledge appeared to be developed and expressed

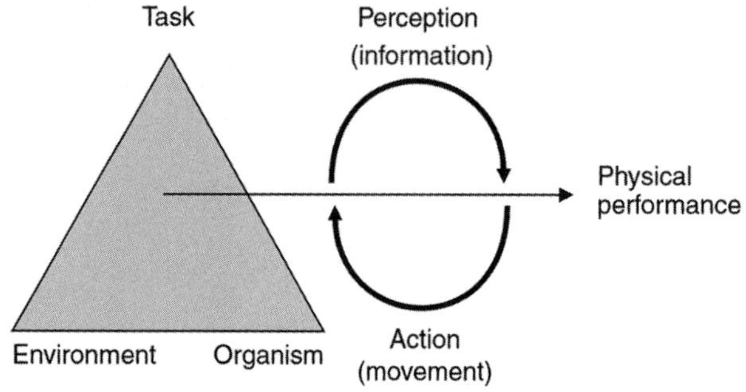

FIG. 28.11 Newell's model of interacting constraints adapted to illustrate the resulting effects of variability of physical performance. *(From Davids K, Glazier P, Araújo D, Bartlett R. Movement systems as dynamical systems: the functional role of variability and its implications for sports medicine. Sports Med. 2003;33(4):247.)*

within the relationship among individual capabilities, the task, and the situated context of game play.[60] With training, the athlete–environment relationship may be altered because of increases in physical capabilities creating different affordances and thus altering perception–action coupling. Understanding that the demands of tennis require the performer to possess sufficient levels of cardiorespiratory fitness, speed, agility, and quickness allows the rehabilitation professional to determine which organismic constraints should be addressed to optimize tennis performance. Furthermore, by considering the environment and task constraints, the rehabilitation professional is able to anticipate how these changes in organismic constraints is likely to alter perception–action coupling. Treatment or training can then be structured by manipulating various task and environmental demands, allowing the athlete opportunities to explore different motor solutions to best optimize performance in given situations.

MECHANICAL CONSTRAINTS IN SENIOR ATHLETES

Sprinting

Running velocity of the different phases of the 100-m sprint decline on average from 5% to 6% per decade in men and 5% to 7% per decade in women.[61] Although the maximal effectiveness of horizontal force application also decreases with age, the decreases experienced with increasing velocity within the sprint acceleration of a 30-m sprint is suggested to be independent of age.[62] Mechanical constraints contributing to the declines in sprinting speed with aging include stride length, ground reaction force (GRF), and leg stiffness. For example, progressive age-related declines in running speed has been demonstrated to be mainly related to a reduction in stride length and an increase in ground contact time with little to no change in stride frequency.[61,63] This results in reductions in the magnitude of the average breaking and push-off resultant GRFs and declines in the rate of GRF development.[63] Leg stiffness of older runners has been reported to be between 10% to 20% lower than that of young runners across the range of speeds and decreases with increased running speed.[64] Age-related decrements in muscle thickness, type II muscle fiber size, and maximal and rapid force-generating capacity of lower limb muscle and muscle thickness (knee extensor and plantar flexor) have been identified as significant predictors of braking force developed during running.[63]

Golf

Older adults account for a large percentage of the total rounds of golf played annually. Cardiorespiratory benefits combined with the low-impact nature of the sport make golf an appealing option for staying physically active as an older adult. The physical demands of golf require intermittent bursts of moderate-intensity activity performed over a period of several hours.[46] The ability to produce high club head velocities enables the golfer to advance the golf ball over greater distances, assuming the ball travels in the intended direction. Declines in maximum club head speed are seen between the ages of 40 and 59 years.[45] The combination of loss in rotational strength and power, flexibility, and balance with aging plays a major role in altered swing biomechanics and the reduction of club head speed, resulting in decreased hitting distance.[45] To minimize the risk of injury and performance decline, it is proposed that a multidisciplinary approach be applied.[46] Strength and flexibility programs have been shown to be beneficial for increasing club head speed, and an appropriately design warm-up is essential for injury prevention.[46]

Swimming

The effects of age on swimming performance is experienced across all events.[65] The impact of age on biomechanical profiles of masters swimmers reveals event specific changes.[65] For example, in male swimmers aged 25 to 75 years, the older swimmers experienced lower stroke frequency and stroke length when competing in the 50-meter event. When comparing the youngest age group (25–29 years) with the oldest age group (+75 years), stroke frequency and stroke length decreased by 21% and 26.7%. In the 200-m freestyle stroke, frequency was more effected than stroke length.[65] In male swimmers, whereas stroke frequency increased 1.8%, stroke length decreased 33.5% from the youngest age group (25–29 years) to the oldest age group (+75 years). Additionally, propelling efficiency decreased 37.5% with aging when comparing the youngest and oldest age. In female swimmers, stroke frequency, stroke length, and propelling efficiency were all shown to decrease with age (15.6%, 31.2%, and 28.6%, respectively).[65] The neuromuscular and cardiorespiratory alterations associated with aging contribute to the declines in swimming performance. Specifically, whereas the reductions in aerobic capacity (i.e., VO_{2max}) has important implications for endurance events, loss of type II muscle fiber atrophy leading to decrements in neuromuscular power impacts sprint events.[65] In the absence of pain or preexisting injury, stretching and strengthening exercises to address ROM deficits and strength imbalances help to maintain appropriate swimming biomechanics and thus reduce the potential for future injury.

SPORT-SPECIFIC TRAINING AND PROGRAMMING CONSIDERATIONS FOR SENIOR ATHLETES

The stress-response theory describes the processes associated with the body's adjustments to a stressor or stimulus.[66] According to the stress-response theory, the presence of a stressor (i.e., exercise) causes disruptions to the body's homeostatic state. Through repeated exposures to a given stressor, the body adapts to be able to overcome such disturbances more efficiently, increasing functional capacity.[66] For example, the metabolic state of skeletal muscle is perturbed at the initiation of running because of the energy required to initiate and sustain muscle contraction. The cardiorespiratory and skeletal muscle bioenergetic systems respond rapidly to replenish the energy deficit experienced. From a treatment and training perspective, the ultimate goal is to enhance the body's ability to respond and adjust to such disturbances, resulting in improve functional capabilities.

The degree to which a training program will benefit a senior athlete's performance is determined by how well the principles of specificity, progressive overload, and variation are incorporated into the training plan (Table 28.4). The response elicited through training should be specific to the demands of the performance of interest. Using the metabolic and running example, the stress imposed on the bioenergetic systems must be specific to the energetic demands of the event. In sprinting events, this means training the glycolytic energy system, but endurance events require sufficient oxidative energetic capabilities. *Progressive overload* refers to the ability of the stimulus to promote the desired response by exposing the system or systems of interest to a stressor of a sufficient intensity (i.e., above a certain threshold).[10] If the stimulus is below the threshold required to promote a given response, homeostasis will not be perturbed, and therefore no adaptation be will be experienced. Last, appropriately placed variation of training stimuli throughout the training period is important for managing the fitness–fatigue relationship.[67] This is reflected by strategically manipulating training frequency, intensity, time, type, volume, pattern, and progression (i.e., FITT principle; see Table 28.4) at specified times within long-term training plans and should coincide with sport-specific activities. For example, as primary competitions near, the training emphasis should be placed on the sport-specific technical and tactical activities while reducing the training volume of general fitness.[67] Theoretically, the incorporation of variation will decrease the likelihood of the presence of fatigue and thus ensure optimization of sport performance at critical times. Furthermore, variation may be necessary to ensure continued adaptation and prevent stagnation over longer training durations.

Two additional principles need consideration when planning and prescribing training programs for athletic performance, the principles of reversibility and individuality. Whereas the stress-response theory explains conceptually the physiological processes leading to physical adaptation, the principle of reversibility suggests that when the specific stress or stimulus is removed for sufficient amounts of time, the adaptation will dissipate, resulting in the gains in functional capacity reverting back toward pretraining levels. Interestingly, the concept of reversibility may explain the decrements in sports performance experienced by senior athletes given the reductions in training workload with age. The principle of individuality refers to the unique individual responses and adaptations experienced across athletes when exposed to the same training stimuli. On a surface level, many responses and adaptations seem predictable. However, for a given training program, the magnitude and time course of adaptations will vary from one athlete to the next because of a variety of factors such as age, training history, genetics, sex, motivation, and so on. Therefore, it should not be assumed that for a given training program, all athletes will benefit equally, highlighting the importance of individualization when planning and programming for senior athletes.

TABLE 28.4 Principles of Exercise Program Design for Optimizing Human Performance and Elements of FITT-VP

Principle	Description
Specificity	Physiological adaptations to exercise are specific to the stressors imposed by the type of exercise performed
Progressive overload	Stressors associated with a type of exercise must be of a sufficient level to elicit homeostatic disturbances to promote physiologic adaptation and must be incrementally increased over time
Variation	Systematic altering of one or more program variable(s) over time to allow for the exercise stimulus to remain challenging while preventing fatigue and stagnation
Reversibility	Removal of the exercise stimulus and physical inactivity will result in performance decrements
Individuality	Individual responses to a given exercise stimulus
FITT-VP	Description
Frequency	How often?
Intensity	How hard?
Time	How long or duration?
Type	What kind of exercise or exercise mode?
Volume	Amount?
Progression	Advancement?

FITT-VP, Frequency, intensity, time, type, volume, and progression.
Principles and descriptions - Data from *ACSM's Exercise Testing and Perscription*, Philadelphia: Wolters-Kluwer; 2018 and Brooks GA. *Exercise Physiology: Human Bioenergetics and Its Applications*. New York: McGraw-Hill; 2005.

Stages of Program Development: Planning versus Programming

The development of sport-specific training programs requires stages of planning and programming. The planning stage considers the objectives of the training program, the timelines to which performance improvements are required, and the fitness outcomes of interest.[67] The

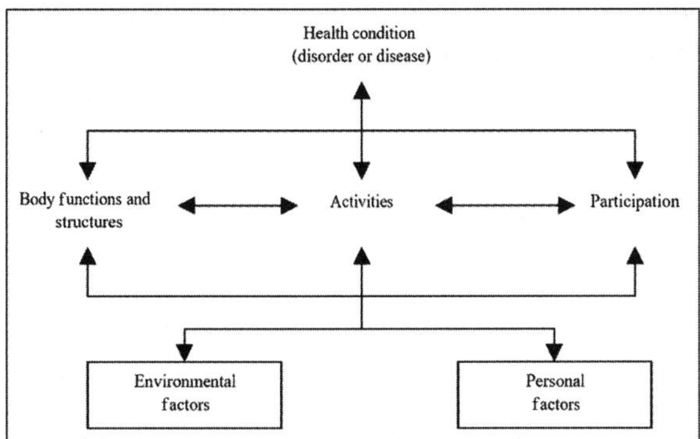

FIG. 28.12 Interactions between the components of the International Classification of Functioning, Disability and Health. *(From World Health Organization. International Classification of Functioning, Disability and Health: ICF. Geneva: World Health Organization; 2001.)*

programming stage is then structured in an attempt to meet the goals of the training plan by identifying strategies for promoting performance enhancements and the training variables to be prescribed.[67] The International Classification of Functioning, Disability and Health (ICF) model provides a framework for understanding health and health-related states, outcomes, and determinants and can be useful to help guide the decision-making process during the planning stage (Fig. 28.12).[68] Here it is proposed that the ICF framework be applied to the senior athlete to aid in understanding performance deficits to which the training plan can then be designed to address. This information is then used to determine which training structure and elements are most appropriate for improving performance goals. However, it is important not to assume that performance of the sporting activity will improve by simply remediating the identified impairments. Rather, by enhancing physiological capacity through impairment remediation, the athlete will need to become accustomed to the new capabilities and how to most effectively use these capabilities within the context of a given sport. Therefore, the combination of the ICF model with the constraints-oriented approach provides a basis for understanding the relationships between impairments and activity limitations and the resulting effects on movement performance.

Components of a Training Program

The components of a single exercise training session should be composed of a warm-up, conditioning or sports-related exercise, cool-down, and stretching.[10] The warm-up is recommended to last at least 5 to 10 minutes using light- to moderate-intensity activity. Sport-specific warm-ups encourage the incorporation of dynamic activities to stimulate neuromuscular and bioenergetic processes emphasized during the conditioning or sports-related portion of the session. The warm-up can also serve as an opportunity to evaluate and instruct foundational motor patterns before the patient-athlete's engaging in more vigorous activities. It is important not to induce fatigue during the warm-up because this may compromise the quality and quantity of work performed during the proceeding segment. Conditioning and sports-related activities include bioenergetic, resistance, technical (i.e., movement technique), and tactical (i.e., sport-specific strategies during competition) exercises specific to enhancing performance. The goal of the cool-down period is to allow for the reestablishment of resting homeostasis through gradual reductions in effort and intensity of dynamic movements. The cool-down period is especially critical when working with older adults with cardiovascular disease.[10] Static stretching after exercise is recommended to improve ROM because of the increased temperature of previously active muscles.[10]

Training to Improve Neuromuscular Impairments

Specific neuromuscular impairments related to the aging process must be considered when determining the most effective approaches for improving athletic performance (see the chapters in this text on muscle function with age and the chapter on exercise for a detailed description). Resistance training is a powerful impetus for enhancing neuromuscular deficits. Factors contributing to the enhancement of the force-generating capacity of the neuromuscular system consist of neurologic and morphological mechanisms.[66] The primary neuromuscular outcomes of interest typically discussed for enhancing force-generating capabilities are hypertrophy, strength, and power. To promote hypertrophy and strength in trained older adults, it is recommended that three or four sets per exercise be performed using slow to moderate lifting velocities with loads corresponding to 60% to 80% of an individual's 1 repetition maximum (1 RM) with rest periods of 1 to 3 minutes between sets (Table 28.5).[69] Dose–response relationships have been identified for training period, intensity, time under tension (i.e., the duration of each repetition), and rest in between sets, highlighting the importance of these variables for promoting muscular strength and morphologic (i.e., cross-sectional area, volume, thickness) adaptations in trained older adults.[70,71] For enhancing lean body mass, whereas programs consisting of higher volume were associated with the greatest increases, maximal strength gains favored training at higher intensities (i.e., 60%–80% 1 RM).[70,71] To improve muscular power, it is recommended that training include one to three sets per exercise performed using high velocities with loads corresponding to 30% to 60% 1 RM for 6-10 repetitions with rest periods of 1 to 3 minutes.[69] However, no consensus regarding optimal loading for the maximization of muscular power in older adults currently exists.

Senior athletes experience the greatest decrements in sport performance with age in events requiring a high

TABLE 28.5 Resistance Exercise Recommendations for Older Adults[a]

Neuromuscular Target	Hypertrophy	Strength	Power
Modality	Free weights; machines	Free weights; machines	Free weights; machines
Frequency	2–3 days/wk on nonconsecutive days	2–3 days/wk on nonconsecutive days	2–3 days/wk on nonconsecutive days
Intensity	60%–80% 1 RM	60%–80% 1 RM	30%–60% 1 RM
Training volume	1–3 sets/exercise; 8-12 repetitions/set	1–3 sets/exercise; 8-12 repetitions/set	1–3 sets/exercise; 6-10 repetitions/set
Contraction velocity	Slow to moderate	Slow to moderate	High
Rest intervals	1–3 min between sets	1–3 min between sets	1–3 min between sets
Additional comments	Multiple- and single-joint exercises	Multiple- and single-joint exercises	Should be conducted in combination with training to improve strength; multiple- and single-joint exercises

1 RM, 1 Repetition maximum
[a]Resistance exercise recommendations for enhancing muscular hypertrophy, strength, and power for older adults as proposed by the American College of Sports Medicine.[69]

degree of force and power involvement.[12] The inability to maintain performance in strength and power events may be caused by the specific neuromuscular alterations associated with aging (see earlier section Effects of Aging on Performance and Physiological Changes in Senior Athletes). Older adults experience reductions in power development caused by decrements in both force and velocity components of the force–velocity relationship (see Fig. 28.5).[28] Force–velocity profiles can be used to determine where an athlete falls on the force–velocity continuum. This information can aid in the training prescription to determine whether to emphasize force-generating capabilities (i.e., neuromuscular strength) or movement velocity (i.e., neuromuscular power).[69] Therefore, resistance exercise programs that focus on increasing force-generating capabilities and muscle contraction velocity independently or concurrently may be advantageous for sport performance in older populations. Currently, the most appropriate sequencing of resistance training variables is unknown for senior athletes.

Training to Improve Cardiorespiratory Limitations

Central and peripheral mechanisms contributing to lactate threshold, VO_{2max}, and exercise economy have been identified as primary factors influencing endurance performance (see Fig. 28.7).[7] Endurance training can be structured to improve specific central and peripheral mechanisms. Commonly observed cardiorespiratory adaptations experienced with endurance training in healthy adults include increases in SV, a-vO_2 diff, and VO_{2max}.[66] However, the magnitude of central and peripheral adaptations is dependent on exercise intensity and duration. Central adaptations can be emphasized using workloads consisting of higher intensities performed over shorter durations, thus resulting in greater increase in cardiac output. Conversely, peripheral adaptations can be promoted with workloads of longer durations performed at lower intensities leading to greater changes in a-vO_2 diff.[66] Furthermore, endurance training can result in faster adjustments of the processes responsible for the delivery and utilization of oxygen (VO_2 on-kinetics) in response to activity initiation.[72]

Current recommendations for maintaining or improving cardiorespiratory fitness suggest engaging 5 days or more per week of moderate-intensity exercise, 3 days per week or more of vigorous exercise, or 3 to 5 days per week or more of any combination moderate and vigorous exercise (Table 28.6).[10] For moderate-intensity

TABLE 28.6 Cardiorespiratory Exercise Recommendations for Older Adults[a]

Frequency (How often?)	Intensity (How hard?)	Time
$\geq$5 days wk^{-1} for moderate intensity $\geq$3 days wk^{-1} for vigorous intensity 3-5 days wk^{-1} for a combination of moderate and vigorous intensity	On a scale of 0–10 for level of physical exertion, 5–6 for moderate intensity, and 7–8 for vigorous intensity	30–60 min/day of moderate-intensity exercise 20–30 min/day of vigorous-intensity exercise Or an equivalent combination of moderate- and vigorous-intensity exercise; may be accumulated in bouts of at least 10 minutes each

[a]Cardiorespiratory exercise recommendations for maintaining and enhancing cardiorespiratory fitness in older adults as proposed by the American College of Sports Medicine.
Data from ACSM's exercise testing and prescription. (Wolters Kluwer, 2018).

exercise bouts, 30 to 60 minutes of exercise is encouraged, and for vigorous exercise, 20 to 30 minutes is used to achieve the greatest cardiorespiratory benefits.[10] According to guidelines provided by Franklin and associates,[73] elite senior athletes should exercise 3 to 5 days per week at intensities of 55% to 90% of HR_{max} or maximum HR reserve for 20 to 60 minutes of continuous or intermittent aerobic activity for developing or maintaining cardiorespiratory fitness.[73] Although these recommendations provide valuable information for promoting or maintaining general cardiorespiratory health, senior athletes may require sport-specific training to maximize performance. Using the principles outlined, endurance training programs can be structured to promote specific central or peripheral adaptations required for a given sport.

Responses to Training

In male cyclists, aged 55 to 79 years, type I fibers and capillarity were significantly associated with training volume, VO_{2max}, oxygen uptake kinetics, and ventilatory threshold.[41] Similarly, male masters athletes between the ages of 40 to 80 years of age experienced declines in weekly training mileage and cardiorespiratory fitness over a 5- to 7-year period.[33] In female cyclists of the same age, only capillarity and training volume were associated. In males, both type II fiber proportion and size were associated with peak power during sprint cycling and with maximal rate of torque development during maximal voluntary isometric contraction. In this cohort of male and female cyclists, there was little evidence of age-related changes in properties of the vastus lateralis; however, some muscle characteristics were correlated with in vivo physiological indices.[41] Katzel and coworkers[39] found no significant changes in VO_{2max} in older athletes with aging when training stimulus was maintained at levels experienced at study initiation. Findings from a longitudinal study over 45 years revealed the ability to blunt the effects of aging on cardiorespiratory fitness as these athletes reported fitness levels near the 95th percentile for population norms.[40] The most active individuals reported exercising between 300 to 600 minutes per week, and all had a VO_{2max} of 45 to 50 mL/kg/min and were older than 66 years old. In contrast, another individual reported exercising only 60 minutes per week and had a VO_{2max} of 32 mL/kg/min.[40]

In a case study of a centenarian cyclist who established the 1-hour cycling record for individuals 100 years of age or older, it was reported that their body weight and lean mass did not change, but maximal oxygen consumption increased from 31 to 35 mL/kg/min (+13%) over a 2-year training period.[8] Peak power increased from 90 to 125 W (+39%) mainly because of increasing pedaling frequency. No changes in maximum HR occurred (134–137 beats/min), but maximal ventilation increased (57–70 L/min; +23%). Training included cycling 5000 km/year at a "light" ($\leq$12) rate of perceived exertion (RPE) for 80% and 20% at "hard" ($\geq$15) RPE at a cadence between 50 and 70 rpm. The results from this case study are quite intriguing and highlight the plasticity of the human body even in this later stage of life. It also provides insight into the benefits of altering between light and vigorous intensity training to improve performance and to increase the likelihood of exercise adherence in senior athletes.

High-intensity interval training (HIIT) has gained popularity as an effective training paradigm in younger athletes; however, limited research has been conducted in aging populations. In one study on 17 male masters athletes (60 $\pm$ 5 years), nine sessions of HIIT consisting of 30-second sprints at 40% peak power output with 3 minutes active recovery increased both absolute and relative peak power output (799 $\pm$ 205 W to 865 $\pm$ 211 W and 10.2 $\pm$ 2.0 W/kg to 11.0 $\pm$ 2.2 W/kg, respectively).[74] Thus, modifications of HIIT to account for reduced tolerability to higher intensity workloads and prolonged recovery times are likely necessary for senior athletes. Although these data provide initial information regarding the potential benefits of HIIT in master athletes, extreme caution should be taken when considering the application of such training for senior athletes.

Nutrition Supplementation

Appropriate timing and dosing of nutrient supplementation can have a profound impact on sport performance through aiding in postexercise recovery and ultimately the exercise-induced adaptations experienced. Of primary interest with aging athletes is the ability to meet or increase daily recommended levels of protein intake. Exercise performed at sufficient intensities to promote muscle damage stimulates the upregulation of protein synthesis. The rate of muscle protein synthesis is blunted in aging athletes (known as anabolic resistance) compared with younger athletes of similar training backgrounds.[75] This is one potential explanation for why the time course of recovery in master athletes is longer than in their younger counterparts. The inability to maintain a positive protein balance throughout training is necessary to prevent skeletal muscle loss. It is recommended that younger athletes consume an estimated 20 g of dietary protein immediately after intense activity to maximize muscle protein recovery.[75] Because of the anabolic resistance experienced by master athletes, greater amounts of dietary protein may be necessary to maximize muscle protein synthesis. Therefore, it is recommended that masters athletes consume 35 to 40 g of leucine-rich whey protein or approximately 0.4 g/kg of body mass after exercise-induced muscle damage.[75] In addition, to maximize muscle protein remodeling, it is encouraged that masters athletes ingest four protein-rich meals of similar quantities evenly spaced throughout the day.[75]

SUMMARY

Information gained from senior athlete performance provides valuable insight into understanding human performance and the physiological changes that occur with successful aging. Specific neuromuscular and cardiorespiratory alterations associated with aging have major implications on rehabilitation and sport performance in senior athletes. Current evidence suggests that senior athletes possess greater health and physical function than their sedentary counterparts. The ability to improve senior athlete performance with training demonstrates that the plasticity of the human body is preserved with aging. As rehabilitation professionals, we are in a position to promote health and wellbeing across the lifespan while assisting in helping senior athletes achieve their sporting goals. To accomplish this, treatment plans must be prescribed to account for the unique characteristics associated with aging athletes.

The constraints-oriented approach provides a framework to understand changes in movement performance in senior athletes. The planning and programming of individualized treatment plans can be developed in accordance with identified constraints limiting performance. Principles of specificity, progressive overload, variation, reversibility, and individuality can be used to guide intervention design to ensure the adaptations pursued meet the physical demands required during activity. Resistance training is an effective approach to combat the neuromuscular declines experienced with aging. Similarly, endurance training provides a potent stimulus to promote improved cardiorespiratory fitness. Current evidence regarding the health and functional benefits of sport participation in the aging population are promising. As the aging population continues to grow, there is a need for future research to better understand the implications of aging on human performance and to determine the most effective approaches to treating and training the senior athlete.

REFERENCES

1. World Health Organization. *World Report on Ageing and Health*. Geneva: World Health Organization; 2015.
2. Tanaka H, Seals DR. Endurance exercise performance in masters athletes: age-associated changes and underlying physiological mechanisms: endurance performance and masters athletes. *J Physiol.* 2008;586:55–63.
3. Tanaka H, Seals DR. Invited review: dynamic exercise performance in masters athletes: insight into the effects of primary human aging on physiological functional capacity. *J Appl Physiol.* 2003;95:2152–2162.
4. Lazarus NR, Harridge SDR. Declining performance of master athletes: silhouettes of the trajectory of healthy human ageing? Ageing and master athletes. *J Physiol.* 2017;595:2941–2948.
5. World Masters Athletics. https://world-masters-athletics.com. Accessed August 2, 2018.
6. United States Master Swimming. http://www.usms.org. Accessed May 1, 2018.
7. Lepers R, Stapley PJ. Master athletes are extending the limits of human endurance. *Front Physiol.* 2016;7:613.
8. Billat V, Dhonneur G, Mille-Hamard L, et al. Case studies in physiology: maximal oxygen consumption and performance in a centenarian cyclist. *J Appl Physiol.* 2017;122:430–434.
9. Centers for Disease Control and Prevention. http://www.cdc.gov. Accessed July 17, 2018.
10. Riebe D, Ehrman JK, Liguori I, Magai M. American College of Sports Medicine. In: *ACSM's Exercise Testing and Prescription*. 10th ed. Philadelphia: Wolters Kluwer; 2018.
11. Trappe S. Marathon runners: how do they age? *Sports Med.* 2007;37:302–305.
12. Baker AB, Tang YQ. Aging performance for masters records in athletics, swimming, rowing, cycling, triathlon, and weightlifting. *Exp Aging Res.* 2010;36:453–477.
13. Akkari A, Machin D, Tanaka H. Greater progression of athletic performance in older masters athletes. *Age Ageing.* 2015;44:683–686.
14. Wright VJ, Perricelli BC. Age-related rates of decline in performance among elite senior athletes. *Am J Sports Med.* 2008;36:443–450.
15. Gava P, Kern H, Carraro U. Age-associated power decline from running, jumping, and throwing male masters world records. *Exp Aging Res.* 2015;41:115–135.
16. Ransdell LB, Vener J, Huberty J. Masters athletes: an analysis of running, swimming and cycling performance by age and gender. *J Exerc Sci Fitness.* 2009;7(suppl):S61–S73.
17. Chakravarty EF. Reduced disability and mortality among aging runners: a 21-year longitudinal study. *Arch Intern Med.* 2008;168:1638.
18. Foster C, Wright G, Battista RA, Porcari JP. Training in the aging athlete. *Curr Sports Med Rep.* 2007;6:200–206.
19. Wroblewski AP, Amati F, Smiley MA, Goodpaster B, Wright V. Chronic exercise preserves lean muscle mass in masters athletes. *Phys Sportsmed.* 2011;39:172–178.
20. Jordre B, Schweinle W, Beacom K, Graphenteen V, Ladwig A. The five times sit to stand test in senior athletes. *J Geriatr Phys Ther.* 2013;36:47–50.
21. Jordre B, Schweinle W, Oetjen S, Dybsetter N, Braun M. Fall history and associated physical performance measures in competitive senior athletes. *Top Geriatr Rehabil.* 2016;32:1–16.
22. Unhjem R, van den Hoven LT, Nygård M, Hoff J, Wang E. Functional performance with age: the role of long-term strength training. *J Geriatr Phys Ther.* 2017;42(3):115–122. https://doi.org/10.1519/JPT.0000000000000141.
23. Power GA, Allen MD, Gilmore KJ, et al. Motor unit number and transmission stability in octogenarian world class athletes: can age-related deficits be outrun? *J Appl Physiol.* 2016;121:1013–1020.
24. Hunter SK, Pereira HM, Keenan KG. The aging neuromuscular system and motor performance. *J Appl Physiol.* 2016;121:982–995.
25. Venturelli M, Reggiani C, Richardson RS, Schena F. Skeletal muscle function in the oldest-old: the role of intrinsic and extrinsic factors. *Exerc Spor Sci Rev.* 2018;46(3):188–194.
26. Mitchell WK, Williams J, Atherton P, Larvin M, Lund J, Narici M. Sarcopenia, dynapenia, and the impact of advancing age on human skeletal muscle size and strength; a quantitative review. *Front Physiol.* 2012;3:260.
27. Raue U, Slivka D, Minchev K, Trappe S. Improvements in whole muscle and myocellular function are limited with high-intensity resistance training in octogenarian women. *J Appl Physiol.* 2009;106:1611–1617.
28. Raj IS, Bird SR, Shield AJ. Aging and the force–velocity relationship of muscles. *Exp Gerontol.* 2010;45:81–90.
29. Reid KF, Fielding RA. Skeletal muscle power: a critical determinant of physical functioning in older adults. *Exerc Spor Sci Rev.* 2012;40:4–12.

30. Gerstner GR, Thompson BJ, Rosenberg JG, et al. Neural and muscular contributions to the age-related reductions in rapid strength. *Med Sci Sports Exerc.* 2017;49(7):1331–1339.
31. Baker AB, Tang YQ, Turner MJ. Percentage decline in masters superathlete track and field performance with aging. *Exp Aging Res.* 2003;29:47–65.
32. Mckendry J, Breen L, Shad BJ, Greig CA. Muscle morphology and performance in master athletes: a systematic review and meta-analyses. *Ageing Res Rev.* 2018;45:62–82.
33. Wiswell RA, Hawkins SA, Dreyer HC, Jaque SV. Maintenance of BMD in older male runners is independent of changes in training volume or VO(2)peak. *J Gerontol A Biol Sci Med Sci.* 2002;57:M203–M208.
34. Nichols JF, Palmer JE, Levy SS. Low bone mineral density in highly trained male master cyclists. *Osteoporos Int.* 2003;14: 644–649.
35. Velez NF, Zhang A, Stone B, Perera S, Miller M, Greenspan SL. The effect of moderate impact exercise on skeletal integrity in master athletes. *Osteoporos Int.* 2008;19:1457–1464.
36. Piasecki J, McPhee JS, Hannam K, et al. Hip and spine bone mineral density are greater in master sprinters, but not endurance runners compared with non-athletic controls. *Arch Osteoporos.* 2018;13(1):72.
37. Fleg JL, Morrell CH, Bos AG, et al. Accelerated longitudinal decline of aerobic capacity in healthy older adults. *Circulation.* 2005;112:674–682.
38. Hawkins SA, Marcell TJ, Victoria Jaque S, Wiswell RA. A longitudinal assessment of change in VO2max and maximal heart rate in master athletes. *Med Sci Sports Exerc.* 2001;33: 1744–1750.
39. Katzel LI, Sorkin JD, Fleg JL. A comparison of longitudinal changes in aerobic fitness in older endurance athletes and sedentary men. *J Am Geriatr Soc.* 2001;49:1657–1664.
40. Everman S, Farris JW, Bay RC, Daniels JT. Elite distance runners: a 45-year follow-up. *Med Sci Sports Exerc.* 2018;50:73–78.
41. Pollock RD, O'Brien KA, Daniels LJ, et al. Properties of the vastus lateralis muscle in relation to age and physiological function in master cyclists aged 55-79 years. *Aging Cell.* 2018;17(2): e12735. https://doi.org/10.1111/acel.12735. Epub 2018 Mar 8.
42. Kettunen JA, Kujala UM, Kaprio J, Sarna S. Health of master track and field athletes: a 16-year follow-up study. *Clin J Sport Med.* 2006;16:142–148.
43. McKean KA, Manson NA, Stanish WD. Musculoskeletal injury in the masters runners. *Clin J Sport Med.* 206;16:149–154.
44. Ganse B, Degens H, Drey M, et al. Impact of age, performance and athletic event on injury rates in master athletics—first results from an ongoing prospective study. *J Musculoskelet Neuronal Interact.* 2014;14(2):148–154.
45. Cabri J, Sousa JP, Kots M, Barreiros J. Golf-related injuries: a systematic review. *Eur J Sport Sci.* 2009;9:353–366.
46. Cann AP, Vandervoort AA, Lindsay DM. Optimizing the benefits versus risks of golf participation by older people. *J Geriatr Phys Ther.* 2005;28:85–92.
47. Matzkin E, Suslavich K, Wes D. Swimmer's shoulder: painful shoulder in the competitive swimmer. *J Am Acad Orthop Surg.* 2016;24(8):527–536.
48. Stocker D, Pink M, Jobe FW. Comparison of shoulder injury in collegiate- and master's-level swimmers. *Clin J Sport Med.* 1995;5:4–8.
49. Weldon EJ, Richardson AB. Upper extremity overuse injuries in swimming. A discussion of swimmer's shoulder. *Clin Sports Med.* 2001;20:423–438.
50. Roberts WO. Running causes knee osteoarthritis: myth or misunderstanding. *Br J Sports Med.* 2018;52(3):142. https://doi.org/10.1136/bjsports-2017-098227.
51. Chakravarty EF, Hubert HB, Lingala VB, Zatarain E, Fries JF. Long distance running and knee osteoarthritis. *Am J Prev Med.* 2008;35(2):133–138.
52. Lefèvre-Colau MM, Nguyen C, Haddad R, et al. Is physical activity, practiced as recommended for health benefit, a risk factor for osteoarthritis? *Ann Phys Rehabil Med.* 2016;59 (3):196–206.
53. Magnusson K, Turkiewicz A, Timpka S, Englund M. A prediction model for the 40-year risk of knee osteoarthritis in adolescent men. *Arthritis Care Res.* 2019;71(4):558–562.
54. Hart LE, Haaland DA, Baribeau DA, Mukovozov IM, Sabljic TF. The relationship between exercise and osteoarthritis in the elderly. *Clin J Sport Med.* 2008;18 (6):508–521.
55. Fransen M, McConnell S, Harmer AR, et al. Exercise for osteoarthritis of the knee. *Cochrane Database Syst Rev.* 2015;(1):CD004376.
56. Fransen M, McConnell S, Hernandez-Molina G, Reichenbach S. Exercise for osteoarthritis of the hip. *Cochrane Database Syst Rev.* 2014;2(4):CD007912.
57. Hulteen RM, Morgan PJ, Barnett LM, Stodden DF, Lubans DR. Development of foundational movement skills: a conceptual model for physical activity across the lifespan. *Sports Med.* 2018;48(7):1533–1540.
58. Davids K, Glazier P, Araújo D, Bartlett R. Movement systems as dynamical systems: the functional role of variability and its implications for sports medicine. *Sports Med.* 2003;33: 245–260.
59. Newell KM. Constraints on the development of coordination. In: Wade MG, Whiting HT, eds. *Motor Development in Children: Aspects of Coordination and Control.* Amsterdam, The Netherlands: Martinus Nijhoff, Dordrecht; 1986: 341–360.
60. Langley DJ, Knight SM. Exploring practical knowledge: a case study of an experienced senior tennis performer. *Res Q Exerc Sport.* 1996;67:433–447.
61. Korhonen MT, Mero A, Suominen H. Age-related differences in 100-m sprint performance in male and female master runners. *Med Sci Sports Exerc.* 2003;35:1419–1428.
62. Pantoja PD, Saez DE Villarreal E, Brisswalter J, Peyré-Tartaruga LA, Morin JB. Sprint acceleration mechanics in masters athletes. *Med Sci Sports Exerc.* 2016;48:2469–2476.
63. Korhonen MT, Mero AA, Alén M, et al. Biomechanical and skeletal muscle determinants of maximum running speed with aging. *Med Sci Sports Exerc.* 2009;41(4):844–856.
64. Beck ON, Kipp S, Roby JM, Grabowski AM, Kram R, Ortega JD. Older runners retain youthful running economy despite biomechanical differences. *Med Sci Sports Exerc.* 2016;48(4):697–704.
65. Ferreira MI, Barbosa TM, Costa MJ, Neiva HP, Marinho DA. Energetics, biomechanics, and performance in masters' swimmers: a systematic review. *J Strength Cond Res.* 2016;30 (7):2069–2081.
66. Brooks GA. *Exercise Physiology: Human Bioenergetics and Its Applications.* New York: McGraw-Hill; 2005.
67. Cunanan AJ, DeWeese BH, Wagle JP, et al. The general adaptation syndrome: a foundation for the concept of periodization. *Sports Med.* 2018;48(4):787–797.
68. World Health Organization. *International Classification of Functioning, Disability and Health: ICF.* Geneva: World Health Organization; 2001.
69. American College of Sports Medicine. American College of Sports Medicine Position Stand. Progression Models in resistance training for healthy adults. *Med Sci Sports Exerc.* 2009;41(3):687–708.
70. Borde R, Hortobágyi T, Granacher U. Dose–response relationships of resistance training in healthy old adults: a systematic review and meta-analysis. *Sports Med.* 2015;45: 1693–1720.
71. Steib S, Schoene D, Pfeifer K. Dose-response relationship of resistance training in older adults: a meta-analysis. *Med Sci Sports Exerc.* 2010;42:902–914.

72. Murias JM, Kowalchuk JM, Paterson DH. Speeding of VO2 kinetics in response to endurance-training in older and young women. *Eur J Appl Physiol.* 2011;111:235–243.
73. Franklin BA, Fern A, Voytas J. Training principles for elite senior athletes. *Curr Sports Med Rep.* 2004;3:173–179.
74. Herbert P, Hayes L, Sculthorpe N, Grace F. HIIT produces increases in muscle power and free testosterone in male masters athletes. *Endocr Connect.* 2017;6:430–436.
75. Doering TM, Reaburn PR, Phillips SM, Jenkins DG. Postexercise dietary protein strategies to maximize skeletal muscle repair and remodeling in masters endurance athletes: a review. *Int J Sport Nutr Exerc Metab.* 2016;26(2): 168–178.
76. Raj IS, Bird SR, Shield AJ. Aging and the force–velocity relationship of muscles. *Exp Gerontol.* 2010;45(2):85.

CHAPTER 29

Health Policy for Physical Therapists and Older Adults

Ellen Strunk

OUTLINE

INTRODUCTION

Physical therapists and physical therapist assistants provide exceptional clinical care to older adults in a variety of settings. The body of clinical knowledge related to this population continues to grow, and as a result, techniques are refined, and new approaches adapted. And yet, a therapist's understanding of how these techniques and approaches are paid for is often seen as less important to obtaining knowledge in specific areas of clinical care. However, over the past decade there has been increased scrutiny of health care services, and physical therapy has not been immune to the scrutiny. Inadequate knowledge of the scope and rules of coverage can result in underpayments and overpayments, which might be perceived as fraudulent or abusive behaviors. A lack of awareness of how reimbursement procedures are developed misses an opportunity to advocate on behalf of patients and the physical therapy profession. The lack of a basic understanding for how physical therapy services are paid for increases the risk of other unintended consequences, namely that the patient beneficiary fails to receive the services they require.

This chapter will help readers understand the health insurance programs for older adults, as well as recent reforms to control costs and improve quality. It is not a primer to the nuances of reimbursement regulations. Application of this knowledge will enable readers to effectively advocate for patients, for older adults as a population, and for policy changes that benefit society as a whole. Health care is a rapidly changing industry, and readers are encouraged to refer to the Centers for Medicare and Medicaid Services (CMS) and the American Physical Therapy Association (APTA) websites to read up-to-date information on legislation, regulatory interpretation, and opportunities for professional legislative advocacy.

PUBLIC POLICY, HEALTH POLICY, AND ADVOCACY

The desired outcome of policy and the advocacy process is to influence decisions aimed to improve the health of individuals that physical therapists serve. Health policy and advocacy are interwoven with policy decisions that determine how health care professionals practice. Physical therapists who provide services to older adults are subject to a number of policies that range from determining the scope of practice through state licensure laws to the payment for services delivered through entitlement programs, such as Medicare and Medicaid. Although it may be challenging to understand the nuances of the different applications of the policies, it is important that health care professionals actively engage in the advocacy process to improve current policies, or to enact new policies to enable physical therapists to better serve this growing population of Americans.

Public policy is the means a government uses, through actions defined by its constitution, to address the needs of its citizens. Public policy is a system of laws, regulatory measures, courses of actions, and functional priorities promulgated by government entities. This definition is an amalgamation of several contemporary definitions and provides a pragmatic approach to a broad and diverse discipline that is without a consensus definition. The Congress of the United States passes national laws, applicable to all U.S. citizens, sometimes called Acts, to address social, health, or economic needs or problems. They become law when the President signs them. Examples include the Social Security Act (SSA) or the Affordable Care Act mentioned later in this chapter. Regulatory agencies are empowered to enforce the Acts and are authorized to adopt the regulations that implement them. For example, the Affordable Care Act gave the Secretary of Health and Human Services (HHS) broad authority in developing, implementing, and monitoring the requirements mandated in the law.

State legislatures are responsible for enacting laws at the state level, and, if passed, apply throughout a state. Many states grant local boards the authority to pass public health rules and regulations. State boards of physical therapy actively promote and protect the citizens of their respective state by regulating the profession of physical therapy. In addition to state statutes or laws, a state or state physical therapy board may have administrative codes that have the force and effect of law and consist of rules and regulations that interpret the requirements of the physical therapy board.

Health policy comprises the choices and decisions a society makes regarding health goals and priorities, and consequently the ways it allocates resources or policies to attain these goals. Health policies can be as basic as handwashing procedures for a restaurant, which is a voluntary health policy based on scientific evidence and backed by public interest, or as complex as payment based on the adherence to clinical guidelines. The Medicare program has policies they call coverage documents. Policies and coverage documents are also used in retrospective review of provider claims or other audits to compare what was provided to what was or should have been paid for. Payers may also issue guidelines or guidance documents to help define terms and/or expectations that are a part of the regulation. For example, the CMS publishes an array of guidance documents including manuals, transmittals, and rulings.

Health policies focus primarily on how to contain the outputs or expenditures. Concerns about the rising costs of federal and state health care programs drive policy. However, these policies can have detrimental impacts on the quality of care or access to services. The major pressure point in health care today are the policies of cost containment and their impact across all domains of health policy. Physical therapists experience cost-containment strategies in two forms: regulations and mechanisms of payment. Regulations that set criteria for what is payable by the government or private insurance help to control costs. These regulations can set criteria for the use of support personnel, set minimum time requirements for certain interventions, and limit what interventions can be utilized for certain diagnoses. Mechanisms of payment are designed to help control costs and manage resource allocation in physical therapy. Mechanisms of payment range from fee-for-service, in which a fee is charged for each intervention utilized, to case-rate payments, in which a single preset fee is paid for a certain clinical condition to cover all services provided, whether the actual cost of care falls within the case rate or not.

Domains of Health Services

Access, quality, and cost are the three major domains that are commonly used to evaluate health services in our country (Fig. 29.1). The first domain, access, encompasses health policies that ensure individuals have accessibility and availability of health care services to meet their own needs and the needs of the broader community in which they live. It is the domain defined first because it is the entry point into the health care delivery system in the United States. Individuals' abilities to access health

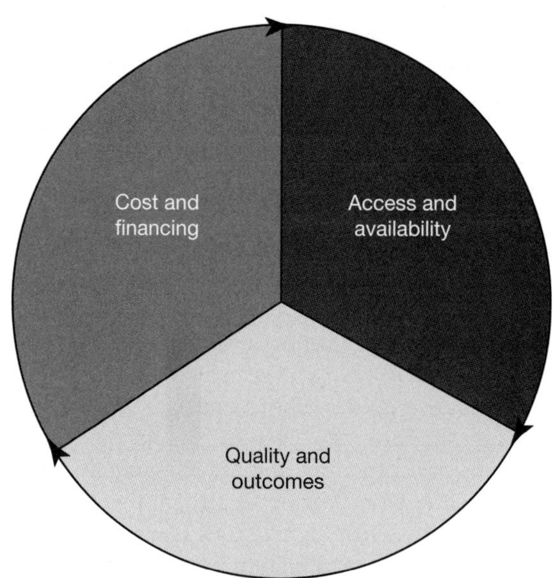

FIG. 29.1 Domains of Health Policy.

care from an available and qualified health care professional is essential to the overarching goal of most health policies, that is, to improve the health status of the population the policy seeks to serve. The second domain of health policy is quality and outcomes. Once an individual can access services from available and qualified health care professionals, policies are needed to ensure that the services meet basic standards for care and do not jeopardize the individual's health, safety, and welfare. The classic Hippocratic Oath "I will do no harm or injustice to them," is the ethical foundation of the charge to health policies to advance quality. The domain of quality is on a continuum that begins with doing no harm and transitions to advancing the health status of a population through evidence and clinical judgment. Quality measurement and outcomes represent a growing area in health policy development, the evaluation of health care professionals and facilities, and resource allocation as discussed later in this chapter. The third domain covers the cost and financing of health policies, or the economics of the decision. This domain is the arena in which the priorities or values on which the policy is based are highly debated. In the United States, the cost and financing of health care has been a long-standing, and often contentious, public debate. Distributing a finite set of resources in a way that is acceptable to the public, health care providers, payers, and policy makers is the primary challenge in health policy today. Balancing the amount of resources with the rising demand on services is critical to our economy and public health. This chapter will explore the primary systems that fund health care.

Further investigation of the three domains of health policy uncovers many examples in the current environment of policies that affect physical therapists and health care providers in each domain. Each domain has specific policy ramifications for the physical therapist whose practice is oriented toward an older adult population. The three domains of health policy are also interrelated; for example, policies that affect accessibility and availability of services have an impact on the quality and cost. Successful health policy systematically balances the three domains to achieve the best possible outcome for the desired population.

Examples of Health Policy Efforts

Therapy Cap. Health policy to eliminate arbitrary limits on benefits is of particular interest to rehabilitation health care professionals that serve a geriatric population. Between 1997 and 2017, a per beneficiary per year financial limitation on therapy services was placed on seniors and individuals with disabilities under the Medicare program. This "therapy cap" in 2017 limited a patient to \$1980 of physical therapy and speech–language pathology services and \$1980 of occupational therapy services per calendar year. Although Congress interceded several times over the 20 years to place a moratorium on therapy caps or to provide a clinically based exceptions process, the policy had significant ramifications for Medicare beneficiaries and their abilities to access clinically appropriate rehabilitation services provided by physical therapists and other rehabilitation health care professionals. Physical therapists and physical therapist assistants, stakeholder advocacy groups, and even Medicare beneficiaries across the country rallied every year in an effort to convince legislators to repeal a health policy that was detrimental to the health and quality of life of older adults. In December 2018, they were successful, and a permanent repeal of the therapy cap was included in the Balanced Budget Act of 2018.

Prevention of Falls. Expanding health care to include prevention and chronic care management programs would have a significant impact on the health policy goal of improving the health status of Americans at a lower per capita or system cost. Policies to prevent falls are another example of increasing the accessibility of prevention services that geriatric physical therapists might provide. The Centers for Disease Control and Prevention report that more than one out of four adults aged 65 years and older fall each year in the United States, but less than half tell their doctor, and that one out of five falls causes a serious injury such as a broken bone or a head injury. They estimate that if rates continue to rise at their current pace, by 2030 there will be 7 deaths every hour caused by falls.[1] A 2018 study found that implementing a single evidence-based fall prevention intervention could prevent up to 45,164 falls per year, resulting in an annual savings of \$94 to \$442 million in medical costs.[2]

To reduce cost and improve health quality, programs and initiatives to reduce falls in older Americans are critical prevention initiatives and health policies for physical therapists who serve this at-risk population. The last piece of federal legislation signed into law addressing falls prevention was the Safe Seniors Act (now Public Law 110-202) that amended the Public Service Act and authorized the Department of HHS to conduct research, implement a national awareness campaign, and improve the diagnosis, treatment, and rehabilitation of individuals at risk for falls or repeat falls.[3] States have also enacted legislation to address falls among older adults as well.[4] California enacted their Osteoporosis Prevention and Education Act that requires the Department of Health Services to develop effective protocols for the prevention of falls and fractures and establish these protocols in community practice to improve the prevention and management of osteoporosis. Florida passed a law that requires the Department of Corrections to establish and operate a geriatric facility where generally healthy older offenders can perform general work appropriate for their physical and mental condition to decrease the likelihood of falls, accidental injury, and other conditions known to be particularly hazardous to older adults. Massachusetts has a law that establishes a commission on falls prevention within the Department of Health. Washington state requires the Department of Social and Health Services to establish a statewide fall prevention program including networking with community services, making affordable senior-based evaluated exercise programs more available, providing consumer education to older adults and the community at large, and conducting professional education on fall risk identification and reduction. Whether at the federal or state levels, physical therapists have an opportunity to influence legislatures to put policies into place to improve the health status of older adults.

Supplemental Benefit Options. The Balanced Budget Act of 2018 and a new guidance letter from the CMS paved the way for Medicare Advantage plans to offer new supplemental benefit options to their enrollees. They will have greater flexibility to offer coverage for nonmedical but health-related services and supports. Therapists can be instrumental in working with Medicare Advantage plans to encourage and recommend coverage for things like home modifications to reduce the risk of falls in the home. The Senior Home Modification Assistance Initiative Act is a piece of bipartisan legislation introduced in the Senate in 2018 that would coordinate, review, and promote the numerous federal home modification programs and resources that are currently available, which would help older adults better access these resources.[5] In April 2018, the Department of Housing and Urban Development and the Department of Veterans Affairs (VA) jointly launched a pilot program to provide $13.7 million in competitive grants to nonprofit organizations that provide nationwide or statewide programs that primarily serve veterans and/or low-income individuals. The grants may be used to modify or rehabilitate eligible veterans' primary residences, recognizing the growing need to fund home adaptations and modifications that can help veterans regain or maintain their independence.[5]

Social Determinants of Health. Access to health care services is further complicated by disparities across racial and ethnic groups and by geographical and socioeconomic factors. In 2017, one out of every four Americans identified themselves as being African American, American Indian/Alaska Native, Asian, Native Hawaiian/Pacific Islander, Hispanic/Latino, or multiracial.[6] Social determinants of health are another area of increasing interest in health policy because of their relationship to health status and access to care. Social determinants include availability of resources to meet daily needs (poverty); access to educational, economic, and job opportunities; access to health care services; transportation options; social support; public safety; and social norms like discrimination and racism.[7] By applying what we know about social determinants of health, physical therapists can seek to improve individual and population health in the communities we serve.

Universal Health Care. Achieving universal coverage in the United States does not guarantee that services will be accessible if a sufficient number of health care providers are not available to provide the services that are now accessible. Compounding the gaps in access for minorities is the corresponding gap in representation of these minorities as health care professionals. Physical therapy is similar to other health professions in that whites continue to represent the vast majority of practicing professionals. This disparity can be a contributing factor to the unavailability of services for underrepresented population subgroups. Directing resources toward the recruitment and retention of underrepresented populations to meet the growing problems of accessibility and availability of health care for racial and ethnic groups as part of a commitment to social justice within the professions is becoming health policy.

Equitable Health Care Access. Where one lives also has a significant effect on one's ability to access health care services. Currently, one in five Americans lives in a rural area.[8] Rural areas have been demonstrated to have higher rates of poverty, a larger percentage of older Americans, and a diminished health status. Not only is access to health services limited in rural areas, these communities have fewer physicians, health care professionals, hospitals, and health resources than urban and suburban areas of the United States.[9] Limited access and scarce available resources and professionals to meet the increasing health care needs in rural areas are a major public health issue for the United States. Health care policy to address this issue should continue to improve accessibility to services. Increasing the availability of health care resources and providers to rural populations is a critical health policy issue because of the poor health status and limited resources available to this population.

Recruiting and retaining qualified health care professionals, such as physical therapists, in rural areas is a policy challenge. Various proposals are examples of health policy whose objective is to ensure accessibility and availability of health care in underserved areas. In 2019, more than 6000 health professional shortage areas exist.[10] If the Physical Therapist Student Loan Repayment Eligibility Act is adopted, physical therapists will be eligible for the National Health Services Corps, a federal program that places qualified health care professionals and physicians in underserved areas. The incentive to recruit and retain health care professionals to this program and to service in underserved areas is student loan repayment. In 2018, a health care professional who is selected and completes the required service in the National Health Service Corps is eligible for up to $60,000 in student loan repayments in return for 2 years commitment.

Access to and the availability of health care services is basic to health policy. Policies to achieve improved access or to increase availability must be balanced to ensure patient safety, enhance quality, and to utilize scarce resources in an efficient and effective manner.

Advocacy

Advocacy plays a key role in building strong health systems. It gives people a voice in decisions that affect their lives and health and helps hold governments accountable for meeting the health needs of all people, including marginalized groups. Health policies developed with broad participation help governments and institutions provide better health care.[11] In the United States, the advocacy process is clearly articulated in the United States Constitution and its First Amendment. The First Amendment, ratified on December 15, 1791, outlines the freedoms of religion, press, and expression, and states:

> *"Congress shall make no law respecting an establishment of religion, or prohibiting the free exercise thereof; or abridging the freedom of speech, or of the press; or the right of the people peaceably to assemble, and to petition the Government for a redress of grievances."*[12]

The right of individuals to bring issues before government entities sets the framework for a majority of health policy initiatives and decisions. Through the process of advocacy, individuals or groups approach recognized individuals, organizations, or governments that are authorized to issue such policies and are empowered to promulgate specific guidelines, rules, regulations, or laws. Advocacy exists at the level of the individual and the group. Self-advocacy is an important personal attribute that is a recognized characteristic of a competent adult. In addition to self-advocacy in which one acts on behalf of oneself, it is also an essential characteristic of health care professionals to advocate as individuals in the best interest of the patient or client. Self-advocacy and patient-focused advocacy are core principles in health care and in physical therapy. APTA's Code of Ethics, Principle 8, states, "Physical therapists shall participate in efforts to meet the health needs of people locally, nationally, or globally." This principle clearly establishes there is an ethical obligation to advocate for changes in laws and regulations that benefit patients.[13] The APTA, and by extension its Sections and Chapters, is the group that advocates on behalf of its members, and by extension for all physical therapy professionals.

Legal, legislative, and regulatory advocacy is the process of educating, implementing, influencing, and enacting policy changes to affect the desired outcome, whether that is to improve health through health policy initiatives or to enable professional advancement. As a health care professional, advocacy is a critical role for physical therapists to provide and is essential for the enactment of policies that enable physical therapists to practice to the full extent of education, experience, and expertise. Advocacy in public or health policy includes the process of setting a plan to influence an authorized body to issue a decision.

Advocacy Process. Advocacy is the process to get to a policy decision. The advocacy process is cyclical and continuous as it depends on the particular policy decision sought and its congruity with shifting priorities for both the advocate and the decision maker. To effectively advocate for changes that match a desired outcome, a systematic plan of action is required. Although there are many different textbooks and articles to assist with formulating an advocacy plan, one approach is outlined in the 6-step advocacy framework (Fig. 29.2). These 6 steps are briefly described next.

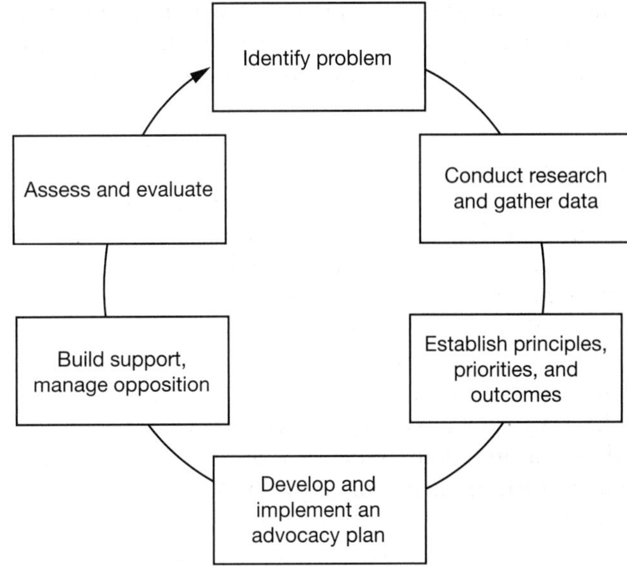

FIG. 29.2 **The 6-Step Advocacy Framework.**

Step 1: problem identification or development of the idea. This step is critical as it defines the deficit that advocacy efforts will seek to correct through policy change. The clear articulation of the problem becomes the case statement and represents step 1 in the 6-step advocacy framework.

Step 2: compile the necessary research, data, and background on the issue. Problem identification only pinpoints the issue an individual or group seeks to change. It is then necessary to collect data and conduct the research to begin to build the case for change. Public health data, consumer opinions, surveys, and other data are needed to build the foundation for the reasons for seeking the change. Defining the issue and supporting it with strong and sound evidence increases the potential for success. One of the essential elements of this second step is identification of the policy that will need to be changed to achieve the desired outcome, and also the venue in which the change can occur. The legislative body is often the venue of last resort. Many times, policies can be changed at the regulatory level, and this is an important assessment of step 2 in the advocacy framework. The regulatory process, although as complex and as difficult to navigate as the legislative process, can make many policy determinations and provide some flexibility in approaches and outcomes.

Step 3: establish principles, priorities and outcomes. This third step can be used to establish short-, intermediate-, and long-range goals. The third step is critical for identifying key advocacy champions and constituencies.

Step 4: develop and implement an advocacy plan. This fourth step articulates what needs to be done to present the case for change to the body that has the authority to make a determination consistent with the desired outcome. This process can involve an in-depth strategic plan or be an informal process. The action plan should consider the individuals or parties involved in making the decision, how the case should be presented to them, a timeline for the desired determination, and the process that the policy will be subject to before it can be issued. The plan should be built on the research and data gathered in step 2, and consistent with the priorities outlined in step 3. This step sets the course for implementing advocacy efforts.

Step 5: build support, manage opposition. Although the fifth step could be a significant part of step 4, it is singled out because of its importance. Broadening the community of advocates behind the action plan is essential. In today's electronic communications world, advocacy plans can be put into action in quick order. Rising above the rank-and-file advocacy initiatives takes a concerted effort to build a community of support and diminish opposition. Coalitions, alliances, and partnerships are as much the fabric of policy development and advocacy world as lobbyists, elected officials, and think tanks. The successful implementation of coalition efforts can build momentum, establish consistency in the plan, and show broad public support. Coalitions, alliances, and partners are the force multiplier in advocacy plans with and without opposition and are a key element to a successful advocacy plan.

Step 6: assess and evaluate. The final step is the assessment and evaluation process and it is essential in a process that is cyclical. The advocacy process never ends at a destination. Although there should be evaluative measures in each step of the advocacy process, there is the need to take the necessary time to assess what worked and what could have been done more effectively or efficiently. This assessment and evaluation will feed into the data collection efforts described in step 2, to inform the next round of advocacy efforts or possibly identify new venues in which to make the case for change.

A good example of the steps in action can be found by reviewing the process used by the National Council on Aging (NCOA) with the Home Safety Council on falls prevention. The recognition that falls prevention programs could improve health outcomes for older adults and other populations served as a catalyst for the development of an advocacy plan. The NCOA and the Home Safety Council built their policy case and priorities around government data on the impact of falls on cost and quality in health care, with a desire to improve access to programs to prevent these adverse events in health care. The NCOA and the Home Safety Council convened stakeholders to develop a national action plan and a corresponding blueprint for health policies to reduce falls and increase falls prevention within the health care system and in the community. These stakeholders developed the plan and built a coalition to implement its objectives, the Falls Free Coalition. This coalition and its advisory committee continue to explore strategies and assess its progress. The coalition has also developed resources to expand their advocacy reach with manuals and guides for state action on falls prevention. The advocacy framework, from problem identification to setting a plan of action to assessing the progress by the NCOA and its partners, provide an effective model for advocacy success.[14] Another example of advocacy in action is the *Jimmo versus Sebelius* case,[15] described in Table 29.1, which changed forever the myth around the "improvement standard" for physical therapy services.

An example of advocacy frequently undertaken by physical therapists is in the realm of payment for services. The Medicare program has two levels of coverage determinations: national coverage determinations (NCDs)

TABLE 29.1 Example of Advocacy: Jimmo versus Sebelius

Identify the problem	Between 1986 and 2009, health care providers identified a longstanding CMS practice called the "improvement standard," whereby an increasing number of processors habitually denied claims for nursing care and therapy services when "significant progress" was not made and/or when beneficiaries' condition was not "improving."
Conduct research and gather data	Stakeholders including the CMA repeatedly appealed these denials through the Office of Medicare Hearing and Appeals, winning some and losing some appeals. On those claims appealed at the federal court level, the government had never appealed, and therefore there was no binding precedent at the circuit court level. Between 2008 and 2010, the CMA undertook serious conversations with the CMS to try to reach a resolution. After exhaustive discussions, the CMA determined the problem was systematic and could be resolved on one-by-one basis.
Establish principles, priorities, and outcomes	The CMA decided to proceed with litigation and engaged in gathering several real-life stories in which patients were denied medically necessary and skilled services. Mrs. Glenda Jimmo was chosen as the lead plaintiff. Ms. Jimmo lived in Vermont, was blind and had her right leg amputated owing to complications from diabetes. She requires a wheelchair and receives multiple home health care visits per week for various treatments for her complex condition. However, Medicare denied coverage for these services, saying that she was unlikely to improve.

Continued

TABLE 29.1	Example of Advocacy: Jimmo versus Sebelius—cont'd
Develop and implement advocacy	The CMA partnered with the Vermont legal aid and filed a federal lawsuit against Kathleen Sebelius, Secretary of Health and Human Services at the time, on behalf of six beneficiary plaintiffs and seven national organization plaintiffs harmed by the improvement standard. The goal was permanent removal of the "improvement" language from Medicare documents.
Build support, manage opposition	In May 2011, the two sides submitted briefs to the court. In June 2011, the federal government attempted to dismiss the case arguing the course lacked jurisdiction over the plaintiff's claims and they had failed to state a claim for which relief could be granted. Numerous advocacy groups including the American Physical Therapy Association, American Occupational Therapy Association, American Speech-Language Pathology Association, and American Association of Retired Persons encouraged members, patients, and caregivers to reach out to the Congressional representatives to put pressure on the CMS to settle the case. On October 25, 2011, the court dismissed the motion, and the case proceeded. While preparing for trial in the spring of 2012, the CMA continued to negotiate with the CMS for a settle agreement that would be fair and just for Medicare beneficiaries. On July 12, 2012, the parties announced they had reached an agreement. On October 16, 2012, the settlement was filed in the federal district court of Vermont, marking a landmark step toward ending the barrier to medically necessary skilled services, and on January 24, 2013, the settlement was officially approved and deemed "fair."
Assess and evaluate	The Department of Health and Human Services agreed to clarify Medicare policy to ensure claims from providers are paid consistently and appropriately and not denied solely based on a "rule-of-thumb" determination that because a beneficiary's condition is not improving, they no longer require skilled medically necessary services. CMS asserts that although maintenance services were always a benefit under Medicare, they will amend language throughout their policy manuals and guidelines to insure these services are available and paid for by the claims processors. Both CMS and CMA issue educational materials and fact sheets. The CMA and health care providers continue to hold CMS accountable to its agreement to insure fair coverage to Medicare beneficiaries.

CMA, Center for Medicare Advocacy; *CMS*, Centers for Medicare and Medicaid Services.
Data from Centers for Medicatre & Medicaid Services. Jimmo Settlement. https://www.cms.gov/Center/Special-Topic/Jimmo-Center.html. Accessed August 3, 2019.

and local coverage determinations (LCDs). Medicare coverage is limited to items and services the CMS determine to be reasonable and necessary for an illness or injury. There are some services for which they have made an NCD, meaning that all Medicare contractors must pay for those services. An example is electrical stimulation for the treatment of stage III and IV chronic pressure ulcers, arterial ulcers, diabetic ulcers, and venous stasis ulcers.[16] If an NCD does not specifically exclude or limit an item or service, or if the item or service is not mentioned in an NCD, a regional Medicare contractor may choose to write an LCD. An LCD contains "reasonable and necessary" information about coverage.[17] Each Medicare contractor has a place on its website that includes information about its LCDs, the process for reviewing LCDs, and how providers can comment on its LCDs. The process provides an opportunity for physical therapists to advocate for improved coverage of existing or new treatment techniques on behalf of their patients.

Summary

Policy and advocacy go hand in hand. To enact or change policy takes a concerted effort to influence the bodies that possess the power to make these changes. Health policy is a complex balancing act of decisions that policy makers must make to improve access, enhance quality, and reduce cost. Understanding health policy will assist understanding the limitations and possibilities of the health care delivery system. Health policies should also outline the need for policy changes to enable all health care professionals to serve to their fullest capabilities and for patients to be assured safety and access. Balancing these policy objectives in health care continues to challenge our policy makers and advocacy organizations.

It is essential regardless of practice setting, political perspective, or policy expertise that physical therapists engage in the health policy and advocacy process. As health care professionals, physical therapists are obligated to comply with existing laws, regulations, and policies. Advocacy is part of their professional responsibility. Competency in health policy and advocacy will only further the professions' ability to serve patients and help them reach their full potential.

FEDERAL AND STATE PAYMENT SYSTEMS FOR OLDER ADULTS

Although the Medicare program is available for people aged 65 years and older, access to all desirable health care services is still a problem for older adults because the Medicare program lacks coverage for many aspects of preventive care, has limits for hospital and skilled nursing facility (SNF) care, and lacks coverage for long-term care provided at home or in nursing homes. Medicare enrollees may choose to obtain supplemental or secondary coverage that will help offset their financial obligations for services provided under the Medicare program or for services that are not covered.

History and Implications of Medicare Program

Franklin Roosevelt passed into law the Social Security Act after extensive study by private groups and in reaction to the Great Depression's effect of a wide-spread unemployment and loss of trust in employer safety nets. What was not popular at the time was a compulsory government health insurance, popular in Europe. In the committee's opinion, the United States was still seen as the land of free enterprise and prosperity, and using the private market for health care reimbursement was the natural choice. Additionally, the American Medical Association and physicians strongly opposed a government solution to health care and was supported by a general lack of interest by the public. These forces influenced the President to postpone a decision to include health insurance legislation as part of the SSA, which was passed on August 14, 1935. The SSA, however, was the first step toward an increased governmental role in social welfare concerns.

During the 1940s, other attempts were made at passing health care insurance legislation, but they did not gain traction largely because of the growth of private insurance plans. However, by 1964, older adults were spending on average between $540 and $600 for hospital care, which was considered high at the time. President Lyndon Johnson made Medicare his number one priority, and in July 1965, both houses of Congress approved a final plan that created Medicare and Medicaid as amendments to the SSA.[18]

Title 18 (Medicare Parts A and B) and Title 19 (Medicaid) was landmark legislation that established a federal health insurance program for older adults that provided for hospital care, posthospital extended care, and home health coverage to almost all Americans aged 65 years or older, and provided states with the option of receiving federal funding for providing health care services to low-income children, their caretaker relatives, the blind, and individuals with disabilities.[18] The success of the program was felt almost immediately. Just 1 year later, more than 19 million persons were enrolled in Medicare.[18] Since 1965, Medicare has been expanded twice to increase access to health care benefits. In 1972, legislation was signed to add people under the age of 65 with permanent disabilities and receiving Social Security Disability Insurance payments and persons with end-stage renal disease to the list of eligible recipients. Additionally, in 2001, Medicare eligibility was again extended to persons with amyotrophic lateral sclerosis (or Lou Gehrig disease).

The Medicare and Medicaid programs are run by the CMS. The CMS is a branch of the Department of HHS, and the Secretary of HHS reports directly to the President of the United States. However, these programs are only two types of programs that provide health insurance to Americans. Others include the Veteran's Administration, employer-based group health insurance plans, concierge health insurance plans, and hundreds of other plans available in the private sector. The mix of private and public financed health care coverage makes the health care system in the United States complex and costly.

The concerns about Medicare spending are nothing new. Since 1970, there have been repeated calls for reforms to the Medicare program because of concerns the Part A program would run out of money. The Medicare program has two trust funds: the Hospital Insurance (HI) Trust Fund and the Supplementary Medical Insurance (SMI) Trust Fund. Medicare Part A is financed mainly through payroll taxes levied on current workers and is accounted for through the HI Trust Fund. Medicare Parts B and D are funded primarily through general revenue and beneficiary premiums and are accounted for through the SMI Trust Fund. Payments to insurance companies for beneficiaries enrolled in Part C programs are made by both the HI and SMI trust funds.[19] Both funds are maintained by the Department of the Treasury and are overseen by the Medicare Board of Trustees, which reports annually to Congress concerning the funds' financial status. Financial projections are made using economic assumptions based on current law, including estimates of consumer price index, workforce size, wage increases, and life expectancy. From the time it was created, the HI Trust Fund has faced projections of eventual insolvency. Because the SMI Trust Fund is funded differently, it is unlikely to become insolvent. Medicare expenditures are significantly affected by a number of factors, such as level of enrollment, the complexity and volume of medical services delivered, health care inflation, and life expectancy. For example, in 1965, when the Medicare program was signed into law, life expectancy for a man was 66.8 years and 73.7 years for a woman.[20] In 2019, those numbers are 84.3 years for a man and 86.7 years for a woman.[21] In other words, Medicare is paying for a beneficiary's health care for potentially 20 years, rather than 2 to 8 years.

The SSA established a Medicare Board of Trustees to oversee the financial operations of the Medicare trust fund. Each year, they issue a report on the solvency of the program. Some years they have projected its insolvency to be only 2 years away, whereas others have estimated it to be much longer. Depending on the Trustees report, legislation has been crafted to modify the Medicare benefit. Whether it passed is dependent on the nation's economy, the Administration and Congress, and the country's willingness to accept change to a program most Americans depend on. Table 29.2 outlines legislative changes to the Medicare program since 1965.[22] In 2018, the Trustees projected the HI Trust Fund to be depleted in 2026.[19]

TABLE 29.2 Legislative Changes to Medicare Program Since 1965

Year	Act	Description
1972	Social Security Act amendments	Allowing persons under the age of 65 years with long-term disabilities and end-stage renal disease to qualify for Medicare coverage. Those with long-term disabilities must wait 2 years before qualifying.
1986	The Emergency Medical Treatment And Active Labor Act	Requires hospitals participating in Medicare to screen and stabilize all persons who use their emergency rooms regardless of their ability to pay.
1997	Balanced Budget Act	Included many changes to how providers are paid in an effort to slow the growth of spending, including mandates for future implementation of prospective payment systems for postacute providers. It established the Medicare + Choice program, later renamed Medicare Advantage in 2003.
2001		Medicare eligibility was extended to persons with amyotrophic lateral sclerosis without having to wait 2 years.
2003	Medicare Drug, Improvement, and Modernization Act	Created a voluntary, subsidized prescription drug benefit under Medicare.
2010	The Patient Protection and Affordable Care Act	Included several provisions that impacted Medicare including: • Preventive services are covered without cost-sharing (flu shots; tobacco cessation counseling; screening for cancer, diabetes, and other chronic diseases; an annual wellness visit). • Created the Center for Medicare and Medicaid Innovation that is tasked with developing, testing, assessing, and disseminating innovations that contribute to improved outcomes, better patient care experiences, and lower costs. Examples include Primary Care Initiatives, Bundled Payments for Care Improvement, and variations on the Accountable Care Organization model. • Created quality reporting programs and value-based purchasing programs designed to implement systems of payment penalties and rewards for outcomes of care. • Reduced prescription drug prices for those who fall in the "donut hole." • Increased payments to primary care physicians and general surgeons for 10 and 5 years, respectively, in an effort to boost the number of providers in these areas. • Added additional funding for scholarships and loan repayments for some health care professions who agree to serve in underserved areas. • Community-Based Care Transitions Program funds community-based organizations to provide transition services to reduce 30-day hospital readmission rates. • CMS Medicare-Medicaid Coordination Office created to integrate dual eligible population benefits. • Extended for 5 years the Money Follows the Person Program that aims to boost access to long-term services and supports at-home care to reduce institutionalization. • Granted the Secretary of Health and Human Services increased authority to set up programs to detect and identify overpayments, as well as prosecute those who commit fraud and abuse. • Increased the burden on providers to self-report any and all overpayments.

CMS, Centers for Medicare and Medicaid Services.
Data from https://www.cms.gov/About-CMS/Agency-Information/History/Downloads/Medicare-and-Medicaid-Milestones-1937-2015.pdf. Accessed January 30, 2019.

Medicare Program

The health care system in the United States is often segmented by funding source as well as the categories of services covered by the funding (Fig. 29.3). Although government funding (i.e., Medicare or Medicaid) is the primary payment vehicle for older adults of all income levels, those adults who continue to work full-time past age 65 years usually have employment-based or private insurance that will have specific coverage and limitations. The Medicare program is funded primarily through general revenues, payroll tax revenues, and premiums paid by some beneficiaries. Fig. 29.4 illustrates payment sources for each part of the Medicare program.[23] Table 29.3 lists coverage under Parts A, B, C, and D of the Medicare program.[24]

At age 65 years, every person has the opportunity to enroll in Medicare Part A. At that time, they can choose which parts to enroll in. As long as they enrolled in Part A at age 65 years, they can opt-in to other parts at later dates. They can stay with original Medicare, meaning they keep their Medicare Part A and Part B benefits, and can choose to join a separate Part D plan, or they can choose a Medicare Advantage plan, also known as Part C (Fig. 29.5).[24] People can also purchase supplemental private insurance known as "Medigap" to help pay for "gaps" in coverage, that is, those services not covered

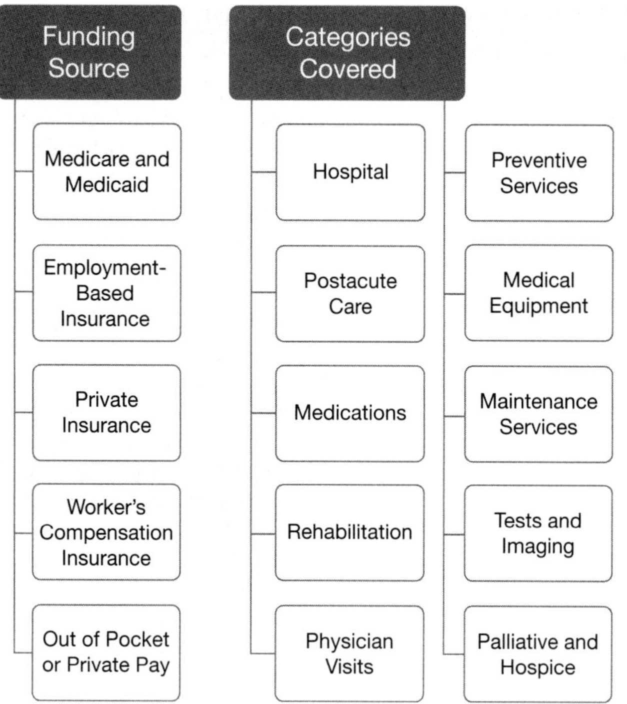

FIG. 29.3 Medicare Funding Sources and Categories.

by Medicare Part A or B and/or those services not completely paid for by Medicare Part A or B.

Medicare Coverage in Different Settings

The Medicare program offers varying coverage in different practice settings for services and durable medical equipment. Medicare pays for hospital care through an inpatient prospective payment system (PPS). Postacute care (PAC) services are currently paid through site-specific PPSs. PAC refers to the constellation of services that beneficiaries receive after (or sometimes in lieu of) an acute care hospital (ACH) stay, and includes services provided in a long-term care hospital (LTCH), an inpatient rehabilitation facility (IRF), an SNF, or by a home health agency (HHA). Outpatient services are generally paid using a fee schedule that pays differently depending on the service provided and the site at which it is delivered. Coverage criteria and payment rates are updated annually through a formal rule-making process.

Prospective Payment Systems. A PPS is a method of reimbursement in which Medicare makes payments based on a predetermined, fixed amount. The payment amount is based on a classification system designed for each

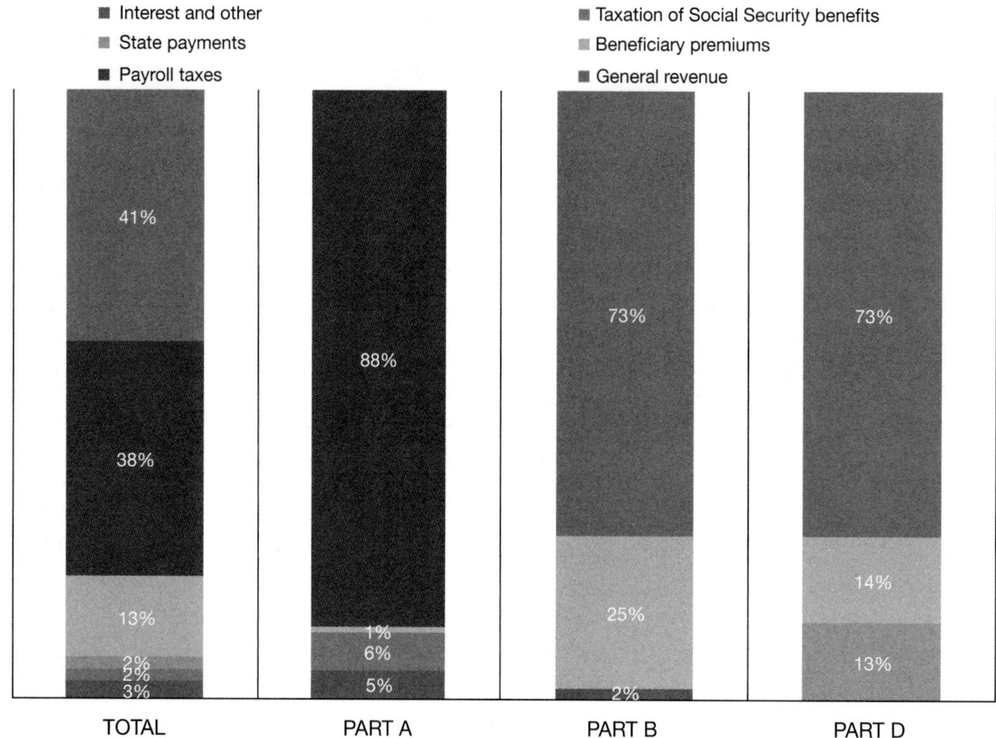

FIG. 29.4 Sources of Medicare Revenue 2013. *(Adapted from the Kaiser Family Foundation based on data from the 2014 Annual Report of the Boards of Trustees of the Federal Hospital Insurance and Federal Supplementary Medical Insurance Trust Funds. A Primer on Medicare, page 32.)*

TABLE 29.3 Medicare Programs A, B, C, and D

Program	Who is Eligible	Basic Coverage	Premium Costs to Beneficiaries
A	• Age 65 years and older if they are U. S. citizens or permanent legal residents with at least 5 years of continuous residence. • Adults under age 65 years with permanent disabilities may be eligible after receiving Social Security Disability Income payments for 24 months. • People with end-stage renal disease or amyotrophic lateral sclerosis are eligible as soon as they begin receiving Social Security Disability Income.	• Inpatient hospital care. • Short-term skilled nursing facility stays. • Hospice care. • Home health care. • Pints of blood received at a hospital or skilled nursing facility.	• Persons age 65 years or older do not pay a premium unless neither they nor their spouse made payroll contributions for 40 or more quarters; if true, then monthly premiums range from $232 to $422 in 2018. • Persons under age 65 years do not pay premiums. • Hospital inpatient: in 2018, $1340 deductible for each benefit period with $0 coinsurance for the first 60 days; between day 61 and day 150 coinsurance rates increase; all costs are the beneficiary's responsibility after lifetime reserve days are used. • Skilled nursing facility: the first 20 days of a stay are paid in full; days 21 to 100, beneficiaries pay up to $167.50/day. • Home health care: no additional costs. • Hospice care: no additional costs.
B Supplementary Medical Insurance program	• Persons eligible for Part A are also eligible for Part B. • Enrollment is voluntary.	• Outpatient hospital care. • Physician visits. • Preventive services, such as mammography and colorectal screening. • Ambulance services. • Clinical laboratory services. • Durable medical equipment. • Kidney supplies and services. • Outpatient mental health care. • Outpatient diagnostic tests. • Free annual comprehensive wellness visit and personalized prevention plan.	• 2018 standard premium is $134.00/month. • Premiums increase for higher income adults to as much as $428.60/month. • Premiums are slightly less for those people receiving Social Security benefits. • 2018 deductible is $183/year. • After the deductible is met, beneficiaries are responsible for 20% of the Medicare-approved amount for doctor services, outpatient therapy, and durable medical equipment.
C	• Persons eligible for Part A and enrolled in Part B may choose to enroll in a Medicare Advantage plan.	• Enrollment period is October 15 to December 7 each year, with benefits taking effect on January 1 of the following year. • All benefits under Medicare Part A (except hospice), Part B, and in most cases, Part D. • Programs are required to provide all Medicare-covered benefits but may vary the benefit design as long as the core benefit package is equivalent to traditional Medicare. • Medicare Part A will still cover hospice care. • Some programs also include extra benefits, such as dental services, eyeglasses, or hearing services.	• Part C plans are administered by private health insurance plans but are required to place a limit on beneficiaries' out-of-pocket expenses for Parts A and B covered services. • Beneficiary may choose to join a Medicare Advantage plan in lieu of traditional Medicare fee-for-service coverage. • Part C monthly premiums vary by plan. • The maximum out-of-pocket spending for enrollees is $6700 in 2018, unless enrollees use out-of-network providers.

Continued

TABLE 29.3 Medicare Programs A, B, C, and D—cont'd

Program	Who is Eligible	Basic Coverage	Premium Costs to Beneficiaries
D	• Persons enrolled in Part A, Part B, or both.	• Enrollment period is October 15 to December 7 each year, with benefits taking effec on January 1 of the following year. • Outpatient prescription drug benefit offered through private plans. • Plans are required to offer a standard benefit but may offer more generous benefits. • Limits are applied annually.	• If enrollment is delayed beyond a person's initial enrollment period, they may be subject to a permanent premium penalty if they choose to enroll in a Part D plan at a later time. • Enrollees pay a monthly premium, along with cost-sharing amounts for each brand-name and generic drug prescription, but premiums and cost-sharing vary by plan. • Enrollees with higher incomes also pay an income-related monthly adjustment amount in addition to the monthly premium charged by their Part D plan. • Most Medicare drug plans have a coverage gap, often referred to as the "donut hole"; e.g., the plan will pay most of the costs of prescription drugs until a certain limit is reached. In 2019, this is $3820 per year. • After exceeding this amount, a beneficiary will pay more for their prescription drugs, but continue to receive some discounts on generic drugs. • In 2019, when a beneficiary reaches $5100 in out-of-pocket costs for covered drugs, he or she will have reached the other end of the "donut hole" and be eligible for catastrophic coverage, and the plan will pay approximately 95% of the cost of all remaining drug costs for that calendar year.

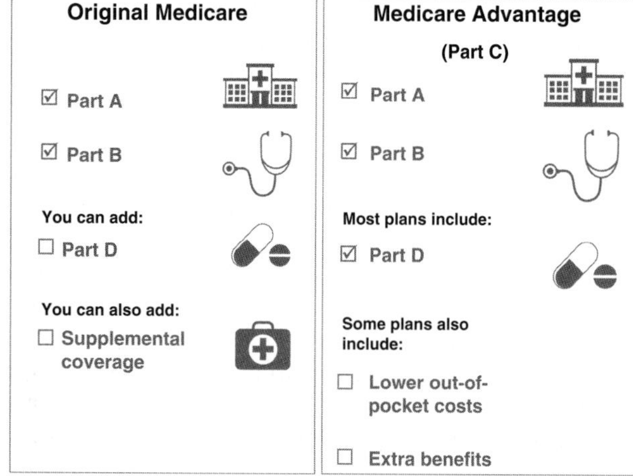

FIG. 29.5 Medicare Advantage Plan. *(From https://www.medicare.gov/sites/default/files/2018-09/10050-medicare-and-you.pdf. Accessed August 3, 2019.)*

setting. Categories or groups are set up around the expected relative cost of treatment for patients in that category or group, and are intended to cover the costs that reasonably efficient providers would incur in furnishing high-quality care. The rates are then adjusted for each local market. PPSs provide an incentive for providers to control costs, either by managing the number and type of services being provided or minimizing the length of stay. The outcome of care could potentially be negatively affected, however, if a provider were to provide insufficient or inadequate care because of reducing the delivery of necessary services with the goal of increasing profit from the prospective payment. Later in this chapter, programs to monitor the quality and outcome of services delivered in all settings will be discussed.

Acute Care Hospital. Medicare Part A covers acute care inpatient hospital stays, and an episode begins when a patient is admitted and ends after they have been out of the hospital (or SNF) for 60 consecutive days.[25] Medicare groups patients with similar clinical problems into Medicare severity diagnosis related groups (MS-DRGs). The MS-DRGs are designed around the expected relative costliness of inpatient treatment for patients in that group and are adjusted higher for hospitals that operate an approved resident training program, that treat a disproportionate share of low-income patients, operate in rural areas, or qualify as low-volume facilities. Generally, the hospital receives the same payment whether the patient stays in the hospital 3 days or 3 weeks (although outlier payments are added for excessively complex patients). An MS-DRG payment model incentivizes providers to control the amount and type of services provided during a hospitalization. The MS-DRG is intended to pay for any services the patient requires and receives. For example, physical therapy services provided to patients who have been admitted to inpatient status in a hospital are not 'billed' separately, and therefore the value in providing physical therapy services in an acute care setting is to prevent complications and insure the patient is transitioned to the next level of care as quickly as indicated.

BOX 29.1 Inpatient Rehabilitation Facilities Qualifying Medical Conditions

- Stroke
- Spinal cord injury
- Congenital deformity
- Amputation
- Major multiple trauma
- Hip fracture
- Brain injury
- Certain neurologic conditions (e.g., multiple sclerosis, Parkinson disease)
- Burns
- Three arthritis conditions (active, polyarticular rheumatoid arthritis, psoriatic arthritis), and seronegative arthropathies resulting in significant functional impairment of ambulation and other activities of daily living for which appropriate, aggressive, and sustained outpatient therapy has failed.
- Hip or knee replacement, when it is bilateral, when the patient's body mass index is $\geq$ 50, or when the patient is aged $\geq$ 85 years.

Inpatient Rehabilitation. IRFs provide intensive services such as physical, occupational, or speech therapy, or orthotics/prosthetics training for patients after surgery, an injury, or illness. To qualify for Medicare coverage, patients must be able to benefit from and tolerate 3 hours of therapy for 5 of 7 days each week or participate in 15 hours of therapy in 7 days. However, they also must require more than one therapy discipline; for example, patients who only need one therapy discipline do not qualify for IRF care.[26]

Reimbursement to IRFs has been under a PPS since 2002. IRFs receive a predetermined per-discharge rate based on information entered into the Patient Assessment Instrument and includes the patient's diagnosis, cognitive status, functional status, market area wages, and a system of case-mix categories that reflects the expected resources needed to provide care. The rate covers all capital and operating costs associated with providing intensive rehabilitation.[27]

The IRF benefit is predicated on the presence of certain diagnoses expected to require an intensive amount of rehabilitation services. The 60% rule (formerly known as the 75% rule) requires that 60% of an IRF's admissions must have one or more of 13 qualifying medical conditions. Box 29.1 lists those conditions as of 2019.[27] The 60% rule intends to promote proper placement of PAC patients into the most cost-effective setting.

Skilled Nursing Facilities/Nursing Facilities. Nursing facilities have evolved to provide a range of services, and most are dually certified, which means they must comply with both Medicare and Medicaid regulations, and in return can admit both Medicare and Medicaid patients to their facility. Medicare pays for 24-hour skilled care, either for short-term skilled nursing and/or rehabilitation care. Medicaid pays for custodial or long-term care. However, residents of a long-term care nursing facility may receive therapy services through Medicaid and/or Medicare Part B, depending on their insurance coverage.

In order for Medicare (and most private insurance) to cover skilled care provided in an SNF, the patient has to have had a 4-day, 3-night qualifying hospital stay or enter the SNF within 30 calendar days of a 4-day, 3-night qualifying hospital stay, and the patient must require daily skilled nursing and/or rehabilitation care for the condition for which they were hospitalized, or a condition that arose while in the SNF for treatment of a condition for which the patient was previously hospitalized.

Reimbursement to SNFs was paid under a PPS between 1999 and October of 2019, that was driven by the volume of services provided to the patient. Over the 20 years, there was a dramatic rise in the amount of physical, occupational, and speech–language therapy services delivered to all patients, regardless of their admitting diagnoses, prior level of function, and/or level of function at admission. Because of the observed trends, the Office of Inspector General released more than one report expressing its concerns that "even though beneficiary characteristics remained largely unchanged," the amount of therapy delivered was driven by the level of reimbursement. Among its recommendations were to change how the CMS paid for therapy in this setting. As a result, the payment model changed drastically on October 1, 2019, from one primarily driven by the number of therapy minutes delivered in a week to a more complex model the CMS named the Patient-Driven Payment Model (PDPM).[28] Under this system, SNFs receive a daily payment that is determined by several components entered into the

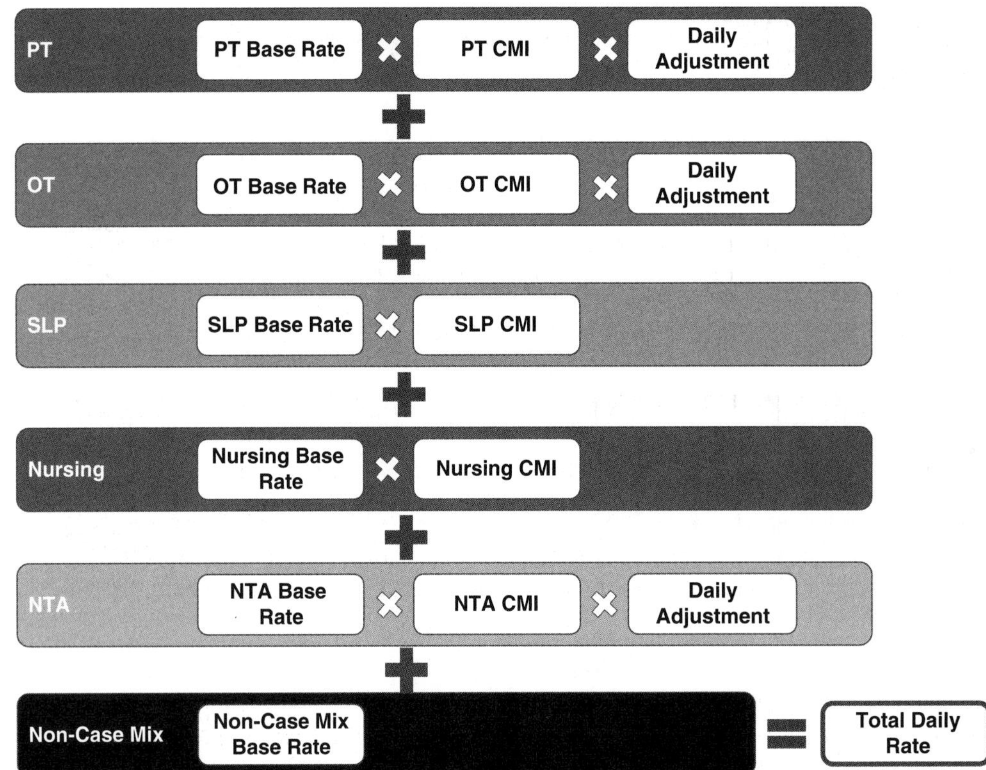

FIG. 29.6 Illustration of Skilled Nursing Facility per Diem Payment Under the Patient-Driven Payment Model. ***CMI*, Case mixed index; *NTA*, nontherapy ancillary services; *PT*, physical therapy; *OT*, occupational therapy; *SLP*, speech–language pathology.**

Minimum Data Set 3.0. Fig. 29.6 provides a diagram of how SNF payments are calculated under the PDPM.[28]

Home Health Services. Medicare beneficiaries who are generally confined to their homes and require skilled care on a part-time or intermittent basis are eligible to receive certain services in their home. To receive Medicare covered home health services, a patient must be confined to his or her home (Box 29.2). This is referred to as the "homebound" requirement. Determining whether a patient is homebound requires the clinician's clinical judgment, clear documentation, and physician certification to support it. For 20 years, the CMS utilized a PPS for home health services. On January 1, 2020, the PPS model for HHAs changed drastically, for the same reasons that the SNF model changed, for example, the utilization of physical, occupational, and speech therapy services has increased without corresponding changes in patient beneficiary characteristics, leading policy makers to conclude the additional therapy is provided just to receive a higher payment. The CMS named the more complex model the Patient-Driven Grouper Model (PDGM), a system that pays HHAs one lump sum payment every 30 days that is determined by several components from the claim and the home health assessment tool, the Outcome and Assessment Information Set (OASIS). Fig. 29.7 provides a diagram of the new payment model. As with the PDPM, the Patient-Driven Grouper Model was intended to remove any incentives to provide an unnecessary amount of physical therapy, occupational therapy, and/or speech–language pathology services, and instead pay HHAs based on the patient's functional and clinical needs.

BOX 29.2 Centers for Medicare and Medicaid Services Homebound Criteria

Step 1: The patient must meet one OR both of the following criteria:

- Because of illness or injury, needs the aid of supportive devices such as crutches, canes, wheelchair, walkers; or the use of special transportation; or the assistance of another person to leave their place of residence

OR

- Have a condition such that leaving his or her home is medically contraindicated

Step 2: After the patient meets one or both of the criteria in Step 1, they must meet BOTH of these criteria:

- There exists a normal inability to leave home

AND

- Leaving the home requires a considerable and taxing effort

Outpatient Therapy Services. Outpatient therapy services include physical therapy, occupational therapy, and speech–language pathology, and can be provided in different settings, including a hospital outpatient department, an SNF, an outpatient rehabilitation agency, a

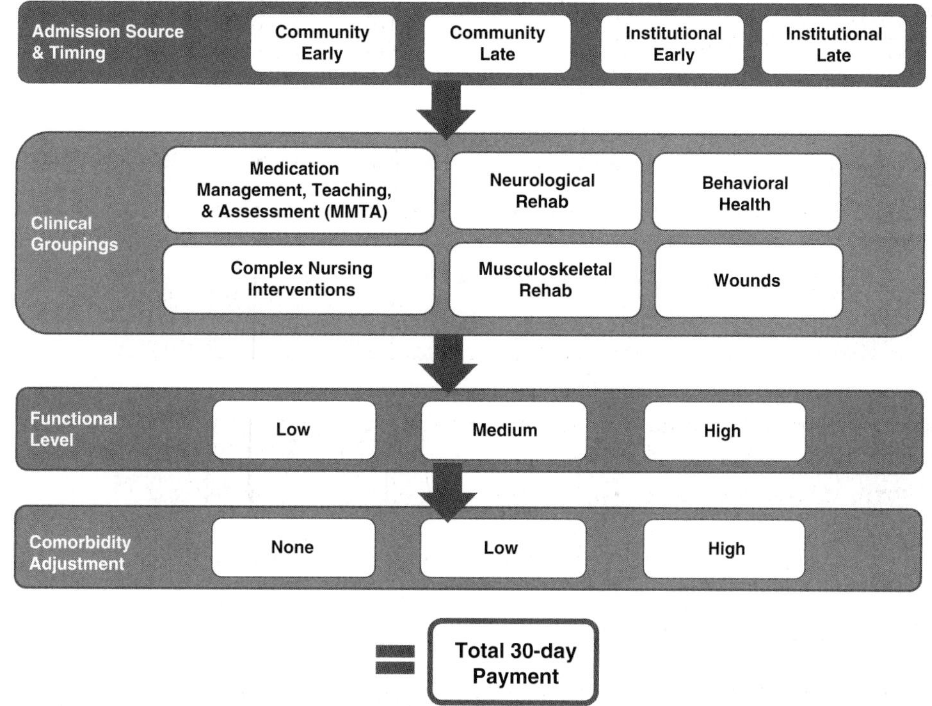

FIG. 29.7 Illustration of Home Health Agency Payment Under the Patient-Driven Grouper Model.

certified outpatient rehabilitation facility, in the patient's home, a physician's office, or a therapist's private practice. Fig. 29.8 illustrates how therapy tends to be distributed by setting.[29] Technically, a referral to therapy from a physician is not required under the Medicare program; however, a physician must certify (e.g., sign) the therapy plan of care within 30 days of the initial therapy evaluation.

In order for Medicare to cover these services, they must be provided by a qualified provider (i.e., a therapist or therapist assistant, but not an aide), be appropriate and effective for a patient's condition, and be reasonable in terms of frequency, intensity, and duration. Medicare will pay for outpatient skilled therapy services to improve a patient's condition, maintain a patient's current condition, or prevent or slow further deterioration of the patient's condition.[30]

Medicare pays for outpatient therapy services using a fee schedule and the unit of payment in each individual therapy service. These are classified using the Healthcare Common Procedure Coding System. Under the fee schedule, each code has a separate payment rate based on a relative weight, or relative value unit. The relative value units account for the relative costliness of providing the service, including the clinicians' work, practice expense, and professional liability insurance.[29] Most of the codes utilized by physical therapists are time-based, and therefore the system is highly scrutinized because, as stated earlier, there is the appearance that it rewards volume of services delivered rather than the quality of care and outcomes of care.

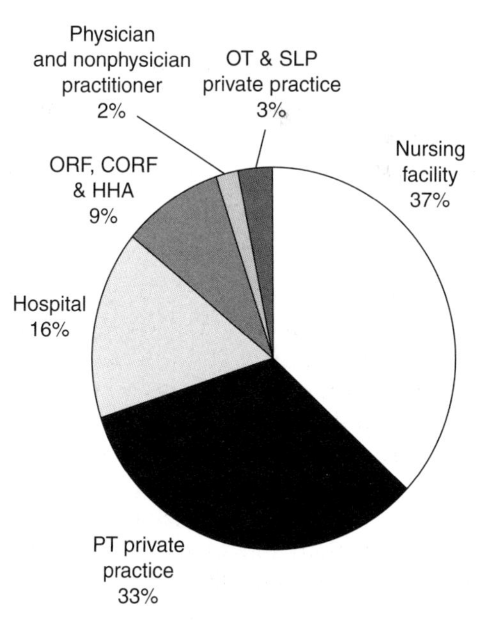

FIG. 29.8 **Distribution of Outpatient Spending by Setting.** *(From http://www.medpac.gov/docs/default-source/payment-basics/medpac_payment_basics_18_opt_final_sec.pdf?sfvrsn=0. Accessed August 3, 2019.)*

Hospice Care. Hospice care gives patients the choice to maintain quality of life, remain alert and pain-free, receive emotional and spiritual support, and to receive end-of-life care at home, in a hospital, or nursing facility. End-of-life care can be costly. Studies have shown approximately 8.5% to 11.2% of Medicare dollars are spent in patients' last year of life, the lowest of any developed country.[31]

Hospice care is routinely considered a lower-cost approach to end-of-life care, although hospice is considered to be expensive, in part because of the escalating utilization.[31] The CMS data show significant growth in the utilization of the hospice benefit since 2000, doubling between 2000 and 2016 to nearly 50%. Public or private hospice organizations provide supportive services and pain relief to terminally ill patients who are expected to live 6 months or less as determined by their physician. Care is provided in the patient's home or in hospice care based in a hospital or nursing facility. Box 29.3 details the services that hospice can provide. Physical, occupational, and speech therapy are covered under Medicare, as are all other services, when treatment is for pain relief and symptom management.[32]

BOX 29.3 Hospice Services Under Medicare

- Skilled nursing services
- Drugs and biologicals for pain control and symptom management
- Physical, occupational, and speech therapy
- Counseling (dietary, spiritual, family bereavement, and other counseling services)
- Home health aide and homemaker services
- Short-term inpatient care
- Inpatient respite care
- Other services necessary for the palliation and management of the terminal illness

Durable Medical Equipment, Prosthetics, Orthotics, and Supplies. Medicare covers equipment a patient needs at home to treat his or her injury or illness under the Durable Medical Equipment, Prosthetics, Orthotics, and Supplies (DMEPOS benefit. DMEPOS is defined as equipment that can withstand repeated use, primarily and usually serves a medical purpose, generally is not useful to a person without an illness or injury, and is appropriate for use in the home.[33] For example, Medicare does not pay for parallel bars that are more suitable to be used in the hospital or SNF, nor does Medicare cover items considered for convenience or comfort, such as grab bars for the bathroom. Table 29.4 shows the categories of coverage under Medicare Part B.[33]

In response to concerns of widespread abuse, the CMS began to implement reforms for DMEPOS providers, and

TABLE 29.4 Durable Medical Equipment, Prosthetics, Orthotics, and Supplies Categories

Category	Definition	Examples
IN: Inexpensive and other routinely purchased items	These items have a purchase price of $150 or less; are generally purchased (as opposed to rented) 75% of the time or more; or are accessories used in conjunction with certain nebulizers, aspirators, and ventilators. If covered, these items can be purchased new or used. They can also be rented, but total payment amounts cannot exceed the purchase-new amount for the item.	Batteries for glucose monitors, tracheal suction tubes, axillary crutch pads, disposable nebulizers, adjustable canes, walkers.
FS: Frequently serviced items	If covered, these items can be rented as long as they are medically necessary.	Home ventilator, continuous passive motion machine.
CR: Capped rental items	These items are not covered in any other durable medical equipment category and are generally expensive items that have historically been rented. If covered, Medicare generally pays for the rental of these items for a period of continuous use not exceeding 13 months. The fee schedule amount is based on the base year purchase price and varies by rental month.	Heavy duty wheeled walker, commode chair with detachable arm, hospital bed, hydraulic patient lift.
OX: Oxygen and oxygen equipment	One bundled monthly payment amount is made for all covered equipment, oxygen, and accessories. Medicare payment for oxygen equipment may not continue beyond 36 months of continuous use. After the 36-month rental cap, Medicare will continue to pay for oxygen and maintenance but not the equipment itself.	Oxygen concentrators, portable oxygen concentrators.
OS: Ostomy, tracheostomy, and urological items	If covered, Medicare pays for the purchase of these supplies.	Ostomy bags, paste, skin barriers.

Continued

TABLE 29.4 Durable Medical Equipment, Prosthetics, Orthotics, and Supplies Categories—cont'd

Category	Definition	Examples
SD: Surgical dressings	If covered, Medicare pays for the purchase of these supplies.	Wound and surgical site dressings.
PD: Prosthetics and orthotics	If covered, Medicare pays for the purchase of these supplies.	Collars, braces, corsets, prosthetics, orthotics.
SU: Supplies	If covered, Medicare pays for the purchase of these supplies.	Casting supplies.
TE: Transcutaneous electrical nerve stimulators	If covered, Medicare pays for the purchase of these supplies.	Transcutaneous electrical nerve stimulators, diabetic shoes, diabetic shoe inserts or molds.

Data from http://www.medpac.gov/docs/default-source/payment-basics/medpac_payment_basics_16_dme_final.pdf. Accessed January 12, 2019.

more regulations for coverage of equipment. Because of the success of a demonstration program piloting a competitive bidding process, Congress passed legislation to mandate the program. Under a competitive bidding program, the CMS determines what supplies or equipment will be put up for bidding. The suppliers operating in that area submit a bid for the selected products. The CMS then evaluates the bids looking at several factors including the supplier's eligibility, their financial stability, the quality of their products, and, of course, their bid price. If chosen, the supplier must agree to accept the assigned payment on all claims for those bid items. The result has been a significant reduction in the cost of durable medical equipment for Medicare and beneficiaries,[33] but may reduce access to adequate provider networks in some areas. Box 29.4 shows the product categories included in the CMS competitive bidding program.[34]

Medicaid

The federal government became involved in health care for individuals with low income through the 1965 congressional enactment of Title 19 of the SSA. Medicaid provides health insurance in all states for some low-income persons, families and children, pregnant women, older adults, and people with disabilities. In 2018, over 66 million individuals were enrolled in Medicaid across the United States,[35] and Medicaid represents $1 out of every $6 spent on health care in the United States.[36] In some states, the program may cover all low-income adults below a certain income level. Table 29.5 outlines legislative changes to the Medicaid program since 1965.[22]

Medicaid is a partnership program between the federal government and the states. Each state is responsible for designing and implementing its own program while the federal government provides financial support and oversight. This gives the states a lot of flexibility in administering their programs. The federal government pays states a portion of their costs by matching the state's spending levels.

Medicaid is financed through the Federal Medical Assistance Percentage (FMAP) in which the federal government guarantees at least $1 in federal funds for every $1 in state spending for qualifying Medicaid expenditures. The FMAP is calculated annually using a formula in the SSA and is based on a state's average personal income relative to the national average. Therefore, states with lower personal incomes have a higher federal match. In 2019, the FMAP ranged from a low of 50% to a high of 76.39%.[37] For example Mississippi, with the lowest per capita income level that year, received $3.24 of federal money for every $1 the state spent on Medicaid, and as a result, a state investment of $100 in Medicaid benefits effectively became $424 they could spend.[37]

The challenge for physical therapists who work with patients receiving Medicaid benefits is that although each state must follow federal guidelines, they can set their own guidelines as to who qualifies for assistance, what services will be paid for, and the amount paid. To receive the federal financial support, called the FMAP, states must provide for certain "mandatory" benefits. These include inpatient and outpatient hospital and x-ray services and home health services. However, other services are considered "optional," and unfortunately, physical, occupational, and speech therapy are included in the list of

BOX 29.4 Product Categories Included in Durable Medical Equipment, Prosthetics, Orthotics, and Supplies (DMEPOS) Competitive Bidding

- Complex rehabilitative power wheelchairs and related accessories
- Continuous positive airway pressure devices/respiratory assist devices and related supplies and accessories
- Enteral nutrients, equipment, and supplies
- General home equipment and related supplies and accessories
- Hospital beds and related accessories
- Mail-order diabetic testing supplies
- Nebulizers and related supplies
- Negative pressure wound therapy pumps and related supplies and accessories
- Oxygen supplies and equipment
- Standard mobility equipment and related accessories
- Standard power wheelchairs, scooters, and related accessories
- Support surfaces
- Transcutaneous electrical nerve stimulation devices and supplies
- Walkers and related accessories

TABLE 29.5 Legislative Changes to Medicaid Program Since 1965

Year	Change
1972	Social Security Income program begins providing cash assistance to elderly and disabled. States are required to cover Social Security Income recipients or apply their 1972 Medicaid eligibility standards for the two groups for coverage under Medicaid.
1981	Federal budget reconciliation (OBRA 81) made several changes: • Requires states to make additional Medicaid payments to hospitals who serve a disproportionate share of Medicaid and low-income patients. • Repeals the requirement that state Medicaid programs pay hospital rates equivalent to those paid by the Medicare program. • Requires states to pay nursing homes at rates that are "reasonable and adequate" under the Boren Amendment. • Establishes two types of Medicaid waivers allowing states to mandate managed care enrollment of certain Medicaid groups and to cover home- and community-based long-term care for those at risk of being institutionalized.
1982	Boren Amendment applied to hospital payments. States allowed to expand Medicaid to children with disabilities who require institutional care but can be cared for at home and would not otherwise qualify for Medicaid if not institutionalized.
1986	Federal budget reconciliation (OBRA 86) allowed state Medicaid programs to pay Medicare premiums and cost sharing for qualified Medicare beneficiaries under 100% of poverty.
1988	Medicare Catastrophic Coverage Act required state Medicaid programs to pay Medicare premiums and cost sharing for qualified Medicare beneficiaries under 100% of poverty.
1990	Federal budget reconciliation (OBRA 90) lowered the requirement for state Medicaid programs to pay Medicare premiums and cost sharing for qualified Medicare beneficiaries to those under 120% of poverty.
1993	The Clinton Administration begins approving Medicaid waivers allowing more statewide expansion demonstrations. Many states turned to managed care for delivery of services and used savings to expand to previously uninsured groups.
1997	Balanced Budget Act of 1997 permits mandatory Medicaid enrollment in managed care and repeals the Boren Amendment.
2006	Deficit Reduction Act of 2005 makes significant changes to Medicaid related to premiums and cost sharing, benefits, and asset transfers.
2010	The Patient Protection and Affordable Care Act included several provisions that impacted Medicaid including: • Expanded eligibility to adults with incomes up to 138% of the federal poverty level; • Required all states to implement recovery audit contractor programs; • Streamlined eligibility, enrollment, and renewal processes.

Data from https://www.cms.gov/About-CMS/Agency-Information/History/Downloads/Medicare-and-Medicaid-Milestones-1937-2015.pdf. Accessed January 30, 2019.

"optional" services. As a result, therapy services outside of a hospital are often the first to be cut (or eliminated) when states are looking for cost savings in their programs.

Beneficiaries who are enrolled in both Medicare and Medicaid are referred to as "dual eligible beneficiaries," and includes beneficiaries receiving full Medicaid benefits and/or assistance with Medicare premiums or cost sharing through one of the Medicare Savings Program categories listed in Box 29.5.[38] These Medicare Savings Programs consider an individual's income, assets, and other resources when determining eligibility; to qualify, older adults have to demonstrate their income is under a certain level—often called a "means test." However, states can raise the qualifying federal income and resources levels in some circumstances to make it more difficult to qualify.

BOX 29.5 Medicare Savings Program Categories

Program	Assistance
Qualified Medicare Beneficiary Program	Assist with premiums, deductibles, coinsurance, and copayments for Part A, Part B, or both
Specified Low-Income Medicare Beneficiary Program	Assists with Part B premium payments
Qualifying Individual Program	Assists with Part B premium payments
Qualified Disabled Working Individual Program	Assists with payments of Part A premium for certain disabled and working beneficiaries

Data from https://www.cms.gov/Outreach-and-Education/Medicare-Learning-Network-MLN/MLNProducts/downloads/Medicare_Beneficiaries_Dual_Eligibles_At_a_Glance.pdf Published May 2018 by US Health and Human Services. Accessed August 2, 2019.

Medicare pays covered medical services for dual eligible beneficiaries first, because Medicaid is generally the payer of last resort. Medicaid may cover medical costs that Medicare may not cover or partially covers (such as nursing home care, personal care, and home- and community-based services). Medicare and Medicaid dual eligible benefits vary by state. Therapists and other providers must be aware of certain billing prohibitions that apply to dual eligible, especially qualified Medicare beneficiaries.[39] Some states offer Medicaid through Medicaid managed care plans, whereas other states provide fee-for-service Medicaid coverage. Other states provide certain dual eligible beneficiary plans that include all Medicare and Medicaid benefits.[38]

Although adults and children make up approximately 77% of enrollees, they utilize only 39% of Medicaid funding. Older adults and those with disabilities make up 23% of enrollees but consume 61% of Medicaid spending. Since 1997, when the Balanced Budget Act permitted mandatory Medicaid enrollment in managed care, the percentage of Medicaid money spent in managed care increased to 49%, whereas fee-for-service payments to long-term care increased only 21%.[36] Because of its size and the amount of federal and state spending, the Medicaid program has become a target for policy makers and legislators focused on controlling health care costs. Section 6411(a) of the Affordable Care Act expanded the Recovery Audit Contractor (RAC) program to Medicaid and required each state Medicaid program to establish an RAC program by January 1, 2012, unless they seek an exception.[40] The RACs scope of work includes identifying overpayments and underpayments by the state's Medicaid program, but are also responsible to educate providers and publicize the areas their audits will focus on. Examples of enforcement actions taken by the states include paying money to physicians in return for referrals, billing for therapy services not provided, and billing for more intensive therapy services than were actually provided. Although 73% of all Medicaid convictions were because of fraud in 2017, the remaining 27% were due to patient abuse or neglect.[41]

The 21st Century Cares Act also included provisions to limit fraud and abuse in the Medicaid fee-for-service and Managed care programs by requiring Medicaid providers to enroll with their state.[42] This enrollment requirement is separate from the Medicare enrollment requirement, adding an additional layer of administrative burden to therapists seeking to provide services to this patient population. Providers should be aware of its state Medicaid RAC program, monitor what they are auditing, and understand the requirements for participation in each state.

Veterans' Affairs and TRICARE

Health care benefits are administered by different agencies for veterans and active military personnel. The Department of VA oversees the program for veterans, for example, those who once served in the military but have now separated from active duty, or retired veterans who meet certain eligibility and health criteria. This program is administered by the Veterans Health Administration. Active Duty service members, National Guard/Reserve members, and their families receive health care benefits through TRICARE, a civilian network, under the Department of Defense when the services cannot be provided at a military treatment facility. Military retirees and their families (spouses and children registered in the Defense Enrollment Eligibility Reporting System) are also eligible for TRICARE.

The VA is required by law to provide hospital care and outpatient care services that are defined as "needed." The VA defines "needed" as care or service that will promote, preserve, and restore health.[43] This includes treatment, procedures, supplies, or services. The decision of need is based on the judgment of the health care provider. In 2014, the Veterans Access, Choice and Accountability Act (Choice Act) provided additional tools and funding to help support and reform the VA system.[44] The bill was created in response to the revelations that veterans had been denied care or were having to wait excessively long periods of time to get an appointment at some VA facilities across the country. The result in some cases was a worsening of their condition up to and including death.[45] The bill authorized medical care to be provided outside of the VA when VA medical facilities are not feasibly available. Eligible non-VA providers can become providers in the Veterans Choice Program by completing an application. Treatment provided by a therapist under these programs does require prior authorization from the Veteran's Administration.

In 2018, the VA announced a new rule, titled "Authority of Health Care Providers to Practice Telehealth," that allows VA doctors, nurses, and other health care providers to administer care to veterans using telehealth, regardless of where in the United States the provider or veteran is located. The rule exercises federal preemption to override state restrictions on licensing and state-specific telehealth laws, and also waives all copays for telehealth services.[46] The rule is expected to especially help veterans living in rural areas who may have to travel long distances or across state lines to receive care. Virtual access to care may also foster timely and critical mental health care. Physical therapists employed by the VA can utilize telehealth in their practice, but they must continue to abide by federal laws and practice acts of the therapist's state of licensure.[47] Unfortunately, the rule does not apply to contracted providers, such as those therapists providing care through the Veterans Choice Program.

Utilization Management and Review

Many commercial payers and Medicare Advantage companies are increasing their use of utilization management and utilization review. It is one method they use to cut health care costs and reduce utilization. Utilization management is defined by URAC, an accreditor of health care organizations, to be "the evaluation of the medical necessity, appropriateness, and efficiency of the use of health care services, procedures, and facilities under the provisions of the applicable health benefits plan, sometimes called 'utilization review.'"[48] There are three types of utilization management used in physical therapy, described in Table 29.6.

Documentation

The medical record serves many purposes, including being a formal record of the patient's status and the services that were provided to the patient. Even more critical and challenging for physical therapists is that the medical record must reflect the decision making of the provider and substantiate the need for skilled care, regardless of what setting the care is provided in. Many payers, including

TABLE 29.6 Types of Utilization Management Reviews

Review	Definition	Purpose	Risk
Prospective Review	Review is conducted prior to services starting or after the initial evaluation; may also be called precertification or prior authorization.	To eliminate or reduce unnecessary services.	The recommended treatment by the physical therapist may be reduced or not authorized at all.
Concurrent Review	Review performed during the course of treatment or episode of care.	Physical therapy is required to update the payer at varied intervals and may include activities such as care coordination, discharge planning, and care transitioning.	May have the impact of shortening an existing episode of care.
Retrospective Review	Conducted after the therapy service or episode of care has been completed.	Assess the appropriateness of the procedures, the intensity delivered, and the duration of care.	May result in a partial or full denial of a claim.

Medicare, have detailed documentation requirements, and the payment for services is often dependent on the information contained in the medical record. The documentation must substantiate the services reported on claim forms and for which the provider was paid. Otherwise, the services are at risk for nonpayment should the documentation be audited.

Medicare has guidance for documentation for therapists in all settings that is located in their set of Internet-Only Manuals.[49] For providers of physical therapy, the Medicare Benefit Policy Manual 100-2 holds most of the information for all settings in which physical therapy professionals practice. However, it is important to note that the Medicare Claims Processing Manual 100-4 contains information about claims processing, and therefore should be familiar to physical therapy professionals who bill Medicare Part B. The Medicare State Operations Manual 100-7 contains information about conditions of participation for hospitals, HHAs, hospices, and rehabilitation agencies as well as the requirements of participation for SNF. Therefore, there could be supplemental requirements for documentation found in these manuals.

The manuals represent another example of advocacy by the physical therapy profession. A significant overhaul of the documentation requirements occurred in 2014, and the APTA was heavily involved with the CMS to craft language that would provide clarity to what was appropriate and sufficient documentation expectations for physical therapy services. The result was that the present manual language has improved a therapists' ability to be compliant with the documentation requirements.

FRAUD, WASTE, AND ABUSE

The cost escalation of health care spending is compelling the federal government to reconsider how to fund health care public programs. However, it is also compelling the federal government, policy makers, and private insurance companies to look closer at what the money is being spent on. Over the past several decades, the amount of time and resources invested in program integrity efforts has consistently increased. As early as 1993, President Clinton addressed Congress about his health care reform efforts, which included cracking down on fraud and abuse that he believed would achieve "large savings" and that could then be put toward providing health care coverage for the unemployed.[50] Table 29.7 defines the terms fraud, abuse, and waste.[51]

Medicare, Medicaid, and private insurance companies each have programs to monitor the integrity of their health insurance programs. The CMS established a program to "address improper payments" and promote "compliance with Medicare coverage and coding rules."[52] The Patient Protection and Affordable Care Act of 2010 (PPACA) granted the Secretary of HHS increased authority to set up programs to detect and identify overpayments, as well as prosecute those who commit fraud and abuse. The amount of money recouped from these kinds of health care investigations has increased year-over-year since 2010, and in 2017 totaled $3.7 billion.[53]

Unfortunately, physical therapy has not been immune. The consequences of improper actions can range from recoupment of money to corporate integrity agreements to civil indictments to criminal indictments and permanent ban from participating in any federal health care insurance program. The downstream effect of this type of publicity is that it breeds public distrust toward health care providers, including physical therapists and physical therapist assistants. It also may cause a decrease in the number of current and/or future professionals from staying in and/or entering the physical therapy profession. It may result in policy makers being reluctant to promote physical therapy services as a cost-effective method of addressing the population's health needs. Each of these effects adds another layer of barrier between the population that can benefit from physical therapy services and those providers who are striving to do the right thing every day.

One of the most basic forms of advocacy is to understand a patient/client's benefits. There are multiple outcomes that result from not understanding a patient's benefits, and they are all negative. Examples include

TABLE 29.7 Definitions of Fraud, Abuse, and Waste

Fraud	Knowingly submitting, or causing to be submitted, false claims or making misrepresentations of fact to obtain a federal health care payment for which no entitlement would otherwise exist. Knowingly soliciting, receiving, offering, and/or paying remuneration to induce or reward referrals for items or services reimbursed by federal health care programs. Making prohibited referrals for certain designated health services.	Submitting claims for more units of service than were actually provided. Paying a physician for every referral he sends to the physical therapist's practice.
Abuse	Practices that are inconsistent with acceptable business of medical practices that either directly or indirectly, result in unnecessary costs to the Medicare Program. It includes any practice inconsistent with providing patients with medically necessary services meeting professionally recognized standards.	A patient in home health lives alone and enjoys having the therapist come regularly to exercise with him. Although the patient could go to outpatient therapy, the therapist continues to see him for a few more visits so he will not be lonely.
Waste	Multidimensional; includes inaccurate payments for services, such as unintentional duplicate payments, excessive administrative costs, and even fraud and abuse.	Submitting claims for services that do not accurately describe what was provided because the therapist did not educate himself on proper billing; e.g., billing Therapeutic Activities (97530) when passive range-of-motion is provided.

Date from https://www.cms.gov/Outreach-and-Education/Medicare-Learning-Network-MLN/MLNProducts/Downloads/Fraud-Abuse-MLN4649244-Print-Friendly.pdf. Accessed August 3, 2019.

providing care that is not covered by the health insurance benefit, providing duplicative care, and/or providing care that uses up the patient/client's benefit. In 2012, the amount of waste in the U.S. health care system was estimated to be as much as 34%, for example, $1 out of every $3 were wasted.[51] Table 29.8 illustrates other forms of waste.[54]

Program Integrity is the name given to the CMS initiative to protect the federal health programs from fraud and abuse. Its primary principle is to pay claims correctly. Contractors with the CMS must have programs in place to insure they are paying the "*right amount to a legitimate provider, for covered, correctly coded and correctly billed services provided to an eligible beneficiary.*"[55] Therefore

TABLE 29.8 Examples of Health Care Waste

	Upstream of Physical Therapy	In Physical Therapy	Downstream of Physical Therapy
Clinical	• Unnecessary procedures • Excessive testing • Medical errors • Delay in referring to physical therapy	• Cursory or incomplete evaluations • Generalized plans of care not focused on function • Unskilled, nonfunctional treatment interventions • Lack of coordination and communication between physical therapist and physical therapist assistants • Lack of coordination and communication between physical therapy and other health care providers	• Fumbled hand-offs • When nonstandardized care is delivered, outcomes of therapy are short-lived • Duplicative physical therapy procedures

Administrative	• Avoidable billing errors
	• Regulations
	• Manual versus automated processes
		• Less than thorough intake procedures results in incomplete and/or inaccurate information
		• Regulations that restrict appropriate care
		• Redundant provider credentialing
		• Variable payer requirements for
		  • Eligibility verification
		  • Claims processing
		  • Documentation
		• Potential mismanagement of patient benefit by upstream providers requires additional appeals and authorizations
		• Manual versus automated processes
			• Potential mismanagement of patient benefit by upstream providers requires additional appeals and authorizations
			• Avoidable billing errors
			• Regulations
			• Manual versus automated processes

Data from *The Healthcare Imperative: Lowering Costs and Improving Outcomes: Workshop Series Summary.* Institute of Medicine (US) Roundtable on Evidence-Based Medicine; Yong PL, Saunders RS, Olsen LA, editors. Washington (DC): National Academies Press (US) 2010. Chapter 3, Inefficiently Delivered Services, Table 3-8.75.[75]

CMS contracts with various contractors to achieve this goal. Types of review entities include Medicare administrative contractors, comprehensive error rate testing contractors, recovery auditors, program safeguard contractors, zone program integrity contractors, and supplemental medical review contractors. Each entity has its own responsibilities in safeguarding all parts of the Medicare trust fund and activities may include things like preventing fraud through effective enrollment of beneficiaries, early detection of billing inaccuracies through medical review, coordination with other contractors and law enforcement, and consistent enforcement policies. More information can be found in the online Medicare Program Integrity Manual.[55]

The CMS also devotes resources to fighting fraud in Medicaid. As a result of the PPACA, states continue to expand Medicaid eligibility. With growth of the program, states must also scale their program integrity efforts to ensure eligibility determinations are accurate, oversight of managed care contractors is intensive, data systems are robust, and beneficiaries receive quality care. Unified Program Integrity Contractors are contracted entities that conduct investigations and audits related to activities in both Medicare and Medicaid programs. They work closely with the CMS on joint projects in addition to partnering with state Medicaid Program Integrity Units. More information can be found in the online Medicaid Integrity Manual.[56]

Potential quality of care issues in the Medicare and Medicaid programs are also of concern to the CMS. Although they are not the responsibility of these review contractors, they are referred to the state licensing/survey and certification agency or the state's quality improvement organization. As the number of people insured by Medicare and Medicaid continues to rise, Americans live longer with more chronic conditions, and payment methods shift from volume-based to value-based, this is an area that will receive more and more attention from medical reviewers.

The Anti-Kickback Statute and the Physician Self-Referral laws are important for all providers to understand. The rationale behind these two statutes is that the government does not want to encourage incentives that would increase inappropriate utilization of services and distort medical decision making. The Anti-Kickback Statute of the SSA makes it a criminal offense to knowingly and willfully "offer, pay, solicit, or receive any remuneration to induce or reward services covered by a federal health care program."[52] Remuneration is anything of value including cash or in-kind services. The criminal penalties are significant for violation of the Anti-Kickback Statute. Besides monetary penalties, a provider can be prohibited from participating in the Medicare program and may be sent to prison. Examples of violations include leasing space to a referral source below market value, discounting or waiving patient copays or deductibles, and giving physicians elaborate gifts such as season tickets to sporting events. Exceptions are in place, but providers need to be aware of these regulations. For example, if a provider fails to collect copays and deductibles after multiple attempts, then an exception might be made. However, the provider should not have a pattern of waiving fees or providing discounts that could be construed as inducement. Providers should have written policies and procedures for these exceptions, and there should be no identifiable pattern of discounting or waiving fees.

The Physician Self-Referral Prohibition statute, sometimes called the "Stark Law," prohibits physicians from referring to designated health services or entities in which the physician or a family member has a financial interest, unless an exception is permitted. Physical therapy is considered a designated health service. However, exceptions have been identified. For example, if the service is being provided by someone who is supervised by that physician, the exception is permissible under the "in office ancillary services" provision. This law applies only to physicians and intent does not have to be apparent. Civil penalties are applied for Stark Law violations and these are less onerous than the criminal penalties under the Anti-Kickback Statute.[52]

Compliance Programs

The CMS encourages providers to conduct regular self-audits to identify coverage and coding errors. The Office of Inspector General publishes guidelines[57] providers can use to assist in developing policies and processes for quality assurance and compliance. Most errors do not represent fraud. Most errors are not acts that were committed intentionally. However, errors are errors and repeatedly submitting claims in error can be perceived as fraud or abuse.

SHIFT TO OUTCOMES, QUALITY, AND VALUE

In 2017, the United States spent 17.9% of its gross domestic product on health care—more than any other industrialized nation in the world.[58] The average amount per individual spent by the United States is $10,224, twice the average of other countries.[59] These costs drive a lot of public and private debate. Medicare costs are projected to grow from 3.7% of the gross domestic product in 2017, to 5.8% by 2038, and gradually increasing thereafter to about 6.2% by 2052.[58] Clearly, the U.S. health care system struggles with quality and value of its health care system.

"Quality is the degree to which health services for individuals and populations increase the likelihood of desired health outcomes and are consistent with current professional knowledge."[60] The United States health care delivery system has been plagued by issues of quality and its impact on the health status of Americans. In 2001, the Institute of Medicine issued a landmark study, *Crossing the Quality Chasm,* and stated "The U.S. health care delivery system does not provide consistent, high quality medical care to all people."[60] This report, along with other health policy studies, indicated a high degree of variance in health care delivery in the United States. For example, before 2010, only half of U.S. adults were receiving key preventative health services.[61] Other studies have found that women, older adults, members of racial and ethnic minorities, poorer, less educated, or uninsured are less likely to receive needed care, largely as a result of a lack of access to care in addition to variance in quality.

The Institute of Medicine in another report, *To Err Is Human*, found that almost 100,000 deaths occur each year in the U.S. health care system as a result of medical errors.[62] The data are clear that we need health policies to reduce the errors and improve the poor quality of health care services in our delivery system. Improving the quality of health care is a multidimensional issue and challenge for health care policy makers. With one of the most expensive health care systems in the world, getting an adequate return on this investment and changing the health status of our population are the key elements of quality in health policy.

Six Dimensions of Quality

The six dimensions of quality or quality improvement in health care as defined by the Institute of Medicine are safety, effectiveness, patient-centeredness, timeliness, efficiency, and equity (Fig. 29.9).[60] Each of these dimensions are described next.

Safety is the practice that ensures patients are not harmed by the health care they receive or where they receive it. Effectiveness is the use of evidence and practice standards to match the care delivered with the best available scientific data with resource allocation and utilization. Patient-centeredness is respect for individuals and their wishes in the health care experience. Timeliness is ensuring that health status is not detrimentally affected by waiting times and delays in access. Efficiency is the reduction of fraud, waste, and abuse in the health care system. Equity is ensuring that disparities in the health care system are reduced.[60]

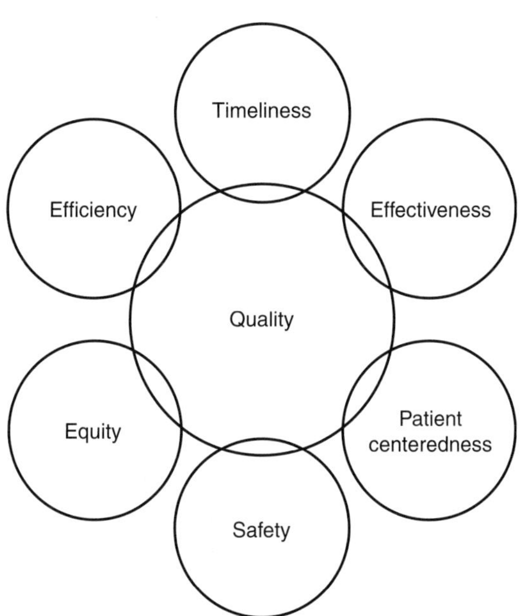

FIG. 29.9 **Dimensions of Quality.**

One dimension especially worth exploration because of its relevance to physical therapy is the dimension of effectiveness. Effectiveness can be divided into the elements of overuse and underuse. The use of interventions in physical therapy that are not proven to provide therapeutic value is a classic overutilization issue. For example, therapeutic exercise that uses less resistance than is required for the functional task and therefore is not challenging to the muscle is not effective. Consistently asking a patient to ride a restorator or recumbent bicycle violates the theory of specificity because pedaling is not a functional activity. The lack of use of interventions for which there is better support leads to underutilization. For example, the lack of incorporating the physical stress theory into the exercise prescription is an example of underutilization of effective therapeutic exercise. Manual therapy and manipulation for individuals with some presentations of low back pain could be considered as examples of underutilization when they are not implemented early enough.

Looking at quality across the six dimensions is critical in health policy as it illustrates the complexity of measuring "quality." These six dimensions also have varying impacts on the other domains of access and cost and must be balanced with these domains. The highest quality might be the most costly and hardest to access. Clinicians would do well to keep these six dimensions in focus as they strive to deliver high-quality care.

Measuring Quality

Measuring quality can proceed along several lines, such as structure, process, and outcome. Structure looks at the system in which the health care experience occurs and those features that enhance quality of care. An example of a structural measure of quality is the use of health information technology. Process measures investigate the method of delivery and assure that critical steps are taken. An example of a process measure of quality can be found in ensuring that a critical question is posed as part of the patient history, such as "Has the patient fallen in the past month?" Outcome measures, the patient-critical level of quality measurement, document the impact of the intervention on the patient's health status. In physical therapy, the functional improvement of the patient is the primary focus of many outcome measures. An example of a treatment outcome measure for population subgroups would be the reduction of falls in patients who have undergone a standardized balance program. The challenge of interpreting outcome measures is that to compare patients with different risk profiles can often complicate interpretation of findings across groups.

Assessment tools and outcome measures in physical therapy have existed in many forms and are important in the direct management of individual patient care as well as providing information about effectiveness of care. Using standardized tests and measures is a method of establishing the baseline status of the patient/client and to be able to quantify change in their functioning. Standard outcome measures provide a common language with which to evaluate the success of physical therapy interventions not just within one episode of care, but also throughout a patient's episode of illness or year over year. Examples of outcome tools used in physical therapy include the APTA's Outpatient Physical Therapy Improvement in Movement Assessment Log,[63] the Uniform Data System of Medical Rehabilitation and its outcome measurement tool, the Functional Independence Measure,[64] the Patient Reported Outcomes Measurement Information System,[65] and the Functional Outcome Measures mandated by the Improving Medicare Post-Acute Care Transformation (IMPACT) Act using the Section GG Self-Care and Mobility Items set. These instruments provide ways for clinicians to measure improvement in patient outcomes following intervention.

Over the past several years, the CMS has put standardized tests and measures front and center. The CMS and other payers are changing the ground rules for what gets paid. Therapy services have been paid on volume for too many years: for example, the number of visits made, the number of minutes provided, the number of codes recorded. However, has that contributed to a better functional outcome for our patient? The unfortunate part is *we do not know*. In every setting where physical therapists work there is a program in place to collect data: ACH, LTCH, IRF, SNF, and HHA all have quality reporting programs (QRPs) and value-based purchasing (VBP) programs mandated by the CMS. Outpatient providers used to have functional limitation reporting but in 2019, the CMS removed that requirement owing to the fact that it was not standardized and therefore did not provide useful information on which to act. The goal of all these programs is, of course, to collect information on patient characteristics, care processes, care variations, and the short- and long-term effects of that care. Collectively, they will allow payers, policy makers, consumers, and health care providers to understand what effective care is and for whom, ultimately improving the health of the population. On a micro-level, they should also inform physical therapists about the quality of the services they deliver and drive improvements in care. However, it may also translate to a time when the effectiveness of our clinical skills in these settings will become more important than how many patients we can see in an 8-hour day.

Quality Reporting Programs

Although private payers have collected a variety of measures for many years, the largest health care provider in the nation—Medicare—has only recently begun to ramp up their implementation requirements that would change the focus of payments from purely quantity to that of incentive payments for quality reporting and performance, efficiency, and eventually value. The Deficit Reduction Act of 2005, the Tax Relief and Health Care Act of 2006, the Medicare Improvements for Patients and Providers Act of 2008, and the PPACA each included key provisions that required the CMS to establish quality reporting mechanisms for all provider types and settings.

Almost 20 years ago, the Department of HHS and the CMS launched their quality initiatives to assure quality health care for all Americans. The goal was to promote accountability among providers and public transparency for the public and consumers. The CMS has a number of quality initiatives touching every aspect of the health care system. Some include publicly reporting quality measures, such as for hospitals, nursing homes, HHAs, and kidney dialysis facilities. Others include utilization and cost data, such as what is reported for physicians and physical therapists practicing under Medicare Part B. This section will touch on some key points of the QRPs where physical therapy professionals practice.

The Hospital Inpatient QRP was originally mandated by Section 501(b) of the Medicare Prescription Drug, Improvement, and Modernization Act of 2003. Section 501(b) authorized the CMS to pay hospitals that successfully report designated quality measures a higher annual update to their payment rates.[66] The amount of that update has been subsequently updated and currently hospitals that do not successfully report can see a reduction of 0.25% of what they would otherwise receive if the QRP requirements were met. The CMS collects quality data from hospitals paid under the inpatient PPS, with the goal of driving quality improvement through measurement and transparency. The data are publicly displayed on the Hospital Compare website[67] to help consumers make more informed decisions about their health care.

In 2007, the SSA was modified to mandate HHAs report quality data. This statute requires that "*each home health agency shall submit to the Secretary such data that the Secretary determines are appropriate for the measurement of health care quality. Such data shall be submitted in a form and manner, and at a time, specified by the Secretary for purposes of this clause.*"[68] The LTCH QRP[69] and the IRF QRP[70] were not mandated until the passage of the PPACA, and in 2014, the SNF QRP[71] was added by the IMPACT Act. Every year, the CMS publishes the quality measures each setting must report to receive their full payment update. Table 29.9 provides a sample of the measures required in each setting in 2019. The penalty for providers in these settings for not reporting all the measures in 2019, is a reduction to all claims billed by 2 percentage

TABLE 29.9 Examples of Measures Included in the Quality Reporting Programs[a]

Measure	Hospital	LTCH	IRF	SNF (for Part A patients)	HH
Survey of Patients' Experiences					
Patients who reported nurses "always" communicated well	X				X
Patients who reported doctors "always" communicated well	X				
Patients who reported the team communicated with patients					X
Patients who reported they were given information about what to do during their recovery at home	X				
Patients who "strongly agree" they understood their care when they left the hospital or facility	X				
Patients who reported YES, they would definitely recommend the hospital or agency	X				X
Timely and Effective Care					
Measures of specific care processes related to sepsis, cataract surgery, colonoscopy, heart attack, emergency room care, preventive care, cancer care, blood clot prevention, pregnancy and delivery	X				
How often care was begun in a timely manner?					X
Percentage of patients whose activities of daily living and thinking skills were assessed and related goals included in their treatment plan		X			
Percentage of patients whose functional abilities were assessed and functional goals included in the treatment plan		X	X	X	
How often patients got better at walking and moving around, getting in and out of bed and better at bathing					X
How often patients had less pain when moving, breathing improved, and wounds healed					X
How often patient/caregivers were taught about their medications					X
How often patients were checked for risk of falling, depression, and were taught about foot care					X
Complications and Deaths					
Surgical complications	X				
Infections	X	X	X		
30-day death rates	X				
Percentage of patients who got antipsychotics for the first time				X	
Percentage of patients who report moderate to severe pain				X	
Rate of pressure ulcers new or worsened		X	X	X	
Percentage of patients who experienced one or more falls with major injury during the stay		X	X	X	
Unplanned Hospital Visits (Return to Hospital Within 30 days of Treatment for…)					
Any condition and/or preventable conditions	X	X	X	X	X
Chronic obstructive pulmonary disease	X				
Heart attack	X				
Heart failure	X				
Pneumonia	X				
Stroke	X				
Coronary artery bypass graft	X				
Hip/knee replacement	X				
Colonoscopy	X				
How often patients had an emergency room visit without hospitalization				X	X
Use of Medical Imaging					
Outpatient with lower back pain who had magnetic resonance imaging before trying physical therapy or other treatment	X				
Outpatient who received double scans	X				
Outpatient who received cardiac imaging stress tests before low-risk outpatient surgery	X				

Continued

TABLE 29.9 Examples of Measures Included in the Quality Reporting Programs—cont'd

Measure	Hospital	LTCH	IRF	SNF (for Part A patients)	HH
Payment and Value of Care					
Medicare spending per beneficiary	X	X	X		
Payment for heart attack patients	X				
Payment for heart failure patients	X				
Payment for hip/knee replacement patients	X				
Payment for pneumonia patients	X				
Rate of successful return to home and community		X	X	X	

[a]This list is not an exhaustive list and is meant to provide context and understanding of the larger quality of care context.
HH, home health; *IRF*, inpatient rehabilitation facility; *LTCH*, long-term care hospital; *SNF*, skilled nursing facility.

points. The information is publicly displayed on the LTCH Compare website,[72] the IRF Compare website[73], the SNF Compare website[74], and the HHA Compare website.[75]

A piece of landmark legislation for therapists working in PAC settings was the IMPACT Act of 2014.[76] PAC is a term that is inclusive of care provided in the LTCH, IRF, SNF, and by HHAs. Patients who are cared for in PAC settings often transition between multiple sites of care, moving among their homes, hospitals, and PAC settings when their health and functional status changes. With almost one in every five Medicare beneficiaries admitted to the hospital each year, approximately 40% are discharged to one of four PAC settings for additional nursing or therapy services.[77] In general, most people assume the four PAC settings differ in the type and intensity of services provided, effectively providing a "continuum of care." After all, that is the way Medicare intended it to be when they set up the conditions of participation for each setting. However, research has shown that the types of patients admitted to these settings and treated by physical therapy professionals do overlap.[78,79] At the same time, there was intense scrutiny on the level of rehabilitation services delivered in all PAC settings. The CMS began to question the value of intense rehabilitation, and the rehabilitation industry struggled with how to justify the services to entities that are primarily interested in the burden of cost it has imposed on the health care system. The challenge facing rehabilitation professionals was that each therapy discipline utilizes standardized clinical performance tools specific to their own professional literature, and some rehabilitation companies have their own proprietary tools, but there was no one tool or measure that all providers had accepted as "the" measure of quality rehabilitative care in these settings. The patients treated in PAC settings are particularly vulnerable and costly to the system, given their clinical complexity and the frequency with which they transition between settings. The CMS recognized that performance measurement across PAC settings had traditionally been fragmented because of the heterogeneity of patient populations, as well as the varying performance measurement obligations and reporting mechanisms across settings.

The IMPACT Act requires the Secretary to implement specified clinical assessment domains using standardized (uniform) data elements to be nested within the assessment instruments currently required for submission by LTCH, IRF, SNF, and HHA providers. The Act further requires that CMS develop and implement quality measures from five quality measure domains using standardized assessment data. In addition, the Act requires the development and reporting of measures pertaining to resource use, hospitalization, and discharge to the community. Through the use of standardized quality measures and standardized data, the intent of the Act, among other obligations, is to enable interoperability and access to longitudinal information for such providers to facilitate coordinated care, improved outcomes, and overall quality comparisons.

One of the domains the IMPACT requires standardization in is function. Using research gathered through the Post-Acute Care Payment Reform Demonstration,[80] the CMS chose 8 items to measure the functional aspects of self-care, 17 items to measure the functional aspects of mobility, and one 6-level rating scale listed in Table 29.10. These items were added to each of the PAC setting assessment tools between April 2016 and January 2019. Although each setting will not collect all the items, each setting will collect a core set of approximately 14 of the same items. Data collected will be calculated and reported back to the provider as a functional outcome measure. Eventually, the CMS will publicly report these measures, which means a consumer of PAC services or a family member looking for the most appropriate care setting for their loved one could access the scores for the specific LTCH, IRF, SNF, or HHA they are considering. It also means that for the first time in the history of the profession, there will be *one* mandated functional instrument for all PAC providers, and it will be used in both process and outcomes measures.[81]

TABLE 29.10 Section GG Self-Care and Mobility Items (included as of January 2019)

Self-Care	LTCH	SNF	IRF	HH	Rating Scale
Eating	X	X	X	X	5 = Set up/clean up
Oral hygiene	X	X	X	X	assistance
Toileting hygiene	X	X	X	X	4 = Supervision or
Wash upper body	X				touching assistance
Shower/bathe self		X	X		3 = Partial/moderate
Upper body dressing		X	X		assistance
Lower body dressing		X	X		2 = Substantial/
Putting on/taking off footwear		X	X		maximal assistance
Mobility					1 = Dependent
Roll left and right		X	X		
Sit to lying	X	X	X	X	
Lying to sitting on side of bed	X	X	X	X	
Sit to stand	X	X	X	X	
Chair/bed to chair transfer	X	X	X	X	
Toilet transfer	X	X	X	X	
Car transfer		X	X		
Walk 10 feet	X	X	X		
Walk 150 feet	X	X	X	X	
Walk 50 feet with two turns	X	X	X	X	
Wheel 50 feet with two turns	X	X	X	X	
Wheel 150 feet	X	X	X	X	
Walk 10 feet on uneven surfaces		X	X		
1 step		X	X		
4 steps		X	X		
12 steps		X	X		
Picking up object		X	X		

HH, home health; *IRF*, inpatient rehabilitation facility; *LTCH*, long-term care hospital; *SNF*, skilled nursing facility.

Does this mean that other functional outcome tools will be unnecessary in these settings? Absolutely not. The primary goal of many LTCH, IRF, SNF, and HHA patients is improvement in function, and physical therapists are accustomed to assessing and documenting patient's functional status at admission and at discharge. Physical therapists also use many assessment tools to identify the underlying impairments that are contributing to the decline in function. The CMS outcome measure, Section GG, will not replace the need to use evidence-based standardized tests and measures that are critical to guiding care plans. However, the measure will be used to evaluate not only the effectiveness of the rehabilitation care provided to individual persons but also the effectiveness of the LTCH, IRF, SNF, and/or HHA.

Value-Based Purchasing Programs

"If you think productivity is threatening, as in, 'How much do you do?' then think about accountability, as in, 'Are you any good?'"[82]

Traditionally, the U.S. health care system has relied on fee-for-service compensation, in which payments to providers are made for each service provided, regardless of the resulting patient outcomes or costs. Today, the U.S. health care system is increasingly rewarding providers for value. This interest comes from the recognition that traditional models of health care delivery, including managed care, have had limited impact on the rising costs and utilization of services in the United States. The PPACA, and the Medicare Access and CHIP Reauthorization Act (MACRA) are two pieces of legislation that solidified the role of value-based payment in Medicare. Many private insurers are also following Medicare's lead. VBP programs aim to link provider payments to their performance in areas such as the cost of care and quality of care they provide. The goal is to incentivize providers to reduce inappropriate care, and identify and reward the best performing providers.[83] Currently, there are many forms of programs built exclusively on shared risk, but there are also models referred to as "pay-for-performance," in which providers are still based on a fee-for-service model, but with payment adjustments up or down based on value

TABLE 29.11	Influences of Value-Based Purchasing
External environment	Regulatory changes, payment policies, patient preferences, and other quality improvement initiatives that can either promote or thwart the potential success of value-based purchasing programs.
Provider characteristics	Structure of the health care system, organizational culture, available resources and capabilities (especially in information technology), and patient population served.
Program features	Defining the targeted patient population, the program goals, measures, financial incentive, and risk structure. Specific program structure considerations include the level at which the data are analyzed and incentives are provided; for example, are the data analyzed and are incentives applied at the individual therapist level, group therapy level, or the entire organization?

Chee TT, Ryan AM, Wasfy JH, Borden WB. Current state of value-based purchasing programs. *Circulation*. 2016;133(22):2197–2205.

metrics. Chee et al.[84] discuss three main influencers to VBP programs (Table 29.11). Next, an overview for some VBP models that physical therapists may encounter is discussed.

As discussed throughout this chapter, the cost of U.S. health care consumes an increasing amount of the country's economy, threatening the resources to be used on important areas such as education, infrastructure, and social security. The PPACA launched unprecedented reforms to put health care value on the fast track. Since that time, a wide spectrum of payment models has been introduced that focus on specific measures, clinical quality, patient experience, and cost (Fig. 29.10).[84] In January 2015, the U.S. Department of HHS announced their intent to shift at least 90% of all traditional Medicare payments to quality or value by the year 2018. In April 2015, MACRA repealed the sustainable growth rate formula for Medicare Part B payments, a constant source of angst for all physical therapy providers because the formula was always forecasting significant cuts in payment and required Congressional intervention to override it. However, MACRA also mandated that a method based on quality be developed that would determine payment updates, which in turn left physical therapists in uncharted territory.[85]

The Hospital VBP program was implemented in 2012, and includes several pieces. One is the Hospital Acquired Conditions (HAC) program. An HAC is a medical condition or complication that was not present when a patient is admitted to the hospital but develops during a hospital stay. In most cases, the CMS believes hospitals can prevent HACs when they use evidence-based care principles. HACs include issues like pressure ulcers, falls in hospital with a hip fracture, postoperative respiratory failure, postoperative pulmonary embolism or deep vein thrombosis, postoperative wound dehiscence, catheter-associated urinary tract infections, and *Clostridium difficile* infections.[86] Another piece of the Hospital VBP program is the Hospital Readmissions Reduction Program, which lowers payments to hospitals with too many readmissions. Readmissions are analyzed at the "all-cause" level, meaning that patients who are readmitted to the same hospital or another applicable ACH for any reason within 30 days of a hospital discharge are counted as a readmission. The CMS also looks at readmission rates for certain high-volume conditions as well, such as acute myocardial infarction, chronic obstructive pulmonary disease, heart failure, pneumonia, coronary artery bypass graft surgery, and elective primary total hip arthroplasty and/or total knee arthroplasty.[87] Finally, hospitals are measured on outcomes such as mortality and complications, health care–associated infections, patient safety, patient experience, process and efficiency, and cost reduction.[88]

The Skilled Nursing Facility VBP Program was mandated by the 2014 Protecting Access to Medicare Act, and SNFs began getting payment rewards or penalties on October 1, 2018, under the SNF VBP. It measures the number of patients who are admitted to an SNF within 24 hours of an inpatient hospital discharge and who are subsequently readmitted to the hospital within 30 calendar days of the SNF admission. Each year, the CMS sets two performance levels for SNFs to achieve. Any SNF with a performance below the first achievement level is likely to get a

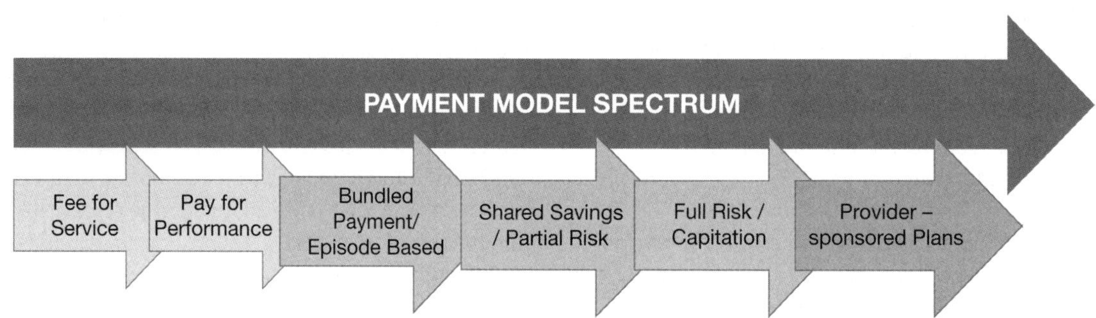

FIG. 29.10 Payment Model Spectrum. *(From Chee TT, Ryan AM, Wasfy JH, Borden WB. Current state of value-based purchasing programs. Circulation.* 2016;133(22):2197–2205.)

payment reduction on every admission in the applicable payment year, whereas SNFs with performance above the first level or even above the second achievement level will receive a positive payment update. The current measure looks at readmissions for any reason, but in the future the CMS plans to replace it with a measure that focuses on potentially preventable readmissions.[89]

Home Health Value-Based Purchasing Model. The Affordable Care Act authorized a Home Health VBP Model be designed and implemented by January 1, 2016. It is designed to leverage the successes and lessons learned from other VBP models and demonstrations in an effort to improve the quality and delivery of home health care services to Medicare beneficiaries. The program began its demonstration on January 1, 2016, in nine states (AZ, FL, IA, MA, MD, NC, NE, TN, and WA) and will run for 5 years. All Medicare-participating HHAs in these states must participate. HHA performance is measured on a number of items, including improvement in dyspnea, improvement in pain interfering with activity, improvement in the management of oral medications, and total change in self-care and mobility function. The results will be analyzed, and if successful, will be rolled out to all HHAs across the country.[90]

The Quality Payment Program (QPP) is the first large scale value-based payment model that will impact outpatient physical therapy providers. The QPP was created to be an alternative to the historical method of providing annual updates to provider payments, effectively changing the way Medicare rewarded clinicians. There are two tracks for participation in the QPP: through the Merit-Based Incentive Payment System (MIPS) and through participation in advanced Alternative Payment Models (APMs). In the first few years, participation for physical therapists might be required, whereas other physical therapists will be eligible to participate if they want to, and still others will not be eligible but could voluntarily participate to gain experience and exposure to the system. Both systems have several components, each requiring successful participation, so therapists will need to do their research to understand their business before choosing whether to participate. In 2019, the program did not provide an avenue of participation for over 50% of therapists who work with Medicare Part B patients. The practical result is that providers not allowed to participate will not receive an update to their payments for at least the next 2 calendar years. The APTA, in conjunction with other stakeholder groups, plan to advocate and collaborate with the CMS to find a way to allow these providers into the program. Fig. 29.11 illustrates the two methods of participation in the QPP. Fig. 29.12 illustrates how participation in each of the programs affects payment in a future year.

An APM is an approach to payment that gives incentive payments to groups of providers who deliver high-quality and efficient care. An APM can be modeled for a specific clinical condition, a category of care episodes, or a population of beneficiaries. An advanced APM allows practices to earn more reward in return for taking on the risk of delivering on patient outcomes. In order for an Alternative Payment Model to be considered "advanced," it must meet three criteria: (1) it requires participants to use certified electronic health record technology; (2) it provides payment for covered professional services based on quality measures, and those measures must be comparable to the ones used in the MIPS; and (3) the APM is either a medical home model expanded under the CMS innovation center or it requires the participants to bear a significant financial risk.[91] In 2019, physical therapists were not eligible to establish an APM. However, physical therapists working in private practice and/or physical therapists working in physician offices could engage with their community partners to participate in these programs. Participating in an advanced APM requires a contract with the participating hospital or convener of the APM. To receive the QPP's financial reward for participating in an advanced APM, the physical therapy practice would have to show that they are receiving a certain percentage of their Medicare Part B payments through this advanced APM (in 2019, the number was 25%) or they are providing care to a minimum percentage of their Medicare beneficiary population through the advanced APM (in 2019, the number was 20%).[92] Table 29.12 provides some examples of Medicare APMs in 2018.

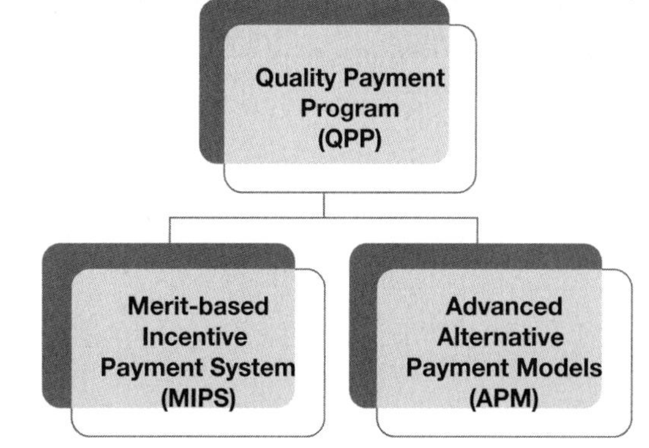

FIG. 29.11 Two Tracks of Participation in the Quality Payment Program.

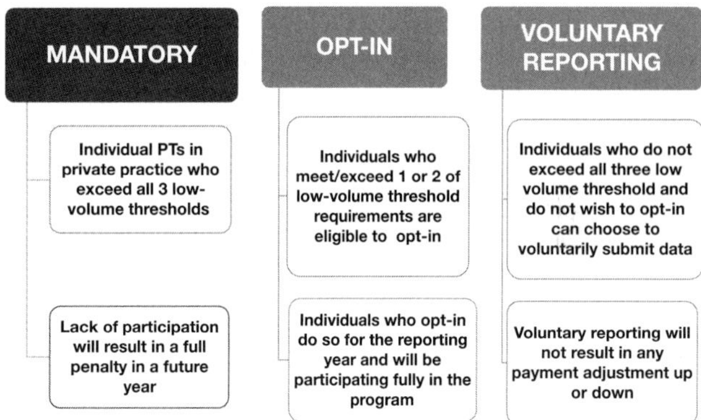

FIG. 29.12 How Quality Payment Program Participation Affects Payment. *PTs*, physical therapists.

TABLE 29.12 2018 Advanced Alternative Payment Models	
Bundled Payments for Care Improvement Advanced (BPCI Advanced) Model	The Bundled Payments for Care Improvement Advanced initiative is a new iteration of bundled payments for 32 clinical episodes. Participating health care providers are held accountable for reducing expenditures and improving quality of care for Medicare beneficiaries. This bundled payment methodology combines the payment for physicians, hospital, and other health care provider services, such as physical therapy, into a single bundled payment amount. The amount is calculated based on expected costs of all items, interventions, and services expected to be furnished to a beneficiary during an episode of care. The model then provides one single bundled payment, and it is up to the health care providers to coordinate care, improve the quality of care, and, of course, share in the payment. Health care providers may realize a gain or a loss based on how successful they are in managing the resources and total costs throughout the episode.[116]
Comprehensive Care for Joint Replacement (CJR) Model (track 1- certified electronic health record [EHR] technology)	The Comprehensive Care for Joint Replacement model aims to support better and more efficient care for beneficiaries undergoing the most common inpatient surgeries for Medicare beneficiaries: hip and knee replacements (also called lower extremity joint replacements). It tests providing one bundled payment to hospitals and downstream providers to encourage hospitals, physicians, postacute care providers, and outpatient providers to work together to coordinate the care and improve quality. These bundles generally provide one lump sum for a 90-day period that starts with the initial hospitalization and continues throughout recovery. Currently, there are 67 metropolitan areas where 465 hospitals are participating.[117] Requires participants to use certified EHR technology.
Comprehensive End-Stage Renal Disease Care (CEC) Model: two-sided risk	The Comprehensive End-Stage Renal Disease Care Model is designed to identify, test, and evaluate new ways to improve care for Medicare beneficiaries with end-stage renal disease. In this model, dialysis clinics, nephrologists, and other providers work together to coordinate care for beneficiaries with whom they are matched. It encourages providers to think beyond their traditional roles in just providing dialysis and instead rewards them for providing patient-centered care that addresses the patients' health needs outside of the dialysis clinic, and thus improve long-term health outcomes. Two-sided risk means the providers must agree to share in any losses on the program, as well as benefit from any savings.[118]
Comprehensive Primary Care Plus (CPC+)	Comprehensive Primary Care Plus is a national advanced primary care medical home model that aims to strengthen primary care. It is unique in that it involves a partnership between both public and private payers. The program provides financial resources and flexibilities to allow practices to innovate and make investments that will reduce the number of unnecessary services their patients receive. The program focuses on access and continuity of care, care management, comprehensiveness and coordination, patient and caregiver engagement, and planned care and population health.[119]
Next Generation Accountable Care Organization (ACO) Model	The Next Generation Accountable Care Organization Model offers an opportunity for groups of doctors, hospitals, and other health care providers, like physical therapists, to participate in an accountable care model for patients with original Medicare benefits. It is generally chosen by those experienced in coordinating care for populations of patients and allows these providers to assume higher levels of financial risk and reward.[120]
Oncology Care Model (OCM): two-sided risk	Under the Oncology Care Model, physician practices have entered into payment arrangements that include financial and performance accountability for episodes of care surrounding chemotherapy administration to cancer patients. Practices participating in this model have agreed to use care coordination, care navigation, and national treatment guidelines in an effort to improve quality and reduce costs. Two-sided risk means the providers must agree to share in any losses on the program, as well as benefit from any savings.[121]
Medicare Shared Savings Program (MSSP)	The Medicare Shared Savings Program offers a basic participation track and an enhanced participation track so Accountable Care Organizations can assume various levels of risk. Each track and level have increasing opportunities to innovate the care delivered. For example, in some tracks, the Accountable Care Organization has the authority to waive the 3-night qualifying hospital stay for skilled nursing facility admission. The result is reducing the costs of a hospital stay when the patient would benefit from an skilled nursing facility stay but does not require 3 nights in a hospital. Another option is to utilize telehealth services in the delivery of services.[122]

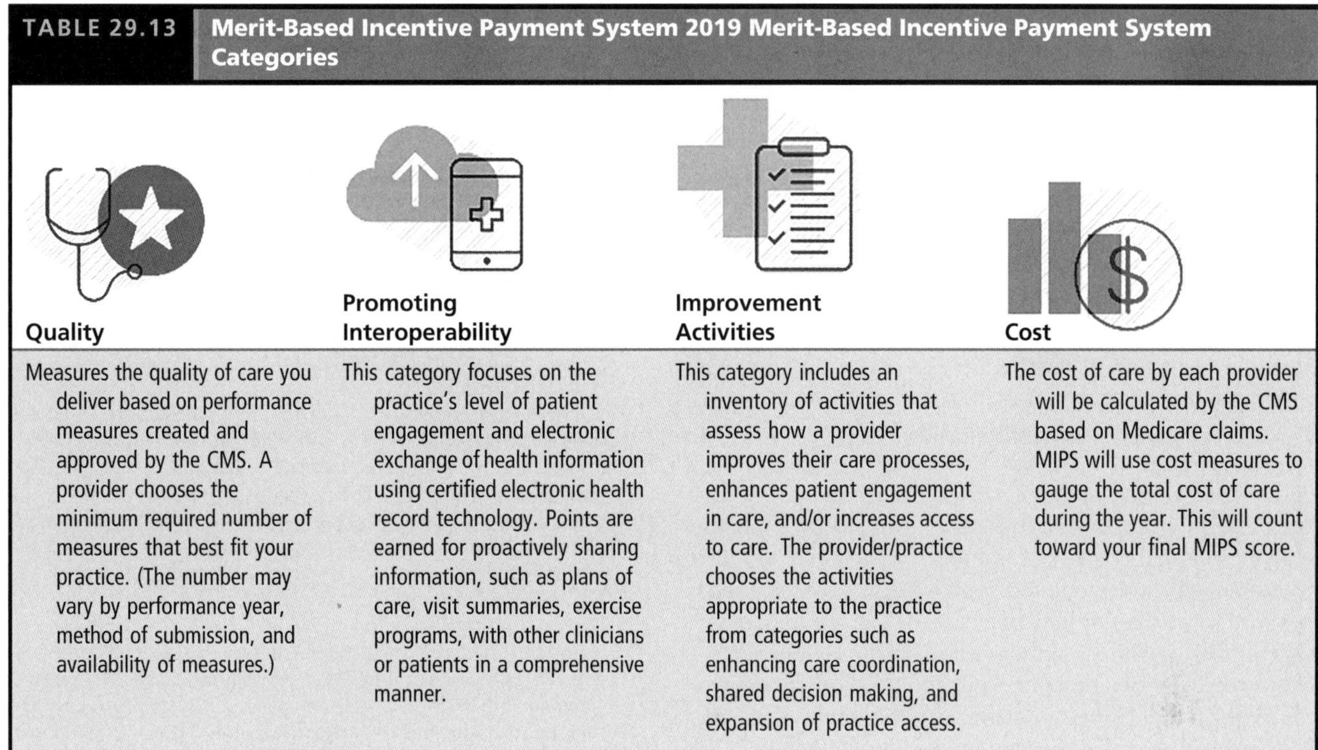

TABLE 29.13 Merit-Based Incentive Payment System 2019 Merit-Based Incentive Payment System Categories

Quality	Promoting Interoperability	Improvement Activities	Cost
Measures the quality of care you deliver based on performance measures created and approved by the CMS. A provider chooses the minimum required number of measures that best fit your practice. (The number may vary by performance year, method of submission, and availability of measures.)	This category focuses on the practice's level of patient engagement and electronic exchange of health information using certified electronic health record technology. Points are earned for proactively sharing information, such as plans of care, visit summaries, exercise programs, with other clinicians or patients in a comprehensive manner.	This category includes an inventory of activities that assess how a provider improves their care processes, enhances patient engagement in care, and/or increases access to care. The provider/practice chooses the activities appropriate to the practice from categories such as enhancing care coordination, shared decision making, and expansion of practice access.	The cost of care by each provider will be calculated by the CMS based on Medicare claims. MIPS will use cost measures to gauge the total cost of care during the year. This will count toward your final MIPS score.

CMS, Centers for Medicare and Medicaid Services; *MIPS*, Merit-Based Incentive Payment System.

The MIPS provides a more direct method of participation in the QPP for most therapists. The program gives providers an opportunity for significant financial incentives, but also for significant financial penalties for noncompliance with the program. There are four categories of participation for the MIPS, and over a calendar year, a physical therapist or physical therapy practice earns an MIPS score that ranges from 0 to 100 points. How many points they earn will determine whether the practice receives an upward payment adjustment, no payment adjustment, or a downward payment adjustment in the subsequent payment year. The four categories of the MIPS are Quality, Promoting Interoperability, Improvement Activities, and Cost (Table 29.13).[93]

The MIPS program focuses on measuring the value of care and care processes physical therapists demonstrate. Examples of quality measures that receive credit for physical therapists are measuring body mass index, pain levels, completing a medication review, and assessing the foot and ankle in a patient with a diagnosis of diabetes. These measures were chosen for the program based on the fact that each of them contributes to a more successful management of chronic disease. For instance, measuring and counseling patients with a high body mass index may reduce obesity. Asking patients about changes in their medication is important for understanding the impact on physical therapy programs, but it also provides an opportunity to identify potential harmful contraindications or identify a patient's lack of adherence to a medication regimen. Assessing the foot and ankle in a patient with diabetes can help prevent costly ulcers and ultimately amputations. Examples of improvement activities that capture points for physical therapists are activities such as utilizing patient-reported outcome tools, collecting and following up on patient experience and satisfaction data, providing self-management materials at an appropriate literacy level and in an appropriate language, regularly assessing your patient's experience of care by implementing surveys or advisory councils, implementing regular care coordination training, and implementing fall screening and assessment programs to identify those at risk but also to address the modifiable risk factors. The CMS updates these activities annually, and therapists can find more information on the APTA website.[94]

In summary, the Medicare program provides access to health care for all older adults. Although there are restrictions in benefits, and cost-sharing with beneficiaries is required for some services, the U.S. health care system is still the most expensive in the world, and only increasing. As a result of the increase in utilization of physical therapy services in all settings, providers are facing increased scrutiny from Medicare, the Office of Inspector General, and the Department of Justice. In 2017, the Justice Department opened over 900 new criminal health care fraud investigations, filed criminal charges in almost half of them, and recovered $4 for every $1 they spent investigating false claims allegations.[95] However, the other side of this issue is a human one. When a patient's Medicare benefit is used for unnecessary or ineffective services, it deprives them of services they need, and for those Medicare benefits that have limitations, it means the patient does not have access to their benefit when they may need services later in the calendar year.

Although the historical focus of the Medicare program has been coverage for illness and injury, the program is beginning to focus attention and resources on prevention services, care coordination, care navigation, and innovative models as a means to improve beneficiary health. Medicare is not the first to use these strategies, and adopted many of them from the commercial insurance market who has been employing them for over 15 years. That is because these same strategies can also contribute to lowering the costs of care. Physical therapy advocacy and research efforts are increasingly turned to focus on demonstrating the value physical therapy can having in cost reductions. Examples include early mobilization in the intensive care unit,[96] the effect of direct access to physical therapy services in reducing the cost of an episode of low back pain,[97] the effect of physical therapy as an alternative or adjunct to short-term opioid use for patients with musculoskeletal pain,[98] and how patients receiving optimal dosages of at-home physical therapy are associated with better long-term outcomes.[99] At this writing, these programs are not fully implemented, so it is unknown whether they will achieve their desired purpose. However, with a focus on outcomes and quality, physical therapists can be important players in delivering high-quality services that demonstrate value throughout the lifespan.

SUMMARY

Policy and advocacy go hand in hand. To enact or change policy takes a concerted effort to influence the bodies that possess the power to make these changes. Health policy is a complex balancing act of decisions that policy makers must make to improve access, enhance quality, and reduce cost. Understanding health policy will assist understanding the limitations and possibilities of the health care delivery system. Health policies should also outline the need for policy changes to enable all health care professionals to serve to their fullest capabilities and for patients to be assured safety and access. Balancing these policy objectives in health care continues to challenge our policy makers and advocacy organizations.

It is essential, regardless of practice setting, political perspective, or policy expertise, that physical therapists engage in the health policy and advocacy process. As health care professionals, physical therapists are obligated to comply with existing laws, regulations, and policies. Advocacy is part of their professional responsibility. Competency in health policy and advocacy will only further the professions' ability to serve patients and help them reach their full potential.

REFERENCES

1. Centers for Disease Control and Prevention. Older Adults Fall. In: *Home and Recreation Safety*. United States Department of Health and Human Services; February 10, 2017. Atlanta, GA, https://www.cdc.gov/HomeandRecreationalSafety/Falls/adultfalls.html. Accessed January 31, 2019.
2. Stevens JA, Lee R. The potential to reduce falls and avert costs by clinically managing fall risk. *AJPM*. 2018; 55(3):290–298. https://www.ajpmonline.org/article/S0749-3797(18)31759-8/fulltext. Accessed January 31, 2019.
3. Public Law – Safe Seniors Act. https://www.congress.gov/110/plaws/publ202/PLAW-110publ202.pdf. Accessed January 30, 2019.
4. National Conference of State Legislatures. Elderly Falls Prevention Legislation and Statutes. http://www.ncsl.org/research/health/elderly-falls-prevention-legislation-and-statutes.aspx; January 2, 2018. Accessed January 30, 2019.
5. Congress.gov. Senior Home Modification Assistance Initiative Act. https://www.congress.gov/bill/115th-congress/senate-bill/913. Accessed January 30, 2019.
6. United States Census Bureau. Quick Facts United States. https://www.census.gov/quickfacts/fact/table/US/PST045217. Accessed January 30, 2019.
7. Centers for Disease Control and Prevention. Social Determinants of Health: Know What Affects Health. https://www.cdc.gov/socialdeterminants/; January 29, 2018. Accessed January 30, 2019.
8. United States Census Bureau. New census data show differences between urban and rural populations. https://www.census.gov/newsroom/press-releases/2016/cb16-210.html; December 8, 2016. Accessed January 30, 2019.
9. Agency for Healthcare Research and Quality. Challenges facing rural health care. https://innovations.ahrq.gov/perspectives/challenges-facing-rural-health-care; March 26, 2014. Accessed January 30, 2019.
10. National Conference of State Legislatures. Health professional shortage areas 2017 postcard. http://www.ncsl.org/research/health/health-professional-shortage-areas-2017-postcard.aspx August 30, 2017. Accessed January 30, 2019.
11. Health Policy Project. Advocacy. http://www.healthpolicyproject.com/index.cfm?ID=topics-Advocacy; 2011. Accessed January 31, 2019.
12. National Constitution Center. Amendment I US Constitution. https://constitutioncenter.org/interactive-constitution/amendments/amendment-i Accessed January 31, 2019
13. American Physical Therapy Association. *Code of Ethics*. Alexandria, VA, https://www.apta.org/uploadedFiles/APTAorg/About_Us/.../Ethics/CodeofEthics.pdf; June 2011. Accessed January 30, 2019.
14. National Council on Aging. Advocacy Toolkit. https://www.ncoa.org/public-policy-action/advocacy-toolkit/toolkits-by-topic/advocacy-toolkit-cdsme-falls-prevention/. Accessed January 30, 2019.
15. Center for Medicare Advocacy. https://www.medicareadvocacy.org/?s=Jimmo&op.x=0&op.y=0. Accessed January 30. 2019.
16. CMS.gov. *Decision Memoir for Electrostimulation for Wounds;* December 13, 2003. Accessed January 30, 2019.
17. CMS.gov. *Local Coverage Determinations*. Updated June 26, 2018, https://www.cms.gov/Medicare/Coverage/DeterminationProcess/LCDs.html. Accessed January 30, 2019.
18. Centers for Medicare and Medicaid Services. Key Milestones in Medicare and Medicaid History, Selected Years 1995–2003. *Health Care Financing Review*. 2005; 27(2):1–3.
19. Davis PA. *Medicare Insolvency Projections. Congressional Research Service. Summary*. https://fas.org/sgp/crs/misc/RS20946.pdf; June 2018. Accessed January 30, 2019.
20. Centers for Disease Control and Prevention. *National Center for Health Statistics. Life Expectancy*. https://www.cdc.gov/nchs/fastats/life-expectancy.htm. Updated May 3, 2017. Accessed January 30, 2019.
21. Social Security Benefits Planner Life Expectancy. https://www.ssa.gov/planners/lifeexpectancy.html. Accessed January 30, 2019.
22. Centers for Medicare & Medicaid Services. Medicare and Medicaid Milestones: 1937–2015. https://www.cms.gov/About-CMS/Agency-Information/History/Downloads/Medicare-and-Medicaid-Milestones-1937-2015.pdf; July 2015. Accessed January 30, 2019.

23. Kaiser Henry J. *Family Foundation. A Primer on Medicare: Key Facts About the Medicare Program and the People it Covers.* https://www.kff.org/medicare/report/a-primer-on-medicare-key-facts-about-the-medicare-program-and-the-people-it-covers/; March 20, 2015. Accessed January 30, 2019.
24. Medicare.gov. *Medicare and You.* https://www.medicare.gov/sites/default/files/2018-09/10050-medicare-and-you.pdf; 2019. Accessed January 31, 2019.
25. MedPAC. Hospital Acute Inpatient Services Payment System. http://www.medpac.gov/docs/default-source/payment-basics/medpac_payment_basics_17_hospital_final65a311adfa9c665e80adff00009edf9c.pdf?sfvrsn=0; October 2017. Accessed January 9, 2019.
26. Medicare Benefit Policy Manual (MBPM). *Chapter 5, Lifetime Reserve Days.* https://www.cms.gov/Regulations-and-Guidance/Guidance/Manuals/Downloads/bp102c05.pdf; October 2003. Accessed January 12, 2019.
27. MedPAC Inpatient Rehabilitation Facilities Payment System. http://www.medpac.gov/docs/default-source/payment-basics/medpac_payment_basics_18_irf_final_sec.pdf?sfvrsn=0; October, 2018. Accessed January 12, 2019.
28. Federal Register. *Medicare Program; Prospective Payment System and Consolidated Billing for Skilled Nursing Facilities (SNF).* https://www.federalregister.gov/documents/2018/08/08/2018-16570/medicare-program-prospective-payment-system-and-consolidated-billing-for-skilled-nursing-facilities; August 8, 2018. Accessed January 30, 2019.
29. MedPAC Outpatient Therapy Services Payment System. http://www.medpac.gov/docs/default-source/payment-basics/medpac_payment_basics_18_opt_final_sec.pdf?sfvrsn=0; Oct 2018. Accessed January 12, 2019.
30. MBPM. *Chapter 15, 220.2 Covered Medical and Other Services.* https://www.cms.gov/Regulations-and-Guidance/Guidance/Manuals/downloads/bp102c15.pdf; November 30, 2018. Accessed January 12, 2019.
31. French EB, McCauley J, Aragon M, et al. End of life medical spending in last twelve months of life is lower than previously reported. *Health Affairs.* 2017; 36(7):1211–1217. https://www.healthaffairs.org/doi/10.1377/hlthaff.2017.0174. Accessed January 30, 2019.
32. MedPAC Hospice Services Payment System. http://www.medpac.gov/docs/default-source/payment-basics/medpac_payment_basics_17_hospice_final4ea311adfa9c665e80adff00009edf9c.pdf?sfvrsn=0; October 2017. Accessed January 12, 2019.
33. MedPAC Durable Medical Equipment Payment System. http://www.medpac.gov/docs/default-source/payment-basics/medpac_payment_basics_16_dme_final.pdf; October 2016. Accessed January 12, 2019.
34. U.S. Centers for Medicare & Medicaid Services. January 2019 DME list. https://www.cms.gov/Medicare/Medicare-Fee-for-Service-Payment/DMEPOSFeeSched/DMEPOS-Fee-Schedule-Items/DME19-A.html. Accessed January 30, 2019.
35. Medicaid.gov. *October 2018 Medicaid & CHIP Enrollment Data Highlights.* https://www.medicaid.gov/medicaid/program-information/medicaid-and-chip-enrollment-data/report-highlights/index.html; October 2018. Accessed January 12, 2019.
36. Henry Kaiser Family Foundation. *Medicaid fact sheet.* http://files.kff.org/attachment/fact-sheet-medicaid-state-US; November 2018. Accessed January 12, 2019.
37. Kaiser Henry J. Family Foundation. Federal Medical Assistance Percentage (FMAP) for Medicaid and Multiplier. https://www.kff.org/medicaid/state-indicator/federal-matching-rate-and-multiplier/?currentTimeframe=0&selectedDistributions=fmap-percentage–multiplier&sortModel=%7B%22colId%22:%22Location%22,%22sort%22:%22asc%22%7D; 2019. Accessed January 12, 2019.
38. CMS.gov. *Dual Eligible Beneficiaries under Medicare and Medicaid.* https://www.cms.gov/.../Medicare.../Medicare_Beneficiaries_Dual_Eligibles_At_a_Gla; May 2018. Accessed January 30, 2019.
39. CMS.gov. *Billing of QMBs is Prohibited by Federal Law.* https://www.cms.gov/Outreach-and-Education/Medicare-Learning.../SE1128.pdf; June 26, 2018. Accessed January 30, 2019.
40. Centers for Medicare and Medicaid. Medicaid RAC FAQ. https://www.cms.gov/Medicare-Medicaid-Coordination/Fraud-Prevention/MedicaidIntegrityProgram/Downloads/Medicaid_RAC_FAQ.pdf; December 2011. Accessed January 12, 2019.
41. U.S. Department of Health and Human Services. Office of Inspector General. Medicaid Fraud Control Units Fiscal Year 2017 Annual Report. Suzanne Murrin. Deputy Inspector General. https://oig.hhs.gov/oei/reports/oei-09-18-00180.pdf. March 2018. OEI-09-18-00180.
42. Medicaid. *Medicaid Provider Enrollment Compendium.* Updated July 24, https://www.medicaid.gov/affordable-care-act/downloads/program-integrity/mpec-7242018.pdf; 2018.
43. Military Advantage. *Veteran's healthcare overview.* https://www.military.com/benefits/veterans-health-care/veterans-health-care-overview.html; 2019. Accessed January 12, 2019.
44. American Physical Therapy Association. *Veteran's Affairs and Tricare.* Updated 12/28/2018, http://www.apta.org/Payment/TRICAREVA/. Accessed January 12, 2019.
45. Department of Veteran's Affairs. Office of Inspector General. Veterans Health Administration. Review of Alleged patient Deaths, Patient Wait Times, and Scheduling Practices at the Phoenix VA Health Care System. https://www.va.gov/oig/pubs/vaoig-14-02603-267.pdf. Published August 26, 2014. Accessed January 30, 2019.
46. US Department of Veterans Affairs. *VA expands telehealth.* https://www.va.gov/opa/pressrel/pressrelease.cfm?id=4054; May 11, 2018. Accessed January 13, 2019.
47. American Physical Therapy Association. PT in Motion. *APTA supported VA change will expand use of telehealth for PT services.* http://www.apta.org/PTinMotion/News/2018/05/11/VATelehealthRule/; May 11, 2018. Accessed January 12, 2019.
48. URAC. *Health Utilization Management Accreditation.* https://www.urac.org/programs/health-utilization-management-accreditation. Accessed January 12, 2019.
49. CMS. *Internet Only Manuals.* 4/04/2012, https://www.cms.gov/Regulations-and-Guidance/Guidance/Manuals/Internet-Only-Manuals-IOMs.html. Accessed January 30, 2019.
50. New York Times. *Clinton's Health Plan._.* https://www.nytimes.com/1993/09/23/us/clinton-s-health-plan-transcript-president-s-address-congress-health-care.html; Sept 23, 1993. Accessed January 13, 2019.
51. CMS. *Medicare Fraud and Abuse.* https://www.cms.gov/Outreach-and-Education/Medicare-Learning-Network-MLN/MLNProducts/downloads/fraud_and_abuse.pdf; September 2017. Accessed January 13, 2019.
52. Medicare Program Integrity Manual. Updated March 7, 2014. 100-08, chapter 1, section 1.3 https://www.cms.gov/Regulations-and-Guidance/Guidance/Manuals/Downloads/pim83c01.pdf. Accessed January 13, 2019.
53. US Department of Justice. *Justice News.* https://www.justice.gov/opa/pr/justice-department-recovers-over-37-billion-false-claims-act-cases-fiscal-year-2017; December 21, 2017. Accessed January 13, 2019.
54. Institute of Medicine (US) Roundtable on Evidence-Based Medicine. In: Yong PL, Saunders RS, Olsen LA, eds. *The Healthcare Imperative: Lowering Costs and Improving Outcomes: Workshop Series Summary. Unnecessary Services.* Washington DC: National Academies Press (US); 2010. https://www.ncbi.nlm.nih.gov/books/NBK53937/. Accessed January 30, 2019.
55. CMS.gov. *Medicare Program Integrity Manual. Chapter 1.* https://www.cms.gov/Regulations-and-Guidance/Guidance/Manuals/.../pim83c04.pdf; April 11, 2003. Accessed January 30, 2019.

56. Centers for Medicare & Medicaid Services. 100-15, https://www.cms.gov/Regulations-and-Guidance/Guidance/Manuals/Internet-Only-Manuals-IOMs-Items/CMS1238527.html?DLPage=2&DLEntries=10&DLSort=0&DLSortDir=ascending. Accessed January 13, 2019.
57. Office of Inspector General. Compliance Guidance. https://oig.hhs.gov/compliance/compliance-guidance/index.asp. Accessed January 30, 2019.
58. US Department of the Treasury. *Medicare Trustees Report.* https://home.treasury.gov/news/press-releases/sm0405; June 2018. Accessed January 9, 2019.
59. Sawyer B, Cox C. *How does health spending in the US compare to other countries? December 7.* https://www.healthsystemtracker.org/chart-collection/health-spending-u-s-compare-countries/#item-relative-size-wealth-u-s-spends-disproportionate-amount-health; 2018 Assessed January 30, 2019.
60. Institute of Medicine (U.S.). *Crossing the quality chasm: a new health system for the 21st century.* Washington, D.C: National Academy Press; 2001. http://www.nationalacademies.org/hmd/~/media/Files/Report%20Files/2001/Crossing-the-Quality-Chasm/Quality%20Chasm%202001%20%20report%20brief.pdf. Accessed January 30, 2019.
61. Centers for Disease Control and Prevention. Nearly half of U.S. adults were not receiving key preventive health services before 2010 June 14, 2012. https://www.cdc.gov/media/releases/2012/p0614_preventive_health.html Accessed January 30, 2019.
62. Kohn LT, Corrigan JM, Donaldson MS. *To err is human: building a safer health system. Institute of Medicine.* Washington DC: National Academies Press; 1999.
63. American Physical Therapy Association. *Optimal 1.1.* http://www.apta.org/OPTIMAL/. Updated Oct 10, 2013. Accessed January 30, 2019.
64. Uniform Data System for Medical Rehabilitation. Functional Indepence Measure. https://www.udsmr.org/. Accessed January 30, 2019.
65. Health Measures. *PROMIS.* http://www.healthmeasures.net/explore-measurement-systems/promis. Accessed January 30, 2019.
66. Centers for Medicare & Medicaid Services. *Hospital Inpatient Quality Reporting Program.* Updated September 19, 2017 https://www.cms.gov/medicare/quality-initiatives-patient-assessment-instruments/hospitalqualityinits/hospitalrhqdapu.html. Accessed January 13, 2019.
67. Medicare.gov. *Hospital compare.* https://www.medicare.gov/hospitalcompare/search.html. Accessed January 13, 2019.
68. Centers for Medicare & Medicaid Services. *Home Health Quality Reporting Requirements.* Updated September 13, 2018, https://www.cms.gov/medicare/quality-initiatives-patient-assessment-instruments/homehealthqualityinits/home-health-quality-reporting-requirements.html. Accessed January 13, 2019.
69. U.S. Centers for Medicare & Medicaid Services. *Long-term Care Hospital (LTCH) Quality Reporting (QRP).* Updated September 28, 2018, https://www.cms.gov/Medicare/Quality-Initiatives-Patient-Assessment-Instruments/LTCH-Quality-Reporting/index.html. Accessed January 13, 2019.
70. Centers for Medicare & Medicaid Services. *Inpatient Rehabilitation Facilities (IRF) Quality Reporting Program (QRP).* Updated October 29, 2018 https://www.cms.gov/Medicare/Quality-Initiatives-Patient-Assessment-Instruments/IRF-Quality-Reporting/index.html. Accessed January 13, 2019.
71. Centers for Medicare & Medicaid Services. *SNF Quality Reporting Program.* Updated August 24, 2018, https://www.cms.gov/Medicare/Quality-Initiatives-Patient-Assessment-Instruments/NursingHomeQualityInits/Skilled-Nursing-Facility-Quality-Reporting-Program/SNF-Quality-Reporting-Program-Overview.html. Accessed January 13, 2019.
72. Medicare.gov. *Long-term care hospital (LTCH) compare.* https://www.medicare.gov/longtermcarehospitalcompare/. Accessed January 13, 2019.
73. Medicare.gov. *Inpatient Rehabilitation Facility (IRF) compare.* https://www.medicare.gov/inpatientrehabilitationfacility compare/. Accessed January 13, 2019.
74. Medicare.gov. *Nursing Home Compare.* https://www.medicare.gov/nursinghomecompare/search.html. Accessed January 13, 2019.
75. Medicare.gov. *Home Health compare.* https://www.medicare.gov/homehealthcompare/search.html. Accessed January 13, 2019.
76. Improving Medicare Post-Acute Care Transformation Act of 2014. https://www.gpo.gov/fdsys/pkg/PLAW-113publ185/pdf/PLAW-113publ185.pdf; Oct 6 2014. Accessed January 13, 2019.
77. Post Acute Care Payment Reform Demonstration Report to Congress Supplement – Interim Report. *RTI International.* CMS contract No. HHSM-500-2005-00029I.
78. Gage B, Morley M, Spain PC, et al. *Examining post-acute care relationships in an integrated hospital system.* Prepared for ASPE.
79. Gage B. Impact of the BBA on post-acute utilization. *Health Care Financing Review.* 1999; 20(4):103–126.
80. Research Triangle Institute. *Post-Acute Care Payment Reform Demonstration Report to Congress Supplement – Interim Report. Prepared for CMS.* https://www.cms.gov/Research-Statistics-Data-and-Systems/Statistics-Trends-and-Reports/Reports/downloads/GAGE_PACPRD_RTC_Supp_Materials_May_2011.pdf; May 2011. Accessed January 13, 2019.
81. Strunk ER. Policy talk: have you heard? Functional outcome measures are here. *GeriNotes.*. 2018; 25(4):9–13.
82. Kovacek P. Productivity. *What We Know and What We Thought We Knew.* Washington DC: APTA Next 2016; 2016. http://www.apta.org/PTinMotion/News/2016/6/14/NEXTProductivity/. Accessed January 30, 2019.
83. healthcare.gov. *Value-based purchasing.* https://www.healthcare.gov/glossary/value-based-purchasing-vbp/. Accessed January 13, 2019.
84. Chee TT, Ryan AM, Wasfy JH, Borden WB. Current state of value-based purchasing programs. *Circulation.* 2016; 133 (22):2197–2205.
85. Congress.gov. *Medicare Access and CHIP Reauthorization Act of 2015. MACRA.* https://www.congress.gov/bill/114th-congress/house-bill/2. Accessed January 30, 2019.
86. Centers for Medicare & Medicaid Services. *Hospital-acquired condition (HAC) reduction program.* Updated July 30, 2018, https://www.cms.gov/Medicare/Quality-Initiatives-Patient-Assessment-Instruments/Value-Based-Programs/HAC/Hospital-Acquired-Conditions.html. Accessed January 13, 2019.
87. Centers for Medicare & Medicaid Services. *Hospital Readmissions Program (HRRP).* Updated December 04, 2018, https://www.cms.gov/Medicare/Quality-Initiatives-Patient-Assessment-Instruments/Value-Based-Programs/HRRP/Hospital-Readmission-Reduction-Program.html. Accessed January 13, 2019.
88. Centers for Medicare & Medicaid Services. *The Hospital value-based purchasing (VBP) program.* Updated August 2, 2018, https://www.cms.gov/Medicare/Quality-Initiatives-Patient-Assessment-Instruments/Value-Based-Programs/HVBP/Hospital-Value-Based-Purchasing.html. Accessed January 13, 2019.
89. Centers for Medicare & Medicaid Services. *The Skilled nursing facility value-based purchasing program (SNF VBP).* Updated October 25, 2018, https://www.cms.gov/Medicare/Quality-Initiatives-Patient-Assessment-Instruments/Value-Based-Programs/Other-VBPs/SNF-VBP.html. Accessed January 13, 2019.

90. Centers for Medicare & Medicaid Services. *Home health value-based purchasing model*. Updated November 29, 2018 https://innovation.cms.gov/initiatives/home-health-value-based-purchasing-model. Accessed January 13, 2019.
91. Centers for Medicare & Medicaid Services. Advanced Alternative Payment Models (APMS). https://qpp.cms.gov/apms/advanced-apms. Accessed January 13, 2019.
92. American Physical Therapy Association. *FAQ: MACRA and Alternative Payment Models*. Updated November, 2016, http://www.apta.org/Payment/Medicare/MACRA/FAQAPMs/. Accessed January 13, 2019.
93. Quality Payment Program. *MIPS Overview*. https://qpp.cms.gov/mips/overview. Accessed January 31, 2019.
94. American Physical Therapy Association. *Participating in MIPS*. Updated January 10, 2019, http://www.apta.org/MIPS/ParticipationOverview/. Accessed January 13, 2019.
95. HHS.gov. *Health and Human Services and the Department of Justice Return $2.6 Billion in Taxpayer Savings from Efforts to Fight Healthcare Fraud*. https://www.hhs.gov/about/news/2018/04/06/hhs-and-department-justice-return-26-billion-taxpayer-savings-efforts-fight-healthcare-fraud.html; April 6, 2018. Accessed January 31, 2019.
96. Adler J, Malone D. Early mobilization in the intensive care unit: a systematic review. *Cardiopulmonary Physical Therapy Journal*. 2012;23(1):5–13.
97. The Moran Company. *Initial Treatment Intervention and Average Total Medicare A/B Costs for FFS Beneficiaries with an Incident Low Back Pain (Lumbago) Diagnosis in CY*. http://www.aptqi.com/Resources/documents/APTQI-Complete-Study-Initial-Treatment-Intervention-Lumbago-May-2017.pdf; 2014 May 2017. Accessed January 31, 2019.
98. Sun E, Moshfegh J, Rishel CA. Association of early physical therapy with long-term opioid use among opioid-naïve patients with musculoskeletal pain. *JAMA Network Open*. 2018;1(8):e185909. https://jamanetwork.com/journals/jamanetworkopen/fullarticle/2718095. Accessed January 31, 2019.
99. University of Colorado. *Home care for knee replacement patients aids in recovery*. https://www.cuanschutztoday.org/study-home-care-for-knee-replacement-patients-aids-in-recovery/; October 23, 2018. Accessed January 31, 2019.

INDEX

Note: Page numbers followed by *f* indicate figures, *t* indicate tables, and *b* indicate boxes.

D

E

F

G

Q

R

S